OKU

4

Orthopaedic Knowledge Update

Shoulder and Elbow

AAOS

AMERICAN ACADEMY OF ORTHOPAEDIC SURGEONS

OKU 4

Orthopaedic Knowledge Update:

Shoulder and Elbow

EDITOR

Gregory P. Nicholson, MD
Midwest Orthopaedics at Rush
Associate Professor
Department of Orthopaedic Surgery
Rush University Medical Center
Chicago, Illinois

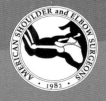

Developed by
the American Shoulder and Elbow Surgeons

AAOS
AMERICAN ACADEMY OF
ORTHOPAEDIC SURGEONS

AAOS

AMERICAN ACADEMY OF ORTHOPAEDIC SURGEONS

Published 2013 by the
American Academy of Orthopaedic Surgeons
6300 North River Road
Rosemont, IL 60018

Copyright 2013
by the American Academy of Orthopaedic Surgeons

ISBN 978-0-89203-955-5
Library of Congress Control Number:
2013940531
Printed in the USA

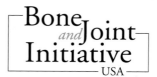

Bone *and* Joint Initiative
USA

Acknowledgments

Contributors

Daniel Aaron, MD
Shoulder Fellow
Department of Orthopaedic Surgery
Mount Sinai School of Medicine
New York, New York

Julie Adams, MD
Assistant Professor
Department of Orthopaedic Surgery
University of Minnesota
Minneapolis, Minnesota

Tjarco Alta, MD
Orthopaedic Fellow
Departments of Orthopaedic Surgery and
*   Sports Traumatology*
L'Archet 2 Hospital
Nice, France

James R. Andrews, MD
Orthopaedic and Medical Director
The Andrews Institute
Gulf Breeze, Florida

Michael E. Angeline, MD
Sports Medicine and Shoulder Surgery Fellow
Hospital for Special Surgery
New York, New York

Daisuke Araki, MD, PhD
Research Fellow
Department of Orthopaedic Surgery
University of Pittsburgh
Pittsburgh, Pennsylvania

Robert A. Arciero, MD
Professor of Orthopaedics
Department of Orthopaedics
University of Connecticut Health Center
Farmington, Connecticut

April D. Armstrong, BSc (PT), MSc, MD,
**   FRCSC**
Associate Professor, Chief Shoulder and Elbow
*   Surgery*
Department of Orthopaedics
Penn State Milton S. Hershey Medical Center
*   Bone and Joint Institute*
Hershey, Pennsylvania

Robert M. Beer, MD
Orthopaedic Trauma Fellow
Department of Orthopaedic Trauma
University of Maryland Shock Trauma Center
Baltimore, Maryland

Knut Beitzel, MA, MD
Orthopedic Resident
Department of Trauma and Orthopedic Surgery
Trauma Center Murnau
Murnau, Germany

John-Erik Bell, MD, MS
Assistant Professor, Orthopaedic Surgery
Department of Orthopaedic Surgery
Dartmouth-Hitchcock Medical Center
Lebanon, New Hampshire

Pascal Boileau, MD
Head of Department, Chair
Department of Orthopaedic Surgery and Sports
*   Traumatology*
L'Archet 2 Hospital
Nice, France

Robert E. Boykin, MD
Sports Medicine Fellow
The Steadman Clinic
Steadman Philippon Research Institute
Vail, Colorado

James P. Bradley, MD
Clinical Professor of Orthopaedic Surgery,
*   Head Team*
Physician, Pittsburgh Steelers
Department of Orthopaedic Surgery
University of Pittsburgh Medical Center
Pittsburgh, Pennsylvania

E. David Bravos, MD
Assistant Professor
Department of Anesthesiology and Critical Care
*   Medicine*
The Johns Hopkins Hospital
Baltimore, Maryland

Stephen S. Burkhart, MD
Fellowship Director
The San Antonio Orthopaedic Group, LLP
San Antonio, Texas

Wayne Z. Burkhead Jr, MD
Clinical Professor
University of Texas Southwestern Medical
School
Department of Orthopaedics
The Carrell Clinic
Dallas, Texas

John A. Carrino, MD, MPH
Associate Professor
The Russell H. Morgan Department of
Radiology and Radiological Science
The Johns Hopkins Hospital
Baltimore, Maryland

Kyle A. Caswell, DO
Orthopaedic Surgeon
The Carrell Clinic
Baylor University Medical Center
Dallas, Texas

Aaron Chamberlain, MD
Shoulder and Elbow Fellow
Department of Orthopaedic Surgery
Washington University School of Medicine
St. Louis, Missouri

Emilie V. Cheung, MD
Assistant Professor
Department of Orthopaedic Surgery
Stanford University
Redwood City, California

Paul J. Christo, MD, MBA
Associate Professor
Division of Pain Medicine
Department of Anesthesiology
Johns Hopkins University School of Medicine
Baltimore, Maryland

Christopher R. Chuinard, MD, MPH
Orthopaedic Surgeon
Great Lakes Orthopaedic Center
Munson Medical Center
Traverse City, Michigan

Brandon Cincere, MD
Sports Fellow
Nirschl Orthopaedic Center
Arlington, Virginia

Brian J. Cole, MD, MBA
Professor
Department of Orthopedics
Rush University Medical Center
Chicago, Illinois

John Costouros, MD
Assistant Professor
Department of Orthopaedic Surgery
Stanford University School of Medicine
Stanford, California

Mark P. Cote, PT, DPT, MSCTR
Sports Medicine Clinical Outcomes Research
Facilitation
Department of Orthopaedic Surgery
University of Connecticut Health Center
Farmington, Connecticut

Lynn Crosby, MD
Chief of Orthopaedic Surgery
Department of Orthopaedic Surgery, Shoulder
Medical College of Georgia
August, Georgia

Richard E. Debski, PhD
Associate Professor
Department of Bioengineering
University of Pittsburgh
Pittsburgh, Pennsylvania

Ruth A. Delaney, MB, BCh, MRCS
Harvard Shoulder Service Fellow
Department of Orthopedic Surgery
Brigham and Women's Hospital
Boston, Massachusetts

Kathleen A. Derwin, PhD
Associate Staff Scientist
Department of Biomedical Engineering
Cleveland Clinic
Cleveland, Ohio

Brian D. Dierckman, MD
Attending Surgeon
American Health Network Bone and Spine
Carmel, Indiana

Joshua S. Dines, MD
Orthopedic Surgeon
Department of Sports Medicine and Shoulder
  Service
The Hospital for Special Surgery
New York, New York

James G. Distefano, MD
Fellow
Department of Orthopedics
Brigham and Women's Hospital
Boston, Massachusetts

Richard E. Duey, MD
Fellow
The San Antonio Orthopedic Group
San Antonio, Texas

Andrew A. Dunkman, BA
Research Assistant
McKay Orthopaedic Research Laboratory
University of Pennsylvania
Philadelphia, Pennsylvania

James M. Dunwoody, MD, FRCSC
Fellow
Department of Surgery
University of Toronto
Toronto, Ontario, Canada

T. Bradley Edwards, MD
Attending Surgeon
Fondren Orthopedic Group
Texas Orthopedic Hospital
Houston, Texas

Kelly Fitzpatrick, DO
Orthopaedic Surgeon
Department of Orthopaedics
Tripler Army Medical Center
Honolulu, Hawaii

Evan Flatow, MD
Lasker Professor and Chairman
Department of Orthopaedic Surgery
Mount Sinai School of Medicine
New York, New York

Mark A. Frankle, MD
Chief of Shoulder and Elbow Surgery
Shoulder and Elbow Specialty
Florida Orthopaedic Institute
Tampa, Florida

Yoshimasa Fujimaki, MD, PhD
Research Fellow
Department of Orthopaedic Surgery
University of Pittsburgh
Pittsburgh, Pennsylvania

Michael J. Gardner, MD
Assistant Professor
Department of Orthopaedic Surgery
Washington University School of Medicine
St. Louis, Missouri

Raffaele Garofalo, MD
Department of Orthopaedics
Shoulder Service
F. Miulli Hospital
Acquaviva delle Fonti-Ba, Italy

Neil Ghodadra, MD
Orthopedic Surgeon
Sports Specialty
Southern California Orthopedic Institute
Van Nuys, California

Reuben Gobezie, MD
Director
Cleveland Shoulder Institute
University Hospitals of Cleveland
Cleveland, Ohio

Andrew Green, MD
Associate Professor, Chief of Division of
  Shoulder and Elbow Surgery
Department of Orthopaedic Surgery
Warren Alpert Brown Medical School
Providence, Rhode Island

Michael J. Griesser, MD
Fellow
Department of Orthopaedic Surgery
The Cleveland Clinic Foundation
Cleveland, Ohio

James Hammond, DO, ATC
Shoulder and Elbow Fellow
Division of Sports Medicine
Rush University Medical Center
Chicago, Illinois

Daniel M. Hampton, MD
Fellow
Department of Orthopedic Surgery
Brigham and Women's Hospital
Boston, Massachusetts

Hill Hastings II, MD
Physician
Indiana Hand to Shoulder Center
Indiana University
Indianapolis, Indiana

Armodios M. Hatzidakis, MD
Orthopaedic Surgeon
Western Orthopaedic PC
Denver, Colorado

Wendell Heard, MD
Department of Orthopedics
Tulane University
New Orleans, Louisiana

Laurence D. Higgins, MD
Chief, Sports Medicine and Shoulder Service
Department of Orthopedic Surgery
Brigham and Women's Hospital
Boston, Massachusetts

James A. Hurt III, MD
Department of Orthopaedic Surgery
Tulane University School of Medicine
New Orleans, Louisiana

Waqas Munawar Hussain, MD
Orthopaedic Surgery Sports Medicine Fellow
Sports Health Center
Cleveland Clinic Foundation
Cleveland, Ohio

Sarah Ilkhani-Pour, MSE
Graduate Student Research Assistant
McKay Orthopaedic Research Laboratory
University of Pennsylvania
Philadelphia, Pennsylvania

Nicholas Jarmon, MD
Department of Orthopaedics
Johns Hopkins University
Baltimore, Maryland

Mark J. Jo, MD
Orthopaedic Trauma Fellow
Department of Orthopaedic Surgery
Washington University School of Medicine
St. Louis, Missouri

Charles M. Jobin, MD
Shoulder and Elbow Surgery Fellow
Department of Orthopedic Surgery
Washington University
St. Louis, Missouri

James A. Johnson, PhD
Director, Biomedical Engineering
Hand and Upper Limb Centre
St. Joseph's Health Centre
London, Ontario, Canada

Jay D. Keener, MD
Assistant Professor
Department of Orthopedic Surgery
Washington University
St. Louis, Missouri

W. Ben Kibler, MD
Medical Director
Shoulder Center of Kentucky
Lexington Clinic
Lexington, Kentucky

Myung-Sun Kim, MD, PhD
Assistant Professor
Department of Orthopaedic Surgery
Chonnam National University College of Medicine
Gwangju, Republic of Korea

Graham J.W. King, MD, MSc, FRCSC
Professor of Surgery
Hand and Upper Limb Centre
St. Joseph's Health Centre, University of Western Ontario
London, Ontario, Canada

Steven Klepps, MD
Orthopedic Surgeon
Ortho Montana
St. Vincent's Hospital
Billings, Montana

David Kovacevic, MD
Resident
Department of Orthopaedic Surgery
Cleveland Clinic
Cleveland, Ohio

Rudy Kovachevich, MD
Fellow
Indiana Hand to Shoulder Center
Indiana University
Indianapolis, Indiana

Sumant G. Krishnan, MD
The Shoulder Service
The Carrell Clinic
Dallas, Texas

Albert Lin, MD
Harvard Shoulder Service
Massachusetts General Hospital
Boston, Massachusetts

Ian K.Y. Lo, MD, FRCSC
Assistant Professor
Department of Surgery
University of Calgary
Calgary, Alberta, Canada

Frank Martetschläger, MD
Department of Orthopaedic Sports Medicine
Clinic rechts der Isar
Technical University
Munich, Germany

Augustus D. Mazzocca, MS, MD
Interim Director
New England Musculoskeletal Institute
Interim Chairman
Department of Orthopaedic Surgery
University of Connecticut Health Center
Farmington, Connecticut

Brett McCoy, MD
Fellow
Orthopaedic Surgery
The Cleveland Clinic Foundation
Cleveland, Ohio

Michael D. McKee, MD, FRCSC
Professor
Surgery
University of Toronto
Toronto, Ontario, Canada

John W. McNeill II, BA
Research Assistant
Orthopaedics
Naval Medical Center San Diego
San Diego, California

Peter J. Millett, MD, MSc
Director of Shoulder Surgery
The Steadman Clinic
Steadman Philippon Research Institute
Vail, Colorado

Anthony Miniaci, MD
Professor
Department of Orthopaedic Surgery
The Cleveland Clinic Foundation
Garfield Heights, Ohio

Todd C. Moen, MD
Attending Surgeon
The Carrell Clinic
Dallas, Texas

Stephanie Muh, MD
Orthopaedic Fellow
Case Shoulder and Elbow Fellowship
University Hospitals of Cleveland
Cleveland, Ohio

Phillip T. Nigro, MD
Shoulder and Elbow Fellow
Florida Orthopedic Institute
Tampa, Florida

Robert P. Nirschl, MD, MS
Nirschl Orthopaedic Center
Arlington, Virginia

Robert V. O'Toole, MD
Assistant Professor
Department of Orthopaedics
University of Maryland School of Medicine
Baltimore, Maryland

Randall J. Otto, MD
Orthopaedics Fellow
Shoulder and Elbow
Florida Orthopaedic Institute
Tampa, Florida

Brett D. Owens, MD
Chief
Orthopaedic Surgery
Keller Army Hospital
West Point, New York

Bradford Parsons, MD
Assistant Professor
Orthopaedic Surgery
Mount Sinai School of Medicine
New York, New York

CDR Matthew T. Provencher, MD, MC USN
Department of Orthopedics
San Diego Naval Academy
San Diego, California

Patric Raiss, MD
Orthopaedic and Trauma Surgeon
Clinic for Orthopaedic and Trauma Surgery
University of Heidelberg
Heidelberg, Germany

D. Nicholas Reed, MD
Fellow
Department of Orthopaedics
University of Connecticut Health Center
Farmington, Connecticut

Eric T. Ricchetti, MD
Associate Staff
Orthopaedic Surgery
Cleveland Clinic
Cleveland, Ohio

David Ring, MD, PhD
Director of Research
Orthopaedic Hand and Upper Extremity
  Service
Massachusetts General Hospital
Boston, Massachusetts

Daniel Rios, MD
Fellow
Sports Medicine
Steadman Philippon Research Institute
Vail, Colorado

Christopher P. Roche, MSBE, MBA
Extremities E&D Manager
Engineering and Development
Exactech, Inc.
Gainesville, Florida

Anthony A. Romeo, MD
Assistant Professor
Orthopedics
Rush University Medical Center
Chicago, Illinois

Glen H. Rudolph, MD
Fellow
Shoulder Service
W.B. Carrell Memorial Clinic
Dallas, Texas

Marc Safran, MD
Professor
Orthopaedic Surgery
Stanford University
Stanford, California

Felix H. Savoie III, MD
Lee C. Schlesinger Professor
Department of Orthopaedic Surgery
Tulane University School of Medicine
New Orleans, Louisiana

Daniel Grant Schwartz, MD
Fellow in Shoulder and Elbow Surgery
Florida Orthopaedic Institute
Tampa, Florida

Douglas Scott, MD
Fellow
Shoulder and Elbow Service
Brown University
Providence, Rhode Island

Benjamin W. Sears, MD
Attending Physician
Synergy Orthopaedics
St. Anthony's North Hospital
Westminster, Colorado

Brett Shore, MD
Orthopaedic Surgeon
Southern California Permanente Medical Group
Kaiser – Panorama City
Panorama City, California

Daniel J. Solomon, MD
Partner
Marin Orthopaedics and Sports Medicine
Novato, California

Louis J. Soslowsky, PhD
Fairhill Professor, Vice Chair for Research, and
*   Center Director*
McKay Orthopaedic Research Laboratory
University of Pennsylvania
Philadelphia, Pennsylvania

Umasuthan Srikumaran, MD
Assistant Professor
Department of Orthopaedic Surgery
Johns Hopkins School of Medicine
Baltimore, Maryland

Mark D. Stanley, MD
Musculoskeletal Radiologist
Department of Radiology
Naval Medical Center San Diego
San Diego, California

Scott P. Steinmann, MD
Professor of Orthopedics
Department of Orthopedic Surgery
Mayo Clinic
Rochester, Minnesota

Hiroyuki Sugaya, MD
Director
Shoulder & Elbow Service
Funabashi Orthopaedic Sports Medicine Center
Funabashi, Japan

Robert Z. Tashjian, MD
Associate Professor
Department of Orthopaedics
University of Utah School of Medicine
Salt Lake City, Utah

Rashmi S. Thakkar, MD
Research Fellow in Musculoskeletal Radiology
The Russell H. Morgan Department of
*   Radiology and Radiological Sciences*
Johns Hopkins University School of Medicine
Baltimore, Maryland

Fotios P. Tjoumakaris, MD
Assistant Professor of Orthopaedic Surgery
Department of Orthopaedic Surgery
Rothman Institute Orthopaedics
Jefferson Medical College
Egg Harbor Township, New Jersey

John Tokish, MD
Orthopaedic Surgery Residency Program
*   Director*
Orthopaedics
Tripler Army Medical Center
Honolulu, Hawaii

Geoffrey S. Van Thiel, MD, MBA
Surgeon
Orthopedics
Rockford Orthopedic Associates
Rockford, Illinois

Gilles Walch, MD
Orthopaedic Surgeon
Centre Orthopédique Santy
Lyon, France

Jon J.P. Warner, MD
Harvard Shoulder Service
Massachusetts General Hospital
Boston, Massachusetts

Brian G. Wilhelmi, MD, JD
Housestaff Faculty
Department of Anesthesiology
Johns Hopkins University School of Medicine
Baltimore, Maryland

Ken Yamaguchi, MD
Sam & Marilyn Fox Distinguished Professor of
  Orthopaedic Surgery
Department of Orthopaedic Surgery
Washington University School of Medicine
St. Louis, Missouri

Albert Yoon, MBChB
Clinical Fellow
Hand and Upper Limb Centre
St. Joseph's Hospital
London, Ontario, Canada

Preface

The field of shoulder and elbow surgery continues to rapidly expand and evolve. This fourth edition of *Orthopaedic Knowledge Update (OKU): Shoulder and Elbow* is focused on the most recent advances in this area of orthopaedics. It is written for practicing orthopaedic surgeons and presents, in a concise yet thorough manner, the most recent literature on the shoulder and the elbow and the advances in all areas of shoulder and elbow surgery. Shoulder and elbow specialists will also find this edition useful, along with residents and fellows, who will benefit from the knowledge and expertise of a world-class group of section editors and authors.

New to this edition is a chapter on the design and biomechanics of reverse shoulder arthroplasty. As all upper extremity surgeons know, pain syndromes, which are difficult to diagnose and treat, can occur. The chapter on complex regional pain syndrome and causalgia provides an update on current terminology, thought, diagnosis, and treatment. A chapter on both basic and advanced elbow arthroscopy is included, along with updated information on acromioclavicular injuries, suprascapular nerve issues, and scapular dysfunction. The section on the rotator cuff includes chapters that discuss treatment and the most recent science on tendon healing and possible augmentation of rotator cuff healing.

The section editors are leaders in their fields and have selected a dedicated team of chapter authors, and they all have done a remarkable job in writing, editing, and preparing *OKU: Shoulder and Elbow 4*. I am deeply grateful for their efforts and contributions to this project. The staff at the American Academy of Orthopaedic Surgeons has been invaluable in moving this project forward and helping me as the editor to bring the fourth edition to publication. I am grateful for the opportunity to be the editor of this project and honored to have been chosen by the American Shoulder and Elbow Surgeons to lead this project. I would like to thank all the authors, section editors, contributors, and AAOS staff for their excellent effort. I hope that the information put forth is a valuable resource for all who treat shoulder and elbow conditions.

Gregory P. Nicholson, MD
Editor

Table of Contents

Section 4: Arthroscopy

Section 5: Arthritis and Arthroplasty

Section 8: Miscellaneous Shoulder and Elbow Topics

Section Editor:
Edward G. McFarland, MD

Basic Science

SECTION EDITOR:
PATRICK J. MCMAHON, MD

Chapter 1

Anatomy and Function of the Shoulder Structures

Yoshimasa Fujimaki, MD, PhD   Daisuke Araki, MD, PhD   Richard E. Debski, PhD

Introduction

The shoulder has a larger range of motion than any other major joint in the musculoskeletal system. This range of motion primarily is attributed to the organization of the bony and soft-tissue structures that provide mobility and stability. Because the bony structures provide minimal stability, the muscles and the passive soft-tissue structures must maintain stability while the muscles move the arm. Shoulder motion involves the entire shoulder complex, including the scapulothoracic joint, which acts as a base for upper extremity motion.

Osseous Anatomy

Humeral Head

The proximal humerus has an ellipsoidal humeral head that forms part of the glenohumeral joint. The humeral head is covered with hyaline articular cartilage, and the anatomic neck of the humerus is marked by a bony transition from cartilage to the metaphyseal border. The retroversion angle of the humeral head is defined as the orientation of the articular surface with respect to the sagittal plane. The most widely used reference is between the transepicondylar axis of the elbow and the anterior-posterior axis at the cartilage or metaphyseal border[1-3] (**Figure 1**). The anatomic neck of the humerus is used as a reference for osteotomy during shoulder arthroplasty; the retroversion angle of the humeral head has been described as having great variability.[4,5]

A three-dimensional study using surface topographic data from 24 humeral heads found that the mean radius of curvature of the articular surface was 23.9 mm (range, 22.5 to 25.8 mm).[2] The deviation from sphericity was 0.2 mm (range, 0.15 to 0.26 mm), which is 0.9% of the radius of curvature. Retroversion of the humeral head at the midpoint between the superior and inferior margins was 18.6° (range, 2.5° to 40°), but the angle varied with the location of the measurement (**Figure 2**). The study concluded that a reference at a central point anteriorly along the cartilage may be a useful landmark for re-creating the version calculated using the centroid of the articular surface.[2]

In throwing athletes, the two shoulders appear to have different glenohumeral ranges of motion. Specifically, a greater external rotation and a loss of internal rotation was found in the dominant shoulder than in the nondominant shoulder.[6] Range of motion and laxity of the glenohumeral joint as well as humeral head and glenoid version in the dominant and nondominant shoulders were studied in 25 professional pitchers and 25 nonthrowing control athletes. Humeral and glenoid retroversion increased in the dominant shoulder of the throwing athletes compared with the nondominant shoulder. External rotation increased in the dominant shoulder at 90° and 45° of abduction and decreased in internal rotation at 90°. The nonthrowing athletes had no significant side-to-side difference in any parameter.

The implication of this altered arc of motion is that a physiologic adaptation of the dominant shoulder as a result of repetitive microtrauma leads to selective stretching of the anterior capsule and tightening of the posterior capsule. Adaptation also can occur in osseous structures because of the applied stresses. Surgeons should carefully examine high-level overhead athletes to determine their side-to-side difference in range of motion and bony characteristics.

Bicipital Groove

The bicipital groove has been used as a landmark during surgical fracture repair or prosthesis alignment during shoulder arthroplasty.[7,8] A morphometric study of 50 dry humeri found an average groove length of 8.1 cm (range, 6.7 to 10.4 cm), which corresponded to 25.4% (range, 16.3% to 32.5%) of the width of the humerus. The width at the midpoint of the groove was 10.1 mm (range, 7.3 to 15.5 mm), which corresponded to 49.7% to 54.5% of the width of the humerus. The 4.0-mm depth of the groove corresponded to 18.8% of the depth of the humerus. The angle formed by the walls of the bicipital groove was 106°. No correlation could be found among these parameters.[9]

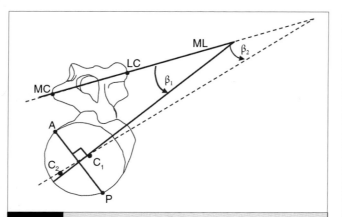

Figure 1 Schematic drawing showing retroversion definition based on the transepicondylar axis and the cartilage-calcar interface in the sagittal plane and the centroid of the articular surface. A to P = axial plane, β_1 = retroversion angle from the cartilage-calcar interface, β_2 = retroversion angle from the centroid of the articular surface, C_1 = centroid of the sphere representing the articular surface, C_2 = centroid of the articular surface, LC = lateral epicondyle, MC = medial epicondyle, ML = transepicondylar line. (Reproduced with permission from Harrold F, Wigderowitz C: A three-dimensional analysis of humeral head retroversion. *J Shoulder Elbow Surg* 2012;21[5]:612-617.)

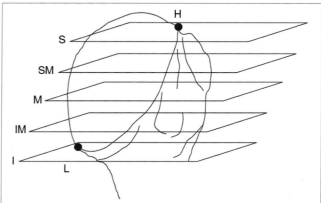

Figure 2 Schematic drawing showing the division of the humeral head into six sections by five parallel planes running orthogonal to the shaft axis. H = superiormost point on the cartilage-calcar interface, I = inferior plane, IM = inferior middle plane, L = inferiormost point on the cartilage calcar interface, M = middle plane, S = superior plane, SM = superior middle plane. (Reproduced with permission from Harrold F, Wigderowitz C: A three-dimensional analysis of humeral head retroversion. *J Shoulder Elbow Surg* 2012;21[5]:612-617.)

Glenoid

The glenoid is a pear-shaped concave projection that extends laterally from the scapular body and acts as the socket of the glenohumeral joint. CT is commonly used to evaluate the effect on glenoid retroversion of scapular rotation in the coronal and sagittal planes. Measurements are made using a coordinate system for each scapula based on three anatomic landmarks: the center of the glenoid fossa, the point on the vertebral border at which the scapular spine intersects the medial border of the scapula, and the most distal point of the inferior scapular angle.[10] The anatomic glenoid version was found to be 2.0° (± 3.8°) when it was evaluated independently from the resting position of the scapula. The difference between anatomic glenoid version and clinical glenoid version was found to depend on the position of the scapula in the original axial CT images, and it averaged 6.9° (range, 0.1° to 22.5°). These results suggest that misalignment of 1° of the scapula in the coronal or the sagittal plane creates inaccuracies in the measurement of glenoid version. The plane of axial reconstruction must be taken into account when CT is used to evaluate glenoid version.[10]

Labral and Capsular Anatomy

Glenoid Labrum

The glenoid labrum is composed of a rim of fibrous tissue with a fibrocartilaginous transition zone that acts as a passive stabilizer by adding depth to the shallow glenoid fossa. It also serves as a primary attachment site for the glenohumeral capsule and the long head of the biceps tendon (LHBT).[11]

The labral outline is ovoid, conforming to the underlying glenoid rim, and is most firmly attached to the glenoid posteroinferiorly.[12] The contributions of the glenoid labrum to glenohumeral joint stability have been well described.[13,14] Superior labrum anterior to posterior (SLAP) lesions increasingly are recognized as a source of pain and instability in the shoulder. Labral lesions such as SLAP lesions are being more commonly diagnosed with MRI or shoulder arthroscopy, and, as a result, an accurate understanding of normal labral variations has become crucial[15] (**Figure 3**).

Several studies suggest that wide variability exists in the anatomy of the anterosuperior portion of the labrum. A clinical study of 546 patients undergoing shoulder arthroscopy found that 73 (13.4%) had an anatomic variation in the anterosuperior labrum, including a sublabral foramen only in 18 patients (3.3%), a sublabral foramen with a cordlike middle glenohumeral ligament in 47 patients (8.6%), and an absence of labral tissue in the anterosuperior portion of the labrum with a cordlike middle glenohumeral ligament in 8 patients (1.5%).[16] The presence of one of these variations was positively associated with anterosuperior labral fraying, an abnormal superior glenohumeral ligament, and increased passive internal rotation with the arm in 90° of abduction (**Figure 4**).

A study of 691 patients found that 98 (14.2%) had one of three distinct anatomic variations in the antero-

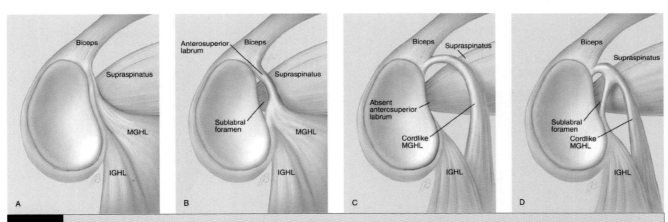

| **Figure 3** | Schematic drawings showing the normal anatomy of the labrum (**A**), an isolated sublabral foramen (**B**), a sublabral foramen with a cordlike middle glenohumeral ligament (**C**), and a cordlike middle glenohumeral ligament without tissue at the anterosuperior labrum (**D**). IGHL = inferior glenohumeral ligament, MGHL = middle glenohumeral ligament. (Reproduced with permission from Moseley H, Overgaard B: The anterior capsular mechanism in recurrent anterior dislocation of the shoulder: Morphological and clinical studies with special reference to the glenoid labrum and gleno-humeral ligaments. *J Bone Joint Surg Br* 1962;44[4]:913-927.) |

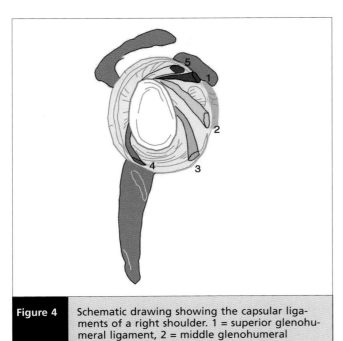

| **Figure 4** | Schematic drawing showing the capsular ligaments of a right shoulder. 1 = superior glenohumeral ligament, 2 = middle glenohumeral ligament, 3 = anterior band of inferior glenohumeral ligament, 4 = posterior band of inferior glenohumeral ligament, 5 = long head of the biceps tendon. |

superior portion of the labrum, classified as a sublabral recess (in 17 patients [2.46%]), a sublabral foramen (in 53 patients [7.67%]), or an absent anterosuperior labrum with a cordlike middle glenohumeral ligament (in 28 patients [4.05%]).[17] Two of the variations, the sublabral foramen and the absent anterosuperior labrum with a cordlike middle glenohumeral ligament, had a significant relationship with a type II SLAP lesion. Even though labral variations do not appear to contribute to instability, they may allow increased inter-

nal rotation and predispose the shoulder to lesions of the superior glenohumeral ligament and the anterosuperior portion of the labrum.

Glenohumeral Capsule

The glenohumeral capsule surrounds the glenohumeral joint, maintains the synovial environment, and provides stability at the extremes of the range of motion.[18,19] Current references describe the superior, middle, and inferior glenohumeral ligaments as thickenings of the anterior joint capsule that reinforce the anteroinferior part of the capsule and directly connect the humeral head to the glenoid fossa (**Figure 5**).

Experimental and computational investigations typically have isolated discrete ligamentous regions, but recent data suggest that the regions of the glenohumeral capsule have significant interactions and function multiaxially.[20-22] Finite element models were used to determine the distribution of maximum principal strain and deformed shape of the glenohumeral capsule at the apprehension position while a 25-N anterior load was applied to the humerus, with and without mechanical connection of the regions.[22] The results suggested that the regions of the capsule commonly described as glenohumeral ligaments have significant interactions when transferring forces between the scapula and humerus. Discrete capsular regions should not be isolated for experimental or computational analysis of glenohumeral capsule function. Instead, the glenohumeral capsule should be evaluated as a continuous sheet of fibrous tissue. The material properties of the glenohumeral capsule were found to be similar in directions parallel and perpendicular to the glenohumeral ligaments.[21] This finding further supported the concept of a continuous sheet of fibrous tissue.

An anatomic study with a histologic examination of 27 specimens concluded that the superior glenohumeral

1: Basic Science

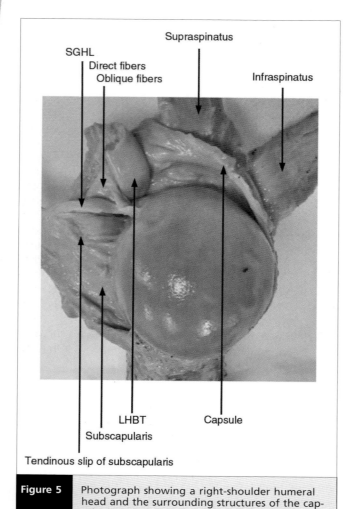

Figure 5 Photograph showing a right-shoulder humeral head and the surrounding structures of the capsule, ligaments, and rotator cuff tendons. LHBT = long head of biceps tendon, SGHL = superior glenohumeral ligament.

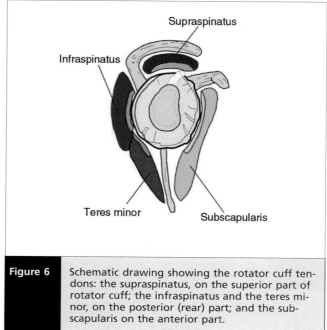

Figure 6 Schematic drawing showing the rotator cuff tendons: the supraspinatus, on the superior part of rotator cuff; the infraspinatus and the teres minor, on the posterior (rear) part; and the subscapularis on the anterior part.

ligament is a constant macroscopic structure consisting of direct and oblique fibers.[23] The study suggested that the function of the superior glenohumeral ligament is not only to connect and stabilize the glenohumeral joint but also to place and stabilize the LHBT from its origin through the insertion into the biceps groove.

Muscle and Tendon Anatomy

Rotator Cuff
The rotator cuff consists of the tendons of the supraspinatus, infraspinatus, subscapularis, and teres minor muscles, which stabilize and move the glenohumeral joint (**Figure 6**). Shoulder stability is one of the primary functions of the rotator cuff muscles. During abduction of the arm, the rotator cuff pulls the humeral head into the glenoid to allow the large deltoid muscle to elevate the arm.[24] This motion is called concavity compression. Without the action of the rotator cuff, the humeral head would translate superiorly out of the glenoid, and

the deltoid would be less efficient. The glenoid fossa is most susceptible to shear force perturbation in the anterior-to-posterior direction because the glenoid fossa is less deep than it is in the superior-to-inferior direction.[25] In a normal shoulder, the combined antagonistic forces of the subscapularis anteriorly and the infraspinatus and teres minor posteriorly function to compress the humeral head onto the glenoid. A cadaver analysis found glenohumeral instability superiorly when rotator cuff paralysis of the infraspinatus, subscapularis, and teres minor tendons was simulated.[26]

Supraspinatus
The supraspinatus arises from the supraspinous fossa above the scapular spine. The accepted belief is that the supraspinatus and other tendons of the rotator cuff insert on the greater and lesser tuberosities lateral to the anatomic neck of the humerus. This pattern has been recently questioned, however. The supraspinatus was found to have a long tendinous portion in the anterior half of the muscle, which always inserted into the anteriormost area of the highest impression on the greater tuberosity; in 21% of the specimens, it also inserted into the superiormost area of the lesser tuberosity.[27] The footprint of the supraspinatus was found to be triangular, with an average maximum medial-to-lateral length of 6.9 mm and an average maximum anterior-to-posterior width of 12.6 mm. In contrast, the infraspinatus had a long tendinous portion in the superior half of the muscle, which was curved anteriorly and extended to the anterolateral area of the highest impression of the greater tuberosity. The footprint of the infraspinatus was trapezoidal, with an average maximum medial-to-lateral length of 10.2 mm and an average maximum anterior-to-posterior width of

32.7 mm. Thus, the footprint of the supraspinatus on the greater tuberosity was found to be much smaller than previously believed; this area of the greater tuberosity actually is occupied by a substantial amount of the infraspinatus. The researchers suggested that rotator cuff tears previously believed to involve only the supraspinatus tendon may have a substantial infraspinatus component.[27]

Contraction of the supraspinatus leads to shoulder abduction at the glenohumeral joint. The supraspinatus is the primary agonist muscle for shoulder abduction during the first 10° to 15° of the arc. Beyond 30° of abduction, the deltoid muscle becomes the main abductor. The supraspinatus muscle helps in resisting the inferior gravitational forces across the shoulder caused by the weight of the upper limb.[28]

Infraspinatus

The infraspinatus muscle is in a thick triangular shape that occupies the infraspinatus fossa on the scapula. The muscle arises by thick fibers from the medial two thirds of the infraspinatus fossa and by tendinous fibers from the ridges on its surface; the muscle also arises from the infraspinatus fascia that covers it and separates it from the teres major and the teres minor.[29] The fibers converge to form a tendon that glides over the lateral border of the spine of the scapula, passes across the posterior region of the glenohumeral capsule, and inserts into the middle impression on the greater tubercle of the humerus.

The primary function of the infraspinatus is to horizontally extend and laterally rotate the humerus at the shoulder joint. When the arm is fixed, the infraspinatus abducts the inferior angle of the scapula. The infraspinatus and the teres minor externally rotate the shoulder and assist in extension of the glenohumeral joint.[29] A recent study examined the instantaneous moment arms of subregions in several muscles that cross the glenohumeral joint in axial rotation of the humerus during coronal plane abduction and sagittal plane flexion.[30] The study found that the inferior infraspinatus and the teres minor were the most important external rotators.

Subscapularis

The subscapularis originates from the anterior surface of the scapula, passing laterally beneath the coracoid and the scapular neck and becoming tendinous at the level of the glenoid. At its insertion, the tendinous portion of the subscapularis blends with the fibers of the glenohumeral capsule and inserts into the lesser tuberosity. The remaining insertion consists of muscle and is below the lesser tuberosity. The morphology of the subscapularis insertion recently was found to be broad proximally and tapered distally in a comma shape.[31] The insertion was found to consist of a proximal tendinous part and a distal muscular part. With the exception of the bare area at the proximal end, the measured values were significantly greater in specimens from men than from women.

The subscapularis muscle is the largest and strongest muscle of the rotator cuff. The subscapularis rotates the head of the humerus medially (in internal rotation). When the arm is raised, the subscapularis draws the humerus forward and downward.[32] The subscapularis also prevents anterior displacement of the humeral head. The inferior subscapularis was found to be the most important internal rotator.[30] The diagnosis of subscapularis injuries can be difficult, and the ability to assess some tears may be limited during arthroscopy or open surgery. An MRI study of subscapularis tendon tears compared with normal anatomy found diagnostic imaging to be important for diagnosing and evaluating the extent of subscapularis injury.[32] Clinicians must understand several unusual types of subscapularis tendon tears, however. A full-thickness tear may be difficult to appreciate because of overlying scar tissue attaching to the greater tuberosity and mimicking intact tendon fibers. Even an extensive subscapularis tendon tear may lack tendon retraction because of the stabilizing effect of the coracohumeral ligament or an intact inferior subscapularis attachment. Scar tissue may prevent leakage of contrast material on magnetic resonance arthrography.

Teres Minor

The upper two thirds of the teres minor arise from the dorsal surface of the axillary border of the scapula. The remaining one third arises from two aponeurotic laminae, one of which separates the teres minor from the infraspinatus muscle, and the other separates it from the teres major muscle. The fibers of the teres minor run obliquely upward and downward into the lowest portion of the greater tuberosity. In 31 cadaver shoulders, approximately half of the shoulders had a distinct fascial compartment surrounding the teres minor muscle, and the other half had a combined fascia surrounding both the infraspinatus and teres minor muscles.[33] All shoulders had a stout fascial sling at the inferior glenoid neck. The primary motor nerve branch to the teres minor always traveled between this sling and the teres minor muscle after making a sharp bend. These findings may have implications for understanding isolated teres minor muscle atrophy.

In addition to their function in adduction, extension, and transverse extension, the infraspinatus and the teres minor work in tandem with the posterior deltoid to externally rotate the humerus.

Biceps

The LHBT originates from the superior glenoid labrum and the supraglenoid tubercle and has an intra-articular portion that passes over the humeral head before leaving the glenohumeral joint through the bicipital groove.[34] The origin is continuous with and contributes to the glenoid labrum. The small head of the biceps originates at the coracoid, and the muscle belly from each origin converges to form the biceps muscle proper.[35]

1: Basic Science

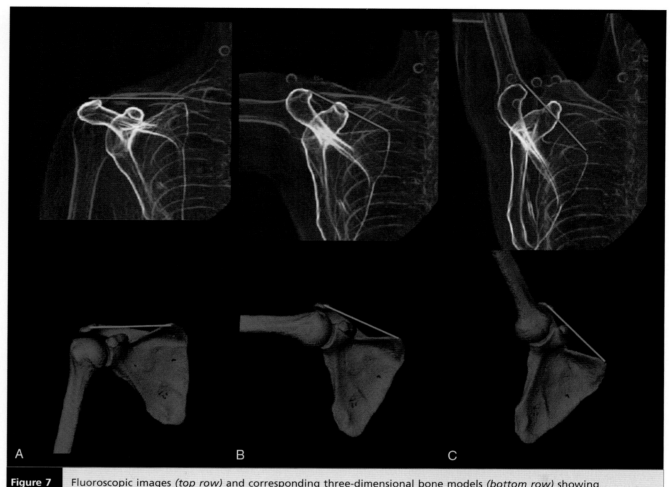

Figure 7 Fluoroscopic images *(top row)* and corresponding three-dimensional bone models *(bottom row)* showing scapulothoracic motion in three positions *(green lines)*: neutral position (**A**), 90° of abduction (**B**), and maximum elevation (**C**).

The origin of the LHBT from the superior glenoid labrum and the supraglenoid tubercle was found to vary in a study of 101 cadaver shoulders.[36] Four origin types were described: entirely posterior, in 28 shoulders; posterior dominant, in 56 shoulders; equal, in 17 shoulders; and entirely anterior, in none of the shoulders. In all shoulders, the LHBT was found to originate from both the glenoid labrum and supraglenoid tubercle. Information from this study can aid clinicians in assessing the origin of the LHBT and treating pathology such as a SLAP lesion.

The size of the LHBT also varies. The intra-articular portion typically is wide and flat, and the extra-articular portion is smaller and rounder. The tendon is approximately 5 to 6 mm in diameter and 9 cm in length.[35] The anterior circumflex humeral artery provides the blood supply of the articular portion of the LHBT. The more distal portion of the tendon is avascular to accommodate its sliding motion within its sheath in the bicipital groove.[37]

From the neutral arm position, the LHBT slides up to 18 mm in and out of the glenohumeral joint during forward flexion and internal rotation.[38] The LHBT functions in shoulder flexion, extension, abduction, internal rotation, external rotation, and anterior stabilization.

Scapulothoracic Joint Function

The scapula serves as a base for glenohumeral joint motion, allowing the rotator cuff to function as a link in the kinematic chain between the thorax and the arm. Humerothoracic motion is generated by both the scapulothoracic and glenohumeral joints (**Figure 7**). Motion of the scapula on the thorax is essential for normal function of the upper extremity.[39] The scapulothoracic joint is not a diarthrodial joint. However, a significant amount of motion occurs between the scapula and the thorax during arm motion. In shoulder abduction, 2° of every 3° occur at the glenohumeral joint and 1° occurs at the scapulothoracic joint.[40] The coordinated motion during arm movement is called the scapulohumeral rhythm.

In a study using electromagnetic motion sensors and surface electrodes to detect muscle activity in 20 healthy subjects, the orientation and the position of the scapula on the thorax were found to be different when the arm was elevated actively rather than passively.[41] Decreased levels of muscle activity during passive elevation resulted in altered scapulothoracic kinematics, including upward rotation and external rotation of the scapula. The greatest effect was noted through the midrange of arm elevation. Significantly more upward rotation of the scapula occurred when the arm was raised actively rather than passively. This finding reinforces the important role of the trapezius and serratus anterior muscles in producing scapular upward rotation, especially throughout the midrange of arm elevation. These muscles and the upward rotation of the scapula, especially in the midrange of arm elevation, should be carefully assessed during physical examination.

An in vivo MRI study assessed the three-dimensional motion of the scapula from 90° of external rotation to 90° of internal rotation with the humerus in 90° of abduction.[42] The scapulothoracic joint was found to contribute approximately 12.5% of the motion during the entire motion. As the arm position changed from 90° of external rotation to 60° of internal rotation, most of the movement was from the glenohumeral joint. At more than 60° of internal rotation, the scapula began to markedly tilt in the anterior direction.[42] These findings reinforce the concept that scapulothoracic motion is important for normal function of the shoulder.

Summary

The shoulder consists of a complex arrangement of osseous and soft-tissue structures that provide a large range of motion and maintain stability. The complex anatomy varies greatly among individuals and must be properly modeled to understand normal and pathologic function. To properly restore normal anatomy and joint function, surgeons must account for a patient's anatomic variability during diagnostic and surgical procedures.

Annotated References

1. Crockett HC, Gross LB, Wilk KE, et al: Osseous adaptation and range of motion at the glenohumeral joint in professional baseball pitchers. *Am J Sports Med* 2002;30(1):20-26.

2. Harrold F, Wigderowitz C: A three-dimensional analysis of humeral head retroversion. *J Shoulder Elbow Surg* 2012;21(5):612-617.

   Surface topography data for 24 cadaver humeral heads were collected using a handheld digitizer and a surface laser scanner to determine variability in retroversion of the cartilage-metaphysis interface in the axial plane. The results suggested that the cartilage-metaphyseal interface has a high degree of variability and is not a suitable landmark for osteotomy procedures.

3. Hill JA, Tkach L, Hendrix RW: A study of glenohumeral orientation in patients with anterior recurrent shoulder dislocations using computerized axial tomography. *Orthop Rev* 1989;18(1):84-91.

4. Robertson DD, Yuan J, Bigliani LU, Flatow EL, Yamaguchi K: Three-dimensional analysis of the proximal part of the humerus: Relevance to arthroplasty. *J Bone Joint Surg Am* 2000;82(11):1594-1602.

5. Pearl ML, Volk AG: Retroversion of the proximal humerus in relationship to prosthetic replacement arthroplasty. *J Shoulder Elbow Surg* 1995;4(4):286-289.

6. Kvitne RS, Jobe FW, Jobe CM: Shoulder instability in the overhand or throwing athlete. *Clin Sports Med* 1995;14(4):917-935.

7. Angibaud L, Zuckerman JD, Flurin PH, Roche C, Wright T: Reconstructing proximal humeral fractures using the bicipital groove as a landmark. *Clin Orthop Relat Res* 2007;458:168-174.

   Three-dimensional geometry of the bicipital groove was quantified in 49 dried humeri. The anterior offset of the bicipital groove was found to be almost constant from proximal to distal relative to the intramedullary axis. The distal bicipital groove at the level of the surgical neck is a reasonable landmark for establishing humeral head retroversion.

8. Itamura J, Dietrick T, Roidis N, Shean C, Chen F, Tibone J: Analysis of the bicipital groove as a landmark for humeral head replacement. *J Shoulder Elbow Surg* 2002;11(4):322-326.

9. Wafae N, Atencio Santamaría LE, Vitor L, Pereira LA, Ruiz CR, Wafae GC: Morphometry of the human bicipital groove (sulcus intertubercularis). *J Shoulder Elbow Surg* 2010;19(1):65-68.

   Morphometric study of the bicipital groove and humerus in 50 dry humeri confirmed the variability of length, thickness, width, and angle measurements of the bicipital groove.

10. Bryce CD, Davison AC, Lewis GS, Wang L, Flemming DJ, Armstrong AD: Two-dimensional glenoid version measurements vary with coronal and sagittal scapular rotation. *J Bone Joint Surg Am* 2010;92(3):692-699.

    Three-dimensional CT scans of 36 cadaver scapulae were evaluated while being rotated in 1° increments in the coronal and sagittal planes to investigate the effect of scapular rotation on glenoid version. Misalignment of 1° or more in the coronal or the sagittal plane created inaccuracy in measurement.

11. Dunham KS, Bencardino JT, Rokito AS: Anatomic variants and pitfalls of the labrum, glenoid cartilage, and glenohumeral ligaments. *Magn Reson Imaging Clin N Am* 2012;20(2):213-228, x.

    Normal glenoid labrum, articular cartilage, and gleno-

1: Basic Science

humeral ligament anatomy and variants were evaluated. Pitfalls were described related to interpreting conventional and arthrographic MRI.

12. Stoller D: *Magnetic Resonance Imaging in Orthopaedics and Sports Medicine.* Philadelphia, PA, Lippincott, Williams & Wilkins, 2007.

13. Moseley H, Overgaard B: The anterior capsular mechanism in recurrent anterior dislocation of the shoulder: Morphological and clinical studies with special reference to the glenoid labrum and gleno-humeral ligaments. *J Bone Joint Surg Br* 1962;44(4):913-927.

14. Pagnani MJ, Deng XH, Warren RF, Torzilli PA, Altchek DW: Effect of lesions of the superior portion of the glenoid labrum on glenohumeral translation. *J Bone Joint Surg Am* 1995;77(7):1003-1010.

15. Powell SN, Nord KD, Ryu RKN: The diagnosis, classification, and treatment of SLAP lesions. *Oper Tech Sports Med* 2012;20:46-56.

    The clinical features of SLAP lesions were reviewed, with mechanism of injury, physical examination, classification, associated lesions, normal and pathologic anatomy, and a treatment algorithm.

16. Rao AG, Kim TK, Chronopoulos E, McFarland EG: Anatomical variants in the anterosuperior aspect of the glenoid labrum: A statistical analysis of seventy-three cases. *J Bone Joint Surg Am* 2003;85(4):653-659.

17. Kanatli U, Ozturk BY, Bolukbasi S: Anatomical variations of the anterosuperior labrum: Prevalence and association with type II superior labrum anterior-posterior (SLAP) lesions. *J Shoulder Elbow Surg* 2010; 19(8):1199-1203.

    Retrospective evaluation of 713 consecutive shoulder arthroscopies for anterosuperior labral variations and coexisting labral pathologies found that some anatomic variants of the anterosuperior labrum were associated with the development of SLAP lesions.

18. Burkart AC, Debski RE: Anatomy and function of the glenohumeral ligaments in anterior shoulder instability. *Clin Orthop Relat Res* 2002;400:32-39.

19. Tischer T, Vogt S, Kreuz PC, Imhoff AB: Arthroscopic anatomy, variants, and pathologic findings in shoulder instability. *Arthroscopy* 2011;27(10):1434-1443.

    Information on shoulder anatomy and pathology related to shoulder stability was synthesized to improve clinical diagnoses and surgical treatment.

20. Moore SM, Stehle JH, Rainis EJ, McMahon PJ, Debski RE: The current anatomical description of the inferior glenohumeral ligament does not correlate with its functional role in positions of external rotation. *J Orthop Res* 2008;26(12):1598-1604.

    The strain distribution in the inferior glenohumeral ligament was observed in five cadaver shoulders at 0°, 30°, and 60° of external rotation while a 25-N anterior load was applied. The complex strain distribu-

tions suggested that the inferior glenohumeral capsule should be treated as a continuous sheet of fibrous tissue.

21. Rainis EJ, Maas SA, Henninger HB, McMahon PJ, Weiss JA, Debski RE: Material properties of the axillary pouch of the glenohumeral capsule: Is isotropic material symmetry appropriate? *J Biomech Eng* 2009; 131(3):031007.

    A combined experimental and computational protocol was used to characterize the mechanical properties of the axillary pouch of the glenohumeral capsule, which were found to be the same in the longitudinal and transverse directions.

22. Moore SM, Ellis BJ, Weiss JA, McMahon PJ, Debski RE: The glenohumeral capsule should be evaluated as a sheet of fibrous tissue: A validated finite element model. *Ann Biomed Eng* 2010;38(1):66-76.

    Finite element models were used to determine the distribution of maximum principal strain and deformed shape of the glenohumeral capsule at the apprehension position. The study concluded that discrete capsular regions should not be isolated for experimental or computational analysis of glenohumeral capsule function.

23. Kask K, Põldoja E, Lont T, et al: Anatomy of the superior glenohumeral ligament. *J Shoulder Elbow Surg* 2010;19(6):908-916.

    Twenty-seven cadaver shoulder specimens were examined to provide a detailed anatomic description of the superior glenohumeral ligament and its relationship to the rotator cuff interval. The superior glenohumeral ligament was found to be a constant macroscopic structure consisting of direct and oblique fibers.

24. Harryman DT II, Sidles JA, Clark JM, McQuade KJ, Gibb TD, Matsen FA III: Translation of the humeral head on the glenoid with passive glenohumeral motion. *J Bone Joint Surg Am* 1990;72(9):1334-1343.

25. Wuelker N, Korell M, Thren K: Dynamic glenohumeral joint stability. *J Shoulder Elbow Surg* 1998;7(1): 43-52.

26. Thompson WO, Debski RE, Boardman ND III, et al: A biomechanical analysis of rotator cuff deficiency in a cadaveric model. *Am J Sports Med* 1996;24(3):286-292.

27. Mochizuki T, Sugaya H, Uomizu M, et al: Humeral insertion of the supraspinatus and infraspinatus: New anatomical findings regarding the footprint of the rotator cuff. *J Bone Joint Surg Am* 2008;90(5):962-969.

    The humeral insertions of the rotator cuff were investigated in 113 cadaver shoulders. The supraspinatus was found to have a long tendinous portion in its anterior half, which always inserted into the anterior-most area of the highest impression on the greater tuberosity.

28. Ackland DC, Pandy MG: Lines of action and stabilizing potential of the shoulder musculature. *J Anat* 2009;215(2):184-197.

The lines of action were determined for 18 major muscles and muscle subregions crossing the glenohumeral joint of the human shoulder. Computer simulations then predicted the contribution of these muscles to joint shear and compression forces during scapular plane abduction and sagittal plane flexion.

29. Clemente C: *Gray's Anatomy of the Human Body,* ed 30. Philadelphia, PA, Lea & Febiger, 1985.

30. Ackland DC, Pandy MG: Moment arms of the shoulder muscles during axial rotation. *J Orthop Res* 2011;29(5):658-667.

The moment arms were determined for 18 major muscle subregions crossing the glenohumeral joint with axial rotation of the humerus during coronal plane abduction and sagittal plane flexion. The inferior infraspinatus and the teres minor were found to be the most important external rotators.

31. Ide J, Tokiyoshi A, Hirose J, Mizuta H: An anatomic study of the subscapularis insertion to the humerus: The subscapularis footprint. *Arthroscopy* 2008;24(7):749-753.

The morphology of the subscapularis insertion to the humerus was elucidated in 40 cadaver shoulders. The insertion site anatomy was broad proximally and tapered distally in a comma shape.

32. Morag Y, Jamadar DA, Miller B, Dong Q, Jacobson JA: The subscapularis: Anatomy, injury, and imaging. *Skeletal Radiol* 2011;40(3):255-269.

Anatomy and MRI findings in injured subscapularis tendons were compared with normal anatomy.

33. Chafik D, Galatz LM, Keener JD, Kim HM, Yamaguchi K: Teres minor muscle and related anatomy. *J Shoulder Elbow Surg* 2013;22(1):108-114.

The complex anatomy surrounding the teres minor muscle was evaluated.

34. Ghalayini SR, Board TN, Srinivasan MS: Anatomic variations in the long head of biceps: Contribution to shoulder dysfunction. *Arthroscopy* 2007;23(9):1012-1018.

Current knowledge of anatomic variants and management of LHBT lesions was discussed, with a report of congenital absence of the LHBT in three patients. A classification system was proposed for symptomatic lesions and congenital absence of the LHBT.

35. Elser F, Braun S, Dewing CB, Giphart JE, Millett PJ: Anatomy, function, injuries, and treatment of the long head of the biceps brachii tendon. *Arthroscopy* 2011;27(4):581-592.

An update was provided on the anatomy and biomechanical properties of the LHBT, with an evidence-based approach to current treatment strategies for disorders of the LHBT.

36. Tuoheti Y, Itoi E, Minagawa H, et al: Attachment types of the long head of the biceps tendon to the glenoid labrum and their relationships with the glenohumeral ligaments. *Arthroscopy* 2005;21(10):1242-1249.

37. Ahrens PM, Boileau P: The long head of biceps and associated tendinopathy. *J Bone Joint Surg Br* 2007;89(8):1001-1009.

Current views on the pathology of LHBT lesions were described. The anterior circumflex humeral artery feeds the articular portion of the LHBT, but the distal portion of the tendon is avascular.

38. Braun S, Millett PJ, Yongpravat C, et al: Biomechanical evaluation of shear force vectors leading to injury of the biceps reflection pulley: A biplane fluoroscopy study on cadaveric shoulders. *Am J Sports Med* 2010;38(5):1015-1024.

The LHBT was evaluated in eight fresh-frozen cadaver shoulders to measure its course in common arm positions. Shear and compressive force vectors as well as the excursion of the tendon also were determined.

39. Kibler WB, McMullen J: Scapular dyskinesis and its relation to shoulder pain. *J Am Acad Orthop Surg* 2003;11(2):142-151.

40. Karduna AR, McClure PW, Michener LA: Scapular kinematics: Effects of altering the Euler angle sequence of rotations. *J Biomech* 2000;33(9):1063-1068.

41. Ebaugh DD, McClure PW, Karduna AR: Three-dimensional scapulothoracic motion during active and passive arm elevation. *Clin Biomech (Bristol, Avon)* 2005;20(7):700-709.

42. Koishi H, Goto A, Tanaka M, et al: In vivo three-dimensional motion analysis of the shoulder joint during internal and external rotation. *Int Orthop* 2011;35(10):1503-1509.

Open MRI was used to examine the right shoulder of 10 healthy volunteers to assess the three-dimensional motion of the scapula from 90° of external rotation to 90° of internal rotation with the humerus in 90° of abduction. The scapulothoracic joint was found to contribute approximately 12.5% of the entire motion.

Chapter 2

Basic Science of Rotator Cuff Tendons and Healing

Sarah Ilkhani-Pour, MSE   Andrew A. Dunkman, BA   Louis J. Soslowsky, PhD

Introduction

The shoulder is one of the most complex regions of the human musculoskeletal system. The ball-and-socket character of the glenohumeral joint allows it to have a greater range of motion than any other joint. The complexity and mobility of the glenohumeral joint suggest the reason the tendons of the rotator cuff are frequently injured, leading to pain, disability, and economic loss. The frequent occurrence of shoulder injury and degeneration provides the impetus for clinicians and scientists to investigate the biology, pathology, and management of these conditions. Recent studies of rotator cuff tendons have focused on molecular events, including the factors that influence biomechanics, the causes of deterioration, and the interactions between biologic structures and mechanical function. Clinical studies, animal model studies, and new imaging techniques are providing insight into rotator cuff tendon healing and guiding the selection of repair techniques, postoperative care, and rehabilitation.

Anatomy, Composition, and Structure of the Rotator Cuff

The four main muscles that make up the rotator cuff are the supraspinatus, the infraspinatus, the teres minor, and the subscapularis. These muscles impart stability to the glenohumeral joint and movement to the arm. Each of the tendons of these muscles inserts into the proximal end of the humerus. Of these tendons, the supraspinatus is most often injured; this fact often is attributed to its vulnerable location under the coracoacromial arch and its poor vascularity. For this reason, most research on rotator cuff tendon healing has focused on the supraspinatus.

Type I collagen is believed to account for 85% of the dry weight of the rotator cuff tendons, with a significant amount of type III collagen in the supraspinatus tendon and a relatively high glycosaminoglycan content. The supraspinatus tendon undergoes significant compression and expresses extracellular matrix proteins often found in cartilage. Investigators have begun to quantify the distributions and locations of specific proteoglycans in the supraspinatus tendon. Sandwich enzyme-linked immunosorbent assays were used to measure decorin, aggrecan, and biglycan levels in the supraspinatus tendon of healthy cadaver shoulders. Decorin, often associated with tension bearing, was found in constant concentrations across six regions. Aggrecan and biglycan, associated with compression and active remodeling, respectively, were found in greater concentrations in the anterior and posterior regions of the tendon. Because the anterior region is the most susceptible to injury, understanding proteoglycan concentrations at this location is particularly valuable.[1]

Most rotator cuff injuries occur at the tendon-to-bone enthesis of the supraspinatus. This region endures significant stress concentrations because of the sharp gradient of material transitioning from tendon to bone. Understanding these properties from an engineering perspective is critical to improving treatments and surgical techniques. Although the insertion site has been characterized as having four distinct zones, the transition is in fact, gradual and continuous. Tendon proper, the zone similar to the midsubstance of the tendon, primarily contains well-aligned type I collagen fibers. Fibrocartilage, the second zone, primarily contains type II and III collagens and exhibits increased proteoglycan concentration. As the enthesis continues, mineralization increases dramatically; the final two zones are described as mineralized fibrocartilage and, ultimately, bone. Researchers recently have used Raman spectroscopy to further investigate this transitional zone. This new method of quantifying mineral composition revealed linear increases in the mineral-to-collagen ratio and crystalline organization across the insertion site[2] (**Figure 1**). The failure of repair and postoperative healing to re-create and restore this gradation contributes to the high rate of retearing.

1: Basic Science

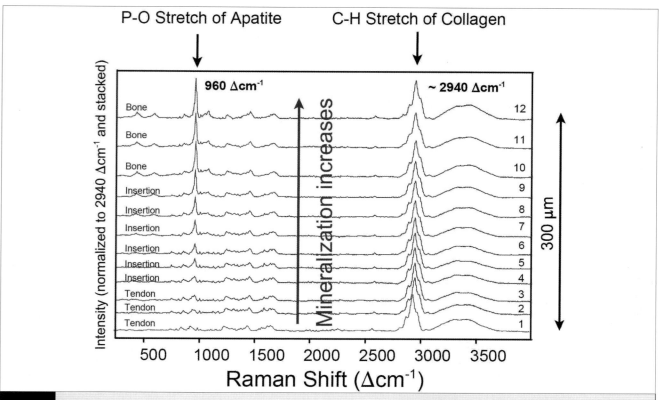

P-O Stretch of Apatite   **C-H Stretch of Collagen**

Figure 1	Diagram showing the use of Raman spectroscopy to quantify mineral composition across the rat shoulder tendon-bone insertion site. All spectra are normalized by the C-H stretch of collagen and then stacked along the y-axis for better comparison. The mineral content, represented by the P-O stretch of apatite at 960 Δcm^{-1}, can be seen to gradually increase along the traverse from tendon to bone. (Reproduced with permission from Wopenka B, Kent A, Pasteris JD, Yoon Y, Thomopoulos S: The tendon-to-bone transition of the rotator cuff: A preliminary Raman spectroscopic study documenting the gradual mineralization across the insertion in rat tissue samples. *Appl Spectrosc* 2008;62[12]:1285-1294.)

Tendon Biomechanics

The main function of the rotator cuff is mechanical and includes primary stabilization of the shoulder joint and secondary movement of the shoulder. Rotator cuff tendons have nonlinear, viscoelastic, and heterogeneous material properties. Understanding these biomechanical properties provides insight into rotator cuff tear prevention, repair, and rehabilitation. Recent advances include technologies to measure in vivo rotator cuff deformation, quantification of uninjured tendon material properties, insights into tear propagation, and appreciation for the effects of systemic alterations on rotator cuff tendon mechanics.

In Vivo Measurements

Noninvasive imaging techniques are useful in evaluating rotator cuff tendon healing. In roentgen stereophotogrammetric analysis, markers inserted into the materials of interest are analyzed using static x-ray image pairs. Stainless steel suture used as a marker in ovine rotator cuff tendon accurately measured migration to approximately 1 mm.[3] This technique may be appropriate for tracking the formation of a gap after surgical re-

pair. Similarly, low-dosage CT was used to measure the position of markers implanted in patients.[4] This technique was accurate to within 0.7 mm; the intermarker distances were influenced by arm position and the location of the bead within the rotator cuff. These methods can be used only with static imaging and cannot be used to assess the functional properties of the tissue. To overcome this limitation, biplane x-ray analysis uses high-speed radiographic images to track implanted tantalum beads and measure dynamic deformation of rotator cuff tissue. In an in vivo canine model, this technique distinguished an intact repair, an unsuccessful repair, and a control infraspinatus.[5] The intact tendon repair contracted approximately 19% and became 70% stiffer over 28 weeks. However, the unsuccessful repair did not contract despite a stiffening of the scar tissue. This system is accurate to within 0.1 mm and is useful for functional analysis of in vivo tissue deformations. Two-dimensional speckle tracking echocardiography has been applied to intact, healthy supraspinatus tendons to determine the in vivo strains.[6] This technique detected differences in strain between the superficial (bursal) and deep (articular) sides of the supraspinatus tendon as well as different responses of the

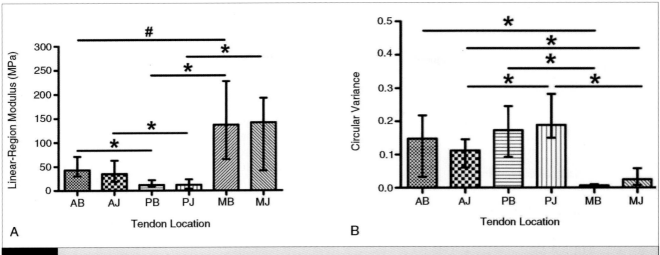

Figure 2 Diagrams depicting regional variations in tensile modulus and collagen organization. Both plots depict median and interquartile ranges. **A,** The elastic modulus of the supraspinatus tendon varies regionally. Posterior samples are consistently lower in modulus than medial and anterior samples. **B,** Circular variance, a measure of the disorganization of collagen fibers, is inhomogeneous across the supraspinatus tendon. The more aligned regions tend to have a higher modulus, whereas the more disorganized regions (with higher circular variance) tend to have lower modulus values. # = trend, * = significant, AB = anterior bursa, AJ = anterior joint, PB = posterior bursa, PJ = posterior joint, MB = medial bursa, MJ = medial joint. (Adapted with permission from Lake SP, Miller KS, Elliott DM, Soslowsky LJ: Effect of fiber distribution and realignment on the nonlinear and inhomogeneous mechanical properties of human supraspinatus tendon under longitudinal tensile loading. *J Orthop Res* 2009;27[12]:1596-1602.)

tendon to isotonic and isometric muscle contractions. These findings may suggest the use of a different technique for repairing delaminated tears.

Material Properties

Finite element models allow computational analysis of the rotator cuff mechanical environment. A three-dimensional finite element model of the supraspinatus tendon was used to determine that maximum tensile stress occurs on the articular side of the anterior edge of the tendon, accounting for the frequency of tears at this site.[7] Although this analysis was the first to use a three-dimensional finite element model of the supraspinatus, it was limited by its assumptions of isotropy and homogeneity. In other studies, in vitro mechanical testing of human cadaver supraspinatus tendon tissue found that it has highly inhomogeneous and nonlinear mechanical properties.[8,9] Including a polarized light setup during mechanical testing allowed collagen fiber alignment to be quantified throughout testing. Tensile modulus is the ratio of stress to strain in the linear region of a stress-strain curve. Tensile moduli values and fiber alignment were region dependent within the tendon during tensile loading, whether longitudinal (in the direction of fibers) or transverse (orthogonal to fibers). In longitudinal loading, samples taken from the posterior portion of the supraspinatus tendon had lower tensile moduli than samples from the anterior or medial tendon; no tensile moduli differences existed between bursal- and articular-side regions. Similarly, fiber alignment was most disorganized in posterior samples and most highly aligned in medial samples (**Figure 2**). Ten-

don material properties also can be used to distinguish between a normal and a torn rotator cuff tendon. Biopsies from patients with a massive rotator cuff tear revealed a significantly lower storage modulus than in normal tendons, when measured using dynamic shear mechanical testing.[10] The storage modulus measures the stored elastic energy in viscoelastic materials. Torn tendons are mechanically weaker, and storage modulus may be a useful parameter for future studies. Decreased mechanical properties may predispose a massive tear to repair failure.

Mechanical Interactions Between Tendons

The progression of rotator cuff tears from small and manageable to massive and subject to repair failure is a major clinical concern. A direct relationship between tear size and tendon strain was established using a sheep cadaver model of an infraspinatus tear. Larger tears failed at a lower load than smaller tears.[11] Tear propagation began at strains of only 1.7%, indicating that even a small tear may propagate. In this study, the infraspinatus tendon was isolated and tested separately from the other rotator cuff tendons. In vivo, however, the rotator cuff tendons work together to provide stability and motion to the glenohumeral joint. For this reason, a set of studies investigated the mechanical interactions between the supraspinatus and infraspinatus tendons. Human cadaver shoulders were dissected, leaving the supraspinatus and infraspinatus tendons intact. Supraspinatus-applied loads and tear sizes, glenohumeral abduction angles, joint rotation angles, and the presence or absence of a supraspinatus repair were

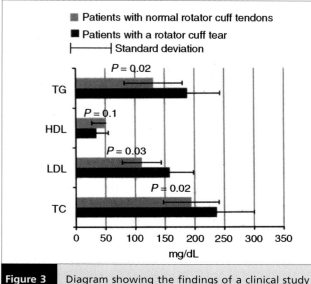

Figure 3 Diagram showing the findings of a clinical study comparing levels of triglyceride (TG), high-density lipoproteins (HDL), low-density lipoproteins (LDL), and total cholesterol (TC) in patients with normal rotator cuff tendons and patients with a rotator cuff tear. The patients with a rotator cuff tear had a higher incidence of hypercholesterolemia than those with normal rotator cuff tendons. (Adapted with permission from Abboud JA, Kim JS: The effect of hypercholesterolemia on rotator cuff disease. *Clin Orthop Relat Res* 2010;468[6]:1493-1497.)

investigated to determine their effect on supraspinatus and infraspinatus tendon strains.[12-14] Multiple regression models using these data found that the glenohumeral abduction angle and the supraspinatus tendon load were significant predictors of infraspinatus and supraspinatus tendon strains.[15] These findings suggest that tear propagation may be reduced by limiting loading and keeping the arm at 30° abduction in neutral rotation. This information has implications for postrepair management.

Systemic Alterations

Researchers have sought to understand the risk factors associated with rotator cuff tendinopathy and tearing. Recently, the role of systemic alterations, including high cholesterol, diabetes, age-related bone loss, and smoking, has been examined. In one clinical study, patients with a rotator cuff tear had significantly higher levels of total cholesterol, triglycerides, and low-density lipoproteins than those who had shoulder pain without a tear (**Figure 3**). Deposits of cholesterol (xanthomata) on the tendon or the extracellular matrix may alter the tendon's mechanics, increasing its susceptibility to injury or impairing its healing. In addition, the well-known restriction of blood flow in patients with hypercholesterolemia may further diminish the poor vascularity of the rotator cuff tendon.[16] This study identified a correlation between high cholesterol and

rotator cuff tears but did not establish causation. Research using animal models suggests that hypercholesterolemia significantly affects the elastic modulus of tendons.[17]

Earlier findings that patients with diabetes have decreased bone mass and diminished fracture healing led researchers to induce hyperglycemia in rats to model the effect of diabetes in tendon-to-bone healing after surgical repair. As anticipated, the repair sites of the hyperglycemic rats appeared qualitatively inferior, had significantly reduced collagen fiber organization and fibrocartilage formation, and failed under approximately half the load of repair sites in control animals. Special consideration therefore may be needed for patients with poorly controlled glycemic levels.[18]

Estrogen deficiency causes greater bone resorption and resultantly less dense bones. Rats that received a bilateral ovariectomy had decreased bone density at the supraspinatus enthesis, but rats that also received bisphosphonate had increased density and a significantly higher failure stress. All estrogen-deficient rats (regardless of whether they received bisphosphonate) had poorer fibrocartilage and insertion-site organization, increased stiffness, and an increased tensile modulus compared with control animals. Increasing a patient's bone density may help prevent repair failure.[19] Recent research has evaluated the effect of nicotine on the mechanical properties of normal supraspinatus tendons in a rat model. The supraspinatus tendons of nicotine-dosed rats had a significantly higher elastic modulus than those of control animals, and the researchers speculated that this factor may be related to the increased risk of tearing among those who smoke tobacco.[20]

Tendon Degeneration and Tears

Animal Models

The rat shoulder is the most widely used animal model of the human rotator cuff. The bony anatomy of the rat shoulder closely mimics that of humans, with the supraspinatus passing underneath the acromion. Rat shoulder function also parallels that of the human shoulder. The placement of the scapula means that forward flexion in the rat shoulder is equivalent to abduction in humans. Supporting this notion, an acute rotator cuff tendon detachment was found to alter rat gait.[21] The decreased stride length at both early and late time points is consistent with reduced supraspinatus function. A second tendon detachment led to additional detrimental effects. This gait analysis technique was modified in a follow-up study to include force plates that measure ground reaction forces during rat locomotion.[22] After unilateral supraspinatus detachment and repair, the alterations in gait were transient; early changes were seen in step length, peak vertical force, peak breaking force, and peak lateral force, but all parameters returned to control levels within 4 weeks of the repair.

The rabbit subscapularis also has been suggested as a model for human rotator cuff pathology.[23] The rabbit acromion has little prominence, but the rabbit subscapularis tendon passes through another bony tunnel consisting of the tuberculum supraglenoidale, coracoid process, tuberculum infraglenoidale, and coracobrachialis muscle.

Chronic Tears

Chronic rotator cuff tears are associated with degenerative changes and atrophy. Tendon biopsy samples from patients with a supraspinatus tear revealed a loss of fiber structure, rounded tenocytes, increased cellularity, increased vascularity, and decreased collagen stainability compared with specimens from unruptured shoulders.[24] These biopsies from the middle portion of the supraspinatus tendon indicate that degeneration occurs throughout the tendon, not only at the torn end. Attenuated total reflectance Fourier transform infrared spectroscopy can distinguish the chemical and structural properties of tendon biopsy samples from different-size rotator cuff tears.[25] Torn tendons had decreased collagen I, II, and III content. The changes in small tears primarily involved lipids and some proteoglycans; massive tears had the greatest change in collagen, with an association between increased tear size and degeneration.

Muscle biopsies from patients with a rotator cuff tear revealed distinct differences that depended on the size of the rupture.[26] Fatty infiltration was the most obvious difference; massive tears had significantly greater lipid accumulation between muscle fibers and within the sarcoplasm of type I muscle fibers in comparison with control muscle samples. Although the term fatty infiltration is commonly used to describe the atrophy of muscle tissue and accompanying fatty deposits, the origin of the adipocytes has not been firmly established. Massive tears had a decreased number of myofibrils and increases in interfiber connective tissue, the mitochondrial content of slow muscle fibers, and the blood vessel supply to the supraspinatus muscle. Fatty atrophy is more common in shoulders with a relatively large tear or a tear of the anterior portion of the supraspinatus tendon.[27] A retrospective analysis revealed that the extent of fatty infiltration is related to patient age, the delay between the onset of symptoms and diagnosis, and the number of involved tendons.[28] Fatty degeneration occurred more quickly and progressed more rapidly if the tear involved more than one tendon. A multiple regression analysis showed that the amount of retraction, abduction torque, and serum calcifediol (vitamin D) levels were independent predictors of supraspinatus fatty degeneration; low levels of serum vitamin D were related to increased fatty degeneration.[29] Expression levels of α-skeletal muscle actin and myosin heavy chain polypeptide-1, two components of the contractile portion of muscle, were correlated with increasing supraspinatus fatty degeneration.[30] This increase in muscle gene expression suggests that fatty changes do not occur because of muscle fiber degeneration but instead because of muscle regeneration failure.

Animal models have been used to investigate degenerative change associated with chronic rotator cuff tears. Historically, it has been difficult to induce fatty infiltration in a rat model. Studies investigating acute transection of the supraspinatus tendon in rats found muscle retraction, sarcomere shortening, muscle atrophy, and tendon degeneration but minimal fatty atrophy.[31,32] Even at an advanced age, rats did not have significant levels of fatty atrophy.[33] Muscular changes were transient, but tendon degeneration progressed over time. Scar formation in rats, unlike humans, reattaches the tendon to the humerus, thereby reestablishing load. The detrimental supraspinatus and infraspinatus tendon changes seen in the rat after a unilateral infraspinatus-supraspinatus detachment are consistent with human chronic tear biopsies; these changes include increased area, percent relaxation (a measure of viscoelasticity that describes the amount the load decreases over time with a given strain), disorganization, cellularity, and rounding of cells.[34] The effects of tendon reattachment decreased with increasing size of injury, thus ensuring that the supraspinatus changes were not transient.

Unlike earlier studies, this study did not find fatty atrophy of the muscle. However, the addition of suprascapular nerve transection did lead to fatty degeneration (increased intramuscular and intramyocellular fat content) as well as muscular atrophy of the infraspinatus and supraspinatus, and adipogenic and myogenic transcription factors were upregulated[35] (**Figure 4**). Similar fatty degeneration, greater than in the rat, was seen in a mouse model. In a rabbit model, subscapularis tendon transection decreased muscle wet mass and muscle fiber cross-sectional area, and it increased the fat content.[36] In contrast with the rat model, these findings were similar between animals with a tendon transection and animals with both tendon and nerve transection. The rat, mouse, and rabbit model studies suggest a role for nerve degeneration in the development of muscle fatty degeneration. An in vivo rat model and an in vitro cell culture study suggested that the role of suppressed Wnt signaling in increasing the expression of adipogenic marker genes causes fat accumulation in the rotator cuff.[37]

Effect of Tears on Remaining Shoulder Structures

Recent studies investigated the effects of a torn rotator cuff on the intact rotator cuff tendons, the biceps tendon, and the coracoacromial ligament. A supraspinatus detachment in a rat model caused increased cross-sectional area and decreased modulus of the remaining infraspinatus, the subscapularis, and the long head of the biceps tendons.[38,39] Two tendon tears were more detrimental than a single tendon tear, and changes were more pronounced over time (**Figure 5**). These damages may result from alterations in the loading patterns of

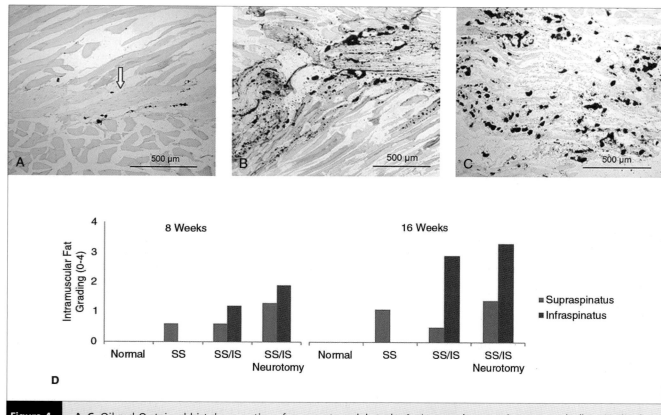

Figure 4   **A–C,** Oil red O stained histology sections from a rat model study. **A,** A normal supraspinatus muscle (longitudinal section in the coronal plane, 10-μm thickness) shows few intramuscular fat deposits and intramyocellular fat droplets. The supraspinatus tendon can be seen at the center of the muscle *(arrow)*, and the muscle fibers can be seen above and below the tendon. **B,** An infraspinatus muscle 16 weeks after tenotomy of the supraspinatus and infraspinatus tendons. Many fat deposits are seen *(red staining)*. **C,** An infraspinatus muscle 16 weeks after tenotomy plus neurotomy shows high levels of intramuscular fat *(red staining)*. **D,** Diagram showing semiquantitative histology grading results for intramuscular fat at 8 and 16 weeks, as seen on oil red O stained histology sections. 0 = no fat deposits, 4 = numerous fat deposits. No fat was seen in normal muscles. The infraspinatus (IS) muscle had more intramuscular fat than the supraspinatus (SS) muscle after tenotomy of the supraspinatus and infraspinatus tendons, with or without neurotomy. The 16-week specimens from each postsurgical group had more intramuscular fat than the 8-week specimens. (Reproduced with permission from Kim HM, Galatz LM, Lim C, Havlioglu N, Thomopoulos S: The effect of tear size and nerve injury on rotator cuff muscle fatty degeneration in a rodent animal model. *J Shoulder Elbow Surg* 2012;21[7]:847-858.

the remaining tendons. Further investigation using a supraspinatus-infraspinatus detachment in a rat model found that biceps alterations began in the intraarticular portion of the tendon before extending to the extra-articular portion.[40] Biopsy specimens from patients with different-size rotator cuff tears contained different levels of matrix metalloproteinases (MMPs) and vascular endothelial growth factor (VEGF).[41,42] MMPs are molecules that degrade extracellular matrix proteins, particularly collagen, and VEGF is associated with angiogenesis. Patients with a rotator cuff tear had increased VEGF, MMP-1, and MMP-9 expression but decreased MMP-3 expression. There were differences between articular-side and bursal-side partial tears. Scanning acoustic microscopy revealed an increased coracoacromial ligament elastic modulus in cadaver specimens with a rotator cuff tear or spur compared with control specimens.[43] These findings of altered compositional, histologic, and mechanical properties in

shoulder structures with a rotator cuff tear have implications for treatment strategies.

Genetics and Biology of Tendon Degeneration

Although the histology of tendon degeneration is well described, the biologic events have only recently gained attention. Samples collected from patients with rotator cuff disease showed angiogenesis- and inflammatory-related imbalances as the degeneration progressed.[44] Hypervascularization occurred later in tendinopathy. Although inflammation is not a characteristic of chronic tendon degeneration, it may exist in early stages. Subscapularis tendon biopsies from patients with a torn supraspinatus tendon had increased staining for macrophages, mast cells, and T cells compared with biopsies from the patient's torn supraspinatus tendon or control subscapularis tendons.[45] The larger the

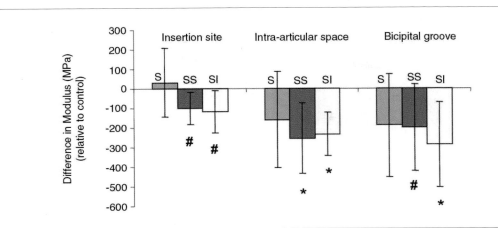

Figure 5 Diagram showing the decrease in the biceps tendon modulus in a rat model between 4 and 8 weeks after supraspinatus and subscapularis detachment (SS) or supraspinatus and infraspinatus detachment (SI), compared with control rats. S = supraspinatus detachment, * = significant difference from control group, # = trend toward difference from control group. (Reproduced with permission from Peltz CD, Perry SM, Getz CL, Soslowsky LJ: Mechanical properties of the long-head of the biceps tendon are altered in the presence of rotator cuff tears in a rat model. *J Orthop Res* 2009;27[3]:416-420.)

supraspinatus tear, the less often inflammatory cell infiltration occurs. The subscapularis tendon in patients with a torn supraspinatus tendon may be a model for early tendinopathy.

The role of apoptosis in rotator cuff disease is debated. Patient biopsies revealed increased numbers of apoptotic cells throughout the torn supraspinatus and paired subscapularis samples.[46] Degenerate supraspinatus tendons from rats as well as humans had increases in heat shock proteins and caspases, with an imbalance between the antiapoptotic (heat shock protein) and proapoptotic (caspase) genes.[47] However, rats trained on a treadmill for as long as 16 weeks had no apoptosis or neovascularization. These rats did have an increase in insulin-like growth factor–1, which affects proliferation, cell survival, and chondrogenesis.[48] Late-stage rotator cuff disease may develop into calcific tendinopathy, in which the altered expression of genes is related to bone development and resorption.[49] These insights into differences between the stages of rotator cuff disease will lead to improvements in diagnosis and treatment.

Mechanical loading affects tendon degeneration. Altered loading on excised rat supraspinatus tendons changed the expression of MMPs and tissue inhibitors of metalloproteases (TIMPs).[50] Tendinopathy is characterized by imbalances in MMPs and TIMPs. Overused rat supraspinatus tendons expressed cartilage markers[51] (**Figure 6**). These cartilage markers and other genes regulated by short-term overuse returned to near baseline levels after rest.[52] In addition, levels of proteoglycan and heparin affine regulatory peptide (a chondrogenesis-promoting factor) increased with overuse[53] (**Table 1**). Tenocytes in rotator cuff tendinopathy may be undergoing a transformation into a chondrocyte phenotype. Although mechanical loading is be-

lieved to be the primary source of rotator cuff disease, evidence also exists for a genetic predisposition.[54] Further work is needed to elucidate the complex interactions among mechanics, genetics, and biology in the onset and the progression of rotator cuff degeneration.

Progression of Tendon Degeneration and Tears

Rotator cuff degeneration can lead to a partial-thickness tear, which can progress to a full-thickness tear and can expand in size. The reasons for this progression have not been fully identified. The stages of degeneration are associated with different levels of hypoxia-inducible factor (HIF)–1α and a trend toward increased apoptosis with increased degeneration.[55] A similar trend occurred with the expression of BNip3, a proapoptotic protein. Alterations in HIF-1α also were seen in retracted torn rotator cuff tendons.[56] Increasing vessel density is related to the amount of retraction, suggesting that neovascularity may be a useful parameter for tracking progression. These degenerated samples also had increased levels of MMP-1 and MMP-9 and decreased levels of MMP-3.[57] Increased MMP-9 expression was correlated with increased retraction. A comparison of full-thickness tears with partial-thickness tears revealed increased proinflammatory cytokines and angiogenesis factors in the synovium.[58] Supraspinatus tendon biopsies revealed increased tissue remodeling and neovascularization with full-thickness tears. Furthermore, subscapularis biopsies from shoulders with a full-thickness supraspinatus tear showed increased degeneration and remodeling compared with shoulders with a partial-thickness tear. These results suggest that greater tear severity leads to greater synovial inflammation, degeneration of the supraspinatus tendon matrix, and subscapularis tendon degeneration (**Figure 7**).

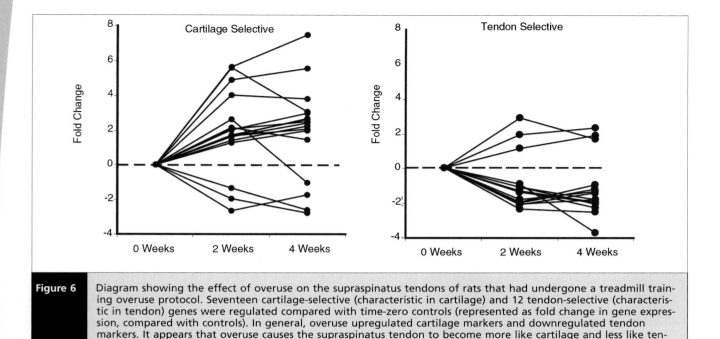

Figure 6 Diagram showing the effect of overuse on the supraspinatus tendons of rats that had undergone a treadmill training overuse protocol. Seventeen cartilage-selective (characteristic in cartilage) and 12 tendon-selective (characteristic in tendon) genes were regulated compared with time-zero controls (represented as fold change in gene expression, compared with controls). In general, overuse upregulated cartilage markers and downregulated tendon markers. It appears that overuse causes the supraspinatus tendon to become more like cartilage and less like tendon. (Reproduced with permission from Archambault JM, Jelinsky SA, Lake SP, Hill AA, Glaser DL, Soslowsky LJ: Rat supraspinatus tendon expresses cartilage markers with overuse. *J Orthop Res* 2007;25[5]:617-624.)

Tendon Healing, Repair, and Treatment

Healing

The basic phases of tendon healing are described as inflammatory, proliferative (fibroplasic), and remodeling (maturing). Recent attention has been focused on the basic science of molecular healing, new imaging techniques for healing tendons, and optimal treatment protocols for obtaining the best results during each of the basic phases. To further the understanding of the molecular processes that occur during tendon healing, an analysis of growth-factor concentrations was completed by taking measurements at multiple postoperative time points. Increased expression of growth factors was observed 1 week after surgical detachment and repair of the supraspinatus tendon in a rat model; by 16 weeks, the levels had gradually tapered to control or undetectable levels. The initial increase may be attributable to the inflammatory response, and the midsubstance-specific increase at 8 weeks may be attributable to the increased loading environment as the tendon heals. This finding provides further evidence that loading influences healing[59] (**Table 2**).

Traditional cast or sling immobilization limits only the gross movement of the shoulder joint. A temporary elimination of strain is suspected to be beneficial in early healing, however. Rat supraspinatus detachment and repair models were used in two studies to evaluate the effect of total muscle paralysis on insertion site healing. One study examined the effects of botulinum toxin A injections after surgical repair of the supraspinatus and found that it negatively influenced the me-

chanical properties of the tendon and the insertion, especially in rats immobilized with a cast.[60] A second study found similar early time point mechanical differences but also found significantly improved collagen fiber organization at 4 weeks, with no significant difference in mechanical properties 24 weeks after surgery.[61]

Contrast-enhanced ultrasound was used to characterize in vivo vascularity of the supraspinatus tendon in human shoulders 3 months after surgical repair. Tendons with a defect had significantly lower vascular volume and lower resting perfusion at the insertion site.[62] This finding suggests that the quality of vascular supply to the region is an important consideration in surgical repair.

Effects of Repair

Although surgery is generally effective for repairing torn supraspinatus tendons, approximately 25% of repairs are unsuccessful. A significant focus of research has been to investigate and better understand what happens in the body after repair, what factors influence such processes, and how the postoperative response can be measured. Multivariate regression was used to analyze factors that may predict functional outcomes following repair. Patient age, long reported to be a determinant of surgical outcome, was not found to be an independent causal factor but merely a correlate of significant factors, including tear retraction, fatty degeneration, and muscle strength.[63] Preoperative scores for muscle atrophy and fatty infiltration in the supraspinatus and infraspinatus were significant predictors of functional outcome, were intercorrelated, and generally worsened with increasing tear size (**Figure 8**). Muscle

Table 1

Genetic and Protein Changes in the Rat Supraspinatus Tendon After a 2- or 4-Week Treadmill Training Overuse Protocol, Compared With Normal Tendon

Molecule	Level of Expression[a]	
	After 2 Weeks	After 4 Weeks
Collagen		
1α1 mRNA	-	--
2 α1 mRNA	+	+
3α1 mRNA	+	=
6α1 mRNA	++	=
Decorin		
mRNA	+	++
Protein	=	++
Biglycan		
mRNA	++	++
Versican		
mRNA	++	++
Protein	=	++
Aggrecan		
mRNA	++	++
Protein	++	++
SOX9		
mRNA	++	+
Glycosaminoglycans		
Total	=	++
Dermatan sulfate	=	++
Chondroitin sulfate	=	+
Heparan sulfate	=	=
Carbohydrate sulfotransferase–14 (involved in dermatan sulfate synthesis)	++	=
Heparin affine regulatory peptide		
mRNA	=	=
Protein	+	++

[a] - decreased expression, -- further-decreased expression, = no difference from control expression, + increased expression, ++ further-increased expression.
Adapted with permission from Attia M, Scott A, Duchesnay A, Carpentier G, Soslowsky LJ, Huynh MB, Van Kuppevelt TH, Gossard C, Courty J, Tassoni MC, Marteli I: Alterations of overused supraspinatus tendon: A possible role of glycosaminoglycans and heparin affine regulatory peptide/pleiotrophin in early tendon pathology. *J Orthop Res* 2012;30(1):61-71.

ful repair. Repair should therefore be performed as early as possible to minimize the influences of fatty infiltration and muscle atrophy.[64]

A novel device to measure in vivo shoulder stiffness in anesthetized rats found that stiffness increased if the rat had been immobilized; however, the difference was transient and not significant after 8 weeks. The use of a human corollary of this device would be helpful for clinical evaluation. A temporary increase in shoulder stiffness with immobilization may be acceptable, given the benefit to the properties of the repaired insertion site.[65]

Using a rabbit model, researchers found that CT can reveal the strength of a surgically repaired tendon-bone construct.[66] Increased blood flow during healing resulted in lower attenuation, and hypoattenuation increased with time after surgery. Most importantly, hypoattenuation seen in early images was correlated with a stronger union and a decreased likelihood of failure. Early CT may be useful for predicting surgical success. Another study used roentgen stereophotogrammetric analysis to measure the migration of the markers. Surgeons embedded metal beads into the greater humeral tuberosity and wire sutures into the supraspinatus tendon of patients during open repair of a rotator cuff tear. After 1 year, intact repairs had moved an average of 6.3 mm; the average movement in completely unsuccessful tears was 23.7 mm. The most movement occurred during the period of active rehabilitation (2 to 3 months after surgery). This timing suggests that the greatest vulnerability to retearing is during this time, possibly as a function of activity levels in physical therapy. Migration was minimal during the period of 3 to 4 months and 1 year after surgery, possibly because the repairs that were intact at the beginning of the period were tolerant of future loading.[67]

Earlier clinical work suggested that partial repair of a massive tear (involving both the infraspinatus and the supraspinatus), in which only the infraspinatus is reattached, may be effective for restoring adequate functionality. Recent research in a rat model used a two-tendon detachment and quantitative ambulatory measures. The results of both partial and complete repair were significantly different from those of no repair; the results of the two-tendon reattachment were not significantly different from those of infraspinatus-only reattachment.[68] These findings support the clinical practice of using a partial repair to restore adequate function. A human cadaver study that sought to evaluate the specific influence of type of repair on the interaction between the supraspinatus and infraspinatus tendons found that so-called transosseous-equivalent arthroscopic techniques have led to decreased interaction at high loads and thereby reduce the ability of the infraspinatus to help the supraspinatus. This finding highlights the possible risk of a partial compared with a traditional open transosseous repair.[69]

atrophy and fatty infiltration scores had not improved 1 year after surgery but instead had worsened if the patient had these conditions at the time of surgery. The progression was worse in shoulders with an unsuccess-

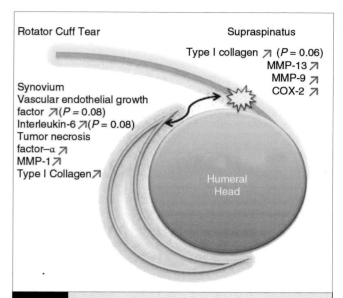

Figure 7 Diagram showing the association of a rotator cuff tear with synovial inflammation. Increased tear size is correlated with a greater proinflammatory response in the synovium. Green arrows indicate increase. (Adapted with permission from Shindle MK, Chen CC, Robertson C, et al: Full-thickness supraspinatus tears are associated with more synovial inflammation and tissue degeneration than partial-thickness tears. *J Shoulder Elbow Surg* 2011;20[6]: 917-927.)

Postoperative and Nonsurgical Treatment

The poor outcome often associated with rotator cuff repair and the treatment of degeneration has stimulated research into treatment techniques. Beyond the specifics of the repair technique, the surgeon can influence patient outcomes through the prescription of rehabilitation protocols. In addition, nontraditional treatment techniques have garnered increasing scientific attention.

A series of experiments using an established rat model investigated the effects of immobilization and exercise at multiple time points after repair. Immobilization resulted in improved collagen organization after 4 weeks but not after 16 weeks. Immobilized rats had better mechanical properties after 16 weeks but not after 4 weeks. It appears that long-term immobilization allowed a more organized repair, which eventually improved mechanical properties.[70] A follow-up study combined immobilization with two distinct passive motion protocols, both of which led to significantly decreased range of motion, probably because of increased subacromial scar formation.[71] A short period of immobilization was followed by either cage activity or treadmill running. The exercised rats had inferior physical and mechanical properties, suggesting that the tissue was disorganized with increased matrix and scar production.[72]

Clinical studies have sought to determine the relative efficacy of aggressive and more limited early passive

Table 2

Growth Factor Concentration (Insertion/Midsubstance) in a Rat Model 1 to 16 Weeks After Surgical Detachment and Repair of the Supraspinatus Tendon

Growth Factor	Nonsurgical Control	Postsurgical Week				
		1	2	4	8	16
Basic fibroblastic growth factor	+/+	+++/+++	++/+++	+/+	++/++	+/–
Bone morphogenetic protein–12	+/+	+++/+++	+/++	+/+	++/++	+/–
Bone morphogenetic protein–13	+/–	++/+++	++/+	++/+	++/+	–/–
Bone morphogenetic protein–14	+/++	++/+++	+/+	+/+	+/++	–/–
Cartilage oligomeric matrix protein	+/+	+++/+++	+/++	++/+	+/+	–/–
Connective tissue growth factor	+/+	+++/++	++/++	+/+	+/++	+/–
Platelet-derived growth factor–B	*/+	*/+++	*/++	*/+	*/+	*/+
Transforming growth factor–β1	+/+	++/++	++/++	–/+	+/++	–/–

Median values of semiquantitative staining intensity: + = low, ++ = moderate, +++ = high, – = trace, * = undetected.
Adapted with permission from Würgler-Hauri CC, Dourte LM, Baradet TC, Williams GR, Soslowsky LJ: Temporal expression of 8 growth factors in tendon-to-bone healing in a rat supraspinatus model. *J Shoulder Elbow Surg* 2007;16(5, suppl):S198-S203.

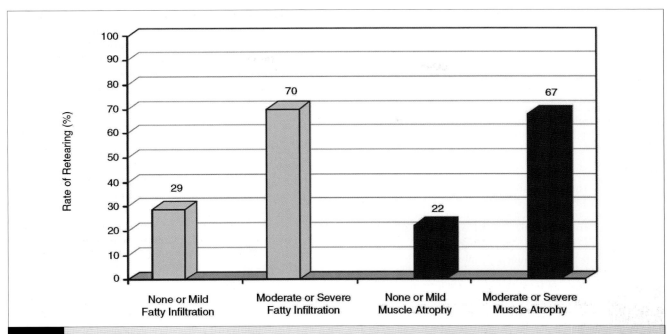

| Figure 8 | Diagram showing the effect of clinically insignificant or significant fatty infiltration or muscle atrophy on the rate of rotator cuff retearing ($P < 0.05$). (Adapted with permission from Gladstone JN, Bishop JY, Lo IK, Flatow EL: Fatty infiltration and atrophy of the rotator cuff do not improve after rotator cuff repair and correlate with poor functional outcome. *Am J Sports Med* 2007;35[5]:719-728.) |

motion rehabilitation protocols. In one study, patients who underwent aggressive rehabilitation received manual therapy twice a day and were instructed to perform pendulum and stretching exercises three times a day.[73] Those who underwent more limited rehabilitation were assisted by a continuous passive motion machine and performed only forward-flexion stretching exercises twice daily. The programs converged after 6 weeks into an active stretching and strengthening protocol. The patients who had been treated aggressively had greater range of motion and better clinical evaluations 3 months after surgery, but these differences were not significant at 1 year. Retearing occurred in 7 of the 30 patients in the aggressive treatment group but only 3 of the 34 patients in the limited treatment group.

A naturopathic treatment protocol was compared with physical exercise in patients with nontear rotator cuff tendinopathy. The naturopathic treatment consisted of anti-inflammatory dietary counseling, the use of a dietary supplement (phlogenzym), and weekly acupuncture. Both groups were provided with a therapeutic doctor-patient relationship, physical therapy, and a pill (placebo for patients in the exercise group). Patients in both groups improved significantly on subjective questionnaires, with those in the naturopathic treatment group improving significantly more than those in the exercise control group. Quantitative measures of range of motion revealed significant improvements in patients in the naturopathic treatment group, in comparison both with baseline and with patients in the exercise group; in contrast, the patients in the exercise group did not improve significantly on the quantitative measures.[74]

Summary

The tendons of the rotator cuff provide crucial stability and enable the shoulder's unique range of motion, but these structures are prone to degeneration and injury. Research continues to explore the molecular anatomy and healing biology of these structures. Progress has been made in identifying and quantifying important molecules and in describing the insertion site in detail. Modeling the mechanics of the joint has led to an improved understanding of the interactions of related structures is improving the understanding of anatomic function. The biology of the progression of tendon pathology is slowly being elucidated, and great strides have been made in novel imaging techniques that allow in vivo measurements. From surgical technique and rehabilitation protocol to genetics and lifestyle, the understanding of the factors that influence degeneration and healing is improving. Future research will continue to elucidate these factors through animal, cadaver, and clinical studies. Advances in biologic augmentation and tissue engineering may offer new hope in treating these challenging tendons.

Annotated References

1. Matuszewski PE, Chen YL, Szczesny SE, et al: Regional variation in human supraspinatus tendon proteoglycans: Decorin, biglycan, and aggrecan. *Connect Tissue Res* 2012;53(5):343-348.

   Enzyme-linked immunosorbent assays of cadaver tissue revealed no regional difference in decorin concentrations, but aggrecan and biglycan were regionally variable.

2. Wopenka B, Kent A, Pasteris JD, Yoon Y, Thomopoulos S: The tendon-to-bone transition of the rotator cuff: A preliminary Raman spectroscopic study documenting the gradual mineralization across the insertion in rat tissue samples. *Appl Spectrosc* 2008;62(12):1285-1294.

   Quantification of mineral content using Raman spectroscopy led to a challenge to the belief that the insertion site should be thought of in terms of distinct zones.

3. Cashman PM, Baring T, Reilly P, Emery RJ, Amis AA: Validation of a new technique to monitor rotator cuff tears. *J Med Eng Technol* 2010;34(3):159-165.

   Steel sutures were used as Roentgen stereophotogrammetric analysis markers to track rotator cuff tissue deformation in an ovine model. Although this technique was less accurate than bone motion tracking, it provided a method to measure soft-tissue migration in vivo.

4. Derwin KA, Milks RA, Davidson I, Iannotti JP, McCarron JA, Bey MJ: Low-dose CT imaging of radioopaque markers for assessing human rotator cuff repair: Accuracy, repeatability and the effect of arm position. *J Biomech* 2012;45(3):614-618.

   This study investigated the accuracy and repeatability of distance measurement between markers in the rotator cuff using CT. Arm position and location of the bead within the rotator cuff affect measurements.

5. Bey MJ, Kline SK, Baker AR, McCarron JA, Iannotti JP, Derwin KA: Estimation of dynamic, in vivo soft-tissue deformation: Experimental technique and application in a canine model of tendon injury and repair. *J Orthop Res* 2011;29(6):822-827.

   Biplane radiographic analysis was used in a canine model to distinguish an intact infraspinatus repair, a failed repair, and a control.

6. Kim YS, Kim JM, Bigliani LU, Kim HJ, Jung HW: In vivo strain analysis of the intact supraspinatus tendon by ultrasound speckles tracking imaging. *J Orthop Res* 2011;29(12):1931-1937.

   Two-dimensional speckle tracking echocardiography showed differences in strain between deep and superficial regions of the supraspinatus tendon as well as differences in isometric and isotonic motions.

7. Seki N, Itoi E, Shibuya Y, et al: Mechanical environment of the supraspinatus tendon: Three-dimensional finite element model analysis. *J Orthop Sci* 2008;13(4):348-353.

   Three-dimensional finite element model analysis of the supraspinatus tendon mechanical environment showed a maximal tensile stress on the articular side of the anterior edge of the supraspinatus tendon.

8. Lake SP, Miller KS, Elliott DM, Soslowsky LJ: Effect of fiber distribution and realignment on the nonlinear and inhomogeneous mechanical properties of human supraspinatus tendon under longitudinal tensile loading. *J Orthop Res* 2009;27(12):1596-1602.

   Longitudinally loaded cadaver supraspinatus tendon specimens varied in moduli values and collagen alignment, depending on the region tested.

9. Lake SP, Miller KS, Elliott DM, Soslowsky LJ: Tensile properties and fiber alignment of human supraspinatus tendon in the transverse direction demonstrate inhomogeneity, nonlinearity, and regional isotropy. *J Biomech* 2010;43(4):727-732.

   This follow-up study investigated transverse loading on cadaver supraspinatus tendon specimens. Differences existed between bursal- and joint-side specimens, with values for the bursal specimens similar to those achieved in longitudinal loading.

10. Chaudhury S, Holland C, Vollrath F, Carr AJ: Comparing normal and torn rotator cuff tendons using dynamic shear analysis. *J Bone Joint Surg Br* 2011;93(7):942-948.

    Dynamic shear analysis was used to determine the storage modulus of biopsy samples taken from healthy and torn rotator cuff tissue. Massive tears had a reduced storage modulus.

11. Andarawis-Puri N, Ricchetti ET, Soslowsky LJ: Rotator cuff tendon strain correlates with tear propagation. *J Biomech* 2009;42(2):158-163.

    In an ovine cadaver model, the principal infraspinatus tendon strains were correlated with tear propagation.

12. Andarawis-Puri N, Ricchetti ET, Soslowsky LJ: Interaction between the supraspinatus and infraspinatus tendons: Effect of anterior supraspinatus tendon full-thickness tears on infraspinatus tendon strain. *Am J Sports Med* 2009;37(9):1831-1839.

    In a human cadaver study, infraspinatus tendon strains increased with supraspinatus tear size and loading. There are mechanical interactions between these two tendons.

13. Andarawis-Puri N, Kuntz AF, Ramsey ML, Soslowsky LJ: Effect of glenohumeral abduction angle on the mechanical interaction between the supraspinatus and infraspinatus tendons for the intact, partial-thickness torn, and repaired supraspinatus tendon conditions. *J Orthop Res* 2010;28(7):846-851.

    In a human cadaver study, the abduction angle affected the interaction between the supraspinatus and infraspinatus tendons. Abduction at 30° decreased supraspinatus and infraspinatus tendon strain.

14. Andarawis-Puri N, Kuntz AF, Kim SY, Soslowsky LJ: Effect of anterior supraspinatus tendon partial-thickness tears on infraspinatus tendon strain through a range of joint rotation angles. *J Shoulder Elbow Surg* 2010;19(4):617-623.

   In a human cadaver study, joint rotation angles affected the interaction between the supraspinatus and infraspinatus tendons.

15. Andarawis-Puri N, Kuntz AF, Jawad AF, Soslowsky LJ: Infraspinatus and supraspinatus tendon strain explained using multiple regression models. *Ann Biomed Eng* 2010;38(9):2979-2987.

   Regression models using data described in earlier studies revealed that the abduction angle and supraspinatus loading are significant predictors of strain in the infraspinatus and supraspinatus tendons. Supraspinatus tear size was not a predictor of infraspinatus strain.

16. Abboud JA, Kim JS: The effect of hypercholesterolemia on rotator cuff disease. *Clin Orthop Relat Res* 2010;468(6):1493-1497.

   Cholesterol levels were measured in 147 patents. Those with a rotator cuff tear were found to have higher cholesterol levels. Age, sex, and body mass index were not found to be predictive of rotator cuff tears.

17. Beason DP, Abboud JA, Kuntz AF, Bassora R, Soslowsky LJ: Cumulative effects of hypercholesterolemia on tendon biomechanics in a mouse model. *J Orthop Res* 2011;29(3):380-383.

   Hypercholesterolemia had a detrimental effect in a mouse model of tendon elastic modulus.

18. Bedi A, Fox AJ, Harris PE, et al: Diabetes mellitus impairs tendon-bone healing after rotator cuff repair. *J Shoulder Elbow Surg* 2010;19(7):978-988.

   Rats with streptozotocin-induced hyperglycemia had poor recovery from supraspinatus repair at 1- and 2-week postoperative time points.

19. Cadet ER, Vorys GC, Rahman R, et al: Improving bone density at the rotator cuff footprint increases supraspinatus tendon failure stress in a rat model. *J Orthop Res* 2010;28(3):308-314.

   Ovariectomy and bisphosphonate administration in rats were used to explore the effects of estrogen deficiency and bone mineral density on the supraspinatus tendon insertion site.

20. Ichinose R, Sano H, Kishimoto KN, Sakamoto N, Sato M, Itoi E: Alteration of the material properties of the normal supraspinatus tendon by nicotine treatment in a rat model. *Acta Orthop* 2010;81(5):634-638.

   The effect of nicotine on the mechanical properties of healthy tendons was investigated. Increased elastic moduli were found in the treated rats.

21. Perry SM, Getz CL, Soslowsky LJ: Alterations in function after rotator cuff tears in an animal model.
J Shoulder Elbow Surg 2009;18(2):296-304.

   Supraspinatus detachment in a rat model altered gait and range of motion. These effects were increased with the addition of a second rotator cuff tendon detachment.

22. Sarver JJ, Dishowitz MI, Kim SY, Soslowsky LJ: Transient decreases in forelimb gait and ground reaction forces following rotator cuff injury and repair in a rat model. *J Biomech* 2010;43(4):778-782.

   Step length and ground reaction forces are altered immediately after rotator cuff injury and repair in a rat model but return to control levels within 4 weeks.

23. Grumet RC, Hadley S, Diltz MV, Lee TQ, Gupta R: Development of a new model for rotator cuff pathology: The rabbit subscapularis muscle. *Acta Orthop* 2009;80(1):97-103.

   The rabbit subscapularis traverses a bony tunnel, in a manner similar to the human supraspinatus tendon. The mechanical properties of the native rabbit subscapularis tendon were quantified.

24. Longo UG, Franceschi F, Ruzzini L, et al: Histopathology of the supraspinatus tendon in rotator cuff tears. *Am J Sports Med* 2008;36(3):533-538.

   Supraspinatus tendon samples taken from patients with a tear had more degeneration than those taken from control subjects.

25. Chaudhury S, Dicko C, Burgess M, Vollrath F, Carr AJ: Fourier transform infrared spectroscopic analysis of normal and torn rotator-cuff tendons. *J Bone Joint Surg Br* 2011;93(3):370-377.

   Fourier transform infrared spectroscopy revealed differences in the chemical and structural composition of normal rotator cuffs and those with a partial, small, medium, large, or massive tear.

26. Steinbacher P, Tauber M, Kogler S, Stoiber W, Resch H, Sänger AM: Effects of rotator cuff ruptures on the cellular and intracellular composition of the human supraspinatus muscle. *Tissue Cell* 2010;42(1):37-41.

   Increased muscle degeneration and fatty tissue were found in massive rotator cuff tear muscle biopsy samples.

27. Kim HM, Dahiya N, Teefey SA, Keener JD, Galatz LM, Yamaguchi K: Relationship of tear size and location to fatty degeneration of the rotator cuff. *J Bone Joint Surg Am* 2010;92(4):829-839.

   Ultrasound of patients with a rotator cuff tear revealed that larger tears and tears located at the anterior portion of the supraspinatus tendon are more likely to result in fatty degeneration of the muscle. Level of evidence: III.

28. Melis B, DeFranco MJ, Chuinard C, Walch G: Natural history of fatty infiltration and atrophy of the supraspinatus muscle in rotator cuff tears. *Clin Orthop Relat Res* 2010;468(6):1498-1505.

   A retrospective review of patients with a rotator cuff

1: Basic Science

tear found a moderate level of fatty infiltration 3 years after symptoms occurred and a severe level by 5 years. Level of evidence: IV.

29. Oh JH, Kim SH, Kim JH, Shin YH, Yoon JP, Oh CH: The level of vitamin D in the serum correlates with fatty degeneration of the muscles of the rotator cuff. *J Bone Joint Surg Br* 2009;91(12):1587-1593.

A lower serum level of vitamin D was associated with increased fatty degeneration of the muscle in patients with a rotator cuff tear.

30. Fuchs B, Zumstein M, Regenfelder F, et al: Upregulation of alpha-skeletal muscle actin and myosin heavy polypeptide gene products in degenerating rotator cuff muscles. *J Orthop Res* 2008;26(7):1007-1011.

Reverse transcription–polymerase chain reaction on patients' supraspinatus tendon biopsies showed upregulation of α-skeletal muscle actin and myosin heavy polypeptide-1 gene transcripts, correlating with fatty degeneration.

31. Ward SR, Sarver JJ, Eng CM, et al: Plasticity of muscle architecture after supraspinatus tears. *J Orthop Sports Phys Ther* 2010;40(11):729-735.

Several changes in supraspinatus muscle occurred after supraspinatus tendon transection in rats. All changes except muscle mass and length returned to control levels within 9 weeks.

32. Buchmann S, Walz L, Sandmann GH, et al: Rotator cuff changes in a full thickness tear rat model: Verification of the optimal time interval until reconstruction for comparison to the healing process of chronic lesions in humans. *Arch Orthop Trauma Surg* 2011; 131(3):429-435.

Muscle and tendon degeneration occurred after detachment of the rat supraspinatus tendon. The 3-week time point mimicked several characteristics of chronic tears in humans.

33. Farshad M, Würgler-Hauri CC, Kohler T, Gerber C, Rothenfluh DA: Effect of age on fatty infiltration of supraspinatus muscle after experimental tendon release in rats. *BMC Res Notes* 2011;4:530.

Significant fatty infiltration could not be found 6 weeks after supraspinatus tendon transection in young and old rats.

34. Dourte LM, Perry SM, Getz CL, Soslowsky LJ: Tendon properties remain altered in a chronic rat rotator cuff model. *Clin Orthop Relat Res* 2010;468(6):1485-1492.

Acute detachment of the supraspinatus and infraspinatus tendons in rats caused degenerative changes similar to those in chronic tears in humans. The severity of the injury ensured that these changes were not transient.

35. Kim HM, Galatz LM, Lim C, Havlioglu N, Thomopoulos S: The effect of tear size and nerve injury on rotator cuff muscle fatty degeneration in a rodent animal model. *J Shoulder Elbow Surg* 2012;21(7):847-858.

The addition of a suprascapular nerve transection to supraspinatus and infraspinatus tendon transections increased the fatty degeneration of the muscles in rats and mice.

36. Rowshan K, Hadley S, Pham K, Caiozzo V, Lee TQ, Gupta R: Development of fatty atrophy after neurologic and rotator cuff injuries in an animal model of rotator cuff pathology. *J Bone Joint Surg Am* 2010; 92(13):2270-2278.

Transection of the subscapularis tendon with the addition of subscapular nerve transection in rabbits resulted in fatty atrophy of the muscle and degeneration of the nerve.

37. Itoigawa Y, Kishimoto KN, Sano H, Kaneko K, Itoi E: Molecular mechanism of fatty degeneration in rotator cuff muscle with tendon rupture. *J Orthop Res* 2011; 29(6):861-866.

Reverse transcription–polymerase chain reaction of rotator cuff muscles with a tendon rupture revealed decreased Wnt10b expression and increased adipogenic marker genes. Wnt signaling may play a role in fatty degeneration.

38. Perry SM, Getz CL, Soslowsky LJ: After rotator cuff tears, the remaining (intact) tendons are mechanically altered. *J Shoulder Elbow Surg* 2009;18(1):52-57.

After detachment of one or two rotator cuff tendons in a rat model, the remaining rotator cuff tendons (infraspinatus, subscapularis) exhibited signs of degeneration.

39. Peltz CD, Perry SM, Getz CL, Soslowsky LJ: Mechanical properties of the long-head of the biceps tendon are altered in the presence of rotator cuff tears in a rat model. *J Orthop Res* 2009;27(3):416-420.

After detachment of one or two rotator cuff tendons in a rat model, the long head of the biceps tendon exhibited signs of degeneration.

40. Peltz CD, Hsu JE, Zgonis MH, Trasolini NA, Glaser DL, Soslowsky LJ: Intra-articular changes precede extra-articular changes in the biceps tendon after rotator cuff tears in a rat model. *J Shoulder Elbow Surg* 2012;21(7):873-881.

After detachment of the supraspinatus and infraspinatus tendons in a rat model, the long head of the biceps tendon first showed signs of degeneration in the intra-articular region. Over time, these changes extended the length of the tendon.

41. Lakemeier S, Schwuchow SA, Peterlein CD, et al: Expression of matrix metalloproteinases 1, 3, and 9 in degenerated long head biceps tendon in the presence of rotator cuff tears: An immunohistological study. *BMC Musculoskelet Disord* 2010;11:271.

Biopsy specimens of the long head of the biceps tendon from patients with a rotator cuff tear showed increased expression of MMP-1 and MMP-9 as well as decreased expression of MMP-3.

42. Lakemeier S, Reichelt JJ, Timmesfeld N, Fuchs-Winkelmann S, Paletta JR, Schofer MD: The relevance of long head biceps degeneration in the presence of rotator cuff tears. *BMC Musculoskelet Disord* 2010; 11:191.

Biopsy specimens of the long head of the biceps tendon from patients with a rotator cuff tear showed increased VEGF expression, vessel size, and vessel density.

43. Kijima H, Minagawa H, Saijo Y, et al: Degenerated coracoacromial ligament in shoulders with rotator cuff tears shows higher elastic modulus: Measurement with scanning acoustic microscopy. *J Orthop Sci* 2009; 14(1):62-67.

Coracoacromial ligaments from cadavers with a rotator cuff tear showed increased elastic modulus as measured with scanning acoustic microscopy.

44. Savitskaya YA, Izaguirre A, Sierra L, et al: Effect of angiogenesis-related cytokines on rotator cuff disease: The search for sensitive biomarkers of early tendon degeneration. *Clin Med Insights Arthritis Musculoskelet Disord* 2011;4:43-53.

Patients with a rotator cuff tear had increased levels of interleukin-1β, interleukin-8, and VEGF in their blood. Angiogenin and interleukin-10 were decreased. Rotator cuff disease causes imbalances in pro- and anti-inflammatory genes and angiogenesis.

45. Millar NL, Hueber AJ, Reilly JH, et al: Inflammation is present in early human tendinopathy. *Am J Sports Med* 2010;38(10):2085-2091.

Subscapularis tendon biopsies from patients with a torn supraspinatus show increased macrophage, mast cell, and T-cell expression. Subscapularis tendons from patients with a torn supraspinatus may be a model for early tendinopathy, and inflammation is present.

46. Lundgreen K, Lian OB, Engebretsen L, Scott A: Tenocyte apoptosis in the torn rotator cuff: A primary or secondary pathological event? *Br J Sports Med* 2011; 45(13):1035-1039.

Supraspinatus and subscapularis tendon biopsy samples from patients with a torn supraspinatus tendon showed an increased apoptotic index. Torn supraspinatus tendons showed an increase in p53, unlike subscapularis tendons, and this finding suggests different apoptotic pathways.

47. Millar NL, Wei AQ, Molloy TJ, Bonar F, Murrell GA: Heat shock protein and apoptosis in supraspinatus tendinopathy. *Clin Orthop Relat Res* 2008;466(7): 1569-1576.

Heat shock protein and apoptotic genes are upregulated in biopsy specimens from patients with torn supraspinatus tendons as well as rats that have undergone a supraspinatus overuse protocol.

48. Scott A, Cook JL, Hart DA, Walker DC, Duronio V, Khan KM: Tenocyte responses to mechanical loading in vivo: A role for local insulin-like growth factor 1 signaling in early tendinosis in rats. *Arthritis Rheum* 2007;56(3):871-881.

Supraspinatus tendons from rats that underwent an overuse protocol exhibited increased local insulin-like growth factor–1 expression and phosphorylation of downstream targets insulin receptor substrate–1 and extracellular signal–related kinases–1/2.

49. Oliva F, Barisani D, Grasso A, Maffulli N: Gene expression analysis in calcific tendinopathy of the rotator cuff. *Eur Cell Mater* 2011;21:548-557.

Biopsy specimens from patients with calcific tendinopathy of the rotator cuff showed increased expression of tissue transglutaminase–2, osteopontin, and cathepsin K as well as decreased bone morphogenetic protein–4 and –6.

50. Thornton GM, Shao X, Chung M, et al: Changes in mechanical loading lead to tendonspecific alterations in MMP and TIMP expression: Influence of stress deprivation and intermittent cyclic hydrostatic compression on rat supraspinatus and Achilles tendons. *Br J Sports Med* 2010;44(10):698-703.

Stress deprivation in excised rat tendons caused increased MMP-13, MMP-3, and TIMP-2 expression. Intermittent cyclic hydrostatic compression caused increased MMP-13 in the excised rat supraspinatus tendon.

51. Archambault JM, Jelinsky SA, Lake SP, Hill AA, Glaser DL, Soslowsky LJ: Rat supraspinatus tendon expresses cartilage markers with overuse. *J Orthop Res* 2007;25(5):617-624.

Supraspinatus tendons from rats that underwent an overuse protocol exhibited increased expression of several cartilage genes.

52. Jelinsky SA, Lake SP, Archambault JM, Soslowsky LJ: Gene expression in rat supraspinatus tendon recovers from overuse with rest. *Clin Orthop Relat Res* 2008; 466(7):1612-1617.

Rest for 2 or 4 weeks after 2 or 4 weeks of an overuse protocol returned gene expression and biochemical composition to near-normal levels in rats. Collagen content remained slightly decreased.

53. Attia M, Scott A, Duchesnay A, et al: Alterations of overused supraspinatus tendon: A possible role of glycosaminoglycans and HARP/pleiotrophin in early tendon pathology. *J Orthop Res* 2012;30(1):61-71.

Sulfated glycosaminoglycans increased after an overuse protocol was used in rats. Heparin affine regulatory peptide, a cytokine that regulates developmental chondrocyte formation, also increased, indicating the change toward a chondrocyte phenotype.

54. Tashjian RZ, Farnham JM, Albright FS, Teerlink CC, Cannon-Albright LA: Evidence for an inherited predisposition contributing to the risk for rotator cuff disease. *J Bone Joint Surg Am* 2009;91(5):1136-1142.

Review of the Utah Population Database revealed that patients diagnosed with rotator cuff disease before age 40 years had relatedness in close and distant relationships, suggesting a genetic predisposition. Level of evidence: III.

1: Basic Science

55. Benson RT, McDonnell SM, Knowles HJ, Rees JL, Carr AJ, Hulley PA: Tendinopathy and tears of the rotator cuff are associated with hypoxia and apoptosis. *J Bone Joint Surg Br* 2010;92(3):448-453.

Biopsies from patients with different stages of rotator cuff impingement or tearing revealed alterations in HIF-1α and BNip3 expression and apoptosis, depending on the stage.

56. Lakemeier S, Reichelt JJ, Patzer T, Fuchs-Winkelmann S, Paletta JR, Schofer MD: The association between retraction of the torn rotator cuff and increasing expression of hypoxia inducible factor 1α and vascular endothelial growth factor expression: An immunohistological study. *BMC Musculoskelet Disord* 2010; 11:230.

Biopsies from patients with a torn rotator cuff revealed increased HIF and VEGF expression, fatty infiltration, and muscular atrophy. Vessel density was correlated with tendon retraction.

57. Lakemeier S, Braun J, Efe T, et al: Expression of matrix metalloproteinases 1, 3, and 9 in differing extents of tendon retraction in the torn rotator cuff. *Knee Surg Sports Traumatol Arthrosc* 2011;19(10):1760-1765.

Biopsy samples from patients with a torn rotator cuff revealed increased MMP-1 and MMP-9 as well as decreased MMP-3. MMP-9 expression was correlated with tendon retraction.

58. Shindle MK, Chen CC, Robertson C, et al: Full-thickness supraspinatus tears are associated with more synovial inflammation and tissue degeneration than partial-thickness tears. *J Shoulder Elbow Surg* 2011; 20(6):917-927.

Samples from patients' synovium, bursa, torn supraspinatus tendon, and subscapularis tendon revealed that synovial inflammation and tissue degeneration increased with tear size.

59. Würgler-Hauri CC, Dourte LM, Baradet TC, Williams GR, Soslowsky LJ: Temporal expression of 8 growth factors in tendon-to-bone healing in a rat supraspinatus model. *J Shoulder Elbow Surg* 2007;16(5, suppl): S198-S203.

Examination of the differential temporal expression of growth factors revealed a peak 1 week postoperatively and a second surge of some factors during remodeling.

60. Galatz LM, Charlton N, Das R, Kim HM, Havlioglu N, Thomopoulos S: Complete removal of load is detrimental to rotator cuff healing. *J Shoulder Elbow Surg* 2009;18(5):669-675.

In a rat model, the use of botulinum toxin A and casting was found to be inferior to botulinum toxin A alone, which was inferior to casting alone.

61. Hettrich CM, Rodeo SA, Hannafin JA, Ehteshami J, Shubin Stein BE: The effect of muscle paralysis using Botox on the healing of tendon to bone in a rat model. *J Shoulder Elbow Surg* 2011;20(5):688-697.

Botulinum toxin A had a positive effect on early collagen alignment but a negative effect on later cross-sectional area and load to failure.

62. Gamradt SC, Gallo RA, Adler RS, et al: Vascularity of the supraspinatus tendon three months after repair: Characterization using contrast-enhanced ultrasound. *J Shoulder Elbow Surg* 2010;19(1):73-80.

A new technique was successful in characterizing blood flow to the region of interest and suggests the importance of vascular considerations during surgery.

63. Oh JH, Kim SH, Kang JY, Oh CH, Gong HS: Effect of age on functional and structural outcome after rotator cuff repair. *Am J Sports Med* 2010;38(4):672-678.

Multivariate regression was used to show that age is merely correlated with poor surgical outcomes and is not necessarily a causal factor. Level of evidence: IV.

64. Gladstone JN, Bishop JY, Lo IK, Flatow EL: Fatty infiltration and atrophy of the rotator cuff do not improve after rotator cuff repair and correlate with poor functional outcome. *Am J Sports Med* 2007;35(5): 719-728.

Multivariate analysis revealed the influence and persistence of fatty deposits and reduced muscularity. Level of evidence: II.

65. Sarver JJ, Peltz CD, Dourte L, Reddy S, Williams GR, Soslowsky LJ: After rotator cuff repair, stiffness—but not the loss in range of motion—increased transiently for immobilized shoulders in a rat model. *J Shoulder Elbow Surg* 2008;17(1, suppl):108S-113S.

A novel device was created for measuring joint stiffness, and the effects of plaster casts were evaluated.

66. Trudel G, Ramachandran N, Ryan SE, Rakhra K, Uhthoff HK: Supraspinatus tendon repair into a bony trough in the rabbit: Mechanical restoration and correlative imaging. *J Orthop Res* 2010;28(6):710-715.

CT was found useful for predicting restoration of mechanical properties shortly after surgery. Given the importance of the rapid healing reaction, minimal postoperative loading is recommended.

67. Baring TK, Cashman PP, Reilly P, Emery RJ, Amis AA: Rotator cuff repair failure in vivo: A radiostereometric measurement study. *J Shoulder Elbow Surg* 2011;20(8):1194-1199.

Metallic bone and tendon marker migration provides new insight into temporal and activity-based rates of retearing.

68. Hsu JE, Reuther KE, Sarver JJ, et al: Restoration of anterior-posterior rotator cuff force balance improves shoulder function in a rat model of chronic massive tears. *J Orthop Res* 2011;29(7):1028-1033.

A new in vivo model of two-tendon repair suggests that in a massive tear, surgical repair of the infraspinatus may be sufficient only for restoring functionality.

69. Andarawis-Puri N, Kuntz AF, Ramsey ML, Soslowsky LJ: Effect of supraspinatus tendon repair technique on

the infraspinatus tendon. *J Biomech Eng* 2011;133(3): 031008.

Cadaver shoulders revealed a decreased recruitment of the infraspinatus at high loads when arthroscopic repair was used, compared with open transosseous repair.

70. Gimbel JA, Van Kleunen JP, Williams GR, Thomopoulos S, Soslowsky LJ: Long durations of immobilization in the rat result in enhanced mechanical properties of the healing supraspinatus tendon insertion site. *J Biomech Eng* 2007;129(3):400-404.

Immobilization was found to lead to early improvement in collagen organization and later improvement in mechanical properties.

71. Peltz CD, Dourte LM, Kuntz AF, et al: The effect of postoperative passive motion on rotator cuff healing in a rat model. *J Bone Joint Surg Am* 2009;91(10):2421-2429.

The negative effect of passive motion on range of motion was attributed to increased scar formation.

72. Peltz CD, Sarver JJ, Dourte LM, Würgler-Hauri CC, Williams GR, Soslowsky LJ: Exercise following a short immobilization period is detrimental to tendon properties and joint mechanics in a rat rotator cuff injury model. *J Orthop Res* 2010;28(7):841-845.

This study provided cautionary evidence about postoperative exercise.

73. Lee BG, Cho NS, Rhee YG: Effect of two rehabilitation protocols on range of motion and healing rates after arthroscopic rotator cuff repair: Aggressive versus limited early passive exercises. *Arthroscopy* 2012; 28(1):34-42.

Early aggressive exercise led to improvement in scores after 3 months but not after 1 year, and it may increase the risk of retearing. Level of evidence: II.

74. Szczurko O, Cooley K, Mills EJ, Zhou Q, Perri D, Seely D: Naturopathic treatment of rotator cuff tendinitis among Canadian postal workers: A randomized controlled trial. *Arthritis Rheum* 2009;61(8):1037-1045.

Acupuncture, diet, and supplements were found to benefit patients with rotator cuff tendinitis. Level of evidence: I.

Chapter 3

Biologic Augmentation of Rotator Cuff Healing

Kathleen A. Derwin, PhD   David Kovacevic, MD   Myung-Sun Kim, MD, PhD   Eric T. Ricchetti, MD

Introduction

Rotator cuff tears affect at least 40% of people older than 60 years and are a common cause of debilitating pain, reduced function, and weakness in the shoulder. More than 250,000 rotator cuff repairs are performed annually in the United States.[1] Despite improvements in the understanding of the disease process and advances in surgical treatment, healing after rotator cuff repair remains a significant clinical challenge. The reported rates of unsuccessful repair range from 20% to 70%,[2-4] depending on patient age, tear size and chronicity, muscle atrophy and degeneration, tendon quality, repair technique, and postoperative rehabilitation. There is a need for strategies to augment the repair by mechanically reinforcing it while biologically enhancing the intrinsic healing potential of the tendon. Tissue-engineering strategies, including the use of scaffolds, platelet-rich plasma (PRP), specific growth factors, and cell seeding, have been investigated for improving the healing of rotator cuff repairs and/or inducing the regeneration of functional tissues.

Scaffold Devices

During the past 10 years, scaffold devices derived from mammalian extracellular matrix (ECM) and/or synthetic polymers have been approved by the FDA and marketed as medical devices for rotator cuff repair in humans. The rationales for using a scaffold device for rotator cuff repair include mechanical augmentation by

Dr. Derwin or an immediate family member has received royalties from the Musculoskeletal Transplant Foundation; has received nonincome support (such as equipment or services), commercially derived honoraria, or other non–research-related funding (such as paid travel) from the Musculoskeletal Transplant Foundation; and serves as a board member, owner, officer, or committee member of the Orthopaedic Research Society. None of the following authors or any immediate family member has received anything of value from or has stock or stock options held in a commercial company or institution related directly or indirectly to the subject of this chapter: Dr. Kovacevic, Dr. Kim, and Dr. Ricchetti.

off-loading the repair immediately and during a period of postoperative healing and/or biologic augmentation by improving the rate and the quality of tendon healing. In particular, ECM-derived scaffolds are believed to provide a chemically and structurally instructive environment for host cells through their natural composition, three-dimensional structure, and remodeling biomolecules.[5,6] Synthetic scaffolds may not influence the biology of repair healing, but their ability to maintain their mechanical properties over time may function to mechanically stabilize the repair construct until host tissue healing can occur.

Commercially Available Scaffold Devices

Synthetic scaffolds and ECM scaffolds derived from nonhuman sources are cleared for use through the 510(k) regulatory process of the FDA as medical devices with no significant risk for use in humans. Devices are cleared through this pathway by demonstrating substantial equivalence to a predicate device in performance, biocompatibility, safety, stability, sterility, and packaging. It is not mandatory to establish proof of efficacy through a preclinical or controlled human clinical study, however. These scaffold devices have been cleared by the FDA as augmentation devices to be used for reinforcing a suture or suture anchor repair during rotator cuff surgery. In contrast, human-derived ECM scaffolds are classified as human tissue for transplantation (21 CFR, Pt. 1270), and they require no FDA clearance for use. The commercially available scaffold devices for rotator cuff repair are listed in Table 1.

Basic Science Studies on the Use of Scaffolds

The basic science studies on the use of scaffolds for rotator cuff repair include evaluations of the host response, remodeling characteristics, biomechanics, and practical applicability using in vitro and animal models.[7] ECM scaffolds elicit distinct histologic and morphologic responses in the recipient. These responses depend on the species of origin, tissue of origin, processing methods, methods of terminal sterilization, and mechanical loading environment. The host immune response, including the macrophage component of the

Table 1

Commercial Scaffold Devices With FDA Clearance for Rotator Cuff Repair

Product	Scaffold Type	Scaffold Material	Commercial Source
Restore Orthobiologic Implant	Extracellular matrix	Porcine small intestinal submucosa	DePuy (Warsaw, IN)
CuffPatch	Extracellular matrix	Porcine small intestinal submucosa (cross-linked)	Organogenesis (Canton, MA)
GraftJacket	Extracellular matrix	Human dermis	Wright Medical (Arlington, TX)
ArthroFlex	Extracellular matrix	Human dermis	Arthrex (Naples, FL)
Conexa	Extracellular matrix	Porcine dermis (αGal-reduced)	Tornier (Montbonnot, France)
Zimmer Collagen Repair	Extracellular matrix	Porcine dermis (cross-linked)	Zimmer (Warsaw, IN)
TissueMend	Extracellular matrix	Bovine dermis (fetal)	Stryker (Mahwah, NJ)
BioBlanket	Extracellular matrix	Bovine dermis (cross-linked)	Kensey Nash (Exton, PA)
OrthADAPT Bioimplant	Extracellular matrix	Equine pericardium (cross-linked)	Pegasus Biologics (Irvine, CA)
OrthADAPT PR Bioimplant	Extracellular matrix + synthetic	Equine pericardium (cross-linked) reinforced with polyether ether ketone fiber	Pegasus Biologics
SportMesh Soft Tissue Reinforcement	Synthetic	Poly(urethaneurea)	Biomet Sports Medicine (Warsaw, IN)
X-Repair	Synthetic	Poly-L-lactide	Synthasome (San Diego, CA)
Biomerix RCR Patch	Synthetic	Polycarbonate polyurethane-urea	Biomerix (Fremont, CA)

immune response, appears to be a critical determinant—and perhaps a predictor of successful and constructive remodeling with the use of small intestinal submucosa (SIS), which is a rapidly resorbing ECM (in days to weeks). Less is known about the role of immune cells with the use of ECM scaffold materials such as dermis, which undergo slower remodeling and to some extent may be incorporated by the host. Cross-linked ECM scaffolds are associated with the presence of foreign-body giant cells; chronic inflammation; and/or the accumulation of dense, poorly organized fibrous tissue. The duration and intensity of the host response to a synthetic scaffold are dictated by its biomaterial composition and morphology (size, shape, porosity, and roughness) and probably by biologic and mechanical factors at the implantation site. Animal studies generally have reported favorable histologic outcomes and tendonlike remodeling using ECM or synthetic scaffold for rotator cuff repair.

The material, geometry, and suture retention properties of a scaffold influence the extent to which the device can augment the mechanical properties of a tendon repair at surgical implantation. The surgical methods of scaffold application, including the number, type, and location of fixation sutures, along with scaffold preten-

sioning at the time of repair, contribute to the mechanical performance of the device. It is important to note that scaffold degradation is expected during the days to weeks after surgical implantation, with the rate and extent depending on the particular scaffold and its remodeling characteristics. Degradation causes loss of mechanical strength, but host tissue deposition and remodeling can concomitantly strengthen the repair. The sequence of remodeling events, including the rate and the extent of scaffold degradation, incorporation, and host tissue deposition is not well established for most scaffold devices.

Clinical Studies on the Use of Scaffolds for Rotator Cuff Repair

The first clinical studies of ECM scaffolds investigated non–cross-linked porcine SIS (Restore Orthobiologic Implant; DePuy).[8-11] In two studies, 20% to 30% of patients had a severe, sterile, postoperative inflammatory reaction.[10,11] Based on this complication, the American Academy of Orthopaedic Surgeons (AAOS) does not recommend the use of Restore for the treatment of rotator cuff tears in humans.[12] Retrospective follow-up studies using non–cross-linked human dermis scaffolds (for example, GraftJacket; Wright Medical) as augmentation and interpositional devices reported improvement compared with patients' preoperative condition, but these studies did not include a comparison with control subjects (patients who received nonaugmented repair)[13-17] (**Table 2**). The clinical use of cross-linked dermis scaffolds (Zimmer Collagen Repair; Zimmer) was reported in two small retrospective case studies that found mixed results[18,19] (**Table 2**). A recent prospective randomized controlled study that investigated the use of GraftJacket for augmentation of chronic two-tendon tears found that patients who received an augmented rotator cuff repair had significantly better scores on the American Shoulder and Elbow Surgeons Shoulder Index and the Constant Shoulder Score and had significantly better healing rates than those who received a nonaugmented repair.[20] Gadolinium-enhanced magnetic resonance arthrography at 1- or 2-year follow-up revealed that 85% of the augmented repairs were intact, compared with 40% of the nonaugmented repairs. No adverse events related to the acellular human dermal matrix were observed. These studies support further investigation of non–cross-linked dermis-derived scaffolds for the treatment of rotator cuff tears.

Only one clinical study on the use of a synthetic scaffold for rotator cuff repair has been reported.[2] The polycarbonate polyurethane-urea Biomerix RCR Patch (Biomerix) was evaluated as an augmentation device in 10 patients undergoing open repair of a full-thickness tear of the supraspinatus or the infraspinatus tendon (mean tear size, 2 cm).[21] At 1-year follow-up, significant improvement in outcome scores were reported. Ultrasound and MRI showed that 10% of the repairs were unsuccessful. However, the lack of a control group for comparison means it is difficult to determine the precise benefit of the graft, particularly in limiting repair failure. The mean tear size in this study represented a small- to medium-size tear, which may not require repair augmentation as commonly as a large or massive tear.

Several scaffold devices are currently available to the orthopaedic surgeon for rotator cuff repair. The unique physical, chemical, and/or biologic characteristics of any given device for rotator cuff repair as well as the manner in which it is used have critical roles in the effectiveness of the device. Only two prospective randomized controlled studies have been performed using any of the available devices,[10,20] and no peer-reviewed clinical data are available for many of the currently available scaffold devices. Because of the paucity of clinical evidence, the AAOS has not made recommendations in favor of or against the use of soft-tissue allografts or other xenografts for treating patients with a rotator cuff tear.[12] Additional well-designed randomized controlled studies are needed to answer the many questions related to these devices, including their indications, surgical application, safety, mechanism of action, and efficacy.

Platelet-Rich Plasma

The clinical interest in a platelet concentrate dates to 1954, when evidence of an antagonist to blood-clotting factors in PRP was reported.[22] Currently, more than 6,000 citations of PRP appear in the National Library of Medicine (PubMed) database, and almost half of this literature has been published within the past 12 years. The recent emphasis has been on the biologic potential of platelet concentrate in healing. This blood product has been used to augment healing after injury and repair in dentistry, oral and maxillofacial surgery, plastic surgery, and orthopaedic surgery.[23-26] The rationale for the widespread use of PRP is to enhance recruitment, proliferation, and differentiation of cells involved in tissue regeneration by concentrating the growth factors believed to be responsible for the healing process and reintroducing them to the site of injury.[27]

Definition and Preparation Considerations

PRP is an autologous blood-derived product that contains at least 1 million platelets per microliter of blood, which is an amount four to seven times greater than normal baseline levels.[28] However, this simple working definition does not accurately reflect the variability among different types of PRP formulations. A recent qualitative classification system allows platelet concentrate preparations to be compared and proposes a consistent terminology.[29] Six categories of platelet concentrate preparation can be defined, depending on leukocyte content, exogenous platelet activation, and the presence of strong fibrin architecture (**Table 3**). The presence of leukocytes signifies that a prepared platelet concentrate contains not only the growth factors responsible for wound healing but also inflammatory cytokines and matrix metalloproteinases.[30] Exogenous application of calcium chloride or thrombin immediately before administration at the site of injury initiates platelet activation, clot formation, and growth factor release through α granules.[28] It is believed that approximately 70% of the stored growth factors are released within 10 minutes, and almost 100% of the growth factors are released within 1 hour.[31] The release of growth factors can be delayed by creating a platelet-rich fibrin (PRF) matrix. A second centrifugation in the presence of calcium chloride converts fibrinogen to fibrin. The dense fibrin matrix traps intact platelets, allowing a slow release of growth factors for approximately 5 to 7 days.[28] An understanding of the cellular composition, growth factor concentrations, and the matrix architecture of a platelet concentrate will allow clinicians and scientists to evaluate commercial formulations and their best clinical applications. For example, a certain type of platelet concentrate formulation may be most effective for treating a specific musculoskeletal pathology.

Table 2

Clinical Studies of Scaffold Devices for Rotator Cuff Repair

Product	Study (Year)	Level of Evidence and Study Type	Tear Size (Number of Patients)	Surgical Procedure Type/Scaffold Application Technique
GraftJacket	Burkhead et al[13] (2007)	IV Retrospective case study	Massive (17)	Open/Augmentation
	Dopirak et al[14] (2007) Bond et al[15] (2008)	IV Retrospective case study	Massive, irreparable (16)	Arthroscopic/Interposition
	Wong et al[16] (2010) (update of Bond et al[15])	IV Retrospective case study	Massive, irreparable (45)	Arthroscopic/Interposition
	Barber et al[20] (2012)	II Prospective randomized controlled study	Chronic two-tendon > 3 cm (augmented, 22; nonaugmented, 20)	Arthroscopic/Augmentation
Acellular human dermal matrix	Rotini et al[17] (2011)	IV Retrospective case study	Large or massive (2) Large or massive (3)	Arthroscopic/Augmentation and interposition Open/Augmentation and interposition
Zimmer Collagen Repair	Soler et al[18] (2007)	IV Retrospective case study	Massive (4)	Open/Interposition
	Badhe et al[19] (2008)	IV Retrospective case study	Large or massive (10)	Open/Interposition
Biomerix RCR Patch	Encalada-Diaz et al[21] (2011)	IV Retrospective case study	Small or medium; mean, 2 cm (10)	Open/Augmentation

Commercially Available Platelet Concentrate Preparation Systems

A platelet concentrate is made by centrifuging a patient's peripheral venous blood to obtain a concentrated platelet preparation suspended in a volume of plasma.[32] More than 16 systems are commercially available.[33] These systems vary in their preparation protocol, platelet capture efficiency, inclusion of leukocytes, use of activators, and growth factor content (Table 4), and their use leads to the preparation of markedly dissimilar platelet concentrate formulations. The inherent biologic variability among individual patients can lead to significant differences in the platelet concentrate preparation produced using one system.[34] Significant temporal variation has been found in the number of platelets and leukocytes in a platelet concentrate prepared with the same system from the same individual, and platelets from some patients fail to concentrate with one preparation system but successfully concentrate with another system.[30,34] The wide variability in

Table 2

Clinical Studies of Scaffold Devices for Rotator Cuff Repair (continued)

Follow-Up Period	Failure Rate on MRI or Ultrasound	Measure[a]: Mean Scores	Outcomes
14 months	3 of 12	UCLA: Preoperative 9.06, follow-up 26.12	No adverse events reported. Scores, strength, range of motion improved. Fourteen of 17 patients satisfied with outcome. Recurrent tears smaller than on preoperative MRI.
12-38 months	3 of 16	UCLA: Preoperative 18.4, follow-up 30.4 Constant: Preoperative 53.8, follow-up 84	No adverse events reported. Scores, pain, strength, range of motion improved. Fifteen of 16 patients satisfied with outcome. Thirteen patients had full incorporation of graft into native tissue on MRI.
24-68 months	3 of 16	UCLA: Preoperative 18.4, follow-up 27.5 WORC: Follow-up 75.2 ASES: Follow-up 84.1	Deep wound infection in 1 (immunocompromised) patient, requiring arthroscopic irrigation and débridement with antibiotics. Long-term neurapraxia in 1 patient, resolved at 1 year. Surgical time consistently less than 3 hours.
12-38 months	Augmented: 3 of 20 Nonaugmented: 9 of 15	UCLA: Augmented at follow-up 28.2, nonaugmented at follow-up 28.3 Constant: Augmented at follow-up 91.9, nonaugmented at follow-up 85.3 ASES: Augmented at follow-up 98.9, nonaugmented at follow-up 94.8	No adverse events reported. Patients with augmentation had significantly better Constant and ASES scores and significantly better healing rate on magnetic resonance arthrogram, compared with patients in the nonaugmented group.
12-18 months	2 of 5	Constant: Preoperative 64, follow-up 88	No adverse events reported. Healed repairs had graft incorporation into native tissue on MRI.
3–6 months	4 of 4	Not reported	Older patient population (71 to 82 years). Graft disruption at 3 to 6 months postoperatively in all patients. Inflammatory reaction in all patients, with graft disintegration and tissue necrosis at revision surgery.
3–5 years	2 of 10	Constant: Preoperative 42, follow-up 62	No adverse events reported. Scores, pain, range of motion, abduction power improved. Nine of 10 patients satisfied with outcome.
12 months	1 of 10	ASES: Preoperative 44, follow-up 73 UCLA: Follow-up 29.2 SST: Preoperative 3.6, follow-up 7.7	Relatively small tears (single-tendon tears of supraspinatus or infraspinatus). No adverse events reported. Scores, pain, range of motion improved.

[a] ASES = American Shoulder and Elbow Surgeons Shoulder Index (100-point scale), Constant = Constant Shoulder Score (100-point scale), SST = Simple Shoulder Test (12-point scale), UCLA = University of California Los Angeles Shoulder Scale (35-point scale), WORC = Western Ontario Rotator Cuff Index (100-point scale).

both platelet concentrate preparation and patient response undoubtedly affect the biologic effect on tissue healing. Researchers and clinicians must seek to identify, quantify, and report the components present in the individual patient's platelet concentrate preparation so that its efficacy as a regenerative therapy for connective tissue healing can be conclusively investigated.

Basic Science Studies on the Use of Platelet Concentrate

The application of a platelet concentrate to augment the local biology of repaired tissues at the time of surgery is appealing because platelets are normally involved in tissue hemostasis and thrombosis during the early inflammatory phase of healing. Platelets contain α

Table 3

Platelet Concentrate Classification System

Platelet Concentrate	Leukocytes	Exogenous Activation	Strong Fibrin Architecture
Pure platelet-rich plasma	No	No	No
Leukocyte- and platelet-rich plasma	Yes	No	No
Pure platelet-rich plasma gel	No	Yes	No
Leukocyte- and platelet-rich plasma gel	Yes	Yes	No
Pure platelet-rich fibrin	No	Yes	Yes
Leukocyte- and platelet-rich fibrin	Yes	Yes	Yes

Data from Dohan Ehrenfest DM, Bielecki T, Mishra A, et al: In search of a consensus terminology in the field of platelet concentrates for surgical use: Platelet-rich plasma (PRP), platelet-rich fibrin (PRF), fibrin gel polymerization and leukocytes. *Curr Pharm Biotechnol* 2012;13(7):1131-1137.

Table 4

Characteristics of Commercially Available Platelet Concentrate Preparation Systems

System (Commercial Source)	Blood Volume (mL)	Procedure	Centrifuge Time/Speed	Final PRP volume (mL)
Cascade Medical FIBRINET (Musculoskeletal Transplant Foundation, Edison, NJ)	9–18	PRP: Single spin PRFM: Double spin	PRP: 6 min/1,100 g PRFM: 6 min/1,100 g + 15 min/1,450 g	4-9
Gravitational Platelet Separation (GPS) III (Biomet)	27-110	Single spin	15 min/1,900 g	3–12
Autologous Conditioned Plasma-Double Syringe (ACP-DS) (Arthrex)	9	Single spin	5 min/1,500 rpm	3
SmartPReP (Harvest Technologies, Plymouth, MA)	20-120	Double spin	14 min/1,000g	3-20
Magellan (Medtronic, Minneapolis, MN)	30-60	Double spin	4-6min/1,200 g	6
Plasma Rich in Growth Factors–Endoret (PRGF-Endoret);(BTI Biotechnology, Blue Bell, PA)	9-72	Single spin	8 min / 580 g	4-32

PRFM = platelet-rich fibrin matrix or membrane (depending on volume of whole blood and duration of second spin cycle), PRP = platelet-rich plasma.

granules, which when degranulated release adhesive proteins, clotting factors, and growth factors. Plasma consists of numerous proteins, electrolytes, and hormones.[27,30] A platelet concentrate contains concentrated levels of growth factors (such as platelet-derived growth factor, vascular-derived growth factor, transforming growth factor–β1, basic fibroblast growth factor, epidermal growth factor, hepatocyte growth factor, and insulin-like growth factor–1) that are known to play a role in cell proliferation and differentiation, chemotaxis, angiogenesis, and ECM production. These factors can be expected to influence tendon healing[27,32,33,35] (Table 4).

Several key basic science findings have emerged regarding the effect of a platelet concentrate on tendon healing. In vitro studies have consistently found that platelet concentrate preparations positively affect gene expression and matrix synthesis in cultured tendon cells.[36-38] In vivo animal studies have found that tendon healing is enhanced by the use of platelet concentrate preparations. In a rat Achilles tenonectomy model, allogeneic PRP gel applied at the defect site led to better mechanical properties at the site of injury compared with platelet-poor plasma or saline.[39,40] In a rabbit model, augmentation of a patellar tendon defect with PRP gel led to more mature and dense neovascularized tissue compared with control treatment.[41] In a dog model, augmentation of the same injury with PRF did not improve the rate or histologic quality of tissue healing.[42] Although the basic science literature generally supports the potential of platelet concentrate preparations to augment tendon healing, many questions remain related to the timing, the concentration, and the formulation necessary to capture the potential benefit of a platelet concentrate in an orchestrated manner.

Table 4

Characteristics of Commercially Available Platelet Concentrate Preparation Systems (continued)

Final Platelet Concentration	Leukocytes	Activator	Anticoagulant	Growth Factor Levels
1-1.5×	No	Calcium chloride	Sodium citrate	PDGF: N/A EGF: 5–10× VEGF: 5–10× TGF-β1: 5-10× IGF-1: 5-10×
3–8×	Yes	Calcium chloride/ autologous thrombin	ACD-A	PDGF: N/A EGF: 3.9× VEGF: 6.2× TGF-β1: 3.6× IGF-1: 1×
2–3×	No	None	ACD-A	PDGF: 25× EGF: 5× VEGF: 11× TGF-β1: 4× IGF-1: 1×
4–6×	Yes	Calcium chloride/ bovine thrombin	ACD-A	PDGF: 4.4× EGF: 4.4× VEGF: 4.4× TGF-β1: 4.4× IGF-1: N/A
3-7×	Yes	Calcium chloride	ACD-A	—
2-3×	No	Calcium chloride	Sodium citrate	—

ACD-A = anticoagulant citrate dextrose solution A, EGF = epidermal growth factor, IGF-1 = insulin-like growth factor–1, N/A = not available, PDGF = platelet-derived growth factor, TGF-β1 = transforming growth factor–β1, VEGF = vascular endothelial growth factor, × = times.
Data from Hall MP, Band PA, Meislin RJ, Jazrawi LM, Cardone DA: Platelet-rich plasma: Current concepts and application in sports medicine. *J Am Acad Orthop Surg* 2009;17(10):602-608; Castillo TN, Pouliot MA, Kim HJ, Dragoo JL: Comparison of growth factor and platelet concentration from commercial platelet-rich plasma separation systems. *Am J Sports Med* 2011;39(2):266-271; Lopez-Vidriero E, Goulding KA, Simon DA, Sanchez M, Johnson DH: The use of platelet-rich plasma in arthroscopy and sports medicine: Optimizing the healing environment. *Arthroscopy* 2010;26(2):269-278.

Table 5

Clinical Studies of Platelet Concentrate in Rotator Cuff Repair

System (Commercial Source)	Study (Year)	Level of Evidence and Study Type	Type of Surgical Repair/Tear Size and Type	Platelet Concentrate Application (Number of Patients)
Cascade Medical FIBRINET (Musculoskeletal Transplant Foundation)	Castricini et al[43] (2011) Arnoczky[47] (2011)	I Prospective randomized controlled study	Arthroscopic double-row Small to medium supraspinatus tears	Control (45) PRF interposed at tendon-bone interface (43)
	Bergeson et al[45] (2012)	III Case-control study	Arthroscopic single- or double-row One- to three-tendon tears ≥ 2 cm	Control (21) Two PRF constructs interposed at tendon-bone interface (16)
	Barber et al[44] (2011)	III Case-control study	Arthroscopic single-row/One- to two-tendon tears, 1–5 cm	Control (20) Two PRF constructs interposed at tendon-bone interface (20)
	Rodeo et al[46] (2012)	I Prospective randomized controlled study	Arthroscopic single- or double-row/Small to large tears	Control (39) PRF interposed at tendon-bone interface (40)
Gravitational Platelet Separation (GPS) II (Biomet)	Randelli et al[48] (2011)	I Prospective randomized controlled study	Arthroscopic single-row/ One- to three-tendon tear	Control (27) PRF injected at tendon-bone repair site (26)
COBE Spectra LRS Turbo (CaridianBCT, Lakewood, CO)	Jo et al[49] (2011)	II Prospective cohort study	Arthroscopic suture bridge technique/ small to massive tears	Control (23) Three leukocyte-poor PRP gels interposed at tendon-bone interface (19)

Clinical Studies on the Use of Platelet Concentrate for Rotator Cuff Repair

An electronic search of the National Library of Medicine and Cochrane Collaboration databases using the search terms *platelet-rich plasma* and *rotator cuff* identified eight clinical studies examining the use of platelet concentrate for augmentation in rotator cuff repair. Six of these studies provided level I, II, or III evidence. The design and the results of these studies are summarized in **Table 5**. Four of the six studies used the Cascade Medical FIBRINET system (Musculoskeletal Transplant Foundation) to create PRF matrix that was interposed at the tendon-bone interface during arthroscopic repair of small to massive rotator cuff tears.[43-46] None of the studies reported better functional outcomes at final follow-up for patients treated with PRF, compared with those treated without PRF. Two studies used MRI or ultrasound to evaluate tendon healing and found no difference in retear rates based on whether patients were treated with PRF.[43,46] One study found a significantly higher retear rate among patients treated with PRF,[45] but another study found a significantly higher retear rate among patients treated without PRF.[44] One study found no between-group difference in final rates of retear but did find a significant improvement in tendon signal intensity in tendons treated with PRF as well as a trend to increased tendon footprint size in intact repairs treated with PRF.[43] These findings suggest that PRF has a positive effect on rotator cuff healing.[47] In

Table 5

Clinical Studies of Platelet Concentrate in Rotator Cuff Repair (continued)

Mean Follow-up (Months)	Failure Rate on MRI or Ultrasound	Measure[a]: Mean Scores at Final Follow-up	Outcomes
20.2 (range, 16-30)	4 of 38 (10.5%) 1 of 40 (2.5%)	Constant: PRF 88.4, C 88.4	No significant between-group differences in Constant scores or retear rates. For intact repairs, MRI signal intensity score significantly better in patients treated with PRF.
27 (range, 18-45) 13 (range, 3-19)	8 of 21 (38%) 9 of 16 (56%)	ASES: PRF 87, C 84 Constant: PRF 73, C 76 UCLA: PRF 29, C 29 WORC: PRF 80, C 82 SANE: PRF 89, C 87	No significant between-group differences on any measures. Retear rate was significantly higher in patients treated with PRF. Two deep infections (*Propionibacterium acnes*) in patients treated with PRF, requiring irrigation and débridement.
33 (range, 24-44) 28.3 (range, 24-44)	12 of 20 (60%) 6 of 20 (30%)	ASES: PRF 95.7, C 94.7 Constant: PRF 88.1, PC 84.7 SST: PRF 11.3, C 11.4 SANE: PRF 94.5, C 93.7 Rowe: PRF 94.9, C 84.8	Patients treated with PRF had significantly higher Rowe scores, but no other significant between-group score differences. Retear rate was significantly higher in control group patients.
12	6 of 31 (19%) 12 of 36 (33%)	ASES: PRF 91.30, C 96.43 L'Insalata: PRF 90.39, C 94.11	No significant between-group differences in any strength measure. No significant between-group differences in retear rates. PRF was a significant predictor of retear by regression analysis.
24	12 of 23 (52%) 9 of 22 (41%)	Constant: PRF 82.4, C 78.7 UCLA: PRF 33.3, C 31.2 SST: PRF 11.3, C 10.9	Patients in the PRF group had significantly reduced pain during the first month after surgery and significant increase in external rotation strength and all scores at 3 months. No significant between-group differences in external rotation strength or any scores at 6-, 12-, and 24-month follow-up. For small tears, patients in the PRF group had significantly increased external rotation strength at 3-, 6-, 12-, and 24-month follow-up. No significant between-group differences in retear rates. Repair integrity was significantly associated with patient age, tear shape, and retraction.
20.3 ± 1.89 18.94 ± 1.63	7 of 17 (41%) 4 of 15 (27%)	ASES: PRP 87.61, C 89.92 Constant: PRP 79.12, C 82.00 UCLA: PRP 31.78, C 30.83 DASH: PRP 13.19, C 8.48 SST: PRP 9.83, C 10.57 SPADI: PRP 12.03, C 10.08	Patients in control group had significantly higher ASES, Constant, and SPADI scores at 3-month follow-up. No significant between-group differences in any measures after 3 months. No significant between-group differences in satisfaction or retear rate.

[a] ASES = American Shoulder and Elbow Surgeons Shoulder Index (100-point scale), Constant = Constant Shoulder Score (100-point scale), C = control; DASH = Disabilities of the Arm, Shoulder and Hand (100-point scale), L'Insalata = L'Insalata Scale (100-point scale), PRP = platelet-rich plasma, PRF = platelet-rich fibrin, Rowe = Rowe Scale (100-point scale), SANE = Single Assessment Numeric Evaluation (100-point scale), SPADI = Shoulder Pain and Disability Index (100-point scale), SST = Simple Shoulder Test (12-point scale), UCLA = University of California Los Angeles Shoulder Scale (35-point scale), WORC = Western Ontario Rotator Cuff Index (100-point scale).

contrast, another study found PRF treatment to be a significant predictor of a tendon defect at 12 weeks, and this finding suggests a negative effect of PRF on rotator cuff tendon healing.[46]

Two of the six studies used a platelet concentrate formulation other than the Cascade Medical FIBRINET system. In a randomized study, PRF prepared with the Gravitational Platelet Separation (GPS) II system (Biomet) was injected at the tendon-bone interface dur-ing arthroscopic repair of one- to three-tendon tears.[48] Patients treated with PRF had earlier improvement in pain scores than those treated without PRF. Strength and functional outcomes scores in patients treated with PRF were better at 3 months but not at 6 months. MRI revealed no between-group difference in rates of retear 2 years after surgery. A prospective cohort study evaluated PRP gel prepared with the COBE Spectra LRS

Turbo system (CaridianBCT, Lakewood, CO).[49] Three PRP gels were interposed at the tendon-bone interface during arthroscopic repair of small to massive tendon tears. Patients in the control group had improved functional outcomes scores at 3 months, but there were no between-group differences in strength, range of motion, or functional outcomes scores after 3 months. There were no between-group differences in overall satisfaction or healing rate at an average 20-month follow-up after surgery.

The available clinical data do not provide conclusive evidence on the efficacy of platelet concentrate as a regenerative therapy for rotator cuff repair. No difference in functional outcome or healing rate has been found at early follow-up as a result of platelet concentrate treatment. However, it is challenging to draw conclusions regarding the efficacy of platelet concentrate treatment from the existing clinical data because of wide variability among studies in tear size, repair technique, platelet concentrate characteristics (platelet concentration, presence of leukocytes, fibrin architecture, growth factor levels), application technique, and rehabilitation protocol. The available studies are limited by relatively small sample sizes, subjective imaging outcomes, variable functional outcome measures, and limited or no characterization of the platelet preparation used. Appropriately powered level I or II studies are needed with documentation and, to the extent possible, control of these variables. Numerous issues remain to be investigated regarding the effect of timing, dosing, the mode of application, and the formulation of the platelet concentrate in the context of rotator cuff repair.

Although clinical studies have reported minimal complications of the use of platelet concentrates, one study reported two cases of deep infection that required reoperation in patients who underwent PRF augmentation during rotator cuff repair.[45] A causal relationship between PRF treatment and infection was not established, and none of the other reviewed studies reported a complication or infection related to platelet concentrate use. Further research is needed to better delineate any risk of infection associated with the use of platelet concentrate to augment rotator cuff repair healing.

Summary

Numerous scaffolds and platelet concentrate products are being used by shoulder surgeons to augment healing after rotator cuff repairs. These strategies are conceptually attractive and supported by basic science investigation, but only limited clinical evidence supports their efficacy in improving healing rates and patient functional outcomes. It is possible that these products may be effective only in particular patient populations and/or surgical indications. Their efficacy may be dependent on the manner in which they are formulated or delivered. To recognize the full therapeutic potential of scaffolds and platelet concentrates, the complexity of these products must be embraced, and researchers and clinicians must continue rigorous scientific investigation regarding their mechanism of action, appropriate indications, and methods of use.

Annotated References

1. Colvin AC, Egorova N, Harrison AK, Moskowitz A, Flatow EL: National trends in rotator cuff repair. *J Bone Joint Surg Am* 2012;94(3):227-233.

   Between 1996 and 2006 there was a significant shift from inpatient to outpatient rotator cuff repair surgery in the United States. The increase in rates of rotator cuff repair was dramatic, particularly for arthroscopically assisted repair.

2. Tashjian RZ, Hollins AM, Kim HM, et al: Factors affecting healing rates after arthroscopic double-row rotator cuff repair. *Am J Sports Med* 2010;38(12):2435-2442.

   A retrospective case study found that older age and longer duration of follow-up were associated with lower healing rates after double-row rotator cuff repair. The biologic limitation at the repair site appears to be the most important factor influencing tendon healing, even with a double-row construct. Level of evidence: IV.

3. Toussaint B, Schnaser E, Bosley J, Lefebvre Y, Gobezie R: Early structural and functional outcomes for arthroscopic double-row transosseous-equivalent rotator cuff repair. *Am J Sports Med* 2011;39(6):1217-1225.

   Short-term results of a retrospective case study suggested that the clinical outcomes and structural integrity of transosseous-equivalent double-row rotator cuff repairs compare favorably with those reported for other double-row suture anchor techniques in rotator cuff repair. Level of evidence: IV.

4. Koh KH, Kang KC, Lim TK, Shon MS, Yoo JC: Prospective randomized clinical trial of single- versus double-row suture anchor repair in 2- to 4-cm rotator cuff tears: Clinical and magnetic resonance imaging results. *Arthroscopy* 2011;27(4):453-462.

   A prospective randomized controlled study found that the clinical results and retear rates of double-row repair with one additional medial suture anchor were not significantly different from those of single-row repair with two lateral suture anchors in patients with a medium to large rotator cuff tear. Level of evidence: I.

5. Reing JE, Zhang L, Myers-Irvin J, et al: Degradation products of extracellular matrix affect cell migration and the proliferation. *Tissue Eng Part A* 2009;15(3):605-614.

   ECM degradation products had chemotactic and mitogenic activities for multipotential progenitor cells, and the same degradation products inhibited both chemotaxis and proliferation of differentiated endothelial cells.

6. Badylak SF, Freytes DO, Gilbert TW: Extracellular matrix as a biological scaffold material: Structure and function. *Acta Biomater* 2009;5(1):1-13.

An overview of the composition and the structure of selected ECM scaffold materials includes the effects of manufacturing methods on structural properties and resulting mechanical behavior of the material and the in vivo degradation and remodeling of ECM scaffolds, with an emphasis on tissue function.

7. Ricchetti ET, Aurora A, Iannotti JP, Derwin KA: Scaffold devices for rotator cuff repair. *J Shoulder Elbow Surg* 2012;21(2):251-265.

The basic science and clinical understanding of commercially available synthetic and ECM scaffolds for rotator cuff repair are reviewed, with an emphasis on host response and scaffold remodeling, mechanical and suture-retention properties, and preclinical and clinical studies.

8. Metcalf MH, Savoie FH III, Kellum B: Surgical technique for xenograft (SIS) augmentation of rotator-cuff repairs. *Oper Tech Orthop* 2002;12:204-208.

9. Sclamberg SG, Tibone JE, Itamura JM, Kasraeian S: Six-month magnetic resonance imaging follow-up of large and massive rotator cuff repairs reinforced with porcine small intestinal submucosa. *J Shoulder Elbow Surg* 2004;13(5):538-541.

10. Iannotti JP, Codsi MJ, Kwon YW, Derwin K, Ciccone J, Brems JJ: Porcine small intestine submucosa augmentation of surgical repair of chronic two-tendon rotator cuff tears: A randomized, controlled trial. *J Bone Joint Surg Am* 2006;88(6):1238-1244.

11. Walton JR, Bowman NK, Khatib Y, Linklater J, Murrell GA: Restore Orthobiologic Implant: Not recommended for augmentation of rotator cuff repairs. *J Bone Joint Surg Am* 2007;89(4):786-791.

A retrospective case-control study reported the open repair of large or massive rotator cuff tears using Restore Orthobiologic Implant. Overall satisfaction and range of motion were not significantly different between groups, but patients who did not receive augmentation had significantly greater strength and sports participation. Four patients who received Restore had a severe postoperative reaction requiring surgical treatment. Level of evidence: III.

12. Pedowitz RA, Yamaguchi K, Ahmad CS, et al; American Academy of Orthopaedic Surgeons: Optimizing the management of rotator cuff problems. *J Am Acad Orthop Surg* 2011;19(6):368-379.

Of 31 recommendations for the optimal management of rotator cuff issues, 19 were determined to be inconclusive, 4 were classified as moderate grade, 6 as weak, and 2 as consensus statements of expert opinion.

13. Burkhead WZ, Schiffern SC, Krishnan SG: Use of Graft Jacket as an augmentation for massive rotator cuff tears. *Semin Arthroplasty* 2007;18:11-18.

A retrospective case-control study reported the open repair of massive rotator cuff tears using GraftJacket. Strength, range of motion, and outcome scores were improved, and no complications were observed. Level of evidence: IV.

14. Dopirak R, Bond JL, Snyder SJ: Arthroscopic total rotator cuff replacement with an acellular human dermal allograft matrix. *Int J Shoulder Surg* 2007;1(1):7-15.

A retrospective case-control study reported the technique and short-term results of arthroscopic repair of irreparable rotator cuff tears using GraftJacket. Strength, pain, range of motion, and outcome scores were improved, and no complications were observed. Level of evidence: IV.

15. Bond JL, Dopirak RM, Higgins J, Burns J, Snyder SJ: Arthroscopic replacement of massive, irreparable rotator cuff tears using a GraftJacket allograft: Technique and preliminary results. *Arthroscopy* 2008;24(4):403-409, e1.

A retrospective case-control study reported the technique and short-term results of arthroscopic repair of irreparable rotator cuff tears using GraftJacket. Strength, pain, range of motion, and outcome scores were improved, and no complications were observed. Level of evidence: IV.

16. Wong I, Burns J, Snyder S: Arthroscopic GraftJacket repair of rotator cuff tears. *J Shoulder Elbow Surg* 2010;19(2, suppl):104-109.

A retrospective case-control study reported the arthroscopic repair of irreparable rotator cuff tears using GraftJacket. Outcome scores were improved, and two complications were observed. The procedure was considered safe and associated with high patient satisfaction, without the morbidity of tendon transfer or arthroplasty. Level of evidence: IV.

17. Rotini R, Marinelli A, Guerra E, et al: Human dermal matrix scaffold augmentation for large and massive rotator cuff repairs: Preliminary clinical and MRI results at 1-year follow-up. *Musculoskelet Surg* 2011; 95(suppl 1):S13-S23.

A retrospective case-control study reported the arthroscopic or open repair of large or massive rotator cuff tears using GraftJacket. Outcome scores were improved, and no adverse events reported. Level of evidence: IV.

18. Soler JA, Gidwani S, Curtis MJ: Early complications from the use of porcine dermal collagen implants (Permacol) as bridging constructs in the repair of massive rotator cuff tears: A report of 4 cases. *Acta Orthop Belg* 2007;73(4):432-436.

A retrospective case-control study reported the open repair of massive rotator cuff tears using Zimmer Collagen Repair. Graft disruption occurred 3 to 6 months postoperatively in all patients. Inflammatory reaction was seen in all patients, with graft disintegration and tissue necrosis observed at revision surgery. Level of evidence: IV.

19. Badhe SP, Lawrence TM, Smith FD, Lunn PG: An assessment of porcine dermal xenograft as an augmentation graft in the treatment of extensive rotator cuff tears. *J Shoulder Elbow Surg* 2008;17(1, suppl): 35S-39S.

    A retrospective case-control study reported the open repair of large or massive rotator cuff tears using Zimmer Collagen Repair. Outcome scores, pain, range of motion, and abduction power improved, and no adverse events were reported. Level of evidence: IV.

20. Barber FA, Burns JP, Deutsch A, Labbé MR, Litchfield RB: A prospective, randomized evaluation of acellular human dermal matrix augmentation for arthroscopic rotator cuff repair. *Arthroscopy* 2012;28(1):8-15.

    A prospective randomized controlled study reported the arthroscopic repair of chronic two-tendon rotator cuff tears with or without GraftJacket augmentation. Patients treated with augmentation had significantly better outcome scores and a significantly better healing rate on magnetic resonance arthrography, compared with those treated without augmentation. No adverse events were reported. Level of evidence: II.

21. Encalada-Diaz I, Cole BJ, Macgillivray JD, et al: Rotator cuff repair augmentation using a novel polycarbonate polyurethane patch: Preliminary results at 12 months' follow-up. *J Shoulder Elbow Surg* 2011; 20(5):788-794.

    A retrospective case-control study reported the open repair of small to medium rotator cuff tears using Biomerix RCR Patch. Pain, range of motion, and outcome scores were improved, and no complications were observed. Level of evidence: IV.

22. Kingsley CS: Blood coagulation: Evidence of an antagonist to factor VI in platelet-rich human plasma. *Nature* 1954;173(4407):723-724.

23. Del Fabbro M, Bortolin M, Taschieri S, Weinstein R: Is platelet concentrate advantageous for the surgical treatment of periodontal diseases? A systematic review and meta-analysis. *J Periodontol* 2011;82(8): 1100-1111.

    PRP may exert a positive adjunctive effect when used in combination with graft materials for the treatment of intrabone defects. No significant benefit of platelet concentrates was found for the treatment of gingival recession.

24. Marx RE, Carlson ER, Eichstaedt RM, Schimmele SR, Strauss JE, Georgeff KR: Platelet-rich plasma: Growth factor enhancement for bone grafts. *Oral Surg Oral Med Oral Pathol Oral Radiol Endod* 1998;85(6): 638-646.

25. Knighton DR, Ciresi KF, Fiegel VD, Austin LL, Butler EL: Classification and treatment of chronic nonhealing wounds: Successful treatment with autologous platelet-derived wound healing factors (PDWHF). *Ann Surg* 1986;204(3):322-330.

26. Sheth U, Simunovic N, Klein G, et al: Efficacy of autologous platelet-rich plasma use for orthopaedic indications: A meta-analysis. *J Bone Joint Surg Am* 2012; 94(4):298-307.

    A meta-analysis of the efficacy of PRP for orthopaedic applications found that PRP provided no significant benefit as late as 24 months across randomized or prospective cohort studies in patients with an orthopaedic injury.

27. Foster TE, Puskas BL, Mandelbaum BR, Gerhardt MB, Rodeo SA: Platelet-rich plasma: From basic science to clinical applications. *Am J Sports Med* 2009; 37(11):2259-2272.

    The basic science of PRP is examined, with a description of current clinical applications in sports medicine. Human studies published in the orthopaedic surgery and sports medicine literature are reviewed and evaluated. The use of PRP in amateur and professional sports is reviewed, and the regulation of PRP by anti-doping agencies is discussed.

28. Civinini R, Macera A, Nistri L, Redl B, Innocenti M: The use of autologous blood-derived growth factors in bone regeneration. *Clin Cases Miner Bone Metab* 2011;8(1):25-31.

    This review describes the biologic properties of platelets and their factors, as well as the methods used for producing PRP, to provide a basic science background and an overview of evidence-based medicine on the clinical application of PRP in bone healing.

29. Dohan Ehrenfest DM, Bielecki T, Mishra A, et al: In search of a consensus terminology in the field of platelet concentrates for surgical use: Platelet-rich plasma (PRP), platelet-rich fibrin (PRF), fibrin gel polymerization and leukocytes. *Curr Pharm Biotechnol* 2012; 13(7):1131-1137.

    A consensus terminology is proposed for characterizing products derived from platelet concentrates.

30. Boswell SG, Cole BJ, Sundman EA, Karas V, Fortier LA: Platelet-rich plasma: A milieu of bioactive factors. *Arthroscopy* 2012;28(3):429-439.

    In addition to platelets, a role is described for growth factors, soluble proteins, electrolytes, plasma hormones, leukocytes, and erythrocytes in the clinical response to PRP. Depending on the specific constituents of a PRP preparation, the clinical use theoretically can be matched to the pathology to improve clinical efficacy.

31. Marx RE: Platelet-rich plasma: Evidence to support its use. *J Oral Maxillofac Surg* 2004;62(4):489-496.

32. Hall MP, Band PA, Meislin RJ, Jazrawi LM, Cardone DA: Platelet-rich plasma: Current concepts and application in sports medicine. *J Am Acad Orthop Surg* 2009;17(10):602-608.

    Current concepts and the use of PRP in sports medicine are reviewed.

33. Castillo TN, Pouliot MA, Kim HJ, Dragoo JL: Comparison of growth factor and platelet concentration

from commercial platelet-rich plasma separation systems. *Am J Sports Med* 2011;39(2):266-271.

Three commercially available PRP separation systems produced single-donor PRP with different compositions and different concentrations of growth factors and white blood cells.

34. Mazzocca AD, McCarthy MB, Chowaniec DM, et al: Platelet-rich plasma differs according to preparation method and human variability. *J Bone Joint Surg Am* 2012;94(4):308-316.

The levels of platelets, growth factors, red blood cells, and white blood cells were quantified across patients using commercially available one-step and two-step separation systems, and intraindividual variability in PRP was determined. Within the evaluated procedures, platelet numbers and the numbers of white blood cells differed significantly in and between individuals.

35. Kobayashi M, Itoi E, Minagawa H, et al: Expression of growth factors in the early phase of supraspinatus tendon healing in rabbits. *J Shoulder Elbow Surg* 2006;15(3):371-377.

36. Schnabel LV, Mohammed HO, Miller BJ, et al: Platelet rich plasma (PRP) enhances anabolic gene expression patterns in flexor digitorum superficialis tendons. *J Orthop Res* 2007;25(2):230-240.

Tendon explants cultured in 100% PRP had enhanced gene expression of three matrix molecules, with no concomitant increase in the catabolic molecules metalloproteinase-3 and -13.

37. de Mos M, van der Windt AE, Jahr H, et al: Can platelet-rich plasma enhance tendon repair? A cell culture study. *Am J Sports Med* 2008;36(6):1171-1178.

In human tenocyte cultures, platelet-rich clot releasate and platelet-poor clot releasate stimulate cell proliferation and total collagen production. Platelet-rich clot releasate, not platelet-poor clot releasate, slightly increases the expression of matrix-degrading enzymes and endogenous growth factors.

38. Jo CH, Kim JE, Yoon KS, Shin S: Platelet-rich plasma stimulates cell proliferation and enhances matrix gene expression and synthesis in tenocytes from human rotator cuff tendons with degenerative tears. *Am J Sports Med* 2012;40(5):1035-1045.

PRP promoted cell proliferation and enhanced gene expression as well as the synthesis of tendon matrix in tenocytes from human rotator cuff tendons with degenerative tears.

39. Virchenko O, Grenegård M, Aspenberg P: Independent and additive stimulation of tendon repair by thrombin and platelets. *Acta Orthop* 2006;77(6):960-966.

40. Aspenberg P, Virchenko O: Platelet concentrate injection improves Achilles tendon repair in rats. *Acta Orthop Scand* 2004;75(1):93-99.

41. Lyras D, Kazakos K, Verettas D, et al: Immunohisto-

chemical study of angiogenesis after local administration of platelet-rich plasma in a patellar tendon defect. *Int Orthop* 2010;34(1):143-148.

PRP gel was applied to a central full-thickness patellar tendon defect in rabbits. Neovascularization was significantly higher in rabbits treated with PRP during the first 2 weeks and was significantly lower during the third and fourth weeks compared with control rabbits. The tissue formed in the PRP-treated rabbits was more mature and dense with less elastic fibers remaining.

42. Visser LC, Arnoczky SP, Caballero O, Gardner KL: Evaluation of the use of an autologous platelet-rich fibrin membrane to enhance tendon healing in dogs. *Am J Vet Res* 2011;72(5):699-705.

PRF membrane was applied to a central full-thickness patellar tendon defect in dogs. There was no significant difference in the histologic quality of the repair tissue in between the control (empty) defects and the PRF membrane–treated defects at 4 or 8 weeks.

43. Castricini R, Longo UG, De Benedetto M, et al: Platelet-rich plasma augmentation for arthroscopic rotator cuff repair: A randomized controlled trial. *Am J Sports Med* 2011;39(2):258-265.

A prospective randomized controlled study reported the arthroscopic repair of small to medium rotator cuff tears with or without PRF matrix. There were no between-group differences in outcome scores or retear rates. The MRI signal intensity score improved in those treated with PRF. Level of evidence: I.

44. Barber FA, Hrnack SA, Snyder SJ, Hapa O: Rotator cuff repair healing influenced by platelet-rich plasma construct augmentation. *Arthroscopy* 2011;27(8):1029-1035.

A case-control study reported the arthroscopic repair of one- or two-tendon rotator cuff tears with or without PRF matrix. There were no differences in outcome scores between groups, other than Rowe scores. The retear rate was significantly lower in those treated with PRF. Level of evidence: III.

45. Bergeson AG, Tashjian RZ, Greis PE, Crim J, Stoddard GJ, Burks RT: Effects of platelet-rich fibrin matrix on repair integrity of at-risk rotator cuff tears. *Am J Sports Med* 2012;40(2):286-293.

A case-control study reported the arthroscopic repair of one- to three-tendon rotator cuff tears with or without PRF matrix. There were no between-group differences in outcome scores. The retear rate was significantly higher in those treated with PRF. Level of evidence: III.

46. Rodeo SA, Delos D, Williams RJ, Adler RS, Pearle AD, Warren RF: The effect of platelet-rich fibrin matrix on rotator cuff tendon healing: A prospective, randomized clinical study. *Am J Sports Med* 2012;40(6):1234-1241.

A prospective randomized controlled study reported the arthroscopic repair of small to large rotator cuff tears with or without PRF matrix. There were no between-group differences in strength, outcome scores,

1: Basic Science

or retear rate. PRF was a significant predictor of a tendon defect at 12 weeks. Level of evidence: I.

47. Arnoczky SP: Platelet-rich plasma augmentation of rotator cuff repair: Letter. *Am J Sports Med* 2011;39(6): NP8-NP9, author reply NP9-NP11.

   A letter to the editor and author reply commented on the MRI findings and conclusions published in Castricini R, Longo UG, De Benedetto M, et al, *Sports Med* 2011;39(2)258-265.

48. Randelli P, Arrigoni P, Ragone V, Aliprandi A, Cabitza P: Platelet rich plasma in arthroscopic rotator cuff repair: A prospective RCT study, 2-year follow-up. *J Shoulder Elbow Surg* 2011;20(4):518-528.

   A prospective randomized controlled study reported the arthroscopic repair of one- to three-tendon rotator cuff tears with or without PRF matrix. There were no between-group differences in healing rates or scores after 6, 12, and 24 months. Subanalysis of small tears showed that patients treated with PRF had increased strength at 3, 6, 12, and 24 months. Level of evidence: I.

49. Jo CH, Kim JE, Yoon KS, et al: Does platelet-rich plasma accelerate recovery after rotator cuff repair? A prospective cohort study. *Am J Sports Med* 2011; 39(10):2082-2090.

   A prospective cohort study reported the arthroscopic repair of small to massive rotator cuff tears with or without leukocyte-poor PRP gels. There were no between-group differences in range of motion or outcome scores, in satisfaction, or retear rates after 3 months. Level of evidence: II.

Chapter 4

Kinematics and Biomechanics of Reverse Shoulder Arthroplasty

Christopher P. Roche, MSBE, MBA   Lynn Crosby, MD

1: Basic Science

Glenohumeral Joint Anatomy

The glenohumeral joint is the most mobile joint in the human body, but its nonconforming articular curvature makes it inherently unstable. The motion patterns of the glenohumeral joint have been described as spinning (in rotation only), sliding (in translation only), and rolling (in rotation and translation).[1,2] The stability of the glenohumeral joint is assisted throughout its range of motion by the coordinated action of muscle contractions and is controlled by ligament and capsular tightening, all of which vary with the joint position and the type of motion. The muscles of the shoulder are required for both mobility and stability.[3]

The deltoid is the largest and most important muscle in the shoulder girdle. This primary mover in the shoulder generates forward elevation in the scapular plane. The three distinct heads of the deltoid are the anterior (the anterior acromion and the clavicle), the middle (the lateral margin of the acromion), and the posterior (scapular spine) deltoid. Together, the three deltoid heads account for approximately 20% of the mass of the shoulder muscles.[4] At low levels of abduction, the wrapping of the middle deltoid around the greater tuberosity of the humeral head generates a stabilizing compressive force; however, this compressive force is small relative to the humeral head compression generated by the rotator cuff.[5,6]

The rotator cuff muscles generate the torque necessary for rotation of the humerus about the glenoid fossa, while they compress the humeral head into the glenoid concavity.[7] The rotator cuff muscles are aligned around the proximal humerus for effective joint compression at all glenohumeral joint positions, allowing the rotator

cuff to dynamically balance the joint, thereby compensating for the lack of osseous constraint in the glenohumeral joint.[8-10] Specifically, the anatomic arrangement of the anterior (subscapularis) and posterior (infraspinatus and teres minor) rotator cuff muscles creates a transverse force couple that in all joint positions approximately centers the humeral head on the glenoid fossa in the anterior and posterior directions.[11-13]

Rotator Cuff Tear Arthropathy

Disruption of rotator cuff integrity, most commonly by a tear in the rotator cuff muscle tendons, can have devastating consequences on glenohumeral joint stability. As the rotator cuff fails to compress the humeral head against the glenoid and balance the forces of the other muscles in the shoulder (primarily the deltoid), the humeral head tends to migrate superiorly and impinge on the undersurface of the acromion. This impingement can lead to further tearing of the rotator cuff, which is associated with fatty infiltration of the cuff muscles and eventually to arthritic changes secondary to increased friction and a lack of nutrients supplied to the cartilage. Continued tearing propagates further compression and results in humeral head collapse; biceps tendon dislocation; and superior glenoid, acromion, and coracoid erosion.[14,15] Neer used the term cuff tear arthropathy to describe this arthritic and eroded or collapsed condition of the glenohumeral joint after prolonged, progressive subacromial compression resulting from massive full-thickness rotator cuff tearing.[14]

The Philosophy and Design History of Reverse Shoulder Arthroplasty

The reverse shoulder implant was devised in the early 1970s for treating patients with cuff tear arthropathy. The use of this device was intended to relieve pain and prevent progressive acromial, coracoid, and glenoid erosion by resisting superior migration of the humeral head.[16] The reverse shoulder implant inverts the anatomic concavities; the glenoid articular component is made convex, and the humeral articular component is made concave, thereby creating a fixed fulcrum that prevents the humerus from migrating superiorly. Because these articulations are conforming, the motion of a reverse shoulder implant is limited to spinning. Several reverse shoulder designs were developed, including the Fenlin, Reeves-Leeds, Kessel, and Neer-Averill shoulders.[17-23] Each of these prostheses had a constrained and conforming articulation whose center of rotation was lateral to the glenoid fossa. These design features generated excessive torque on the glenoid bone-implant interface that compromised fixation and caused mechanical failure. As a result, these early designs were removed from the US market.[16,23]

In 1987 Grammont introduced a reverse shoulder design consisting of a 42-mm convex glenoid component whose thickness formed approximately two thirds of a sphere and a concave humeral component whose depth was approximately one third of a sphere. This early design also was associated with glenoid failure, and in 1991 it was redesigned for noncemented fixation with a fixed central peg to include divergent locking and compression screws. In addition, the thickness of the convex glenoid was decreased to half the diameter of the sphere so that the joint center of rotation would be placed medially on the glenoid fossa.[16,24-26]

The Grammont reverse shoulder implant medialized the joint center of rotation, thus minimizing the torque on the glenoid bone-implant interface and increasing the moment arm lengths of the abductor muscles. All contemporary reverse shoulder implant designs are derived from the Grammont design. Although lateralizing the center of rotation (relative to the Grammont) has been suggested as a means of reducing the risk of scapular notching, the preferred mitigation strategy (first recommended by Nyffeler et al[27]) is to position the glenoid component along the inferior glenoid rim, with or without an inferior tilt. This positioning has the additional benefit of inferiorly shifting the joint center of rotation, thus elongating the deltoid and improving its resting tone and tension.

The Biomechanics and Kinematics of Reverse Shoulder Arthroplasty

Muscles generate straight-line forces that are converted to torque in proportion to the perpendicular distance between the joint center of rotation and the muscle's line of action.[3,28] This perpendicular distance is called the muscle moment arm; thus, a 50% larger moment arm implies that a 50% lower force is required by a muscle to induce a specific torque or motion. The location of the moment arm relative to the joint center of rotation determines the type of motion the muscle will create. In the shoulder, the motions are abduction-adduction (in the scapular, coronal, and/or transverse planes), internal-external rotation (of the long axis of the humerus), and flexion-extension (in the sagittal plane). Muscles can induce force only in tension, which

can be generated either by contraction (muscle shortening) or stretching beyond resting length (muscle lengthening). Motion thus can result from muscle shortening, muscle lengthening, or no change in muscle length. Motion with no change in muscle length occurs when the line of action coincides with the joint center of rotation.[28] In other words, contraction of a muscle can either cause or stabilize motion, depending on the muscle's line of action relative to the center of rotation. Some muscles can function as an agonist (causing motion), antagonist (stabilizing motion), or both (biphasic functioning as both agonist and antagonist, depending on the specific joint position during a range of motion).[3,28] The greater the muscle's moment arm, the greater the capacity the muscle has to generate the torque required for motion and support external loads. The trade-off for a larger moment arm is that the muscle requires a greater excursion (more muscle shortening is required to generate a given amount of motion). A muscle's moment arm is only one component of its ability to generate torque; the other components include the muscle's physiologic cross-sectional area, architecture, neural activity, and length-tension relationship.[3]

The inversion of the anatomic concavities and the inferior and medial shift of the center of rotation in the contemporary reverse shoulder designs dramatically alter the relationship of each shoulder muscle to its normal physiologic function. Medially shifting the center of rotation both elongates and increases the length of the abduction moment arms of the anterior, middle, and posterior heads of the deltoid, allowing them to contribute more toward abduction.[5,29-32] These larger abductor moment arms enhance the capacity of the deltoid to elevate the arm in the scapular and coronal planes, compensating for the impaired function of the supraspinatus and the superior portions of the subscapularis and infraspinatus rotator cuff muscles, which typically are involved in the pathology. Medially shifting the center of rotation also translates the humerus medially, increasing the laxity of any remaining rotator cuff muscles and leads to impingement of the humerus when the scapular neck is at low elevation (scapular notching).[33,34]

The inferior shifting of the center of rotation with reverse shoulder arthroplasty elongates the deltoid in comparison with a normal shoulder. Elongating the deltoid 10% to 20% improves its resting tone and tension and may increase its strength and improve the overall stability of the joint. With the arm at 0° of abduction, different reverse shoulder implant designs were found to elongate the deltoid between 13% and 17% (compared with the normal shoulder).[5,29] Optimal tension was found to be based on humeral lengthening; arm lengthening of more than 2.5 cm was recommended as the surgical objective because it was associated with greater active elevation.[35,36] In contrast, shortening of the humerus was associated with increased risk of dislocation. However, increased deltoid elongation modi-

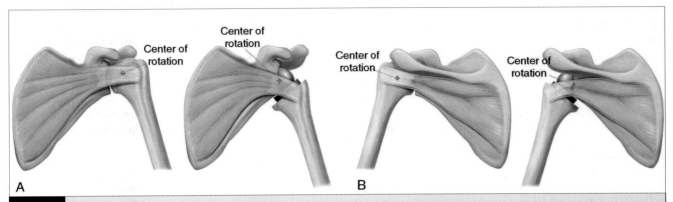

Figure 1 Drawings comparing the positioning of the subscapularis tendon (**A**) and the infraspinatus tendon (**B**) relative to the center of rotation in a normal shoulder *(left)* and a shoulder with a reverse prosthesis *(right)*.

Table 1

Studies on the Joint Center of Rotation in Shoulders With a Reverse Prosthesis

Study (Year)	Reverse Shoulder Prosthesis	Shift in Center of Rotation (Relative to Normal Shoulder)	
		Medial (mm)	**Inferior (mm)**
Boileau et al[26] (2005)	36-mm Grammont (DePuy, Warsaw, IN)	19.0 ± 9.9	Not reported
Henninger et al[37] (2012)	36-mm Grammont (Tornier, Montbonnot, France)	17.3 ± 1.8	9.7 ± 3.5
Saltzman et al[39] (2010)	36-mm Grammont (DePuy)	28.3	11.1
	Reverse (DJO Medical, Austin, TX)	17.2	15.3
Jobin et al[29] (2011)	Grammont (DePuy and Tornier) and Zimmer (Warsaw, IN)	18 ± 7	Not reported
Ackland et al[32] (2010)	Zimmer	20.9 ± 3.9	9.5 ± 4.1
De Wilde et al[5] (2004)	Grammont (DePuy)	28.6	Not reported
	Reverse (DJO Medical)	16.5	Not reported

fies the normal deltoid contour, which decreases its wrapping angle around the greater tuberosity and thus reduces stability. In addition, deltoid elongation creates cosmetic concerns.[5,6,33] Increased humeral lengthening may lead to an acromial stress fracture and brachial plexopathy.[37,38] Restoring the lateral position of the humeral tuberosities is important for tensioning the remaining rotator cuff muscles in a relatively natural physiologic manner to restore rotational strength.[33,34] Although overtensioning these muscles can improve resting tone and tension, it may increase the difficulty of repair after subscapularis tenotomy. Inferiorly shifting the center of rotation also alters the point at which the subscapularis and the infraspinatus muscles convert from adductors at low elevation to abductors at high elevation. In the normal shoulder, the subscapularis and

infraspinatus tendons span the center of rotation. As the center of rotation becomes inferiorly shifted with reverse shoulder arthroplasty, the subscapularis tendon and infraspinatus tendon become positioned below the joint center of rotation; as a result, the muscles act largely as adductors throughout arm elevation (**Figure 1**). In some patients, these muscles may altogether lose their biphasic function, with important implications for both mobility and stability.[30,33]

The parameters of the reverse shoulder design and the positioning of the implant in the scapula and the humerus can affect how the joint center of rotation changes relative to the normal shoulder (**Table 1**). Several studies reported that the Grammont device is associated with an 18-mm medial shift in the joint center of rotation, but other studies reported a 28-mm medial

1: Basic Science

Table 2

Studies Comparing Abductor Moment Arms in Normal Shoulders and Shoulders With a Reverse Prosthesis When the Humerus is Abducted in the Scapular Plane

Study (Year)	Moment Arms	
	Normal Shoulder	Shoulder With a Reverse Prosthesis
Poppen and Walker[50] (1978)	Middle deltoid abductor moment arms increased from 18 to 30 mm between 30° and 150° abduction. Anterior deltoid abductor moment arms increased from 5 to 45 mm between 30° and 150° abduction. Posterior deltoid converted from adductor to abductor at 60° abduction with a maximum abductor moment arm of 20 mm at 150° abduction. Subscapularis converted from adductor to abductor at 90° abduction with a maximum abductor moment arm of 10 mm at 120° abduction.	Not compared or evaluated
Otis et al[28] (1994)	Middle deltoid abductor moment arm was 18 mm at 0° abduction and 30 mm at 60° abduction. Anterior deltoid abductor moment arm was −8 mm at 0° abduction, converted from adductor to abductor at 15° abduction, and was 21 mm at 60° abduction. Posterior deltoid abductor moment arm was −55 mm at 0° abduction and −15 mm at 60° abduction.	Not compared or evaluated
Jobin et al[29] (2012)	Middle deltoid abductor moment arm was 18 mm ± 6 mm at 0° abduction	Middle deltoid abductor moment arm was 36 ± 6 mm at 0° abduction (average, Grammont [DePuy/Tornier] and Zimmer prostheses).
Kontaxis and Johnson[30] (2009)	Middle deltoid abductor moment arm was at its maximum 35 mm at 0° abduction. Anterior deltoid was −30 mm at 0° abduction, converted from adductor to abductor at 40° abduction, and had a maximum abductor moment arm of 40 mm at 150° abduction. Posterior deltoid was −25 mm at 0° abduction, converted from adductor to abductor at 75° abduction, and had a maximum abductor moment arm of 20 mm at 150° abduction. Infraspinatus converted from adductor to abductor at 25° abduction; its moment arm ranged from −3.6 to 17.9 mm between 0° and 150° abduction. Subscapularis converted from adductor to abductor at 25° abduction; its moment arm ranged from −4.0 to 15.7 mm between 0° and 150° abduction.	Middle deltoid abductor moment arm was 40 mm at 0° abduction and 55 mm at 90° abduction (Grammont prosthesis). Anterior deltoid converted from adductor to abductor at 5° abduction and had a maximum abductor moment arm of 40 mm at 150° abduction. Posterior deltoid converted from adductor to abductor at 15° abduction and had a maximum abductor moment arm of 21 mm at 150° abduction. Infraspinatus acted as an adductor throughout range of motion; its moment arm ranged from −16.8 to −1.5 mm between 0° and 150° abduction. Subscapularis converted from adductor to abductor at 120° abduction; its moment arm ranged from −20.2 to 4.5 mm between 0° and 150° abduction.
Terrier et al[31] (2008)	Middle deltoid abductor moment arm was at its maximum 35 mm at 15° abduction.	Middle deltoid abductor moment arm was 38 mm at 15° abduction and reached a maximum 48 mm at 110° abduction. It was 20 mm larger than the normal shoulder at 90° abduction (36-mm Grammont prosthesis).

Table 2

Studies Comparing Abductor Moment Arms in Normal Shoulders and Shoulders With a Reverse Prosthesis When the Humerus Is Abducted in the Scapular Plane (continued)

Study (Year)	Moment Arms	
	Normal Shoulder	**Shoulder With a Reverse Prosthesis**
	Anterior deltoid was 0 mm at 15° abduction and reached a maximum 28 mm at 150° abduction.	Anterior deltoid was 20 mm at 15° abduction and reached a maximum 38 mm at 125° abduction.
	Posterior deltoid was –25 mm at 15° abduction, converted from adductor to abductor at 90° abduction, and had a maximum abductor moment arm of 25 mm at 150° abduction.	Posterior deltoid was –10 mm at 15° abduction, converted from adductor to abductor at 45° abduction, and had a maximum abductor moment arm of 30 mm at 150° abduction.
Ackland et al[32] (2010)	With an anatomic total shoulder arthroplasty, the middle deltoid abductor moment arm was 9 mm at 0° abduction and reached a maximum moment arm of 26 mm between 80° and 100° abduction.	Middle deltoid abductor moment arm was 30 mm at 0° abduction and reached a maximum moment arm of 45 mm at 90° abduction (Zimmer prosthesis).
	Anterior deltoid abductor moment arm was 1 mm at 0° abduction and reached a maximum moment arm of 27 mm at 95° abduction.	Anterior deltoid abductor moment arm was 16 mm at 0° abduction and reached a maximum moment arm of 35 mm at 95° abduction.
	Posterior deltoid abductor moment arm was –18 mm at 0° abduction and reached a maximum moment arm of 2 mm at 120° abduction.	Posterior deltoid abductor moment arm was 0 mm at 0° abduction and reached a maximum moment arm of 12 mm at 120° abduction.

shift.[5,26,29,32,37,39] This apparent discrepancy primarily reflects differences in measurement techniques; studies that found smaller medial shifts in general measured joint center of rotation directly from preoperative and postoperative patient radiographs, and the studies that found larger differences used computer models and simulations. Although measurements acquired directly from patients take into account the natural anatomic variation of the proximal humerus (such as humeral head diameter, neck angle, offset, and thickness), the data may be confounded by the collapsed condition of the humeral head often associated with cuff tear arthropathy and by variations in methods of surgical preparation and implantation (such as differences in humeral neck cuts, stem positioning, and glenoid reaming).[34] In **Table 2**, abductor moment arms for the normal shoulder and the shoulder with a reverse prosthesis are compared when the humerus is abducted in the scapular plane; a positive moment arm value indicates abduction, and a negative moment arm indicates adduction.

The Grammont reverse shoulder implant is effective in restoring active abduction and forward flexion but is less effective in restoring active internal and external rotation in patients with a deficient rotator cuff and a functioning deltoid.[40-42] Lateralizing the joint center of rotation relative to the Grammont design has been proposed as a method for improving active internal and external rotation, strength, and stability.[33] By lateralizing the joint center of rotation, the humerus is lateralized, the remaining rotator cuff muscles are tensioned, and impingement of the humeral component along the inferior scapular neck is minimized. Lateralizing the joint center of rotation also increases the torque on the glenoid bone-implant interface and decreases the lengths of the deltoid abductor moment arms.[5,37] Because the deltoid abductor moment arms are decreased as the center of rotation is lateralized, the deltoid becomes less effective as an abductor, and a greater force is required to elevate the arm in the scapular or coronal planes.[37] These elevated loads and torques can have negative implications for prosthesis fixation, patient rehabilitation, muscle fatigue, and stress fracture. The humerus can be lateralized without lateralizing the joint center of rotation, however. Doing so has the advantage of restoring the anatomic rotator cuff muscle length and tension while maintaining the Grammont abductor moment arm lengths and minimizing the torque on the glenoid-bone interface. The humerus can be lateralized to place the tuberosities in a more anatomic position while minimizing humeral liner impingement along the inferior scapular neck;[43,44] this can be accomplished by decreasing the humeral neck angle from the Grammont humeral neck angle of 155°, proportionally increasing the Grammont glenosphere diameter and thickness, decreasing the humeral liner constraint, and/or increasing the medial offset of the

1: Basic Science

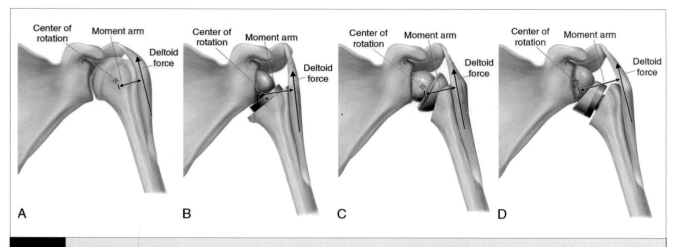

Figure 2	Drawings comparing the center of rotation, deltoid moment arm, direction of deltoid elongation (deltoid force), and humeral position in a normal shoulder (**A**) and in three reverse shoulder prostheses positioned along the inferior glenoid rim at 0° tilt. All drawings show abduction to 15° in the scapular plane. **B,** The 36-mm Grammont (DePuy; medialized center of rotation and medialized humeral component). **C,** The 32-mm Reverse (DJO Medical; lateralized center of rotation and medialized humeral component). **D,** The 38-mm Equinoxe (Exactech, Gainesville, FL; medialized center of rotation and lateralized humeral component).

humeral liner–humeral stem. Increasing the medial offset of the humeral stem in total shoulder arthroplasty was found to increase the middle deltoid moment arm as well as the middle deltoid–wrapping angle about the greater tuberosity and thus to help stabilize the joint by compressing the humeral head into the glenoid fossa.[6] **Figure 2** illustrates the effect of reverse shoulder arthroplasty design on humeral positioning by depicting a normal shoulder relative to three commercially available prostheses.

Although increased stability can be achieved by the compensatory action of muscles with smaller moment arms or by the combined force generated by two opposing muscle lines of action positioned about a joint, each of these methods increases the overall joint reaction force.[45] For these reasons, the repair of the subscapularis–lesser tuberosity in reverse shoulder arthroplasty is controversial. When the subscapularis functions as an adductor, its line of action opposes the deltoid at low- and mid-humeral elevation in the scapular and coronal planes, and this opposing force requires the deltoid to generate a larger force to achieve a given motion.[30,32,46] These opposing forces increase joint stability and perhaps counteract the deltoid's induced torque on the glenoid bone-implant interface. The question of subscapularis–lesser tuberosity repair is even more relevant if the patient has weak external rotators. A study using a shoulder controller found a subscapularis release required less force to be generated by the deltoid and the posterior rotator cuff in abduction.[46] With repair of the subscapularis–lesser tuberosity, the joint reaction force increased 426%, the required deltoid force increased 132% at 15°, and the required posterior rotator cuff force increased 460% at 15°. These increased forces are problematic because in many patients, the posterior rotator cuff is compro-

mised by tearing or fatty infiltration, and it may not be able to support elevated loads. Some recommend repairing the subscapularis–lesser tuberosity if possible because the repair was associated with a lower dislocation rate when the Grammont prosthesis was used.[47] However, this observation may not be applicable to the use of reverse shoulder prosthesis designs that do not translate the humerus medially (increasing the laxity of any remaining rotator cuff muscles).[33,34] Each of these factors should be accounted for when subscapularis–lesser tuberosity repair is being considered with reverse shoulder arthroplasty because repair may not be necessary with all prothesis designs or in all clinical situations.

A loss of external rotation and excessive internal rotation impair the patient's ability to maintain the arm in neutral rotation when the arm is elevated (a positive hornblower sign). The patient is unable to perform numerous activities of daily living, such as drinking, eating, hair washing, and hand shaking.[40-42] The internal rotator muscles predominate in a normally functioning shoulder. There are four internal rotators (subscapularis, teres major, pectoralis major, and latissimus dorsi) and only two external rotators (infraspinatus and teres minor). External rotation deficiency therefore is more debilitating to a patient's activities of daily living than internal rotation deficiency, particularly when the arm is elevated.[40,41] The posterior deltoid alone is insufficient to restore active external rotation, even with a lateralized reverse shoulder design. Therefore, muscle transfers often are recommended in reverse shoulder arthroplasty if the patient has an external rotation deficiency. In general, one or more of the internal rotation muscles, which attach to the anterior side of the humerus, are transferred across the joint center of rotation to the posterior side of the humerus, where their contraction will now cause external rotation. The latissimus dorsi is the muscle most commonly transferred in reverse shoulder arthroplasty; it is detached from the anterior shaft of the humerus and reattached to the greater tuberosity.[48] Another common muscle transfer method is a modification of the L'Episcopo method, in which both the latissimus dorsi and the teres major are transferred to the greater tuberosity. Although muscle transfers have been shown to restore active external rotation, they should not be performed if the teres minor is functional.[40,41] In addition, it should be recognized that such procedures limit active internal rotation and further alter the relationship of each shoulder muscle relative to its normal physiologic function.

Scapular morphology alters kinematics after reverse shoulder arthroplasty. Abnormal glenoid wear patterns and the strategies used to prepare the glenoid and position the prosthesis to minimize the complication of scapular notching (such as a 10° to 15° inferior tilt) can affect the joint center of rotation, muscle moment arms, muscle lengths, and muscle lines of action. As the prosthesis is further medialized and inferiorly tilted, the middle deltoid wrapping around the greater tuberosity is greatly diminished. In addition, severe glenoid wear medializes the joint line and increases the laxity of the muscles in the shoulder girdle. With a sufficient amount of glenoid wear, the humerus can become so medialized that the deltoid generates a distraction force that can result in instability.[49]

Summary

Reverse shoulder arthroplasty is effective for relieving pain and restoring active abduction and forward flexion in patients with a deficient rotator cuff and a functioning deltoid. The inversion of the anatomic concavities restores stability to the unstable shoulder, and the inferior and medial shift in the joint center of rotation (compared with a normal shoulder) lengthens the abductor moment arms and elongates the deltoid to facilitate improvements in function and mobility. Reverse shoulder kinematics can be affected by prosthesis design parameters, prosthesis positioning on the scapula, and abnormal scapular morphology–glenoid wear patterns. Future work should focus on methods that optimize these kinematic parameters, thereby increasing the overall function of the shoulder and facilitating the patient's ability to conduct activities of daily living.

Acknowledgments

The authors express their appreciation to Matt Hamilton, PhD, and Phong Diep for their contributions to the manuscript.

Annotated References

1. Morrey BF: *The Shoulder*, ed 2. Philadelphia, PA, WB Saunders, 1998, pp 233-276.

2. Yu J, McGarry MH, Lee YS, Duong LV, Lee TQ: Biomechanical effects of supraspinatus repair on the glenohumeral joint. *J Shoulder Elbow Surg* 2005;14(1, suppl S):65S-71S.

3. Kuechle DK, Newman SR, Itoi E, Morrey BF, An KN: Shoulder muscle moment arms during horizontal flexion and elevation. *J Shoulder Elbow Surg* 1997;6(5): 429-439.

4. Lee SB, An KN: Dynamic glenohumeral stability provided by three heads of the deltoid muscle. *Clin Orthop Relat Res* 2002;400:40-47.

5. De Wilde LF, Audenaert EA, Berghs BM: Shoulder prostheses treating cuff tear arthropathy: A comparative biomechanical study. *J Orthop Res* 2004;22(6): 1222-1230.

6. Lemieux PO, Hagemeister N, Tétreault P, Nuño N: Influence of the medial offset of the proximal humerus on the glenohumeral destabilising forces during arm elevation: A numerical sensitivity study. *Comput Methods Biomech Biomed Engin* 2013;16(1):103-111.

   A computer model study assessed the influence of humeral head medial offset on joint stability. Varying the medial offset influenced the destabilizing action of the middle deltoid, where a larger medial offset increased the middle deltoid wrapping around the tuberosity.

7. Lippitt SB, Vanderhooft JE, Harris SL, Sidles JA, Harryman DT II, Matsen FA III: Glenohumeral stability from concavity-compression: A quantitative analysis. *J Shoulder Elbow Surg* 1993;2(1):27-35.

8. Sharkey NA, Marder RA: The rotator cuff opposes superior translation of the humeral head. *Am J Sports Med* 1995;23(3):270-275.

9. Parsons IM, Apreleva M, Fu FH, Woo SL: The effect of rotator cuff tears on reaction forces at the glenohumeral joint. *J Orthop Res* 2002;20(3):439-446.

10. Mura N, O'Driscoll SW, Zobitz ME, et al: The effect of infraspinatus disruption on glenohumeral torque and superior migration of the humeral head: A biomechanical study. *J Shoulder Elbow Surg* 2003;12(2): 179-184.

11. Burkhart SS, Nottage WM, Ogilvie-Harris DJ, Kohn HS, Pachelli A: Partial repair of irreparable rotator cuff tears. *Arthroscopy* 1994;10(4):363-370.

12. Halder AM, Zhao KD, O'Driscoll SW, Morrey BF, An KN: Dynamic contributions to superior shoulder stability. *J Orthop Res* 2001;19(2):206-212.

13. Labriola JE, Lee TQ, Debski RE, McMahon PJ: Stability and instability of the glenohumeral joint: The role of shoulder muscles. *J Shoulder Elbow Surg* 2005; 14(1, suppl S):32S-38S.

14. Neer CS II, Craig EV, Fukuda H: Cuff-tear arthropathy. *J Bone Joint Surg Am* 1983;65(9):1232-1244.

15. Visotsky JL, Basamania C, Seebauer L, Rockwood CA, Jensen KL: Cuff tear arthropathy: Pathogenesis, classification, and algorithm for treatment. *J Bone Joint Surg Am* 2004;86-A(2, suppl 2):35-40.

16. Flatow EL, Harrison AK: A history of reverse total shoulder arthroplasty. *Clin Orthop Relat Res* 2011; 469(9):2432-2439.

    A literature review described the evolution of reverse shoulder prosthesis design, focusing on the challenges of historical designs and describing the influence of the Grammont prosthesis on current designs.

17. Fenlin JM Jr: Semi-constrained prosthesis for the rotator cuff deficient patient. *Orthop Trans* 1985;9:55.

18. Redfern TR, Wallace WA: *Joint Replacement in the Shoulder and Elbow.* Oxford, United Kingdom, Butterworth and Heinemann, 1998, pp 6-16.

19. Reeves B, Jobbins B, Dowson D, Wright V: A total shoulder endoprosthesis. *Eng Med* 1974;1:64-67.

20. Bayley I, Kessel L: *The Kessel Total Shoulder Replacement: Shoulder Surgery.* New York, NY, Springer Verlag, 1982.

21. Broström LA, Wallensten R, Olsson E, Anderson D: The Kessel prosthesis in total shoulder arthroplasty: A five-year experience. *Clin Orthop Relat Res* 1992;277: 155-160.

22. Wretenberg PF, Wallensten R: The Kessel total shoulder arthroplasty: A 13- to 16-year retrospective followup. *Clin Orthop Relat Res* 1999;365:100-103.

23. Neer CS II: *Shoulder Reconstruction.* Philadelphia, PA, WB Saunders, 1990.

24. Grammont P, Trouillod P, Laffay JP, Deries X: Etude et Realisation D'une Novelle Prosthese D'Paule. *Rhumatologie* 1987;39:17-22.

25. Grammont PM, Baulot E: Delta shoulder prosthesis for rotator cuff rupture. *Orthopedics* 1993;16(1): 65-68.

26. Boileau P, Watkinson DJ, Hatzidakis AM, Balg F: Grammont reverse prosthesis: Design, rationale, and biomechanics. *J Shoulder Elbow Surg* 2005;14(1, suppl S):147S-161S.

27. Nyffeler RW, Werner CM, Gerber C: Biomechanical relevance of glenoid component positioning in the reverse Delta III total shoulder prosthesis. *J Shoulder Elbow Surg* 2005;14(5):524-528.

28. Otis JC, Jiang CC, Wickiewicz TL, Peterson MG, Warren RF, Santner TJ: Changes in the moment arms of the rotator cuff and deltoid muscles with abduction and rotation. *J Bone Joint Surg Am* 1994;76(5): 667-676.

29. Jobin CM, Brown GD, Bahu MJ, et al: Reverse total shoulder arthroplasty for cuff tear arthropathy: The clinical effect of deltoid lengthening and center of rotation medialization. *J Shoulder Elbow Surg* 2012; 21(10):1269-1277.

    Forty-nine consecutive patients who underwent reverse shoulder arthroplasty for cuff tear arthropathy were prospectively studied to correlate functional outcomes with deltoid lengthening and center of rotation medialization. Deltoid lengthening was found to be correlated with active forward elevation.

30. Kontaxis A, Johnson GR: The biomechanics of reverse anatomy shoulder replacement—a modelling study. *Clin Biomech (Bristol, Avon)* 2009;24(3):254-260.

    A computer modeling study quantified deltoid abductor moment arm and muscle forces associated with a normal shoulder and a Delta reverse shoulder prosthesis. Impingement and scapular notching were simulated under various conditions.

31. Terrier A, Reist A, Merlini F, Farron A: Simulated joint and muscle forces in reversed and anatomic shoulder prostheses. *J Bone Joint Surg Br* 2008;90(6): 751-756.

    A computer modeling study quantified deltoid abductor moment arms and forces in the reverse shoulder prosthesis compared with an anatomic prosthesis. The reverse prosthesis was evaluated under two conditions: with only a deficient supraspinatus and with no rotator cuff.

32. Ackland DC, Roshan-Zamir S, Richardson M, Pandy MG: Moment arms of the shoulder musculature after reverse total shoulder arthroplasty. *J Bone Joint Surg Am* 2010;92(5):1221-1230.

    Cadaver shoulders were used to measure muscle moment arms with anatomic and reverse shoulder arthroplasty. Increases in the length of the moment arms were observed for the major abductors, flexors, adductors, and extensors with reverse shoulder arthroplasty.

33. Frankle M, Siegal S, Pupello D, Saleem A, Mighell M, Vasey M: The Reverse Shoulder Prosthesis for glenohumeral arthritis associated with severe rotator cuff deficiency: A minimum two-year follow-up study of sixty patients. *J Bone Joint Surg Am* 2005;87(8):1697-1705.

34. Herrmann S, König C, Heller M, Perka C, Greiner S: Reverse shoulder arthroplasty leads to significant biomechanical changes in the remaining rotator cuff. *J Orthop Surg Res* 2011;6:42.

1: Basic Science

Subscapularis and teres minor rotation moment arms and muscle lengths were calculated from CT reconstructions of seven cadavers with reverse shoulder arthroplasty. The rotation moment arms and muscle lengths were decreased compared with those of the anatomic shoulder.

35. Lädermann A, Walch G, Lubbeke A, et al: Influence of arm lengthening in reverse shoulder arthroplasty. *J Shoulder Elbow Surg* 2012;21(3):336-341.

    Radiographic measurements of humeral lengthening were made from 183 reverse shoulder arthroplasties. At a minimum 1-year follow-up, lengthening of the humerus was evaluated relative to the contralateral side. Shortening of the arm reduced active anterior elevation.

36. Lädermann A, Williams MD, Melis B, Hoffmeyer P, Walch G: Objective evaluation of lengthening in reverse shoulder arthroplasty. *J Shoulder Elbow Surg* 2009;18(4):588-595.

    A technique was proposed to preoperatively plan adequate deltoid tensioning using radiographic measurements from the contralateral arm.

37. Henninger HB, Barg A, Anderson AE, Bachus KN, Burks RT, Tashjian RZ: Effect of lateral offset center of rotation in reverse total shoulder arthroplasty: A biomechanical study. *J Shoulder Elbow Surg* 2012; 21(9):1128-1135.

    A shoulder controller was used to evaluate cadaver shoulders before and after reverse shoulder arthroplasty, with spacers added to laterally shift the center of rotation. Center of rotation lateralization had no influence on adduction or external rotation but increased abduction and dislocation forces because of smaller moment arms.

38. Gallo RA, Gamradt SC, Mattern CJ, et al: Instability after reverse total shoulder replacement. *J Shoulder Elbow Surg* 2011;20(4):584-590.

    After 57 reverse shoulder arthroplasties, instability occurred in 9 shoulders within the first 6 months. All 9 patients had a compromised subscapularis tendon, and 5 had a questionable glenosphere position.

39. Saltzman MD, Mercer DM, Warme WJ, Bertelsen AL, Matsen FA III: A method for documenting the change in center of rotation with reverse total shoulder arthroplasty and its application to a consecutive series of 68 shoulders having reconstruction with one of two different reverse prostheses. *J Shoulder Elbow Surg* 2010;19(7):1028-1033.

    The change in center of rotation on preoperative and postoperative radiographs is quantified using two different reverse shoulder implants. The position of the center of rotation was found to be significantly different after surgery and between the two implant designs.

40. Boileau P, Chuinard C, Roussanne Y, Bicknell RT, Rochet N, Trojani C: Reverse shoulder arthroplasty combined with a modified latissimus dorsi and teres major tendon transfer for shoulder pseudoparalysis associated with dropping arm. *Clin Orthop Relat Res* 2008;466(3):584-593.

    A prospective study of 11 patients with a combined loss of active elevation and external rotation found that reverse shoulder arthroplasty and latissimus dorsi and teres major transfer restored both active elevation and external rotation.

41. Boileau P, Rumian AP, Zumstein MA: Reversed shoulder arthroplasty with modified L'Episcopo for combined loss of active elevation and external rotation. *J Shoulder Elbow Surg* 2010;19(2, suppl):20-30.

    A study of 17 patients with a combined loss of active elevation and external rotation found that reverse shoulder arthroplasty and latissimus dorsi and teres major transfer restored both active elevation and external rotation.

42. Favre P, Loeb MD, Helmy N, Gerber C: Latissimus dorsi transfer to restore external rotation with reverse shoulder arthroplasty: A biomechanical study. *J Shoulder Elbow Surg* 2008;17(4):650-658.

    A biomechanical analysis quantified external rotation moment arms after latissimus dorsi transfer and reverse shoulder arthroplasty using two different humeral cup designs.

43. Roche C, Flurin PH, Wright T, Zuckerman J: An evaluation of the relationship between prosthetic design parameters and clinical failure modes. *Proceedings of the 19th Annual Symposium.* Auburn, CA, International Society for Technology in Arthroplasty, 2006, p. 288. http://www.instaonline.org. Accessed July 19, 2012.

44. Roche C, Flurin PH, Wright T, Crosby LA, Mauldin M, Zuckerman JD: An evaluation of the relationships between reverse shoulder design parameters and range of motion, impingement, and stability. *J Shoulder Elbow Surg* 2009;18(5):734-741.

    A computer modeling study modified the Grammont reverse shoulder prosthesis and made recommendations to minimize impingement and improve stability. Subtle changes in design parameters were found to minimize impingement and offer potential for dramatic functional improvements in range of motion and jump distance.

45. Bergmann G, Graichen F, Bender A, Kääb M, Rohlmann A, Westerhoff P: In vivo glenohumeral contact forces—measurements in the first patient 7 months postoperatively. *J Biomech* 2007;40(10):2139-2149.

    Glenohumeral forces and moments were presented at 7-month follow-up of a patient who received an instrumented shoulder implant with telemetric data transmission. The maximum reported force was 150% of body weight.

46. Onstot BR, Suslak AG, Colley R, Jacofsky MC, Otis JC, Hansen ML: Consequences of concomitant subscapularis repair with reverse total shoulder arthroplasty. *Transactions of the 58th Annual Meeting.* Rosemont, IL, Orthopaedic Research Society, 2012, paper 297.

1: Basic Science

A shoulder controller study evaluated the impact of subscapularis repair on reverse shoulder biomechanics in a cadaver scapula. Repair of the subscapularis increased the deltoid force, the joint reaction force, and the posterior rotator cuff force compared with an unrepaired cadaver specimen.

47. Edwards TB, Williams MD, Labriola JE, Elkousy HA, Gartsman GM, O'Connor DP: Subscapularis insufficiency and the risk of shoulder dislocation after reverse shoulder arthroplasty. *J Shoulder Elbow Surg* 2009; 18(6):892-896.

A prospective study of Grammont reverse shoulder arthroplasty in 138 patients found that the subscapularis was reparable in 62 patients and irreparable in 76 patients. All 7 dislocations occurred in patients whose subscapularis was irreparable. Repair of the subscapularis is recommended whenever possible.

48. Gerber C, Maquieira G, Espinosa N: Latissimus dorsi transfer for the treatment of irreparable rotator cuff tears. *J Bone Joint Surg Am* 2006;88(1):113-120.

49. Norris TR, Kelly JD: Management of glenoid bone defects in revision shoulder arthroplasty: A new application of the reverse total shoulder prosthesis. *Tech Shoulder Elbow Surg* 2007;8(1):37-46.

A one-stage method is presented for treating patients with severe glenoid wear who are in need of reverse shoulder arthroplasty. Clinical challenges and surgical technique are discussed.

50. Poppen NK, Walker PS: Forces at the glenohumeral joint in abduction. *Clin Orthop Relat Res* 1978;135: 165-170.

Chapter 5

Biomechanics of Elbow Arthroplasty

James A. Johnson, PhD   Graham J.W. King, MD, MSc, FRCSC

Introduction

It is well established that the elbow may be subjected to forces that exceed body weight. Research on the biomechanics of elbow arthroplasty during the past several decades has focused on load transfer and stress analysis of the implant-bone construct. Significant attention has been directed toward the kinematics and stability of the implant-reconstructed ulnohumeral and radiocapitellar joints. Recent research advances have led to an improved understanding of the biomechanics of radial head arthroplasty, particularly with respect to head shape and placement, implant design, and stem fixation. Implant alignment has been found to be important for load transfer, particularly on the ulnohumeral side, and novel computer-assisted techniques have been developed to optimize surgical placement. There has been recent interest in hemiarthroplasty systems for the capitellum and coronoid.

Radial Head Replacement

From a biomechanical perspective, the two principal features of radial head implants are the articulating region that replaces the radial head and the stem that is inserted into the canal of the radial neck to achieve fixation to host bone.

Kinematics and Stability

It is becoming increasingly clear that the design of the radial head implant has important implications for sta-

Dr. King or an immediate family member serves as a board member, owner, officer, or committee member of the American Shoulder and Elbow Surgeons; has received royalties from Wright Medical Technology, Tornier, and Tenet Medical; is a member of a speakers' bureau or has made paid presentations on behalf of Wright Medical Technology; and serves as a paid consultant to or is an employee of Wright Medical Technology. Neither Dr. Johnson nor any immediate family member has received anything of value from or has stock or stock options held in a commercial company or institution related directly or indirectly to the subject of this chapter.

bility. Significant effort has been directed toward determining the biomechanical characteristics of bipolar radial head implants compared with monopolar systems. When a benchtop cadaver-based model was used to compare radiocapitellar joint stability in bipolar and monopolar radial head prostheses, the monopolar prosthesis conferred stability against subluxation similar to that of the native elbow, but the bipolar device facilitated subluxation and thereby probably compromised concavity compression.[1] In an unstable elbow model, a somewhat similar experimental model tested the resistance to posterior translation of the native articulation as well as radial head implant shapes and designs including monopolar and bipolar devices.[2] Although the ability of the bipolar radial head implant to tilt was believed to be advantageous for tracking and joint contact, the researchers found that the tilting action of the head decreased the force needed for subluxation, and therefore the bipolar had lower stability than the monopolar implant or native elbow. Interestingly, a radial head implant with an anatomic shape had similar stability to that of a native radial head and was more stable than a circular head, with a more shallow concavity of the articular surface possibly explaining this observation. An experimental study found that bipolar devices were quite adaptable for ensuring that articular contact was not affected by joint position but that there was a tendency toward abnormal positioning of the implant.[3] In another in vitro study, bipolar implants offered advantages with respect to self-alignment, which did not occur with a rigidly fixed monoblock implant.[4] This consideration may be particularly important if implant alignment is not properly achieved at surgery, as is not uncommon.

Researchers also have focused on the geometric characteristics of the radial head dish. In a study of the influence of the depth and radius of curvature of the articular dish of a monopolar design on stability, the stability of a deeper dished anatomic implant was found to match that of the native head, but the stability of a shallow-dished circular implant with a larger radius of curvature did not[5] (**Figure 1**). Work is likely to continue on developing new and innovative shapes and designs of radial head articular surfaces in an effort to optimize load transfer and reduce capitellar cartilage wear.

Soft tissues provide an important constraint to both the intact and implant-reconstructed elbow. Much of the stability of the radiocapitellar joint arises from the concavity compression of the dish of the implant, with additional stability provided from the collateral ligaments, annular ligament, and capsule. A benchtop model was used to determine the effect of soft tissues in resisting posterior translation under loading.[6] Soft-tissue restraint was found to be most important with the use of a bipolar implant. The soft tissues had a less important role for the native or monopolar radial head, whose stability is chiefly provided by the concavity compression of the radial dish with the capitellum.

The kinematics and stability of the elbow improve after metallic radial head arthroplasty but do not return to normal, probably because an exact restoration of both articular congruity and axial height is difficult to achieve with conventional surgical techniques.[7] Joint laxity clearly will increase if the implant height is less than that of the native structure. Conversely, when the implant height is greater than that of the native structure, some overstuffing of the joint will occur, reducing laxity and probably causing a detrimental increase in joint contact stress and capitellar wear as well as alterations in the congruity of the ulnohumeral articulation. The difficulty in diagnosing overlengthening of a radial head implant was recently reported.[8] A cadaver model with muscle loading and plain radiographs was used to evaluate ulnohumeral joint congruity for overlengthening of the radial head implant in increments of 2 mm. Incongruity was radiographically apparent only after overlengthening of at least 6 mm (**Figure 2**). Changes in articular contact stress and tracking probably result in much smaller changes in articular height, but these have not yet been established. Research is needed to determine the optimal design and placement of a radial head implant to restore lateral column height and ensure optimal load transfer between the ulnohumeral and radiocapitellar articulations.

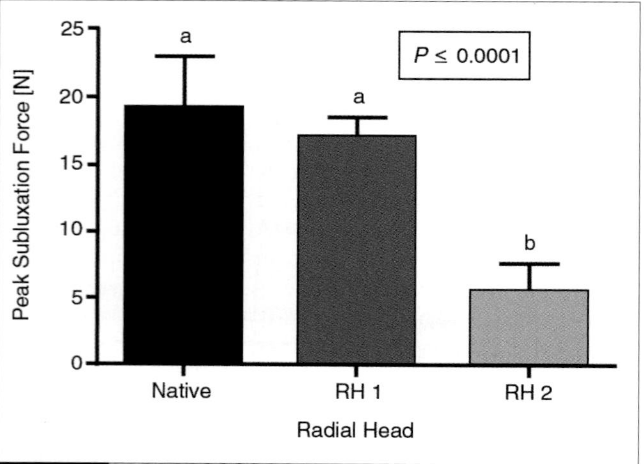

Figure 1 Graph comparing mean peak subluxation forces in the native radial head and two radial head prostheses (RH 1 = anatomic radial head, RH 2 = circular radial head). (Adapted with permission from Chanlalit C, Shukla DR, Fitzsimmons JS, An KN, O'Driscoll SW: Influence of prosthetic design on radiocapitellar concavity-compression stability. *J Shoulder Elbow Surg* 2011;20:885-890.)

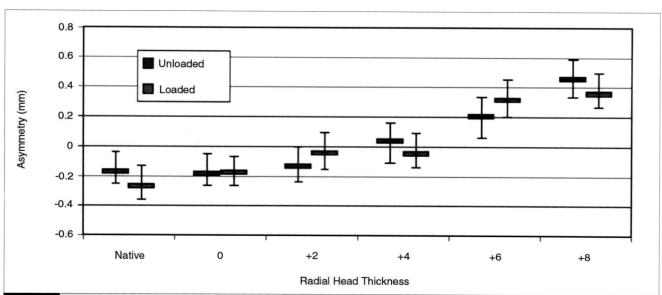

Figure 2 Graph showing the increased asymmetry of the medial ulnohumeral joint with progressive increases (overlengthening) in the thickness of the radial head implant. 0 = an implant of the correct size. (Adapted with permission from Frank SG, Grewal R, Johnson J, Faber KJ, King GJ, Athwal GS: Determination of correct implant size in radial head arthroplasty to avoid overlengthening. *J Bone Joint Surg Am* 2009;91[7]:1738-1746.)

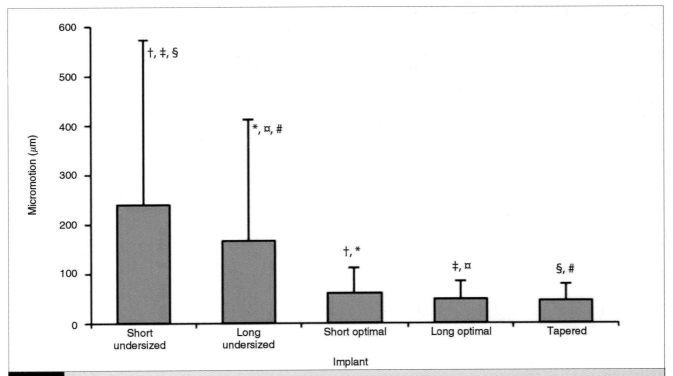

Figure 3 Graph showing implant motion for each of the five tested implants (pooled data). Motion significantly increased with the use of an undersized implant ($P < 0.02$). There were no significant differences between the short and long undersized implants or among the short optimal, long optimal, and tapered implants. Matching symbols imply significant difference. (Adapted with permission from Ferreira LM, Stacpoole RA, Johnson JA, King GJ: Cementless fixation of radial head implants is affected by implant stem geometry: An in vitro study. *Clin Biomech [Bristol, Avon]* 2010;25[5]:422-426.)

Fixation

The optimal technique for fixing the stem of a radial head implant remains unknown. Stem fixation techniques are highly dependent on the morphology of the head. It is well established that the native radial head is somewhat elliptical and eccentric to the shaft of the neck. Thus, uncemented fixation can be used for an axisymmetric implant to permit toggling of the stem in the canal, or a bipolar implant can be used to ensure congruent tracking of the radial dish with the native capitellum. One commercially available implant design attempts to replicate the asymmetric shape of the proximal radius. Rigid stem fixation is a prerequisite for this design concept, however, to ensure correct implant orientation and avoid maltracking on the capitellum. Rigid fixation can be achieved by cementation of the stem or porous surfaces with osseointegration.

Successful ingrowth or ongrowth of an uncemented stem requires minimal interface micromotion after implantation. Little is known about this mode of fixation for radial head implants, although it is generally accepted that oversizing of the stem relative to the canal may be advantageous to achieve a solid press fit. There is a risk of fracture, however, as in intramedullary stem insertion of an uncemented device into the femur or humerus. The risk is exacerbated by the tapered shape of

the stem and/or the host canal. A cadaver study of the effect of stem size on initial stability focused on oversizing and bone fracture caused by hoop stresses.[9] The researchers concluded that small fractures from hoop stresses in the cortical shell did not result in excessive micromotion and loss of stability and may be clinically acceptable. Another study found that the initial stability of a radial head stem with a partially grit-blasted surface was comparable to that of a fully grit-blasted device.[10] This finding suggests that the partially grit-blasted device may be preferable because of its advantages related to stem removal and stress shielding. A cadaver model was used to investigate the effect of stem size, length, and shape (straight or tapered) on the stability of radial head implants when subjected to an eccentric axial load.[11] Complete canal filling was found to be the most important parameter affecting initial stability; stem length and shape did not have a significant effect (**Figure 3**). A benchtop model also was used to determine the micromotion of press-fit radial head implant stems, with a focus on rasp size and insertion force.[12] These experiments found that micromotion was minimized by enlarging the canal and using a larger diameter stem. Micromotion was lower with larger insertion forces and may be a useful intraoperative metric for judging stem fixation. Collectively, these studies suggest that initial fixation of an uncemented press-fit

1: Basic Science

radial head implant is best achieved by choosing a stem size that optimizes canal filling, particularly with respect to stem diameter. Clinical studies are needed to determine the longer-term effect of stem size on implant fixation and performance.

Total Elbow Arthroplasty

The most common causes of failure of total elbow arthroplasty are implant loosening and material wear. Almost all elbow implants are fixed with acrylic bone cement between the implant and the surrounding cortical bone. Loss of fixation at the implant-cement and cement-bone interfaces can be caused by altered motion patterns and loading across the joint. The characteristics of the articulation and alignment are the two most significant factors affecting the load and stresses borne by the implant-cement-bone composite structures of the humerus and ulna.

The Ulnohumeral Articulation

A linked total elbow implant often is called a semiconstrained or sloppy hinge joint because it permits small secondary motions, such as varus-valgus or internal-external rotation of the ulna, as well as the primary flexion-extension motion. The amount of secondary motion permitted is considered a design feature, and most linked total elbow implants incorporate some varus-valgus and rotational laxity. Overconstraint of the linkage mechanism results in the transfer of greater loads through the bone-implant interface, which can lead to mechanical loosening. Underconstraint leads to elbow instability.

In a linked total elbow implant, the constraint between the ulnar and humeral components provides increased stability and prevents dislocation, but it probably is an important source of increased stress at the implant-cement interface. There is a theoretic advantage to using an unlinked device designed to decrease loading and wear on the implant, but instability has occurred in some patients because of difficulty in achieving secure ligament fixation or use of antirheumatic medications that retard healing.

One recent experimental study with a companion finite element study examined the bone stresses of the unlinked iBP prosthesis (Biomet, Warsaw, IN).[13] Strain gauges on synthetic humeri and ulnae were used, and measurements were taken before and after replacement. Bone strains adjacent to the implant tip were found to be greatly increased in the humerus and ulna. Decreased epiphyseal cancellous bone strain was measured in the humerus and ulna and compared with intact bones. It was concluded that the unlinked elbow prosthesis may carry a risk of bone fatigue failure, particularly in the ulna. Moreover, stress shielding in the epiphyseal regions may promote bone resorption. This behavior may be similar to that of linked prostheses. Modifications in stem shape, length, and materials

should be considered to reduce the extent of stress shielding and improve load transfer to bone.

Implant Alignment

If alignment of the humeral and ulnar components is not ideal, the additional constraint imposed by the linkage may increase wear and stresses at the implant-cement interface, possibly leading to component loosening and mechanical failure. The primary cause of changes in kinematics and load transfer is improper joint positioning and alignment. With respect to the ulnohumeral articulation, failure to align the mechanical axis of the component to the anatomic flexion-extension axis changes the normal motion characteristics of the joint. These abnormal motion pathways alter ligament and capsule tension as well as muscle moment arms and lines of action. Changes in joint kinematics result in altered forces in the implant and subsequent abnormal forces in the implant-bone structure. Most recent biomechanical studies in total elbow arthroplasty have focused on the alignment of the ulnohumeral articulation, with a focus on reestablishing the flexion-extension axis.

The positioning of the humeral stem is based on the alignment of the articulation hinge with the elbow's flexion-extension axis. It is well established that this alignment can be achieved by using the shape of the capitellum and the trochlea to determine the center of each, which defines the anatomic axis. However, it is difficult to determine the flexion-extension axis intraoperatively. The estimation of the orientation of the axis in a series of distal humeri by three subspecialty-trained orthopaedic surgeons led to alignment errors as large as 10° in either direction[14] (Figure 4). Hence, better surgical cutting guides should be developed to improve the alignment of the components or navigation systems used in elbow arthroplasty systems. A later study investigated methods for achieving optimal alignment of the ulnar component.[15] Increased knowledge of the position and orientation of the center of the radial head was found to improve accuracy not only in matching the center and orientation of the central prominence of the greater sigmoid notch of the ulna (the guiding ridge) with the corresponding axis of the ulnar component articulation, but also in predicting the kinematics-derived flexion-extension axis. This finding suggests that the surgeon (or the computerized guidance system) should take the position and orientation of the radial head into account, if possible, when orienting the ulnar component during elbow arthroplasty. Ulnar cutting guides also should exploit the characteristics of the radial head to improve the accuracy of ulnar component positioning.

The effect of humeral implant malalignment on loading was recently investigated in an in vitro biomechanical study.[16] The load on an optimally positioned implant was shown to be significantly lower than on an anterior-positioned or malrotated implant (Figure 5). These increased loads, and in particular varus-valgus

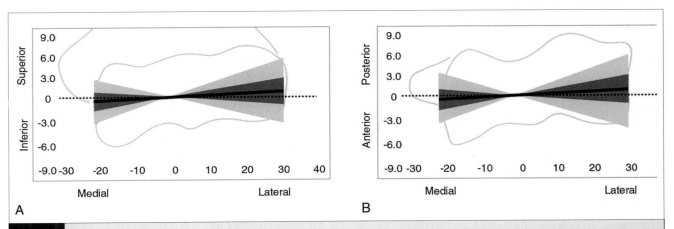

Figure 4 Graph showing varus-valgus and internal rotation–external rotation error in flexion-extension axis determination. The varus-valgus (frontal plane) view **(A)** and the internal rotation–external rotation (coronal plane) view **(B)** were generated from unit-vector analysis for all specimens. Dashed line = horizontal axis (0°), solid line = the mean angle (1.5° valgus and 1.6° external rotation), dark gray area = the area within 1 SD of the mean line (4.5° valgus to 1.5° varus, 4.9° external rotation to 1.7° internal rotation), light gray area = remaining values (9.6° valgus to 6.3° varus, 10.2° external rotation to 8.3° internal rotation). Proximal, anterior, and medial were considered positive directions. (Adapted with permission from Brownhill JR, Furukawa K, Faber KJ, Johnson JA, King GJ: Surgeon accuracy in the selection of the flexion-extension axis of the elbow: An in vitro study. *J Shoulder Elbow Surg* 2006;15[4]:451-456.)

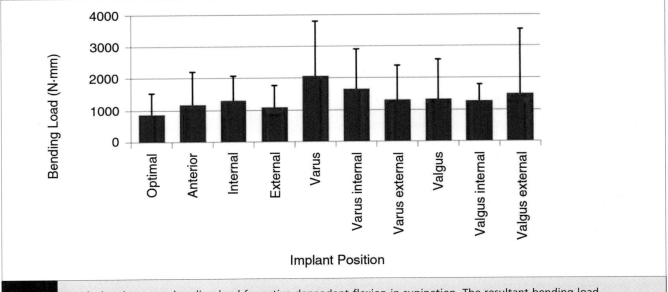

Figure 5 Graph showing mean bending load for active-dependent flexion in supination. The resultant bending load (mean + SD) of the entire flexion range is shown for each of 10 tested implant positions. (Adapted with permission from Brownhill JR, Pollock JW, Ferreira LM, Johnson JA, King GJ: The effect of implant malalignment on joint loading in total elbow arthroplasty: An in vitro study. *J Shoulder Elbow Surg* 2012;21[8]:1032-1038.)

bending and internal-external torsion, are likely to result in increased wear on the polyethylene linkage mechanism, thereby increasing the likelihood of loosening.

Reestablishing the native position of the articulation with the implant appears to be important for minimizing loading and damage, but it may be difficult to achieve with current implant systems because of stem abutment within the medullary canal. Recent studies examined the morphology of the bone and the relationships between joint position and intramedullary canal offset. A CT study examined the relationship of the medullary canal axis and the flexion-extension axis in 40 distal humeri.[17] The anterior offset and cubital angle between the two axes also were quantified. The anterior offset of the flexion-extension axis from canal axis was found to be proportional to the canal length. No relationship was established among the width of the ar-

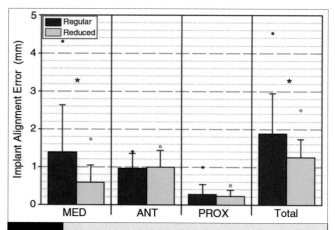

Figure 6 Graph showing implant alignment error in translation (mean + 1 SD). For each error, the three directional components (medial-lateral [MED], anterior-posterior [ANT], and proximal-distal [PROX]) and the total error are provided. Circle = the maximum error for each translational component of error (in mm). * = significance (P < 0.05). (Adapted with permission from McDonald CP, Peters TM, Johnson JA, King GJ: Stem abutment affects alignment of the humeral component in computer-assisted elbow arthroplasty. *J Shoulder Elbow Surg* 2011;20[6]:891-898.)

ticular surface, cubital angle, and anterior-posterior and canal curvature. The researchers suggested that the use of modular humeral implants that allow for the variability in the natural anterior bow and articular offset of the distal humerus may improve the restoration of the flexion-extension axis. A more recent study by the same researchers used CT of 31 proximal ulnae to determine the shape of the medullary canal relative to the articular surface.[18] Posterior and lateral offsets were found to increase distally from the articulation center. The average valgus angulation was 8° (± 4°) in men and 7.2° (± 3.1°) in women. The researchers concluded that ulnar implants with longer stems may need to be modular to accommodate the variable offsets of the canal to the articular axes.

In recent years there has been substantial progress in exploring image- and computer-assisted procedures for total elbow arthroplasty. This logical approach has the potential to greatly diminish the number of implant placement errors based on visual landmark identification. Success in hip and knee arthroplasties has prompted exploration of similar techniques for the upper limb. An initial study investigated the possibility of using a surface-based registration technique.[19] With the use of a handheld laser scanner and conventional paired-point registration of the distal articular surfaces of cadaver specimens, registration error ranged between 1 and 2 mm. Implementation of surface-based registration should produce a more accurate determination of the target axes than the surgeon's visual estimation. The effect of distal humeral landmark selection

and bone loss on the accuracy of image-guided registration was investigated using cadaver specimens.[20] The study found that, even in the setting of substantial bone loss, only the limited remaining anatomic landmarks were needed to register surfaces accurately to a preoperative CT scan; the errors were approximately 1 mm in translation and 0.5° in rotation. Good alignment of a CT scan with intraoperative surface digitizations can be achieved using only the relatively small portion of the periarticular region of distal humerus that is available during surgery. The use of appropriate tracking technology and imaging can allow accurate implant alignment, based on imaging of the uncompromised contralateral elbow. In a subsequent study, the researchers verified that the variations in anatomy of the distal humerus from side to side were on the order of 0.5 mm and 1.0°, and therefore were within an acceptable range for image- and computer-assisted implant reconstruction from the contralateral side.[21] The accuracy of a computer-assisted implant alignment technique for the humeral stem recently was evaluated in cadaver specimens.[22] With an implant with a reduced stem (to minimize medullary canal impingement), the alignment error was 1.3 mm (± 0.5 mm) in translation and 1.2° (± 0.4°) in rotation. However, when a full, regular stem was used, the errors were 1.9 mm (± 1.1 mm) in translation and 3.6° (± 2.1°) in rotation (**Figure 6**). It was concluded that a humeral component with a fixed valgus angulation is difficult to position to accurately restore the alignment of the flexion-extension axis; the use of implant systems offering more variability in valgus angulations may be warranted.

Although significant knowledge has recently been gained on in vitro implant alignment at the ulnohumeral articulation, further work is needed to translate these findings into improved prosthesis positioning in patients.

Other Implant Systems

Recently, interest has emerged in the development of implants for capitellar deficiency resulting from arthritis, fracture, or osteochondritis dissecans. In a CT-based morphologic investigation of 50 cadaver specimens, the capitellar surface was quantified in both the sagittal and transverse planes.[23] The sagittal and transverse radii of curvatures were 11.6 mm (± 1.4 mm) and 14 mm (± 3 mm; range, 9.6 to 20.9 mm), respectively. These findings indicate that the capitellum is not spherical. Substantial variability was found in the various morphologic measurements; this finding suggests that replication with an off-the-shelf implant may not be optimal. A significant concern with any hemiarthroplasty is the change in contact mechanics with the native cartilaginous surface. This concept was investigated in a comparison of the joint contact area of spherical and elliptical metal capitellar implants to the native radial head in cadaver specimens.[24] The joints

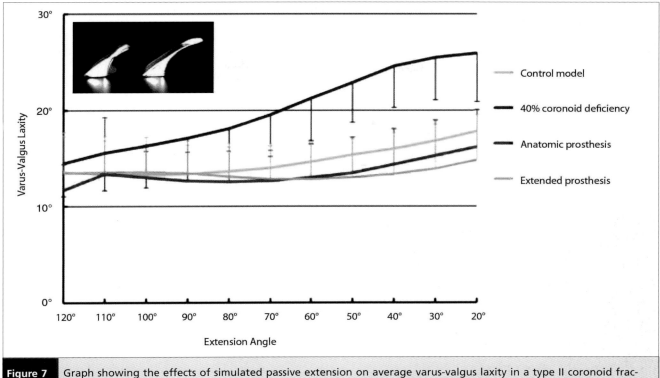

| **Figure 7** | Graph showing the effects of simulated passive extension on average varus-valgus laxity in a type II coronoid fracture with the forearm in supination, after repair of collateral ligaments and prosthetic replacement. A 40% coronoid deficiency increases elbow laxity relative to the native coronoid. Prosthetic replacement with an anatomic or extended-length implant creates elbow stability similar to that of the native coronoid. Error bars indicate the SD. Inset: Lateral-view photograph of an anatomic prosthesis *(left)* and an extended-length prosthesis *(right)*. (Adapted with permission from Alolabi B, Gray A, Ferreira LM, Johnson JA, Athwal GS, King GJ: Reconstruction of the coronoid using an extended prosthesis: An in vitro biomechanical study. *J Shoulder Elbow Surg* 2012;21[7]:969-976.) |

were loaded in compression, and a specialized impression material was used to quantify the contact area. The contact areas for the anatomic and spherical hemiarthroplasties were markedly lower (59% and 51%, respectively) than those of the native articulation. The same study found that two capitellar implant shapes had similar contact areas against an ultra-high–molecular-weight polyethylene radial head in unicompartmental arthroplasty. This finding suggests that although the native capitellum is elliptical, a spherical capitellar implant should suffice in clinical implant designs. The decrease in contact area probably is related to the stiffness of the metallic implant, and further studies are needed to find alternative materials for joint hemiarthroplasties. An elbow simulator was used in an investigation of spherical and elliptical implants in cadaver arms during a variety of activities.[25] Excision of the capitellum resulted in an increase in varus-valgus laxity of 3.1° and an increase in external ulnar rotation of 1.5°; both implant designs corrected the instability. Collectively, these studies support the effectiveness of a spherical implant to manage capitellar deficiency.

The concept of a coronoid implant was recently explored.[26] A metal coronoid implant was developed based on detailed anthropometric studies. Using an upper limb joint motion simulator, varus-valgus laxity was quantified for intact, coronoid-deficient, and implant-reconstructed cadaver specimens. Both the standard-size and extended coronoid implants restored joint stability so that it was similar to that of the intact state (**Figure 7**). The extended coronoid implant achieved better stability than the standard-size implant in the setting of deficient collateral ligaments. This finding suggests that coronoid implants, which are not commercially available, may have an important role in the future management of unreconstructable comminuted coronoid fractures.

Although these novel hemiarthroplasty systems are in their infancy, significant advances in their design and development may be forthcoming. It is likely that other minimally invasive implant designs will emerge in the future.

Summary

Within the past 5 years, several significant advances have been made in the study of radial head implant design, sizing, and canal fixation. In particular, important new knowledge has been developed on the anatomic characteristics of radial head arthroplasty, with a focus on stability and kinematics. Studies of total elbow arthroplasty implant design and alignment have emphasized image- and computer-assisted surgery to improve implant placement. It is becoming increasingly clear that the design of elbow implants needs to accommodate the wide range and unique features of the intramedullary canals of the humerus and ulna, particularly if joint position is to be restored to the anatomic state. Some early studies on specialized small implants for the capitellum and coronoid have been reported, and additional systems for hemiarthroplasty and minimally invasive procedures are likely to be developed in the future.

Annotated References

1. Moon JG, Berglund LJ, Zachary D, An KN, O'Driscoll SW: Radiocapitellar joint stability with bipolar versus monopolar radial head prostheses. *J Shoulder Elbow Surg* 2009;18(5):779-784.

   An experimental cadaver study examined the stability of radial head components. A monopolar prosthesis is more effective in stabilizing the radiocapitellar joint than a bipolar prosthesis. The bipolar device has a compromising effect on the concavity compression stability of the radiocapitellar joint.

2. Chanlalit C, Shukla DR, Fitzsimmons JS, An KN, O'Driscoll SW: The biomechanical effect of prosthetic design on radiocapitellar stability in a terrible triad model. *J Orthop Trauma* 2012;26(9):539-544.

   In an in vitro model of a terrible triad injury, two monopolar radial head implants conferred greater radiocapitellar stability than bipolar implants. The anatomic prosthesis provided more stability than the nonanatomic prosthesis.

3. Moungondo F, El Kazzi W, van Riet R, Feipel V, Rooze M, Schuind F: Radiocapitellar joint contacts after bipolar radial head arthroplasty. *J Shoulder Elbow Surg* 2010;19(2):230-235.

   Molding techniques were used to determine radiocapitellar contact before and after radial head replacement, using the bipolar design of the Judet device. Contact area averaged 44% and 33% in the intact and implant-reconstructed elbows, respectively. Because of intraprosthetic mobility, contact areas were not dependent on elbow position when the bipolar implant was used. This factor led to abnormal positioning of the prosthesis with supination, causing subluxation over the trochlea lateral margin.

4. Yian E, Steens W, Lingenfelter E, Schneeberger AG: Malpositioning of radial head prostheses: An in vitro study. *J Shoulder Elbow Surg* 2008;17(4):663-670.

   An in vitro study analyzed the ability to perform anatomic radial head replacement and to study radiocapitellar prosthetic subluxation under unstable conditions. Anatomic alignment of radial head implants was difficult to consistently achieve. Bipolar implants offer better self-alignment, which can be difficult to achieve with rigid implants. Posterolateral stress produced radiocapitellar subluxation in the rigid but not the bipolar implants.

5. Chanlalit C, Shukla DR, Fitzsimmons JS, An KN, O'Driscoll SW: Influence of prosthetic design on radiocapitellar concavity-compression stability. *J Shoulder Elbow Surg* 2011;20(6):885-890.

   An experimental study examined the influence of the shape of the articular dish of a monopolar radial head implant on joint stability. An implant that more closely matches the normal anatomy is more effective than a shallow implant with a longer-than-normal radius of curvature.

6. Chanlalit C, Shukla DR, Fitzsimmons JS, Thoreson AR, An KN, O'Driscoll SW: Radiocapitellar stability: The effect of soft tissue integrity on bipolar versus monopolar radial head prostheses. *J Shoulder Elbow Surg* 2011;20(2):219-225.

   An in vitro model was used to measure the effects of the soft tissues on radiocapitellar stability in monopolar and bipolar radial head prostheses. Stability was better with a monopolar radial head prosthesis, particularly in the absence of soft-tissue support.

7. Beingessner DM, Dunning CE, Gordon KD, Johnson JA, King GJ: The effect of radial head excision and arthroplasty on elbow kinematics and stability. *J Bone Joint Surg Am* 2004;86-A(8):1730-1739.

8. Frank SG, Grewal R, Johnson J, Faber KJ, King GJ, Athwal GS: Determination of correct implant size in radial head arthroplasty to avoid overlengthening. *J Bone Joint Surg Am* 2009;91(7):1738-1746.

   The purpose of this biomechanical study was to identify clinical and radiographic features that may be used to diagnose overlengthening of the radius intraoperatively and on postoperative radiographs. Radial head implants of different thicknesses were implanted into cadaver specimens and assessed radiographically. Incongruity of the medial ulnohumeral joint can be radiographically assessed only after overlengthening of the radius by at least 6 mm.

9. Chanlalit C, Shukla DR, Fitzsimmons JS, An KN, O'Driscoll SW: Effect of hoop stress fracture on micromotion of textured ingrowth stems for radial head replacement. *J Shoulder Elbow Surg* 2012;21(7):949-954.

   Grit-blasted radial head prosthetic stems of increasing sizes were implanted into cadaver specimens. Insertion forces and implant micromotion were measured. A small radial neck fracture occurred with a stem oversized by 1 mm, but it did not compromise stability or micromotion.

10. Chanlalit C, Fitzsimmons JS, Moon JG, Berglund LJ, An KN, O'Driscoll SW: Radial head prosthesis micromotion characteristics: Partial versus fully grit-blasted stems. *J Shoulder Elbow Surg* 2011;20(1):27-32.

    This in vitro study found that the stability of a radial head stem partially grit blasted at the proximal end was similar to that of a stem grit blasted along the full length.

11. Ferreira LM, Stacpoole RA, Johnson JA, King GJ: Cementless fixation of radial head implants is affected by implant stem geometry: An in vitro study. *Clin Biomech (Bristol, Avon)* 2010;25(5):422-426.

    This experimental study examined the effects of radial head stem geometry on the initial stability of uncemented implants of various geometries and lengths. Filling the diameter of the canal was found to be more relevant than filling the length. A canal-filling stem reduced implant micromotion to less than 50 microns.

12. Moon JG, Berglund LJ, Domire Z, An KN, O'Driscoll SW: Stem diameter and micromotion of press fit radial head prosthesis: A biomechanical study. *J Shoulder Elbow Surg* 2009;18(5):785-790.

    This experimental study determined the effect of the stem diameter and insertion force on stability with a press-fit radial head designed for bone ingrowth. The greatest stability in the press-fit implant was achieved by maximizing sizing in the neck canal.

13. Completo A, Pereira J, Fonseca F, Ramos A, Relvas C, Simões J: Biomechanical analysis of total elbow replacement with unlinked iBP prosthesis: An in vitro and finite element analysis. *Clin Biomech (Bristol, Avon)* 2011;26(10):990-997.

    This experimental and computational study quantified strains and stresses in bone and cement around humeral and ulnar implant stems. In the epiphyseal region, a strain reduction was observed relative to the intact bones, but strains increased markedly at the tip.

14. Brownhill JR, Furukawa K, Faber KJ, Johnson JA, King GJ: Surgeon accuracy in the selection of the flexion-extension axis of the elbow: An in vitro study. *J Shoulder Elbow Surg* 2006;15(4):451-456.

15. Brownhill JR, Ferreira LM, Pichora JE, Johnson JA, King GJ: Defining the flexion-extension axis of the ulna: Implications for intra-operative elbow alignment. *J Biomech Eng* 2009;131(2):021005.

    An in vitro study determined the relationship of various kinematically and anatomically derived flexion axes of the ulna, with a focus on the accuracy of implant positioning. The most accurate technique was found to be an anatomic-based measurement that used the guiding ridge of the greater sigmoid notch of the ulna and the radial head.

16. Brownhill JR, Pollock JW, Ferreira LM, Johnson JA, King GJ: The effect of implant malalignment on joint loading in total elbow arthroplasty: An in vitro study. *J Shoulder Elbow Surg* 2012;21(8):1032-1038.

    An in vitro study used load sensors in the ulnohumeral articulation to determine the effect of implant alignment on joint loading in cadaver-based testing. Loading increased with malaligned implant positions, but combinations of internal-external and varus-valgus malrotations that tended to preserve the line of action of the elbow flexors were less aggressive.

17. Brownhill JR, King GJ, Johnson JA: Morphologic analysis of the distal humerus with special interest in elbow implant sizing and alignment. *J Shoulder Elbow Surg* 2007;16(3, suppl):S126-S132.

    The relationship between the medullary canal axis and the flexion-extension axis of the distal humerus was examined as they relate to implant selection and design for elbow arthroplasty. The anterior offset of the flexion-extension axis relative to the medullary canal axis was proportional to the length of canal proximally that was used to determine the alignment of the stem.

18. Brownhill JR, Mozzon JB, Ferreira LM, Johnson JA, King GJ: Morphologic analysis of the proximal ulna with special interest in elbow implant sizing and alignment. *J Shoulder Elbow Surg* 2009;18(1):27-32.

    A CT-based study assessed the shape of the medullary canal relative to the articular surface. Both the posterior and lateral offsets increased distally from the articulation center. The average valgus angulation was 8° in men and 7.2° in women. It was suggested that longer stemmed ulnar implants may require a modular design to meet anatomic constraints during implant positioning.

19. McDonald CP, Brownhill JR, King GJ, Johnson JA, Peters TM: A comparison of registration techniques for computer- and image-assisted elbow surgery. *Comput Aided Surg* 2007;12(4):208-214.

    An experimental study compared the alignment of the flexion-extension axis of a surface-based registration technique (using a handheld laser scanner) to a conventional paired-point registration. Registration was better by a factor of approximately 2 for the surface-based technique.

20. McDonald CP, Beaton BJ, King GJ, Peters TM, Johnson JA: The effect of anatomic landmark selection of the distal humerus on registration accuracy in computer-assisted elbow surgery. *J Shoulder Elbow Surg* 2008;17(5):833-843.

    An in vitro study determined the anatomic landmarks needed to successfully register surface digitizations to a preoperative image of the distal humerus. It was shown that close alignment can be achieved using a portion of the distal humerus that is measurable intraoperatively, even with major loss of articular structures.

21. McDonald CP, Peters TM, King GJ, Johnson JA: Computer assisted surgery of the distal humerus can employ contralateral images for pre-operative planning, registration, and surgical intervention. *J Shoulder Elbow Surg* 2009;18(3):469-477.

    A study determined whether the contralateral side can be used to determine implant position in the setting of bone loss. In CT scans of paired distal humeri, the anthropometric features were similar, with side-to-side differences in the range of 1.0° and 0.5 mm. The geometry found on preoperative imaging of the contralateral normal elbow may be used for referencing anatomic landmarks on the surgical side.

22. McDonald CP, Peters TM, Johnson JA, King GJ: Stem abutment affects alignment of the humeral component in computer-assisted elbow arthroplasty. *J Shoulder Elbow Surg* 2011;20(6):891-898.

An in vitro study used computer-assisted alignment (based on a preoperative image) of the implant axis with the humeral flexion-extension axis for a regular and a reduced-length humeral implant. Implant alignment was markedly improved in the reduced-length stem. Because of impingement with the regular stems, it was concluded that a humeral component with a fixed valgus angulation cannot be reproducibly positioned if maintenance of the flexion-extension axis is required.

23. Sabo MT, McDonald CP, Ng J, Ferreira LM, Johnson JA, King GJ: A morphological analysis of the humeral capitellum with an interest in prosthesis design. *J Shoulder Elbow Surg* 2011;20(6):880-884.

The purpose of this CT-based study was to quantify the anthropometric features of the capitellum in an effort to enhance implant design. The capitellum was found not to be spherical in shape, and there is substantial variability in the relationship between its height and width and between the radii of curvature in the sagittal and transverse planes. These variations may result in challenges in the design of implants that match the anatomic characteristics.

24. Sabo MT, Shannon H, Ng J, Ferreira LM, Johnson JA, King GJ: The impact of capitellar arthroplasty on elbow contact mechanics: Implications for implant design. *Clin Biomech (Bristol, Avon)* 2011;26(5):458-463.

An experimental study used a casting technique to assess the contact mechanics of both a spherical and an anatomic-based capitellar implant against the native radius and a unicompartmental design. Relative to the native state, both capitellar implants resulted in large decreases in contact area, suggesting that the radial head cartilage would have increased contact pressures. The contact areas for the anatomic and spherical hemiarthroplasties were not significantly different, nor were those for the unicompartmental devices.

25. Sabo MT, Shannon HL, Deluce S, et al: Capitellar excision and hemiarthroplasty affects elbow kinematics and stability. *J Shoulder Elbow Surg* 2012;21(8):1024, e4.

An evaluation of the effect of capitellar excision, with and without implant replacement, on stability using cadaver specimens in a testing simulator found that the capitellum has a role as a stabilizer to valgus and external rotation ulnohumeral articulation. These instabilities were corrected by capitellar hemiarthroplasty.

26. Alolabi B, Gray A, Ferreira LM, Johnson JA, Athwal GS, King GJ: Reconstruction of the coronoid using an extended prosthesis: An in vitro biomechanical study. *J Shoulder Elbow Surg* 2012;21(7):969-976.

Using an elbow simulator and cadaver limbs, varus-valgus laxity was measured in intact, coronoid-deficient, and coronoid-restored states using both an anatomic and an extended prosthesis. The anatomic device with ligament repair restores stability to the intact state relative to the coronoid-deficient state. With ligament insufficiency, the extended device produces greater stability than the anatomic implant, although stability remains less than that of the intact elbow.

Section 2

Instability and Athletic Injuries

SECTION EDITOR:
CDR Matthew T. Provencher, MD, MC, USN

Chapter 6

Clinical Assessment, Imaging, and Classification of Glenohumeral Instability

Brett D. Owens, MD

1: Basic Science

Introduction

Glenohumeral instability is common among athletes and young, active patients. Its incidence is second only to that of acromioclavicular injury among athletes, and it leads to more severe disability and a greater likelihood of surgical intervention than other shoulder injuries.[1-3] In a patient younger than 25 years with glenohumeral symptoms, the default diagnosis should be instability, until another diagnosis is proven.

The treatment of shoulder instability hinges on proper classification and patient risk profiling. The identification of instability requires a subjective sense that the glenohumeral joint is moving beyond its physiologic limits, whereas laxity is an objective measurement of the amount of motion, as identified by the examiner. Symptomatic instability, physiologic and/or pathologic laxity, and imaging findings are key to ensuring appropriate treatment.

Clinical Assessment

Patient History

Obtaining a high-quality patient history is critical to evaluating a patient with suspected shoulder instability. Complete glenohumeral dislocation is easier to diagnose than subluxation because most patients will have undergone a manual reduction maneuver. Reduction in an emergency department is typical, and as a result, prereduction and postreduction radiographs often are available for assessment. Reduction outside of an emergency department also is common, such as by an athletic trainer, and communication with the person who

provided the reduction can yield information on the injury and ease of reduction. Patients with chronic instability may report self-reduction.

There may be more variability in reports of subluxation because a manual reduction maneuver is not required. Patients typically describe their shoulder as "slipping out, and then going back in." These events may include a dislocation that spontaneously reduces (called a transient luxation event).[4] At the opposite end of the instability spectrum, microinstability may be similarly described by a patient who is a throwing or other overhead athlete. Therefore, it is critical to assess the patient's injury mechanism and sports activity in as much detail as can be obtained. Patients with both anterior and posterior instability events may report a fall onto an outstretched arm; posterior events often occur with the arm at 90° of forward flexion, and anterior events often occur as the arm moves rapidly into a position of extreme forward flexion and/or abduction.

If the patient has chronic, recurrent instability, an attempt should be made to determine the number of earlier events. A history of multiple events should alert the clinician to the possibility of bone loss. Determining the activities associated with these events also can provide insight. The presence of voluntary instability may suggest significant capsular laxity.[5] Instability during sleep may be associated with glenohumeral bone loss or soft-tissue deficiency.

Before revision surgery, a complete surgical history should be obtained including surgical reports and any available arthroscopic images. The earlier use of a thermal probe for capsulorrhaphy should alert the surgeon to the possibility that soft-tissue deficiency will be encountered during surgery and that capsular augmentation may be needed.

The patient history should include the patient's athletic goals. A young athlete who is planning to return to an intercollegiate contact sport is at a significantly higher risk of recurrence than a less active patient. The patient should be appropriately counseled on the risk of recurrence as well as the surgical treatment options.

Dr. Owens or an immediate family member serves as a paid consultant to the Musculoskeletal Transplant Foundation and serves as a board member, owner, officer, or committee member of the American Orthopaedic Society for Sports Medicine and the Society of Military Orthopaedic Surgeons.

Physical Examination

The patient history may guide the examiner to focus on specific aspects of the physical examination, but a general upper extremity examination is important to avoid missing a contributing pathology that is absent from the history. The physical examination for shoulder instability follows the routine of a thorough musculoskeletal examination and includes inspection, palpation, range-of-motion assessment, testing of motor strength, neurovascular examination, and specialized tests. The examination should be conducted with both shoulders completely exposed. Each phase of the examination should begin with the asymptomatic shoulder to provide an understanding of the patient's normal laxity and to build the patient's trust in the examiner.

During inspection of the shoulder girdle, the muscular contour should be evaluated for any asymmetry indicating atrophy of the deltoid, supraspinatus, or infraspinatus. Squaring of the lateral shoulder border with a prominent acromion may represent deltoid atrophy from an axillary nerve injury. The scapular body position should be assessed for scapular winging. The skin around the shoulder should be inspected for evidence of previous surgical incisions, thin atrophic skin, or excessive scar widening that may indicate a collagen disorder. Palpation of the entire shoulder girdle can be helpful to rule out concomitant pathology and determine the need for specialized testing and imaging.

Range of Motion

After sites of tenderness are recorded, the shoulder is taken through a full active range of motion. It is helpful to record maximal active forward flexion, internal rotation in adduction and 90° of abduction, and external rotation in adduction and 90° of abduction. Internal rotation in adduction is recorded relative to the nearest vertebral level. Throwing athletes commonly have an increased ability to externally rotate their dominant extremity, with a concomitant loss of internal rotation that leaves the total arc of motion symmetric to that of the contralateral extremity. A glenohumeral internal rotation deficit may exist if the total arc of motion is more than 25° less than that of the contralateral shoulder, and it may predispose the patient to internal impingement or labral pathology.

The examiner should determine whether a patient with an active motion deficit has full passive motion. Importantly, a patient with a locked posterior shoulder dislocation has a loss of external rotation actively and passively on the affected side. A large rotator cuff tear initially may appear as a loss of active external rotation while full passive motion is maintained. The patient is observed from behind during forward flexion and abduction to detect scapular asymmetry or winging during motion. Medial or lateral scapular winging may be attributable to long thoracic or cranial nerve XI palsy but also can be caused by scapular dyskinesis in a patient who is a throwing athlete or has multidirectional instability.

Muscular Strength Testing

During active motion testing, it is important to record general muscle strength in shoulder abduction, elbow flexion and extension, and wrist flexion and extension. The strength of the hand intrinsic muscles also should be recorded. Muscle strength grading is imperfect because the examination is subjective and measures only static muscle strength, but it is important to provide a baseline reference, usually in comparison with the contralateral extremity.

The rotator cuff muscles should be specifically assessed for strength. The Jobe empty can test isolates the supraspinatus muscle. The test is performed with the arm flexed to 90° in the scapular plane and the thumb pointed downward while the examiner applies a downward force. Pain or weakness as the downward pressure is resisted may indicate pathology in the supraspinatus muscle-tendon unit. Resisted external rotation at the side and in 90° of abduction tests the strength of the posterior rotator cuff.

Independent assessment of subscapularis function is critical in a patient with instability, especially a patient with a history of open surgery. In the lift-off test, the patient lifts the hand away from its position over the lumbar spine. The examiner can perform this test as a lag test by passively lifting the hand away from the back and asking the patient to hold the position. An inability to hold the position suggests subscapularis dysfunction. The examination may be difficult if pain in internal rotation prevents the patient from comfortably placing the hand over the lumbar spine. A false negative test may result if the patient uses the triceps muscle to move the hand away from the back. The belly-press test is used if the patient is unable to perform the lift-off test because of internal rotation contracture. In the belly-press test, the hand is on the abdomen with the wrist in neutral position and the elbow in the plane of the body. If the subscapularis is intact, the patient is able to apply pressure to the abdomen with internal rotation of the shoulder. A patient with subscapularis dysfunction is unable to internally rotate and flex the wrist or to move the elbow posteriorly to press on the abdomen. The belly-off test is similar, with the examiner passively holding the affected arm at the elbow in slight flexion and internal rotation and using the other hand to passively place the patient's hand onto the abdomen. The examiner instructs the patient to hold the maximally internally rotated position and releases the hand. In a positive test for subscapularis dysfunction, the hand rises off the patient's abdomen when released. The bear-hug test is performed with the arm in 90° of forward flexion. The elbow is flexed and held as far anterior to the body as possible, and the hand is placed on the contralateral shoulder. The examiner attempts to lift the hand away from the shoulder while the patient resists. An electromyelographic evaluation study revealed that all portions of the subscapularis are tested when the bear-hug, lift-off, and belly-press tests are used.[6]

Neurovascular Examination

Neurologic injuries are common in a shoulder dislocation, and it is important to document the initial neurologic examination. A recent study found a 13.5% incidence of neurologic deficit in 3,633 patients with dislocation.[7] The axillary nerve can be assessed in terms of sensation over the lateral shoulder. Axillary nerve motor function can be tested by resisted shoulder abduction and by watching and feeling the deltoid fire. Although axillary nerve injury is most common after shoulder dislocation, a neurologic examination of the median, ulnar, radial, and musculocutaneous nerves should be documented.

The vascular examination should begin with a simple inspection of the extremity to note skin pallor, trophic skin changes, venous engorgement, or hair loss. Palpation of the radial and ulnar pulses and observation of capillary refill should be compared in the affected and contralateral extremities.

Anterior Instability

Traumatic anterior instability is most common in young athletes, but it does not always occur in isolation. Combined instability patterns therefore are important to discover. The most commonly used test for elucidating anterior instability is the apprehension test, typically performed with the patient seated or supine with the scapula supported by the edge of the bed[8] The arm is placed in 90° of abduction, and the elbow is flexed and held by the examiner's right hand for a right shoulder examination. The arm is externally rotated, and an anteriorly directed force is applied when the examiner's left thumb presses the posterior aspect of the humeral head. Pain or apprehension with this maneuver is associated with an injury to the anterior labrum. The augmentation test can be applied if anterior instability is suspected despite the patient's equivocal response to the apprehension test. The augmentation test is performed in the same position of apprehension, abduction, and maximal external rotation, with the examiner placing an anteriorly directed force on the proximal humerus. The relocation test is performed with the patient in the same position, with the arm in the position of apprehension; a posteriorly directed force is applied to the proximal humerus, and relief of apprehension or pain is a positive test result.[9] Relief of shoulder pain with the relocation test has been associated with a superior labrum anterior to posterior (SLAP) lesion. The release (or surprise) test is performed after the relocation test by removing the posteriorly directed force on the proximal humerus.[10] A positive test result is the return of pain and apprehension in the shoulder.

The load-and-shift test is the preferred test for determining passive translation of the humeral head on the glenoid. The test can be done with the patient seated or supine and with the arm abducted 20° and held in slight flexion in the plane of the scapula. To examine the right shoulder, the examiner grasps the patient's right forearm with the right hand and applies a compressive force to center the humeral head on the glenoid. The examiner grasps the proximal humerus with the left thumb and index finger around the humeral head and applies an anteriorly directed force. The force then should be applied posteriorly and inferiorly. The load-and-shift translation test is graded based on the amount of humeral head translation, using the modified Hawkins scale: grade I is minimal translation along the glenoid fossa, grade II is translation to or over the glenoid rim with reduction once the force is removed, and grade III is translation over the glenoid rim that remains dislocated once the force is removed.[11]

The Gagey hyperabduction test assesses the integrity of the inferior glenohumeral ligament.[12] The test is performed with the patient seated and the examiner positioned behind the patient. The elbow is positioned at 90°, and the arm is in neutral rotation. One hand of the examiner pushes down on the shoulder girdle, and the other hand lifts the relaxed upper extremity. Passive abduction of more than 105° indicates laxity of the inferior glenohumeral ligament (**Figure 1**). In the initial report of the maneuver, 85% of patients with shoulder instability had passive abduction of more than 105°; abduction was limited by apprehension and pain in the remaining 15% of patients.[12]

Posterior Instability

The posterior load-and-shift test is performed with the patient's arm placed in the plane of the scapula, abducted to 45°, and in neutral rotation. The examiner stands to the side of the seated or supine patient. One hand controls the arm by grasping the elbow and gently loads the humerus into the glenoid while the other hand grasps the humerus near the deltoid insertion and applies a posterior force. The arm is moved into progressive internal rotation to increase the tension of the posterior capsuloligamentous structures and decrease translation. The scoring system is the same as for the load-and-shift translation test. As much as 50% displacement of the humeral head can be considered normal, but the result always should be compared with that of the contralateral shoulder to detect asymmetric increases in translation.

The posterior stress (or posterior apprehension) test is performed with the patient seated or supine; the arm is forward flexed to 90° and maximally internally rotated.[10] The examiner places a posteriorly directed force through the elbow, with the other hand held posterior to the shoulder to palpate a subluxation of the humeral head. The test is positive with palpable subluxation or dislocation, apprehension of a pending dislocation, or pain that reproduces the patient's symptoms. The jerk test is performed with the patient seated on the examination table. The patient's arm is forward flexed to 90° and placed in maximal adduction and internal rotation. The examiner applies a posterior directed force through the elbow. A dislocated or subluxated arm in this position indicates posterior instability. While maintaining the posteriorly directed force, the

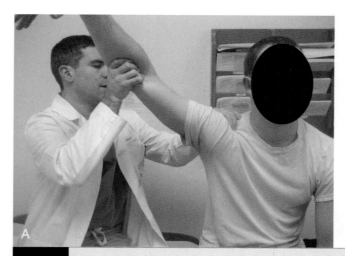
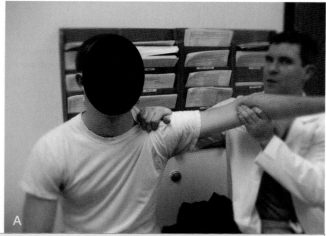

Figure 1 Clinical photographs of a 20-year-old man with anteroinferior instability. A positive Gagey test on the right side (**A**) is compared with the normal left side (**B**). A humeral avulsion of the glenohumeral ligament was detected on MRI.

examiner slowly takes the arm out of adduction; a "clunk" or "jerk" is seen and/or felt as the humeral head reduces into the glenoid.

Inferior and Multidirectional Instability

To quantify inferior laxity, the sulcus sign is elicited with the patient seated and the arms relaxed by the side in neutral rotation. The examiner places a downward distraction force onto the distal humerus while monitoring the lateral acromial edge. Inferior instability allows formation of a sulcus, which can be measured in centimeters, in the deltoid muscle inferior to the lateral acromion. The test is repeated in maximal external rotation, which places the anterior capsule and rotator cuff interval under tension. A sulcus sign that persists in external rotation may indicate incompetence of the rotator cuff interval.

A patient with multidirectional instability may have any of the physical examination findings for instability. Many such patients have signs of ligamentous laxity in multiple joints, including the contralateral shoulder. General articular mobility can be assessed using the Beighton scoring system, in which a score higher than 3 or 4 on a scale of 0 to 9 is associated with general hypermobility in a skeletally mature adult.[13] One point is assigned if the patient is able to perform each of nine maneuvers: metacarpophalangeal hyperextension beyond 90° in the left and/or right small finger, touching of the left and/or right thumb to the volar forearm, hyperextension of the left and/or right elbow more than 10°, hyperextension of the left and/or right knee beyond 10°, and placing of the palms of the hands flat on the floor with the knees fully extended. A score of 4 or higher is associated with a diagnosis of general ligamentous laxity. In addition, a score of 2 or higher is associated with a history of glenohumeral instability.[14]

Biceps and SLAP Lesions

Superior labral detachment may be associated with glenohumeral instability and often is associated with another intra-articular pathology. A comprehensive shoulder evaluation should include testing of the superior labrum. In the active compression test, the examiner stands behind the patient while the patient forward flexes the arm to 90°, adducts the arm 15° across the body, and maximally internally rotates the shoulder to point the thumb toward the floor.[15] The patient resists a downward force applied by the examiner and reports the location of pain. The examination is repeated in maximal supination. Relief of deep pain inside the shoulder when the palm faces upward is a positive test for superior labral pathology. The active compression test has been shown to be the most sensitive test for SLAP lesions (at 47%).[16] Pain on top of the shoulder probably represents acromioclavicular joint pathology or impingement syndrome. The so-called SLAPrehension test also uses traction on the biceps insertion and is performed with cross-chest adduction of the affected shoulder, with the elbow extended and forearm pronated. A positive test result occurs with pain in the bicipital groove, an audible or palpable click, or apprehension. The crank test is performed with the arm elevated to 160° in the scapular plane, axial compression applied by the examiner, and the shoulder passively rotated through full internal and external rotation. This examination is of uncertain usefulness in a patient with previous glenohumeral dislocation because of its similarity to the apprehension position. The anterior slide test is performed with the patient's hands on the hips with the thumbs posterior. The examiner stands behind the patient and places one hand on the patient's superior shoulder and the other hand on the elbow. The examiner places a slightly anterosuperior force on the shoulder to load the biceps anchor.[17] A

Table 1

Plain Radiographic Views for the Detection of Shoulder Lesions

Shoulder Lesion	Radiographic View(s) for Best Visualization	Imaging Technique
Bony Bankart	West Point axillary	Patient prone with arm abducted to 90° in neutral rotation, cassette placed superior to shoulder, beam directed from axilla with a 25° cephalad tilt (Figure 2)
	Bernageau	Patient standing with arm abducted and hand on head, cassette placed over axilla, beam directed at posterior shoulder with a 30° caudal tilt
	Garth	Patient standing, cassette placed behind shoulder, beam directed with a 45° caudal tilt
Glenohumeral dislocation	Axillary lateral	Patient supine with arm abducted, cassette placed superior to shoulder, beam directed into axilla
Hill-Sachs	AP internal rotation	Patient standing or supine with arm internally rotated, cassette placed posterior to shoulder, beam directed posteriorly from front of shoulder
	Garth	Patient standing, cassette placed behind shoulder, beam directed with a 45° caudal tilt
	Stryker notch	Patient supine with hand placed on head and elbow pointing superior, cassette placed posterior to shoulder, beam directed 10° cephalad and aiming at coracoids (Figure 3)

positive test result consists of pain in the anterior shoulder, a palpable click in the anterior shoulder region, or a reproduction of the symptoms that occur with overhead activities. The anterior slide test has been shown to be the most specific test for a SLAP lesion (at 84%).[16] A patient with a SLAP tear also may have pain with a classic biceps provocation maneuver such as the Speed or Yergason test. In the Speed test, the patient forward flexes the arm with the elbow at 30° of flexion and the forearm supinated. In the Yergason test, the patient performs resisted supination with the elbow flexed to 90°. In both examinations, pain in the bicipital groove is a positive test result.

Imaging

Plain Radiography

Imaging studies are critical for the optimal management of shoulder instability (**Table 1**). The evaluation typically begins with plain orthogonal radiographs. The standard AP and axillary are two typical views of the shoulder. The West Point axillary view can be used to improve the ability to see the anteroinferior glenoid rim and assess bony avulsions[18] (**Figure 2**). An AP view in internal rotation or a Stryker notch view can improve the ability to see a Hill-Sachs lesion (**Figure 3**). The Bernageau view can facilitate appreciation of glenoid bone loss.[19]

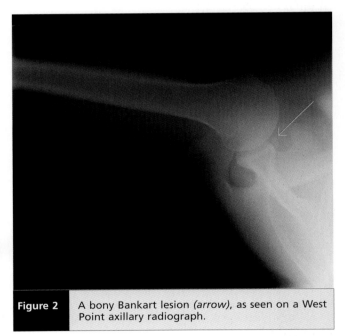

Figure 2 A bony Bankart lesion (*arrow*), as seen on a West Point axillary radiograph.

Magnetic Resonance Imaging

MRI is indicated for all patients with shoulder instability. The quality of MRI studies can vary among facilities, and indirect or direct gadolinium enhancement may facilitate the assessment of labral and capsular injury patterns as well as capsular volume. A Bankart lesion is present in a high proportion of young athletes with traumatic glenohumeral dislocation or sublux-

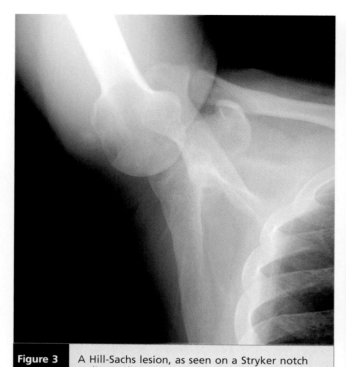

Figure 3   A Hill-Sachs lesion, as seen on a Stryker notch radiograph.

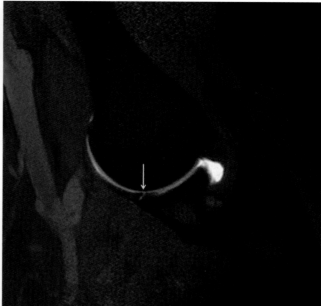

Figure 4   Magnetic resonance arthrogram of the shoulder of a 21-year-old collegiate football player with recurrent subluxation events. No labral pathology was noted on axial or coronal views, but a nondisplaced tear in the anteroinferior labrum *(arrow)* is visible in the abduction–external rotation view. This finding was corroborated by arthroscopic examination.

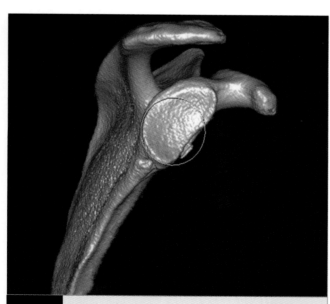

Figure 5   Three-dimensional CT reconstruction with the humeral head subtracted (en face view) showing glenoid bone loss *(circled)* in a 23-year-old patient. The patient had no history of dislocation but reported having experienced many subluxation events.

ation. This pathology often is best seen on axial and coronal views but also can be seen in abduction–external rotation views[4,20] (**Figure 4**). An anterior labral periosteal sleeve avulsion (ALPSA lesion) can be seen on MRI. The ALPSA lesion has been linked to chronic re-

current instability and inferior outcomes of surgical repair.[21,22]

A humeral avulsion of the glenohumeral ligament (HAGL lesion) is best seen with gadolinium enhancement and on coronal views. HAGL lesions can be difficult to classify based on imaging alone, but it is important to determine whether the anterior or posterior bands of the inferior glenohumeral ligament are intact or torn because this factor can influence the choice of repair technique.[23]

Computed Tomography

Although bone loss can be seen on MRI, most surgeons recommend CT if bone loss is suspected or revision surgery is being considered. The current methods of measuring bone loss incorporate three-dimensional CT reconstruction, with humeral head subtraction for glenoid assessment.

Glenoid Bone Loss

Glenoid bone loss increasingly is appreciated as a factor in shoulder instability. The presence of bone loss may be associated with a high rate of recurrence after arthroscopic repair alone.[24] Bone loss can be present even in a patient who reports only subluxation events (**Figure 5**). Bone loss may be attritional or involve a bony Bankart lesion. A recent study found some level of bone loss in 72% of patients with instability who

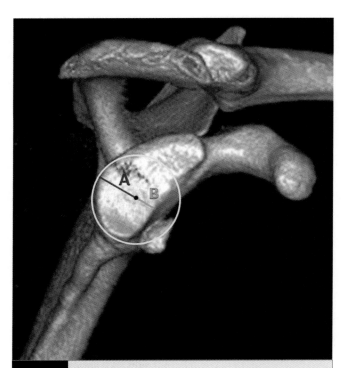

Figure 6 Three-dimensional CT reconstruction showing the anterior-posterior distance method of measuring glenoid bone loss from the bare area *(dot)* to the edge of defect *(A)* and from the posterior rim to the bare area *(B)*. The amount of bone loss is calculated as B − A) / 2B × 100%.

underwent stabilization, with severe bone loss (more than 20%) in 7.5%.[25] The amount of bone loss that necessitates a bone augmentation procedure is debatable. However, there is consensus that a loss of 0 to 15% is acceptable but that a loss of 20% to 30% is significant, and a bone procedure is recommended.[26]

One challenge of radiographically measuring glenoid bone loss is the absence of clear data as to the normal size of the glenoid. Some researchers recommend comparison imaging of the contralateral shoulder.[27] Glenoid bone loss can be measured on the ipsilateral three-dimensional CT reconstruction en face view by using a best-fit circle overlay.[28] With specialized computer software, researchers were able to digitally establish the area of the defect and to calculate the percentage of loss. Other reported methods of measuring bone loss also involve the use of three-dimensional CT with humeral head subtraction and a superimposed circle over the lower glenoid in the en face view, as shown in **Figure 6**.[26] In one measurement technique, the length of the lesion is directly compared with the radius of the lower glenoid. When the length of the lesion is longer than that of the radius, the resistance to dislocation is less than 70% of that of the intact joint.[29]

Neither the optimal method of measurement nor the critical amount of bone loss has been determined. The threshold should be low for obtaining CT to evaluate bone loss preoperatively. If the measured bone loss is

more than 20%, the surgeon should consider an alternative to an arthroscopic Bankart repair or an augmentative procedure and should counsel the patient about the risk of recurrence.

Humeral Head Bone Loss

Humeral head bone loss can be of concern whether it occurs in isolation or in conjunction with glenoid bone loss. The Hall measurement technique remains an excellent way to estimate the percentage of bone loss. Although plain radiographs were originally used for the Hall technique, axial MRI or CT is now used. The angle formed by the defect is measured and divided by the total 180° arc of the articular surface.[30] A Hill-Sachs defect as large as 25% may not require treatment.[31,32] In addition to lesion size, the concept of engagement is important. An engaging Hill-Sachs lesion comes into contact with the anteroinferior glenoid during a physiologic range of motion and has been shown to lead to failure of an arthroscopic soft-tissue repair.[24] An engaging Hill-Sachs lesion is best appreciated during an arthroscopic examination.

Classification

Many classification systems for shoulder instability have been proposed, but there is no universally accepted system. Most systems incorporate similar characteristics: direction, the distinction between traumatic and atraumatic instability, and ligamentous laxity.

Direction was among the earliest means of differentiating shoulder instability, with most dislocations classified as anterior. In early research, posterior instability was found to constitute only 4% of all dislocations.[33] Classification by direction has been consistent over time, with a relatively recent prospective cohort study finding that 5% of dislocations in young athletes were posterior in direction.[34] Complete instability events (dislocations) in the posterior direction are rare, but posterior subluxation events are more common, constituting 11% of all subluxation events.[34]

The most commonly used dichotomy in both dislocation and subluxation instability events is related to mechanism of injury. When dislocations were first classified as traumatic or atraumatic, a higher recurrence rate was found in patients with atraumatic dislocation.[35] A classification of subluxations as traumatic, atraumatic, or voluntary found good results when atraumatic or voluntary instability was nonsurgically managed.[36,37] In the most widely used system, two shoulder instability categories broadly define diagnosis and management. Atraumatic, multidirectional, bilateral shoulder instability (the AMBRI category) initially is treated with rehabilitation or an inferior capsular shift. The second broad category (TUBS) includes patients with traumatic dislocation, unilateral direction, and, commonly, a Bankart lesion requiring surgery. The AMBRI and TUBS categories accurately describe two

1: Basic Science

Table 2

The Instability Severity Index Score[a]

Prognostic Factor	Points
Age	
Younger than 20 years	2
Older than 20 years	0
Preoperative level of sports participation	
Competitive	2
Recreational or none	0
Preoperative type of sport	
Contact or forced overhead	1
Other	0
Shoulder hyperlaxity	
Anterior or inferior hyperlaxity	1
Normal laxity	0
Hill-Sachs lesion on AP radiograph	
Visible in external rotation	2
Not visible in external rotation	0
Glenoid contour on AP radiograph	
Loss of contour	2
No loss of contour	0
Total	10

[a]Risk of recurrence after arthroscopic repair = 10% if total score is ≤ 6, 70% if total score is ≥ 7.
(Adapted from Balg F, Boileau P: The instability severity index score: A simple pre-operative score to select patients for arthroscopic or open shoulder stabilization. J Bone Joint Surg Br 2007;89[11]:1470-1477.)

ables into consideration, including age, activity level, and pathologic changes, with a score assigned to six specific risk factors. A score of 6 or lower predicts a 10% recurrence risk after arthroscopic stabilization, compared with a 70% recurrence rate in patients with a score of 7 or higher[42] (**Table 2**).

Summary

Shoulder instability is common among young athletes. In such patients, shoulder symptoms should be considered to represent instability until proven otherwise. The diagnosis hinges on a combination of a thorough history, a physical examination, and imaging. Plain radiographs and MRI are routinely used to identify the labral and osteochondral lesions commonly seen with both complete dislocation and subluxation events. CT should be obtained if there is any concern about glenoid bone loss, which has been linked to inferior outcomes after arthroscopic soft-tissue stabilization alone. Instability can be classified in many ways, but an understanding of its direction, severity, and possible traumatic nature can be useful in risk stratification and planning of the optimal surgical stabilization technique.

Annotated References

1. Zacchilli MA, Owens BD: Epidemiology of shoulder dislocations presenting to emergency departments in the United States. *J Bone Joint Surg Am* 2010;92(3): 542-549.

   An epidemiologic study of emergency department visits for glenohumeral dislocation found an incidence that was higher than previously reported in the United States but consistent with European literature. The highest incidence was in men and boys in the second or third decade of life.

2. Kaplan LD, Flanigan DC, Norwig J, Jost P, Bradley J: Prevalence and variance of shoulder injuries in elite collegiate football players. *Am J Sports Med* 2005; 33(8):1142-1146.

3. Headey J, Brooks JH, Kemp SP: The epidemiology of shoulder injuries in English professional rugby union. *Am J Sports Med* 2007;35(9):1537-1543.

   An epidemiologic study of English rugby union players found that glenohumeral dislocation led to more time lost from sport (81 days) than any other shoulder injury.

4. Owens BD, Nelson BJ, Duffey ML, et al: Pathoanatomy of first-time, traumatic, anterior glenohumeral subluxation events. *J Bone Joint Surg Am* 2010;92(7): 1605-1611.

   A high rate of Bankart and Hill-Sachs lesions was found in patients who underwent early imaging after a first traumatic anterior glenohumeral subluxation. The term transient luxation was introduced for sublux-

ends of the instability spectrum but not the gradations between them.[38]

Another classification is based on whether shoulder instability is static, dynamic, or voluntary.[29] The static category is subdivided by directionality, and the dynamic category is subdivided based on the presence or absence of ligamentous laxity. A recent system takes a scientific approach to the classification of instability.[39] Its four components include frequency within a 1-year period (one, two to five, or more than five occurrences), etiology (traumatic or atraumatic), direction (anterior, inferior, or posterior), and severity (subluxation or dislocation). This comprehensive FEDS system appears to encompass all possible instability patterns within its 36 possible classes and was shown to be reproducible at one institution.[40]

These classification systems may become important research tools, but they do little to help the surgeon make an appropriate treatment decision. One recent study used published recurrence data for a decision analysis of treatment after an initial anterior dislocation event and may be useful for surgeons in counseling patients on expected risks.[41] The recently introduced instability severity index score takes several patient variation with significant pathology. A high index of suspicion and early imaging were recommended for young athletes.

5. Neer CS II, Foster CR: Inferior capsular shift for involuntary inferior and multidirectional instability of the shoulder: A preliminary report. *J Bone Joint Surg Am* 1980;62(6):897-908.

6. Pennock AT, Pennington WW, Torry MR, et al: The influence of arm and shoulder position on the bearhug, belly-press, and lift-off tests: An electromyographic study. *Am J Sports Med* 2011;39(11):2338-2346.

   An electromyelographic study of tests for subscapularis function found that all tests are effective for determining subscapularis deficiency but do not allow differentiation between upper and lower subscapularis function.

7. Robinson CM, Shur N, Sharpe T, Ray A, Murray IR: Injuries associated with traumatic anterior glenohumeral dislocations. *J Bone Joint Surg Am* 2012;94(1):18-26.

   Review of a large trauma database found 3,633 patients with anterior glenohumeral dislocation, of whom 13.5% had a neurologic deficit after reduction and 33.4% had a rotator cuff tear or an avulsion fracture.

8. Rowe CR, Zarins B: Recurrent transient subluxation of the shoulder. *J Bone Joint Surg Am* 1981;63(6):863-872.

9. Jobe FW, Kvitne RS, Giangarra CE: Shoulder pain in the overhand or throwing athlete: The relationship of anterior instability and rotator cuff impingement. *Orthop Rev* 1989;18(9):963-975.

10. Silliman JF, Hawkins RJ: Classification and physical diagnosis of instability of the shoulder. *Clin Orthop Relat Res* 1993;291:7-19.

11. McFarland EG, Tanaka MJ, Papp DF: Examination of the shoulder in the overhead and throwing athlete. *Clin Sports Med* 2008;27(4):553-578.

    Current shoulder examination techniques and their clinical efficacy are described.

12. Gagey OJ, Gagey N: The hyperabduction test. *J Bone Joint Surg Br* 2001;83(1):69-74.

13. Moriatis Wolf J, Cameron KL, Owens BD: Impact of joint laxity and hypermobility on the musculoskeletal system. *J Am Acad Orthop Surg* 2011;19(8):463-471.

    Ligamentous laxity is reviewed, with its effect on the musculoskeletal system and shoulder-specific concerns. The routine use of a Beighton score assessment is recommended.

14. Cameron KL, Duffey ML, DeBerardino TM, Stoneman PD, Jones CJ, Owens BD: Association of generalized joint hypermobility with a history of glenohumeral joint instability. *J Athl Train* 2010;45(3):253-258.

    A correlation was found between an elevated Beighton score for ligamentous laxity and a history of glenohumeral instability in young athletes.

15. O'Brien SJ, Pagnani MJ, Fealy S, McGlynn SR, Wilson JB: The active compression test: A new and effective test for diagnosing labral tears and acromioclavicular joint abnormality. *Am J Sports Med* 1998;26(5):610-613.

16. McFarland EG, Kim TK, Savino RM: Clinical assessment of three common tests for superior labral anterior-posterior lesions. *Am J Sports Med* 2002;30(6):810-815.

17. Kibler WB, McMullen J: Scapular dyskinesis and its relation to shoulder pain. *J Am Acad Orthop Surg* 2003;11(2):142-151.

18. Rokous JR, Feagin JA, Abbott HG: Modified axillary roentgenogram: A useful adjunct in the diagnosis of recurrent instability of the shoulder. *Clin Orthop Relat Res* 1972;82:84-86.

19. Bernageau J, Patte D, Debeyre J, Ferrane J: Intérêt du profil glénoïdien dans les luxations récidivantes de l'épaule. *Rev Chir Orthop Reparatrice Appar Mot* 1976;62(2, suppl)142-147.

20. Taylor DC, Arciero RA: Pathologic changes associated with shoulder dislocations: Arthroscopic and physical examination findings in first-time, traumatic anterior dislocations. *Am J Sports Med* 1997;25(3):306-311.

21. Ozbaydar M, Elhassan B, Diller D, Massimini D, Higgins LD, Warner JJ: Results of arthroscopic capsulolabral repair: Bankart lesion versus anterior labroligamentous periosteal sleeve avulsion lesion. *Arthroscopy* 2008;24(11):1277-1283.

    Patients with an ALPSA lesion had a higher rate of recurrent instability after arthroscopic soft-tissue repair than those with a Bankart lesion.

22. Kim DS, Yoon YS, Yi CH: Prevalence comparison of accompanying lesions between primary and recurrent anterior dislocation in the shoulder. *Am J Sports Med* 2010;38(10):2071-2076.

    A review found a higher rate of Bankart lesions, ALPSA lesions, Hill-Sachs lesions, and glenoid bone loss after arthroscopic soft-tissue repair in patients with recurrent anterior instability than in patients with a single anterior dislocation.

23. Bui-Mansfield LT, Banks KP, Taylor DC: Humeral avulsion of the glenohumeral ligaments: The HAGL lesion. *Am J Sports Med* 2007;35(11):1960-1966.

    The literature on HAGL lesions is reviewed, and a comprehensive classification system is presented.

24. Burkhart SS, De Beer JF: Traumatic glenohumeral bone defects and their relationship to failure of arthroscopic Bankart repairs: Significance of the inverted-pear glenoid and the humeral engaging Hill-Sachs lesion. *Arthroscopy* 2000;16(7):677-694.

25. Milano G, Grasso A, Russo A, et al: Analysis of risk factors for glenoid bone defect in anterior shoulder instability. *Am J Sports Med* 2011;39(9):1870-1876.

    CT evaluation of patients with instability showed that glenoid bone loss was correlated with the number of dislocation events.

26. Piasecki DP, Verma NN, Romeo AA, Levine WN, Bach BR Jr, Provencher MT: Glenoid bone deficiency in recurrent anterior shoulder instability: Diagnosis and management. *J Am Acad Orthop Surg* 2009; 17(8):482-493.

    A comprehensive review of glenoid bone deficiency includes the relevant literature and guidelines for the clinician. A method of bone loss measurement is presented for use in CT or arthroscopy.

27. Baudi P, Righi P, Bolognesi D, et al: How to identify and calculate glenoid bone deficit. *Chir Organi Mov* 2005;90(2):145-152.

28. Sugaya H, Moriishi J, Dohi M, Kon Y, Tsuchiya A: Glenoid rim morphology in recurrent anterior glenohumeral instability. *J Bone Joint Surg Am* 2003;85(5): 878-884.

29. Gerber C, Nyffeler RW: Classification of glenohumeral joint instability. *Clin Orthop Relat Res* 2002;400:65-76.

30. Hall RH, Isaac F, Booth CR: Dislocations of the shoulder with special reference to accompanying small fractures. *J Bone Joint Surg Am* 1959;41(3):489-494.

31. Sekiya JK, Jolly J, Debski RE: The effect of a Hill-Sachs defect on glenohumeral translations, in situ capsular forces, and bony contact forces. *Am J Sports Med* 2012;40(2):388-394.

    A cadaver laboratory study found that the presence of a 25% humeral head defect did not significantly increase glenohumeral translation if the capsule was intact.

32. Skendzel JG, Sekiya JK: Diagnosis and management of humeral head bone loss in shoulder instability. *Am J Sports Med* 2012; 40(11):2633-2644.

    A thorough overview of the literature on humeral head bone loss in patients with shoulder instability is presented, with clinical treatment guidelines.

33. McLaughlin HL, MacLellan DI: Recurrent anterior dislocation of the shoulder: II. A comparative study. *J Trauma* 1967;7(2):191-201.

34. Owens BD, Duffey ML, Nelson BJ, DeBerardino TM, Taylor DC, Mountcastle SB: The incidence and characteristics of shoulder instability at the United States Military Academy. *Am J Sports Med* 2007;35(7):1168-1173.

    A prospective study of shoulder instability epidemiology in a high-risk population found that 85% of all events were subluxations and confirmed earlier findings that 80% of events were anterior.

35. Rowe CR: Prognosis in dislocations of the shoulder. *J Bone Joint Surg Am* 1956;38-A(5):957-977.

36. Rockwood CA Jr: Subluxation of the shoulder: The classification, diagnosis, and treatment. *Orthop Trans* 1979;3:306.

37. Burkhead WZ Jr, Rockwood CA Jr: Treatment of instability of the shoulder with an exercise program. *J Bone Joint Surg Am* 1992;74(6):890-896.

38. Thomas SC, Matsen FA III: An approach to the repair of avulsion of the glenohumeral ligaments in the management of traumatic anterior glenohumeral instability. *J Bone Joint Surg Am* 1989;71(4):506-513.

39. Kuhn JE: A new classification system for shoulder instability. *Br J Sports Med* 2010;44(5):341-346.

    The FEDS classification system was introduced. This comprehensive system has 36 possible categories of instability and may be better suited to research than clinical use.

40. Kuhn JE, Helmer TT, Dunn WR, Throckmorton V TW: Development and reliability testing of the frequency, etiology, direction, and severity (FEDS) system for classifying glenohumeral instability. *J Shoulder Elbow Surg* 2011;20(4):548-556.

    The FEDS system was found to be reproducible in a single-institution evaluation.

41. Mather RC III, Orlando LA, Henderson RA, Lawrence JT, Taylor DC: A predictive model of shoulder instability after a first-time anterior shoulder dislocation. *J Shoulder Elbow Surg* 2011;20(2):259-266.

    A decision-tree analysis based on published recurrence rates was intended to provide clinicians with a means of counseling patients on recurrence risk based on their demographic characteristics.

42. Balg F, Boileau P: The instability severity index score: A simple pre-operative score to select patients for arthroscopic or open shoulder stabilisation. *J Bone Joint Surg Br* 2007;89(11):1470-1477.

    The instability severity index score is a clinical tool for risk stratifying patients with instability based on their age, activity level, and clinical presentation. This tool appears to be best for guiding clinicians as to the risk of recurrence after soft-tissue repair and determining whether a patient can benefit from an augmented repair.

Chapter 7

Acute and Chronic Shoulder Dislocations

Geoffrey S. Van Thiel, MD, MBA   Wendell Heard, MD   Anthony A. Romeo, MD
CDR Matthew T. Provencher, MD, MC, USN

Introduction

The glenohumeral joint allows a tremendous range of motion, but it also is the most commonly dislocated large joint. The stability of the glenohumeral joint is provided by static and dynamic restraints, negative intra-articular pressure, and concavity compression. A true glenohumeral dislocation is a complete instability event that results in the loss of contact between the humeral head and the glenoid. The humeral head rests in a dislocated position, requiring manual reduction to restore anatomy. Spontaneous reduction is possible, particularly if there is glenoid or combined glenoid and humeral head bone loss.

The overall incidence of shoulder dislocation in the United States was estimated at 23.9 per 100,000 population in 2010.[1] Men accounted for 72% of all dislocations, and individuals age 15 to 29 years accounted for 47%. The age distribution is bimodal, with peaks among younger adults and adults older than 70 years.

Dr. Romeo or an immediate family member has received royalties from Arthrex; is a member of a speakers' bureau or has made paid presentations on behalf of Arthrex, DJ Orthopaedics, and the Joint Restoration Foundation; serves as a paid consultant to Arthrex; has received research or institutional support from Arthrex and DJ Orthopaedics; has received nonincome support (such as equipment or services), commercially derived honoraria, or other non–research-related funding (such as paid travel) from Arthrex and DJ Orthopaedics; and serves as a board member, owner, officer, or committee member of the American Orthopaedic Society for Sports Medicine, American Shoulder and Elbow Surgeons, and the Arthroscopy Association of North America. Dr. Provencher or an immediate family member serves as a board member, owner, officer, or committee member of the American Academy of Orthopaedic Surgeons; American Orthopaedic Society for Sports Medicine; American Shoulder and Elbow Surgeons; Arthroscopy Association of North America; International Society of Arthroscopy, Knee Surgery, and Orthopaedic Sports Medicine; San Diego Shoulder Institute, and the Society of Military Orthopaedic Surgeons. Neither of the following authors nor any immediate family member has received anything of value from or owns stock in a commercial company or institution related directly or indirectly to the subject of this chapter: Dr. Van Thiel and Dr. Heard.

In a study of 4,141 students, 18 dislocations occurred, 17 of which had an anterior direction.[2] This finding corresponded to previously reported values.

Acute Anterior Shoulder Dislocation

Pathoanatomy and Associated Injuries

The age of the patient is the factor that best predicts the anatomic pathology, possible complications, and the prognosis of an anterior shoulder dislocation. Patients younger than 40 years are more likely than older patients to have a ligamentous injury of the labrum and capsule. Patients age 40 years or older are more likely to have associated injuries of the rotator cuff, proximal humerus, or surrounding neurovascular structures.

Arthroscopic examination after acute anterior shoulder dislocation may show capsulolabral injury such as an anterior labral tear, anterior capsular insufficiency, or humeral avulsion of the glenohumeral ligaments (**Figure 1**). Three patterns of injury were identified in

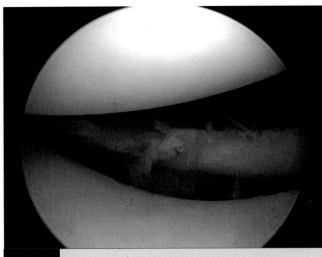

Figure 1   Arthroscopic image showing a Bankart injury to the anterior labrum after a primary dislocation, as seen from the posterior portal.

1990: a capsular tear without a labral lesion, seen in 13% of patients, was considered stable; a capsular tear with partial labral detachment, seen in 24% of patients, was considered mildly unstable; and a capsular tear with complete labral detachment, seen in 62% of patients, was considered grossly unstable.[3] A biomechanical study found that an anteroinferior labral detachment alone does not result in glenohumeral dislocation.[4] Extension of the Bankart lesion to the superoposterior labrum was required for the tensioning mechanism to fail in external rotation and abduction, producing an anterior dislocation.

Rotator cuff injury becomes more common with increasing patient age. An anterior shoulder dislocation can cause an avulsion of the posterosuperior rotator cuff or a subscapularis tendon tear. A rotator cuff tear was found in 49% of patients older than 60 years with an anterior shoulder dislocation.[5] The rotator cuff should be evaluated during the physical examination of patients who have an anterior shoulder dislocation. Advanced imaging can help in the diagnosis.

Fractures of the glenoid, the proximal humerus, or the coracoid can occur with anterior shoulder dislocation. Anterior glenoid rim fracture occurs as a bony avulsion of the anteroinferior capsulolabral structures. Greater tuberosity fracture occurs in as many as one third of dislocations and becomes more common with advancing patient age. Hill-Sachs lesions are often seen in association with anterior shoulder dislocation, but their true clinical significance and management continue to be debated.

Patient History

After an acute anterior shoulder dislocation, the patient is usually evaluated in the field, the training room, or the emergency department. The classic mechanism of injury is a combination of abduction, extension, and a posteriorly directed force applied to the arm. The patient's history of shoulder injury should be determined. If the patient is being seen for follow-up, it is useful to obtain a history of events, including the mechanism of injury, the necessity for reduction, and the time and the place of reduction; prereduction and postreduction imaging; and episodes of recurrence since the initial dislocation.

Physical Examination

A systematic examination of the upper extremity is useful for eliminating the possibility of associated pathology in a patient with anterior shoulder dislocation. The patient often holds the arm against the body using the contralateral arm. The shoulder girdle should be inspected for muscle contour, taking note of a prominent acromion or the presence of the humeral head anteriorly, which suggests an unreduced anterior dislocation. Palpation should include the sternoclavicular joint, the coracoid, the long head of the biceps tendon, the acromioclavicular joint, and the greater tuberosity. The inferior acromial border can be palpated to assess the po-

sition of the humeral head relative to the glenoid. A hollow sulcus may be palpable inferior to the lateral border of the acromion after an anterior glenohumeral dislocation. The scapula should be palpated in its entirety.

The active and passive range of motion should be evaluated in a patient with a dislocated shoulder that has been reduced, keeping in mind that a large rotator cuff tear may be observed as a loss of external rotation with full passive range of motion. Scapular motion can be observed from behind during active forward flexion and abduction. Strength testing should be tested in the affected extremity and compared with the contralateral limb. It is important to perform a complete strength examination, including the hand intrinsic muscles, the flexors and the extensors of the wrist and elbow, the shoulder abductors, and the individual muscles of the rotator cuff.

A complete neurologic and vascular examination should be performed and carefully documented. Neurologic injury is most common among older patients and patients with associated fractures. The axillary nerve is susceptible to injury because it is tethered anterior and posterior to the glenohumeral joint and has limited excursion. If a reduction maneuver is to be performed, it is important to perform neurovascular examinations before and after the reduction.

Special tests for anterior instability may be difficult and unnecessary in a recently reduced shoulder. The apprehension test, the augmentation test, and the relocation test all can suggest anterior labral injury. The load-and-shift test evaluates passive translation of the humeral head on the glenoid. The Gagey hyperabduction test assesses the integrity of the inferior glenohumeral ligament.

Closed Reduction

If the patient has an acute dislocation, the treating physician must make a decision about the timing of reduction. Reduction without first obtaining a radiograph, as on the field or in the training room, is controversial. Some physicians believe that reducing the shoulder immediately is preferable because muscle spasm has not yet set in, so the maneuver can be performed without conscious sedation. The athlete must not be allowed to return to play after an on-field reduction, and postreduction radiographs must be obtained to confirm the reduction and assess the bony structures. For a patient in the emergency department, it is likely that the onset of muscle guarding and pain will prevent a reduction without conscious sedation or an intra-articular anesthetic.

The Stimson technique for the reduction of an anterior shoulder dislocation is safe and effective.[6] An intra-articular injection of lidocaine is used. The patient is placed prone, with the arm hanging down, and traction and rotation of the humerus reduces the shoulder. In the traction-countertraction technique, the patient is supine and traction is applied in the direction of the deformity while countertraction is applied using a sheet placed around the chest. In the Milch technique, the physician places one hand in the axilla of the dislocated shoulder while the other hand holds the patient's hand. Pressure is applied to the humeral head as the arm is gently abducted. When the arm has been fully abducted, it is externally rotated, and traction is applied to reduce the humeral head. The external rotation method for closed reduction of anterior shoulder dislocation, was successfully used with minimal premedication in 29 of 40 patients.[7] The so-called FARES (fast, reliable, safe) was found to be effective without the use of anesthetic agents.[8] The patient is supine with the forearm in neutral rotation, the elbow extended, and the arm at the side. The physician stands on the side of the affected extremity and applies a gentle longitudinal traction to gradually move the arm into greater abduction while performing continuous short-range vertical oscillating arm movements. At 90° of abduction, the arm is brought into external rotation. Most reductions were found to occur at approximately 120° of abduction.[8]

Imaging

Prereduction radiographs determine the direction of the dislocation and may show associated fracture. Postreduction radiographs confirm the reduction, and the restoration of normal glenohumeral anatomy may expose associated injury not evident on prereduction imaging. An AP radiograph in slight internal rotation can show a greater tuberosity fracture. A true AP view can show a glenoid fracture. A Bankart lesion, anterior glenoid deficiency, or bony avulsion of the inferior glenohumeral ligament attachment can be seen on a West Point modified axillary view. The Stryker notch view can show a Hill-Sachs defect in the posterosuperior humeral head. If further bony imaging is required, CT can be particularly helpful in evaluating anterior glenoid bone loss or a Hill-Sachs lesion. MRI is helpful in assessing pathology associated with anterior shoulder dislocation. A Bankart lesion, a labral tear, a rotator cuff tear, humeral avulsion of the glenohumeral ligaments, or an articular cartilage defect can be well defined with MRI.

Nonsurgical Management

Treatment after the reduction of an anterior shoulder dislocation is tailored to the individual patient. For many years, sling immobilization with the shoulder in internal rotation was the accepted treatment of patients with a first-time anterior shoulder dislocation. The sling was removed when the discomfort resolved. Immobilization of the arm in external rotation was investigated in an arthroscopic evaluation of 25 patients.[9] The best reduction of the labrum occurred when the arm was held in 30° of abduction and 60° of external rotation. The study conclusion was that immobilization with the shoulder in internal rotation contributes to the incidence of recurrent instability. A prospective ran-

domized study compared immobilization in internal and external rotation in 40 patients.[10] At 15-month follow-up, no recurrences had occurred in the patients treated with external rotation, but those treated with internal rotation had a 30% recurrence rate. Follow-up analysis did not support these findings, however.[11]

An in-season dislocation in an athlete who wishes to continue competing poses a treatment dilemma. Twenty-six of 30 athletes with an anterior shoulder dislocation were able to return to sport for the remainder of the season by using a protocol including early range of motion with no restrictions, strengthening with a 1-lb weight, and a shoulder brace restricting abduction and external rotation.[12] Patients were allowed to return to sport when they had symmetric strength and a functional range of motion that would allow full participation at the specific playing position. Two basketball players and one hockey player were unable to return to sport. One patient was able to return to sport but was unable to complete the season because of recurrent instability. Two patients returned to play immediately following the reduction and missed no days of participation. Of the 26 patients who returned to complete the season, 12 (46%) underwent surgical stabilization at the end of the season. Sixteen of the original 30 patients (53%) underwent surgical stabilization at some point.[12]

In general, patients who are treated nonsurgically for an anterior shoulder dislocation are able to return to sport when they have achieved full active range of motion and normal side-to-side upper extremity muscle strength. If the patient is to return to a contact or collision sport, an adjustable brace is used to prevent injury to the vulnerable shoulder.

Surgical Management

Interest in surgical management of acute anterior shoulder dislocations has increased because of high recurrence rates in younger patients coupled with improvements in the success of arthroscopic repairs. A 25-year follow-up study on nonsurgical treatment of anterior shoulder dislocations reported a recurrence in 72% of patients age 12 to 22 years, 56% of patients age 23 to 29 years, and 27% of patients older than 30 years.[13] A meta-analysis of five studies of acute anterior shoulder dislocation in a total of 239 patients found that surgically treated young patients had significantly lower rates of recurrent instability and dislocation or subluxation than nonsurgically treated young patients, despite their highly demanding physical activity.[14]

A prospective nonrandomized study of arthroscopic and nonsurgical treatment of acute traumatic anterior shoulder dislocation in young patients, most of whom were rugby players, found more favorable outcomes after surgical treatment.[15] The rate of recurrent dislocation within 18 months of the first injury was 94.5% in the nonsurgically treated patients. In the surgically treated patients, only one patient had a recurrent dislocation, and 96% had an excellent result. A small prospective randomized study comparing arthroscopic stabilization and nonsurgical management for first-time acute traumatic anterior shoulder dislocations found a recurrent dislocation in one of the nine patients treated surgically and 9 of the 12 patients treated nonsurgically.[16]

Arthroscopic management of anterior instability is contraindicated and an open procedure is preferred in certain situations, the most important of which is the presence of significant bone loss.[17,18] Some surgeons recommend arthroscopic repair for a humeral avulsion of the glenohumeral ligaments (a rare variant in traumatic anterior instability), but most recommend open repair. Repair of subscapularis tendon rupture in association with primary dislocation and revision of an earlier unsuccessful instability surgery also may be more effectively done with an open procedure.

Bone Loss With Anterior Shoulder Dislocation

Glenohumeral instability in the presence of glenoid bone loss is difficult to treat and important to recognize. The biomechanical stability of the glenohumeral joint changes as the amount of glenoid bone loss approaches 15% to 20% of the glenoid surface.[19] The current techniques for managing anterior glenoid bone defects include several types of coracoid transfer as well as fresh distal tibia osteochondral allograft and iliac crest autograft.[20-23]

Several studies have described the contribution of a Hill-Sachs defect to recurrent instability. The presence of a large humeral head defect in patients who underwent arthroscopic stabilization was associated with surgical failure and recurrent instability.[24,25] A biomechanical study suggested that defects as small as 12.5% of the humeral head can affect joint stability, and defects of 37.5% to 50% may benefit from osteoarticular allograft transplantation to help restore stability.[26]

Acute Posterior Shoulder Dislocation

Posterior shoulder dislocation is relatively rare and accounts for 2% to 5% of all traumatic glenohumeral dislocations.[27] However, posterior dislocation represents a much higher percentage of so-called missed shoulder dislocations because it is difficult to detect and is associated with distracting high-energy trauma and seizure.[28,29] As many as 79% of posterior dislocations were found to be initially overlooked by the treating physician.[30] More recently, 50% of posterior shoulder dislocations were found to be initially misdiagnosed.[31] However, a review of all available literature found an overall rate of only 24%.[32] This initial oversight can lead to a delay in the diagnosis and ultimately influences the treatment algorithm.

The largest epidemiologic study on acute posterior shoulder dislocation reported an incidence of 1.1 per 100,000 population, with higher rates in men age 20 to 49 years and individuals older than 70 years.[33] The cause was trauma in 67% of the dislocations and a seizure caused by epilepsy or substance withdrawal in 31%. Six percent of the patients had an associated rotator cuff tear, always involving the subscapularis. These patients were age 54 to 75 years; two of them required rotator cuff repair. A small (less than 1.5 cm³) reverse Hill-Sachs lesion was found in 58% of the patients, and a large Hill-Sachs lesion was found in 42%.

Rates of recurrent instability recently have been reported in the orthopaedic literature, but these data are limited by the rarity of posterior dislocation. At 2-year follow-up, 19% of the shoulders had a recurrence of instability.[33] In 16 of these 23 shoulders, the initial dislocation resulted from a seizure, and most of these recurrences occurred within 8 months of the initial dislocation. The identified risk factors included age younger than 40 years (a 30% rate of recurrence), dislocation resulting from seizure (a 42% rate), and a Hill-Sachs lesion larger than 1.5 cm³ (a 50% rate). These risk factors are additive, and each increases the risk of recurrence. In patients with no risk factors, the redislocation rate was only 3%.

Associated injuries can play a important role in the management of an acute posterior dislocation. The incidence of injuries associated with a posterior dislocation was reported to be 65%.[32] Fracture was present with 34% of the dislocations, a reverse Hill-Sachs lesion with 29%, and a rotator cuff tear with 13%. Further analysis showed that the rate of rotator cuff tears increased fivefold in the presence of a posterior dislocation without a fracture or a Hill-Sachs lesion. Thus, a posterior dislocation often occurs in association with other pathology and with distracting injuries.

Patient History

Posterior dislocation can be present in the setting of significant trauma and has been reported with humeral shaft and distal humeral fractures. In three patients, a missed posterior dislocation was diagnosed after intramedullary treatment of a humeral shaft fracture.[34] The posterior dislocation can be difficult to diagnose because of not only the distracting trauma but also the sling position in which the arm is held.

In a seizure, it is believed that the relatively powerful posterior cuff muscles cause the shoulder to dislocate with forceful contraction. Bilateral dislocations have been reported secondary to seizure or electrocution. Nonetheless, the patient's history may not include a traumatic event with a known dislocation but instead may include a single significant event unrelated to the shoulder.

Physical Examination

The classic physical examination findings for a posteriorly dislocated shoulder include an inability to externally rotate the glenohumeral joint with limited flexion and abduction. Essentially, the arm is held in the sling position because the humeral head is fixed on the posterior glenoid. However, in some chronic dislocations

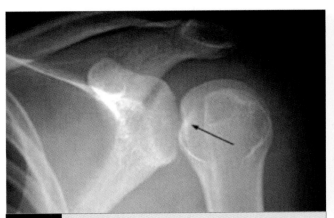

Figure 2   AP radiograph showing a posterior dislocation with a slight overlap of the humeral head and the glenoid and a loss of tuberosity contour creating the appearance of a light bulb in a humeral head defect *(arrow)*. (Reproduced from Johnson TR, Steinbach LS, eds: Glenohumeral instability, in *Essentials of Musculoskeletal Imaging*. Rosemont, IL, American Academy of Orthopaedic Surgeons, 2004, pp 196-201.)

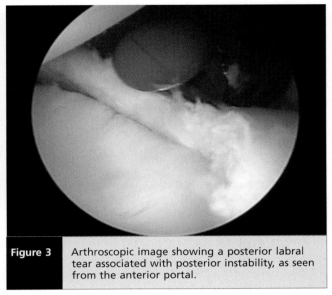

Figure 3   Arthroscopic image showing a posterior labral tear associated with posterior instability, as seen from the anterior portal.

the patient can maintain flexion and abduction of 80° to 90°. A flattening of the anterior shoulder and a prominence of the coracoid also can occur.

Imaging

An adequate axillary radiograph can be painful and difficult to obtain if the patient has a posterior dislocation, but often this is the most valuable diagnostic view. If there is concern about bony involvement, CT can provide the information necessary to guide treatment. Although earlier studies reported 50% to 79% rates of missed diagnosis, a rate of only 9% was reported in a contained population at one trauma center.[33] The protocol in this study used orthogonal shoulder views with either a Velpeau or a modified axial view.

An AP radiograph shows a few signs characteristic of a posterior dislocation, including the light bulb sign, in which a loss of the normal tuberosity outline caused by internal rotation is seen (**Figure 2**); and a break in the Moloney line, which is analogous to the Shenton line in the hip. These can be subtle findings, however. To improve visualization, ultrasonography was used to diagnose a posterior dislocation in a small case study of two patients who could not tolerate an axial radiograph.[35] This technique requires further analysis in a controlled setting before it can be recommended for use.

MRI can provide additional information in a patient with posterior dislocation. A retrospective MRI review of 36 patients with a first-time posterior dislocation found that 31 (86%) had a reverse Hill-Sachs lesion and 11 (31%) had a reverse osseous Bankart lesion.[36] Seven patients (19%) had a full-thickness rotator cuff tear (four supraspinatus, three infraspinatus, and five subscapularis tears), and 21 (58%) had a posterior cap-

sulolabral complex tear (10 posterior labral sleeve avulsions and 11 reverse Bankart lesions; **Figure 3**).

Treatment Decision Making

A large spectrum of treatments is available for a posterior dislocation. The decision is predicated on the answers to several questions: Is the dislocation reduced? How long has the shoulder been dislocated? How often does dislocation occur? How does dislocation occur? Is there a bone lesion on the humeral head or the glenoid? What is the patient's functional level?

Certain patient characteristics can influence treatment decisions and outcomes. For example, contact athletes have a higher than average recurrence of posterior instability.[37] A retrospective review found that patients treated within the first 4 weeks of dislocation had significantly better outcome scores than those treated after 4 weeks.[31] This finding underscores the necessity of early diagnosis and treatment, although the definition of early treatment has not been clearly defined. Some experts define the duration of acute dislocation and early treatment as less than 3 weeks, and others believe that 6 weeks is a more appropriate cutoff point. Decisions must be made on a case-by-case basis.

Closed or Arthroscopic Reduction

Reduction is an important first step in the management of a posterior shoulder dislocation. If necessary, general anesthesia is administered. The presence of a bony lesion should be determined ahead of time. Closed reduction was highly successful under general anesthesia in seven patients with a humeral head defect as large as 30%.[38] The technique for reducing a posterior dislocated shoulder involves cross-body traction of a flexed, adducted, and internally rotated arm. Gentle posterior manipulation of the head can guide it over the posterior aspect of the glenoid. All 120 posterior shoulder

2: Instability and Athletic Injuries

dislocations that were diagnosed within 10 days of injury could be reduced by closed means.[33]

If closed reduction cannot be achieved, an arthroscopic reduction can be attempted.[39] A switching stick is brought in posteriorly and placed superomedial to the head. The anterior glenoid rim is used as a fulcrum, with the force placed through the rotator cuff rather than the humeral articular surface.

Nonsurgical Management

Nonsurgical management is the treatment of choice in the absence of significant osseous pathology or if the patient has low functional demands. A retrospective review of 35 patients with a posterior dislocation found that the 6 patients who were nonsurgically treated had significantly higher outcome scores than those who were surgically treated.[31] This study has an inherent bias because the more severe injuries were treated surgically, but the good outcome scores of the patients who were nonsurgically treated nonetheless provide an important piece of information.

Nonsurgical management should be the first-line treatment of a patient with an acute shoulder dislocation. In one protocol for a reduced posterior shoulder dislocation, patients were maintained in a sling that created slight abduction and neutral rotation.[33] Pendulum exercises were done for 20 minutes per day for the first 4 weeks, after which the use of the sling was discontinued and physical therapy was initiated. The patients had only slight deficits in internal rotation at 2-year follow-up.

Surgical Management

If nonsurgical care of a posterior dislocation is unsuccessful, surgical intervention should be considered. The first decision point involves an analysis of humeral head and glenoid bone loss. The humeral head defect has a larger role in recurrent instability after a posterior dislocation than after an anterior dislocation. The size of the defect must be evaluated to determine the appropriate treatment. If a patient experiences a symptomatic or recurrent posterior dislocation and there is no bone loss, a primary soft-tissue reconstruction can be completed, as for an anterior dislocation. Good results were reported when arthroscopic posterior shoulder stabilization involved a vertical shift of the posterior capsule and an anatomic repair of the labrum.[40] Commonly, however, a bone lesion is present and must be treated using one of the following techniques: elevation of the humeral defect, allograft replacement of the defect, tendon augmentation, or arthroplasty.

Elevation of the Humeral Defect

The humeral head defect can have an important role in the pathologic instability of a posterior dislocation. The choice of procedure is influenced by the percentage of the humeral head affected. Some experts have suggested that defects smaller than 25% to 30% can be treated with humeral head defect elevation, and those that involve 25% to 40% can be treated with allograft reconstruction. Larger defects should be treated with shoulder arthroplasty. However, there are no definitive studies to support such algorithms. Case studies have reported the use of a variety of treatment modalities in a wide range of defect sizes using multiple techniques involving arthroscopy, subscapularis takedown, or visualization through the rotator cuff interval. For example, good results were reported when an open approach was used for defects larger than 40%, in the absence of other pathology.[41] Transhumeral bioabsorbable screw fixation was visualized through the open rotator cuff interval after reduction of an impression fracture involving 50% of the humeral head.[42] The two patients had a good clinical result with no radiographic signs of osteoarthritis or necrosis at a mean 26-month follow-up.

These reduction techniques for large defects do have the potential to fail, however. In a patient with a posterior dislocation, the 40% humeral head defect was elevated arthroscopically, packed with bone allograft, and fixed with two cancellous screws.[43] Initial postoperative imaging studies showed good restoration of the humeral articular surface; however, at 6-month follow-up resorption of the graft and depression of the defect had occurred, necessitating humeral head replacement.

After elevation and reduction of the articular segment, a variety of constructs can be used to support the reduction. Autograft iliac crest was used to support an unstable articular reduction of an acute locked posterior dislocation.[44] The articular segment was prepared with chondral flakes and fixed with resorbable polydioxanone pins and fibrin glue. Six patients with a posterior shoulder dislocation and an impression fracture of 20% to 40% were treated by elevating the cartilage in one piece and filling the defect with cancellous bone (from the iliac crest alone or in combination with cancellous allograft).[45] The cartilage was fixed with suture anchors implanted under the affected area. At 63-month follow-up, two patients had an excellent result, and four had a good result. One patient had a redislocation, which was treated with the same method. Other options to support the articular segment include the use of cancellous screws, bioabsorbable screws, allograft, and bone cement.

Allograft Replacement of Defect

Allograft replacement is the treatment of choice for a large humeral defect or comminuted articular segments, if the humeral head is viable. A wedge resection in the afflicted region is replaced by a size-matched wedge from a humeral or a femoral head allograft. In six patients who underwent allograft reconstruction of a 40% humeral head defect, the dislocation was caused by a seizure in three patients and by trauma in three patients.[46] Five of the dislocations were initially reduced but recurred. A matched segment of an allograft humeral head was used in all patients 7 to 8 weeks after injury. At final follow-up of 62 months, no patients had recurrent instability. Four patients had full, pain-free motion, but two patients continued to have decreased motion and pain.

Although a humeral head defect is more common with posterior dislocation, a glenoid defect also can be successfully managed with an allograft, in a manner similar to the bone-block techniques for anterior instability. An open posterior approach to the glenoid with detachment of the deltoid was used in eight patients, with tricortical iliac crest bone grafting to the posteroinferior glenoid.[47] At 34-month follow-up, none of the patients had a recurrence of instability, although all patients continued to have intermittent pain. Three patients required a secondary operation for screw removal or reattachment of the deltoid. An arthroscopic technique has been used for placing a posterior bone block through the rotator cuff interval.[48] Thus, allograft can be used as needed for both humeral and glenoid defects.

Tendon Augmentation

Subscapularis augmentation of an anterior humeral head defect was first described in 1952.[49,50] Through multiple modifications over the years, this technique has evolved into an arthroscopic approach that does not require transection of the subscapularis. However, the use of both types of procedures has significantly decreased in recent years because of the success of bone reconstruction. A retrospective comparison found that tendon augmentation with anatomic allograft or autograft reconstruction led to consistently inferior outcomes; this finding was consistent with previously reported results.[31]

Arthroplasty

Primary arthroplasty for a posterior shoulder dislocation can be an effective option for patients with a large humeral head defect as well as patients who are older than approximately 60 years and have a low activity level. Encouraging functional improvement results have been reported for these patients, but the results continue to be inferior to those of primary arthroplasty for patients with osteoarthritis.[51]

The patient may have multiple areas of pathology. A 77-year-old man with an atraumatic posterior shoulder dislocation had a 40% humeral head defect and 30% loss of the posteroinferior glenoid. He was treated with hemiarthroplasty and a posterior glenoid bone block created from the resected humeral head. A deltopectoral approach was used, with percutaneously placed posterior screws.[52]

Chronic Shoulder Dislocations

Researchers have used different time points to define chronic dislocation, ranging from 24 hours to 6 weeks. The recommended definition is 3 weeks after initial dislocation.[53] Unrecognized glenohumeral dislocation leading to chronic dislocation is relatively uncommon, although fracture often is present. A review of 61 chronic dislocations found that 50% had an associated fracture, 33% had neurologic injury, and 28% were posterior.[54] Other studies found that a chronic dislocation had been seen by 50% of the orthopaedic surgeons in practice 5 to 10 years, 70% of those in practice for 10 to 20 years, and 90% of those in practice more than 20 years.[30,54] Although chronic dislocation is rare, the orthopaedic surgeon should be knowledgeable about the diagnosis and the management options.

Any concomitant shoulder pathology must be recognized in a chronic shoulder dislocation. Often there is degeneration of the humeral head articular cartilage. Significant soft-tissue contractures can develop, with adhesions between the humeral head and the adjacent neurovascular structures in an anterior dislocation. A concomitant rotator cuff tear (sometimes massive) may influence shoulder stability, and a subscapularis rupture with biceps dislocation also can occur. Glenohumeral bone deficiency can significantly influence joint stability; anteroinferior glenoid bone loss is common in anterior dislocation, and anterosuperior humeral defect is common with posterior dislocation. These defects in the humeral head and the glenoid can create engaging lesions that make reduction difficult. In general, a chronic shoulder dislocation is challenging to treat. The patient's functional status, surgical morbidity, and coexisting pathology are used to define the treatment plan.

Chronic Posterior Dislocation

Many patients with a chronic posterior dislocation are addicted to alcohol or are older than approximately 70 years. The patient's inability to provide a clear history may contribute to an initial misdiagnosis. In addition, a patient with a history of seizures or with multitrauma should be thoroughly evaluated. Other medical issues, functional status, and expectations should be determined because they will factor into the eventual treatment plan. The patient may describe initial shoulder pain that dissipated and allowed resumption of waist-level activity. However, the patient will continue to lack external rotation. The physical examination findings are similar to those for an acute posterior dislocation. However, in a chronic dislocation, the humeral head may have remodeled sufficiently to allow a functional range of motion (**Figure 4**).

The imaging studies are the same as for acute dislocations. The axillary lateral view provides important information on the amount of glenoid involvement and any impaction of the humeral head. The extent of impaction can be quantified by estimating the size of the defect and comparing it to the arc of the articular surface. All images should be examined to detect fracture. If osseous involvement is detected, CT is recommended to evaluate the amount and the location of bony destruction.

2: Instability and Athletic Injuries

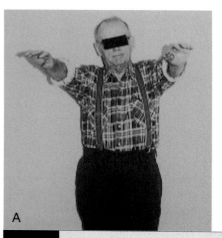 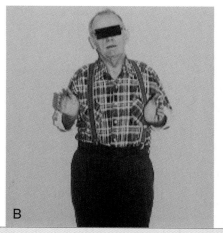 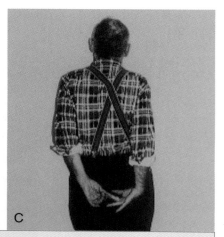

Figure 4 Photographs showing a 60-year-old man with chronic bilateral posterior dislocation. He had a functional range of motion with limitations in forward flexion (**A**), external rotation (**B**), and internal rotation (**C**). (Adapted with permission from Zuckerman JD: *Comprehensive Care of Orthopaedic Injuries in the Elderly.* Baltimore, MD, Urban & Schwarzenberg, 1990, pp 287-288.)

Management

Despite the anatomic deformity and severe loss of glenohumeral rotation, a chronic posterior dislocation can be surprisingly well tolerated, especially in a patient who is older than 70 years or debilitated. Such a patient may regain a range of motion sufficient for performing activities of daily living with minimal pain. It is important to balance the surgical morbidity with the expected outcomes. Nonsurgical management should be considered for a patient who has uncontrolled seizures, a patient who will be unable or unwilling to undergo postoperative rehabilitation, or a patient who is free of pain and has low functional demands. For these patients, the risks of surgery exceed the potential benefit of an improved outcome.

Numerous soft-tissue, osseous, and prosthetic procedures are available for a patient who is able to benefit from surgical intervention. The choice of procedure is influenced by several patient factors and the concomitant pathology: patient age, functional demands, time since injury, glenoid bone quality and loss, and humeral bone quality and loss. Time since injury and the type of operation were found to be the most important predictors of the outcome.[31] Patients treated within 4 weeks of the initial dislocation had relatively high outcome scores, as did patients treated with an anatomic restoration (humeral head elevation or allograft). However, this study had inherent bias, in that patients with severe injury often received a hemiarthroplasty and were not good candidates for allograft reconstruction.

Closed Reduction

Closed reduction can be done if the dislocation is less than 3 weeks old, the humeral head impaction is less than 25%, and there are no other humeral fractures. Some experts believe that reduction can be attempted if the dislocation is less than 6 weeks old and radiographs show a humeral head defect of less than 20% of the articular surface.[55] In one study, reduction was successful in 19 of 30 dislocations no more than 4 weeks old, but it was successful in only 1 of 10 dislocations older than 4 weeks.[54]

An attempted reduction should be gentle because of the chronicity of the injury. General anesthesia should be used for complete relaxation. Controlled internal rotation helps stretch the posterior capsule, and lateral traction allows the humeral head to unlock from the glenoid rim. The glenohumeral joint then can be reduced with controlled external rotation. The arm is braced in slight external rotation (approximately 20°). The point of instability should be noted, and this position should be avoided by using a brace. External rotation is allowed beginning in the early postreduction period.

Surgical Options

Disimpaction and bone grafting of the humeral head defect can be considered if the patient has a relatively acute injury, less than 50% humeral head involvement, and viable articular cartilage.[56] The procedure requires an access window for elevation of the articular segment and support with autograft or allograft.

The currently used procedure for transfer of the subscapularis tendon, which leaves the subscapularis attached to its lesser tuberosity insertion, can be considered if the patient has a relatively small humeral defect (less than 40%).[57,58] This procedure is no longer commonly performed, however, because of superior results when patients are treated with a bony reconstruction procedure.

Allograft reconstruction is the preferred method of treating a defect in a viable humeral head, especially in a relatively young patient. A sized-matched fresh-frozen humeral or femoral head allograft is required for the

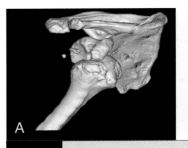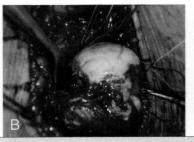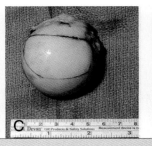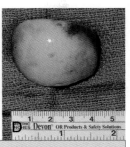

Figure 5 **A,** Three-dimensional CT reconstruction showing a locked anterior dislocation. **B,** Intraoperative photograph showing a large Hill-Sachs defect. **C,** Photograph showing an allograft humeral head. **D,** Photograph showing the allograft segment removed from the humeral head.

reconstruction. Good outcomes were reported at a mean 54-month follow-up in 13 patients with a defect of 25% to 50%.[56]

The indications for shoulder arthroplasty include a defect of more than 50% of the humeral head, severe articular damage, and significant osteopenia. The choice among hemiarthroplasty, total shoulder arthroplasty, and surface replacement can be difficult and must be made on a case-by-case basis. A study of 12 shoulders with a chronic locked posterior dislocation treated with shoulder arthroplasty found that that the 11 patients had improved range of motion after surgery but an average Constant Shoulder Score of 59.4.[51] One patient required revision, and another had severe humeral head elevation.

Chronic Anterior Dislocations

Inspection of the affected and unaffected shoulders in a patient with a chronic anterior dislocation can reveal a loss of the deltoid prominence and squaring of the posterior acromion. A chronic anterior dislocation typically limits the amount of rotation to a significant extent. The arm is held away from the body in external rotation. The amount of pain varies, with only mild pain possible in a patient with a long-standing dislocation. A complete neurovascular examination should be completed and documented to evaluate any axillary nerve or artery injury.

As with a posterior dislocation, several factors influence the indications for surgery, including the presence of a bone defect. In contrast to posterior dislocations, in which the glenoid commonly maintains its structural integrity, a chronic anterior dislocation often is associated with anteroinferior glenoid bone loss. An acute fracture can occur at the time of the dislocation, or progressive attritional bone loss can occur later. The anterior capsular structures often are torn, and reattachment is required to achieve a stable shoulder.

Surgical Treatment

The neurovascular structures must be carefully evaluated during any surgical approach for a chronic anterior dislocation. Often, these structures are adhering to scar tissue, making the dissection difficult. The axillary

nerve should be identified and protected, and a vascular surgeon should be available in case axillary artery injury develops. As for a chronic posterior dislocation, multiple treatment options are available.

Labral repair almost always is a focus in managing an acute anterior dislocation and can be an important component in managing a chronic anterior dislocation. Unreduced chronic shoulder dislocations with a Hill-Sachs lesion of less than 40% were evaluated in eight patients an average 10 weeks after the injury.[59] All patients were treated with open reduction and labral repair using transglenoid suturing. At final follow-up, the average Rowe-Zarin score was 86, and the average losses in forward flexion and external rotation were 18° and 17.5°, respectively. Good results were reported after the same repair was completed arthroscopically.[60]

The glenoid often is involved in a chronic anterior dislocation. If glenoid bone loss is less than 20%, a Bankart repair can be completed, with or without bony augmentation. However, a bony augmentation should be used if the glenoid bone loss is greater than 20%. An autograft, an allograft, or a coracoid transfer can be used.

A lesion involving less than 25% of the humeral head often does not require treatment after reduction, if the shoulder remains stable. A defect larger than 25% should be treated, however. Disimpaction of the defect can be considered if the lesion is smaller than 50%, the articular cartilage remains viable, and the bone stock is good. If the articular segment is not viable, an allograft reconstruction can be considered.[61] In a dislocation of more than 6 months' duration, the bone quality often is poor, and arthroplasty should be considered. A large exposure is required for an allograft reconstruction of a posterolateral humeral head defect from an anterior approach (**Figure 5**). The subscapularis must be completely detached, and maintenance of the anterior humeral circumflex artery to the humeral head is essential.

Any dislocation of more than 6 months' duration may involve irreversible damage to the articular surface. Thus, arthroplasty should be considered if a patient with such a dislocation has a humeral head defect larger than 50%, poor bone quality, or low functional demands. The surgeon should ensure that appropriate

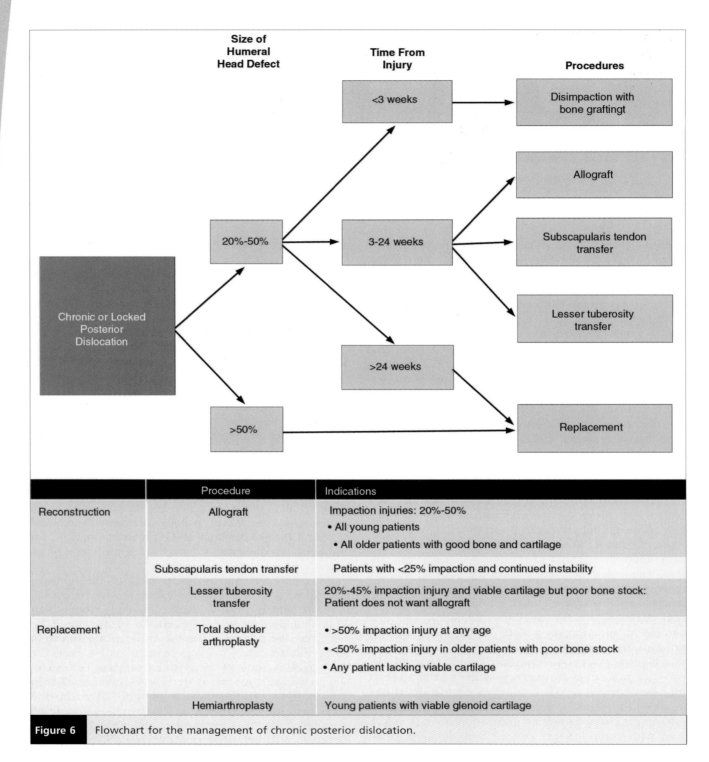

Size of Humeral Head Defect	Time From Injury	Procedures
	<3 weeks	Disimpaction with bone graftingt
20%-50%	3-24 weeks	Allograft
		Subscapularis tendon transfer
		Lesser tuberosity transfer
	>24 weeks	Replacement
>50%		Replacement

Chronic or Locked Posterior Dislocation

	Procedure	Indications
Reconstruction	Allograft	Impaction injuries: 20%-50% • All young patients • All older patients with good bone and cartilage
	Subscapularis tendon transfer	Patients with <25% impaction and continued instability
	Lesser tuberosity transfer	20%-45% impaction injury and viable cartilage but poor bone stock: Patient does not want allograft
Replacement	Total shoulder arthroplasty	• >50% impaction injury at any age • <50% impaction injury in older patients with poor bone stock • Any patient lacking viable cartilage
	Hemiarthroplasty	Young patients with viable glenoid cartilage

Figure 6   Flowchart for the management of chronic posterior dislocation.

retroversion (approximately 30°) is maintained to prevent further anterior instability. Furthermore, with the increase in literature supporting reverse total shoulder arthroplasty in the management of acute proximal humeral fractures, a reverse replacement total shoulder arthroplasty can be considered in the setting of a chronic anterior dislocation. This implant can be especially effective in the setting of significant anterior glenoid bone

loss and subscapularis insufficiency. However, there are no reported results in the contemporary literature of this technique for a chronic anterior dislocation.

In general, the management of chronic dislocations can involve complex algorithms, and multiple patient and injury factors must be considered. The question of which treatment option is best for a particular patient has not been definitely answered. Algorithms for the

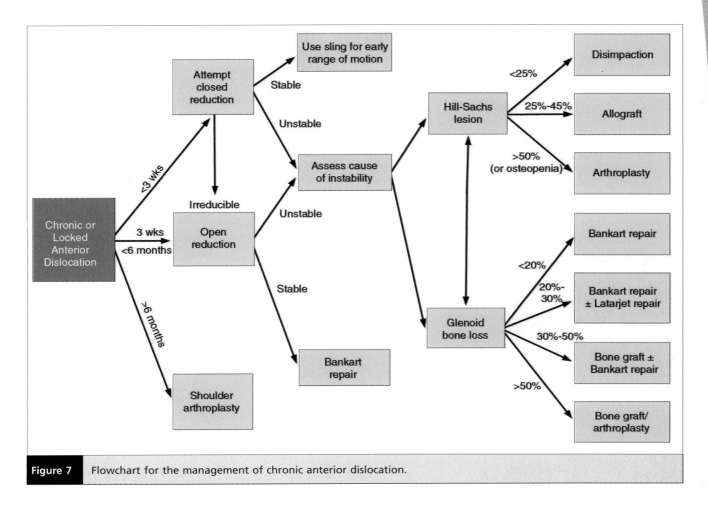

Figure 7   Flowchart for the management of chronic anterior dislocation.

management of a chronic posterior or anterior dislocation (**Figures 6 and 7**) are based on the currently available evidence.

Summary

Acute and chronic shoulder dislocations are complex, and no single paradigm applies to all such conditions. However, some general points can be made. Evidence is building that patients younger than approximately 25 years have a high rate of recurrence after a primary anterior dislocation. As a result, some experts recommend repair after the first event, but others have reported good results after nonsurgical management with a variety of rehabilitation and immobilization protocols. Anterior glenoid and humeral head bone constraints must be evaluated when surgical treatment is considered for anterior instability. If there is significant bone loss, an arthroscopic soft-tissue procedure is likely to fail and the bone lesion may need to be treated.

The available treatment options are significantly different for chronic shoulder dislocations. The percentage of involvement and viability of the humeral head and glenoid must be taken into account. Allograft replacement can be considered if the remaining bone will survive and

support the graft. Many such injuries require prosthetic replacement to achieve functional improvement.

Annotated References

1. Zacchilli MA, Owens BD: Epidemiology of shoulder dislocations presenting to emergency departments in the United States. *J Bone Joint Surg Am* 2010;92(3): 542-549.

   The overall incidence of shoulder dislocations seen in US emergency departments was 23.9 per 100,000. Male sex and young age were the most important risk factors for injury.

2. Owens BD, Duffey ML, Nelson BJ, DeBerardino TM, Taylor DC, Mountcastle SB: The incidence and characteristics of shoulder instability at the United States Military Academy. *Am J Sports Med* 2007;35(7):1168-1173.

   A descriptive epidemiologic study found that traumatic glenohumeral instability events are common in young athletes, and 85% of these events are subluxations.

3. Baker CL, Uribe JW, Whitman C: Arthroscopic evaluation of acute initial anterior shoulder dislocations. *Am J Sports Med* 1990;18(1):25-28.

2: Instability and Athletic Injuries

4. Pouliart N, Marmor S, Gagey O: Simulated capsulo-labral lesion in cadavers: Dislocation does not result from a bankart lesion only. *Arthroscopy* 2006;22(7): 748-754.

5. Shin SJ, Yun YH, Kim DJ, Yoo JD: Treatment of traumatic anterior shoulder dislocation in patients older than 60 years. *Am J Sports Med* 2012;40(4):822-827.

   More than half of the patients older than 60 years with traumatic anterior shoulder dislocation had a rotator cuff tear or an anterior capsulolabral injury. Clinical outcomes were satisfactory with early detection of abnormalities and treatments tailored to associated injuries.

6. Miller SL, Cleeman E, Auerbach J, Flatow EL: Comparison of intra-articular lidocaine and intravenous sedation for reduction of shoulder dislocations: A randomized, prospective study. *J Bone Joint Surg Am* 2002;84(12):2135-2139.

7. Eachempati KK, Dua A, Malhotra R, Bhan S, Bera JR: The external rotation method for reduction of acute anterior dislocations and fracture-dislocations of the shoulder. *J Bone Joint Surg Am* 2004;86(11):2431-2434.

8. Sayegh FE, Kenanidis EI, Papavasiliou KA, Potoupnis ME, Kirkos JM, Kapetanos GA: Reduction of acute anterior dislocations: A prospective randomized study comparing a new technique with the Hippocratic and Kocher methods. *J Bone Joint Surg Am* 2009;91(12): 2775-2782.

   The authors introduced the FARES method for reducing an anterior shoulder dislocation and compared it with the Hippocratic and Kocher methods in 154 patients. The FARES method was found to be more effective, less time consuming, less painful, and effective when performed by one person. Level of evidence: I.

9. Hart WJ, Kelly CP: Arthroscopic observation of capsulolabral reduction after shoulder dislocation. *J Shoulder Elbow Surg* 2005;14(2):134-137.

10. Itoi E, Hatakeyama Y, Kido T, et al: A new method of immobilization after traumatic anterior dislocation of the shoulder: A preliminary study. *J Shoulder Elbow Surg* 2003;12(5):413-415.

11. Liavaag S, Brox JI, Pripp AH, Enger M, Soldal LA, Svenningsen S: Immobilization in external rotation after primary shoulder dislocation did not reduce the risk of recurrence: A randomized controlled trial. *J Bone Joint Surg Am* 2011;93(10):897-904.

    Anterior shoulder dislocation in 188 patients was treated with bracing in internal or external rotation. The rate of recurrence was not lower with immobilization in external rotation. Level of evidence: I.

12. Buss DD, Lynch GP, Meyer CP, Huber SM, Freehill MQ: Nonoperative management for in-season athletes with anterior shoulder instability. *Am J Sports Med* 2004;32(6):1430-1433.

13. Hovelius L, Olofsson A, Sandström B, et al: Nonoperative treatment of primary anterior shoulder dislocation in patients forty years of age and younger: A prospective twenty-five-year follow-up. *J Bone Joint Surg Am* 2008;90(5):945-952.

    At 25-year follow-up, half of the 257 nonsurgically treated anterior shoulder dislocations in patients age 12 to 25 years had not recurred or had become stable.

14. Handoll HH, Almaiyah MA, Rangan A: Surgical versus non-surgical treatment for acute anterior shoulder dislocation. *Cochrane Database Syst Rev* 2004;1: CD004325.

15. Larrain MV, Botto GJ, Montenegro HJ, Mauas DM: Arthroscopic repair of acute traumatic anterior shoulder dislocation in young athletes. *Arthroscopy* 2001; 17(4):373-377.

16. Bottoni CR, Wilckens JH, DeBerardino TM, et al: A prospective, randomized evaluation of arthroscopic stabilization versus nonoperative treatment in patients with acute, traumatic, first-time shoulder dislocations. *Am J Sports Med* 2002;30(4):576-580.

17. Balg F, Boileau P: The instability severity index score: A simple pre-operative score to select patients for arthroscopic or open shoulder stabilisation. *J Bone Joint Surg Br* 2007;89(11):1470-1477.

    In a prospective study of 131 consecutive patients with recurrent anterior shoulder instability who underwent arthroscopic Bankart repair, the risk factors for recurrent instability after surgery were age younger than 20 years, competitive or contact athletic participation, hyperlaxity, a Hills-Sachs lesion, or loss of the sclerotic inferior glenoid contour. A scoring system helped determine whether arthroscopic treatment would be sufficient.

18. Porcellini G, Campi F, Pegreffi F, Castagna A, Paladini P: Predisposing factors for recurrent shoulder dislocation after arthroscopic treatment. *J Bone Joint Surg Am* 2009;91(11):2537-2542.

    In a study of 385 patients who underwent a single arthroscopic Bankart repair, 13% of the patients younger than 22 years and 6.3% of the older patients had a recurrence at 36-month follow-up. The risk factors were age at the time of the first dislocation, male sex, and the time from the first dislocation until surgery. Level of evidence: II.

19. Itoi E, Lee SB, Berglund LJ, Berge LL, An KN: The effect of a glenoid defect on anteroinferior stability of the shoulder after Bankart repair: A cadaveric study. *J Bone Joint Surg Am* 2000;82(1):35-46.

20. Provencher MT, Ghodadra N, LeClere L, Solomon DJ, Romeo AA: Anatomic osteochondral glenoid reconstruction for recurrent glenohumeral instability with glenoid deficiency using a distal tibia allograft. *Arthroscopy* 2009;25(4):446-452.

    A novel technique for the management of glenoid bone loss used a fresh osteochondral distal tibia allograft.

The advantages included improved graft availability compared with fresh glenoid specimens, a cartilaginous interface, excellent conformity of the graft, and no requirement for presurgical sizing. Studies are needed to evaluate long-term efficacy.

21. Warner JJ, Gill TJ, O'Hollerhan JD, Pathare N, Millett PJ: Anatomical glenoid reconstruction for recurrent anterior glenohumeral instability with glenoid deficiency using an autogenous tricortical iliac crest bone graft. *Am J Sports Med* 2006;34(2):205-212.

22. Hovelius L, Sandström B, Olofsson A, Svensson O, Rahme H: The effect of capsular repair, bone block healing, and position on the results of the Bristow-Latarjet procedure (study III): Long-term follow-up in 319 shoulders. *J Shoulder Elbow Surg* 2012;21(5): 647-660.

    The results of the May modification of the Bristow-Latarjet procedure were evaluated in 319 shoulders. The procedure yielded consistently good results, with bony fusion in 83%. Recurrent instability was more likely if the coracoid was placed 1 cm or more medial to the rim. The addition of a horizontal capsular shift to the coracoid transfer improved the recurrence rate and the subjective results.

23. Hovelius L, Vikerfors O, Olofsson A, Svensson O, Rahme H: Bristow-Latarjet and Bankart: A comparative study of shoulder stabilization in 185 shoulders during a seventeen-year follow-up. *J Shoulder Elbow Surg* 2011;20(7):1095-1101.

    Subjective patient evaluations and postoperative stability were better after Bristow-Latarjet repair in 88 consecutive shoulders than after Bankart repair with anchors in 97 shoulders.

24. Boileau P, Villalba M, Héry JY, Balg F, Ahrens P, Neyton L: Risk factors for recurrence of shoulder instability after arthroscopic Bankart repair. *J Bone Joint Surg Am* 2006;88(8):1755-1763.

25. Burkhart SS, De Beer JF: Traumatic glenohumeral bone defects and their relationship to failure of arthroscopic Bankart repairs: Significance of the inverted-pear glenoid and the humeral engaging Hill-Sachs lesion. *Arthroscopy* 2000;16(7):677-694.

26. Sekiya JK, Wickwire AC, Stehle JH, Debski RE: Hill-Sachs defects and repair using osteoarticular allograft transplantation: Biomechanical analysis using a joint compression model. *Am J Sports Med* 2009;37(12): 2459-2466.

    A controlled laboratory study quantified data on the critical defect size of Hill-Sachs lesions requiring surgical repair and the ability of allograft transplantation to restore joint stability. Defects measuring 12.5% of the humeral head have biomechanical effects that may affect joint stability, and defects of 37.5% may benefit from osteoarticular allografting.

27. Kowalsky MS, Levine WN: Traumatic posterior glenohumeral dislocation: Classification, pathoanatomy, diagnosis, and treatment. *Orthop Clin North Am* 2008;

39(4):519-533, viii.

    The classification, pathoanatomy, diagnosis, and treatment of traumatic posterior glenohumeral dislocation were reviewed in detail.

28. Cicak N: Posterior dislocation of the shoulder. *J Bone Joint Surg Br* 2004;86(3):324-332.

29. Kayali C, Agus H, Kalenderer O, Turgut A, Imamoglu T: Overlooked posterior shoulder dislocation: Preoperative and postoperative CT studies (a case report). *Ortop Traumatol Rehabil* 2009;11(2):177-182.

    A sustained posterior shoulder dislocation initially was overlooked. The patient later was treated with a modified McLaughlin procedure.

30. Rowe CR, Zarins B: Chronic unreduced dislocations of the shoulder. *J Bone Joint Surg Am* 1982;64(4): 494-505.

31. Schliemann B, Muder D, Gessmann J, Schildhauer TA, Seybold D: Locked posterior shoulder dislocation: Treatment options and clinical outcomes. *Arch Orthop Trauma Surg* 2011;131(8):1127-1134.

    In a review of 35 patients with a locked posterior shoulder dislocation, the shoulder remained stable after closed reduction in 6 patients, and the treatment was nonsurgical. The treatment was surgical in 29 patients. The patients treated nonsurgically had a slightly better outcome. There was a high correlation between the time to correct diagnosis and outcome.

32. Rouleau DM, Hebert-Davies J: Incidence of associated injury in posterior shoulder dislocation: Systematic review of the literature. *J Orthop Trauma* 2012;26(4): 246-251.

    Of 475 patients (543 shoulders) with posterior shoulder dislocation, 34% had seizures. Injury was associated with 65% of dislocations. Fractures were most common, followed by reverse Hill-Sachs injuries and rotator cuff tears. In the absence of fracture or a reverse Hill-Sachs injury, the risk of rotator cuff tear increased almost fivefold.

33. Robinson CM, Seah M, Akhtar MA: The epidemiology, risk of recurrence, and functional outcome after an acute traumatic posterior dislocation of the shoulder. *J Bone Joint Surg Am* 2011;93(17):1605-1613.

    Posterior glenohumeral dislocations were retrospectively reviewed in 112 patients treated nonsurgically. Survival analysis revealed that recurrent instability occurred within the first year in 17.7%. On multivariable analysis, age younger than 40 years, dislocation during a seizure, and a reverse Hill-Sachs lesion larger than 1.5 cm^3 were predictive of recurrent instability.

34. Singh S, Tan CK, Sinopidis C, Frostick S, Brownson P: Missed posterior dislocation of the shoulder after intramedullary fixation of humeral fractures: A report of three cases. *J Shoulder Elbow Surg* 2009;18(3): e33-e37.

    Three patients had a posterior shoulder dislocation after humeral nailing.

35. Yuen CK, Chung TS, Mok KL, Kan PG, Wong YT: Dynamic ultrasonographic sign for posterior shoulder dislocation. *Emerg Radiol* 2011;18(1):47-51.

    Bedside ultrasonography was used for diagnosing posterior shoulder dislocation. The dynamic ultrasonographic sign of posterior shoulder dislocation is described.

36. Saupe N, White LM, Bleakney R, et al: Acute traumatic posterior shoulder dislocation: MR findings. *Radiology* 2008;248(1):185-193.

    MRI of traumatic posterior shoulder dislocation revealed a reverse Hill-Sachs lesion in 86% of the patients and a posterocaudal labrocapsular lesion in almost 60%. A full-thickness rotator cuff tear occurred in approximately 20%.

37. Bradley JP, Baker CL III, Kline AJ, Armfield DR, Chhabra A: Arthroscopic capsulolabral reconstruction for posterior instability of the shoulder: A prospective study of 100 shoulders. *Am J Sports Med* 2006;34(7): 1061-1071.

38. Duralde XA, Fogle EF: The success of closed reduction in acute locked posterior fracture-dislocations of the shoulder. *J Shoulder Elbow Surg* 2006;15(6):701-706.

39. Verma NN, Sellards RA, Romeo AA: Arthroscopic reduction and repair of a locked posterior shoulder dislocation. *Arthroscopy* 2006;22(11):e1-e5.

40. Savoie FH III, Holt MS, Field LD, Ramsey JR: Arthroscopic management of posterior instability: Evolution of technique and results. *Arthroscopy* 2008;24(4): 389-396.

    In 136 shoulders surgically treated for primary posterior instability, no essential lesion was found for posterior instability. Multiple varied pathologies can be present in a shoulder with posterior instability.

41. Gerber C, Lambert SM: Allograft reconstruction of segmental defects of the humeral head for the treatment of chronic locked posterior dislocation of the shoulder. *J Bone Joint Surg Am* 1996;78(3):376-382.

42. Assom M, Castoldi F, Rossi R, Blonna D, Rossi P: Humeral head impression fracture in acute posterior shoulder dislocation: New surgical technique. *Knee Surg Sports Traumatol Arthrosc* 2006;14(7):668-672.

43. Moroder P, Resch H, Tauber M: Failed arthroscopic repair of a large reverse Hill-Sachs lesion using bone allograft and cannulated screws: A case report. *Arthroscopy* 2012;28(1):138-144.

    A reverse Hill-Sachs lesion affecting more than 40% of the articulating surface was treated arthroscopically using retrograde elevation, bone allografting, and cannulated screw insertion. Postoperative radiographs showed successful reduction of the impacted articulating surface of the humeral head. At 6-month follow-up, the patient had pain and symptoms of a frozen shoulder. Cross-sectional imaging showed necrosis, partial absorption, and loss of reduction of the for-

    merly elevated segment, requiring humeral head replacement.

44. Khayal T, Wild M, Windolf J: Reconstruction of the articular surface of the humeral head after locked posterior shoulder dislocation: A case report. *Arch Orthop Trauma Surg* 2009;129(4):515-519.

    An acute locked posterior shoulder dislocation was successfully treated by reconstructing the articular surface of the humeral head with autologous bone graft from the iliac crest.

45. Bock P, Kluger R, Hintermann B: Anatomical reconstruction for reverse Hill-Sachs lesions after posterior locked shoulder dislocation fracture: A case series of six patients. *Arch Orthop Trauma Surg* 2007;127(7): 543-548.

    In six patients at an average 62-month follow-up, anatomic head reconstruction using spongiotic autograft or allograft proved to be valid for restoring shoulder function and stability.

46. Martinez AA, Calvo A, Domingo J, Cuenca J, Herrera A, Malillos M: Allograft reconstruction of segmental defects of the humeral head associated with posterior dislocations of the shoulder. *Injury* 2008;39(3): 319-322.

    Six men with posterior dislocation of the humeral head underwent surgical allograft treatment for a defect involving at least 40% of the articular surface. At discharge, four patients had no pain, instability, clicking or catching; two had pain, clicking, catching, and stiffness.

47. Barbier O, Ollat D, Marchaland JP, Versier G: Iliac bone-block autograft for posterior shoulder instability. *Orthop Traumatol Surg Res* 2009;95(2):100-107.

    Eight patients with recurrent posterior shoulder instability were treated with a posterior iliac bone-block procedure. All patients recovered normal joint range of motion in abduction and anterior elevation. In three patients, external rotation was limited an average of 20° compared with the opposite side. Only four patients were able to return to their preoperative sports activity level. At a mean 3-year follow-up, 80% had a satisfactory result.

48. Barth J, Grosclaude S, Lädermann A, Denard PJ, Graveleau N, Walch G: Arthroscopic posterior bone graft for posterior instability: The transrotator interval sparing cuff technique. *Tech Shoulder Elbow Surg* 2011;12(3):67-71.

    In a new arthroscopic technique, the bone graft is passed through an anatomic portal, that is, the rotator cuff interval. One patient had a good result after bone graft was passed through the rotator cuff interval before being secured to the posterior glenoid.

49. McLaughlin HL: Posterior dislocation of the shoulder. *J Bone Joint Surg Am* 1952;24-A(3):584-590.

50. McLaughlin HL: Locked posterior subluxation of the shoulder: Diagnosis and treatment. *Surg Clin North*

Am 1963;43:1621-1622.

51. Gavriilidis I, Magosch P, Lichtenberg S, Habermeyer P, Kircher J: Chronic locked posterior shoulder dislocation with severe head involvement. *Int Orthop* 2010;34(1):79-84.

    Retrospective review of 12 shoulder arthroplasties (11 patients) for a locked dislocation found a significant improvement in range of motion for flexion, abduction, and external rotation at a mean 37-month follow-up. There was a negative correlation between the Constant Shoulder Score and number of previous operations, pain, and duration of symptoms.

52. Riggenbach MD, Najarian RG, Bishop JY: Recurrent, locked posterior glenohumeral dislocation requiring hemiarthroplasty and posterior bone block with humeral head autograft. *Orthopedics* 2012;35(2):e277-e282.

    A 77-year-old man with a recurrent posterior shoulder dislocation was treated with humeral hemiarthroplasty and reconstruction of a large posteroinferior glenoid defect using a bone block created from humeral head autograft.

53. Griggs SM, Holloway B, Williams GR Jr, Iannotti JP: *Disorders of the Shoulder Diagnosis and Management.* Philadelphia, PA, Lippincott, Williams & Wilkins, 2006, pp 461-486.

    Chronic dislocations of the shoulder and associated techniques are described.

54. Schulz TJ, Jacobs B, Patterson RL Jr: Unrecognized dislocations of the shoulder. *J Trauma* 1969;9(12):1009-1023.

55. Loebenberg MI, Cuomo F: The treatment of chronic anterior and posterior dislocations of the glenohumeral joint and associated articular surface defects. *Orthop Clin North Am* 2000;31(1):23-34.

56. Diklic ID, Ganic ZD, Blagojevic ZD, Nho SJ, Romeo AA: Treatment of locked chronic posterior dislocation of the shoulder by reconstruction of the defect in the humeral head with an allograft. *J Bone Joint Surg Br* 2010;92(1):71-76.

    At a mean 54-month follow-up after humeral head reconstruction with femoral head allograft, 9 of 13 patients (10 men, 3 women; mean age, 42 years) had no pain or restriction of activities of daily living. No patient had symptoms of shoulder instability. The mean Constant-Murley Shoulder Score was 86.8 (range, 43 to 98).

57. Spencer EE Jr, Brems JJ: A simple technique for management of locked posterior shoulder dislocations: Report of two cases. *J Shoulder Elbow Surg* 2005;14(6):650-652.

58. Delcogliano A, Caporaso A, Chiossi S, Menghi A, Cillo M, Delcogliano M: Surgical management of chronic, unreduced posterior dislocation of the shoulder. *Knee Surg Sports Traumatol Arthrosc* 2005;13(2):151-155.

59. Rouhani A, Navali A: Treatment of chronic anterior shoulder dislocation by open reduction and simultaneous Bankart lesion repair. *Sports Med Arthrosc Rehabil Ther Technol* 2010;2:15.

    Eight patients with a chronic anterior shoulder dislocation underwent open reduction and capsulolabral complex repair an average 10 weeks after injury. Four shoulders were graded as excellent, three as good, and one as fair. All patients were able to perform daily activities with mild or no pain. Outcomes were found to be more favorable than with earlier methods.

60. Galano GJ, Dieter AA, Moradi NE, Ahmad CS: Arthroscopic management of a chronic primary anterior shoulder dislocation. *Am J Orthop (Belle Mead NJ)* 2010;39(7):351-355.

    A 70-year-old woman underwent arthroscopic reduction and labral fixation of a chronically dislocated shoulder.

61. Mehta V: Humeral head plasty for a chronic locked anterior shoulder dislocation. *Orthopedics* 2009;32(1):52.

    A 52-year-old man had a chronic anterior shoulder dislocation with a massive Hill-Sachs lesion. The Hill-Sachs lesion was managed with humeral headplasty performed with an 8-mm anterior cruciate ligament guide adjacent to the lesser tuberosity. The Hill-Sachs lesion was tamped out to restore the contour of the humeral head and backfilled with allograft.

2: Instability and Athletic Injuries

Chapter 8

Recurrent Anterior Shoulder Instability

Brian D. Dierckman, MD   Neil Ghodadra, MD   Daniel J. Solomon, MD   Mark D. Stanley, MD
John W. McNeil II, BA, CDR Matthew T. Provencher, MD, MC, USN

Introduction

The glenohumeral joint is the most commonly dislocated joint in the body. The limited bony constraints of the glenohumeral joint allow a wide range of shoulder motion at the inherent risk of instability. The static and dynamic restraints of the glenohumeral joint provide stability through complex musculoskeletal interactions, and injury to one or more of these restraints tilts the delicate balance of shoulder stability toward instability. Many patients who sustain a first anterior shoulder dislocation regain shoulder stability and do not experience another instability event.[1] However, some patients go on to develop recurrent anterior shoulder instability; young male contact athletes are the most susceptible subset of patients.

The critical role of bone loss in recurrent instability has been elucidated in recent years. This chapter discusses the pathophysiology, the evaluation, and the management of recurrent anterior shoulder instability, with a focus on glenoid and humeral bone loss. The exact roles of glenoid and/or humeral bone loss in recurrent instability are still being defined.

Pathophysiology

With first-time anterior shoulder dislocation, the most common anatomic injury is an avulsion of the anteroinferior labrum and the capsular attachments from the glenoid rim (a Bankart lesion)[2] (**Figure 1**). Concurrently, most patients have a compression fracture of the posterosuperolateral aspect of the humeral head (a

The views expressed in this article are those of the authors and do not reflect the official policy or position of the Department of the Navy, Department of Defense, or United States Government. Neither of the following authors nor any immediate family member has received anything of value from or owns stock in a commercial company or institution related directly or indirectly to the subject of this chapter: Dr. Dierckman, Dr. Ghodadra, Dr. Solomon, Dr. Stanley, Dr. McNeil II, and Dr. Provencher.

Hill-Sachs lesion) as the head forcibly collides with the harder bone of the anteroinferior glenoid rim.[3] However, most initial Hill-Sachs lesions are small, shallow, and not clinically significant (**Figure 2**).

In recurrent instability, the further compromise of the static and dynamic stabilizers of the shoulder contributes to a downward spiral of bone and cartilage loss, often leading to degenerative changes. Several factors in addition to the typical Bankart lesion contribute to recurrent instability, to a varying extent. Glenoid and humeral head bone loss have been recognized as key pathologic features in most patients with recurrent instability. In each dislocation, the humeral head collides with the anterior glenoid, leading to attritional bone loss in the glenoid as well as enlargement of the Hill-Sachs lesion. The inferior glenohumeral ligament (IGHL) complex is further stretched and attenuated, leading to plastic deformation and further weakening of the shoulder's static restraints.[4]

Certain uncommon anatomic findings are seen with relative frequency during imaging evaluation or arthroscopic visualization of patients with recurrent anterior shoulder instability. These include an anterior labral periosteal sleeve avulsion (ALPSA) lesion, a humeral avulsion of the glenohumeral ligament (HAGL), a circumferential or extensive labral tear, and a glenoid labral articular damage (GLAD) lesion.

ALPSA Lesions

As the humeral head dislocates anteriorly, the capsulolabral complex is stripped away from the anteroinferior glenoid. In a typical Bankart lesion the capsulolabral complex detaches from the surrounding periosteum, but in an ALPSA lesion, the capsulolabral complex remains attached to the periosteum, and the entire sleeve of tissue is peeled back medially along the neck of the glenoid. The injured soft tissues heal in a more medial position along the glenoid neck[5] (**Figure 3**).

ALPSA lesions are uncommon with an initial dislocation. One study found that 78% of the patients with an acute dislocation had a Bankart lesion, and 97% of the patients with recurrent dislocation had either a Bankart or an ALPSA lesion.[6] Only patients with recurrent dislocation had an ALPSA lesion.

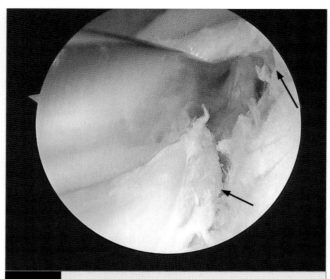

Figure 1 Arthroscopic image of a right shoulder from the anterosuperior portal, with the patient in the lateral decubitus position, showing a typical Bankart (anterior labral) tear *(arrows)*, from approximately the 6 o'clock position inferiorly to the 3 o'clock position anteriorly.

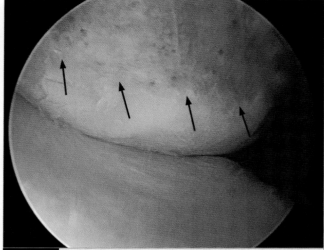

Figure 2 Arthroscopic image of a right shoulder from the posterior portal, with the patient in the beach chair position, showing a Hill-Sachs lesion *(arrows)* that is moderate in size and engages the glenoid with anterior translation and approximately 30° of external rotation.

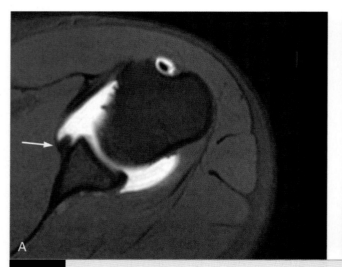

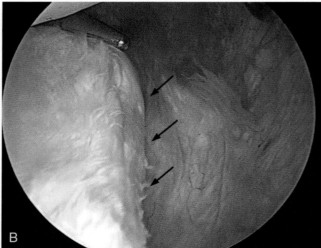

Figure 3 Axial MRA **(A)** and an arthroscopic image from the anterosuperior portal **(B)** showing the same ALPSA lesion *(arrows)*.

HAGL Lesions

The IGHL and the labrum detach from the glenoid as a capsulolabral complex in almost all anterior shoulder dislocations. Uncommonly, the IGHL instead avulses from its attachment onto the humeral neck.[7] The HAGL lesion often is missed and therefore is not appropriately treated. This pattern recently was recognized as a relatively common cause of arthroscopic stabilization surgery failure (**Figure 4**).

Extensive Labral Tears

Recurrent anterior dislocation can cause extensive labral tears as the tear propagates around the glenoid from repetitive trauma.[8] Uncommonly, these extensive lesions result from both anterior and posterior instability events. Initial posterior instability also can lead to circumferential labral tearing. These tears may even propagate around the glenoid to eventually involve the superior labrum, or a superior labrum anterior to posterior (SLAP) lesion may occur at the time of initial injury (**Figure 5**).

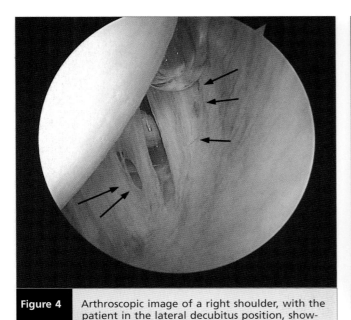

Figure 4 Arthroscopic image of a right shoulder, with the patient in the lateral decubitus position, showing a HAGL tear of the anteroinferior capsule *(arrows)*.

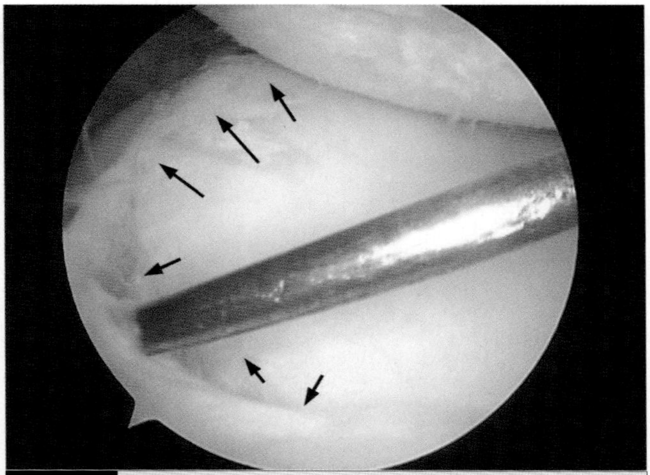

Figure 5 Arthroscopic image of a right shoulder from the posterior portal showing an extensive 180° labral tear. Arrows = anterior labrum, arrowheads = posterior labrum.

GLAD Lesions

Some surgeons believe GLAD lesions form early in the spectrum of osteochondral injuries to the anteroinferior glenoid. If a sufficient adduction force is present when the humeral head dislocates anteriorly, the humeral head is compressed into the glenoid, leading to a glenoid rim fracture. A GLAD lesion involves a sheer force more than a compressive force to the chondrolabral junction, and the result is cartilage loss rather than a bony fracture (**Figure 6**). The original description of GLAD lesions was that of an anterior labral-articular cartilage injury without associated anterior instability. It is important to recognize that a capsulorrhaphy should be avoided if the shoulder otherwise is stable; anterior labral repair with treatment of chondral pathology is preferable.

Bone Loss

A patient with recurrent shoulder instability almost always has osseous injury to the glenoid and/or the humeral head. Understanding and appropriately treating irregularities in the osseous architecture of the glenohumeral joint are critical to the overall success of surgical treatment of glenohumeral instability. Bone loss in recurrent anterior instability must be considered a bipolar phenomenon because most patients have varying bone loss in both the glenoid and the humeral head.

Glenoid Bone Loss

The integrity of the glenoid osseous architecture is one of the most critical factors affecting the outcome of shoulder instability surgery. Anteroinferior glenoid bone loss decreases the contact area between the humeral head and the glenoid, diminishing the ability of

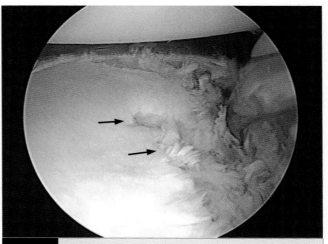

Figure 6 Arthroscopic image of a right shoulder from the anterosuperior portal, with the patient in the lateral decubitus position, showing a GLAD lesion *(arrows)*.

the glenoid to resist humeral head shear forces.[9] Anterior bone loss also reduces the concave morphology of the glenoid, further diminishing the stabilizing forces of concavity-compression as well as the buttress effect of the glenoid.[9,10]

Several different glenoid injury patterns have been reported, and no distinct glenoid bone loss model has been established. Acute glenoid injury can range from a large fracture resulting from a significant axial loading injury to a small bony avulsion occurring as the labroligamentous complex displaces from the glenoid during

2: Instability and Athletic Injuries

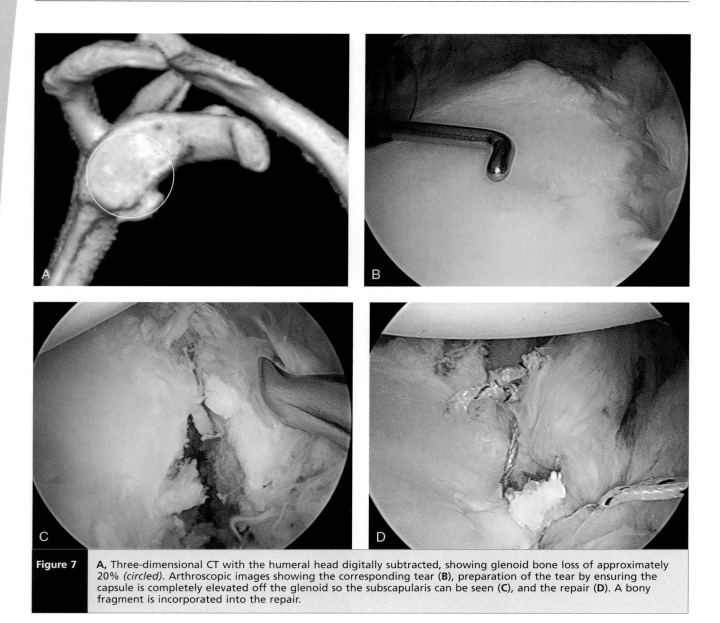

Figure 7 A, Three-dimensional CT with the humeral head digitally subtracted, showing glenoid bone loss of approximately 20% *(circled)*. Arthroscopic images showing the corresponding tear (**B**), preparation of the tear by ensuring the capsule is completely elevated off the glenoid so the subscapularis can be seen (**C**), and the repair (**D**). A bony fragment is incorporated into the repair.

a rotational shear injury. Chronic, attritional bone loss also occurs in different ways, from blunting or smoothing of the anterior rim after a compression injury to repetitive shearing and erosion of the anterior edge of the glenoid. One study reported that more than 50% of the patients had erosive glenoid bone loss without visible bone fragments only 15 months after an initial dislocation.[11]

Regardless of the mechanism of injury, recurrent dislocation compromises the already-limited bony constraints of the shoulder. Several studies have found that glenoid bone loss is the most common cause of failure in arthroscopic shoulder stabilization.[9,12] This finding serves to emphasize the importance of recognizing glenoid bone loss in developing and executing an appro-

priate surgical plan. Repetitive injury can lead to flattening or even reversal of the shape of the glenoid cavity and the creation of an inverted pear appearance of the glenoid (**Figure 7**). One study reported a significant increase in the failure rate of arthroscopic repair in patients who had an inverted pear glenoid.[9] The rate was 89% in a subgroup of young contact athletes.

Hill-Sachs Lesions

Hill-Sachs lesions occur as the relatively soft cancellous bone of the posterosuperolateral humeral head contacts the hard cortical bone of the anteroinferior glenoid during an anterior instability event. The Hill-Sachs lesion is common in recurrent anterior shoulder dislocation; in one study, it was found in 100% of the patients.[2]

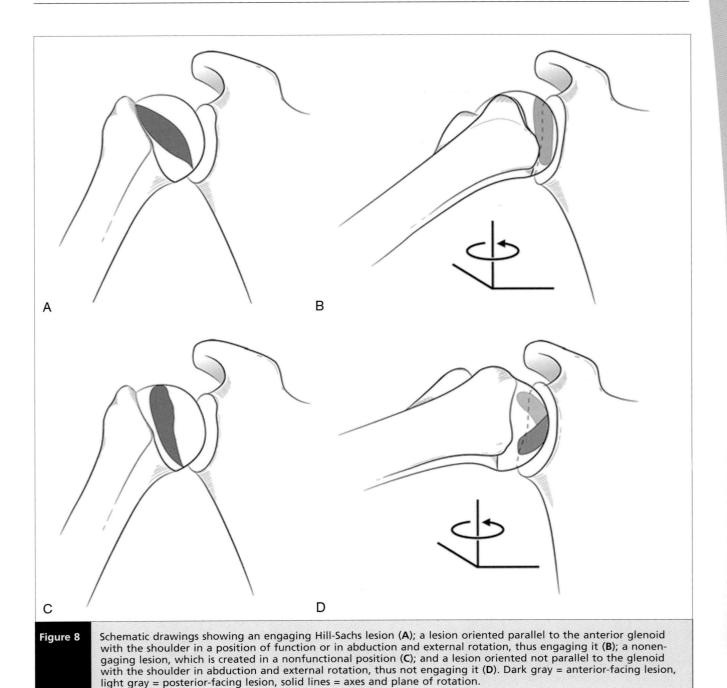

| Figure 8 | Schematic drawings showing an engaging Hill-Sachs lesion (**A**); a lesion oriented parallel to the anterior glenoid with the shoulder in a position of function or in abduction and external rotation, thus engaging it (**B**); a nonengaging lesion, which is created in a nonfunctional position (**C**); and a lesion oriented not parallel to the glenoid with the shoulder in abduction and external rotation, thus not engaging it (**D**). Dark gray = anterior-facing lesion, light gray = posterior-facing lesion, solid lines = axes and plane of rotation. |

Most Hill-Sachs lesions are not clinically problematic, but a limited number will contribute to instability. Lesion size and engagement are widely considered the two most important factors in the treatment of Hill-Sachs lesions.[9] Deep and/or broad lesions are most likely to require treatment.[3] Lesion location and orientation also should be considered (**Figure 8**). Several classification systems have been described, but none has been validated or recognized as the most clinically relevant (**Table 1**).

The concept of the glenoid track recently was introduced.[13] In a cadaver model, the contact area between the humeral head and the glenoid was measured at different degrees of abduction and external rotation. Based on the results, the researchers described an area on the humeral head that contacts the glenoid during abduction and external rotation maneuvers. If the Hill-Sachs lesion lies within this glenoid track, it will contact the glenoid and not engage. With glenoid bone loss, the glenoid track decreases in size and the Hill-Sachs lesion is more likely to be outside the track and at increased risk of engagement, leading to instability. Clinical studies are needed to validate this promising theory.

Table 1

Classification Systems for Hill-Sachs Lesions

System	Visualization	Description
Rowe et al[53]	Axillary radiograph	Mild: 2 cm long, ≤ 0.3 cm deep Moderate: 2 to 4 cm long, 0.3 to 1 cm deep Severe: 4 cm long, ≥ 1 cm deep
Calandra et al[54]	Direct	Grade I: confined to articular cartilage Grade II: extension into subchondral bone Grade III: large subchondral defect
Franceschi et al[55]	Direct	Grade I: cartilaginous Grade II: bony scuffing Grade III: hatchet fracture
Flatow and Warner[29]	Direct	Grade I: clinically insignificant, < 20% Grade II: variably significant, 20% to 40% Grade III: clinically significant, > 40%
Hall et al[56]	Stryker notch radiograph	Extent of 180° articular arc involvement (percentage)
Richards et al[57]	Axillary MRI	Extent of axillary degree involvement (anterior articular margin = 0°)

Clinical Evaluation of Recurrent Anterior Instability

A thorough patient history is critical for characterizing the etiology of instability and selecting the ideal treatment. Clues are provided as to the anatomic cause of the instability by the type and the magnitude of the initial injury (for example, a football injury or a ground-level fall) and subsequent instability events, the trend of these events (are they becoming more frequent or initiated by a lower energy mechanism?), the position of the arm at the time of injury, and the ease of relocation (is self-reduction possible or is emergency department reduction required?). A patient whose shoulder initially was dislocated during football playing but now dislocates during sleep or a patient who has instability symptoms during midranges of motion is likely to have significant glenoid and/or humeral bone loss.

History

Relatively young age is a significant risk factor for recurrence. Patients younger than 30 years have a much higher rate of subsequent dislocation than older patients.[14] A 55.7% recurrence rate within the first 2 years of an initial dislocation was reported in a study of 252 patients age 15 to 35 years, and boys at age 15 years had an 86% probability of recurrence.[15] A study of 105 patients found that 64% of the patients younger than 20 years but only 6% of the patients older than 40 years had a redislocation within 6 years.[16] A Markov decision model recently was used to predict shoulder stability after an initial anterior shoulder dislocation.[17] The model was internally and externally validated against high-level clinical studies and was found to predict that an 18-year-old man has a 77% chance of de-

veloping recurrent instability within 1 year and a 32% chance of stability at 10 years. Patients who underwent surgical intervention were included in the model.

Certain activities substantially increase the risk of shoulder dislocation, including contact sports such as football, rugby, basketball, lacrosse, and martial arts; military training such as hand-to-hand drills and obstacle course training; climbing; whitewater kayaking; and other sports or activities during which the patient's arm may be forcibly abducted and externally rotated.[18] Population studies have reported annual incidence rates widely ranging from 8.2 per 100,000 to 28.3 per 1,000. The overall incidence of dislocation in a select group of young, active individuals (active-duty US military personnel) was 1.69 per 1,000 person-years.[19] The incidence in men was 1.82 compared with 0.90 for women. An earlier study of US Military Academy cadets found that the incidence of instability events (subluxations and dislocations) was 28.3 per 1,000.[14] All initial anterior shoulder dislocations were recorded over a 10-year period in a more heterogeneous population composed of the residents of Olmstead County, Minnesota.[20] The overall incidence was 8.2 per 100,000 person years.

Physical Examination

A standard shoulder examination for laxity and instability should be performed. Specific attention should be given to findings that suggest significant instability and bone loss, including midrange apprehension (at 45° abduction with initiation of external rotation), apprehension at lower degrees of abduction with external rotation beyond 30°, a shoulder that is easily dislocated but requires reduction force during examination under anesthesia, a palpable clunk or catching sensation (suggesting Hill-Sachs lesion engagement), or a shoulder

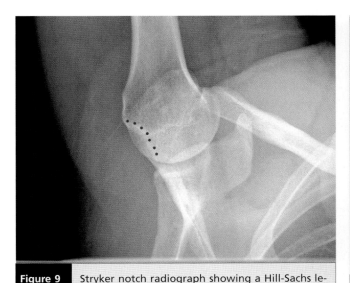

| Figure 9 | Stryker notch radiograph showing a Hill-Sachs lesion *(dotted line)*. |

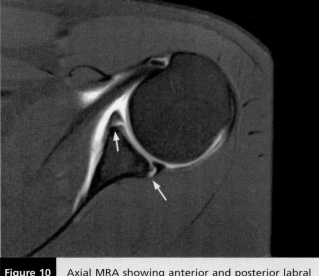

| Figure 10 | Axial MRA showing anterior and posterior labral tears *(arrows)*. |

with more than 90° of external rotation with the arm at the side (usually bilateral and often associated with generalized ligamentous laxity).

Scapular dynamics should be carefully evaluated because many patients have poor scapular control after repetitive shoulder injury. If scapular mechanics are not restored, surgical repair will be futile. Positional or volitional dislocation also must be identified because surgical repair of a lesion is unlikely to withstand the substantive muscular forces, leading to instability in such a patient.

Shoulder instability may develop in a patient with greater than normal shoulder laxity, often resulting from a trivial injury. These patients have a relatively high risk of recurrence after an initial dislocation.[12] The surgeon should suspect and evaluate for hyperlaxity (often bilateral) in a patient whose initial dislocation occurred with minimal trauma.[12] Before surgery is considered, the patient should undergo appropriate rehabilitation that focuses on strengthening the dynamic stabilizers, including the rotator cuff and the periscapular musculature. The surgeon may consider using the Gagey hyperabduction assessment, which suggests inferior capsular attenuation from recurrent dislocations.[21]

Imaging

Bone loss of the glenoid and/or the humeral head almost always is seen in a patient with recurrent shoulder instability and is the most common cause of failure in arthroscopic stabilization procedures. Radiologic and arthroscopic methods of measuring glenoid bone loss have been reported. It is preferable to assess the amount of glenoid bone loss before surgery, using radiography as well as advanced imaging modalities, to allow appropriate preoperative planning and coordination of care. If significant bone loss is detected, the planned surgery is likely to be changed to a bone-restorative procedure (such as a Latarjet, a distal tibial allograft, or an iliac crest allograft procedure).

Radiographs

Standard radiographs (AP, axillary, and scapular Y views) should be obtained for every patient. The West Point and Stryker notch views also may be helpful. The West Point view improves visualization of the anteroinferior glenoid. Some surgeons believe that radiographs are sufficient to screen for glenoid bone loss.[18] Any abnormalities should be further evaluated with advanced studies, however. Humeral bone loss also can be assessed with radiographs, specifically with an AP external rotation view of the shoulder.[12] The Stryker notch view provides improved visualization of a Hill-Sachs lesion (**Figure 9**).

Magnetic Resonance Imaging

High-quality MRI, with or without magnetic resonance arthrography (MRA), is helpful for imaging the capsule, the labrum, and the rotator cuff. Specific lesions of the capsule, including HAGL lesions and capsular redundancy, also can be identified. MRA is especially beneficial if a SLAP lesion or an extensive labral tear is suspected or after an unsuccessful stabilization procedure or recurrence of dislocation (**Figure 10**). Glenoid and humeral head bone loss can be seen on MRI but is more accurately assessed with CT.[22]

Computed Tomography

CT with three-dimensional reconstruction and humeral head subtraction is the gold standard imaging study for evaluating glenoid bone loss.[23] MRI and MRA may not provide optimal differentiation between labrum and bone, leading to underestimation of the amount of

2: Instability and Athletic Injuries

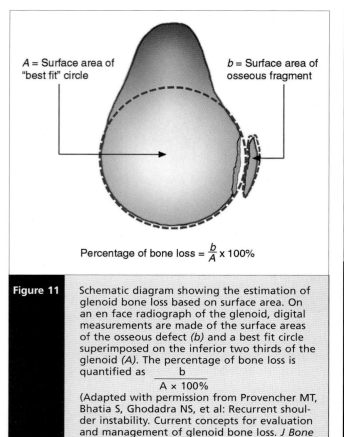

$$\text{Percentage of bone loss} = \frac{b}{A} \times 100\%$$

Figure 11	Schematic diagram showing the estimation of glenoid bone loss based on surface area. On an en face radiograph of the glenoid, digital measurements are made of the surface areas of the osseous defect (b) and a best fit circle superimposed on the inferior two thirds of the glenoid (A). The percentage of bone loss is quantified as $\frac{b}{A} \times 100\%$ (Adapted with permission from Provencher MT, Bhatia S, Ghodadra NS, et al: Recurrent shoulder instability. Current concepts for evaluation and management of glenoid bone loss. J Bone Joint Surg Am 2010;92(suppl 2);133-151.)

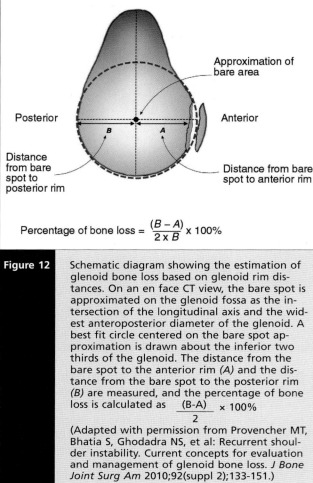

$$\text{Percentage of bone loss} = \frac{(B - A)}{2 \times B} \times 100\%$$

Figure 12	Schematic diagram showing the estimation of glenoid bone loss based on glenoid rim distances. On an en face CT view, the bare spot is approximated on the glenoid fossa as the intersection of the longitudinal axis and the widest anteroposterior diameter of the glenoid. A best fit circle centered on the bare spot approximation is drawn about the inferior two thirds of the glenoid. The distance from the bare spot to the anterior rim (A) and the distance from the bare spot to the posterior rim (B) are measured, and the percentage of bone loss is calculated as $\frac{(B-A)}{2} \times 100\%$ (Adapted with permission from Provencher MT, Bhatia S, Ghodadra NS, et al: Recurrent shoulder instability. Current concepts for evaluation and management of glenoid bone loss. J Bone Joint Surg Am 2010;92(suppl 2);133-151.)

bone loss. CT also allows more accurate evaluation of glenoid version and dysplasia, which are uncommon causes of shoulder instability but should be screened for in a patient who has undergone an unsuccessful procedure or has bilateral instability.

Several methods of assessing glenoid bone loss on CT and with arthroscopy have been published, but no method has been widely accepted over others. It is important to understand the limitations of these methods. The use of arthroscopic assessment of bone loss prevents precise preoperative planning because the surgeon must be prepared to immediately treat the pathology with the appropriate arthroscopic or open technique.

A cadaver study found that the inferior two thirds of the glenoid has the shape of a true circle, and subsequent methods of bone loss measurement have been based on this model.[24] The center of the circle is roughly correlated with the anatomic bare spot. The most precise method for determining the percentage of glenoid bone loss is based on surface area measurements[25] (Figure 11). Using digital imaging software, the area of the osseous defect is divided by the total surface area of the true circle. Although accurate, this method is not commonly used. Most surgeons (including the authors of this chapter) prefer to use the glenoid rim measurement method for CT and arthroscopic measurement[26] (Figure 12). The distances from the bare

spot to the anterior rim and the posterior rim are measured, and the anterior-rim distance is subtracted from the posterior-rim distance. This figure is divided by the diameter of the circle to determine the percentage of bone loss. Recent work has shown that the bare spot is slightly anterior to the exact center of the true circle, so this method may overestimate bone loss.[27] Other techniques are being investigated, including a model based on the secant chord theory.[28]

The measurement and the classification of humeral head defects have been less thoroughly investigated. The most commonly used system grades the severity of the lesion based on the percentage of articular surface involved.[29] A grade I lesion involves less than 20%, a grade II lesion involves 20% to 40%, and a grade III lesion involves more than 40% of the articular surface.

Treatment and Outcomes

The ultimate goal of surgery is to provide the patient with a stable and functional shoulder, with minimal risk of arthropathy and a safe return to desired activities. The patient's age, anticipated postoperative activity level, and extent of glenoid and/or humeral bone loss are three of the most important factors to consider when developing a patient-specific treatment plan.

Nonsurgical Management

Nonsurgical management is of limited benefit for most patients with recurrent instability. Nonetheless, surgery may not be the preferred treatment in a patient who is older than approximately 50 years and has low physical demands, has a significant medical comorbidity such as uncontrolled seizures, or will be unable to complete the tedious postoperative rehabilitation process. Also, it is important to evaluate for a rotator cuff tear in any patient older than 40 years who has shoulder instability. Nonsurgical treatment should focus on strengthening the dynamic stabilizers of the shoulder, including the rotator cuff and the periscapular muscles.

In-season athletes are a unique and challenging group of patients. These patients often desire to return to competitive play as quickly as possible and are willing to risk redislocation. They can be successfully treated with a brace to limit at-risk external rotation positions, with surgery delayed until the off-season.[30]

Surgical Management

No clear algorithm has been developed to treat the wide range of pathology in recurrent dislocation, but general guidelines aid in selecting specific treatment based on the patient's unique history, examination, and imaging findings. Instability resulting from bone loss of the glenoid and the humeral head should be considered as a continuum because these conditions commonly occur in combination and not as isolated lesions. One patient may have a small, shallow Hill-Sachs lesion combined with 30% attritional glenoid bone loss; another patient may have only minimal glenoid bone loss but a large, engaging Hill-Sachs lesion; and a third patient may have 20% glenoid bone loss with a medium-size engaging Hill-Sachs lesion. Each patient with recurrent anterior shoulder instability must be carefully and individually assessed to determine the cause of the instability, and the clues will help in formulating a patient-specific surgical plan. This approach can optimize patient outcomes while avoiding overtreatment or undertreatment, which can result if a nonspecific algorithm is followed. Every patient should receive a thorough and detailed examination under anesthesia. The ease and the direction of humeral head translation should be carefully assessed in the anterior, inferior, and posterior directions.

Most surgeons prefer to use an arthroscopic rather than an open approach for most patients.[31-33] Arthroscopy allows better visualization and more complete capsular plication and shifting in a posterior-to-anterior direction. Arthroscopy also avoids the complications and other issues associated with open surgical dissection. Relatively recent studies have found that recurrence rates after arthroscopy are equivalent to or lower than those after traditional open surgery.[31-33] It is important to note that most recent arthroscopic studies excluded patients with significant bone loss. It is well established that arthroscopic treatment of these patients carries a considerable risk of failure.

Some surgeons recommend using the Instability Severity Index Score to help determine whether an open repair should be considered in lieu of an arthroscopic repair.[18] The Instability Severity Index Score was developed based on prospective identification of several patient risk factors for recurrent anterior instability: age younger than 20 years at the time of surgery, participation in a competitive or a contact sport or a sport involving forced overhead activity, shoulder hyperlaxity, and the presence of a Hill-Sachs lesion and/or loss of the sclerotic inferior glenoid contour on an AP radiograph of the shoulder in external rotation. These factors were integrated into a 10-point score that was retrospectively tested in the same population. Patients with a preoperative score higher than 6 points had an unacceptable 70% recurrence risk ($P < 0.001$).

Revision Surgery

An arthroscopic stabilization procedure can fail for a variety of reasons, and the treating surgeon must identify the cause to decide on an appropriate revision treatment. Bone loss, whether glenoid or humeral head, is the primary reason arthroscopic stabilization procedures fail. Other factors include a return to a contact sport in a young patient, shoulder hyperlaxity and forced overhead activity, and the use of three or fewer anchors during the repair.[12,18,34]

If the patient has an isolated engaging Hill-Sachs lesion, a revision arthroscopic Bankart repair combined with arthroscopic remplissage may be adequate.[35] Some surgeons believe that an open glenoid bone restorative procedure will restore the functional arc and shoulder stability in such patients without directly treating the humeral head defect.[36] No clearly defined algorithms are available. The surgeon should carefully define all pathology and choose the safest, most effective available procedure.

Specific Lesions

Proper identification of an ALPSA lesion is the key to its treatment. No examination findings specifically distinguish an ALPSA lesion from a Bankart lesion. On imaging studies, the labrum may not be well visualized because it is medialized and adhering to the glenoid neck. During arthroscopy, the labrum must be located (it is best seen through the anterosuperior portal) and carefully mobilized back to the glenoid rim to restore its anatomic location. Capsular plication while leaving the labrum in a medialized, unreduced position creates a high risk of failure. Some surgeons believe that ALPSA lesions are a result of recurrent dislocation and that arthroscopic repair of an ALPSA lesion is less predictably successful than that of a standard Bankart lesion.[37]

2: Instability and Athletic Injuries

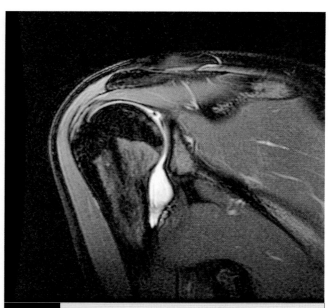

Figure 13 | Coronal MRA showing intra-articular gadolinium leakage inferiorly down the humeral shaft, indicating a HAGL tear.

A HAGL lesion similarly cannot be reliably distinguished from a Bankart lesion on the basis of the patient history or examination. MRI and especially MRA can be helpful in identifying a HAGL lesion. The most reliable imaging finding is the absence of the teardrop shape of the capsule and the IGHL on coronal MRI studies (**Figure 13**). To treat a HAGL lesion, the patient is best placed in the lateral decubitus position with balanced traction to provide access to the inferior glenohumeral joint. A HAGL lesion can be challenging to treat arthroscopically, and the surgeon should be prepared for an open HAGL repair if arthroscopic repair is not feasible.

The GLAD lesion is of unclear significance, but most experts believe that efforts should be made to sufficiently mobilize the labrum to cover exposed bone or create fibrocartilage along the deficient area of the glenoid with microfracture.

Recurrent anterior dislocation can cause extensive labral tearing as the tear propagates around the glenoid. Patients often describe numerous low-energy dislocation events as well as significant pain, which is uncommon with more isolated labral tears. Provocative testing is likely to reveal both posterior and anterior apprehension or instability and may suggest the presence of a SLAP lesion. MRA can increase diagnostic specificity, especially in evaluating for a SLAP lesion, which can be critical for optimal planning before surgical intervention. Given the need for circumferential access to the glenoid, lateral positioning of the patient is preferred. This challenging surgery must be carefully planned, with an appropriate number of anchors and tools to allow for a circumferential labral repair.[8,38]

Bone Loss

In recurrent anterior instability, bone loss must be considered as a bipolar phenomenon. Treating one lesion without considering the other can lead to surgical failure. Nonetheless, most patients with both glenoid and humeral head bone loss are successfully treated when only the glenoid bone loss is directly treated. By restoring the relatively normal morphology of the anterior glenoid, the glenoid arc is effectively lengthened, and engagement of the Hill-Sachs lesion is prevented.[4]

Glenoid Bone Loss

Glenoid bone loss in the setting of recurrent instability can be surgically treated with several well-described techniques. Several factors must be considered when selecting the appropriate bone restorative procedure. Although no algorithm for clinical decision making has been validated, a comprehensive review of glenoid bone loss in recurrent anterior shoulder instability has provided general guidelines that depend on the amount of bone loss.[22] Based on other researchers' biomechanical and clinical research, the review concluded that anterior glenoid bone loss of more than 25% to 30% significantly increases the risk of instability events.[9,39-41] Lesions smaller than 15% rarely are significant, and those between 15% and 25% must be carefully assessed on an individual basis.

Coracoid Transfer (Latarjet Procedure)

Coracoid transfer is the most common procedure to restore glenoid bone stock. In the United States, it is typically performed if a patient has more than 25% glenoid bone loss or after unsuccessful arthroscopic stabilization in a patient with less than 25% bone loss. With both glenoid and humeral head bone deficiency, some surgeons still believe that the humeral head defect will no longer engage when the glenoid bony morphology is reestablished.[36] Several clinical studies found that the Latarjet procedure has excellent results in the setting of combined glenoid and humeral head bone loss.[42-44] One study even suggested that the Latarjet procedure will lead to a stable shoulder in patients with a large, engaging Hill-Sachs lesion without glenoid bone loss.[36] These researchers stated that the block of bone extends the glenoid arc to the point that the humeral head cannot externally rotate and anteriorly translate sufficiently for the Hill-Sachs lesion to engage over the front of the bone block.

Coracoid transfer procedures are invasive and not free of complications.[44] If the graft is malpositioned, further chondral injury can occur.[45] The recently described arthroscopic coracoid transfer procedures are challenging and require extensive initial laboratory experience.[46,47]

Alternative sources of bone graft for glenoid deficiency have been investigated because a coracoid transfer does not completely re-create the normal anatomy and contour of the anterior glenoid. These glenoid

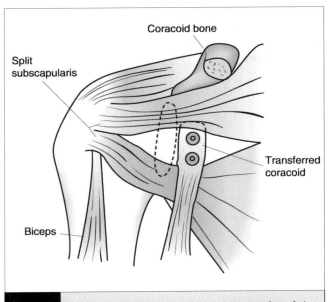

Figure 14 The Latarjet procedure involves a transfer of the coracoid process to the medial glenoid via a split of the subscapularis. The coracoid provides for glenohumeral stability by augmenting the anterior glenoid rim, whereas the conjoined tendon acts as a stabilizer with the arm abducted and externally rotated. (Reproduced from Burns JP, Snyder SJ: Shoulder instability, in Fischgrund JS, ed: *Orthopaedic Knowledge Update 9.* Rosemont, IL, American Academy of Orthopaedic Surgeons, 2008, pp 301-311.)

bone graft options include autograft or allograft iliac crest, allograft glenoid, and, most recently, distal tibial allograft[48] (**Figure 14**).

Humeral Head Bone Loss (Hill-Sachs Lesions)

Most Hill-Sachs lesions are small (less than 20% of the articular surface), shallow, and not clinically significant. A lesion larger than 40% of the articular surface almost always is clinically significant and must be directly treated. The challenge is to decide whether a lesion between 20% and 40% of the articular surface is clinically significant enough to treat directly or whether it can be rendered insignificant by appropriate treatment of glenoid bone loss.

The treatment should be aimed at restoring a stable arc of motion. In many patients, restoration of the glenoid side alone may be sufficient because it restores the normal glenoid track and reduces the risk of Hill-Sachs lesion engagement. It is especially important in this setting to understand that bone loss is a bipolar phenomenon; glenoid bone loss can potentiate a medium-size Hill-Sachs lesion and increase the risk of instability. Without glenoid bone loss, the Hill-Sachs lesion may not engage on the anterior glenoid. With glenoid bone loss, less anterior translation or external rotation is needed for the humeral head lesion to engage. Several techniques have been described to treat the humeral head defect, each of which has a role.

Remplissage

Arthroscopic remplissage (translated from French as "filling") was developed as a means of filling the humeral head defect to render the lesion extra-articular and therefore nonengaging. The open version of this technique, known as the Connolly procedure, was described in 1972 and involves transferring part of the greater tuberosity into the defect, along with the infraspinatus tendon. The arthroscopic technique, described in 2007, involves a posterior capsulodesis and an infraspinatus tenodesis.[49] Although the exact indications for remplissage have yet to be defined, it may be best used in patients with a medium-size or large, shallow, engaging Hill-Sachs lesion and less than 20% glenoid bone loss.

Early promising results for arthroscopic remplissage have been published, with 98% stability reported in one study.[35,50] It is important to note that the patients were carefully selected and had limited glenoid bone loss and a large Hill-Sachs lesion. Remplissage alone probably would be insufficient in patients with more than 25% glenoid bone loss, and strong consideration should be given to a glenoid-based bony procedure for these patients.

Bone Grafting

Bone-grafting procedures have been used in an attempt to restore the bony architecture of the humeral head to prevent lesion engagement. Bone grafting typically is indicated in the uncommon setting of a large Hill-Sachs lesion (more than 40% of the articular surface) with minimal glenoid bone loss. Filling the defect and restoring normal anatomy reestablishes the articular arc of the humeral head, thus preventing lesion engagement. Both autograft and allograft bone plug techniques have been described, and fresh-frozen osteoarticular allografts also have been used.[4,51] Reasonable outcomes have been reported, although one study reported that 8 of 18 patients had a complication.[52] These procedures are technically challenging, and the risk of disease transmission with allograft use must be considered.

Disimpaction of a Hill-Sachs compression fracture is a relatively new procedure with little available clinical or biomechanical data.[4] Several different techniques have been reported, all of which involve elevating the compression fracture and applying bone graft to support the elevated bone. The clinical application of this procedure has not been defined, but it may be best suited for an acute lesion involving less than 40% of the articular surface.

Resurfacing

Partial resurfacing, complete resurfacing, and hemiarthroplasty are used to restore a more normal articular arc to the humeral head. These procedures should be used cautiously in young, active patients because of the risks of hardware loosening and glenoid wear. The indications are unclear, but the use of implants is best suited for patients who are older, have lower physical demands, or have a lesion larger than 40% of the articular surface. One definitive surgery typically is preferred for a patient older than approximately 50 to 60 years, and therefore hemiarthroplasty or total shoulder arthroplasty may be chosen over a resurfacing procedure.

Summary

Several factors commonly contribute to recurrent anterior shoulder instability. As with most orthopaedic conditions, a complete history and physical examination provide the keys to a correct diagnosis. Advanced imaging studies are desirable for every patient with recurrent instability. MRA can be useful to delineate a SLAP lesion or more extensive or subtle labral pathology. If glenoid bone loss or a significant Hill-Sachs lesion is suspected, three-dimensional CT is the preferred imaging modality. Bone loss in the glenoid and/or humeral head is present in almost all patients with recurrent instability, and it must be recognized and appropriately treated to minimize further injury to the joint. Proper diagnosis leads to appropriate patient counseling and the selection of the ideal technique.

Annotated References

1. Hovelius L, Augustini BG, Fredin H, Johansson O, Norlin R, Thorling J: Primary anterior dislocation of the shoulder in young patients: A ten-year prospective study. *J Bone Joint Surg Am* 1996;78(11):1677-1684.

2. Taylor DC, Arciero RA: Pathologic changes associated with shoulder dislocations: Arthroscopic and physical examination findings in first-time, traumatic anterior dislocations. *Am J Sports Med* 1997;25(3):306-311.

3. Armitage MS, Faber KJ, Drosdowech DS, Litchfield RB, Athwal GS: Humeral head bone defects: Remplissage, allograft, and arthroplasty. *Orthop Clin North Am* 2010;41(3):417-425.

   A comprehensive literature review was provided for remplissage, allograft reconstruction, and arthroplasty in the treatment of Hill-Sachs lesions, with a useful algorithm based on lesion size and patient factors.

4. Provencher MT, Frank RM, Leclere LE, et al: The Hill-Sachs lesion: Diagnosis, classification, and management. *J Am Acad Orthop Surg* 2012;20(4):242-252.

   The diagnosis, classification, and management of the Hill-Sachs lesion in anterior shoulder instability were discussed.

5. Neviaser TJ: The anterior labroligamentous periosteal sleeve avulsion lesion: A cause of anterior instability of the shoulder. *Arthroscopy* 1993;9(1):17-21.

6. Yiannakopoulos CK, Mataragas E, Antonogiannakis E: A comparison of the spectrum of intra-articular lesions in acute and chronic anterior shoulder instability. *Arthroscopy* 2007;23(9):985-990.

   A case study compared arthroscopic findings during treatment of acute and chronic instability. ALPSA lesions, Bankart lesions, and inverted pear glenoids were found significantly more often in patients with chronic instability.

7. Wolf EM, Cheng JC, Dickson K: Humeral avulsion of glenohumeral ligaments as a cause of anterior shoulder instability. *Arthroscopy* 1995;11(5):600-607.

8. Tokish JM, McBratney CM, Solomon DJ, Leclere L, Dewing CB, Provencher MT: Arthroscopic repair of circumferential lesions of the glenoid labrum. *J Bone Joint Surg Am* 2009;91(12):2795-2802.

   Thirty-nine shoulders with a circumferential labral lesion were prospectively followed for a mean 31.8 months. Significant improvements in functional and pain scores were reported, and only two shoulders developed recurrent instability.

9. Burkhart SS, De Beer JF: Traumatic glenohumeral bone defects and their relationship to failure of arthroscopic Bankart repairs: Significance of the inverted-pear glenoid and the humeral engaging Hill-Sachs lesion. *Arthroscopy* 2000;16(7):677-694.

10. Lazarus MD, Sidles JA, Harryman DT II, Matsen FA III: Effect of a chondral-labral defect on glenoid concavity and glenohumeral stability: A cadaveric model. *J Bone Joint Surg Am* 1996;78(1):94-102.

11. Mologne TS, Provencher MT, Menzel KA, Vachon TA, Dewing CB: Arthroscopic stabilization in patients with an inverted pear glenoid: Results in patients with bone loss of the anterior glenoid. *Am J Sports Med* 2007;35(8):1276-1283.

    Outcomes of arthroscopic stabilization were reviewed in 21 patients with significant glenoid bone loss. Three patients developed recurrent instability, and patients with attritional bone loss had lower outcomes scores than those with a bony fragment.

12. Boileau P, Villalba M, Héry JY, Balg F, Ahrens P, Neyton L: Risk factors for recurrence of shoulder instability after arthroscopic Bankart repair. *J Bone Joint Surg Am* 2006;88(8):1755-1763.

13. Yamamoto N, Itoi E, Abe H, et al: Contact between the glenoid and the humeral head in abduction, external rotation, and horizontal extension: A new concept of glenoid track. *J Shoulder Elbow Surg* 2007;16(5):649-656.

    The authors present a novel concept known as the glenoid track, based on cadaver data. The glenoid track represents the area on the humeral head that makes contact with the glenoid when the shoulder is in various abduction–external rotation positions.

14. Owens BD, Duffey ML, Nelson BJ, DeBerardino TM, Taylor DC, Mountcastle SB: The incidence and characteristics of shoulder instability at the United States Military Academy. *Am J Sports Med* 2007;35(7):1168-1173.

All shoulder instability events at the US Military Academy were prospectively captured during an 8-month period. In 4,141 students, 117 events occurred, yielding a 1-year incidence of 2.8%.

15. Robinson CM, Howes J, Murdoch H, Will E, Graham C: Functional outcome and risk of recurrent instability after primary traumatic anterior shoulder dislocation in young patients. *J Bone Joint Surg Am* 2006;88(11):2326-2336.

16. te Slaa RL, Wijffels MP, Brand R, Marti RK: The prognosis following acute primary glenohumeral dislocation. *J Bone Joint Surg Br* 2004;86(1):58-64.

17. Mather RC III, Orlando LA, Henderson RA, Lawrence JT, Taylor DC: A predictive model of shoulder instability after a first-time anterior shoulder dislocation. *J Shoulder Elbow Surg* 2011;20(2):259-266.

A Markov decision model was created to predict the long-term outcome of initial anterior shoulder dislocation, with internal and external validation.

18. Balg F, Boileau P: The instability severity index score: A simple pre-operative score to select patients for arthroscopic or open shoulder stabilisation. *J Bone Joint Surg Br* 2007;89(11):1470-1477.

Several factors were correlated with the recurrence of instability in initial anterior dislocation and were combined into a 10-point preoperative Instability Severity Index Score. A score greater than 6 was correlated with a recurrence rate of 70%.

19. Owens BD, Dawson L, Burks R, Cameron KL: Incidence of shoulder dislocation in the United States military: Demographic considerations from a high-risk population. *J Bone Joint Surg Am* 2009;91(4):791-796.

The overall incidence of anterior shoulder instability in military personnel was 1.69 dislocations per 1,000 person-years. White men younger than 30 years with a junior rank in the US Army were identified as being at highest risk.

20. Simonet WT, Melton LJ III, Cofield RH, Ilstrup DM: Incidence of anterior shoulder dislocation in Olmsted County, Minnesota. *Clin Orthop Relat Res* 1984;186:186-191.

21. Gagey OJ, Gagey N: The hyperabduction test. *J Bone Joint Surg Br* 2001;83(1):69-74.

22. Piasecki DP, Verma NN, Romeo AA, Levine WN, Bach BR Jr, Provencher MT: Glenoid bone deficiency in recurrent anterior shoulder instability: Diagnosis and management. *J Am Acad Orthop Surg* 2009;17(8):482-493.

A detailed review was presented of the diagnosis and management of glenoid bone loss in recurrent anterior shoulder instability.

23. Rerko MA, Pan X, Donaldson C, Jones GL, Bishop JY: Comparison of various imaging techniques to quantify glenoid bone loss in shoulder instability. *J Shoulder Elbow Surg* 2012.

Radiographs, MRI, CT, and three-dimensional CT were compared for the detection of various-size glenoid defects in cadaver shoulders. Three-dimensional CT was found to be the most accurate of the four modalities.

24. Huysmans PE, Haen PS, Kidd M, Dhert WJ, Willems JW: The shape of the inferior part of the glenoid: A cadaveric study. *J Shoulder Elbow Surg* 2006;15(6):759-763.

25. Sugaya H, Moriishi J, Dohi M, Kon Y, Tsuchiya A: Glenoid rim morphology in recurrent anterior glenohumeral instability. *J Bone Joint Surg Am* 2003;85(5):878-884.

26. Sugaya H, Kon Y, Tsuchiya A: Arthroscopic repair of glenoid fractures using suture anchors. *Arthroscopy* 2005;21(5):635.

27. Kralinger F, Aigner F, Longato S, Rieger M, Wambacher M: Is the bare spot a consistent landmark for shoulder arthroscopy? A study of 20 embalmed glenoids with 3-dimensional computed tomographic reconstruction. *Arthroscopy* 2006;22(4):428-432.

28. Detterline AJ, Provencher MT, Ghodadra N, Bach BR Jr, Romeo AA, Verma NN: A new arthroscopic technique to determine anterior-inferior glenoid bone loss: Validation of the secant chord theory in a cadaveric model. *Arthroscopy* 2009;25(11):1249-1256.

The traditional method of measuring glenoid bone loss based on distance from the bare spot was compared with a new model based on secant chord theory in cadaver specimens. The secant chord theory model was more accurate but required more complex mathematical calculations.

29. Flatow EL, Warner JI: Instability of the shoulder: Complex problems and failed repairs. Part I: Relevant biomechanics, multidirectional instability, and severe glenoid loss. *Instr Course Lect* 1998;47:97-112.

30. Buss DD, Lynch GP, Meyer CP, Huber SM, Freehill MQ: Nonoperative management for in-season athletes with anterior shoulder instability. *Am J Sports Med* 2004;32(6):1430-1433.

31. Archetti Netto N, Tamaoki MJ, Lenza M, et al: Treatment of Bankart lesions in traumatic anterior instability of the shoulder: A randomized controlled trial comparing arthroscopy and open techniques. *Arthroscopy* 2012;28(7):900-908.

Forty-two patients were randomly assigned to open or arthroscopic treatment of anterior shoulder instability with an isolated Bankart lesion. At 37.5-month follow-up, there was no clinical difference in recurrence or outcome scores between the two groups.

32. Zaffagnini S, Marcheggiani Muccioli GM, Giordano G, et al: Long-term outcomes after repair of recurrent post-traumatic anterior shoulder instability: Comparison of arthroscopic transglenoid suture and open Bankart reconstruction. *Knee Surg Sports Traumatol Arthrosc* 2012;20(5):816-821.

 The outcomes of 110 consecutive patients treated with open or arthroscopic stabilization for recurrent anterior shoulder instability were retrospectively reviewed. There were no differences in recurrence rates or outcomes scores between groups.

33. Petrera M, Patella V, Patella S, Theodoropoulos J: A meta-analysis of open versus arthroscopic Bankart repair using suture anchors. *Knee Surg Sports Traumatol Arthrosc* 2010;18(12):1742-1747.

 This meta-analysis found no overall difference in recurrence rates between open and arthroscopic stabilization for recurrent anterior shoulder instability. When studies more recent than 2002 were compared, arthroscopically treated patients were found to have lower recurrence rates.

34. Calvo E, Granizo JJ, Fernández-Yruegas D: Criteria for arthroscopic treatment of anterior instability of the shoulder: A prospective study. *J Bone Joint Surg Br* 2005;87(5):677-683.

35. Boileau P, O'Shea K, Vargas P, Pinedo M, Old J, Zumstein M: Anatomical and functional results after arthroscopic Hill-Sachs remplissage. *J Bone Joint Surg Am* 2012;94(7):618-626.

 The authors' early experience with remplissage was reported for the treatment of Hill-Sachs lesions as part of anterior shoulder instability. At a mean 24-month follow-up, 98% of the patients had a stable shoulder, and 74% of the patients had more than 75% filling of the defect.

36. Burkhart SS, De Beer JF, Barth JR, Cresswell T, Roberts C, Richards DP: Results of modified Latarjet reconstruction in patients with anteroinferior instability and significant bone loss. *Arthroscopy* 2007;23(10):1033-1041.

 The results of the Latarjet procedure in patients with recurrent anterior shoulder instability and an inverted pear glenoid were presented. The overall recurrence rate was 4.9% at a mean 59-month follow-up.

37. Ozbaydar M, Elhassan B, Diller D, Massimini D, Higgins LD, Warner JJ: Results of arthroscopic capsulolabral repair: Bankart lesion versus anterior labroligamentous periosteal sleeve avulsion lesion. *Arthroscopy* 2008;24(11):1277-1283.

 A retrospective study found that patients with an ALPSA lesion were more likely to have dislocation before arthroscopic capsulolabral repair and had a higher recurrence rate after surgery than those with a traditional Bankart lesion.

38. Lo IK, Burkhart SS: Triple labral lesions: Pathology and surgical repair technique-report of seven cases. *Arthroscopy* 2005;21(2):186-193.

39. Itoi E, Lee SB, Berglund LJ, Berge LL, An KN: The effect of a glenoid defect on anteroinferior stability of the shoulder after Bankart repair: A cadaveric study. *J Bone Joint Surg Am* 2000;82(1):35-46.

40. Greis PE, Scuderi MG, Mohr A, Bachus KN, Burks RT: Glenohumeral articular contact areas and pressures following labral and osseous injury to the anteroinferior quadrant of the glenoid. *J Shoulder Elbow Surg* 2002;11(5):442-451.

41. Lo IK, Parten PM, Burkhart SS: The inverted pear glenoid: An indicator of significant glenoid bone loss. *Arthroscopy* 2004;20(2):169-174.

42. Neyton L, Young A, Dawidziak B, et al: Surgical treatment of anterior instability in rugby union players: Clinical and radiographic results of the Latarjet-Patte procedure with minimum 5-year follow-up. *J Shoulder Elbow Surg* 2012;21(12):1721-1727.

 Retrospective review of 34 rugby players (37 shoulders) found that no patients reported recurrence of instability at a mean 12-year follow-up after the Latarjet-Patte procedure for recurrent anterior shoulder instability.

43. Hovelius L, Vikerfors O, Olofsson A, Svensson O, Rahme H: Bristow-Latarjet and Bankart: A comparative study of shoulder stabilization in 185 shoulders during a seventeen-year follow-up. *J Shoulder Elbow Surg* 2011;20(7):1095-1101.

 Retrospective review of 185 consecutive patients who underwent Bankart repair or the Bristow-Latarjet procedure for recurrent shoulder instability found that patients treated with the Bristow-Latarjet procedure reported better functional outcomes and lower recurrence rates at a mean 17-year follow-up.

44. Shah AA, Butler RB, Romanowski J, Goel D, Karadagli D, Warner JJ: Short-term complications of the Latarjet procedure. *J Bone Joint Surg Am* 2012;94(6):495-501.

 Short-term complications associated with the Latarjet procedure were studied in 45 patients (48 shoulders). Five procedures (10%) resulted in neurologic injury, four procedures (8%) in recurrent instability, and three procedures (6%) in a superficial infection.

45. Ghodadra N, Gupta A, Romeo AA, et al: Normalization of glenohumeral articular contact pressures after Latarjet or iliac crest bone-grafting. *J Bone Joint Surg Am* 2010;92(6):1478-1489.

 A cadaver study evaluated the effect of iliac crest bone graft or coracoid piece positioning on level and location of peak contact pressures in a Latarjet procedure. Placing the graft flush with the native glenoid and using the inferior portion of the coracoid as the glenoid face are recommended.

46. Boileau P, Mercier N, Roussanne Y, Thélu CÉ, Old J: Arthroscopic Bankart-Bristow-Latarjet procedure: The development and early results of a safe and reproducible technique. *Arthroscopy* 2010;26(11):1434-1450.

    Retrospective review of an all-arthroscopic Latarjet procedure in 47 consecutive patients found good results in most patients, although there were seven migrations and one bone block fracture.

47. Lafosse L, Boyle S: Arthroscopic Latarjet procedure. *J Shoulder Elbow Surg* 2010;19(2, suppl):2-12.

    Of the first 100 patients treated with an all-arthroscopic Latarjet procedure, 91 had an excellent result, but 11 had a complication.

48. Provencher MT, Bhatia S, Ghodadra NS, et al: Recurrent shoulder instability: Current concepts for evaluation and management of glenoid bone loss. *J Bone Joint Surg Am* 2010;92(suppl 2):133-151.

    A comprehensive review of the evaluation and the management of recurrent anterior shoulder instability focused on the role of glenoid bone loss.

49. Purchase RJ, Wolf EM, Hobgood ER, Pollock ME, Smalley CC: Hill-Sachs "remplissage": An arthroscopic solution for the engaging Hill-Sachs lesion. *Arthroscopy* 2008;24(6):723-726.

    An arthroscopic technique based on the Connolly open infraspinatus tenodesis technique was described for the treatment of an engaging Hill-Sachs lesion in patients with anterior shoulder instability.

50. Franceschi F, Papalia R, Rizzello G, et al: Remplissage repair—new frontiers in the prevention of recurrent shoulder instability: A 2-year follow-up comparative study. *Am J Sports Med* 2012;40(11):2462-2469.

    Retrospective review of 50 patients with an engaging Hill-Sachs lesion found recurrent instability in 20% of the patients treated with a traditional arthroscopic Bankart repair alone but none in patients treated with arthroscopic Bankart repair combined with remplissage.

51. Diklic ID, Ganic ZD, Blagojevic ZD, Nho SJ, Romeo AA: Treatment of locked chronic posterior dislocation of the shoulder by reconstruction of the defect in the humeral head with an allograft. *J Bone Joint Surg Br* 2010;92(1):71-76.

    Retrospective review of 13 patients treated with humeral head allograft reconstruction for a locked chronic posterior shoulder dislocation found that 9 patients had no pain or restriction of activities of daily living. Good overall functional outcomes were reported.

52. Miniaci A, Gish MW: Management of anterior glenohumeral instability associated with large Hill-Sachs defects. *Tech Shoulder Elbow Surg* 2004;5:170-175.

53. Rowe CR, Zarins B, Ciullo JV: Recurrent anterior dislocation of the shoulder after surgical repair: Apparent causes of failure and treatment. *J Bone Joint Surg Am* 1984;66(2):159-168.

54. Calandra JJ, Baker CL, Uribe J: The incidence of Hill-Sachs lesions in initial anterior shoulder dislocations. *Arthroscopy* 1989;5(4):254-257.

55. Franceschi F, Longo UG, Ruzzini L, Rizzello G, Maffulli N, Denaro V: Arthroscopic salvage of failed arthroscopic Bankart repair: A prospective study with a minimum follow-up of 4 years. *Am J Sports Med* 2008;36(7):1330-1336.

    A prospective study of 10 carefully selected patients found that arthroscopic revision surgery for a Bankart lesion was successful at an average 68-month follow-up.

56. Hall RH, Isaac F, Booth CR: Dislocations of the shoulder with special reference to accompanying small fractures. *J Bone Joint Surg Am* 1959;41(3):489-494.

57. Richards RD, Sartoris DJ, Pathria MN, Resnick D: Hill-Sachs lesion and normal humeral groove: MR imaging features allowing their differentiation. *Radiology* 1994;190(3):665-668.

Chapter 9

Multidirectional and Posterior Shoulder Instability

Fotios P. Tjoumakaris, MD   James P. Bradley, MD

Introduction

Posterior instability and multidirectional instability of the shoulder are overlapping conditions. Most patients have ill-defined symptoms, and the diagnosis is challenging. The management of patients with posterior or multidirectional instability of the shoulder has evolved considerably in the past several years. With advanced imaging and arthroscopic techniques, surgical management has vastly improved, and better patient outcomes are being reported.

Clinical Evaluation

Patient History

Traumatic dislocation is seldom reported by patients with posterior or multidirectional instability of the shoulder. Posterior shoulder dislocation classically occurs in a patient who has experienced electrocution, seizure, or a posteriorly directed blow to the shoulder (typically in a contact sport or a motor vehicle crash). These patients report pain with attempted range of motion, have difficulty externally rotating the arm, and require emergency closed reduction of the humeral head within the glenoid fossa. Frequently, these patients are most comfortable with the arm resting in a sling in internal rotation. Patients with posterior instability report less severe symptoms than patients with a posterior dislocation and have difficulty correlating their symptoms with a particular event or injury. In these patients, certain arm positions or motions, such as cross-body adduction or overhead throwing, can precipitate pain or other symptoms. In many of these patients, the probable cause is recurrent posterior subluxation; patients may report pain, fatigue in the shoulder, or loss

of velocity when throwing. When the symptoms become pervasive, the patient may report numbness in the upper extremity or the feeling that the arm is "going dead." Patients with multidirectional instability also report pain in the shoulder, may have difficulty using the arm during activities of daily living, and often report bilateral symptoms. Identifying a particular arc of motion or a causative mechanism can be challenging because the patient's symptoms often are vague and may mimic those of rotator cuff impingement (**Table 1**).

Physical Examination

The clinician should carefully assess the cervical spine and its contribution to shoulder and upper extremity pain. The cervical spine assessment includes palpation, range of motion, and provocative testing (the Spurling test) to evaluate for radiculopathy that could be contributing to pain around the shoulder and scapula. A thorough shoulder examination is required in all patients with shoulder pain and dysfunction. Strength testing and assessment for atrophy, passive and active range of motion, and scapular rhythm and synchronization should be an integral part of the examination and may be useful in detecting concomitant pathology. Provocative maneuvers, such as the jerk and Kim tests, can help to elicit instability and pain as the humeral head glides over the posterior glenoid rim.[1,2]

The jerk test is a true test of posterior instability and is performed while the patient is seated. The scapula is stabilized, and the arm is taken horizontally across the body from a position of abduction and internal rota-

Table 1

Common Symptoms of Patients With Recurrent Posterior Subluxation

Pain

Fatigue

Loss of throwing velocity

Weakness ("dead arm")

Numbness, paresthesias

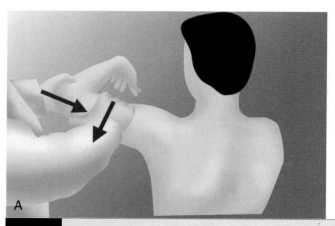 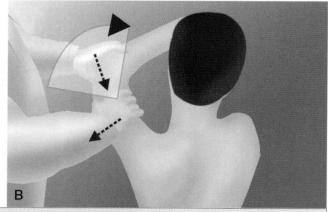

Figure 1	Drawings showing the Kim test. **A,** With the arm in 90° of abduction, the examiner applies an axial and downward force to the proximal arm *(arrows)*. **B,** With the abducted arm elevated 45°, the examiner applies a posterior force with axial compression *(arrows)* while the arm is adducted across the body *(arrowhead)*. If pain is elicited with this maneuver, the test is considered positive and highly suggestive of a posteroinferior labral lesion. (Adapted with permission from Kim SH, Park JS, Jeong WK, Shin SK: The Kim test: A novel test for posteroinferior labral lesion of the shoulder: A comparison to the jerk test. *Am J Sports Med* 2005;33[8]:1188-1192.)

tion while a posteriorly directed force is applied to the affected arm. The shoulder can be heard (as a clunking sound) and is seen to subluxate posteriorly off the glenoid. A second clunking sound can be elicited when the shoulder is taken back across the body as the humeral head reduces within the glenoid fossa. The Kim test is performed with the patient seated and the arm in 90° of abduction. The examiner holds the proximal arm and applies an axial and posterior-directed force while elevating the arm upward by 45°. Pain with this maneuver indicates a posteroinferior labral lesion, which can contribute to posterior instability (**Figure 1**). Load-and-shift testing can help to define the extent of shoulder joint laxity, and an apprehension sign can be elicited to evaluate for subjective instability anteriorly. Alleviation of the apprehension sign with a relocation test can further define the direction of instability. In patients undergoing shoulder surgery, the ability to subluxate the shoulder over the glenoid rim was found to be common, and only higher degrees of laxity were correlated with clinical instability of the shoulder.[3] Ligamentous laxity should be generally assessed by evaluating elbow and knee hyperextension, patellar mobility, metacarpophalangeal joint hyperextension, and the sulcus sign off the anterolateral edge of the acromion with an inferiorly applied force. A sulcus sign value that is greater than 2 cm and does not diminish in external rotation is regarded as pathologic in a patient with symptoms and may imply rotator cuff interval laxity. In a recent cross-sectional study, the presence of the sulcus sign was correlated with a history of shoulder instability in healthy patients.[4] A thorough neurovascular examination of both upper extremities is performed to evaluate for differences in pulse or nerve function that might suggest thoracic outlet syndrome or a brachial plexopathy. Patients with multidirectional instability of the shoulder may have increased translation with load-and-shift testing, a positive sulcus sign, a positive ap-

prehension sign, and positive jerk and Kim tests. Positive results on multiple tests indicate capsular laxity that is more global in nature. Patients with posterior instability are most likely to have these findings when the posterior capsule and labrum are stressed (by the posterior load-and-shift, jerk, or Kim tests), indicating an isolated spectrum of injury. Substantial overlap may exist, however, and this factor makes optimal management of these patients challenging.

Epidemiology

Posterior shoulder instability represents 5% of all incidences of shoulder instability.[5] Approximately 50% of the patients with posterior instability may have a traumatic etiology. In most patients with dislocation, the reported cause is trauma; in the remaining patients, the cause is a seizure disorder or electrical shock. The reported incidence of posterior dislocation is 1.1 per 100,000 population per year, with peaks in men age 20 to 49 years and in men and women older than 70 years. Young age at initial dislocation, the presence of a seizure disorder, and the presence of a large reverse Hill-Sachs lesion are correlated with recurrence. Almost 20% of patients have a recurrence during the first year after a posterior shoulder dislocation.[6]

Multidirectional instability occurs more often in patients in the second or third decade of life and may be most prevalent in athletes who engage in overhead repetitive arm use, as in volleyball, swimming, or gymnastics.[7] Instability patterns in two planes are required for a diagnosis of multidirectional instability. The diagnosis often is challenging, and a misdiagnosis of unidirectional instability may lead to failure of the initial treatment. The epidemiologic characteristics of these patients are difficult to quantify because precise diag-

Table 2

Anatomic Determinants of Posterior or Multidirectional Instability of the Shoulder

Anatomic Determinant	Pathology
Static Restraint	
Humeral head	Reverse Hill-Sachs lesion
	Increased humeral retroversion
Glenoid	Posterior glenoid fracture or deficiency
	Increased glenoid retroversion
Labrum	Labral tear
	Increased chondrolabral retroversion
	Kim lesion
	Posterior labrocapsular periosteal sleeve avulsion
Capsule	Capsular tear
	Capsular insufficiency or laxity
	Posterior avulsion of the inferior glenohumeral ligament and reverse humeral avulsion of the glenohumeral ligament
Dynamic Restraint	
Muscular control	Rotator cuff tear
	Weakness of scapular stabilizing muscles (rhomboid, pectoralis minor, serratus anterior)
Neuromuscular control	Forceful internal rotation from seizure disorder or electrocution

nostic criteria do not exist in the orthopaedic literature. Whether to include patients who have had unidirectional dislocation but exhibit signs of laxity in other planes is a source of ongoing debate.

Anatomic Considerations

The glenohumeral joint relies on static restraints to stability (the capsule, labrum, and glenoid or chondrolabral version) as well as dynamic stabilizers (the rotator cuff, scapular and thoracic musculature, and neuromuscular control (**Table 2**). In a patient with posterior dislocation from trauma or a seizure disorder, the bony architecture of the humeral head or glenoid may be compromised, resulting in a posterior glenoid fracture or deficiency or an impaction fracture of the anterior humeral head (a reverse Hill-Sachs lesion). In such a patient, the extent of bone loss may substantially contribute to the recurrence of instability. Because the humeral head is internally rotated, the lesion can engage and cause a recurrence of subluxation or dislocation. Relative glenoid or chondrolabral retroversion may be a risk factor or the result of recurrent instability and recurrent posterior subluxation. Labral injury from repet-

itive posterior loading or instability can range from a posterior labral crack to a Kim lesion (an incomplete, concealed avulsion of the posteroinferior labrum) to a reverse Bankart lesion. Capsular tearing, posterior labrocapsular periosteal sleeve avulsion, or humeral avulsion of the posteroinferior glenohumeral ligament also can occur and contribute to recurrence of posterior instability.[8-12] Altered scapular kinematics, including reduced serratus activation, increased trapezius activity, and short resting length of the pectoralis minor, have been shown to alter the stability of the glenohumeral joint; cadaver studies found that posterior instability increases when posterior scapular tilt is increased more than 15°.[13,14] The rotator cuff also plays a critical role in dynamic joint stability and can be torn in patients who sustain a posterior dislocation at any age. Loss of concavity compression and recurrence of instability may occur despite normal bone and ligamentous architecture. In patients with recurrent posterior subluxation, there may be associated rotator cuff pathology from abnormal glenohumeral joint translations. A high level of suspicion on the part of the treating clinician, with careful scrutiny of advanced imaging, is important for an accurate diagnosis and treatment plan.

Imaging

Routine radiographs may be diagnostic in the setting of trauma or a suspected acute dislocation. Plain radiographs typically are obtained in three views (AP, scapular Y, and axillary). In a patient with a posterior dislocation, obtaining an axillary radiograph may be challenging because of the characteristic inability to externally rotate the arm. In such a patient, the AP radiograph may reveal a lightbulb sign, in which the glenoid fossa is relatively empty and the proximal humerus has the shape of a lightbulb secondary to internal rotation (**Figure 2**). A Velpeau axillary view sometimes is helpful if a traditional axillary view cannot be obtained. The radiographs are inspected for a bone defect of the posterior glenoid rim as well as a reverse Hill-Sachs lesion on the anterior humeral head. The radiographs also should be reviewed for associated fractures of the tuberosities, surgical neck, or humeral head, any of which may affect surgical treatment.[15] CT may be helpful for further defining the osseous injury pattern, especially if the plain radiographs are nondiagnostic. CT is beneficial for determining the size of an associated Hill-Sachs lesion, the extent of bone deficiency of the posterior glenoid rim, and the degree of glenoid retroversion, which may contribute to recurrent instability.

Magnetic resonance arthrography (MRA) and MRI are the best imaging modalities for identifying lesions within the posterior capsulolabral complex. Axial images may reveal posterior translation of the humeral head relative to the glenoid, a posterior labrocapsular avulsion, a posterior labral tear with paralabral cyst formation, or humeral avulsion of the posteroinferior glenohumeral ligament complex.[16] A concealed lesion

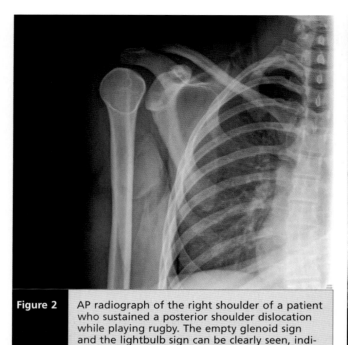

Figure 2 AP radiograph of the right shoulder of a patient who sustained a posterior shoulder dislocation while playing rugby. The empty glenoid sign and the lightbulb sign can be clearly seen, indicating dislocation of the glenohumeral joint.

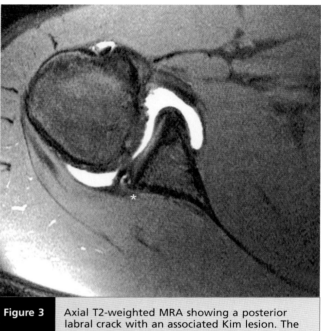

Figure 3 Axial T2-weighted MRA showing a posterior labral crack with an associated Kim lesion. The patient's symptoms were consistent with recurrent posterior subluxation. * = area of labral crack.

(Kim lesion or incomplete to near-complete labral crack), a posterior periosteal sleeve avulsion, or increased chondrolabral retroversion also can be seen and quantified on axial MRI or MRA studies (**Figure 3**). A rotator cuff tear, bone edema, an impaction fracture, and an articular cartilage abnormality can be further evaluated with MRI and may be seen in a large number of patients. A recent study found that positioning the arm in flexion, adduction, and internal rotation during MRA further defined the injury to the postero-inferior labrum in patients for whom more subtle abnormalities to the posterior capsule and the labrum were identified.[17] Patients with multidirectional instability typically do not have specific labral pathology, but they may have characteristic morphologic osseous changes of instability, such as increased chondrolabral retroversion and a patulous posterior capsule.[18]

Treatment Considerations

Nonsurgical Treatment

The treatment of patients with posterior or multidirectional instability of the shoulder has evolved considerably in the past decade. For patients with acute dislocation and fracture contributing to instability, closed reduction and fracture fixation often are necessary to restore stability to the glenohumeral joint. In patients with recurrent posterior subluxation or signs of multidirectional instability, physical therapy is the preferred first-line treatment. Despite aggressive therapy and strengthening, nonsurgical management is unsuccessful for many patients, and surgical intervention is re-

quired.[19] A recent study of patients with multidirectional instability found that a combination of capsular shift and physical therapy was superior to physical therapy alone in restoring normal kinematics and muscle activation of the glenohumeral joint.[20] This finding underscores the difficulty of nonsurgical treatment of patients with instability. Nonetheless, many patients, especially those who do not have optimal function of the periscapular musculature, benefit from an initial nonsurgical approach and may be able to avoid surgical intervention.

Surgical Treatment

Arthroscopic surgery has become the gold standard for patients who require surgical treatment for posterior or multidirectional instability of the shoulder without associated osseous defects (**Figure 4**). Historically, many patients with posterior instability were treated with an open posterior stabilization procedure, with recurrence rates ranging from 0% to 40%. Few patients returned to their previous level of activity or sport.[21-27] High recurrence rates as well as patient dissatisfaction with open surgery increased interest in arthroscopic management of the condition. With the use of current arthroscopic techniques, the average recurrence rate is close to 5%, with a range of 0% to 10% in most recent studies. A high percentage of patients return to their previous level of activity or sport.[28] A comparative study of arthroscopic and open techniques found that arthroscopically treated patients had superior functional outcomes.[29] A cadaver biomechanics study found that open bone block procedures overcorrected posterior

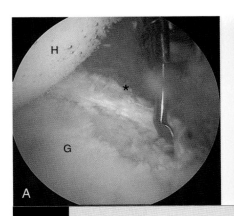
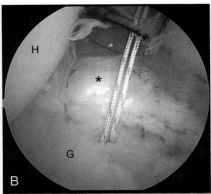
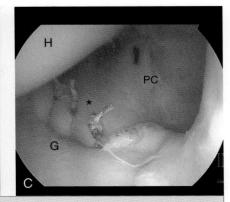

Figure 4 Arthroscopic photographs showing a posterior labral repair from the anterior portal. The patient is in the lateral decubitus position. **A,** The posterior labrum is detached from the posterior glenoid margin, with loss of articular cartilage on the glenoid from recurrent posterior subluxation. **B,** Anchor placement to secure the posterior labrum and capsule back to the glenoid margin. **C,** The final repair. The posterior portal has been repaired to prevent capsular insufficiency through the defect. * = labrum, G = glenoid, H = humeral head, PC = posterior capsule.

translation and did not restore inferior stability as effectively as arthroscopic posterior Bankart repair.[30] The failure rates in high-demand throwing athletes have remained relatively low (5% to 10%) when modern arthroscopic techniques are used.[31-35] In these retrospective studies, failure to plicate the posterior capsule with suture anchors may have been a factor in the relatively few unsuccessful procedures.[36]

Open capsular shift has provided solid long-term results for most patients with multidirectional instability. However, in recent studies, arthroscopic techniques have had equal rates of success, with a trend toward better rates of return to sport in patients treated arthroscopically.[37] A recent cadaver study found that capsular volume was reduced more with arthroscopic plication than with a traditional open technique, further validating the shift toward an arthroscopic approach to treatment.[38] A study of high-demand athletes with multidirectional instability found that 91% of the patients had full or satisfactory range of motion, and 86% were able to return to their previous level of competition.[39] The advantages of an arthroscopic technique over traditional open methods include the ability to treat concomitant pathology (such as a superior labrum anterior to posterior tear, global capsular laxity, or a rotator cuff tear) and anterior and posterior capsular laxity, as well as a reduction in the morbidity of an open approach.[36]

In patients with an osseous defect from a locked posterior dislocation, pathologic glenoid retroversion, or bone deficiency or avulsion of the glenohumeral ligaments from the humerus, open surgery may be the preferred method of treatment. For a patient with a large humeral head defect from a reverse Hill-Sachs lesion, the preferred option may be an osteoarticular allograft reconstruction, a humeral head arthroplasty, or a lesser tuberosity transfer (the McLaughlin procedure).[40] For patients with increased glenoid or humeral retrover-

sion, glenoid osteotomy and humeral osteotomy can provide stability, but these procedures have fallen from favor in recent years.

Arthroscopic Surgery for Posterior Instability

In most patients with posterior instability or recurrent posterior subluxation, arthroscopic surgery with posterior labral or capsular repair can achieve an excellent outcome with low rates of recurrence and complications. The recommended technique described here may be varied as indicated and still achieve a favorable outcome. Lateral decubitus patient positioning typically is used, with a beanbag to avoid pressure injury and interscalene block and general anesthesia to achieve complete muscle relaxation. The affected arm is placed in balanced arm traction in 45° of abduction and slight forward flexion using 10 to 15 lb of weight.

A single posterior portal is preferred for anchor placement and suture management and is created first, in line with the lateral edge of the acromion. This portal should allow for an anchor placement trajectory of 45° relative to the glenoid face (**Figure 5**). If the trajectory of the posterior portal is not optimal for inferior anchor placement, an accessory lateral portal may provide better access to the 7-o'clock position of the glenoid. The anterior portal is made in the rotator cuff interval just inferior to the biceps tendon. A 5.75-mm clear cannula is placed anteriorly for arthroscopic visualization, and an 8.25-mm clear cannula is placed posteriorly for use as the working portal. After identification of the labral and capsular pathology, the labrum is elevated off the posterior glenoid margin with a periosteal elevator. The posterior rim of the glenoid is débrided with a motorized burr or a shaver device (**Figure 6**). Often, it is more useful to introduce the elevator and the shaver from the anterior portal than to work exclusively from the posterior portal. The arthroscope

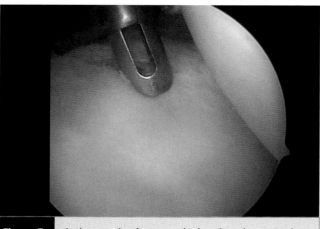

Figure 5 Arthroscopic photograph showing the posterior portal created in line with the lateral edge of the acromion. This placement facilitates anchor placement through a single posterior portal by allowing a 45° trajectory of the anchor drill guide.

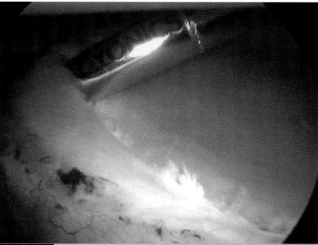

Figure 6 Arthroscopic photograph showing a motorized shaver used to débride the posterior glenoid and the labrum. The shaver has been brought in from the anterior portal and is used to create an optimal healing environment.

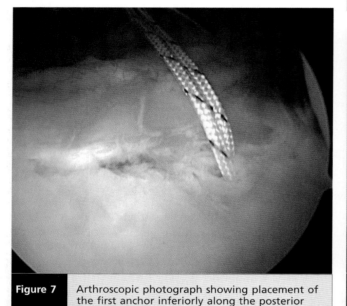

Figure 7 Arthroscopic photograph showing placement of the first anchor inferiorly along the posterior glenoid surface.

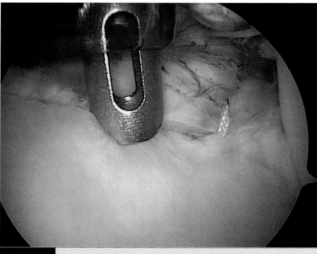

Figure 8 Arthroscopic photograph showing typical anchor spacing (3 to 5 mm apart) to avoid fragmentation of the posterior glenoid bone.

then can be placed in the anterior portal for anchor placement and suture management. A 70° arthroscope in the anterior portal can be useful for visualizing of the posterior and inferior glenoid rim. Anchors typically are placed along the posterior glenoid margin, starting inferiorly and progressing superiorly, as needed (**Figure 7**). Biocomposite anchors with a 2- to 2.4-mm diameter are recommended; they should be spaced 3 to 5 mm apart to avoid fragmentation of the posterior glenoid bone and prevent later glenoid fracture (**Figure 8**). The posterior suture limb of the anchor (most distant from the glenoid) is shuttled around the labrum and capsule slightly inferior and lateral to the anchor to achieve capsular plication. In a patient for whom plica-

tion should be avoided (for example, a high-level throwing athlete), the suture can be shuttled around the labrum at the location of anchor placement to prevent excessive tightening of the posterior capsule. A suture hook is used to assist with suture passage, and the sutures are tied in an inferior-to-superior direction (**Figure 9**). When shuttling sutures through a single posterior cannula, it is important to retrieve the suture limb and the shuttling suture (typically PDS; Ethicon, Somerville, NJ) at the same time to avoid crossing the sutures (**Figure 10**). The sutures are then tied; to allow the knot to be placed away from the glenohumeral joint, the suture that has been passed through the capsule and labrum (most distant from the glenoid) is used as the post limb

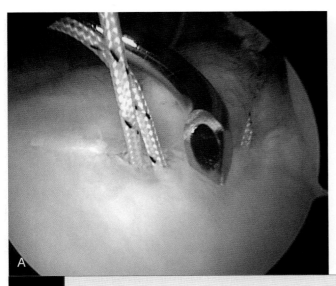

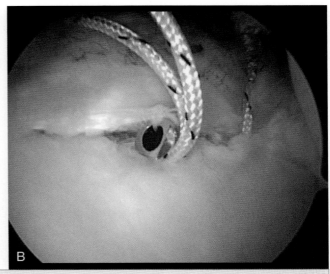

Figure 9 Arthroscopic photographs showing the use of a suture hook to shuttle sutures through the posterior labrum and capsule complex, as seen from the anterior viewing portal. **A,** A short curved suture hook is brought in through the posterior portal. **B,** The suture hook is passed around the labrum and capsule complex at the level of the anchor, or slightly inferior to the anchor if a capsular plication is performed.

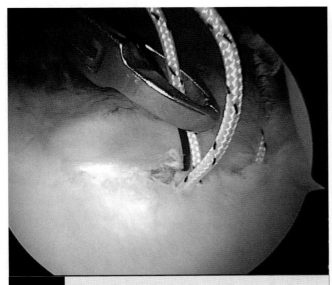

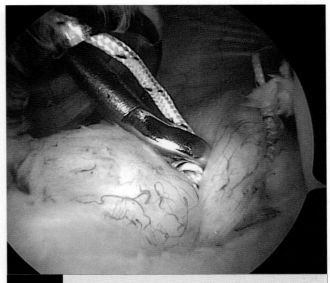

Figure 10 Arthroscopic photograph showing the suture shuttle and suture from the anchor grasped together to avoid suture entanglement. When a single posterior portal is used, this step facilitates passage and prevents early knot formation.

Figure 11 Arthroscopic photograph showing the shuttled suture limb used as the post limb during knot tying to place the knot away from the glenohumeral joint and prevent impingement.

(**Figure 11**). For a labral tear that extends to the superior labrum, 2-mm anchors loaded with No. 1 suture can be used, or a knotless 2.9-mm anchor can be used to avoid abrasion of the knot against the posterosuperior rotator cuff during glenohumeral motion. When all of the anchors have been placed, the posterior portal typically is closed to prevent stress-riser formation within the posterior capsule. Closure of the capsule also allows the surgeon to titrate the repair after the labrum has been anatomically restored to the glenoid rim. The posterior cannula is withdrawn to a level just posterior to the capsule. A crescent suture hook loaded with suture is used to penetrate one side of the portal incision, and the suture is retrieved from the opposite side with a penetrating grasper (**Figure 12**). The suture then can be tied just beyond the posterior capsule (**Figure 13**). Varying the distance of the suture from the portal incision allows additional tension to be applied to the posterior capsule. The repair is complete when

2: Instability and Athletic Injuries

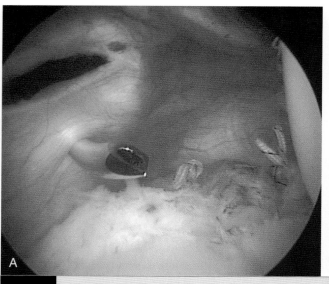
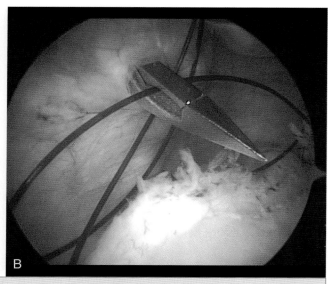

Figure 12 Arthroscopic photographs showing the closure of the posterior portal after completion of the labral repair. **A,** The posterior cannula is backed up just posterior to the posterior portal. On one side of the portal, a crescent suture hook is used to penetrate the posterior capsule. **B,** A penetrating grasper is used to grasp the shuttled blue suture on the opposite side of the posterior portal arthrotomy to allow closure.

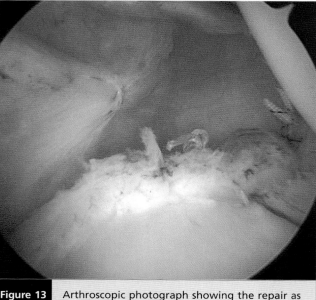
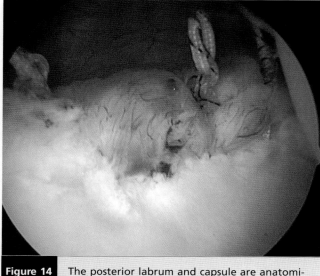

Figure 14 The posterior labrum and capsule are anatomically restored to the posterior glenoid rim.

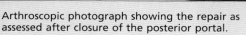

Figure 13 Arthroscopic photograph showing the repair as assessed after closure of the posterior portal.

all of the sutures have been tied and the posterior portal is closed, preventing pathologic posterior glenohumeral translation (**Figure 14**).

An abduction sling is used postoperatively, and passive range-of-motion exercises can begin the day after surgery. Neutral external rotation and 90° of forward elevation are allowed by 4 weeks after surgery. At 6 weeks, sling use can be discontinued, and the patient begins active-assisted range-of-motion exercises with a slow progression to active motion without motion constraints. At 4 months, the shoulder often is pain free

and has a near-normal range of motion. Rotator cuff strengthening and conditioning are started at this stage. At 5 months, isokinetic and isotonic exercises are advanced. Patients are assessed for return to play at 6 months, depending on the particular sport or activity. An overhead or throwing athlete may begin a throwing program at this stage of rehabilitation.

Summary

Posterior and multidirectional instability of the shoulder represent a complex injury pattern whose etiology often is multifactorial. Anatomic variations in glenoid and humeral retroversion, capsular deficiency, labral injury, osseous defects from acute injury, and dynamic muscle control can contribute to the instability pattern. MRI and MRA have improved the sensitivity and the specificity available for the diagnosis of these conditions. Imaging findings should be correlated with physical examination findings for a tailored treatment approach. If nonsurgical management is unsuccessful, arthroscopic surgery often is the first-line surgical treatment and can be used to treat a variety of pathologies, with low rates of recurrence and high rates of patient satisfaction.

Annotated References

1. Kim SH, Park JC, Park JS, Oh I: Painful jerk test: A predictor of success in nonoperative treatment of posteroinferior instability of the shoulder. *Am J Sports Med* 2004;32(8):1849-1855.

2. Kim SH, Park JS, Jeong WK, Shin SK: The Kim test: A novel test for posteroinferior labral lesion of the shoulder. A comparison to the jerk test. *Am J Sports Med* 2005;33(8):1188-1192.

3. Jia X, Ji JH, Petersen SA, Freehill MT, McFarland EG: An analysis of shoulder laxity in patients undergoing shoulder surgery. *J Bone Joint Surg Am* 2009;91(9): 2144-2150.

   Shoulder laxity was correlated with pathologic instability in patients undergoing surgery. Greater laxity while under anesthesia was significantly correlated with shoulder instability.

4. Owens BD, Duffey ML, Deberardino TM, Cameron KL: Physical examination findings in young athletes correlate with history of shoulder instability. *Orthopedics* 2011;34(6):460.

   A cross-sectional study evaluated more than 700 healthy patients using physical examination techniques. Patients with a history of instability were more likely to have increased posterior translation, an apprehension sign, a sulcus sign, and a positive relocation sign.

5. Robinson CM, Aderinto J: Recurrent posterior shoulder instability. *J Bone Joint Surg Am* 2005;87(4): 883-892.

6. Robinson CM, Seah M, Akhtar MA: The epidemiology, risk of recurrence, and functional outcome after an acute traumatic posterior dislocation of the shoulder. *J Bone Joint Surg Am* 2011;93(17):1605-1613.

   A retrospective review defined the epidemiology of posterior shoulder dislocation. Recurrence was found in 17.7% of the patients within the first year after injury. Recurrence of instability was associated with age younger than 40 years, a seizure-associated dislocation, and a large reverse Hill-Sachs lesion.

7. Gaskill TR, Taylor DC, Millett PJ: Management of multidirectional instability of the shoulder. *J Am Acad Orthop Surg* 2011;19(12):758-767.

   The authors discuss the diagnosis and treatment of multidirectional shoulder instability.

8. Kim SH, Noh KC, Park JS, Ryu BD, Oh I: Loss of chondrolabral containment of the glenohumeral joint in atraumatic posteroinferior multidirectional instability. *J Bone Joint Surg Am* 2005;87(1):92-98.

9. Kim SH, Ha KI, Yoo JC, Noh KC: Kim's lesion: An incomplete and concealed avulsion of the posteroinferior labrum in posterior or multidirectional posteroinferior instability of the shoulder. *Arthroscopy* 2004;20(7): 712-720.

10. Safran O, Defranco MJ, Hatem S, Iannotti JP: Posterior humeral avulsion of the glenohumeral ligament as a cause of posterior shoulder instability: A case report. *J Bone Joint Surg Am* 2004;86-A(12):2732-2736.

11. Shah AA, Butler RB, Fowler R, Higgins LD: Posterior capsular rupture causing posterior shoulder instability: A case report. *Arthroscopy* 2011;27(9):1304-1307.

    A 20-year-old man had successful arthroscopic repair of a posterior capsular rupture that resulted in posterior instability of the shoulder.

12. Bokor DJ, Fritsch BA: Posterior shoulder instability secondary to reverse humeral avulsion of the glenohumeral ligament. *J Shoulder Elbow Surg* 2010;19(6): 853-858.

    A retrospective review of 19 patients diagnosed with posterior capsular disruption after a traumatic injury to the shoulder found a high number of associated lesions: labral tear (more than 50%), reverse Bankart lesion (26%), chondral injury (21%), rotator cuff tear (21%), and extension of the tear into the posterior band of the inferior glenohumeral ligament (11%).

13. Ludewig PM, Reynolds JF: The association of scapular kinematics and glenohumeral joint pathologies. *J Orthop Sports Phys Ther* 2009;39(2):90-104.

    The role of scapular kinematics specific to shoulder pathology is outlined. Reduced serratus activation and pectoralis minor contracture were associated with rotator cuff impingement and instability in the cited studies.

14. Kikuchi K, Itoi E, Yamamoto N, et al: Scapular inclination and glenohumeral joint stability: A cadaveric study. *J Orthop Sci* 2008;13(1):72-77.

    Nine cadavers were studied by loading the glenohumeral joint in different directions with alterations in scapular inclination. Posterior and inferior stability increased with an anterior tilt of more than 5° and a superior tilt of 10°. This study shows the importance of the scapular position in maintaining glenohumeral joint stability.

15. Robinson CM, Akhtar A, Mitchell M, Beavis C: Complex posterior fracture-dislocation of the shoulder: Epidemiology, injury patterns, and results of operative treatment. *J Bone Joint Surg Am* 2007;89(7):1454-1466.

Epidemiologic data were obtained from a study of 26 patients with complex posterior fracture-dislocation of the shoulder. The incidence of this injury was determined to be 0.6 per 100,000 per year. Most injuries occurred secondary to a seizure or a fall from height in middle-aged men. Surgical results and outcomes generally are favorable after open reduction and internal fixation.

16. Tung GA, Hou DD: MR arthrography of the posterior labrocapsular complex: Relationship with glenohumeral joint alignment and clinical posterior instability. *AJR Am J Roentgenol* 2003;180(2):369-375.

17. Chiavaras MM, Harish S, Burr J: MR arthrographic assessment of suspected posteroinferior labral lesions using flexion, adduction, and internal rotation positioning of the arm: Preliminary experience. *Skeletal Radiol* 2010;39(5):481-488.

Diagnostic confidence for detecting posterior labral pathology was increased in nine patients when MRA in flexion, adduction, and internal rotation was used.

18. Jana M, Gamanagatti S: Magnetic resonance imaging in glenohumeral instability. *World J Radiol* 2011;3(9):224-232.

MRI findings consistent with instability are outlined. Cited studies of multidirectional instability show that labral pathology often is absent. Increased chondrolabral retroversion is a more characteristic finding in these patients.

19. Misamore GW, Sallay PI, Didelot W: A longitudinal study of patients with multidirectional instability of the shoulder with seven- to ten-year follow-up. *J Shoulder Elbow Surg* 2005;14(5):466-470.

20. Nyiri P, Illyés A, Kiss R, Kiss J: Intermediate biomechanical analysis of the effect of physiotherapy only compared with capsular shift and physiotherapy in multidirectional shoulder instability. *J Shoulder Elbow Surg* 2010;19(6):802-813.

In a prospective study, the kinematic patterns in patients with multidirectional instability who were treated with physical therapy only or with physical therapy and capsular shift were compared with those of healthy control subjects. Surgery and physical therapy led to the more close approximation of normal shoulder kinematics, with a durable outcome at 4 years.

21. Tibone JE, Bradley JP: The treatment of posterior subluxation in athletes. *Clin Orthop Relat Res* 1993;291:124-137.

22. Hawkins RJ, Janda DH: Posterior instability of the glenohumeral joint: A technique of repair. *Am J Sports Med* 1996;24(3):275-278.

23. Bigliani LU, Pollock RG, McIlveen SJ, Endrizzi DP, Flatow EL: Shift of the posteroinferior aspect of the capsule for recurrent posterior glenohumeral instability. *J Bone Joint Surg Am* 1995;77(7):1011-1020.

24. Fronek J, Warren RF, Bowen M: Posterior subluxation of the glenohumeral joint. *J Bone Joint Surg Am* 1989;71(2):205-216.

25. Misamore GW, Facibene WA: Posterior capsulorrhaphy for the treatment of traumatic recurrent posterior subluxations of the shoulder in athletes. *J Shoulder Elbow Surg* 2000;9(5):403-408.

26. Meuffels DE, Schuit H, van Biezen FC, Reijman M, Verhaar JA: The posterior bone block procedure in posterior shoulder instability: A long-term follow-up study. *J Bone Joint Surg Br* 2010;92(5):651-655.

At 18-year follow-up after the posterior bone block procedure for posterior shoulder instability, 36% of the patients had a recurrence of dislocation, and almost 50% would not have the surgery a second time. More than one third of the patients had evidence of osteoarthritis, with deteriorating outcomes over the study period.

27. Rhee YG, Lee DH, Lim CT: Posterior capsulolabral reconstruction in posterior shoulder instability: Deltoid saving. *J Shoulder Elbow Surg* 2005;14(4):355-360.

28. Bahk MS, Karzel RP, Snyder SJ: Arthroscopic posterior stabilization and anterior capsular plication for recurrent posterior glenohumeral instability. *Arthroscopy* 2010;26(9):1172-1180.

At midterm follow-up, 29 patients had a good result after arthroscopic posterior stabilization with a balanced capsular plication. However, patients with supplemental anterior plication reported more pain, and this adjunctive procedure probably is unnecessary.

29. Bottoni CR, Franks BR, Moore JH, DeBerardino TM, Taylor DC, Arciero RA: Operative stabilization of posterior shoulder instability. *Am J Sports Med* 2005;33(7):996-1002.

30. Wellmann M, Bobrowitsch E, Khan N, et al: Biomechanical effectiveness of an arthroscopic posterior Bankart repair versus an open bone block procedure for posterior shoulder instability. *Am J Sports Med* 2011;39(4):796-803.

A cadaver study compared an arthroscopic posterior repair to a capsular repair with a bone block procedure after the creation of a posterior capsulolabral injury. The bone block procedure was found to overcorrect posterior translation and did not reduce inferior translation. The arthroscopic technique more effectively restored normal joint kinematics.

31. Williams RJ III, Strickland S, Cohen M, Altchek DW, Warren RF: Arthroscopic repair for traumatic posterior shoulder instability. *Am J Sports Med* 2003;31(2): 203-209.

32. Mair SD, Zarzour RH, Speer KP: Posterior labral injury in contact athletes. *Am J Sports Med* 1998;26(6): 753-758.

33. Radkowski CA, Chhabra A, Baker CL III, Tejwani SG, Bradley JP: Arthroscopic capsulolabral repair for posterior shoulder instability in throwing athletes compared with nonthrowing athletes. *Am J Sports Med* 2008;36(4):693-699.

    A prospective study compared the results of arthroscopic posterior repair for athletes in throwing and nonthrowing sports. The overall results were favorable and comparable in approximately 90% of patients. Nonthrowing athletes were more likely to return to their previous level of sport (71%) than throwing athletes (55%).

34. Seroyer S, Tejwani SG, Bradley JP: Arthroscopic capsulolabral reconstruction of the type VIII superior labrum anterior posterior lesion: Mean 2-year follow-up on 13 shoulders. *Am J Sports Med* 2007; 35(9):1477-1483.

    All patients with a type VIII superior labrum anterior and posterior lesion were able to return to sports at a minimum 2-year follow-up, and 69% were able to compete at their previous level of play.

35. Bradley JP, Baker CL III, Kline AJ, Armfield DR, Chhabra A: Arthroscopic capsulolabral reconstruction for posterior instability of the shoulder: A prospective study of 100 shoulders. *Am J Sports Med* 2006;34(7): 1061-1071.

36. Tjoumakaris FP, Bradley JP: The rationale for an arthroscopic approach to shoulder stabilization. *Arthroscopy* 2011;27(10):1422-1433.

    A rationale is presented for using arthroscopic techniques for most incidences of shoulder instability. The results of recent studies of arthroscopic results are similar or superior to those of earlier studies.

37. Jacobson ME, Riggenbach M, Wooldridge AN, Bishop JY: Open capsular shift and arthroscopic capsular plication for treatment of multidirectional instability. *Arthroscopy* 2012;28(7):1010-1017.

    A systematic review of level IV studies found that the results of arthroscopic surgery and open capsular shift were similar for the treatment of multidirectional shoulder instability with regard to recurrent instability, loss of external rotation, return to sport, and overall complications.

38. Sekiya JK, Willobee JA, Miller MD, Hickman AJ, Willobee A: Arthroscopic multi-pleated capsular plication compared with open inferior capsular shift for reduction of shoulder volume in a cadaveric model. *Arthroscopy* 2007;23(11):1145-1151.

    A study of seven cadavers assessed the extent of volume reduction with arthroscopic capsular plication compared with an open capsular shift. The authors found that capsular volume was reduced with both techniques, but the arthroscopic technique was slightly superior (58% versus 45% reduction).

39. Baker CL III, Mascarenhas R, Kline AJ, Chhabra A, Pombo MW, Bradley JP: Arthroscopic treatment of multidirectional shoulder instability in athletes: A retrospective analysis of 2- to 5-year clinical outcomes. *Am J Sports Med* 2009;37(9):1712-1720.

    After arthroscopic surgery for multidirectional instability in 43 patients, 91% had full or satisfactory range of motion, 98% had normal or slightly decreased strength, and 86% were able to return to their previous level of sport.

40. Hawkins RJ, Neer CS II, Pianta RM, Mendoza FX: Locked posterior dislocation of the shoulder. *J Bone Joint Surg Am* 1987;69(1):9-18.

2: Instability and Athletic Injuries

Chapter 10

Arthroscopic Reconstruction for Recurrent Shoulder Instability

Robert A. Arciero, MD   D. Nicholas Reed, MD

2: Instability and Athletic Injuries

Introduction

The glenohumeral joint is one of the least constrained joints, and its stability depends on a delicate balance of dynamic and static constraints. Injury to any of the constraints can lead to an array of conditions, from frank dislocation to repetitive microinstability or atraumatic instability. Most shoulder instability is anterior, and early and appropriate treatment often is necessary to avoid recurrence. Advances in understanding pathology, imaging, and surgical techniques have led to the success of arthroscopic reconstruction for treating recurrent instability, all in the hands of an experienced orthopaedic surgeon.

Clinical Evaluation

History

A thorough patient history should be obtained for preoperative and intraoperative decision making (Table 1). The patient's age, sex, hand dominance, medical conditions (such as seizures, hyperlaxity, or alcohol use), occupation, activity level, and expectations after surgery should be included. Age at initial dislocation should be included because a relatively young age is associated with an increased risk for recurrence.[1] The exact etiology should be defined by investigating the patient's history of trauma, microtrauma, or hyperlaxity as well as the extent of trauma; each of these will affect preoperative planning. For defining the direction of instability, the exact position of the arm at the time of the dislocation or the subluxation should be determined, as should the arm position that re-creates the symptoms. The patient should be asked about the frequency of in-

stability symptoms, the ease of re-creating symptoms, any instability during sleep, and whether it is becoming easier to subluxate the shoulder. The answers may provide insight into the severity of the soft-tissue and bony deficiency. Also important is whether the initial episode required a manual reduction. The need for a manual reduction typically indicates a major soft-tissue injury, possibly with a bony injury. Surgical notes and radiographs related to any earlier treatment should be reviewed for their effect on the surgical plan. Any history of voluntary instability or psychiatric disorder should be documented because an affected patient may be best treated nonsurgically.

Physical Examination

A detailed physical examination should be performed on both shoulders to allow a side-to-side comparison (Table 2). The involved and noninvolved shoulders should be inspected both anteriorly and posteriorly to detect any asymmetry or surgical scarring. The passive and active range of motion should be documented as well as rotator cuff strength; weakness has been associated with recurrent anterior instability.[2] If the patient has undergone an open procedure, the integrity of the subscapularis must be documented using the belly press and lift-off tests. The arm position that produces the instability should be noted. Instability in a position of abduction and external rotation suggests anterior instability. The exact degrees of abduction and external rotation should be noted because instability with relatively little abduction and external rotation suggests bony deficiency. Forward flexion, adduction, and internal rotation re-creating pain or instability suggests posterior instability. A sulcus sign with internal or external rotation should be documented and compared with the contralateral side. A detailed neurologic examination should be performed, with particular attention to the axillary nerve.

When the initial examination is complete, provocative testing should be performed. The apprehension and relocation tests should be used to assess anterior instability, and the jerk test should be used to detect posterior instability. The load-and-shift test should be used to detect anterior or posterior instability. Patients with a history of recurrent instability are more likely to have

Dr. Arciero or an immediate family member is a member of a speakers' bureau or has made paid presentations on behalf of Arthrex; has stock or stock options held in Soft Tissue Regeneration; and has received research or institutional support from Arthrex. Neither Dr. Reed nor any immediate family member has received anything of value from or owns stock in a commercial company or institution related directly or indirectly to the subject of this chapter.

Table 1

Patient History Findings Relevant to Instability

Finding	Significance
Age at initial dislocation	The risk for recurrence is increased in younger patients (especially those younger than 25 years).
Medical conditions (eg, seizures or electrical shock)	The risk for posterior dislocation or posterior instability is increased.
Trauma or manual reduction	A significant trauma or a manual reduction suggests a relatively severe soft-tissue injury or possible bony injury of the glenoid or the humeral head.
Activity level (sports participation)	Contact athletes may be at increased risk for recurrence.
Arm position at time of initial event	Anterior instability is suggested by a position of abduction and external rotation. Posterior instability is suggested by a position of forward flexion, adduction, and internal rotation.
Hyperlaxity	Multidirectional instability should be suspected.
Frequency of instability	Relative frequency may be related to bony deficiency.
Instability during sleep	Bony deficiency should be suspected.
Ease of re-creating symptoms or instability	Symptoms that can be re-created at progressively lower levels of abduction and external rotation suggest worsening bony involvement.

Table 2

Physical Examination Findings Relevant to Instability

Finding	Significance
Scars or asymmetry	Surgical scarring can provide information on earlier surgeries or trauma. Asymmetry can provide information on muscular atrophy secondary to muscle or tendon injury or neurologic injury.
Shoulder range of motion	Loss of full range of motion compared with contralateral side can signify adhesive capsulitis or bony or soft-tissue blocks.
Rotator cuff testing	A patient older than 40 years often has a rotator cuff injury with dislocation. Rotator cuff weakness may occur with recurrent instability. The subscapularis should be evaluated closely.
Arm position that re-creates symptoms or instability	Anterior instability is suggested by a position of abduction and external rotation. Posterior instability is suggested by a position of forward flexion, adduction, and internal rotation.
Provocative testing (apprehension, relocation, jerk tests)	Test results can provide information on the direction of instability.
Neurologic examination	The axillary and musculocutaneous nerves should be checked because of possible injury during earlier surgery or dislocation.
Hyperlaxity (elbow recurvatum, thumb-to-forearm test, sulcus sign)	Hyperlaxity suggests multidirectional instability.
Cervical spine evaluation	A full evaluation can rule out cervical pathology mimicking shoulder pain.

positive apprehension, relocation, and sulcus signs as well as greater posterior translation on the involved side than on the contralateral side.[3] Joint hyperlaxity should be determined by assessing elbow recurvatum, metacarpophalangeal hyperlaxity, and the thumb-to-forearm sign; affected patients may benefit from rehabilitation rather than surgery. A comprehensive shoulder examination should include a full neck evaluation to rule out cervical pathology as a cause of shoulder symptoms.

Imaging

The initial imaging should include standard trauma radiographs, including the true AP, scapular Y, and axillary lateral views. Specialized views that should be ob-

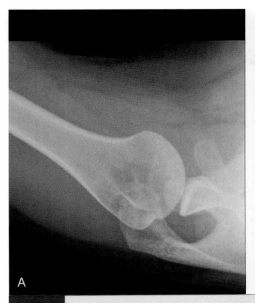
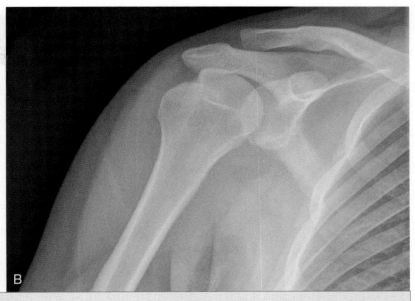

Figure 1 | **A,** West Point radiograph showing an anterior glenoid rim defect in the shoulder of a patient with recurrent anterior instability. The anterior contour of the glenoid is abnormal compared with the well-defined posterior glenoid rim. **B,** Stryker notch radiograph showing a Hill-Sachs lesion in the right humeral head of a patient with a traumatic dislocation. The abnormal contour of the humeral head can be seen laterally.

tained include the West Point modified axillary view to detect glenoid bone deficiency and the Stryker notch view to detect a humeral head (Hill-Sachs) lesion[4] (**Figure 1**).

MRI is useful for evaluating recurrent instability because of its superiority to other imaging modalities in assessing soft-tissue pathology. In patients with traumatic anterior instability, the most frequently diagnosed lesion is the Bankart lesion, which is an anteroinferior capsulolabral disruption.[5] Patients with recurrent shoulder instability have more posterior labral tears, superior labrum anterior to posterior (SLAP) tears, and rotator cuff pathology than patients with a first dislocation.[6] MRI also allows visualization of a humeral-sided avulsion of the glenohumeral ligaments (HAGL lesion), capsular tearing or attenuation, and bony edema. Preoperative recognition of additional pathology allows the surgeon to be prepared to treat all conditions during surgery and thereby improve the outcome.[7,8]

MRI is less useful than CT for detecting a bony defect. CT allows accurate assessment of bony injuries of both the glenoid and the humeral head. Bony defects are important to recognize and treat appropriately because treating only soft-tissue pathology leads to a high risk that arthroscopic stabilization will fail.[9,10] It is important to understand that as many as 90% of patients with recurrent instability have a glenoid rim defect, and as many as 100% have a Hill-Sachs lesion.[11,12] Three-dimensional CT can allow accurate assessment of a Hill-Sachs lesion or glenoid deficiency by digital subtraction of the humeral head so the glenoid can be viewed en face[13] (**Figure 2**). Many techniques exist for

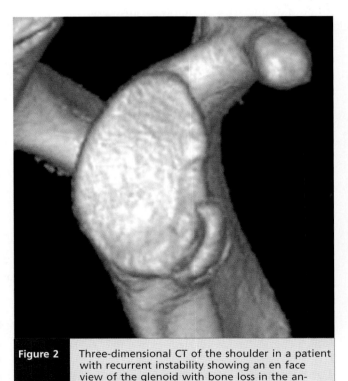

Figure 2 | Three-dimensional CT of the shoulder in a patient with recurrent instability showing an en face view of the glenoid with bone loss in the anteroinferior quadrant.

accurately calculating the percentage of bone loss on both the humeral and glenoid sides, and the surgeon should thoroughly understand the use of one of these methods[14-16] (**Table 3, Figure 3**). The threshold should be low for ordering three-dimensional CT before surgi-

2: Instability and Athletic Injuries

Table 3

Common Methods of Evaluating Glenoid Bone Loss

Method	Rationale
Plain radiography, including trauma-series and specialized views (West Point, apical oblique)	Useful for detecting bony abnormalities but not the percentage of bone loss. The West Point view is most precise.
MRI	Useful for evaluating soft-tissue injuries but not the percentage of bone loss.
Three-dimensional CT	Useful for measuring glenoid bone loss. The simplest methods are as follows: • Measure the glenoid bone loss. A measurement of 6 to 8 mm is approximately equivalent to a 25% loss. • Identify the bare area on an en face view of the glenoid. (The bare area is the center of the true circle of the inferior glenoid, and the distance to the anterior and posterior rims should be equal.) Measure from the bare area to the anterior rim of the intact glenoid (A) and from the bare area to the posterior glenoid (B). The percentage of bone loss is calculated as ([B − A] / 2B) × 100.
Arthroscopy	Glenoid bone loss should be estimated before arthroscopy but can be calculated intraoperatively by identifying the bare area, measuring from the bare area to the anterior (A) and posterior (B) glenoid rims, and using the equation ([B − A] / 2B) × 100.

cal intervention for recurrent instability. Preoperative CT also may be necessary if the patient has significant trauma at the time of initial dislocation, radiographs suggesting bony changes, a history of multiple earlier reductions, increasingly frequent instability, an instability sensation created with decreasing levels of force, instability with minimal abduction and external rotation, instability during sleep, glenoid dysplasia, abnormal version, or unsuccessful instability surgery.

Pathoanatomy

Bony Deficiency

Instability surgery is unlikely to succeed if a bony deficiency is not adequately treated.[9,10] The patient's history and physical examination should provide insight into glenoid- or humeral-side bony deficiency. Both the prevalence and the size of glenoid defects increase with recurrent dislocations. The likelihood of a so-called critical defect (involving more than 20% of the inferior glenoid) is associated with a higher number of dislocations and a younger age at the time of first dislocation.[17] The patient should undergo appropriate preoperative imaging to define the amount of bone loss, which can influence surgical planning.

Labrum and Glenohumeral Ligaments

The labrum is a fibrocartilaginous structure that encircles the glenoid, increasing its surface area and depth and acting as a buttress to translation of the humerus on the glenoid. The inferior glenohumeral ligament (IGHL) complex is a large ligament consisting of an anterior and posterior band connected by a capsular pouch. The IGHL complex is confluent with the labrum and can easily be identified arthroscopically.

The IGHL complex resists anterior translation of the humerus on the glenoid when the arm is in 90° of abduction and external rotation. A detachment of the anteroinferior labrum and the IGHL is called a Bankart lesion. A persistent Bankart lesion can lead to recurrent anterior instability of the shoulder (**Figure 4**). In a patient with recurrent instability, plastic deformation or attenuation of the IGHL occurs. Successful arthroscopic repair requires the labrum to be reattached to the glenoid face and the IGHL complex to have its tension restored.

In patients with recurrent instability, the detached labrum and the IGHL complex can heal in a medial position on the glenoid neck. This condition is called an anterior labroligamentous periosteal sleeve avulsion (ALPSA) lesion (**Figure 5**). An ALPSA lesion results in loss of tension of the IGHL complex and loss of the labrum as a bumper, leading to continued instability. Patients with recurrent instability and an ALPSA lesion typically have had more dislocations and are less likely to have successful surgery than patients who have only a Bankart lesion.[18]

Patients with recurrent instability may also have superior extension of labral pathology leading to a SLAP lesion. Patients with a SLAP lesion typically have more dislocations before surgery than patients with only a Bankart lesion. In contrast to patients with an ALPSA lesion, however, those with a SLAP lesion are no different from those with a Bankart lesion with respect to recurrence and function after surgery.[19] A HAGL lesion or a lateral detachment of the IGHL also can be a cause of recurrent instability (**Figure 6**). A HAGL lesion must be recognized before surgery and treated through an open or arthroscopic procedure. Recurrent instability almost always leads to capsular plastic deformation or attenuation. Failure to restore capsular tension can lead

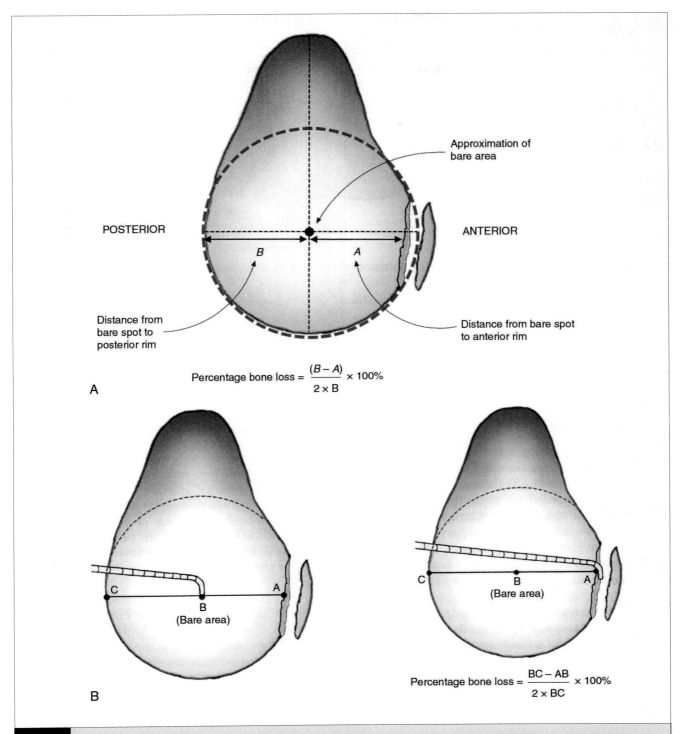

POSTERIOR

ANTERIOR

Approximation of
bare area

Distance from
bare spot to
posterior rim

Distance from bare spot
to anterior rim

$$\text{Percentage bone loss} = \frac{(B - A)}{2 \times B} \times 100\%$$

A

B
(Bare area)

B
(Bare area)

$$\text{Percentage bone loss} = \frac{BC - AB}{2 \times BC} \times 100\%$$

B

Figure 3 Schematic drawings showing the estimation of bone loss based on glenoid rim distances (**A**) and the glenoid bare-spot method (**B**). (Reproduced with permission from Provencher MT, Bhatia S, Ghodadra NS, et al: Recurrent shoulder instability: Current concepts for evaluation and management of glenoid bone loss. *J Bone Joint Surg Am* 2010; 92[suppl 2]:133-151.)

to failure of the surgery. Capsular plication of 1 cm in line with the fibers of the anterior band of the IGHL can reduce laxity and restore appropriate tension to the capsule.[20]

The Rotator Cuff Interval

The rotator cuff interval consists of the superior and middle glenohumeral ligaments, the long head of the biceps tendon, the coracohumeral ligament, and the

2: Instability and Athletic Injuries

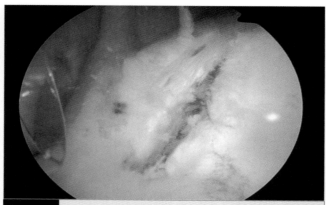

Figure 4 Arthroscopic image taken from the anterosuperior portal, showing a bony Bankart lesion in a patient with anterior instability. Detachment of the bony rim with the labrum attached can be seen. The anterior IGHL is attached to the labrum.

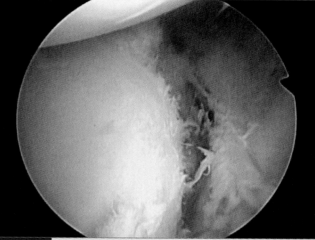

Figure 5 Arthroscopic image taken from the anterosuperior portal, showing an ALPSA lesion in a patient with recurrent instability. The loss of the labrum can be seen at the anterior cartilage rim. The labrum can be seen in a scarred, medialized position on the neck of the glenoid.

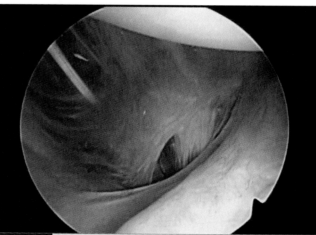

Figure 6 Arthroscopic image showing a HAGL lesion in a patient with recurrent instability. The retracted IGHL complex can be seen, as well as the muscular fibers of the subscapularis adjacent to the humeral head.

capsule. Controversy surrounds the risks and the benefits of rotator cuff interval closure in patients with anterior instability. Closure can improve anterior stability but result in a loss of external rotation, which can lead to loss of motion and the possible progression of osteoarthritis.[21,22]

The Rotator Cuff

Injury to the rotator cuff is rare in patients with a shoulder dislocation who are younger than 40 years. Patients older than 40 years have an increased risk of rotator cuff injury with shoulder dislocation, and rotator cuff injury should be suspected if the patient continues to have pain and weakness more than 3 weeks after the dislocation.

Treatment Planning

Nonsurgical Treatment

Most patients with recurrent instability require surgical intervention. The exception is the patient with multidirectional instability, who should undergo nonsurgical treatment before surgery is considered. Nonsurgical treatment also may be appropriate for a patient who has a significant medical comorbidity, low physical demands, a seizure disorder, or a psychiatric illness; who voluntarily dislocates for secondary gain; or who is unable or unwilling to complete postsurgical rehabilitation. Nonsurgical treatment typically involves a period of immobilization followed by rotator cuff and periscapular strengthening.

An in-season athlete can be treated nonsurgically with a brief period of immobilization followed by rotator cuff strengthening and the use of a protective brace or harness. However, as many as 37% of such athletes were found to have recurrence, and 50% required surgical intervention.[23]

Acute dislocation is treated with sling immobilization. There is controversy regarding the type of sling use after an initial acute dislocation. Some studies found that immobilization in external rotation may reduce the risk of recurrent anterior instability after a single dislocation episode, but other studies challenged this finding.[24] A recent meta-analysis found no benefit to immobilization for longer than 1 week, a greater incidence of recurrence if the patient was younger than 30 years, and no difference in recurrence rates based on whether traditional sling immobilization or immobilization in external rotation was used.[24]

Surgical Treatment

The role of arthroscopic reconstruction for recurrent shoulder instability continues to evolve. A review of data from the American Board of Orthopaedic Surgery reveals a trend toward arthroscopic stabilization and away from open repair as well as a decreasing number of complications among all-arthroscopically treated patients.[25] Arthroscopic procedures can be as successful as open procedures if the surgeon is able to recognize all underlying soft-tissue and bony deficiency and treat them appropriately using modern techniques and devices.[26] Two recent meta-analyses confirmed earlier findings that arthroscopic repair of a Bankart lesion using suture anchors is equivalent to open repair.[27,28] However, the open Bankart repair remains a time-tested standard procedure for achieving a stable, well-functioning shoulder joint.[5] The requirements for a successful arthroscopic reconstruction are to recognize and treat bony deficiency, recognize and treat all concomitant soft-tissue pathology, use an appropriate surgical procedure and technique, and determine whether the patient is at high risk for recurrence.

Glenoid Deficiency

The ability to recognize a glenoid defect before surgery and treat it appropriately during an open or an arthroscopic procedure is crucial to surgical success. If glenoid deficiency is missed before surgery, the surgeon can use the bare spot on the glenoid to measure the defect intraoperatively. However, every attempt should be made to identify significant bone loss on the humerus or the glenoid before surgery so that the patient can be adequately counseled as to the options and a definitive plan can be made before surgery. A 6- to 8-mm defect anteriorly rather than posteriorly means that 25% of the glenoid is missing, and the surgical plan must be changed accordingly. Surgical failure rates as high as 80% have been associated with glenoid bone loss in the anteroinferior region.[9] The extent of bone loss for which an open repair should be performed is debatable, but most experts agree that open repair is required for bone loss greater than 20% to 25%.[29,30] However, all-arthroscopic repair of a bony Bankart lesion with a retained fragment, with incorporation of the bony fragment in the repair, has had acceptable results (failure rates of less than 10%).[31,32] These studies highlight the importance of the glenoid bone stock in glenohumeral stability. If glenoid bone loss is greater than 20% to 25% and there is no bony fragment, an open procedure should be performed to restore the functional arc of the glenoid.

Open procedures, such as iliac crest bone grafting, tibial allograft bone grafting, the Bristow procedure (transfer of the tip of the coracoid), and the Latarjet procedure (transfer of the entire coracoid base with the coracoacromial ligament and the conjoined tendon), have yielded good results in terms of recurrence. A recent review of the Bristow-Latarjet procedure revealed good and consistent results, with bony fusion in 83% of the patients; recurrence rates were lower when the coracoid was placed less than 1 cm medial to the glenoid rim and a horizontal capsular shift was added to the transfer.[33]

Humeral Head Lesions

A defect in the articular surface of the humeral head (a Hill-Sachs lesion) can be found in almost every patient with recurrent instability. Most defects are small and have little effect on the stability of the shoulder. Surgery for a Hill-Sachs lesion that is associated with glenoid bone loss or engages on the glenoid rim with abduction and external rotation (a so-called engaging Hill-Sachs lesion) is likely to fail if only soft tissue is treated.[9,12] Most such lesions require treatment of only the glenoid defect; doing so increases the arc of rotation and prevents the Hill-Sachs lesion from engaging, which can lead to recurrence. However, large defects of the humeral head (more than 30%) may require treating the humeral head directly.[34] Three-dimensional CT can be useful in quantifying the defect. The arm can be placed in abduction and external rotation intraoperatively to determine whether the Hill-Sachs lesion is engaging; if so, it must be treated.

Arthroscopic remplissage (capsulotenodesis of the posterior capsule and infraspinatus tendon into the Hill-Sachs defect) is an emerging treatment option that avoids the potential morbidity of an open procedure and may reduce the ability of the humeral head to engage on the glenoid. Several studies have shown that a large or an engaging Hill-Sachs lesion can be treated with arthroscopic Bankart repair and remplissage with no alteration in range of motion; the recurrence rates were similar to those of open procedures.[35-37] However, as many as 33% of patients have experienced postero-superior pain after remplissage.[38] Open procedures for treating Hill-Sachs lesions are still widely used and reliable. These procedures include elevation of the defect and bone grafting, articular allograft, metal resurfacing, rotational osteotomy, and hemiarthroplasty.

Soft-Tissue Pathology

Arthroscopic reconstruction allows direct visualization of all bony and soft-tissue injures in a patient with recurrent instability. Patients with prolonged recurrent instability typically have extensive soft-tissue injuries, which must be appropriately treated to ensure a successful outcome. The Bankart lesion must be identified and mobilized, and appropriate tension and placement of the labrum and the IGHL complex must be restored on the glenoid face. It is important to carefully visualize the entire labrum and treat any posterior labral tear or SLAP lesion. An ALPSA lesion is best identified from the anterosuperior portal, and it must be mobilized and appropriately tensioned on the face of the glenoid to ensure success. A HAGL lesion typically is identified on preoperative MRI but can be seen arthroscopically. Although experienced surgeons have repaired HAGL lesions arthroscopically, an open subscapularis tendon–

sparing approach should be considered. Patients who have capsular deficiency as a result of recurrent instability or earlier surgery are challenging to treat. Allograft reconstruction of anterior capsulolabral structures had promising results at 2-year follow-up and is a viable alternative to arthrodesis in young patients.[39]

The rotator cuff interval structures continue to be a source of controversy in arthroscopic instability surgery. Closure of the rotator cuff interval can improve anterior instability at the cost of external rotation. Rotator cuff interval closure has been suggested for patients with hyperlaxity and recurrent instability, patients with a positive sulcus sign that does not correspond to the contralateral side or cannot be corrected by external rotation with the arm at the side, patients undergoing revision surgery, and athletes in collision sports who consider stability more important than range of motion.[40] Rotator cuff interval closure also has been used for posterior instability; good results have been achieved without closure, however, and the improvement in posterior stability with closure has been called into question.[22]

Patient Selection

To maximize the likelihood of surgical success, an appropriate history and physical examination should be used to select patients for arthroscopic reconstruction. Success is most likely if the patient meets several criteria: no bone defect larger than 20% to 25%, no engaging Hill-Sachs lesion, a well-defined Bankart lesion with good tissue, no other concomitant soft-tissue injuries, no identifiable hyperlaxity, and an initial dislocation. Favorable indicators for an athlete include participation in an overhead sport (or in a noncollision sport if the patient is older than 20 years).

Surgical Technique

The diagnosis and the surgical plan should be established before surgery. Every patient should be examined under anesthesia to confirm the diagnosis and ensure that no abnormalities were missed preoperatively. The patient is positioned according to the surgeon's preference. The lateral decubitus position with longitudinal traction allows excellent visualization and access to the inferior glenoid. Portal placement is important in instability repair. The posterior portal should be placed in line with the glenoid face; this positioning is more lateral than the traditional posterior portal. The anterior portal should be placed using an outside-in technique to ensure appropriate placement and avoid articular injury. The anterosuperior portal should be placed high in the rotator cuff interval, and the anteroinferior portal should be placed just above the subscapularis. The portals should allow access to the inferior recess.

Visualization of all bony and soft-tissue injuries is critical. All associated injuries must be treated. The Bankart lesion can be seen through the posterior portal,

and the anterosuperior portal is used to ensure that an ALPSA lesion is not missed. The Bankart lesion is mobilized in preparation for tensioning and repair. Capsulolabral release is considered adequate when the surgeon can see the muscle fibers of the subscapularis. The glenoid should be prepared by removing all soft tissue from the intended repair site. After mobilization and preparation, the surgeon determines whether anchors or sutures will be placed first. The anchors should be placed at the glenoid face at the level of the articular cartilage and the scapular neck junction. The anchors must not be placed too medial because appropriate tension will not be restored, and they must not be placed too close to the face because of the risk of injury to articular cartilage and subsequent malreduction of the capsulolabral complex.

Proper anchor placement on the glenoid face should begin between the 5-o'clock and 6-o'clock positions with a minimum of three or four anchors.[9,41] The surgeon should ensure that the anchors are adequately seated to avoid postoperative impingement on the humeral head. Multiple studies have evaluated different anchors and sutures; recent studies have found that capsulolabral height can be restored and outcomes are similar regardless of whether the traditional or newer knotless anchor system is used.[42-46] The next step is to restore tension to the IGHL complex. The sutures for tensioning should be placed 5 to 10 mm caudal to the corresponding anchors to allow appropriate tension. For example, an anchor placed in the 5-o'clock position should have a corresponding tension suture placed around 1 cm of capsulolabral and IGHL complex soft tissue at the 6-o'clock position. The soft tissue should be brought to the 5-o'clock anchor, moving all soft tissue within the tension suture cephalad by 5 to 10 mm to create appropriate tensioning (**Figure 7**). Any capsular redundancy noted before or during surgery should be treated to prevent recurrence. This capsular tissue can be included in the repair by placing sutures in the capsule 1 cm lateral to the labrum using the anchor placed for labral repair. Abrasion of the capsule can enhance capsular healing to the labrum.

The repair should be inspected after it is completed to ensure restoration of tension and the bumper effect (**Figure 8**). If needed, a posterior labral anchor can be placed for a posteriorly directed tear, and the rotator cuff interval can be closed if the surgeon decided to do so before surgery. However, rotator cuff interval closure should not be routinely done (**Figure 9**).

Complications and Controversies

The risk of complications after arthroscopic stabilization, including recurrence, can be minimized by following preoperative and intraoperative recommendations and techniques. Patients such as those with a bone or soft-tissue deficiency should not be treated arthroscopically if their condition is better suited to an open pro-

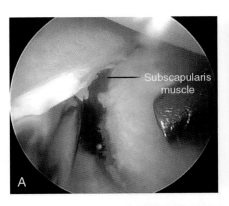

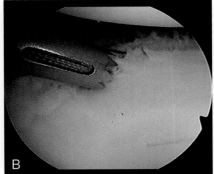

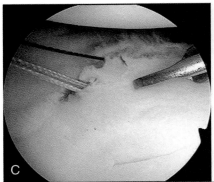

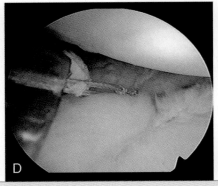

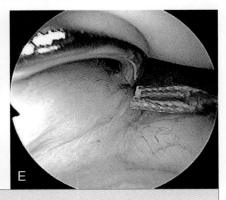

Figure 7 Arthroscopic images showing the surgical technique and placement of anchors for the treatment of anterior instability. **A,** Adequate mobilization is achieved when the muscular fibers of subscapularis are identified. The probe is located between the glenoid rim and the labrum, and the subscapularis muscle belly is identified deep. **B,** Anchors are placed after mobilization is complete. The anchor is in the 5:30 clock position on the anterior glenoid face. **C,** The suture-passing shuttle wire exits inferior to the sutures. The entry site for capsule penetration is 1 cm below the exit site to allow adequate retensioning of the IGHL complex. **D,** Both suture limbs have been passed and tied in horizontal mattress fashion. The knot is off the articular surface, and the bumper effect and tension on the IGHL complex have been restored with the initial anchor. **E,** The suture has been tied inferiorly, and the crescent hook is being used to grasp tissue for the next anchor, placed above the earlier anchor. The amount of capsulolabral tissue obtained for tensioning can be seen. (Reproduced with permission from Arciero RA, Mazzocca A: Arthroscopic treatment of anterior instability: Surgical technique, in Provencher MT, Romeo AA, eds: *Shoulder Instability: A Comprehensive Approach.* Philadelphia, PA, Elsevier-Saunders, 2012, pp 126-146.)

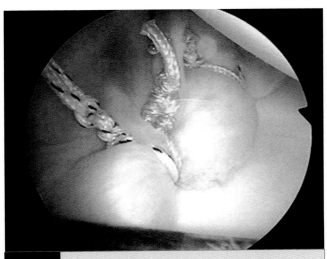

Figure 8 Arthroscopic image of a completed Bankart repair, showing the restoration of the bumper effect and tension on the IGHL.

cedure. Complications such as postoperative stiffness can be avoided if only the injured tissue is treated and a strict postoperative rehabilitation regimen is followed. The risk of chondrolysis can be decreased by avoiding thermal ablation and the use of indwelling pain pumps.

Patients at High Risk

A patient who is at high risk for recurrence must be identified before surgery. A preoperative instability severity index score has been created to help surgeons identify such patients. The system is based on a 10-point scale in which 2 points are assigned if the patient is younger than 20 years, is a competitive athlete, has a Hill-Sachs lesion as noted in external rotation on an AP radiograph, or has any change of the glenoid contour on an AP radiograph; 1 point is assigned if the patient has hyperlaxity or is an athlete in a contact or an overhead sport. Patients with a combined score higher than 6 were found to have a 70% recurrence risk, and those with a score of 6 or less had a 10% risk.[10] Other studies found that male sex, age younger than 22 years, and

2: Instability and Athletic Injuries

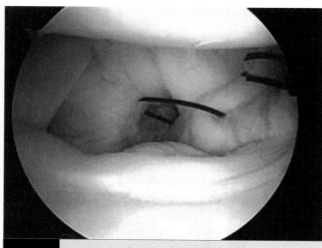

Figure 9 | Arthroscopic image showing rotator cuff interval closure in a patient with multidirectional instability.

recurrent instability are risk factors for arthroscopic surgical failure, and such patients also should be closely evaluated.[47,48]

Controversies

There are multiple controversies related to arthroscopic instability surgery. In particular, the treatment of athletes in contact sports continues to be a source of controversy. Some surgeons support open repair for these athletes, and others support arthroscopic repair. Both sides of the controversy are supported by research.[49-52]

Summary

The indications for arthroscopic reconstruction of recurrent instability continue to evolve. Arthroscopic reconstruction can have excellent results in terms of recurrence and function if close attention is paid to all of its preoperative and intraoperative aspects.

Annotated References

1. Robinson CM, Howes J, Murdoch H, Will E, Graham C: Functional outcome and risk of recurrent instability after primary traumatic anterior shoulder dislocation in young patients. *J Bone Joint Surg Am* 2006;88(11):2326-2336.

2. Edouard P, Degache F, Beguin L, et al: Rotator cuff strength in recurrent anterior shoulder instability. *J Bone Joint Surg Am* 2011;93(8):759-765.

   Internal and external rotator cuff weakness was associated with recurrent anterior instability.

3. Owens BD, Duffey ML, Deberardino TM, Cameron KL: Physical examination findings in young athletes correlate with history of shoulder instability. *Orthopedics* 2011;34(6):460.

   One hundred patients with a history of shoulder instability were compared with healthy control subjects. The patients were more likely to have increased posterior translation and positive apprehension, relocation, and sulcus signs.

4. Itoi E, Lee SB, Amrami KK, Wenger DE, An KN: Quantitative assessment of classic anteroinferior bony Bankart lesions by radiography and computed tomography. *Am J Sports Med* 2003;31(1):112-118.

5. Gill TJ, Micheli LJ, Gebhard F, Binder C: Bankart repair for anterior instability of the shoulder: Long-term outcome. *J Bone Joint Surg Am* 1997;79(6):850-857.

6. Gutierrez V, Monckeberg JE, Pinedo M, Radice F: Arthroscopically determined degree of injury after shoulder dislocation relates to recurrence rate. *Clin Orthop Relat Res* 2012;470(4):961-964.

   Patients with recurrent shoulder dislocation had more soft-tissue injury, including posterior labral tears, SLAP tears, and rotator cuff pathology, compared with patients having a first episode of shoulder dislocation. Level of evidence: II.

7. Porcellini G, Paladini P, Campi F, Paganelli M: Shoulder instability and related rotator cuff tears: Arthroscopic findings and treatment in patients aged 40 to 60 years. *Arthroscopy* 2006;22(3):270-276.

8. Rhee YG, Ha JH, Park KJ: Clinical outcome of anterior shoulder instability with capsular midsubstance tear: A comparison of isolated midsubstance tear and midsubstance tear with Bankart lesion. *J Shoulder Elbow Surg* 2006;15(5):586-590.

9. Burkhart SS, De Beer JF: Traumatic glenohumeral bone defects and their relationship to failure of arthroscopic Bankart repairs: Significance of the inverted-pear glenoid and the humeral engaging Hill-Sachs lesion. *Arthroscopy* 2000;16(7):677-694.

10. Balg F, Boileau P: The instability severity index score: A simple pre-operative score to select patients for arthroscopic or open shoulder stabilisation. *J Bone Joint Surg Br* 2007;89(11):1470-1477.

    A 10-point preoperative instability severity index was created and evaluated through retrospective review of 131 patients. Points were assigned for age, sports participation, hyperlaxity, and bony deficiency. Patients with a score higher than 6 had a recurrence risk of 70%.

11. Piasecki DP, Verma NN, Romeo AA, Levine WN, Bach BR Jr, Provencher MT: Glenoid bone deficiency in recurrent anterior shoulder instability: Diagnosis and management. *J Am Acad Orthop Surg* 2009; 17(8):482-493.

    An excellent review of glenoid bone loss is presented, with its relationship to recurrent shoulder instability and an algorithm for diagnosis and treatment.

12. Cetik O, Uslu M, Ozsar BK: The relationship between Hill-Sachs lesion and recurrent anterior shoulder dislocation. *Acta Orthop Belg* 2007;73(2):175-178.

    In 30 patients with recurrent anterior dislocation, a positive correlation was found between a greater number of dislocations and greater extent and depth of a Hill-Sachs lesion.

13. Provencher MT, Bhatia S, Ghodadra NS, et al: Recurrent shoulder instability: Current concepts for evaluation and management of glenoid bone loss. *J Bone Joint Surg Am* 2010;92(suppl 2):133-151.

    An update is provided on the evaluation, diagnosis, and treatment of patients with glenoid bone loss and recurrent shoulder instability.

14. Sugaya H, Moriishi J, Dohi M, Kon Y, Tsuchiya A: Glenoid rim morphology in recurrent anterior glenohumeral instability. *J Bone Joint Surg Am* 2003; 85(5):878-884.

15. Cho SH, Cho NS, Rhee YG: Preoperative analysis of the Hill-Sachs lesion in anterior shoulder instability: How to predict engagement of the lesion. *Am J Sports Med* 2011;39(11):2389-2395.

    A review of 107 shoulders after arthroscopic Bankart repair for traumatic anterior shoulder instability used three-dimensional CT to evaluate Hill-Sachs lesions. Engaging Hill-Sachs lesions were larger and more horizontally oriented. Level of evidence: II.

16. Chuang TY, Adams CR, Burkhart SS: Use of preoperative three-dimensional computed tomography to quantify glenoid bone loss in shoulder instability. *Arthroscopy* 2008;24(4):376-382.

    Recurrent instability and glenoid bone loss were reviewed with three-dimensional CT in 25 patients. Patients could be identified as needing an open procedure based on glenoid bone loss.

17. Milano G, Grasso A, Russo A, et al: Analysis of risk factors for glenoid bone defect in anterior shoulder instability. *Am J Sports Med* 2011;39(9):1870-1876.

    In a review of 161 patients with anterior shoulder instability, the number of dislocations and age at first dislocation were the most significant predictors of glenoid bone loss in anterior shoulder instability.

18. Ozbaydar M, Elhassan B, Diller D, Massimini D, Higgins LD, Warner JJ: Results of arthroscopic capsulolabral repair: Bankart lesion versus anterior labroligamentous periosteal sleeve avulsion lesion. *Arthroscopy* 2008;24(11):1277-1283.

    In a review of 93 shoulders with recurrent anterior shoulder instability, patients with an ALPSA lesion had more recurrent dislocations and a higher failure rate after arthroscopic capsulolabral repair than patients with a Bankart lesion alone.

19. Hantes ME, Venouziou AI, Liantsis AK, Dailiana ZH, Malizos KN: Arthroscopic repair for chronic anterior shoulder instability: A comparative study between patients with Bankart lesions and patients with combined Bankart and superior labral anterior posterior lesions. *Am J Sports Med* 2009;37(6):1093-1098.

    A review of 63 patients with anterior shoulder instability found no difference at 2-year follow-up in stability or function based on whether the patient had Bankart repair alone or combined Bankart and SLAP repair. Level of evidence: II.

20. Shapiro TA, Gupta A, McGarry MH, Tibone JE, Lee TQ: Biomechanical effects of arthroscopic capsulorrhaphy in line with the fibers of the anterior band of the inferior glenohumeral ligament. *Am J Sports Med* 2012;40(3):672-680.

    A cadaver study evaluated intact shoulders, shoulders with anterior instability, and arthroscopically plicated shoulders. A 10-mm arthroscopic plication in line with the fibers of the anterior band of the IGHL complex effectively reduced capsular laxity without overconstraining the joint.

21. Randelli P, Arrigoni P, Polli L, Cabitza P, Denti M: Quantification of active ROM after arthroscopic Bankart repair with rotator interval closure. *Orthopedics* 2009;32(6):408.

    Rotator cuff interval closure can provide anterior stability but results in a reduction of external rotation.

22. Mologne TS, Zhao K, Hongo M, Romeo AA, An KN, Provencher MT: The addition of rotator interval closure after arthroscopic repair of either anterior or posterior shoulder instability: Effect on glenohumeral translation and range of motion. *Am J Sports Med* 2008;36(6):1123-1131.

    Rotator cuff interval closure can improve anterior shoulder stability, but posterior stability is not improved.

23. Buss DD, Lynch GP, Meyer CP, Huber SM, Freehill MQ: Nonoperative management for in-season athletes with anterior shoulder instability. *Am J Sports Med* 2004;32(6):1430-1433.

24. Paterson WH, Throckmorton TW, Koester M, Azar FM, Kuhn JE: Position and duration of immobilization after primary anterior shoulder dislocation: A systematic review and meta-analysis of the literature. *J Bone Joint Surg Am* 2010;92(18):2924-2933.

    A meta-analysis found no benefit to conventional sling immobilization of longer than 1 week for the treatment of primary anterior shoulder dislocation in relatively young patients. Bracing in external rotation may be less effective than believed.

25. Owens BD, Harrast JJ, Hurwitz SR, Thompson TL, Wolf JM: Surgical trends in Bankart repair: An analysis of data from the American Board of Orthopaedic Surgery certification examination. *Am J Sports Med* 2011;39(9):1865-1869.

    Data show that the number of arthroscopic shoulder stabilization procedures is increasing and the number of open repairs is decreasing. The overall rate of complications was lower overall after arthroscopic stabilization.

26. Mahiroğulları M, Ozkan H, Akyüz M, Uğraş AA, Güney A, Kuşkucu M: Comparison between the results of open and arthroscopic repair of isolated traumatic anterior instability of the shoulder. *Acta Orthop Traumatol Turc* 2010;44(3):180-185.

   Open and arthroscopic Bankart repairs for recurrent anterior shoulder instability were compared. The average follow-up was 26.1 months, and metal anchors were used in all patients. The results of both were similar in terms of recurrence and patient satisfaction.

27. Petrera M, Patella V, Patella S, Theodoropoulos J: A meta-analysis of open versus arthroscopic Bankart repair using suture anchors. *Knee Surg Sports Traumatol Arthrosc* 2010;18(12):1742-1747.

   A meta-analysis found that arthroscopic Bankart repair had better results than open repair in terms of recurrence in studies published later than 2002.

28. Hobby J, Griffin D, Dunbar M, Boileau P: Is arthroscopic surgery for stabilisation of chronic shoulder instability as effective as open surgery? A systematic review and meta-analysis of 62 studies including 3044 arthroscopic operations. *J Bone Joint Surg Br* 2007;89(9):1188-1196.

   A systematic literature search identified 62 studies of Bankart lesions treated arthroscopically or open. When the newest and most effective techniques were used, failure rates were similar at 2-year follow-up.

29. Yamamoto N, Itoi E, Abe H, et al: Effect of an anterior glenoid defect on anterior shoulder stability: A cadaveric study. *Am J Sports Med* 2009;37(5):949-954.

   In a laboratory cadaver study, 2-mm increments of glenoid bone were removed and stability was checked. A 20% loss at the 3-o'clock position significantly decreased anterior stability.

30. Sugaya H, Moriishi J, Kanisawa I, Tsuchiya A: Arthroscopic osseous Bankart repair for chronic recurrent traumatic anterior glenohumeral instability: Surgical technique. *J Bone Joint Surg Am* 2006;88(suppl 1, Pt 2):159-169.

31. Zhu YM, Jiang CY, Lu Y, Xue QY: Clinical results after all arthroscopic reduction and fixation of bony Bankart lesion. *Zhonghua Wai Ke Za Zhi* 2011;49(7):603-606.

   Forty patients with a bony Bankart lesion were treated all-arthroscopically using suture anchors, and the bony lesion was included in the repair. The recurrence rate was 8.9%.

32. Ikeda H: "Rotator interval" lesion. Part 1: Clinical study. *Nihon Seikeigeka Gakkai Zasshi* 1986;60(12):1261-1273.

33. Hovelius L, Sandström B, Olofsson A, Svensson O, Rahme H: The effect of capsular repair, bone block healing, and position on the results of the Bristow-Latarjet procedure (study III): Long-term follow-up in 319 shoulders. *J Shoulder Elbow Surg* 2012;21(5):647-660.

   A review of the open Bristow-Latarjet procedure with long-term follow-up found consistently good results, with fusion in 83% of the patients. A medially placed coracoid (more than 1 cm) led to relatively poor results.

34. Millett PJ, Clavert P, Warner JJ: Open operative treatment for anterior shoulder instability: When and why? *J Bone Joint Surg Am* 2005;87(2):419-432.

35. Park MJ, Tjoumakaris FP, Garcia G, Patel A, Kelly JD IV: Arthroscopic remplissage with Bankart repair for the treatment of glenohumeral instability with Hill-Sachs defects. *Arthroscopy* 2011;27(9):1187-1194.

   A review of 20 patients who underwent arthroscopic Bankart repair with remplissage for recurrent anterior glenohumeral instability and a Hill-Sachs defect involving more than 25% of the humeral head found that 85% of the patients had a satisfactory result. Level of evidence: IV.

36. Haviv B, Mayo L, Biggs D: Outcomes of arthroscopic "remplissage": Capsulotenodesis of the engaging large Hill-Sachs lesion. *J Orthop Surg Res* 2011;6:29.

   A review of 11 patients who underwent arthroscopic surgery with remplissage for recurrent instability with a large engaging Hill-Sachs lesion found that the technique was effective with respect to recurrence, motion, and function.

37. Zhu YM, Lu Y, Zhang J, Shen JW, Jiang CY: Arthroscopic Bankart repair combined with remplissage technique for the treatment of anterior shoulder instability with engaging Hill-Sachs lesion: A report of 49 cases with a minimum 2-year follow-up. *Am J Sports Med* 2011;39(8):1640-1647.

   A review of 49 patients with an engaging Hill-Sachs lesion who underwent arthroscopic Bankart repair and remplissage found a failure rate of 8.2% at a mean 29-month follow-up, with no significant impairment of shoulder function. Level of evidence: IV.

38. Nourissat G, Kilinc AS, Werther JR, Doursounian L: A prospective, comparative, radiological, and clinical study of the influence of the "remplissage" procedure on shoulder range of motion after stabilization by arthroscopic Bankart repair. *Am J Sports Med* 2011;39(10):2147-2152.

   Patients with Bankart repair alone and patients with Bankart repair and remplissage had identical recurrence rates and no difference in shoulder range of motion. One third of the patients had posterosuperior pain. Level of evidence: II.

39. Dewing CB, Horan MP, Millett PJ: Two-year outcomes of open shoulder anterior capsular reconstruction for instability from severe capsular deficiency. *Arthroscopy* 2012;28(1):43-51.

   Allograft reconstruction of anterior capsulolabral structures for capsular deficiency was performed on 22 shoulders. Outcomes were satisfactory in terms of recurrence and function. Level of evidence: IV.

40. Chechik O, Maman E, Dolkart O, Khashan M, Shabtai L, Mozes G: Arthroscopic rotator interval closure in shoulder instability repair: A retrospective study. *J Shoulder Elbow Surg* 2010;19(7):1056-1062.

There was an additive effect on shoulder stability in 37 patients who underwent arthroscopic rotator cuff interval closure in addition to arthroscopic Bankart repair. Systemic hyperlaxity was associated with recurrent dislocation and poor outcome.

41. van der Linde JA, van Kampen DA, Terwee CB, Dijksman LM, Kleinjan G, Willems WJ: Long-term results after arthroscopic shoulder stabilization using suture anchors: An 8- to 10-year follow-up. *Am J Sports Med* 2011;39(11):2396-2403.

Sixty-eight shoulders treated for anterior instability with arthroscopic Bankart repair were followed for 8 to 10 years. The presence of a Hill-Sachs defect and the use of more than three anchors increased the risk of recurrence. Level of evidence: IV.

42. Milano G, Grasso A, Santagada DA, Saccomanno MF, Deriu L, Fabbriciani C: Comparison between metal and biodegradable suture anchors in the arthroscopic treatment of traumatic anterior shoulder instability: A prospective randomized study. *Knee Surg Sports Traumatol Arthrosc* 2010;18(12):1785-1791.

Arthroscopic stabilization was performed in 78 patients with recurrent anterior shoulder instability. Patients were compared based on the use of metal or biodegradable anchors. At 2-year follow-up, there was no difference in recurrence rates.

43. Slabaugh MA, Friel NA, Wang VM, Cole BJ: Restoring the labral height for treatment of Bankart lesions: A comparison of suture anchor constructs. *Arthroscopy* 2010;26(5):587-591.

The Bio-Suture Tak (Arthrex, Naples, FL) and Push-Lock (Arthrex) suture anchors were compared for Bankart lesion restoration in 10 cadaver glenoids. A three-dimensional digitizer was used to measure restored labral height after fixation. No difference was noted.

44. Oh JH, Lee HK, Kim JY, Kim SH, Gong HS: Clinical and radiologic outcomes of arthroscopic glenoid labrum repair with the BioKnotless suture anchor. *Am J Sports Med* 2009;37(12):2340-2348.

Arthroscopic glenoid labral repair was performed with the BioKnotless anchor (DePuy, Warsaw, IN) in 97 patients who were followed for a mean 34.1 months. The anchors were found to be comparable to standard metal anchors without knot tying. Level of evidence: IV.

45. Thal R, Nofziger M, Bridges M, Kim JJ: Arthroscopic Bankart repair using Knotless or BioKnotless suture anchors: 2- to 7-year results. *Arthroscopy* 2007;23(4): 367-375.

Arthroscopic Bankart repair was performed in 73 patients using knotless or BioKnotless suture anchors. At a minimum 2-year follow-up, the recurrence rate was 6.9%, and all patients had a reliable return of function.

46. Monteiro GC, Ejnisman B, Andreoli CV, de Castro Pochini A, Cohen M: Absorbable versus nonabsorbable sutures for the arthroscopic treatment of anterior shoulder instability in athletes: A prospective randomized study. *Arthroscopy* 2008;24(6):697-703.

Anchors with absorbable and nonabsorbable suture were compared in the treatment of arthroscopic Bankart repair. No differences were found between the two types of anchors at a minimum 24-month follow-up.

47. Yan H, Cui GQ, Wang JQ, Yin Y, Tian DX, Ao YF: Arthroscopic Bankart repair with suture anchors: Results and risk factors of recurrence of instability. *Zhonghua Wai Ke Za Zhi* 2011;49(7):597-602.

Arthroscopic Bankart repair with suture anchors was performed in 259 patients with recurrent shoulder instability. At a minimum 1-year follow-up, patients younger than 20 years and athletes were at high risk for recurrence.

48. Porcellini G, Campi F, Pegreffi F, Castagna A, Paladini P: Predisposing factors for recurrent shoulder dislocation after arthroscopic treatment. *J Bone Joint Surg Am* 2009;91(11):2537-2542.

A review of 385 patients who underwent arthroscopic Bankart repair for unidirectional instability found that age younger than 22 years, age at time of first dislocation, and male sex were risk factors for recurrence at 36-month follow-up.

49. Uhorchak JM, Arciero RA, Huggard D, Taylor DC: Recurrent shoulder instability after open reconstruction in athletes involved in collision and contact sports. *Am J Sports Med* 2000;28(6):794-799.

50. Pagnani MJ, Dome DC: Surgical treatment of traumatic anterior shoulder instability in American football players. *J Bone Joint Surg Am* 2002;84-A(5):711-715.

51. Ide J, Maeda S, Takagi K: Arthroscopic Bankart repair using suture anchors in athletes: Patient selection and postoperative sports activity. *Am J Sports Med* 2004; 32(8):1899-1905.

52. Mazzocca AD, Brown FM, Carreira DS, Hayden J, Romeo AA: Arthroscopic anterior shoulder stabilization of collision and contact athletes. *Am J Sports Med* 2005;33(1):52-60.

2: Instability and Athletic Injuries

Chapter 11

Injuries to the Throwing Shoulder

John Tokish, MD   Kelly Fitzpatrick, DO

Introduction

The treatment of the shoulder in a throwing athlete continues to be challenging. The high forces and the kinematic requirements of overhead throwing produce a unique pathophysiology that is most evident in elite throwing athletes. The throwing shoulder exerts a rotational velocity of as much as 7,000° per second, which is reportedly the fastest movement in sports.[1] Throwing shoulders have been found to adapt by increasing external rotation, decreasing internal rotation, increasing humeral and glenoid retroversion, and developing anterior capsular laxity. With each pitch, the soft-tissue envelope surrounding the shoulder is loaded to levels that approach ultimate failure. The combination of the adaptations and the demands on the throwing shoulder means that it is vulnerable to common pathologic conditions such as a partial-thickness rotator cuff tear, anterior capsular laxity or pseudolaxity, posteroinferior capsular contracture, posterior or posterosuperior labral injury, biceps tendon pathology, and scapular dyskenesis.[2]

One of the most difficult challenges in treating a patient with a disabled throwing shoulder is to distinguish a pathologic entity from a normal adaptation. A "fix everything" approach can lead to an inability to return to the previous level of throwing. It is therefore critical that the entire surgical team is cautious during the preoperative evaluation, is meticulous in surgical technique, and uses a comprehensive postoperative rehabilitation program for an athlete who hopes to return to demanding activity.

Biomechanics

A dilemma known as the thrower's paradox ensues as a pitcher pushes for more and more velocity. Although an extreme range of motion at the possible highest force is required to reach maximum velocity, the shoulder must retain enough stability to keep itself centered and create

a stable fulcrum for the motion. The mechanics of throwing occur in six separate phases (**Figure 1** and **Table 1**). In the first phase, the windup, the body initiates force from the legs, trunk, and core and begins the transfer of energy to the shoulder. Very little stress is placed on the glenohumeral joint during this phase. The early cocking phase ensues with the arm in abduction and external rotation. As maximal external rotation is achieved during the late cocking phase and the arm begins to move toward the target, the anterior structures are tensioned and the rotator cuff generates forces as high as 650 N.[3] The acceleration phase is initiated as the arm begins internal rotation, and it ends with the release of the ball. This phase marks the greatest velocity in the upper extremity. Most of the energy is transferred to the ball in this phase, and little stress is imposed on the glenohumeral joint. However, multiple vectors of force are directed within the shoulder and the surrounding tissues during the deceleration phase immediately following release. The shoulder can undergo distraction forces as high as 950 N, compressive forces greater than 1,000 N, and posterior shear forces as high as 400 N.[3,4] During the follow-through phase, the internal forces begin to return to normal, with compression force decreasing to 400 N.

The failure load of the native capsule is 800 to 1,200 N in young individuals. Therefore, it is understandable why throwing athletes are prone to injury and why optimal throwing mechanics are important. A study of young pitchers found that those with proper mechanics had less humeral internal rotation torque, lower elbow valgus load, and more efficiency than pitchers with poor mechanics.[5]

The Disabled Throwing Shoulder

Multiple theories have been presented concerning the etiology of the dysfunctional throwing shoulder. The understanding of contributing pathologies has evolved with improvements over time in diagnostic and surgical technologies. In 1959, a posteroinferior glenoid exostosis was described as the inciting pathology for pain in the professional pitcher, secondary to repetitive traction on the posterior capsule and the triceps tendon.[6] This theory later fell out of favor, although more recently the importance of posterior capsular pathology has again been recognized. Impingement syndrome was

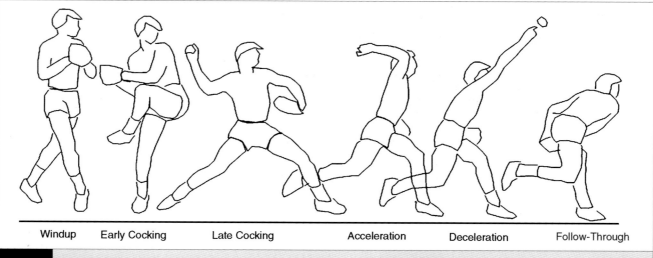

| Windup | Early Cocking | Late Cocking | Acceleration | Deceleration | Follow-Through |

Figure 1   Phases of the baseball pitch. (Reproduced from McMahon PJ, Debski RE: Kinematics and kinesiology of the shoulder, in Galatz LM, ed: *Orthopaedic Knowledge Update: Shoulder and Elbow*, ed 3. Rosemont, IL, American Academy of Orthopaedic Surgeons, 2007, p 47.)

described in 1972 and initially gained a following as an explanation for the painful throwing shoulder.[7] The symptoms and physical examination findings of a painful throwing shoulder overlapped those of impingement, and it was clear that the rotator cuff often was involved. However, a 1985 study of patients treated with acromioplasty for impingement found that only 4 of 18 athletes returned to throwing, despite good pain relief.[8]

During the 1990s, the theory of secondary impingement was developed, in which anterior shoulder instability brought on by repetitive stretching of the anterior capsule was believed to cause the impingement. Reducing the capsular volume of the joint through a subscapularis-splitting approach led to excellent pain relief, but return to throwing at a high level remained elusive.[9]

By the late 1990s, arthroscopy had become an important adjunctive tool for evaluating the throwing shoulder. Impingement of the rotator cuff on the posterosuperior glenoid, called internal impingement, was attributed to anterior laxity or microinstability resulting from repetitive forces in an abducted and maximally externally rotated position. Anterior instability was found to be common in throwing athletes and contributed to internal impingement.[10,11] However, an arthroscopic examination of 16 throwing athletes with internal impingement but no instability found that the rotator cuff impinged in an abducted and externally rotated position, leading to partial-thickness cuff tears and posterior capsular lesions.[12] A study of tennis players confirmed that symptomatic internal impingement can occur in the dominant shoulder without anterior instability or laxity.[13] Laxity continues to be a factor in the disabled throwing shoulder and recently has been implicated as a potential source of vascular compromise.[14] When the effects of throwing on upper extremity arterial blood flow were measured before and after a 50-pitch workout, professional pitchers with laxity had only a 35% increase in blood flow, compared with a 115% increase in pitchers without signs of laxity.

In 2003, there was a challenge to the idea that internal impingement itself is a pathologic rather than a physiologic occurrence secondary to contracture of the posteroinferior capsule.[2] Thickening of the posterior capsule recently was found to be an adaptation in the throwing shoulders of elite pitchers.[15] This contracture is believed to shift the humerus posterosuperiorly, precipitating the contact that leads to pathology in the rotator cuff and the labrum, as seen in the disabled throwing shoulder.[2] The resulting glenohumeral internal rotation deficit (GIRD) is the hallmark of the at-risk throwing shoulder. Other studies have confirmed the high prevalence of GIRD in throwing shoulders, its association with shoulder pathology, and the resolution of symptoms with the correction of GIRD.[2,16,17] However, evidence contrary to this concept also exists. In 2006, the researchers who performed the biomechanical study that initially supported GIRD revised their model and found that obligate translation with simulated posterior capsular contracture was, in fact, anteroinferior and occurred during the follow-through phase, not the cocking phase.[18] In addition, GIRD was found to be present in as many as 40% of the asymptomatic throwers.[19] Recent evidence suggests that excessive horizontal abduction is a critical component of internal impingement.[20] In fact, the disabled throwing shoulder may represent a spectrum of conditions resulting from the adaptations required when an individual's anatomy and physiology are subjected to the extreme demands of throwing an object beyond the individual's physiologic limits.

© 2013 American Academy of Orthopaedic Surgeons

Table 1

Phases of a Baseball Pitch (Right-Handed Pitcher)

Phase	Description	Comments
Windup	The hands are together holding the ball. The body is aligned in good balance. The pitcher takes a small, comfortable step back with the left leg, in line with home plate. The right foot is then positioned parallel to the rubber. (Some coaches have the pitcher wedge the foot so that the lateral half is on top of the rubber.) The left lower extremity is picked up in a controlled, active fashion, and the hips remain level while pointing toward home plate. As the hips begin to move forward, a V is formed in which the hips are the apex and the torso and right leg form the two sides. The hips point toward the batter. The right hand comes out of the glove holding the ball.	These are the components of all successful pitches, although a pitcher's windup phase has individual stylistic adaptations that raise the center of gravity. The shoulders are relatively uninvolved. They move slowly, the hands are together, and the muscle activity is low.
Early cocking	The hand stays on top of the ball as it comes out of the glove. The shoulder is then elevated approximately 100° in the scapular plane and is externally rotated to approximately 45°. The V becomes more pronounced as the hips continue to move forward toward home plate. The hips stay level; rotation of the hips is delayed as long as possible. The ball is hidden from the batter, who cannot yet determine the type of pitch to be delivered. The left leg slowly, easily, and comfortably comes down until the foot reaches the mound.	The initial position of the hand helps the shoulder stay in internal rotation, which is a safer position for the glenohumeral joint. The deltoid and the supraspinatus act together to abduct the humerus. The other rotator cuff muscles are not active.
Late cocking	The left foot makes contact with the mound, landing within the width of the right foot and pointing toward home plate. The pitcher's center of gravity has been lowered, releasing energy. The pitcher's weight is evenly distributed between the two legs, and the legs are firm. The torso is balanced between the legs in an upright position. The pitcher delays trunk rotation as long as possible.	The goal is to move the humerus into maximum external rotation. The humerus maintains its level of elevation in the scapular plane and externally rotates from 46° to 170°. Deltoid and supraspinatus activity diminishes, but the other rotator cuff muscles' activity increases for joint stability. The middle portion of the trapezius, rhomboids, levator scapulae, and serratus anterior muscles are active so that the scapula can provide an effective base for the humeral head.
Acceleration	The acceleration phase is initiated when the humerus begins to internally rotate. In approximately 1/20th of a second, the ball is released from the hand at a speed as high as 100 miles per hour. Both feet are on the mound. The acceleration of the arm coincides with the deceleration of the rest of the body, producing efficient transfer of energy to the upper extremity and the ball.	The motion occurs on the very firm base provided by the lower extremities. Synchronous muscular contraction about the glenohumeral joint and scapulothoracic articulation provides both stability and rapid motion of the upper extremity.
Deceleration	The right hip is brought up and over the left leg after the ball is released. The right foot disengages from the mound, and the body goes into a controlled forward fall.	The kinetic energy not transferred to the ball is dissipated by large muscle activity, beginning with the arm.
Follow through	The arm is brought down.	The forces affecting the arm decrease.

(Adapted with permission from McMahon PJ, Tibone JE, Pink MM: Functional anatomy and biomechanics of the shoulder, in Delee JC, Drez D Jr, Miller MD, eds: *Delee and Drez's Orthopaedic Sports Medicine: Principles and Practice*, ed 2. Philadelphia, PA, Saunders, 2003, p 850.)

Common Pathologic Sequelae

Regardless of their etiology, injuries to the throwing shoulder share many final sequelae, including superior labrum anterior to posterior (SLAP) tears, proximal biceps pathology, partial-thickness rotator cuff tears, and scapular dyskinesia. Superior labral tears in the throwing shoulder originally were described in 1985, when tensile failure at the biceps was postulated as the mechanism of injury, and the primary treatment was débridement.[21] A contrasting theory was that these superior labral tears (later called SLAP tears) were generated from a so-called peel-back mechanism in which the externally rotating shoulder forced an obli-

2: Instability and Athletic Injuries

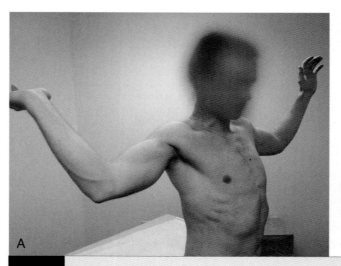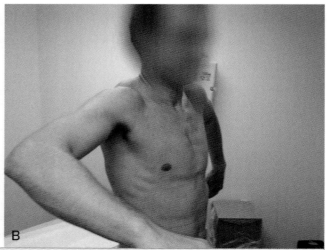

| **Figure 2** | Clinical photographs showing glenohumeral internal rotation deficit. **A,** Increased external rotation of the right shoulder as compared with the contralateral shoulder. **B,** Decreased internal rotation on the right shoulder as evident with glenohumeral internal rotation deficit. |

gate stress of the biceps anchor, leading to the tear that was called the coup de grace of the disabled throwing shoulder.[2,22]

Rotator cuff damage is perhaps the most common pathology in the throwing shoulder. Full-thickness tears are uncommon, but partial-thickness articular-sided tears are almost ubiquitous in throwing athletes and are believed to result from acute tension and/or repetitive microtrauma from eccentric failure. These tears have been described as occurring posterosuperiorly at the junction of the infraspinatus and supraspinatus insertions, as the result of internal impingement.[12,23]

As understanding of the mechanics in the shoulder has evolved, glenoid positioning has become an important consideration when evaluating shoulder pain in the throwing athlete. The concept of scapular dyskinesis has been studied clinically and found to play a role in patients with impingement and anterior instability.[24] The term SICK scapula refers to the phenomenon of *s*capular malposition, *i*nferior medial border prominence, *c*oracoid pain and malposition, and dys*k*inesis of scapular movement.[25] Scapular dyskinesis probably results from periscapular muscular imbalance, fatigue, or nerve injury, and several recent studies have implicated muscular deficits as a risk factor for scapular dyskinesis in the disabled throwing shoulder. Adolescent pitchers with a history of throwing-related pain were found to have a weaker middle trapezius and supraspinatus than their counterparts who did not have pain.[26] Another study found a similar pattern in professional pitchers. Pitchers with preseason weakness of the external rotators and the supraspinatus had a higher risk of in-season throwing-related injury requiring surgical intervention than pitchers without preseason weakness.[27] Pitching itself may contribute to the weakness. A decrease in volitional strength of the external rotators in pitchers was found when a single-performance fatigue

model was used.[28] The study concluded that rehabilitation strategies to prevent fatigue and enhance neuromuscular activation may prevent injury in throwing athletes.

Clinical Evaluation

History and Physical Examination
Patients with a dysfunctional throwing shoulder most often have posterior shoulder pain during the cocking or follow-through phase of the throwing motion. Some patients may describe a loss of control or velocity or a feeling of a "dead arm." Physical examination may reveal tenderness to palpation, increased external rotation and decreased internal rotation, instability or laxity, and positive posterior impingement tests, as well as more traditional impingement signs.[29,30] An internal rotation decrease of more than 20° compared with the contralateral side (measured with the glenohumeral joint abducted to 90°), especially in the setting of a decreased total arc of motion, suggests GIRD (**Figure 2**). In such a patient, the examiner must pay particular attention to the core strength of the athlete, the scapula, and any associated shoulder pathology. SICK scapula syndrome or scapular dyskinesis usually is seen as static and dynamic scapular malposition evident when the patient repeatedly raises and lowers the arms or engages the dynamic stabilizers of the scapula.[25] Other key physical examination findings include a positive relocation test for pain (suggesting shoulder microinstability), a positive active compression test (suggesting a SLAP tear), and pain during a sleeper stretch.

Imaging
Standard radiographs should be included in the workup for a disabled throwing shoulder, but often

Table 2

Pitching Kinematics and the Nonsurgical Management of Deficits

Point of Breakdown in Kinetic Chain	Result	Treatment
Premature forward motion during windup or stride	Arm lags behind body	Strengthen core muscles
Stride foot landing in closed position	Decreased pelvis-trunk rotation Pitcher must throw across body, decreasing force generation in kinetic chain	Strengthen hip external rotators
Stride foot landing in open position	Premature pelvic rotation Uncoupled kinetic chain Arm lags behind body Shoulder must generate increased forces to maintain velocity	Strengthen hip internal rotators
Throwing from an upright position (diminished forward trunk tilt)	Acceleration forces act on ball over shorter distances Less velocity generated	Strengthen core muscles
Increased lead knee flexion at ball release	Less force generated by torso flexing and rotating over front side	Stretch hamstrings
Diminished internal rotation	Acceleration forces act on ball over shorter distance	Perform sleeper stretch
Scapular dyskinesis	Diminished external rotation in late cocking phase (decreased scapular retraction) Subacromial impingement	Stabilize scapula

they are normal. The cornerstone of radiographic evaluation remains MRI or magnetic resonance arthrography, which has greater accuracy for detecting labral pathology, rotator cuff and biceps pathology, capsular thickening, bursal pathology, and bony edema. CT is not standard but may be indicated if there is a bony abnormality on the initial radiographic evaluation.

Treatment

Nonsurgical Management

Because there is a spectrum of adaptations and pathologies among pitchers, surgical treatment of the throwing shoulder does not lend itself to well-controlled study. Nonsurgical management is successful in preventing the need for surgery in many of these athletes. The throwing action is the culmination of multiple energy transfers from the proximal to the distal kinetic chain (**Table 2**). Deficits anywhere along this chain can be translated into a more distal injury. Therefore, successful nonsurgical management of the disabled throwing shoulder must involve all aspects of the kinetic chain, as well as the shoulder itself. Hip and leg strength must be maintained, and core strengthening cannot be overemphasized. The scapular platform must be optimized because it forms the critical transfer point between the power created in the core and the speed generated in the shoulder. Rehabilitation specific to the shoulder includes treatment of the scapular and dynamic stabilizers as well as posterior capsular stretch-

ing. SICK scapula syndrome can be effectively treated with retraining of scapular mechanics.[25]

Rotator cuff weakness is common in the painful throwing shoulder, and strengthening of the rotator cuff is a mainstay of any nonsurgical treatment of the throwing shoulder. Posterior capsular tightness is among the most detrimental adaptations in the throwing athlete, but resolution of its symptoms can be achieved by using stretching exercises, such as the sleeper stretch (**Figure 3**). Pitchers who participated in an internal rotation stretching program for several years had better internal rotation and total arc of motion than those in shorter structured stretching programs.[31]

In most patients, the disabled throwing shoulder responds to this comprehensive approach. A recent report described the researchers' experience with a major league baseball team over 3 years.[17] Many of the pitchers exhibited signs and symptoms of GIRD, but almost all were resolved with a supervised athletic training program. Only 3 of the 40 pitchers with GIRD eventually required surgery. Another study found that nonsurgical management focused on sleeper stretches and scapulothoracic rehabilitation was 100% effective in returning the shoulders of 96 athletes to throwing.[25]

Surgical Management

Surgical intervention is indicated if the patient's throwing shoulder has not responded to adequate nonsurgical management. Injury-specific rehabilitation should be attempted before surgical intervention is considered

2: Instability and Athletic Injuries

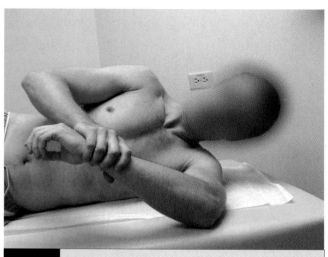

Figure 3 Clinical photograph showing the sleeper stretch, in which the patient lies in the lateral position, with the affected side downward, and manually pushes the arm to the floor. For a patient with GIRD, this movement emphasizes stretching on the posterior capsule.

(**Table 3**). Examination under anesthesia should be performed on both the affected and the unaffected shoulder. Care should be taken to note differences in laxity as well as range of motion. Of particular interest is internal and external rotation at 90° of abduction with scapular stabilization because the presence of GIRD can be detected on this examination. When the examination is complete, the patient is positioned and the shoulder is prepared and draped.

A standard posterior portal is placed approximately 2 cm inferior and medial to the posterolateral border of the acromion. A standard anterior portal is established in the rotator cuff interval under direct visualization. Placement of this portal high in the rotator cuff interval allows easy access to the posterosuperior glenoid and the rotator cuff. A probe is used to evaluate for pathology often seen in the throwing shoulder. The biceps tendon and its attachment, as well as the superior labrum, are noted. It is important to differentiate between a normal labral recess and a SLAP tear. The anterior and posterior labrum should be carefully probed if instability is suspected (**Figure 4**). The undersurface

Table 3

Comprehensive Management of the Throwing Athlete

Diagnosis	Physical Examination Finding	Nonsurgical Management	Surgical Management
Microinstability	Apprehension	Scapular stabilization	Limited capsular shift
Internal impingement	Positive impingement signs	Scapular stabilization Rotator cuff strengthening Sleeper stretch	Rotator cuff débridement (+/- SLAP débridement) or repair
SLAP tear	Positive active compression test	Rest	SLAP débridement or repair
GIRD	Pain with decreased internal rotation	Sleeper stretch	Limited posterior capsular release
Partial-thickness articular-sided rotator cuff tear	Pain or weakness with rotator cuff testing	Rotator cuff strengthening	Débridement or repair

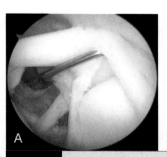
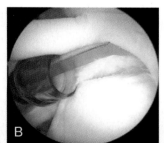
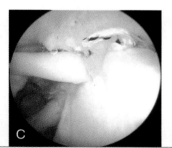
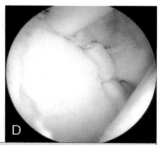

Figure 4 Arthroscopic images showing a SLAP repair. **A,** Abnormal detachment and mobility of the biceps anchor. **B,** Preparation of the superior glenoid with a liberator or a shaver to promote bleeding. **C,** Posterior view of the repair with knots off the face of the glenoid to avoid causing cartilage abrasion with shoulder motion. **D,** Anterior view of the repair. (Reproduced from Keener KD, Brophy RH: Superior labral tears of the shoulder: Pathogenesis, evaluation, and treatment. *J Am Orthop Surg* 2009;17:627-637.)

of the supraspinatus and the infraspinatus is inspected because a partial-thickness tear is a classic finding in the injured throwing shoulder. It is critical to repeat the evaluation in a dynamic examination that includes the abducted, externally rotated position (the position of internal impingement). Contact between the posterosuperior glenoid and the posterior aspect of the rotator cuff often is pathologic, and a possible peel-back effect of the biceps off the posterosuperior labrum should be carefully considered. These hallmarks of internal impingement can be treated with débridement or repair, depending on the extent of the lesion.

A partial-thickness articular-sided rotator cuff tear is more posterior than a classic rotator cuff tear and can be seen by bringing the arm out of traction and into an abducted, externally rotated position. The treatment most often includes débridement (**Figure 5**), although one study reported that in situ repair had good results in returning athletes to throwing.[11] The repair of full-thickness tears has not consistently allowed pitchers to return to throwing, and caution should be exercised against overly aggressive débridement or conversion of a partial- to a full-thickness tear repair. Return-to-throwing rates ranging from 25% to 87% have been reported, with better results after treatment of combined pathology[21,32,33] (**Table 4**).

SLAP tears that extend posterior to the biceps root often are seen in a disabled throwing shoulder. Care must be taken to differentiate between a true pathologic SLAP tear and a labral separation that occurred as an adaptive change with peel-back. The genesis of the SLAP tear is still debated, but it can be a pain generator, create a sense of instability, and affect a thrower's speed and accuracy.

Varied surgical techniques have been reported for optimal repair of a SLAP tear. A basic approach begins with diagnostic arthroscopy (**Figure 4**). A probe is used to assess the integrity of the superior labrum and distinguish between a labral recess and a true SLAP tear. A true tear will extend medial to the cartilaginous portion of the glenoid and have abnormal mobility. The glenoid is prepared by using an arthroscopic shaver or liberator to remove fibrinous cartilage and obtain a healthy bleeding bed, which will promote healing of the repair. A suture passer or similar device is used to establish a simple or a mattress suture into the superior labrum. An unstable SLAP tear should be repaired, but incarceration by overtightening the biceps must be avoided. No attempt should be made to bring the biceps anchor onto the face of the glenoid, as might be done in a labral repair to treat instability. Especially in a throwing athlete, the repair should be made off the face. The surgeon should consider removing a small portion of the impinging glenoid and using a low-profile technique, such as a knotless or a mattress repair. Failure to follow these principles may result in contact between the suture material and the rotator cuff insertion.

There are only sparse reports of SLAP tear repair in overhead throwing athletes (**Table 5**). The initial study reported a 100% rate of good to excellent results, with 87% of the athletes returning to the previous level of play, but these results were not reproduced in other studies.[34,35] A recent systematic review evaluated five studies that included baseball throwers and reported a

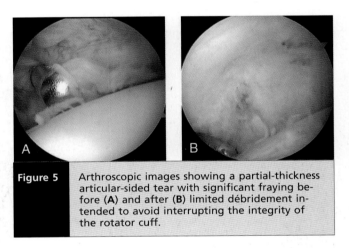

Figure 5 Arthroscopic images showing a partial-thickness articular-sided tear with significant fraying before (**A**) and after (**B**) limited débridement intended to avoid interrupting the integrity of the rotator cuff.

Table 4			
Studies of Rotator Cuff Pathology in Overhead Throwing Athletes			
Study (Year)	**Patient Description (Number)**	**Procedure**	**Outcomes**
Reynolds et al[33] (2008)	Competitive baseball pitchers (82)	Débridement of partial-thickness rotator cuff tear	55% returned to previous level of play
Andrews et al[21] (1985)	Throwing athletes (36, including 23 baseball pitchers	Débridement of partial-thickness articular-sided rotator cuff tear	85% of athletes returned to play; 76% returned to previous level of play
Conway[11] (2001)	Baseball players (9)	Repair of intratendinous rotator cuff tear	89% returned to same or higher level of play
Ferrari et al[32] (1994)	Competitive baseball pitchers (7)	Débridement of rotator cuff tear with or without labrum	85% returned to premorbid activity

Table 5

Studies of SLAP Tear Repair in Overhead Throwing Athletes

Study (Year)	Patient Description (Number)	Procedure	Outcomes
Morgan et al[35] (1998)	Throwing athletes (102, including 37 baseball pitchers)	SLAP repair	87% returned to previous level of play
Kim et al[37] (2002)	Overhead athletes (18)	SLAP repair	Only 22% returned to previous level of play
Reinold et al[38] (2003)	Overhead athletes (130, including 105 baseball pitchers)	SLAP repair with thermal capsular shrinkage	87% returned to play; the results were better after thermal capsular shrinkage and repair than after repair alone
Ide et al[39] (2005)	Baseball pitchers (19)	SLAP repair	63% returned to previous level of play; the results were worse in pitchers than in other overhead athletes
Neuman et al[40] (2011)	Overhead athletes (30)	SLAP repair	84% returned to preinjury level of play; 93% satisfaction rate

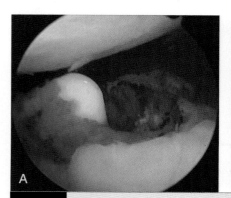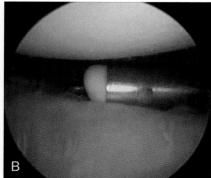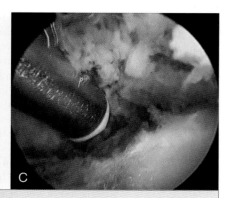

Figure 6 Arthroscopic images showing posterior capsule release. **A,** The capsule is released with electrocautery. The characteristic thickened posterior capsule can be seen. **B,** A hook probe can be used for a more precise capsular release. **C,** Release in close proximity to the glenoid is done to avoid injury to the axillary nerve.

return-to-play rate ranging from 22% to 64% after SLAP repair.[34]

If a patient has GIRD that has not responded to nonsurgical management, the posterior capsule should be carefully evaluated at arthroscopy for thickening (**Figure 6**). In rare patients, a posterior capsular release can be considered to help restore recalcitrant internal rotation. This release should be done with extreme caution, especially inferiorly, where the axillary nerve is at risk. The use of electrocautery may provide a margin of safety because proximity to the nerve should result in contraction of the deltoid musculature and may provide a warning. An arthroscopic biter also can be cautiously used to perform selective capsular release at the capsulolabral junction. Regardless of the method, the release should be done close to the glenoid because this location offers the best buffer to the axillary nerve. Posterior capsular release for GIRD in throwing athletes has rarely been reported in the peer-reviewed literature. Reliable pain relief with less reliable return to throwing was reported when this approach was used.[36] Eleven of 16 athletes (69%) returned to their preinjury performance level. Only 4 of these patients had isolated posteroinferior capsular tightness; this finding highlights the complexity of the pathology of the throwing shoulder.[36]

Rehabilitation

The postoperative program must be tailored to the surgical procedure for the throwing shoulder. Communica-

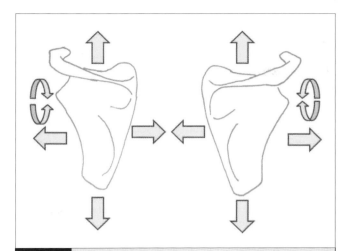

Figure 7	Schematic drawings showing the action of the major scapular muscles during scapular platform retraining. Lateral-medial arrows represent protraction-retraction of the serratus anterior, pectoralis minor, trapezius, and rhomboids muscles. Superior-inferior arrows represent elevation-depression of the trapezius, levator scapulae, pectoralis minor, and latissimus dorsi muscles. Circular arrows represent superoinferior rotation of the trapezius, serratus anterior, levator scapulae, rhomboids, and pectoralis minor muscles.

tion between the surgeon and the athletic trainer is of paramount importance to ensure the soft tissue is protected during early motion and re-engagement of muscular rhythm and strength. The athlete's maintenance core-strengthening program should continue unaffected by the surgery. Scapular platform retraining is begun immediately and should include a program of scapular protraction-retraction, elevation-depression, and inward-outward rotation (**Figure 7**). If the surgical correction did not include repair, the patient is encouraged to move the arm back to full range of active and passive motion as quickly as possible. The motion is supervised to ensure proper stabilization of the scapular musculature. After early motion in the correct rhythm is obtained, the progression of loads and speeds is started and the link between the central core and the scapular platform is reestablished. The progression begins with low loads at low speeds with a stable platform in one plane of motion and continues to higher and faster loads in multiple planes that eventually simulate the sport-specific environment. Endurance must not be neglected because fatigue can lead to poor mechanics and is detrimental to return to sport.

When the athlete has regained a solid core, a full range of motion, functional strength, and proper scapular rhythm, a return-to-throwing program is started under the supervision of the athletic training staff. Initially, the athlete must demonstrate the ability to simulate a pitch at slow speed as well as attainment of the proper functional range of motion, core strength, and scapular stability.

The return-to-throwing program embodies the same principles of progression as the earlier phases. Throwing is started at slow speeds with a light ball tossed for short distances. Any deficits in throwing mechanics halt the progression. As the athlete progresses, distance, speed, and the number of repetitions are increased until the ability to perform specific sport mechanics is regained. At this point, the number of repetitions is increased until the athlete is ready to return to competition. This program must be individualized, any labral or rotator cuff repair must be protected until healed, and the necessary restrictions must be accommodated.

Summary

The throwing shoulder remains a therapeutic challenge. Multiple pathologies commonly occur, including labral and rotator cuff tears, pathologic laxity, and posterior capsular tightness. Nonsurgical management is effective for most patients. When surgical treatment is necessary, the surgeon must take care to distinguish between an anatomic adaptation and a pathologic condition. Return to throwing never is accomplished in the operating room alone. It requires a dedicated team to place the repaired shoulder within a properly rehabilitated kinetic chain that can withstand the extreme demands inherent to the throwing shoulder.

Annotated References

1. Fleisig GS, Andrews JR: *The Athlete's Shoulder*. New York, NY, Churchill Livingstone, 1994, pp 360-365.

2. Burkhart SS, Morgan CD, Kibler WB: The disabled throwing shoulder: Spectrum of pathology. Part I: Pathoanatomy and biomechanics. *Arthroscopy* 2003; 19(4):404-420.

3. Fleisig GS, Andrews JR, Dillman CJ, Escamilla RF: Kinetics of baseball pitching with implications about injury mechanisms. *Am J Sports Med* 1995;23(2): 233-239.

4. Kuhn J, Lindholm SR, Huston LJ: Failure of the biceps superior labral complex (SLAP lesion) in the throwing athlete: A biomechanical model comparing maximal cocking to early deceleration. *J Shoulder Elbow Surg* 2000;9(463):463.

5. Davis JT, Limpisvasti O, Fluhme D, et al: The effect of pitching biomechanics on the upper extremity in youth and adolescent baseball pitchers. *Am J Sports Med* 2009;37(8):1484-1491.
   Quantitative motion analysis and high-speed video were used to assess baseball pitching mechanics based on biomechanical parameters (hip, hand, arm, shoulder, and foot position) in 169 pitchers age 9 to 18 years. Pitchers with three or more correct parameters had lower humeral internal rotation torque, lower elbow valgus load, and greater pitching efficiency.

6. Bennett GE: Elbow and shoulder lesions of baseball players. *Am J Surg* 1959;98:484-492.

7. Neer CS II: Anterior acromioplasty for the chronic impingement syndrome in the shoulder: A preliminary report. *J Bone Joint Surg Am* 1972;54(1):41-50.

8. Tibone JE, Jobe FW, Kerlan RK, et al: Shoulder impingement syndrome in athletes treated by an anterior acromioplasty. *Clin Orthop Relat Res* 1985;198: 134-140.

9. Jobe FW, Giangarra CE, Kvitne RS, Glousman RE: Anterior capsulolabral reconstruction of the shoulder in athletes in overhand sports. *Am J Sports Med* 1991; 19(5):428-434.

10. Paley KJ, Jobe FW, Pink MM, Kvitne RS, ElAttrache NS: Arthroscopic findings in the overhand throwing athlete: Evidence for posterior internal impingement of the rotator cuff. *Arthroscopy* 2000;16(1):35-40.

11. Conway JE: Arthroscopic repair of partial-thickness rotator cuff tears and SLAP lesions in professional baseball players. *Orthop Clin North Am* 2001;32(3): 443-456.

12. Walch G, Boileau P, Noel E, Donell ST: Impingement of the deep surface of the supraspinatus tendon on the posterosuperior glenoid rim: An arthroscopic study. *J Shoulder Elbow Surg* 1992;1(5):238-245.

13. Sonnery-Cottet B, Edwards TB, Noel E, Walch G: Results of arthroscopic treatment of posterosuperior glenoid impingement in tennis players. *Am J Sports Med* 2002;30(2):227-232.

14. Bast SC, Weaver FA, Perese S, Jobe FW, Weaver DC, Vangsness CT Jr: The effects of shoulder laxity on upper extremity blood flow in professional baseball pitchers. *J Shoulder Elbow Surg* 2011;20(3):461-466.

    Eighteen male professional baseball pitchers were examined for signs of shoulder laxity (positive sulcus sign or relocation test), and a vascular examination was performed before and after a 50-pitch session. The 10 pitchers without a sign of laxity had an average arterial volume flow increase of 115%, but the pitchers who had a laxity sign had only a 35% increase in blood flow.

15. Thomas SJ, Swanik CB, Higginson JS, et al: A bilateral comparison of posterior capsule thickness and its correlation with glenohumeral range of motion and scapular upward rotation in collegiate baseball players. *J Shoulder Elbow Surg* 2011;20(5):708-716.

    Posterior capsular thickness was measured in both shoulders of baseball players. The authors found a significantly greater thickness in the dominant throwing arm, which was negatively correlated with internal rotation.

16. Verna C: Shoulder flexibility to reduce impingement. *3rd PBATS Book of Abstracts*. Ellicott City, MD, Professional Baseball Athletic Trainer Society, 1991, abstract 18.

17. Wilk KE, Macrina LC, Fleisig GS, et al: Correlation of glenohumeral internal rotation deficit and total rotational motion to shoulder injuries in professional baseball pitchers. *Am J Sports Med* 2011;39(2):329-335.

    Signs of GIRD were assessed in 122 professional pitchers in three consecutive preseasons. The 40 pitchers with GIRD were almost twice as likely to be injured as those without GIRD ($P = 0.17$).

18. Huffman GR, Tibone JE, McGarry MH, Phipps BM, Lee YS, Lee TQ: Path of glenohumeral articulation throughout the rotational range of motion in a thrower's shoulder model. *Am J Sports Med* 2006;34(10): 1662-1669.

19. Tokish J, Curtin MS, Kim YK, Hawkins RJ: Glenohumeral internal rotation deficit in the asymptomatic professional pitcher and its relationship to humeral retroversion. *J Sports Sci Med* 2008;7:78-83.

20. Mihata T, Gates J, McGarry MH, Lee J, Kinoshita M, Lee TQ: Effect of rotator cuff muscle imbalance on forceful internal impingement and peel-back of the superior labrum: A cadaveric study. *Am J Sports Med* 2009;37(11):2222-2227.

    A cadaver study assessed the rotator cuff and the effect of muscle imbalance during the late cocking phase of throwing. Decreased subscapularis muscle strength resulted in increased maximum external rotation and increased glenohumeral contact pressure, possibly leading to rotator cuff or labral pathology.

21. Andrews JR, Broussard TS, Carson WG: Arthroscopy of the shoulder in the management of partial tears of the rotator cuff: A preliminary report. *Arthroscopy* 1985;1(2):117-122.

22. Burkhart SS, Morgan CD, Kibler WB: The disabled throwing shoulder: Spectrum of pathology. Part II: Evaluation and treatment of SLAP lesions in throwers. *Arthroscopy* 2003;19(5):531-539.

23. Jobe CM: Posterior superior glenoid impingement: Expanded spectrum. *Arthroscopy* 1995;11(5):530-536.

24. Warner JJ, Micheli LJ, Arslanian LE, Kennedy J, Kennedy R: Scapulothoracic motion in normal shoulders and shoulders with glenohumeral instability and impingement syndrome: A study using Moiré topographic analysis. *Clin Orthop Relat Res* 1992;285: 191-199.

25. Burkhart SS, Morgan CD, Kibler WB: The disabled throwing shoulder: Spectrum of pathology. Part III: The SICK scapula, scapular dyskinesis, the kinetic chain, and rehabilitation. *Arthroscopy* 2003;19(6): 641-661.

26. Trakis JE, McHugh MP, Caracciolo PA, Busciacco L, Mullaney M, Nicholas SJ: Muscle strength and range

of motion in adolescent pitchers with throwing-related pain: Implications for injury prevention. *Am J Sports Med* 2008;36(11):2173-2178.

Adolescent pitchers with or without shoulder pain were compared with respect to range of motion and posterior muscular strength. There was no significant difference in range of motion, but pitchers with pain had significantly weaker posterior musculature.

27. Byram IR, Bushnell BD, Dugger K, Charron K, Harrell FE Jr, Noonan TJ: Preseason shoulder strength measurements in professional baseball pitchers: Identifying players at risk for injury. *Am J Sports Med* 2010;38(7): 1375-1382.

Shoulder strength in prone internal and external rotation and seated external rotation was examined in professional pitchers during spring training over 5 years. A statistically significant correlation was found between weakened supraspinatus strength in external rotation and in-season throwing injury requiring surgery.

28. Gandhi J, ElAttrache NS, Kaufman KR, Hurd WJ: Voluntary activation deficits of the infraspinatus present as a consequence of pitching-induced fatigue. *J Shoulder Elbow Surg* 2012;21(5):625-630.

High school baseball pitchers' external rotation strength was measured before and after simulated pitching. Significant fatigue and weakness were noted. Voluntary infraspinatus muscle activation appears to contribute to external rotation muscle weakness in a fatigued pitcher.

29. Myers JB, Laudner KG, Pasquale MR, Bradley JP, Lephart SM: Glenohumeral range of motion deficits and posterior shoulder tightness in throwers with pathologic internal impingement. *Am J Sports Med* 2006;34(3):385-391.

30. Meister K, Buckley B, Batts J: The posterior impingement sign: Diagnosis of rotator cuff and posterior labral tears secondary to internal impingement in overhand athletes. *Am J Orthop (Belle Mead NJ)* 2004; 33(8):412-415.

31. Lintner D, Mayol M, Uzodinma O, Jones R, Labossiere D: Glenohumeral internal rotation deficits in professional pitchers enrolled in an internal rotation stretching program. *Am J Sports Med* 2007;35(4): 617-621.

The effectiveness of the sleeper stretch was assessed by comparing pitchers based on length of participation in a stretching program. Pitchers with at least 3 years' participation had 20° more internal rotation and a 23° greater total arc of motion compared with those having less lengthy participation.

32. Ferrari JD, Ferrari DA, Coumas J, Pappas AM: Posterior ossification of the shoulder: The Bennett lesion. Etiology, diagnosis, and treatment. *Am J Sports Med* 1994;22(2):171-176.

33. Reynolds SB, Dugas JR, Cain EL, McMichael CS, Andrews JR: Débridement of small partial-thickness rotator cuff tears in elite overhead throwers. *Clin Orthop Relat Res* 2008;466(3):614-621.

Data obtained for 67 of 82 professional pitchers after débridement of a partial-thickness rotator cuff tear revealed a 76% rate of return to competition and a 55% rate of return to the same or a higher level of competition.

34. Gorantla K, Gill C, Wright RW: The outcome of type II SLAP repair: A systematic review. *Arthroscopy* 2010;26(4):537-545.

A systematic review assessed the arthroscopic repair of type II SLAP lesions at a minimum 2-year follow-up. Outcomes varied dramatically, with return to play ranging from 20% to 94% (from 22% to 64% in baseball players). No prospective studies have assessed these outcomes. The repair of type II SLAP lesions does not appear to have a predictable outcome.

35. Morgan CD, Burkhart SS, Palmeri M, Gillespie M: Type II SLAP lesions: Three subtypes and their relationships to superior instability and rotator cuff tears. *Arthroscopy* 1998;14(6):553-565.

36. Yoneda M, Nakagawa S, Mizuno N, et al: Arthroscopic capsular release for painful throwing shoulder with posterior capsular tightness. *Arthroscopy* 2006; 22(7):e1-e5.

37. Kim SH, Ha KI, Kim SH, Choi HJ: Results of arthroscopic treatment of superior labral lesions. *J Bone Joint Surg Am* 2002;84-A(6):981-985.

38. Reinold MM, Wilk KE, Hooks TR, Dugas JR, Andrews JR: Thermal-assisted capsular shrinkage of the glenohumeral joint in overhead athletes: A 15- to 47-month follow-up. *J Orthop Sports Phys Ther* 2003; 33(8):455-467.

39. Ide J, Maeda S, Takagi K: Sports activity after arthroscopic superior labral repair using suture anchors in overhead-throwing athletes. *Am J Sports Med* 2005; 33(4):507-514.

40. Neuman BJ, Boisvert CB, Reiter B, Lawson K, Ciccotti MG, Cohen SB: Results of arthroscopic repair of type II superior labral anterior posterior lesions in overhead athletes: Assessment of return to preinjury playing level and satisfaction. *Am J Sports Med* 2011; 39(9):1883-1888.

A retrospective review of arthroscopically repaired SLAP tears in throwing athletes found that at midterm follow-up, patients believed they had returned to approximately 84.1% of preinjury level of function. The overall satisfaction rate was 93%.

2: Instability and Athletic Injuries

Chapter 12
Complications of Instability Repair

James G. Distefano, MD   Albert Lin, MD   Jon J.P. Warner, MD   Laurence D. Higgins, MD

Introduction

Instability of the glenohumeral joint is a broad term that encompasses numerous distinct pathologic processes and conditions. Patients may have a spectrum of symptoms as the result of traumatic insult to the shoulder or innate general joint laxity. The goals of surgery for shoulder instability are to restore static and dynamic balance to allow activities of daily living, a return to work, and participation in athletic competition. The important patient factors that must be considered include age, hand dominance, smoking status, general joint hypermobility, participation in a contact or overhead throwing sport, and the presence of a genetic condition such as Ehlers-Danlos or Marfan syndrome.[1-3] The anatomic deformations can involve a range of combinations and severity of soft-tissue and bony injury. The surgeon must understand the complex interaction of patient and surgical factors to predict the risk of complications related to instability surgery and must choose a treatment strategy that will minimize risk.

Anatomic Factors

Numerous injuries to normal shoulder anatomy can lead to clinical instability. An understanding of the variety of anatomic features in patients with instability is

Dr. Warner or an immediate family member has received nonincome support (such as equipment or services), commercially derived honoraria, or other non–research-related funding (such as paid travel) from Arthrocare, DJ Orthopaedics, Arthrex, Mitek, and Bret, Smith & Nephew: Fellowship Support. Dr. Higgins or an immediate family member serves as a board member, owner, officer, or committee member of the American Shoulder and Elbow Surgeons Value Committee, Membership Committee, and Program Planning Committee; the Arthroscopy Association of North America Education Committee; the American Academy of Orthopaedic Surgeons Patient Safety and Value Committee; and Advocacy for Improvement in Mobility (AIM); and has received nonincome support (such as equipment or services), commercially derived honoraria, or other non–research-related funding (such as paid travel) from Arthrex Smith & Nephew: Fellowship Support, Breg, and DePuy. Neither of the following authors nor any immediate family member has received anything of value from or has stock or stock options held in a commercial company or institution related directly or indirectly to the subject of this chapter: Dr. Distefano and Dr. Lin.

paramount to understanding the disease process, treatment options, and the causes of failure. In traumatic anterior dislocation, the classic disruption is the Bankart lesion, which represents a detachment of the anteroinferior labrum (**Figure 1**). However, surgical detachment of the anteroinferior labrum alone does not produce instability in cadaver models. Frank instability requires an additional injury to the glenohumeral ligaments, capsule, or bony architecture.[4]

A bony defect of the glenoid rim and/or humeral head, called a Hill-Sachs lesion or a reverse Hill-Sachs lesion, is frequently formed at the time of dislocation. A significantly higher incidence of inferior or middle glenohumeral lesions or Hill-Sachs lesions was found during surgery for anterior instability dislocation in patients who had a recurrent dislocation, compared with those who had a first dislocation.[5]

To minimize the risk of recurrent instability, the pathology must be properly identified before a treatment option is selected. For example, a posterior labral tear, capsular tear, glenoid rim defect, or reverse Hill-Sachs defect can be present in combination with posterior instability. It is important to examine for concomitant superior labrum anterior to posterior (SLAP) or rotator cuff pathology, which contribute to the instability spectrum. Biomechanical studies found that the creation of a SLAP tear increased anterior humeral translation, and the repair of a SLAP tear at the same time as a Bankart repair had favorable results.[6,7] The role of the rotator cuff interval in the treatment of shoulder instability remains controversial, with experts presenting contradictory opinions.

Surgical Intervention

The surgical treatment options for shoulder instability can be divided into those that target soft-tissue structures, bony defects, or both. Within each category are procedures developed for arthroscopic as well as open approaches. The soft-tissue procedures include labral repair, glenohumeral ligament repair, rotator cuff repair, and capsular plication. The bony procedures include bony Bankart repair; the Bristow, Latarjet, and Putti-Platt procedures; and other variations of autograft or allograft reconstruction.

Complications from surgical intervention for shoulder instability can occur during the procedure, the im-

2: Instability and Athletic Injuries

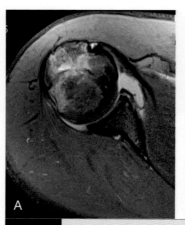
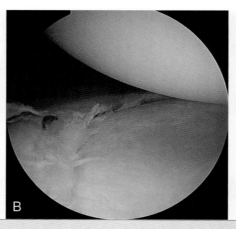
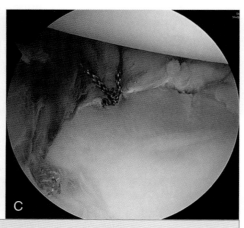

Figure 1 **A,** Axial MRI of a right shoulder showing a Bankart tear with a detached anterior labrum. Arthroscopic images from the posterior portal showing a Bankart tear before (**B**) and after (**C**) suture anchor repair.

mediate perioperative period, or the years that follow. Recurrence is the most common complication of instability surgery. Hardware breakage or disengagement, postoperative shoulder stiffness, residual pain, neurologic injury, infection, and osteoarthritis also occur.

Causes of Instability Recurrence

There are numerous causes for the failure of instability surgery leading to a recurrent subluxation or dislocation event. The surgeon must have a thorough understanding of the normal shoulder anatomy and its variants to properly diagnose all of a patient's pathologic lesions and make the proper treatment choice.[8] Surgical failures can be broadly attributed to diagnosis and treatment choice, surgical technique, or an unavoidable cause.

Diagnosis and Treatment Choice

One of the most common causes of failure after surgical treatment of shoulder instability involves failure to identify the full scope of clinical features and anatomic deformations present. A thorough preoperative workup begins with a patient history to identify the direction(s), the frequency, and the severity of symptoms. Pathologic laxity that causes pain or dysfunction must be differentiated from a functional supraphysiologic range of motion that does not interfere with normal activities and can contribute to sports performance (as in gymnastics). Patients must be screened for psychiatric disease or voluntary dislocation related to drug- or attention-seeking behavior.

The physical examination should include particular attention to the detection of general ligamentous laxity or multidirectional instability, both of which affect the treatment choice and outcomes. Range of motion can provide information about any secondary pathologic process. For example, greater external rotation com-

pared with the contralateral side may indicate subscapularis incompetence. A thorough neurovascular examination must be performed, with particular attention to the axillary and musculocutaneous nerves.

When pathologic laxity is diagnosed, the focus turns to diagnostic studies to determine the extent to which the shoulder anatomy has been affected. The commonly obtained radiographic views include the Grashey scapular AP, scapular Y, axillary, West Point, Hill-Sachs, and Stryker notch views (**Table 1**). Such studies confirm that the shoulder is congruent and provide information about glenoid and humeral bony impaction lesions and bone loss.

A pathologic lesion implicated in instability may be overlooked during both the radiographic workup and surgery. A poor outcome can follow failure to recognize poor-quality capsular tissue, a soft-tissue or bony Bankart lesion, glenohumeral ligament disruption, scapular winging, critical bone loss, or a rotator cuff interval lesion. Failure to recognize and treat glenohumeral ligament pathology is a significant cause of recurrent instability. A 9.3% incidence of humeral avulsion of the glenohumeral ligament (HAGL) was found in 64 shoulders with anterior instability.[4] More recently, additional ligament avulsions have been identified, including the reverse HAGL, the bony HAGL, and glenoid-side avulsion.[9,10] The combination of a HAGL lesion and a Bankart tear is called a floating lesion.

Another area of tissue pathology that affects the recurrence of instability involves differentiation of a Bankart tear from an anterior labral periosteal sleeve avulsion (ALPSA; **Figure 2**). At a minimum 2-year follow-up after arthroscopic stabilization with suture anchors, a study of 93 shoulders with traumatic anterior shoulder instability found a recurrence rate of 7.4% in shoulders with an isolated Bankart lesion and a 19.2% rate in those with an ALPSA tear.[11] The average number of dislocation-subluxation events was 12.3 in patients with an ALPSA tear compared with 4.9 in

Table 1

Diagnostic Radiography for Recurrent Shoulder Instability

Radiographic View	Acquisition Technique	Key Features
Shoulder AP	The x-ray beam is directed at a right angle to the coronal plane of the body.	General overview of the shoulder
Scapular AP (Grashey, true AP)	The patient is externally rotated 35° to 40° to the ipsilateral side to focus the beam tangential to the scapular body.	Loss of inferior glenoid rim (representing bone loss)
Scapular Y (lateral view of the scapula)	Standing with the lateral shoulder against the film, the patient rotates 35° to 40° forward. The beam is directed through the medial aspect of the scapula.	Acromion and coracoid forming the Y
Axillary	The film cassette is superior to the shoulder, and the arm is abducted. The beam is directed into the axillae.	Anterior or posterior subluxation or dislocation Hill-Sachs or reverse Hill-Sachs lesion Glenoid version
West Point	The patient is prone. The beam is angled 25° cephalad and 25° medial toward the coracoid.	Anteroinferior glenoid rim
Stryker notch	The patient is supine, with the hand on the back of the head and the elbow pointing to the ceiling. The beam is angled 10° cephalad.	Posterior humeral impaction Hill-Sachs lesion

(Adapted with permission from Egol K, Koval K, Zuckerman J: *The Handbook of Fractures*, ed 4. Philadelphia, PA, Lippincott, Williams, and Wilkins, 2010.)

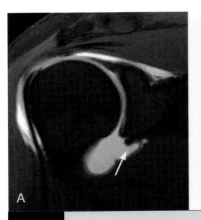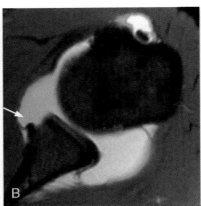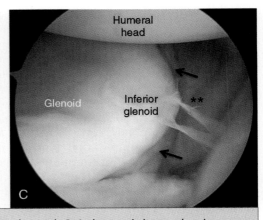

Figure 2 Coronal (**A**) and axial (**B**) MRI of a right shoulder with an ALPSA tear *(arrows)*. **C**, Arthroscopic image showing an ALPSA tear *(arrows)* in a right shoulder, with detachment and medial displacement of the labrum. ** = inferior glenohumeral ligament.

those with a Bankart lesion. Therefore, it was suggested that recurrent events lead to a decrease in tissue quality and a less durable repair.

Although most patients' instability occurs in the anterior direction, posterior instability does occur. Rates of recurrence after posterior surgical stabilization range from 0% to 12%.[12] A retrospective review of 27 shoulders that underwent arthroscopic posterior labral repair for symptomatic unidirectional instability found that 92% of the patients were pain free and had no recurrence of instability at an average 5.1-year follow-up.[13] The causes of failure after posterior surgery include failure to recognize additional directions of

instability or treat redundant or poor-quality capsular tissue. After posterior instability surgery, overhead throwing athletes have relatively low rates of return to sport, and contact athletes have a risk of redislocation.[2] As a result, it has been recommended that the surgeon err toward undertightening in an overhead throwing athlete and overtightening in a contact athlete.[12]

Failure to recognize additional posterior and/or inferior instability in patients with anterior laxity leads to a poor outcome. The factors contributing to a relatively high rate of recurrence after surgery for multidirectional instability include accompanying general ligamentous laxity, a dysplastic glenoid, a rotator cuff in-

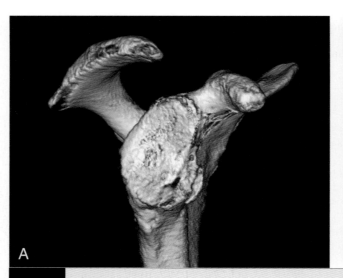

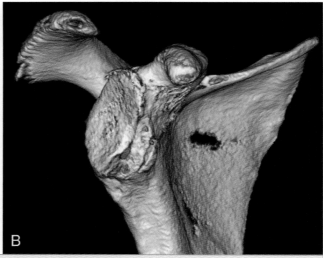

| **Figure 3** | A bony Bankart lesion in a right shoulder, as seen in a three-dimensional CT reconstruction with humeral subtraction (**A**) and in an oblique view showing medial displacement of the lesion (**B**). |

terval lesion, and circumferential labral tearing.[14] Open surgery involving pancapsular shifting has been the classic treatment of multidirectional instability, but arthroscopic procedures have gained favor and have had comparable results.[15]

The role of surgical technique for rotator cuff interval closure in correcting instability has been the subject of much debate. Closure can be performed with an arthroscopic or an open approach. The open technique often involves a medial-to-lateral tissue plication that may improve both posterior and inferior glenohumeral translation. A comparison of arthroscopic and open rotator cuff interval closure in cadaver shoulders found no improvement in posterior translation with either method, and only open plication improved inferior stability.[16] However, anterior translation was improved with both open and arthroscopic rotator cuff interval closure. Open plication primarily improved translation in the neutral position. The effects of arthroscopic closure were most pronounced with the arm abducted and externally rotated.

Numerous studies have focused on methods for radiographically characterizing the extent of bone loss. Three-dimensional CT of the glenoid and the humeral head is recommended if bone loss is suspected. The methods for quantifying glenoid bone defects using CT commonly involve approximating the inferior two thirds of the glenoid as a circle and directly measuring different parameters of the defect for comparison with the contralateral shoulder. CT with three-dimensional reconstruction was found to correctly predict the requirements for bone grafting in 96% of patients[17] (**Figure 3**).

Arthroscopic assessment of glenoid bone loss can be difficult. Characterization of an oblong and irregular surface is required. The established method for measuring the bare spot involves using the glenoid bare spot to represent midline and comparing the amount of bone anterior and posterior. However, an anatomic study questioned whether the bare spot actually represents the anatomic center of the glenoid.[18] Cadaver shoulders were used to create bone loss models at 45° and 0° to the long axis of the glenoid.[19] The arthroscopic bare spot model was found to accurately depict bone loss in the 0° model but overestimated bone loss in the 45° model. The secant chord theory method of measuring glenoid bone loss approximates a perfect inferior glenoid circle by obtaining arthroscopic measurements at unaffected and affected bone areas and comparing the values using geometric calculations.[20] This method was found to be more accurate than the bare spot method but still had a 4% error.

If all anatomic factors were properly identified, a failure related to treatment choice is challenging to analyze. It is clear that numerous anatomic factors contribute to shoulder instability, but determining their relative contributions is particularly difficult. For example, research clearly shows that in the absence of glenoid or humeral bone loss and with adequate tissue, a well-performed open or arthroscopic soft-tissue procedure can lead to a good outcome (**Table 2**). However, glenoid and humeral bone loss can occur independently as well as together and with varying degrees of severity. Thus, it becomes more difficult to determine the definition of critical bone loss and whether the definition changes based on the collective extent of loss.

Humeral-side bone loss occurs at the time of dislocation when the humeral head impacts against the glenoid rim. With recurrent subluxation or dislocation events, the defect can progressively erode and enlarge. After 194 arthroscopic Bankart repairs, the recurrence rate was 4% if no significant bone defects were present but was 67% if the glenoid was classified as inverted-pear shaped or if a so-called engaging Hill-Sachs lesion

Table 2

Recurrence Rates After Anterior Shoulder Instability Recurrence, as Reported in Recent Studies

Study (Year)	Type of Procedure	Number of Patients	Mean Follow-up (Years)	Sports Involvement	Recurrence Rate
Bonnevialle et al[77] (2009)	Open	79	7.1	83%	12.6%
Elmlund et al[78] (2008)	Arthroscopic	84	8.2	87%	11%
Fabre et al[79] (2010)	Open	50	28	73%	16%
Law et al[80] (2008)	Arthroscopic	38	2.3	100%	5.2%
Ogawa et al[56] (2010)	Open	167	8.7	—	4.8%
Oh et al[38] (2009)	Arthroscopic	37	3	40.5%	5.4%
Porcellini et al[81] (2009)	Arthroscopic	385	3	—	8.1%
Thal et al[82] (2007)	Arthroscopic	73	>2	—	6.9%
Thomazeau et al[42] (2010)	Arthroscopic	125	1.5	73%	3.2%
Voos et al[23] (2010)	Arthroscopic	83	2.75	46%	18%

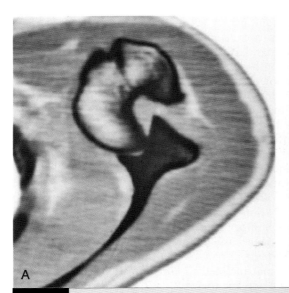
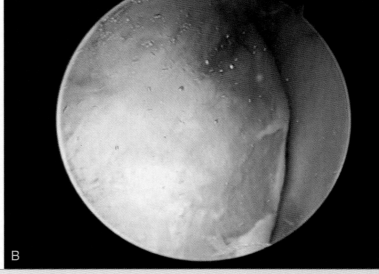

Figure 4 **A,** Axial CT of a left shoulder with a large Hill-Sachs lesion. **B,** Arthroscopic image of the same shoulder showing engagement of the Hill-Sachs lesion.

was present[21] (**Figure 4**). Humeral bone loss can be classified by size (small or large), the percentage of the humeral head involved, the depth of the defect, or the volume of the defect. Significant bone loss requiring surgical treatment has been defined as involving more than 25% to 45% of the humeral head.[22] A prospective review of 83 arthroscopic Bankart repairs found an 18% recurrence rate at a minimum 2-year follow-up.[23] A Hill-Sachs lesion larger than 250 mm³, patient age younger than 20 years, and ligamentous laxity were significantly associated with recurrence. Cadaver shoulders were studied in maximal external rotation and at various abduction angles to evaluate the size of a Hill-Sachs lesion that engages the glenoid rim.[24] Engage-

ment occurred if the diameter from the edge of the rotator cuff to the medial bony lesion was more than 84% of the glenoid width.

A significant engaging Hill-Sachs lesion commonly is treated with an open surgical procedure. Allograft, osteochondral bone graft, metallic resurfacing, and arthroscopic remplissage can be used. Remplissage (meaning "to fill" in French) involves tenodesis of the posterior rotator cuff tendons into the humeral bone defect to prevent it from engaging. This procedure allows arthroscopic treatment of recurrent instability or instability with a humeral bone defect.[25]

Biomechanical studies have classified the range of critical glenoid bone loss as approximately 20% to

2: Instability and Athletic Injuries

30%.[26,27] Anterior defects have been more extensively studied than posterior defects.[28] Options for reconstructing the glenoid after bone loss from recurrent instability include iliac crest autografting, transfer of part or all of the coracoid process, and placement of allograft bone. Arthroscopic techniques have been developed for both glenoid bone grafting and Latarjet reconstruction.[29] Arthroscopic reconstruction is technically demanding and has not been found superior to its open counterparts, although it offers the general benefits of arthroscopic over open surgery.[27] Distal tibial allograft for augmentation of a glenoid defect closely matches the native curvature of the glenoid.

Both the Bristow and the Latarjet procedures provide good results in patients with glenoid bone loss.[30,31] A study of cadaver shoulders with a 45° defect model found that Latarjet reconstruction better limited glenohumeral translation at several arm positions compared with bone grafting.[32] The suggested mechanism of stability in Latarjet reconstruction includes bone augmentation of the deficient glenoid, capsular closure, and the sling effect of the conjoined tendon in abduction and external rotation.[33] The bone block effect was questioned in a prospective study of 26 patients who underwent a Latarjet procedure.[30] CT was used to evaluate for graft osteolysis. Although an average of almost 60% of the coracoid had undergone osteolysis, there were no recurrences at a mean 17.5-month follow-up. A review of 319 shoulders that had undergone a Bristow stabilization procedure found a 5% redislocation rate and a 13% subluxation rate.[31] Medial positioning or displacement of the bone more than 1 cm from the glenoid rim resulted in an increased rate of redislocation.

Despite the potential for improved shoulder stability after coracoid transfer, recurrences have been documented. A review of 46 patients after an unsuccessful Latarjet procedure followed by revision using iliac crest bone graft (a modified Eden-Hybinette procedure) found that only 4 patients had a recurrence at an average 6.8-year follow-up.[34]

An osseous Bankart lesion is a rim fracture that occurs anteriorly (the bony Bankart lesion) or posteriorly (the reverse bony Bankart lesion), based on the anterior or the posterior force of dislocation. In these glenoid bone deficits, the labrum and thr capsule usually remain connected to the osseous fragment. Depending on the size of the osseous fragment, bony Bankart injuries have classically been treated with open repair and possibly with bone grafting. Good results have been reported with the application of arthroscopic techniques. The treatment of bony Bankart injuries was compared in 41 patients with acute injury who were treated within 3 months and 27 patients with chronic injury who were treated more than 3 months after injury.[35] Only 3 patients were missing at 4-year follow-up. Although there was only one redislocation in each group of patients, the preoperative and postoperative Rowe scores were significantly lower in patients with a chronic injury.

Surgical Technique

Improper surgical technique leading to recurrence is related to the surgeon's the surgeon's skills and surgical decision making in open or arthroscopic surgery. Initially, open surgery was the mainstay treatment of shoulder instability, but there has been a progressive increase in the use of arthroscopic surgery by both sports- and non–sports-trained surgeons.[35] Early arthroscopic techniques have evolved with improvements in bone anchor technology, understanding of tissue pathology, and surgeon skill. Both arthroscopic and open repair techniques have been found to produce comparable results.

Arthroscopic techniques for repair of the labrum and capsule use transglenoid sutures as well as various types of bone anchors. Factors influencing the failure rate include anchor design, number, material, size, and location. Glenoid suture anchors are made from metal, biocomposite, and bioabsorbable materials. Osteolysis can occur with the use of bioabsorbable as well as metallic anchors.[36] Resorption of bone adjacent to the anchors can lead to glenoid rim fracture in a traumatic environment, such as a contact sport.[37]

Anchors can be preloaded with suture material or knotless. Standard bone anchors and those with knotless fixation have comparable redislocation rates.[38] Recurrence of dislocation is more likely if fewer than three anchors are used.[39] It is very important to adequately mobilize the capsulolabral tissue and prepare the bone bed for reattachment. In addition, the surgeon must sufficiently plicate the capsule to reduce volume and shift the tissue superiorly. Capsular stretching and redundancy must be treated with plication in addition to restoration of the labral bumper.

Placing anchors for repair of the labrum in a more medial position below the rim cannot restore the appropriate bumper effect of the labrum. For isolated traumatic instability, one technique is to place three anchors below the 3-o'clock position, 2 mm onto the glenoid rim, and inclined to enter the bone at 45°.[40] The ability to place anchors with the proper trajectory and inferiorly on the glenoid is affected by portal placement. Although cannulas are commonly used in instability surgery, noncannulated portals can be established through the subscapularis muscle to help achieve a more inferior anchor placement between the 5-o'clock and 6-o'clock positions. It is particularly important to make sure the anchor is buried below the chondroosseus level to prevent third-body chondral damage to the humeral head (**Figure 5**).

For a patient with recurrent instability after surgical stabilization, additional soft-tissue procedures can be considered if there is no significant bone loss. The ideal candidates include patients with traumatic redislocation after successful stabilization or with pathology not treated during the index procedure. Arthroscopy can contribute to failure of an open procedure. A retrospective review evaluated 22 patients who underwent arthroscopy after unsuccessful earlier open surgery. The

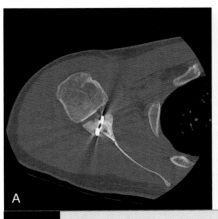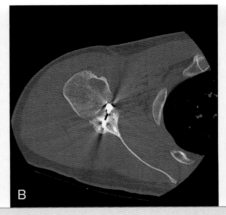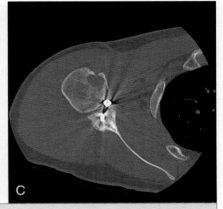

Figure 5 **A** and **B,** Serial axial CT showing the interarticular placement of screws for Laterjet fixation in a right shoulder. **C,** CT showing the humeral defect that subsequently developed.

patients had undergone a Latarjet, an Eden-Hybinette, or a Bankart repair and capsular shift.[41] They were treated with arthroscopic soft-tissue repair, selective removal of hardware, and, in 4 patients, additional rotator cuff interval closure. At an average 43-month follow-up, 1 patient had recurrent subluxation, and 2 had a subjective sense of apprehension but were satisfied with the results of the procedure.

Unavoidable Factors

Some surgical failures result from factors that the surgeon cannot directly control, even after perfect diagnosis and the execution of surgical techniques. One of the more challenging factors is patient noncompliance, which includes a lack of adherence to postoperative restrictions regarding sling wear, activity, physical therapy, and follow-up medical visits. The result can be retearing of Bankart, capsular, or subscapularis repair failure of a lesser tuberosity osteotomy or bone cutout through a coracoid transfer or bone graft. Some patient-related factors are unavoidable, such as disruption from a fall, seizure activity, infection, or overly aggressive physical therapy.

Neither the surgeon nor the patient has control over the patient's genetic composition. In a patient with a condition such as Ehlers-Danlos syndrome, Marfan syndrome, or generalized joint hypermobility, altered tissue elasticity can contribute to recurrent joint hyperlaxity after instability surgery. Conversely, a propensity to develop exuberant scar tissue after surgery can predispose a patient to postoperative stiffness. It is important to identify such factors before surgery so that surgical decision making and postoperative rehabilitation can be adjusted as necessary.

Risk Prediction for Redislocation

A case-control study evaluated 131 arthroscopic Bankart repairs for recurrent shoulder instability.[3] The overall recurrence rate was 13% at a mean 31-month follow-up. Six factors were used to create the 10-point

Table 3	
The Instability Severity Index Score for Assessing the Risk of Recurrent Anterior Instability After Soft-Tissue Repair	
Preoperative Risk Factor	**Score**
Younger than 20 years	2
Participation in competitive sports	2
Participation in a contact or an overhead sport	1
Anterior or inferior hyperlaxity	1
Radiographically visible Hill-Sachs lesion	2
Radiographically visible loss of normal interior glenoid contour	2
Total Possible Score	**10**
Score	**Risk of Recurrence**
< 3	5%
3–6	10%
> 6	70%

(Adapted with permission from Balg F, Boileau P: The instability severity index score: A simple pre-operative score to select patients for arthroscopic or open shoulder stabilisation. *J Bone Joint Surg Br* 2007;89[11]:1470-1477.)

instability severity index score (**Table 3**). If the patient's score was higher than 6, an open non–soft-tissue procedure was indicated to minimize the risk of recurrence.

Short-term outcomes were reported in a prospective multicenter observational study of anterior arthroscopic stabilization procedures in patients with an instability severity index score of 4 or fewer points.[42] At 18-month follow-up, 4 of the 125 patients who met the inclusion criteria (3.2%) had a recurrence.

2: Instability and Athletic Injuries

Types of Complications

Stiffness

The goal of instability surgery is to reconstitute shoulder stability while maintaining a functional range of motion. Numerous factors affect postoperative shoulder motion, including the type of procedure, length of shoulder immobilization, physical therapy protocol, and underlying capacity for scar tissue formation. Patients undergoing stabilization surgery for recurrent traumatic anterior shoulder instability commonly have restricted motion compared with the unaffected contralateral shoulder. External rotation loss is most common, averaging 8° to 33.6° with the arm at the side and 6° to 24.4° with the arm in 90° of abduction.[43] In one study, internal rotation loss averaged 19.2° with 90° of abduction. Such loss of motion was not found to independently influence the development of arthropathy in the long term.[44]

Postoperative management involves sling immobilization of the shoulder for 4 to 6 weeks, followed by progressive active-assisted and active range-of-motion exercises in a structured physical therapy program. The goal commonly is full passive range of motion within 2 to 3 months after surgery.[38] One protocol limits shoulder motion to less than 90° of elevation-abduction and 30° of external rotation until 3 months after surgery and then progresses to full motion.[45] A similar protocol initially uses a gunslinger-type brace to prevent the arm from internally rotating to the body.[46]

Posterior stabilization with capsular plication and labral repair represents fewer than 10% of instability procedures. A postoperative protocol similar to that for anterior instability involves sling immobilization for 6 weeks to limit extreme internal rotation and minimize stress on the posterior repair.[47] After discontinuation of the abduction sling, gentle passive and active motion is advanced until progression to strengthening 4 to 6 months after surgery. A retrospective review of 112 patients with posterior shoulder dislocation treated with arthroscopic stabilization found a 12% decrease in internal rotation at 90° abduction compared with the contralateral arm, in addition to a 17.7% redislocation rate within the first year after surgery.[48] External rotation with the arm at the side or in 90° abduction decreased 8.7% or 5.4%, respectively.

The primary criticism of the remplissage procedure is that an accompanying loss of external rotation has been seen in biomechanical studies.[49] A comparison of patients undergoing arthroscopic Bankart repair with or without remplissage found no difference in postoperative range of motion.[50] However, 33% of the patients who underwent a Bankart repair with remplissage reported a novel posterosuperior pain 2 years after surgery, possibly related to partial or incomplete healing of the defect. Whether rotator cuff tenodesis into the bony defect produces a satisfactory functional result has not yet been determined.

Pain

Pain is a common complication after a shoulder stabilization procedure.[40,43] One study reported an almost 50% incidence of pain in 60 patients at a more than 10-year follow-up after Bankart repair.[51] Postoperative pain after shoulder stabilization may be a sign of remaining pathologic tissue, whether untreated at the time of surgery or resulting from postoperative failure of fixation. Postoperative pain most commonly is multifactorial. It may be secondary to concomitant pathology, such as rotator cuff or biceps tendinopathy, chondral injury, postoperative idiopathic capsulitis, loss of muscle strength or endurance, or a combination of factors.[52]

Early pain also may occur with the development of degenerative glenohumeral arthritis with chondrolysis related to the prominence of suture anchors within the joint, thermal capsulorraphy, or the use of an intra-articular pain catheter.[53-55] Infection is rare but may be a source of early or late pain. Pain after surgery can be a particularly vexing challenge, particularly when no further instability persists and repeat examination and imaging reveal no structural correlation. In this scenario, the initial treatment almost always is nonsurgical. Physical therapy to restore range of motion and strength is supplemented by the use of anti-inflammatory medications.

An 11.3% incidence of arthritic changes was found on radiographs, and a 31.2% incidence was found on CT in 282 patients younger than 40 years with traumatic anterior instability.[56] Most of the identified arthritis was mild or undetectable on radiographs. This study improved the understanding of baseline changes at the time of stability surgery. Chondral lesions were found in 55 of 87 patients (63%) during arthroscopic stabilization.[57] In studies with a 20-year follow-up, the incidence of arthritis ranged from 35% to 71%.[58,59] The likelihood of developing arthritis reportedly is correlated with older age at the time of dislocation, a greater number of dislocations before surgery, greater time between initial dislocation and surgery, and worse degeneration of the labrum.[53,60] At 25-year follow-up after instability surgery in 257 shoulders, 44% of shoulders were radiographically normal, 29% had mild changes, 9% had moderate changes, and 17% had severe changes.[61]

Open reconstructive surgery of a humeral or a glenoid deficiency involves contouring bone graft material to match the defect size and radius and can be technically challenging. Anteroinferior glenoid defects created in cadaver shoulders were reconstructed using a Latarjet or an iliac crest bone graft procedure.[62] Tekscan pressure sensors were used to determine that the contact pressure was best reconstituted when grafts were flush with the surface and the Latarjet graft was rotated so that the inferior surface was congruent with the glenoid. Alterations in the distribution of contact pressure in the long term may contribute to the development of joint arthrosis and the disastrous effects of a

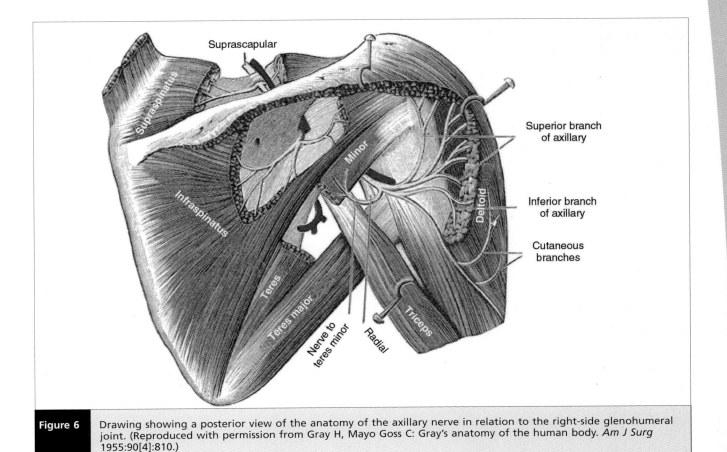

| Figure 6 | Drawing showing a posterior view of the anatomy of the axillary nerve in relation to the right-side glenohumeral joint. (Reproduced with permission from Gray H, Mayo Goss C: Gray's anatomy of the human body. *Am J Surg* 1955:90[4]:810.) |

prominent laterally placed graft.

Neurologic Injury

Neurologic injury can occur with a dislocation event or a shoulder stabilization procedure. In 3,633 consecutive patients with traumatic anterior glenohumeral dislocation, the incidence of neurologic deficit was 13.5% after reduction.[63] Of the 210 patients with neurologic deficit, the axillary nerve was involved in 73.8%, the ulnar nerve in 10.5%, the median nerve in 3.8%, the radial nerve in 1.4%, and the musculocutaneous nerve in 1%. Multiple nerves or the brachial plexus was involved in 9.5% of the injuries. The likelihood of neurologic injury was greatest in patients with a concomitant rotator cuff tear or a greater tuberosity fracture.

Nerve injury can occur with open or arthroscopic stabilization, although most available studies reported nerve injury after an open procedure. The estimated incidence of nerve injury ranges from 1% to 8%, with one study reporting an 8.2% incidence of both sensory and sensorimotor neuropathies in 282 patients after open anterior stabilization.[64,65] The most commonly affected nerves in both open and arthroscopic procedures are the axillary nerve and the musculocutaneous nerve because of their proximity to the glenohumeral joint.[40] Anatomic cadaver studies found that the axillary nerve is 1 to 1.5 cm below the inferior glenohumeral liga-

ment, with the sensory branch closest to the glenoid rim, and the musculocutaneous nerve is approximately 5 cm inferior to the coracoid process after it pierces the coracobrachialis.[66,67] These locations may have particular relevance for an anterior stabilization procedure with inferior capsular shift, which risks injury to the axillary nerve, and an open procedure during the placement of retractors and surgical instrumentation, which risks injury to both nerves (**Figure 6**). Arthroscopic nerve injuries may result from improper placement of an inferior portal, patient malpositioning, manipulation, or traction on the arm, which causes strain on the brachial plexus.[40,68] An anatomic study found the brachial plexus to be only 5 mm from the glenoid rim in some patients, and retractors placed along the scapular neck can make contact with the plexus.[69] However, most nerve injuries are transient neurapraxias as a result of traction, and they seldom are from direct laceration.[69]

The increasing popularity of coracoid transfer and bone block procedures for significant glenoid bone loss has increased the awareness of other nerve complications, such as damage to the suprascapular nerve. In addition to brachial plexus traction injury and musculocutaneous nerve palsy, suprascapular nerve palsy has been reported after an open Latarjet procedure, probably because of the proximity of the suprascapular nerve to the posterior glenoid rim, which puts it at particular risk during screw insertion.[70] The risk can be extrapolated to any bone block procedure requiring screw fixation with penetration through the posterior glenoid.

Some studies have focused on preventing nerve damage during arthroscopic or open stabilization. A subscapularis-splitting approach for open anterior stabilization was used in 128 patients, of whom only 1 (0.8%) had paresthesias in the axillary nerve distribution, with complete resolution and no further intervention.[71] A prospective study followed 20 consecutive patients who received nerve monitoring during arthroscopic shoulder stabilization.[72] In the 11 patients who underwent thermal capsulorrhaphy, four procedures were altered because monitoring revealed an impending nerve injury. None of the patients experienced any clinical deficits. Although this study reported on capsulorrhaphy, a procedure that appears to be losing popularity, neuromonitoring may be helpful for preventing impending nerve injuries, particularly in open procedures such as Latarjet reconstruction, in which the anatomic proximity of nerves to instrumentation and retractors may be a concern.

Infection

Although infection can occur with any type of surgery, it is relatively rare after shoulder stabilization.[40] The estimated incidence of infection ranges from 0% to 6% after open stabilization and from 0.04% to 0.23% after arthroscopic stabilization.[73,74] Over a 21-year study period, only six patients who underwent shoulder instability surgery were treated for infection with *Propionibacterium acnes,* the most common offending organism.[75] There should be a high index of suspicion for a nidus of late infection surrounding nonabsorbable sutures. There are sporadic case reports of unusual infections, one of which occurred around a metallic suture anchor in an arthroscopic Bankart repair.[76] When infection occurs after shoulder instability surgery, general orthopaedic principles of prompt recognition, thorough irrigation and débridement, and the use of intravenous antibiotics should be followed. Elective culturing with a relatively long incubation period should be used to look specifically for the fastidious *P acnes* organism if infection occurs after shoulder stabilization.[75]

Summary

The most common complications after instability surgery involve recurrence, shoulder stiffness, pain, neurovascular injury, and infection. There are numerous factors that contribute to adverse outcomes, such as inaccurate or incomplete preoperative identification of the pathology. In particular, it is important to perform a thorough clinical and radiograph workup to determine the direction(s) of instability, assess the quality of soft-tissue restraints, and determine if significant glenoid and/or humeral bone loss is present. After select-

ing the appropriate surgery, suboptimal execution can result in hardware prominence, failure of fixation, cartilage damage, or injury to adjacent neurovascular structures. A balance must be achieved for postoperative care between the development of stiffness and the recurrence of joint laxity. As in all other areas of orthopaedics, patient noncompliance and secondary traumatic events can have a devastating effect on treatment results.

Annotated References

1. Cho NS, Hwang JC, Rhee YG: Arthroscopic stabilization in anterior shoulder instability: Collision athletes versus noncollision athletes. *Arthroscopy* 2006;22(9):947-953.

2. Balg F, Boileau P: The instability severity index score: A simple pre-operative score to select patients for arthroscopic or open shoulder stabilisation. *J Bone Joint Surg Br* 2007;89(11):1470-1477.

   A prospective case control study of 131 patients with recurrent anterior shoulder instability who underwent suture anchor stabilization found a 14.5% recurrence rate. Significant factors were used to create a 10-point predictive scoring system.

3. Radkowski CA, Chhabra A, Baker CL III, Tejwani SG, Bradley JP: Arthroscopic capsulolabral repair for posterior shoulder instability in throwing athletes compared with nonthrowing athletes. *Am J Sports Med* 2008;36(4):693-699.

   In a cohort study, 107 shoulders in athletes with isolated posterior shoulder instability underwent arthroscopic stabilization. The results were comparable in throwing and nonthrowing athletes, except there was a lower rate of return to preinjury competition level in throwing athletes (55% versus 71%).

4. Wolf EM, Cheng JC, Dickson K: Humeral avulsion of glenohumeral ligaments as a cause of anterior shoulder instability. *Arthroscopy* 1995;11(5):600-607.

5. Spatschil A, Landsiedl F, Anderl W, et al: Posttraumatic anterior-inferior instability of the shoulder: Arthroscopic findings and clinical correlations. *Arch Orthop Trauma Surg* 2006;126(4):217-222.

6. Cho HL, Lee CK, Hwang TH, Suh KT, Park JW: Arthroscopic repair of combined Bankart and SLAP lesions: Operative techniques and clinical results. *Clin Orthop Surg* 2010;2(1):39-46.

   A retrospective cohort study compared arthroscopic repair of an isolated Bankart tear and a combined Bankart and SLAP tear in 47 patients. Both groups had improvement, but return of range of motion was slower after the combined repair.

7. Hantes ME, Venouziou AI, Liantsis AK, Dailiana ZH, Malizos KN: Arthroscopic repair for chronic anterior shoulder instability: A comparative study between pa-

tients with Bankart lesions and patients with combined Bankart and superior labral anterior posterior lesions. *Am J Sports Med* 2009;37(6):1093-1098.

A prospective cohort study of 38 patients with arthroscopic isolated Bankart tear repair and 25 with combined Bankart and SLAP tear repair found comparably improved Constant and Rowe scores. There was a single redislocation in each group at 2-year follow-up.

8. Tischer T, Vogt S, Kreuz PC, Imhoff AB: Arthroscopic anatomy, variants, and pathologic findings in shoulder instability. *Arthroscopy* 2011;27(10):1434-1443.

The literature on normal, pathologic, and variant arthroscopic anatomy is reviewed.

9. Hill JD, Lovejoy JF Jr, Kelly RA: Combined posterior Bankart lesion and posterior humeral avulsion of the glenohumeral ligaments associated with recurrent posterior shoulder instability. *Arthroscopy* 2007;23(3): e1-e3.

In a case report of recurrent of posterior glenohumeral instability caused by a posterior Bankart lesion and a posterior HAGL lesion, both were treated arthroscopically with suture anchors.

10. Wolf EM, Siparsky PN: Glenoid avulsion of the glenohumeral ligaments as a cause of recurrent anterior shoulder instability. *Arthroscopy* 2010;26(9):1263-1267.

Three patients with recurrent anterior shoulder instability caused by avulsion of the glenohumeral ligaments had arthroscopic repair.

11. Ozbaydar M, Elhassan B, Diller D, Massimini D, Higgins LD, Warner JJ: Results of arthroscopic capsulolabral repair: Bankart lesion versus anterior labroligamentous periosteal sleeve avulsion lesion. *Arthroscopy* 2008;24(11):1277-1283.

Of 99 patients with anterior instability who underwent arthroscopic stabilization, the 67 with an isolated Bankart tear had a recurrence rate of 7.4% at an average 5-year follow-up, compared with a 19.2% rate in the 26 patients with an ALPSA lesion.

12. Bradley JP, Tejwani SG: Arthroscopic management of posterior instability. *Orthop Clin North Am* 2010; 41(3):339-356.

The literature on posterior instability was reviewed, with pathoanatomy, history, physical examination factors, imaging, treatment options, and postoperative rehabilitation.

13. Williams RJ III, Strickland S, Cohen M, Altchek DW, Warren RF: Arthroscopic repair for traumatic posterior shoulder instability. *Am J Sports Med* 2003;31(2): 203-209.

14. Schenk TJ, Brems JJ: Multidirectional instability of the shoulder: Pathophysiology, diagnosis, and management. *J Am Acad Orthop Surg* 1998;6(1):65-72.

15. Alpert JM, Verma N, Wysocki R, Yanke AB, Romeo AA: Arthroscopic treatment of multidirectional shoulder instability with minimum 270 degrees labral repair: Minimum 2-year follow-up. *Arthroscopy* 2008; 24(6):704-711.

A retrospective study of 13 patients who underwent arthroscopic stabilization for multidirectional instability involving labral tears larger than 270° found a 15% recurrence rate. Eighty-five percent of the patients were completely or mostly satisfied with the results at average 56-month follow-up.

16. Provencher MT, Mologne TS, Hongo M, Zhao K, Tasto JP, An KN: Arthroscopic versus open rotator interval closure: Biomechanical evaluation of stability and motion. *Arthroscopy* 2007;23(6):583-592.

A basic science biomechanical study tested stability and range of motion after arthroscopic and open rotator cuff interval closure. Neither technique improved posterior stability, and both resulted in significant loss of external rotation. Only the open rotator cuff interval closure improved sulcus stability.

17. Chuang TY, Adams CR, Burkhart SS: Use of preoperative three-dimensional computed tomography to quantify glenoid bone loss in shoulder instability. *Arthroscopy* 2008;24(4):376-382.

The glenoid index was calculated in a retrospective study of 25 patients with anterior instability who underwent bilateral preoperative CT. A level of 0.75 corresponded to arthroscopic findings guiding toward a soft-tissue or bony stabilization procedure.

18. Kralinger F, Aigner F, Longato S, Rieger M, Wambacher M: Is the bare spot a consistent landmark for shoulder arthroscopy? A study of 20 embalmed glenoids with 3-dimensional computed tomographic reconstruction. *Arthroscopy* 2006;22(4):428-432.

19. Provencher MT, Detterline AJ, Ghodadra N, et al: Measurement of glenoid bone loss: A comparison of measurement error between 45 degrees and 0 degrees bone loss models and with different posterior arthroscopy portal locations. *Am J Sports Med* 2008;36(6): 1132-1138.

A basic science study of 14 cadaver shoulders evaluated the ability of the arthroscopic bare spot method to determine the extent of anterior-inferior bone loss in 12.5% and 25% models and at two angles relative to the long axis of the glenoid. The bare spot method was found to be accurate in the 0° model and overestimated bone loss in the 45° model.

20. Detterline AJ, Provencher MT, Ghodadra N, Bach BR Jr, Romeo AA, Verma NN: A new arthroscopic technique to determine anterior-inferior glenoid bone loss: Validation of the secant chord theory in a cadaveric model. *Arthroscopy* 2009;25(11):1249-1256.

A basic science study of seven cadaver shoulders compared the ability of the arthroscopic bare spot and secant chord theory methods to evaluate glenoid bone loss. Regardless of the amount of bone loss or the portal position, the scant chord theory was more accurate,

2: Instability and Athletic Injuries

although more extensive mathematical calculations were required.

21. Burkhart SS, De Beer JF: Traumatic glenohumeral bone defects and their relationship to failure of arthroscopic Bankart repairs: Significance of the inverted-pear glenoid and the humeral engaging Hill-Sachs lesion. *Arthroscopy* 2000;16(7):677-694.

22. Cetik O, Uslu M, Ozsar BK: The relationship between Hill-Sachs lesion and recurrent anterior shoulder dislocation. *Acta Orthop Belg* 2007;73(2):175-178.

    A correlation was found between the number of dislocations and the extent and the depth of a Hill-Sachs lesion. A patient with recurrent anterior shoulder dislocation should receive early surgical treatment to prevent lesion progression.

23. Voos JE, Livermore RW, Feeley BT, et al; HSS Sports Medicine Service: Prospective evaluation of arthroscopic bankart repairs for anterior instability. *Am J Sports Med* 2010;38(2):302-307.

    A study of 83 patients with anterior shoulder instability who underwent arthroscopic Bankart repair found an 18% recurrence rate. The identified risk factors included age younger than 25 years, general ligamentous laxity, and a Hill-Sachs lesion larger than 250 mm^3.

24. Yamamoto N, Itoi E, Abe H, et al: Contact between the glenoid and the humeral head in abduction, external rotation, and horizontal extension: A new concept of glenoid track. *J Shoulder Elbow Surg* 2007;16(5): 649-656.

    A basic science biomechanical study of nine cadaver shoulders tested stability after simulated Hill-Sachs lesions at maximal external rotation and with 0°, 30°, and 60° of abduction. There was an increased risk of engagement when the width of the lesion was more than 84% of the glenoid width.

25. Park MJ, Tjoumakaris FP, Garcia G, Patel A, Kelly JD IV: Arthroscopic remplissage with Bankart repair for the treatment of glenohumeral instability with Hill-Sachs defects. *Arthroscopy* 2011;27(9):1187-1194.

    A case study of 20 patients with recurrent anterior shoulder instability and a large Hill-Sachs defect who underwent arthroscopic Bankart repair with remplissage found a 15% recurrence rate at a mean 2-year follow-up. Range of motion was not reported.

26. Itoi E, Lee SB, Berglund LJ, Berge LL, An KN: The effect of a glenoid defect on anteroinferior stability of the shoulder after Bankart repair: A cadaveric study. *J Bone Joint Surg Am* 2000;82(1):35-46.

27. Provencher MT, Ghodadra N, LeClere L, Solomon DJ, Romeo AA: Anatomic osteochondral glenoid reconstruction for recurrent glenohumeral instability with glenoid deficiency using a distal tibia allograft. *Arthroscopy* 2009;25(4):446-452.

    This is a case study and a description of the technique for using fresh distal tibial osteochondral allograft for reconstructing three shoulders with anterior instability and glenoid bone loss averaging 30%.

28. Yamamoto N, Muraki T, Sperling JW, et al: Stabilizing mechanism in bone grafting of a large glenoid defect. *J Bone Joint Surg Am* 2010;92(11):2059-2066.

    A basic science biomechanical study used 13 cadaver shoulders to create anterior-inferior glenoid defects at increasing 2-mm increments. There was a significant decrease in the force required to translate the humeral head at defects larger than 19% of the glenoid length.

29. Lafosse L, Lejeune E, Bouchard A, Kakuda C, Gobezie R, Kochhar T: The arthroscopic Latarjet procedure for the treatment of anterior shoulder instability. *Arthroscopy* 2007;23(11):e1-e5.

    The background and the indications for the Latarjet procedure are reviewed, with the technique for the arthroscopic procedure. At 8-month follow-up of 62 patients, the results were 98% excellent or good, with an average return to sport 10 weeks after surgery.

30. Di Giacomo G, Costantini A, de Gasperis N, et al: Coracoid graft osteolysis after the Latarjet procedure for anteroinferior shoulder instability: A computed tomography scan study of twenty-six patients. *J Shoulder Elbow Surg* 2011;20(6):989-995.

    In a prospective study, 26 patients underwent Latarjet reconstruction followed by CT. At a mean 17.5-month follow-up, an average of 60% of the coracoid had undergone osteolysis, but 69.2% of the patients had an excellent Rowe score.

31. Hovelius L, Sandström B, Olofsson A, Svensson O, Rahme H: The effect of capsular repair, bone block healing, and position on the results of the Bristow-Latarjet procedure (study III): Long-term follow-up in 319 shoulders. *J Shoulder Elbow Surg* 2012;21(5): 647-660.

    A combined retrospective and prospective study involved 319 patients treated with the Bristow-Latarjet procedure, in three groups. The overall recurrence rate was 5%. Placement of the coracoid more than 1 cm medial to the glenoid rim predisposed the shoulder to redislocation. Bony fusion occurred in 83% of the patients.

32. Wellmann M, Petersen W, Zantop T, et al: Open shoulder repair of osseous glenoid defects: Biomechanical effectiveness of the Latarjet procedure versus a contoured structural bone graft. *Am J Sports Med* 2009;37(1):87-94.

    A basic science biomechanical study compared shoulder stability after Latarjet and bone-grafting procedures in cadavers. The Latarjet procedure better restricted anterior and anteroinferior translation, particularly at 60° of abduction.

33. Wellmann M, de Ferrari H, Smith T, et al: Biomechanical investigation of the stabilization principle of the Latarjet procedure. *Arch Orthop Trauma Surg* 2012; 132(3):377-386.

    A basic science biomechanical study of 12 cadaver

shoulders tested the contributions of the Latarjet procedure to humeral translation. The conjoined tendon, the coracoacromial ligament, capsular reconstruction, and subscapularis integrity all contribute to the stabilizing mechanism of the Latarjet reconstruction.

34. Lunn JV, Castellano-Rosa J, Walch G: Recurrent anterior dislocation after the Latarjet procedure: Outcome after revision using a modified Eden-Hybinette operation. *J Shoulder Elbow Surg* 2008;17(5):744-750.

In a study of 46 patients after a failed Latarjet procedure reconstructed with the Eden-Hybinette operation, 34 patients were followed for a mean 6.8 years. There were four redislocations, and 13 patients had persistent apprehension. Nonetheless, 79% of the patients had a good or an excellent result at final follow-up.

35. Owens BD, Harrast JJ, Hurwitz SR, Thompson TL, Wolf JM: Surgical trends in Bankart repair: An analysis of data from the American Board of Orthopaedic Surgery certification examination. *Am J Sports Med* 2011;39(9):1865-1869.

In a descriptive epidemiology study, American Board of Orthopaedic Surgery data showed a trend toward arthroscopic shoulder stabilization over time, compared with open repair. The overall reported complications were lower after arthroscopic stabilization than after open surgery.

36. Athwal GS, Shridharani SM, O'Driscoll SW: Osteolysis and arthropathy of the shoulder after use of bioabsorbable knotless suture anchors: A report of four cases. *J Bone Joint Surg Am* 2006;88(8):1840-1845.

37. Banerjee S, Weiser L, Connell D, Wallace AL: Glenoid rim fracture in contact athletes with absorbable suture anchor reconstruction. *Arthroscopy* 2009;25(5):560-562.

A rim fracture was reported in three athletes with recurrent dislocation after labral repair using absorbable sutures. Fractures in the area of the sutures were noted as well as the possibility of absorbable sutures playing a role in weakening bone substance at the fracture site.

38. Oh JH, Lee HK, Kim JY, Kim SH, Gong HS: Clinical and radiologic outcomes of arthroscopic glenoid labrum repair with the BioKnotless suture anchor. *Am J Sports Med* 2009;37(12):2340-2348.

Clinically and radiologically, the knotless anchor appears to be an acceptable alternative for arthroscopic labral repair, and it avoids certain drawbacks of the conventional knot-tying suture anchor. Level of evidence: IV.

39. Boileau P, Villalba M, Héry JY, Balg F, Ahrens P, Neyton L: Risk factors for recurrence of shoulder instability after arthroscopic Bankart repair. *J Bone Joint Surg Am* 2006;88(8):1755-1763.

40. Kang RW, Frank RM, Nho SJ, et al: Complications associated with anterior shoulder instability repair. *Arthroscopy* 2009;25(8):909-920.

A review categorized complications of anterior shoulder instability surgery and summarized the treatment options.

41. Boileau P, Richou J, Lisai A, Chuinard C, Bicknell RT: The role of arthroscopy in revision of failed open anterior stabilization of the shoulder. *Arthroscopy* 2009; 25(10):1075-1084.

Arthroscopic revision of failed open anterior shoulder stabilization provided satisfactory results in a selected patient population. The main advantage of the arthroscopic approach is avoiding of anterior dissection and axillary nerve injury, although persistent pain and osteoarthritis progression remain concerns. Level of evidence: IV.

42. Thomazeau H, Courage O, Barth J, et al; French Arthroscopy Society: Can we improve the indication for Bankart arthroscopic repair? A preliminary clinical study using the ISIS score. *Orthop Traumatol Surg Res* 2010;96(8, suppl):S77-S83.

A multicenter study found that an Instability Severity Index Score equal to or less than 4 can be predictive of a successful outcome after arthroscopic Bankart repair. Level of evidence: IV.

43. Pelet S, Jolles BM, Farron A: Bankart repair for recurrent anterior glenohumeral instability: Results at twenty-nine years' follow-up. *J Shoulder Elbow Surg* 2006;15(2):203-207.

44. Hovelius L, Saeboe M: Neer Award 2008: Arthropathy after primary anterior shoulder dislocation—223 shoulders prospectively followed up for twenty-five years. *J Shoulder Elbow Surg* 2009;18(3):339-347.

A 25-year prospective study of 227 patients with radiographic imaging of 225 shoulders found that age at primary dislocation, recurrence, high-energy sports, and alcohol abuse were associated with the development of arthropathy. The absence of a recurrence also was associated with arthropathy.

45. Robinson CM, Jenkins PJ, White TO, Ker A, Will E: Primary arthroscopic stabilization for a first-time anterior dislocation of the shoulder: A randomized, double-blind trial. *J Bone Joint Surg Am* 2008;90(4):708-721.

A prospective randomized double-blind study compared primary arthroscopic stabilization for a first-time anterior dislocation with arthroscopy and lavage. There was a marked treatment benefit from primary arthroscopic repair of a Bankart lesion. Level of evidence: I.

46. Savoie FH III, Holt MS, Field LD, Ramsey JR: Arthroscopic management of posterior instability: Evolution of technique and results. *Arthroscopy* 2008;24(4):389-396.

No essential lesion is present in posterior instability. Attention and treatment of all contributing lesions leads to successful outcomes after arthroscopic repair of posterior instability. Level of evidence: IV.

47. Bradley JP, Forsythe B, Mascarenhas R: Arthroscopic management of posterior shoulder instability: Diagnosis, indications, and technique. *Clin Sports Med* 2008; 27(4):649-670.

    The diagnosis, evaluation, and management of posterior instability are reviewed, with nonsurgical and surgical treatment approaches.

48. Robinson CM, Seah M, Akhtar MA: The epidemiology, risk of recurrence, and functional outcome after an acute traumatic posterior dislocation of the shoulder. *J Bone Joint Surg Am* 2011;93(17):1605-1613.

    A retrospective study found that the prevalence of posterior dislocation was relatively low. The most common complication was recurrent instability, which occurred in 17.7% of shoulders within the first year after dislocation. The risk was highest in patients who were younger than 40 years, sustained the dislocation during a seizure, and had a large humeral head defect. Level of evidence: IV.

49. Giles JW, Elkinson I, Ferreira LM, et al: Moderate to large engaging Hill-Sachs defects: An in vitro biomechanical comparison of the remplissage procedure, allograft humeral head reconstruction, and partial resurfacing arthroplasty. *J Shoulder Elbow Surg* 2012;21(9):1142-1151.

    A biomechanical study of cadaver shoulders found that all procedures improved stability. Shoulders that had undergone humeral head or partial-resurfacing arthroplasty resembled intact shoulders, but those that had undergone remplissage did not. Remplissage improved stability and eliminated engagement but caused a reduction in range of motion. Humeral head and partial-resurfacing arthroplasty reestablished full range of motion, but partial-resurfacing arthroplasty could not fully prevent engagement.

50. Nourissat G, Kilinc AS, Werther JR, Doursounian L: A prospective, comparative, radiological, and clinical study of the influence of the "remplissage" procedure on shoulder range of motion after stabilization by arthroscopic Bankart repair. *Am J Sports Med* 2011; 39(10):2147-2152.

    A prospective cohort study compared arthroscopic Bankart repair alone and in conjunction with remplissage. The remplissage technique did not alter the range of motion of the shoulder compared with the Bankart procedure alone. One third of the patients experienced posterosuperior pain. Level of evidence: II.

51. Gill TJ, Micheli LJ, Gebhard F, Binder C: Bankart repair for anterior instability of the shoulder: Long-term outcome. *J Bone Joint Surg Am* 1997;79(6):850-857.

52. Wall MS, Warren RF: Complications of shoulder instability surgery. *Clin Sports Med* 1995;14(4):973-1000.

53. Franceschi F, Papalia R, Del Buono A, Vasta S, Maffulli N, Denaro V: Glenohumeral osteoarthritis after arthroscopic Bankart repair for anterior instability. *Am J Sports Med* 2011;39(8):1653-1659.

    Degenerative joint disease of the glenohumeral joint was associated with older age at first dislocation, increased time from the first episode to surgery, increased number of preoperative dislocations, increased number of anchors used at surgery, and more degenerated labrum at surgery. The number of anchors and the state of the labrum were most associated with a risk of radiographic degenerative changes. Level of evidence: IV.

54. Good CR, Shindle MK, Kelly BT, Wanich T, Warren RF: Glenohumeral chondrolysis after shoulder arthroscopy with thermal capsulorrhaphy. *Arthroscopy* 2007; 23(7):e1-e5.

    In a retrospective study, eight patients had chondrolysis after shoulder arthroscopy. Five had undergone thermal capsulorrhaphy. Level of evidence: IV.

55. Rapley JH, Beavis RC, Barber FA: Glenohumeral chondrolysis after shoulder arthroscopy associated with continuous bupivacaine infusion. *Arthroscopy* 2009;25(12):1367-1373.

    A retrospective study compared patients receiving a continuous infusion of 0.5% bupivacaine without epinephrine at different rates and into the glenohumeral joint or the subacromial space. The risk of developing chondrolysis depended on the device and rate, location, and length of infusion. Level of evidence: III.

56. Ogawa K, Yoshida A, Ikegami H: Osteoarthritis in shoulders with traumatic anterior instability: Preoperative survey using radiography and computed tomography. *J Shoulder Elbow Surg* 2006;15(1):23-29.

57. Hayes ML, Collins MS, Morgan JA, Wenger DE, Dahm DL: Efficacy of diagnostic magnetic resonance imaging for articular cartilage lesions of the glenohumeral joint in patients with instability. *Skeletal Radiol* 2010;39(12):1199-1204.

    A retrospective MRI study used intraoperative findings as the gold standard. MRI had high sensitivity and specificity for diagnosing articular cartilage injury in patients with glenohumeral instability and was equally reliable with or without intra-articular contrast medium. Level of evidence: IV.

58. Ogawa K, Yoshida A, Matsumoto H, Takeda T: Outcome of the open Bankart procedure for shoulder instability and development of osteoarthritis: A 5- to 20-year follow-up study. *Am J Sports Med* 2010;38(8): 1549-1557.

    A prospective study examined the risk of progression to osteoarthritis after open Bankart surgery. Most postoperatively detected osteoarthritis had developed before surgery. The role of surgery in osteoarthritis was inconclusive. Level of evidence: III.

59. Castagna A, Markopoulos N, Conti M, Delle Rose G, Papadakou E, Garofalo R: Arthroscopic Bankart suture-anchor repair: Radiological and clinical outcome at minimum 10 years of follow-up. *Am J Sports Med* 2010;38(10):2012-2016.

    A study of the long-term outcomes of arthroscopic

Bankart suture-anchor repair found that the recurrence rate declined over time. Involvement in contact sports or overhead activities appeared to be a risk factor. Degenerative changes of the glenohumeral joint were noted but had no significant effect on clinical outcomes. Level of evidence: IV.

60. Cameron ML, Kocher MS, Briggs KK, Horan MP, Hawkins RJ: The prevalence of glenohumeral osteoarthrosis in unstable shoulders. *Am J Sports Med* 2003; 31(1):53-55.

61. Hovelius L, Saeboe M: Documentation of dislocation arthropathy of the shoulder "area index": A better method to objectify the humeral osteophyte? *J Shoulder Elbow Surg* 2008;17(2):197-201.

    A radiographic study defined a method of interpreting and quantifying dislocation arthropathy of the glenohumeral joint.

62. Ghodadra N, Gupta A, Romeo AA, et al: Normalization of glenohumeral articular contact pressures after Latarjet or iliac crest bone-grafting. *J Bone Joint Surg Am* 2010;92(6):1478-1489.

    A biomechanical cadaver study examined the effect on articular contact pressures of graft position in iliac crest bone grafting of the glenoid and the Latarjet procedure. Glenohumeral contact pressure was optimally restored with a flush iliac crest bone graft or a flush Latarjet bone block in which the inferior aspect of the coracoid became the glenoid surface.

63. Robinson CM, Shur N, Sharpe T, Ray A, Murray IR: Injuries associated with traumatic anterior glenohumeral dislocations. *J Bone Joint Surg Am* 2012;94(1): 18-26.

    A prospective study analyzed traumatic anterior glenohumeral dislocation in 3,633 patients. Rotator cuff tears, greater tuberosity fractures, and neurologic deficits were found to be more common than previously believed.

64. Boardman ND III, Cofield RH: Neurologic complications of shoulder surgery. *Clin Orthop Relat Res* 1999; 368:44-53.

65. Ho E, Cofield RH, Balm MR, Hattrup SJ, Rowland CM: Neurologic complications of surgery for anterior shoulder instability. *J Shoulder Elbow Surg* 1999;8(3): 266-270.

66. Loomer R, Graham B: Anatomy of the axillary nerve and its relation to inferior capsular shift. *Clin Orthop Relat Res* 1989;243:100-105.

67. Eglseder WA Jr, Goldman M: Anatomic variations of the musculocutaneous nerve in the arm. *Am J Orthop (Belle Mead NJ)* 1997;26(11):777-780.

68. Carter CW, Moros C, Ahmad CS, Levine WN: Arthroscopic anterior shoulder instability repair: Techniques, pearls, pitfalls, and complications. *Instr Course Lect* 2008;57:125-132.

Arthroscopic techniques for anterior shoulder instability were outlined, with complications and tips for avoiding them.

69. McFarland EG, Caicedo JC, Guitterez MI, Sherbondy PS, Kim TK: The anatomic relationship of the brachial plexus and axillary artery to the glenoid: Implications for anterior shoulder surgery. *Am J Sports Med* 2001; 29(6):729-733.

70. Maquieira GJ, Gerber C, Schneeberger AG: Suprascapular nerve palsy after the Latarjet procedure. *J Shoulder Elbow Surg* 2007;16(2):e13-e15.

    After a Latarjet procedure, a patient had suprascapular nerve palsy resulting from a posteriorly proud screw entering the suprascapular notch.

71. McFarland EG, Caicedo JC, Kim TK, Banchasuek P: Prevention of axillary nerve injury in anterior shoulder reconstructions: Use of a subscapularis muscle-splitting technique and a review of the literature. *Am J Sports Med* 2002;30(4):601-606.

72. Esmail AN, Getz CL, Schwartz DM, Wierzbowski L, Ramsey ML, Williams GR Jr: Axillary nerve monitoring during arthroscopic shoulder stabilization. *Arthroscopy* 2005;21(6):665-671.

73. McFarland EG, O'Neill OR, Hsu CY: Complications of shoulder arthroscopy. *J South Orthop Assoc* 1997; 6(3):190-196.

74. Mair SD, Hawkins RJ: Open shoulder instability surgery; Complications. *Clin Sports Med* 1999;18(4): 719-736.

75. Sperling JW, Cofield RH, Torchia ME, Hanssen AD: Infection after shoulder instability surgery. *Clin Orthop Relat Res* 2003;414:61-64.

76. Ticker JB, Lippe RJ, Barkin DE, Carroll MP: Infected suture anchors in the shoulder. *Arthroscopy* 1996; 12(5):613-615.

77. Bonnevialle N, Mansat P, Bellumore Y, Mansat M, Bonnevialle P: Selective capsular repair for the treatment of anterior-inferior shoulder instability: Review of seventy-nine shoulders with seven years' average follow-up. *J Shoulder Elbow Surg* 2009;18(2): 251-259.

    A retrospective study found a 90% satisfaction rate and 80% good to excellent results at midterm follow-up of patients who underwent selective capsular repair for posttraumatic anterior glenohumeral instability. Level of evidence: IV.

78. Elmlund A, Kartus C, Sernert N, Hultenheim I, Ejerhed L: A long-term clinical follow-up study after arthroscopic intra-articular Bankart repair using absorbable tacks. *Knee Surg Sports Traumatol Arthrosc* 2008;16(7):707-712.

    At a mean 8-year follow-up, arthroscopic repair with absorbable tacks led to a stable shoulder with good function in most of the 73 patients. Dislocation or subluxation had occurred in 19%.

79. Fabre T, Abi-Chahla ML, Billaud A, Geneste M, Durandeau A: Long-term results with Bankart procedure: A 26-year follow-up study of 50 cases. *J Shoulder Elbow Surg* 2010;19(2):318-323.

At a follow-up more than 20 years in 49 patients, including 36 contact athletes, after an open Bankart procedure for recurrent shoulder instability, most patients had a stable shoulder and had returned to their previous level of sports activity. Radiographic osteoarthritis was found in 69% of the patients.

80. Law BK, Yung PS, Ho EP, Chang JJ, Chan KM: The surgical outcome of immediate arthroscopic Bankart repair for first time anterior shoulder dislocation in young active patients. *Knee Surg Sports Traumatol Arthrosc* 2008;16(2):188-193.

At a mean 28-month follow-up, an immediate Bankart repair and accelerated rehabilitation program were found to be an effective method of treating young, active patients with traumatic anterior shoulder dislocation.

81. Porcellini G, Campi F, Pegreffi F, Castagna A, Paladini P: Predisposing factors for recurrent shoulder dislocation after arthroscopic treatment. *J Bone Joint Surg Am* 2009;91(11):2537-2542.

A 36-month study found that the risk of redislocation after arthroscopic repair of an anterior shoulder dislocation can be determined based on patient sex, age, and elapsed time from first dislocation to surgery.

82. Thal R, Nofziger M, Bridges M, Kim JJ: Arthroscopic Bankart repair using Knotless or BioKnotless suture anchors: 2- to 7-year results. *Arthroscopy* 2007;23(4):367-375.

A retrospective study of 73 patients found a 6.9% recurrence rate 2 to 7 years after arthroscopic Bankart repair using knotless suture anchors. There were minimal loss of motion and good function, even among contact athletes. Level of evidence: IV.

The Rotator Cuff

Section Editor:
Sumant G. Krishnan, MD

Anatomy, Pathogenesis, Natural History, and Nonsurgical Treatment of Rotator Cuff Disorders

Hiroyuki Sugaya, MD

Introduction

The term rotator cuff disease includes partial-thickness and full-thickness rotator cuff tears as well as tendinitis. It is not easy to determine whether a rotator cuff disorder itself is responsible for a patient's shoulder pain and disability. MRI and ultrasound often show an anatomic disorder of the rotator cuff in patients older than 65 to 70 years. Some patients who report shoulder pain have no evidence of an anatomic rotator cuff disorder, and others have no symptoms despite the presence of a rotator cuff tear on imaging studies.[1] The presence or the absence of shoulder symptoms appears to be affected by physiologic and psychological factors; for example, it is generally believed that the surgical outcomes of patients with a workers' compensation claim tend to be inferior to those of other patients.[2,3]

Surgeons must assess functional as well as anatomic factors. Rotator cuff function, scapular position and mobility, posture, spine mobility and pelvic inclination, and lower extremity function are among the factors that affect shoulder symptoms. The susceptibility of the shoulder to functional disorders is largely attributable to unique features of the shoulder girdle. The rotator cuff connects the scapula and the humeral head as well as the capsule and the biceps tendon. The scapula and upper extremities form a unit that is connected to the trunk and the clavicle only by the acromioclavicular and sternoclavicular joints. In other words, most of the structures connecting the scapula and upper extremity unit to the trunk are periscapular muscles. Scapula position is greatly affected by posture and lower extremity function, and incorrect posture restricts scapular mobil-

ity. A functionally deteriorated scapula can easily cause symptoms around the shoulder girdle.[4] Correcting morbid scapulothoracic function is the first-choice nonsurgical treatment of a patient with shoulder symptoms.[5]

Anatomy of the Rotator Cuff

The anatomy of the shoulder girdle is relatively complex. The scapula is connected to the trunk anteriorly by the serratus anterior and the pectoralis minor and posteriorly by the upper and lower trapezius, rhomboids, levator scapulae, and latissimus dorsi. The muscular tone and flexibility of these structures greatly affect scapular function.[4] The deltoid muscle encases the shoulder. The deltoid originates anteriorly from the medial half of the clavicle and the anterolateral aspect of the acromion, continues posteriorly along the scapular spine, and inserts distally into the proximal third of the humerus at the deltoid tubercle. Thus, the deltoid is the main source of power for shoulder abduction, with the help of rotator cuff function.

Supraspinatus and Infraspinatus

The rotator cuff is formed by the tendinous insertions of the subscapularis, the supraspinatus, the infraspinatus, and the teres minor. The traditional understanding is that the supraspinatus muscle originates from the suprascapular fossa and inserts onto the superior facet of the greater tuberosity, and the infraspinatus muscle originates from the scapular fossa and inserts onto the posterior aspect of the humeral head at the middle facet of the greater tuberosity.[6,7] However, recent anatomic studies by shoulder surgeons and anatomists revealed that the supraspinatus inserts onto the limited anteriormost portion of the superior facet and even onto the lesser tuberosity and that the infraspinatus inserts onto the middle facet and almost half of the superior facet[8,9]

Dr. Sugaya or an immediate family member is a member of a speakers' bureau or has made paid presentations on behalf of Mitek and Smith & Nephew and serves as an unpaid consultant to Mitek and Smith & Nephew.

3: The Rotator Cuff

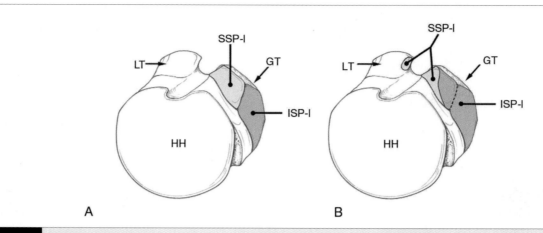

Figure 1   Schematic drawings of the superior aspect of the right humerus showing the humeral insertions of the supraspinatus and the infraspinatus. **A,** The generally accepted belief is that the supraspinatus inserts into the highest impression of the greater tuberosity, and the infraspinatus inserts into the middle impression. **B,** Recent research indicates that the insertion area of the infraspinatus occupies approximately half of the highest and all of the middle impression of the greater tuberosity. The insertion area of the supraspinatus is in the anteromedial region of the highest impression and sometimes in the superiormost area on the lesser tuberosity. GT = greater tuberosity, HH = humeral head, ISP-I = insertion area of the infraspinatus, LT = lesser tuberosity, SSP-I = insertion area of the supraspinatus. (Reproduced with permission from Mochizuki T, Sugaya H, Uomizu M, et al: Humeral insertion of the supraspinatus and infraspinatus: New anatomical findings regarding the footprint of the rotator cuff. *J Bone Joint Surg Am* 2008;90[5]:962-969.)

(**Figure 1**). These studies found that the infraspinatus is divided into two parts: the oblique fibers, which originate from the scapular fossa and insert on the middle and superior facet of the greater tuberosity; and the transverse fibers, which originate from the inferior aspect of the scapula spine and insert onto the tendinous portion of the oblique fibers[10] (**Figure 2**). The glenohumeral capsular insertion has a broad footprint, especially at the tendinous insertion between the infraspinatus and the teres minor[11] (**Figure 3**). Presumably, this thick capsule can function as a tendon along with the tendinous insertion of the infraspinatus and the teres minor, and it may be related to the delamination that is frequently observed during surgery for a large or massive rotator cuff tear.[11]

Subscapularis

The subscapularis is the only anteriorly located rotator cuff muscle, and it has the greatest muscular volume. The development of arthroscopic technology has recently allowed the importance of subscapularis tendon tears to be recognized. Their prevalence appears to be much greater than earlier reports indicated.[12-14]

Several intramuscular tendons can be observed in the subscapularis muscle. The most cranial tendinous portion was found to be longer and thicker than any other tendinous structure inside the subscapularis.[12] The most proximal insertion of the subscapularis tendon was found to be derived from this long, thick intramuscular tendinous portion. The insertion of this portion was widely located on the most proximal upper limit of the lesser tuberosity. The remainder of the subscapularis tendon inserted onto the anteromedial por-

tion of the lesser tuberosity. The insertion of the subscapularis muscle became narrower in the more distal portion, where the muscle fibers came close to the humeral bone and tendon tissue was very short (**Figure 4**). The most proximal insertion of the subscapularis tendon extended as a thin tendinous slip that attached to the fovea capitis of the humerus. The primary function of this tendinous slip was described as providing a greater insertion area for the subscapularis tendon and the smooth floor of the bicipital groove to stabilize the long head of the biceps (LHB) tendon and prevent it from dislocating[15] (**Figure 5**). The most cranial part of the tendon insertion was described as the strongest and the clinically most important, and it has the broadest footprint, along with the tendinous slip.[15]

Some of the intratendinous fibers from the supraspinatus were found to insert onto the lesser tuberosity beyond the LHB tendon, and these fibers reinforce the most cranial insertion of the subscapularis from above the LHB tendon.[8,9] The fibers that insert into the lesser tuberosity can be strongly related to the comma sign, which is an important landmark in full-thickness anterosuperior rotator cuff tears.[16] During surgery, footprint reconstruction repair is strongly recommended to increase the initial fixation strength, especially in the cranial portion of a subscapularis tear.

Teres Minor

The teres minor has a smaller volume than the other rotator cuff muscles, and it inserts immediately inferior to the infraspinatus insertion at the greater tuberosity[11] (**Figure 3**). The tendinous insertion of the teres minor usually remains intact, even in a massive three-tendon

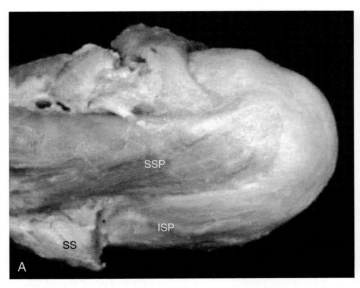

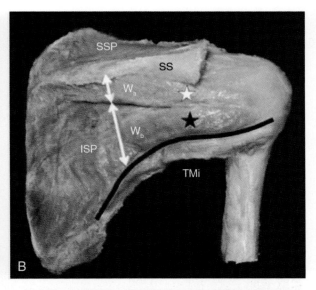

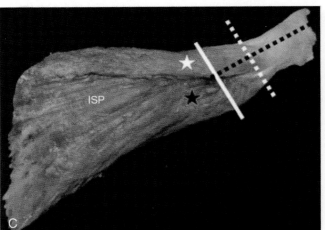

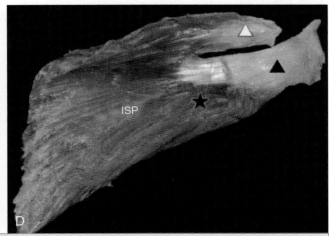

Figure 2 Photographs showing the muscular and tendinous geometry of the supraspinatus and the infraspinatus. **A,** The superior aspect of a right shoulder, showing the myotendinous unit of the supraspinatus and the infraspinatus. **B,** The dorsal aspect of a right shoulder, showing the myotendinous unit of the infraspinatus, composed of a transverse part *(white star)* and an oblique part *(black star)*. The border between the infraspinatus and the teres minor is shown *(black line)*. **C,** The dorsal aspect of the infraspinatus separated from the scapula and the greater tuberosity of the humerus. The transverse *(white star)* and oblique *(black star)* parts can easily be seen. Longitudinal *(black line)* and transverse histologic sections *(white lines)* are shown. **D,** The dorsal aspect of the infraspinatus muscle, showing the separation of the transverse part *(black star)* from the oblique part. The transverse part has a long, thick tendinous portion *(black triangle)* attached to the greater tuberosity. The transverse part has a thin and short tendinous membrane *(white triangle)* attached only to the tendinous portion of the oblique part and not reaching the tuberosity. ISP = infraspinatus, SS = scapular spine, SSP = supraspinatus, TMi = teres minor, W_a = width of the transverse part at the midpoint of the scapula spine, W_b = width of the oblique part at the midpoint of the scapula spine. (Reproduced with permission from Arai R, Mochizuki T, Yamaguchi K, et al: Functional anatomy of the superior glenohumeral and coracohumeral ligaments and the subscapularis tendon in view of stabilization of the long head of the biceps tendon. *J Shoulder Elbow Surg* 2010;19[1]:58-64.)

tear. However, the muscular volume of the teres minor is relevant for surgical decision making because it may predict the prognosis after surgical intervention for a massive rotator cuff tear. The teres minor is innervated by the axillary nerve along with the deltoid muscle. In contrast, the suprascapular nerve passes through the suprascapular notch and innervates the supraspinatus before coursing inferiorly to innervate the infraspinatus.

Physical Examination

A detailed clinical history is particularly important for a precise diagnosis of the cause of shoulder symptoms. The patient should be questioned regarding the onset, duration, and nature of symptoms as well as traumatic episodes, provocative and alleviating factors, earlier treatment, and response to treatment. If pain is an important symptom, it is important to learn whether the

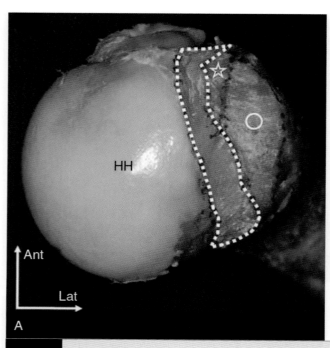
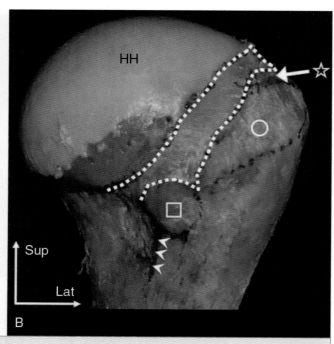

Figure 3 Photographs of the superior (**A**) and posterior (**B**) aspects of the humerus, showing the attachment area of the articular capsule *(white dashed line)*. Also shown are the insertion areas of the supraspinatus *(star, black dashed lines)* and infraspinatus *(circle)* and the tendinous portion *(square)* and muscular portion of the teres minor *(arrowheads)*. HH = humeral head, Ant = anterior, Lat = lateral, Sup = superior. (Reproduced with permission from Nimura A, Kato A, Yamaguchi K, et al: The superior capsule of the shoulder joint complements the insertion of the rotator cuff. *J Shoulder Elbow Surg* 2012;21[7]:867-872.)

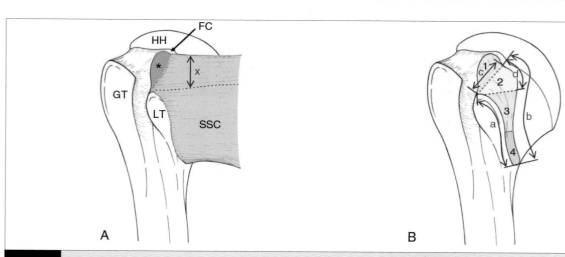

Figure 4 Schematic drawings showing the insertion and the footprint of the subscapularis in a right shoulder. **A**, The superiormost part of the intramuscular tendons is inserted into the uppermost margin of the lesser tuberosity, and the remainder of the subscapularis tendon is inserted into the anteromedial portion of the lesser tuberosity. The superiormost insertion—the lateral portion of the cranial part of the intramuscular tendons—and the tendinous slip make up a structure that is in direct contact with the inferior side of the long head of the biceps tendon at its corner portion. The longitudinal diameter *(x)* of the cranial part of intramuscular tendons was found to be long enough to decrease the curvature of the biceps tendon. **B**, The subscapularis footprint is made up of the attaching area of the tendinous slip *(1)*, insertion of the superiormost part of the intramuscular tendon *(2)*, another tendinous insertion *(3)*, muscular insertion *(4)*. The dimensions of the subscapularis footprint were defined in terms of the lateral margin *(a)*, the medial margin *(b)*, the superiormost lateral margin *(c)*, and the superiormost medial margin *(d)*. The superiormost lateral margin *(c)* is long enough to support the biceps tendon. HH = humeral head, FC = fovea capitis of the humerus, GT = greater tuberosity, LT = lesser tuberosity, SSC = subscapularis muscle. (Reproduced with permission from Arai R, Sugaya H, Mochizuki T, Nimura A, Moriishi J, Akita K: Subscapularis tendon tear: An anatomic and clinical investigation. *Arthroscopy* 2008;24[9]:997-1004.)

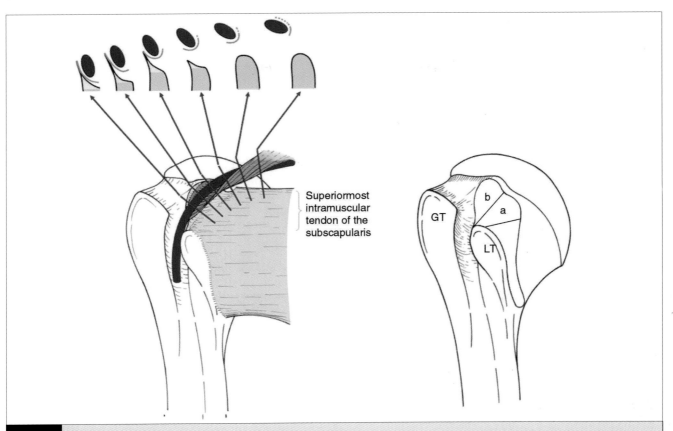

Figure 5 Schematic drawings showing two views of the positional relationships among the LHB tendon *(red)*, the superiormost intramuscular tendon of the subscapularis *(gray)*, the superior glenohumeral ligament (SGHL; *green*), and the tendinous slip of the subscapularis insertion *(yellow)*. The superiormost insertion point of the subscapularis is the wide attachment of the superiormost intramuscular tendon of the subscapularis on the upper margin of the lesser tuberosity *(area a)*. This insertion sends a thin tendinous slip to the fovea capitis of the humerus *(area b)*. The SGHL branches off from the internal wall of the glenohumeral joint near the glenoid in a folded shape, runs laterally to wrap around the LHB in a spiral fashion, and attaches to the tendinous slip of the subscapularis insertion. The area where the SGHL originates is ambiguous. The superiormost insertion of the subscapularis supports the LHB from behind the SGHL. The SGHL and the coracohumeral ligament are continuous, and the tension of the coracohumeral ligament, which covers the whole glenohumeral joint, is considered to be conveyed to the SGHL because the two ligaments form an identical loose connective tissue. This tension may be advantageous for the ability of the SGHL to withstand the dislocation stress of the LHB. GT = greater tuberosity, LT = lesser tuberosity. (Reproduced with permission from Arai R, Sugaya H, Mochizuki T, Nimura A, Moriishi J, Akita K: Subscapularis tendon tear: An anatomic and clinical investigation. *Arthroscopy* 2008;24[9]:997-1004.)

pain is present at night and/or with the arm in a resting position. Pain at rest probably results from inflammation of the glenohumeral joint or the subacromial bursa.[17]

Plain radiographs are routinely obtained to help identify rotator cuff tear arthropathy and other shoulder conditions, such as calcific tendinitis, primary osteoarthritis, and simple superior migration of the humeral head. The physical examination should be based on the information obtained through the clinical history and plain radiographs. The physical examination of a patient with rotator cuff disease has four parts: inspection and palpation plus evaluations of strength, scapulothoracic function, and active and passive range of motion with concomitant scapular movement.

To predict scapulothoracic kinematics, postural alignment and scapular position should be assessed by inspection with the patient standing. Scapular malposition, including protraction, anterior tilt, downward rotation, and depression (in comparison with the contralateral side), is a significant indicator of scapular dyskinesis.[4,5] Tenderness at the coracoid process often is prominent in such a shoulder. Assessment of both active and passive range of motion, beginning with the painful arc test, also is done with the patient standing. If the patient cannot fully elevate the affected arm, the clinician must assess whether the restriction of motion is caused by pain, stiffness, or scapular dysfunction. Forward flexion, abduction, external rotation at the side, external and internal rotation at 90° of shoulder abduction, and the highest spine level the thumb can reach are assessed on both sides. Especially during the eccentric phase of lowering the arm from forward flexion or internal rotation at 90° of abduction, the clinician can observe pain provocation and abnormal scapular motion; these are typical in a patient with subacromial pain, regardless of the presence of a rotator cuff tear.

For suspected rotator cuff disease without stiffness, several strength tests are routinely done on both sides with the patient seated or standing, including abduction strength with the shoulder at 30° and 90° of abduction in the scapular plane (the Jobe test), forward flexion strength with the shoulder at 90° and 120° of horizontal flexion (the Whipple test), and external rotation strength with the arm at the side. Weakness of external rotation and/or an external rotation lag sign are decisive indicators of a large posterosuperior rotator cuff tear. In addition, all patients should be tested for subscapularis strength using the bear hug and belly press tests because subscapularis tears are reported to have a prevalence as high as 27% to 37%.[12-14]

The combined abduction and horizontal flexion test is used to assess scapular dyskinesis with the patient supine.[18] Many provocative maneuvers for specific shoulder conditions have been described, but for the sake of an efficient examination, clinicians must identify the tests they can use most productively.

Pathogenesis of Rotator Cuff Tears

Although tendon fiber failure is the final pathology for all rotator cuff tears, there is no unified theory of the etiology and pathogenesis of atraumatic rotator cuff disease. The causes are multifactorial and generally are divided into intrinsic elements, including age-related tendon degeneration, and extrinsic factors, which are represented by mechanical impingement.[19]

Intrinsic Factors

The rate of both symptomatic and asymptomatic rotator cuff tears increases with age. There is a 50% likelihood that a patient older than 66 years with unilateral shoulder pain has bilateral rotator cuff tears.[20] This fact clearly indicates that tendon degeneration progresses during normal aging. Recent histopathologic studies revealed signs of preexisting age-related tendon degeneration. Macroscopically intact residual tendon tissue from partial articular-side rotator cuff tears in patients with a mean age of 60 years had moderate histopathologic degeneration.[21] In a study of the medial stumps of torn rotator cuff tendon tissue, the frequency and the distribution of thin and disoriented collagen fibers, myxoid degeneration, and hyaline degeneration suggested early degenerative processes in the torn tendons. The main causes of rotator cuff tears appeared to be microtrauma and preexisting degenerative change in the middle and deep layers of the tendon.[22] Intratendinous vascular patterns were studied in patients with or without a rotator cuff tear, using enhanced ultrasound after intravenous injection of a contrast agent. Older patients had a significantly decreased blood flow in the intratendinous region compared with younger patients, regardless of the presence of a rotator cuff tear.[23]

Age-related tendon degeneration leads to swelling and thickening of the tendon and thereby narrows the subacromial space, which has already degenerated because of age-related spur formation and bursal tissue thickening. Arm motion can easily cause rotator cuff tearing from the bursal side, especially if scapular mobility is restricted because of scapulothoracic inflexibility. In addition, partial articular-side rotator cuff tearing appears to occur primarily through intrinsic cuff degeneration, without the strong involvement of extrinsic factors.[24] In shoulders with a full-thickness rotator cuff tear, the population of fibroblasts and inflammatory cells decreases as the size of a tear increases; this finding suggests alteration in the healing ability of torn tendons.[25] Also, a progressive decrease in the number of blood vessels and vascularity is observed as the size of the rotator cuff tear increases.[25,26] Cigarette smoking negatively affects the vascularity of the rotator cuff tendons.[27] A dosage-dependent and time-dependent relationship was observed between smoking and rotator cuff tears, which suggests that smoking is an important risk factor for the development of rotator cuff tears.[28]

The development of rotator cuff tendon pathologies and symptoms is partly genetic.[20,29] Familial clustering was found in a study of patients with diagnosed rotator cuff disease and a known genealogy.[30] The risk to both close and distant relatives of patients was significantly elevated. The study findings strongly supported a heritable predisposition to rotator cuff disease. There is increasing evidence to suggest that several gene pathways related to the composition of rotator cuff tendons are altered in rotator cuff disease, affecting the extracellular matrix, vasculature, and intracellular signaling mechanisms.[31] Further studies are required to clarify the genetic and biologic factors involved in rotator cuff tears.

Extrinsic Factors

Extrinsic factors include anatomic variables such as acromial morphologic characteristics, os acromiale, and acromial spurs that compress the rotator cuff by bony impingement or direct pressure from the surrounding soft tissue. Primary subacromial impingement, as originally described by Neer, occurs when the acromiohumeral space is restricted or when a prominent, hooked anterior and lateral acromion or hypertrophied coracoacromial ligament abrades the rotator cuff if the arm is elevated. Constitutional morphologic features seem less likely to cause rotator cuff tearing. In fact, a recent study revealed that acromial morphology and the acromion index (a large lateral extension of the acromion proposed as a significant causative factor for full-thickness rotator cuff tearing[32]) were not reliably relevant to rotator cuff disease, but the presence of an acromial spur was highly associated with a full-thickness rotator cuff tear in both symptomatic and asymptomatic patients.[33] A functionally deteriorated scapula caused by scapular dyskinesis is the most likely extrinsic cause of rotator cuff tearing, especially if significant aging-related acromial spur formation is present.[4,5,33] Surgeons should recognize that a dynamic factor, such as loss of complementary scapula motion because of malposition or dyskinesis during arm motion, is an important extrinsic factor for rotator cuff tearing in comparison with static morphologic changes.

Another extrinsically generated cuff pathology results from internal impingement with repetitive microtrauma. This condition is caused by repetitive overhead throwing, which causes articular-side partial-thickness tearing, especially in the presence of scapular dyskinesis. Although the etiology is still controversial, a patient with internal impingement may have a tight posterior capsule or a loose anterior band of the glenohumeral ligament in association with tight posterior musculature, causing impingement between the medial rotator cuff footprint area of the greater tuberosity and the posterosuperior glenoid during the late cocking and acceleration phases of throwing. The repetitive motion contributes to partial-thickness articular-side tearing of the posterior supraspinatus and the anterior infraspinatus in addition to adjacent posterosuperior glenolabral tearing.

Natural History of Rotator Cuff Tears

Although partial-thickness and small rotator cuff tears may have potential for spontaneous healing, it is generally believed that a tear will progress over time. Some rotator cuff tears do not cause any shoulder-related symptoms, however. This fact suggests that rotator cuff tearing sometimes may be necessary in people older than approximately 65 to 70 years who have functionally altered scapulothoracic articulation resulting from inflexibility and kyphotic deformity of the thoracic spine. It is important for surgeons to understand the natural history of asymptomatic rotator cuff tears when choosing a treatment.

Symptomatic Alteration of an Asymptomatic Tear

The differences between symptomatic and asymptomatic shoulders with a rotator cuff tear are not well understood.[34,35] However, tear progression appears to be one of the factors in symptomatic alteration of full-thickness asymptomatic rotator cuff tears.[36] The longitudinal natural history of asymptomatic rotator cuff tears was studied over 5 years by reviewing consecutive sonograms in 58 patients with unilateral symptoms who had an asymptomatic contralateral rotator cuff tear.[37] Fifty-one percent of the previously asymptomatic shoulders became symptomatic over a mean 2.8 years. Tear size progression was associated with the development of symptoms, including a significant increase in pain and a decrease in the ability to perform activities of daily living. Bilateral rotator cuff disease, either symptomatic or asymptomatic, was common in patients who initially had unilateral shoulder pain.[20]

Progression of Symptomatic Tears

In a prospective study, patients age 60 years or younger with a relatively small full-thickness rotator cuff tear were treated nonsurgically.[38] At a mean 29-month follow-up, the size of the tear had increased in 49%, not changed in 43%, and decreased in 8%. There was a correlation between the existence of considerable pain at the time of the follow-up ultrasound and a clinically significant increase in tear size. A retrospective investigation found that the factors associated with rotator cuff tear progression were age older than 60 years, a full-thickness tear, and fatty infiltration of the rotator cuff muscles.[39] However, small, symptomatic full-thickness tears did not invariably progress over a limited period of time in a study of clinical and structural outcomes in 24 consecutive patients.[40] These patients had declined repair of a symptomatic isolated full-thickness supraspinatus tear. At a median 42-month follow-up after diagnosis, the average tear size had not changed on standardized MRI. The patients had a surprisingly high level of satisfaction.

Tear progression appears to be the most important factor affecting the outcome of nonsurgical treatment of shoulders with a small, symptomatic rotator cuff tear. The factors related to successful outcome of nonsurgical treatment were investigated in 123 shoulders with a full-thickness rotator cuff tear diagnosed by high-resolution MRI with a microscopy coil.[41] The integrity of the intramuscular tendon of the supraspinatus was found to be the most significant factor affecting the outcome. In the anatomic footprint of the supraspinatus, the main part of the intramuscular tendon of the supraspinatus inserts into the anteriormost portion of the superior facet; tear progression may be related to whether this portion is disrupted, even in a small tear[8,9,11] (**Figures 1 and 3**). If the anteriormost intramuscular tendon insertion is disrupted, tear progression can occur, and an asymptomatic shoulder eventually becomes symptomatic, or a symptomatic shoulder remains symptomatic.

Fatty Infiltration and Massive Rotator Cuff Tears

Fatty infiltration can progress with an increase in tear size, the number of involved tendons, or the time after the tendon rupture. In a retrospective review of 1,688 patients who underwent surgical repair of a rotator cuff tear, moderate (Goutallier grade 2) supraspinatus fatty infiltration appeared at an average of 3 years after the onset of symptoms, and severe (Goutallier grade 3 or 4) fatty infiltration appeared at an average of 5 years.[42] A positive tangent sign appeared at an average of 4.5 years after the onset of symptoms. In the same patients, infraspinatus fatty infiltration increased significantly with multiple tendon tears and increasing patient age.[43] Goutallier grade 2 fatty infiltration ap-

3: The Rotator Cuff

peared at an average of 2.5 years after symptom onset, and grade 3 or 4 fatty infiltration appeared at an average of 4 years. In the subscapularis, Goutallier grade 2 fatty infiltration appeared at an average of 2.5 years after symptom onset, and grade 3 or 4 appeared at an average of 5 years.[44] The researchers suggested that surgical repair should be done before moderate (grade 2) fatty infiltration and atrophy (a positive tangent sign) appear, especially if the tear involves multiple tendons.

Some patients with multiple tendon tears remain asymptomatic or moderately symptomatic. Eventually, however, the tear and fatty infiltration progress to the irreparable level. In a study of 19 consecutive patients with a massive rotator cuff tear who underwent nonsurgical treatment, satisfactory shoulder function was maintained for at least 4 years despite significant progression of degenerative structural joint changes, including glenohumeral osteoarthritis and fatty infiltration.[45]

Nonsurgical Management

There is no consensus on the best treatment for a rotator cuff tear. The treatment is selected on the basis of the patient's symptoms.[46] A patient with a symptomatic rotator cuff tear may have inflammatory pain and a functional deficit, such as scapular dyskinesis, in addition to a lack of anatomic structural integrity. Successful surgery can resolve only the anatomic issues. Considering the absence of an explicit difference between symptomatic and asymptomatic shoulders with a rotator cuff tear, it is important to attempt to relieve pain and improve functional impairment before surgery is undertaken.

Pain Management

Pain is the initial symptom of most patients. It is important to control the patient's pain early in the treatment process, especially if inflammatory pain is present, even at rest and at night, regardless of arm position. Although the use of ice, rest, NSAIDs, and activity modification is the first treatment for the inflammatory pain, a steroid injection to the glenohumeral joint or the subacromial bursa may be the most effective, reliable treatment.[17,47,48] Pain associated only with a specific arm motion (a painful arc or an impingement sign) is considered to be mechanical or functional, and the treatment is surgery or physical therapy to correct scapular dyskinesis. Relieving inflammatory pain early in the treatment process is of particular importance for the effectiveness of physical therapy or surgery to relieve morbidity.

Physical Therapy

In a middle-aged or older patient with a rotator cuff tear, scapular motion normally is restricted because of the inflexibility of muscles and surrounding structures, along with kyphotic deformity of the thoracic spine.[4,5]

Therefore, the most important first step is restoration of scapular and trunk mobility, before proceeding to activation of the remaining rotator cuff function and scapular stabilization. The restoration of normal shoulder girdle mechanics progresses from proper rotator cuff function and scapular stabilization for lifting and reaching to trunk and lower extremity core stabilization for more complex activities. Although a self-guided exercise program directed at stretching and strengthening the rotator cuff and periscapular muscles can be efficacious, a formal program of physical therapy is strongly recommended if the patient has an inflexible upper spine.[49,50]

Annotated References

1. Yamamoto A, Takagishi K, Kobayashi T, Shitara H, Osawa T: Factors involved in the presence of symptoms associated with rotator cuff tears: A comparison of asymptomatic and symptomatic rotator cuff tears in the general population. *J Shoulder Elbow Surg* 2011; 20(7):1133-1137.

   In 211 patients, 283 shoulders had a full-thickness rotator cuff tear, but approximately two thirds of the shoulders did not have symptoms. The factors in symptomatic shoulders with a rotator cuff tear were a positive impingement sign, weakness in external rotation, and a tear in the dominant arm.

2. Holtby R, Razmjou H: Impact of work-related compensation claims on surgical outcome of patients with rotator cuff related pathologies: A matched case-control study. *J Shoulder Elbow Surg* 2010;19(3): 452-460.

   The surgical outcomes of patients with a work-related compensation claim were compared with those of a historical control group based on age, sex, and level of pathology. Both groups improved significantly. At baseline and 1 year after surgery, the patients with a claim had a significantly higher level of disability.

3. Cuff DJ, Pupello DR: Prospective evaluation of postoperative compliance and outcomes after rotator cuff repair in patients with and without workers' compensation claims. *J Shoulder Elbow Surg* 2012;21(12): 1728-1733.

   Compliance and outcomes of rotator cuff repair were compared in patients with or without a workers' compensation claim. Patients with a claim had a higher rate of postoperative noncompliance (52% versus 4%). Patients with a claim who had no evidence of noncompliance had significantly more improvement and a more favorable outcome than patients with a claim who were noncompliant.

4. Kibler WB, Sciascia A, Wilkes T: Scapular dyskinesis and its relation to shoulder injury. *J Am Acad Orthop Surg* 2012;20(6):364-372.

   The scapula plays a key role in almost every aspect of normal shoulder function. Patients with shoulder impingement, rotator cuff disease, labral injury, clavicle fracture, acromioclavicular joint injury, or multidirectional instability should be evaluated for scapular dyskinesis and treated accordingly.

5. Kibler WB: The scapula in rotator cuff disease. *Med Sport Sci* 2012;57:27-40.

    The scapula serves as the platform or the base for the muscles of the rotator cuff, and scapular dyskinesis is frequently identified in rotator cuff disease. Careful examination for scapular dyskinesis and its causative mechanisms should be part of the comprehensive evaluation of patients with rotator cuff disease.

6. Curtis AS, Burbank KM, Tierney JJ, Scheller AD, Curran AR: The insertional footprint of the rotator cuff: An anatomic study. *Arthroscopy* 2006;22(6):e1.

7. Dugas JR, Campbell DA, Warren RF, Robie BH, Millett PJ: Anatomy and dimensions of rotator cuff insertions. *J Shoulder Elbow Surg* 2002;11(5):498-503.

8. Mochizuki T, Sugaya H, Uomizu M, et al: Humeral insertion of the supraspinatus and infraspinatus: New anatomical findings regarding the footprint of the rotator cuff. *J Bone Joint Surg Am* 2008;90(5):962-969.

    In 113 cadaver specimens, the footprint of the supraspinatus on the greater tuberosity was found to be much smaller than previously believed. This area of the greater tuberosity is occupied by a substantial amount of the infraspinatus.

9. Mochizuki T, Sugaya H, Uomizu M, et al: Humeral insertion of the supraspinatus and infraspinatus: New anatomical findings regarding the footprint of the rotator cuff. Surgical technique. *J Bone Joint Surg Am* 2009;91(suppl 2, pt 1):1-7.

    Surgical techniques were recommended based on anatomic study of the footprint of the supraspinatus and the infraspinatus in 113 cadaver specimens.

10. Kato A, Nimura A, Yamaguchi K, Mochizuki T, Sugaya H, Akita K: An anatomical study of the transverse part of the infraspinatus muscle that is closely related with the supraspinatus muscle. *Surg Radiol Anat* 2012;34(3):257-265.

    A cadaver study found that the infraspinatus is composed of oblique and transverse parts according to muscle fiber direction. Both parts have a partially independent morphology. The transverse part inserts into the main tendinous portion of the oblique part as a thin tendinous membrane.

11. Nimura A, Kato A, Yamaguchi K, et al: The superior capsule of the shoulder joint complements the insertion of the rotator cuff. *J Shoulder Elbow Surg* 2012; 21(7):867-872.

    The attachment of the articular capsule of the shoulder joint was found to occupy a substantial area of the greater tuberosity. At the border between the infraspinatus and the teres minor, the very thick attachment of the articular capsule compensated for the lack of attachment of muscular components.

12. Arai R, Sugaya H, Mochizuki T, Nimura A, Moriishi J, Akita K: Subscapularis tendon tear: An anatomic and clinical investigation. *Arthroscopy* 2008;24(9): 997-1004.

    The subscapularis insertion anatomy was investigated in view of the stabilizing function of the long head of the biceps tendon. The prevalence of subscapularis tendon tears was evaluated by reviewing surgical records and videotapes.

13. Adams CR, Schoolfield JD, Burkhart SS: Accuracy of preoperative magnetic resonance imaging in predicting a subscapularis tendon tear based on arthroscopy. *Arthroscopy* 2010;26(11):1427-1433.

    The diagnostic accuracy of MRI of subscapularis tendon tears was studied by comparing preoperative MRI interpretations by radiologists with arthroscopic evaluations of the same shoulders.

14. Garavaglia G, Ufenast H, Taverna E: The frequency of subscapularis tears in arthroscopic rotator cuff repairs: A retrospective study comparing magnetic resonance imaging and arthroscopic findings. *Int J Shoulder Surg* 2011;5(4):90-94.

    A medical chart review of 348 consecutive arthroscopic rotator cuff repairs found subscapularis tears in 129 (37%). Good agreement was found with supraspinatus MRI results, but MRI often failed to reveal subscapularis and infraspinatus tears.

15. Arai R, Mochizuki T, Yamaguchi K, et al: Functional anatomy of the superior glenohumeral and coracohumeral ligaments and the subscapularis tendon in view of stabilization of the long head of the biceps tendon. *J Shoulder Elbow Surg* 2010;19(1):58-64.

    Twelve cadaver shoulders were used to study the anatomy of the lateral rotator cuff interval and the most cranial subscapularis tendon insertion area.

16. Lo IK, Burkhart SS: The comma sign: An arthroscopic guide to the torn subscapularis tendon. *Arthroscopy* 2003;19(3):334-337.

17. Gialanella B, Prometti P: Effects of corticosteroids injection in rotator cuff tears. *Pain Med* 2011;12(10): 1559-1565.

    A randomized controlled study found that intraarticular injection of triamcinolone improved pain relief for 3 months. The drug action was not prolonged or potentiated by two injections at a 21-day interval.

18. Pappas AM, Zawacki RM, McCarthy CF: Rehabilitation of the pitching shoulder. *Am J Sports Med* 1985; 13(4):223-235.

19. Maffulli N, Longo UG, Berton A, Loppini M, Denaro V: Biological factors in the pathogenesis of rotator cuff tears. *Sports Med Arthrosc* 2011;19(3):194-201.

    The biologic factors involved in the pathogenesis of rotator cuff tears were investigated. An understanding of the mechanism of rotator cuff pathology could guide the design, the selection, and the implementation of treatment strategies, such as biologic modulation and preventive measures.

3: The Rotator Cuff

20. Yamaguchi K, Ditsios K, Middleton WD, Hildebolt CF, Galatz LM, Teefey SA: The demographic and morphological features of rotator cuff disease: A comparison of asymptomatic and symptomatic shoulders. *J Bone Joint Surg Am* 2006;88(8):1699-1704.

21. Yamakado K: Histopathology of residual tendon in high-grade articular-sided partial-thickness rotator cuff tears (PASTA lesions). *Arthroscopy* 2012;28(4): 474-480.

    More than 90% of the macroscopically intact residual tendon tissue of partial articular-surface tendon avulsion tears in 30 patients (mean age, 60 years) had moderate histopathologic degeneration.

22. Hashimoto T, Nobuhara K, Hamada T: Pathologic evidence of degeneration as a primary cause of rotator cuff tear. *Clin Orthop Relat Res* 2003;415:111-120.

23. Funakoshi T, Iwasaki N, Kamishima T, et al: In vivo visualization of vascular patterns of rotator cuff tears using contrast-enhanced ultrasound. *Am J Sports Med* 2010;38(12):2464-2471.

    Enhanced ultrasound images were used to investigate the vascularity of intact and torn rotator cuffs. There was a significant age-related decrease in blood flow in the intratendinous region but not in bursal tissue. Blood flow in ruptured rotator cuffs did not differ from that in intact rotator cuffs.

24. Modi CS, Smith CD, Drew SJ: Partial-thickness articular surface rotator cuff tears in patients over the age of 35: Etiology and intra-articular associations. *Int J Shoulder Surg* 2012;6(1):15-18.

    Partial-thickness articular-side tears were common in patients older than 35 years who required arthroscopic surgery for rotator cuff pathology, probably reflecting injury to an already-degenerated rotator cuff. This finding supports the theory of intrinsic degeneration of the tendon in this age group and probably represents an etiology different from that of young athletes.

25. Longo UG, Berton A, Khan WS, Maffulli N, Denaro V: Histopathology of rotator cuff tears. *Sports Med Arthrosc* 2011;19(3):227-236.

    Tendon abnormalities of the rotator cuff include alteration of collagen fiber structure, tenocytes, cellularity, and vascularity. Ruptured tendons have marked collagen degeneration and disordered arrangement of collagen fibers. Fibroblast population decreases as the size of the rotator cuff tear increases.

26. Hegedus EJ, Cook C, Brennan M, Wyland D, Garrison JC, Driesner D: Vascularity and tendon pathology in the rotator cuff: A review of literature and implications for rehabilitation and surgery. *Br J Sports Med* 2010;44(12):838-847.

    Studies reflecting recent improvements in design and technology support that increased vascularity is a normal response to a small tear. As tear size increases, the healing response fails and vascularity decreases.

27. Carbone S, Gumina S, Arceri V, Campagna V, Fagnani C, Postacchini F: The impact of preoperative smoking habit on rotator cuff tear: Cigarette smoking influences rotator cuff tear sizes. *J Shoulder Elbow Surg* 2012;21(1):56-60.

    A correlation was found among cigarette smoking, rotator cuff tearing, and tear size. Increasing tear size corresponded to increasing numbers of daily and lifetime cigarettes smoked.

28. Baumgarten KM, Gerlach D, Galatz LM, et al: Cigarette smoking increases the risk for rotator cuff tears. *Clin Orthop Relat Res* 2010;468(6):1534-1541.

    A questionnaire was administered to 586 consecutive patients age 18 years or older with a diagnostic shoulder ultrasound for unilateral, atraumatic shoulder pain and no history of shoulder surgery. A dosage- and time-dependent relationship was found between smoking and rotator cuff tears.

29. Gwilym SE, Watkins B, Cooper CD, et al: Genetic influences in the progression of tears of the rotator cuff. *J Bone Joint Surg Br* 2009;91(7):915-917.

    Genetic factors were found to have a role in the development and the progression of full-thickness rotator cuff tears in a comparison study involving patients' siblings.

30. Tashjian RZ, Farnham JM, Albright FS, Teerlink CC, Cannon-Albright LA: Evidence for an inherited predisposition contributing to the risk for rotator cuff disease. *J Bone Joint Surg Am* 2009;91(5):1136-1142.

    A population-based resource combining genealogic data and clinical data was used in finding a significantly elevated risk of rotator cuff disease in second- and third-degree relatives of patients diagnosed with rotator cuff disease before age 40 years.

31. Chaudhury S, Carr AJ: Lessons we can learn from gene expression patterns in rotator cuff tears and tendinopathies. *J Shoulder Elbow Surg* 2012;21(2): 191-199.

    Genetic predisposition to rotator cuff tears was reviewed, with gene changes related to rotator cuff tears, cellular dysregulation, metaplasia, and modulation or manipulation of gene expression.

32. Nyffeler RW, Werner CM, Sukthankar A, Schmid MR, Gerber C: Association of a large lateral extension of the acromion with rotator cuff tears. *J Bone Joint Surg Am* 2006;88(4):800-805.

33. Hamid N, Omid R, Yamaguchi K, Steger-May K, Stobbs G, Keener JD: Relationship of radiographic acromial characteristics and rotator cuff disease: A prospective investigation of clinical, radiographic, and sonographic findings. *J Shoulder Elbow Surg* 2012; 21(10):1289-1298.

    The presence of an acromial spur was associated with the presence of a full-thickness rotator cuff tear. The acromial morphology classification system is an unreliable method of assessing the acromion, and the acromial index shows no association with the presence of rotator cuff disease.

34. Keener JD, Steger-May K, Stobbs G, Yamaguchi K: Asymptomatic rotator cuff tears: Patient demographics and baseline shoulder function. *J Shoulder Elbow Surg* 2010;19(8):1191-1198.

When asymptomatic, a rotator cuff tear is associated with a clinically insignificant loss of shoulder function compared with an intact rotator cuff. The presence of pain is important for creating a measurable loss of shoulder function in rotator cuff–deficient shoulders. Hand dominance appears to be an important risk factor for pain.

35. Moosmayer S, Tariq R, Stiris MG, Smith HJ: MRI of symptomatic and asymptomatic full-thickness rotator cuff tears: A comparison of findings in 100 subjects. *Acta Orthop* 2010;81(3):361-366.

Tear characteristics were compared in 50 patients with an asymptomatic full-thickness rotator cuff tear and 50 patients with a symptomatic tear. Statistically significant associations were found between symptoms and tear size exceeding 3 cm in the mediolateral plane, a positive tangent sign, and fatty degeneration exceeding grade 1 in the supraspinatus and infraspinatus muscles.

36. Mall NA, Kim HM, Keener JD, et al: Symptomatic progression of asymptomatic rotator cuff tears: A prospective study of clinical and sonographic variables. *J Bone Joint Surg Am* 2010;92(16):2623-2633.

Pain in a shoulder with an asymptomatic rotator cuff tear is associated with an increase in tear size. A large tear is more likely to become painful in the short term than a small tear.

37. Yamaguchi K, Tetro AM, Blam O, Evanoff BA, Teefey SA, Middleton WD: Natural history of asymptomatic rotator cuff tears: A longitudinal analysis of asymptomatic tears detected sonographically. *J Shoulder Elbow Surg* 2001;10(3):199-203.

38. Safran O, Schroeder J, Bloom R, Weil Y, Milgrom C: Natural history of nonoperatively treated symptomatic rotator cuff tears in patients 60 years old or younger. *Am J Sports Med* 2011;39(4):710-714.

In a prospective study, patients age 60 years or younger were treated nonsurgically for a relatively small full-thickness rotator cuff tear. No correlation was found between considerable pain at the time of the follow-up ultrasound (mean, 29 months) and a clinically significant increase in tear size.

39. Maman E, Harris C, White L, Tomlinson G, Shashank M, Boynton E: Outcome of nonoperative treatment of symptomatic rotator cuff tears monitored by magnetic resonance imaging. *J Bone Joint Surg Am* 2009;91(8):1898-1906.

A retrospective study of 54 patients (mean age, 58.8 years) with a nonsurgically treated rotator cuff tear found that the factors associated with progression were age older than 60 years, a full-thickness tear, and fatty infiltration of the rotator cuff muscles.

40. Fucentese SF, von Roll AL, Pfirrmann CW, Gerber C, Jost B: Evolution of nonoperatively treated symptom-

atic isolated full-thickness supraspinatus tears. *J Bone Joint Surg Am* 2012;94(9):801-808.

Twenty-four consecutive patients were offered repair of an isolated, symptomatic, small, full-thickness supraspinatus tear. Those who refused surgical treatment had surprisingly high satisfaction. There was no increase in the average rotator cuff tear size 3.5 years after surgical repair was recommended.

41. Tanaka M, Itoi E, Sato K, et al: Factors related to successful outcome of conservative treatment for rotator cuff tears. *Ups J Med Sci* 2010;115(3):193-200.

The success of nonsurgical treatment was significantly affected by the integrity of the intramuscular tendon of the supraspinatus, as determined by high-resolution MRI with a microscopy coil, supraspinatus muscle atrophy, the impingement sign, and the external rotation angle.

42. Melis B, DeFranco MJ, Chuinard C, Walch G: Natural history of fatty infiltration and atrophy of the supraspinatus muscle in rotator cuff tears. *Clin Orthop Relat Res* 2010;468(6):1498-1505.

A retrospective review of 1,688 patients with a rotator cuff tear found that moderate supraspinatus fatty infiltration, a positive tangent sign, and severe fatty infiltration appeared at an average of 3 years, 4.5 years, and 5 years, respectively, after the onset of symptoms.

43. Melis B, Wall B, Walch G: Natural history of infraspinatus fatty infiltration in rotator cuff tears. *J Shoulder Elbow Surg* 2010;19(5):757-763.

Moderate and severe infraspinatus fatty infiltration appeared an average of 2.5 years and 4 years, respectively, after the onset of symptoms. A relatively large tendon tear, a longer delay after tendon rupture, and older patient age were associated with more common and severe fatty infiltration.

44. Melis B, Nemoz C, Walch G: Muscle fatty infiltration in rotator cuff tears: Descriptive analysis of 1688 cases. *Orthop Traumatol Surg Res* 2009;95(5):319-324.

The mean time from tendon rupture to grade 2 fatty infiltration was 3 years for the supraspinatus and 2.5 years for the infraspinatus or the subscapularis. The mean time to grade 3 or 4 fatty infiltration was 5, 4, or 3 years for the supraspinatus, the infraspinatus, or the subscapularis, respectively.

45. Zingg PO, Jost B, Sukthankar A, Buhler M, Pfirrmann CW, Gerber C: Clinical and structural outcomes of nonoperative management of massive rotator cuff tears. *J Bone Joint Surg Am* 2007;89(9):1928-1934.

At a mean 48-month follow-up after nonsurgical treatment of 19 consecutive patients with a massive rotator cuff tear, shoulder function, including active range of motion, was almost maintained despite significant progression of degenerative structural joint changes.

46. Longo UG, Franceschi F, Berton A, Maffulli N, Droena V: Conservative treatment and rotator cuff tear progression. *Med Sport Sci* 2012;57:90-99.

3: The Rotator Cuff

There is no definite consensus on the best management for patients with a rotator cuff tear. Few randomized controlled studies are available on nonsurgical management.

47. Hong JY, Yoon SH, Moon J, Kwack KS, Joen B, Lee HY: Comparison of high- and low-dose corticosteroid in subacromial injection for periarticular shoulder disorder: A randomized, triple-blind, placebo-controlled trial. *Arch Phys Med Rehabil* 2011;92(12):1951-1960.

The efficacy of corticosteroid (triamcinolone acetonide) was compared at the two most widely used dosages (40 mg and 20 mg) for subacromial injection in patients with a periarticular shoulder disorder. Because no significant difference was found, the initial use of the lower dosage was preferred.

48. Zufferey P, Revaz S, Degailler X, Balague F, So A: A controlled trial of the benefits of ultrasound-guided steroid injection for shoulder pain. *Joint Bone Spine* 2012;79(2):166-169.

Local steroid injection for shoulder pain led to significant improvement in pain and function for as long as 12 weeks. Ultrasound examination to define the origin of shoulder pain and guide injection can provide as much as 6 weeks of significant additional benefit.

49. Bennell K, Wee E, Coburn S, et al: Efficacy of standardised manual therapy and home exercise programme for chronic rotator cuff disease: Randomised placebo controlled trial. *BMJ* 2010;340:c2756.

A standard program of manual therapy and home exercise did not confer immediate improvement in pain and function compared with a realistic placebo treatment in middle-aged and older adults with chronic rotator cuff disease. Greater improvement was apparent at follow-up, however, particularly in shoulder function and strength. This finding suggests that the benefit of active treatment requires time to manifest.

50. Başkurt Z, Başkurt F, Gelecek N, Özkan MH: The effectiveness of scapular stabilization exercise in the patients with subacromial impingement syndrome. *J Back Musculoskelet Rehabil* 2011;24(3):173-179.

A randomized study found that adding scapular stabilization exercises to stretching and strengthening exercises increased the effectiveness of physical therapy in increasing muscle strength, developing joint position sense, and decreasing scapular dyskinesis in patients with subacromial impingement syndrome.

Chapter 14

Partial-Thickness Rotator Cuff Tears

Ian K.Y. Lo, MD, FRCSC

Introduction

Although partial-thickness rotator cuff tears (PTRCTs) are common, their optimal treatment remains controversial. Most publications on rotator cuff tears have focused on full-thickness rotator cuff tears (FTRCTs), and most of the available studies of PTRCTs have focused on surgical outcome or technique. Few studies have looked at the etiologic factors or the nonsurgical treatment of PTRCTs. The relatively poor understanding of the natural history of the disease compounds the debate over optimal treatment.

Relevant Anatomy

The rotator cuff tendon classically is described as a complex coalescence of the supraspinatus, infraspinatus, teres minor, and subscapularis tendons into a multilayered structure that inserts into the humeral head.[1] Several cadaver studies have evaluated the gross anatomy of the rotator cuff tendon insertion. One study measured the medial-to-lateral width and the anterior-to-posterior length of each footprint and found a wide range of widths and lengths for each insertion[2] (**Table 1**). Another study found the supraspinatus tendon to have a mean width of 12.1 mm (range, 9 to 15 mm) and a mean length of 25.0 mm (range, 19 to 27 mm).[3]

A cadaver study led to an alternative interpretation of the rotator cuff tendon insertion[4] (**Figure 1**). A long trapezoid-shaped insertion of the infraspinatus tendon was described, with an anterior curve. The infraspinatus tendon was found to occupy a large portion of the

Dr. Lo or an immediate family member serves as a board member, owner, officer, or committee member of the Arthroscopy Association of North America; has received royalties from Arthrex, Arthrocare, and Lippincott; is a member of a speakers' bureau or has made paid presentations on behalf of Arthrocare and Arthrex; serves as a paid consultant to or is an employee of Arthrocare; serves as an unpaid consultant to Tenet Medical and Smith & Nephew; has received research or institutional support from Arthrocare, Arthrex, Linvatec, and Smith & Nephew; and has stock or stock options held in Tenet Medical.

lateral aspect of the superior facet of the greater tuberosity; this area previously was assigned to the supraspinatus tendon. In contrast, the supraspinatus tendon insertion was described as small, triangle shaped, and on the most anterior aspect of the greater tuberosity; in 21% of the specimens, some fibers inserted into the lesser tuberosity. These anatomic findings require further investigation. It should be noted, however, that the clinical algorithms for treating a PTRCT (defined as a tear of no more than 50% of tendon thickness) are based on classic descriptions of the rotator cuff tendon insertion.

Incidence, Etiology, and Pathogenesis

Cadaver and imaging studies have found a prevalence of PTRCTs ranging from 13% to 32%.[5-8] An MRI study of asymptomatic individuals found an overall prevalence of 20%.[8] Prevalence was highly age related; 26% of those older than 60 years but only 4% of those younger than 40 years had a PTRCT. Clearly, many PTRCTs are asymptomatic and probably are secondary to age-related degenerative changes. Therefore, it is important to correlate clinical and imaging findings.

Several etiologic factors in isolation or combination can result in the anatomic lesion of a PTRCT. Intrinsic factors include age-related alterations in microscopic anatomy (for example, decreased cellularity, fascicular thinning or disruption, or granulation tissue), metabolic anatomy, and vascular anatomy (for example, decreased vascularity or a hypovascular zone). These factors create a predisposition to degenerative tearing or alterations in intratendinous sheer stress. Extrinsic factors include classic subacromial (outlet) impingement, internal impingement, and glenohumeral instability and/or laxity, which can contribute to the development of a PTRCT. Traumatic events, whether single or repetitive (for example, from overhead throwing) can lead to tensile overload and fiber failure.

Although several general etiologic factors have been identified, certain factors are likely to predispose the rotator cuff to particular types of tearing. A PTRCT in an older patient commonly occurs on the articular surface just posterior to the biceps tendon and is

3: The Rotator Cuff

Table 1

Medial-to-Lateral Width and Anterior-to-Posterior Length of the Rotator Cuff Tendon Insertions

Rotator Cuff Tendon	Mean Medial-Lateral Width, in mm (Range)	Mean Anterior-Posterior Length, in mm (Range)
Supraspinatus	16 (12-20)	23 (18-33)
Infraspinatus	18 (12-24)	28 (20-45)
Teres minor	21 (10-33)	29 (20-40)
Subscapularis	20 (15-25)	40 (35-55)

(Adapted with permission from Curtis AS, Burbank KM, Tierney JJ, Scheller AD, Curran AR: The insertional footprint of the rotator cuff: An anatomic study. *Arthroscopy* 2006;22[6]:603-609.)

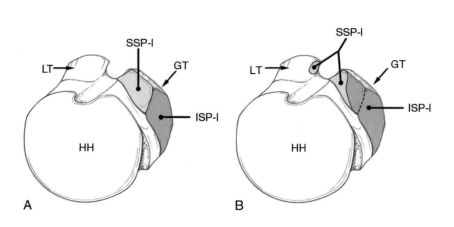

Figure 1   Schematic drawings of the superior aspect of the right humerus, showing the humeral insertions of the supraspinatus and the infraspinatus. **A,** The generally accepted concept of the anatomy of humeral insertions, in which the supraspinatus inserts into the highest impression and the infraspinatus inserts into the middle impression of the greater tuberosity. **B,** An alternative concept, in which the insertion area of the infraspinatus occupies approximately half of the highest impression and all of the middle impression of the greater tuberosity. The insertion area of the supraspinatus is in the anteromedial region of the highest impression and sometimes also in the superior-most area of the lesser tuberosity. GT = greater tuberosity, HH = humeral head, ISP-I = insertion area of the infraspinatus, LT = lesser tuberosity, SSP-I = insertion area of the supraspinatus. (Reproduced with permission from Mochizuki T, Sugaya H, Uomizu M, et al: Humeral insertion of the supraspinatus and infraspinatus: New anatomic findings regarding the footprint of the rotator cuff. *J Bone Joint Surg Am* 2008;90:962-969.)

secondary to age-related degenerative changes. In contrast, a PTRCT in a young overhead athlete commonly occurs near the confluence of the supraspinatus and infraspinatus tendons. This characteristic suggests a different etiologic factor in young overhead athletes (for example, excessive twisting or torsional stress of the rotator cuff fibers or internal impingement), which leads to a more posterior, articular-surface tear.[9]

The natural history of PTRCTs remains unclear, and published studies are rare. At a mean 1.1-year follow-up, 80% of PTRCTs had increased in size, and 28% of patients had full-thickness progression of their PTRCTs.[10] Several relatively recent studies suggested that the natural history of PTRCTs is not so negatively

defined.[11-13] Overall, serial ultrasonography revealed progression to an FTRCT in 4 of 30 patients (13%).[11] In 20 patients who remained asymptomatic, no PTRCT progressed to an FTRCT. Another recent study evaluated 37 patients with a PTRCT using serial MRI or magnetic resonance arthrography (MRA).[13] At a mean 4.4-year follow-up, 28 patients (76%) had no significant PTRCT progression, 6 (16%) had an increase in tear size, and 3 (8%) had progression to an FTRCT. PTRCTs involving at least 50% of the tendon thickness were most likely to progress. Fifty-five percent of such tears progressed compared with 14% of tears involving less than 50% of the tendon thickness.

Table 2

Classification of Partial-Thickness Rotator Cuff Tears

Location

Articular

Bursal

Intratendinous

Grade	Size of Tear (Percentage of Tendon Thickness)
I	< 3 mm (< 25%)
II	3-6 mm (25%-50%)
III	> 6 mm (> 50%)

(Adapted with permission from Ellman H: Diagnosis and treatment of incomplete rotator cuff tears. *Clin Orthop Relat Res* 1990;254:64-74.)

Diagnostic Imaging

The value of ultrasonography for detecting and quantifying PTRCTs and FTRCTs continues to evolve. Ultrasonography has had accuracy similar to that of MRI for detecting FTRCTs, but its use in detecting and quantifying PTRCTs in a community setting is controversial.[14,15] Ultrasonography continues to be limited by its observer-dependent reliability and its limited ability to detect significant glenohumeral pathology. In a meta-analysis of 65 studies evaluating the diagnostic imaging of rotator cuff tears, ultrasonography was found to have sensitivity (66.7%) and specificity (93.5%) similar to that of MRI (sensitivity, 63.6%; specificity, 91.7%) for detecting PTRCTs.[16]

MRA is considered the imaging modality of choice for evaluating PTRCTs, particularly articular-surface tears. MRA has a mean sensitivity of 85.9% and a mean specificity of 96%, and it is significantly more accurate than ultrasonography or MRI for detecting PTRCTs.[16] The addition of an abduction–external rotation view can improve the sensitivity of MRA for detecting articular-surface PTRCTs.[17,18]

Classification

PTRCTs can be generally classified by anatomic location (bursal surface, articular surface, or insubstance), tendon involvement (supraspinatus, infraspinatus, teres minor, or subscapularis), and/or area of involvement and depth (percentage of tendon thickness torn).[19,20] The most commonly used classification is based on anatomic location and the depth of tendon tearing[19] (Table 2). This classification system fails to recognize several factors, including the extent of sagittal-plane tearing, the area of tearing, tissue quality, and etiology.

The interobserver reliability of rotator cuff classification systems recently has been questioned. Ten fellowship-trained orthopaedic shoulder surgeons evaluated 27 MRI studies from patients with a surgically confirmed rotator cuff tear.[21] Interobserver agreement was high for distinguishing between FTRCTs and PTRCTs and for identifying the location of a PTRCT (bursal or articular), but it was poor for identifying the grade of PTRCTs. In a similar study using videotaped arthroscopy, interobserver agreement also was poor for grading PTRCTs.[22]

Nonsurgical Treatment

PTRCTs can be nonsurgically treated using various modalities, including physical therapy, steroid injection, and anti-inflammatory or pain medication. Nonsurgical treatment may be more acceptable for PTRCTs than for FTRCTs because the risk of muscular atrophy, fatty infiltration, or catastrophic tear extension is minimal in PTRCTs. A recent study specifically evaluated the success of nonsurgical treatment of PTRCTs in 76 consecutive patients.[13] Approximately 50% of the patients initially were successfully treated nonsurgically, and 91% were satisfied with their treatment at a mean 46-month follow-up after initial assessment. Patients with an atraumatic onset involving the nondominant extremity and a tear involving less than 50% of the tendon were more likely to be successfully treated without surgery.

Surgical Treatment

Indications

The indications for surgically treating PTRCTs are poorly defined but are based on patient factors (age, activity level, occupation, and sports involvement), clinical factors (traumatic history, severity of pain, weakness, and response to nonsurgical treatment), and pathologic factors (bursal or articular surface and the percentage of tendon thickness torn). Patients with a chronic tear and mild symptoms generally are initially treated nonsurgically. Surgical management should be considered for a young patient with a traumatic PTRCT involving more than 50% of the tendon or for a patient who has undergone adequate but unsuccessful nonsurgical treatment.

Rationale for the 50% Rule

The surgical options for treating a PTRCT include débridement or repair, with or without concurrent subacromial decompression. In general, débridement (with or without subacromial decompression) can be used for a patient with a PTRCT involving less than 50% of the tendon. Rotator cuff repair (with or without subacromial decompression) should be considered for a patient with a PTRCT involving more than 50% of the tendon. The rationale for surgically repairing PTRCTs involv-

3: The Rotator Cuff

ing more than 50% of the tendon thickness is largely based on a single retrospective study of 65 patients with a PTRCT involving more than 50% of the tendon thickness.[23] Thirty-two of the patients underwent an arthroscopic acromioplasty, and 33 patients were treated with arthroscopic acromioplasty followed by miniopen rotator cuff repair. The treatment was not randomly assigned but was chosen based on a preoperative discussion with the patient. At 2- to 7-year follow-up, the mean score on the University of California, Los Angeles (UCLA) Shoulder Rating Scale was 22.7 for patients who underwent arthroscopic acromioplasty and 31.6 for those who underwent arthroscopic acromioplasty and miniopen rotator cuff repair.

This study had several weaknesses (for example, it was nonrandomized and retrospective), but several biomechanical studies also have supported the so-called 50% rule. In a cadaver study, articular-surface PTRCTs of varying severity were subjected to cyclic load.[24] A significant increase in strain on the residual adjacent rotator cuff fibers occurred only if an articular-surface PTRCT was greater than 50% of the tendon thickness. Repair of the PTRCT returned the strain to its normal state. Another cadaver study created progressively larger bursal-surface PTRCTs in the supraspinatus tendon.[25] The strain in the intact tendon increased when the bursal-surface tear was more than 50% of the tendon thickness. As the depth of the tear increased, the stress on the residual intact tendon increased nonlinearly.

Although the percentage of torn tendon thickness is a factor in determining the surgical procedure, other significant variables (patient, clinical, and pathologic factors) also should be considered before making a decision.

Arthroscopic Débridement and Subacromial Decompression

Arthroscopic débridement commonly is performed for a PTRCT involving less than 50% of the tendon thickness (a grade I or II tear), with good to excellent results as measured using validated shoulder-specific scales.[26-32] The addition of subacromial decompression has not been shown to significantly improve symptoms.[33] Although arthroscopic débridement (with or without acromioplasty) can lead to good results, one study found that certain tears are relatively likely to fail after arthroscopic débridement.[27] At a mean 52-month follow-up, more than 90% of the patients had a good outcome, but the procedure was considered a failure in 8% of the patients, most of whom had a bursal-surface PTRCT. The risk of failure was 29% after arthroscopic débridement and acromioplasty in patients with a bursal-surface PTRCT and 38% in those with more extensive bursal-surface tearing. The study results suggested that repair should be considered for a bursal-surface PTRCT, even if the tear involves less than 50% of the tendon.

The long-term results of arthroscopic débridement are unclear. At a mean 101-month follow-up, patients had a mean Constant score of 65 for the treated shoulder, which was approximately 20 points lower than the score for the contralateral shoulder.[28] After arthroscopic débridement, only 57% of the patients were able to return without symptoms to their preoperative level of sports; 20% were able to return to sports at a lower level because of ongoing symptoms, and 22% were unable to participate in sports.[26] In even higher-level overhead athletes, there was a 55% return-to-play rate at the same level or higher.[31]

Arthroscopic débridement (with or without decompression) does not appear to heal a PTRCT or prevent its progression. At a mean 8.4-year follow-up after arthroscopic acromioplasty and débridement, 9 of 26 patients had ultrasonographically detected progression to an FTRCT.[28] Similarly, at a mean 4.2-year follow-up after arthroscopic acromioplasty and débridement in 46 patients with an articular-surface PTRCT, ultrasonography revealed progression to an FTRCT in 3 patients (6.5%).[29] However, only one patient had a poor result.

Arthroscopic Repair

Several surgical techniques have been described for the repair of PTRCTs, including in situ techniques and conversion of the partial tear to an FTRCT. Conversion to a FTRCT is advantageous because it allows standard arthroscopic techniques to be used for repair. In situ techniques, such as transtendon or all–intra-articular repair, maintain the integrity of at least a portion of the intact rotator cuff. In situ techniques are particularly relevant for articular-surface PTRCTs, in which maintaining the intact lateral rotator cuff can be considered. Maintenance of a viable and robust lateral tendon may allow a more anatomic reconstruction of the rotator cuff footprint.

The biomechanical performance of techniques for repairing a PTRCT has been evaluated in several studies. Transtendon repair was compared with full-thickness conversion followed by double-row repair for 50% articular-surface PTRCTs.[34] Under cyclic loading, gap formation was significantly less, and ultimate failure strength was significantly greater after the transtendon repair. In an ovine model of PTRCT, the footprint contact pressure and the strength of various repair techniques were evaluated.[35] Transtendon repair and double-row repair had similar contact pressures, but transtendon repair had a significantly higher ultimate load to failure.

Although there may be theoretic advantages to maintaining the intact portion of the rotator cuff, clinical studies have not clearly shown a substantial superiority of transtendon repair over conversion to an FTRCT and the subsequent repair[36-47] (Table 3). Most clinical studies of PTRCT conversion to FTRCT have reported excellent results, with rates of patient satisfaction greater than 90%.[36-39] Rotator cuff healing has been shown to occur in most patients after PTRCT conversion to FTRCT. In 42 consecutive patients (mean age, 53 years) at a mean 39-month follow-up, the mean

Table 3

Clinical and Anatomic Results of Arthroscopic Repair of Partial-Thickness Rotator Cuff Tears

Study	Number of Patients	Type of Repair	Clinical Outcomes		Anatomic Outcome (Imaging Method)
			Preoperative→ Postoperative Follow-up Scores (Measure)	Percentage of Patients Satisfied	
Porat et al[36]	36	Conversion to FTRCT	17.2 → 31.5 (UCLA)		
Deutsch[37]	41	Conversion to FTRCT	42 → 93 (ASES)	98%	
Kamath et al[38]	42	Conversion to FTRCT	46.1 → 82.1 (ASES)	93%	88% intact (ultra-sonography)
Iyengar et al[39]	22	Conversion to FTRCT	19.1 → 32.9 (UCLA)		82% intact (MRI)
Waibl and Buess[40]	22	Transtendon	17.1 → 31.2 (UCLA)	91%	
Ide et al[41]	17	Transtendon	17.3 → 32.9 (UCLA)		
Castagna et al[42]	54	Transtendon	45.3 → 90.6 (Constant) 14.1 → 32.9 (UCLA)	98%	
Castricini et al[43]	31	Transtendon	44.4 → 91.6 (Constant)	93%	100% intact (MRI)
Seo et al[44]	24	Transtendon double-row	38 → 89 (ASES)	92%	
Tauber et al[45]	16	Transosseous	15.8 → 32.8 (UCLA)	94%	
Spencer[46]	20	Intra-articular	74 → 92 (Penn)		

FTRCT = full-thickness rotator cuff tear; ASES = American Shoulder and Elbow Surgeons Disability Index; UCLA = University of California, Los Angeles; Penn = Penn Shoulder Score

American Shoulder and Elbow Surgeons (ASES) Shoulder Pain and Disability Index score improved from 46.1 to 82.1.[38] At a mean 11 months after surgery, ultrasonography showed that 88% of the repairs were intact. There was no significant difference in clinical outcomes between patients with a recurrent tear or a healed tendon. Patients with a recurrent tear tended to be older than those with an intact repair.

At a minimum 2-year follow-up after the full-thickness conversion technique was used for 22 patients, UCLA scores had improved from 19.4 to 32.9.[39] On MRI, 18 patients (82%) had intact rotator cuffs, and 4 (18%) had recurrent tearing that was full thickness or approaching full thickness. Although there was no correlation between tendon integrity and the postoperative UCLA score, the patients with an intact rotator cuff repair had significantly more score improvement than the patients with a rotator cuff defect.

Transtendon rotator cuff repair has had excellent results, with significant improvement in shoulder-specific scores and patient satisfaction rates greater than 90%[40-44] (**Table 3**). Careful evaluation has shown that many patients experience residual symptoms, however, even with an excellent outcome as measured using a shoulder-specific rating scale. At a mean 2.7-year follow-up after arthroscopic transtendon rotator cuff repair, a review of 54 patients found that 98% were

satisfied with the procedure, with significant improvements in UCLA, Constant, and Simple Shoulder Test scores.[42] On closer evaluation, 41% of the patients were found to have occasional residual shoulder discomfort at extremes of range of motion, particularly with activities of daily living or sports activity requiring abduction and internal rotation. In patients who had relatively great tendon retraction with minimal exposed footprint, particularly older patients with an atraumatic onset, the likelihood of residual symptoms was significantly higher. Despite the absence of control subjects or an alternative procedure in this study, the results suggest that transtendon repair may not be the ideal method of fixation for such patients.

The clinical and anatomic results of transtendon rotator cuff repair were reported in 31 patients at a mean 33-month follow-up.[43] The mean Constant score increased from 44.4 to 91.6 points, with an excellent result in 93% of the patients. Follow-up MRI showed no recurrent rotator cuff tears, and the tuberosity coverage was considered optimal in all patients. Patients were able to return to work at a mean 3.5 months after surgery.

Only one study has compared the clinical results of arthroscopic transtendon rotator cuff repair with those of tear completion followed by arthroscopic repair.[47] Seventy-four patients were randomly assigned to trans-

3: The Rotator Cuff

tendon repair or to conversion to an FTRCT before repair. At minimum 2-year follow-up, patients in both groups had significant improvement in Constant scores (from 62.5 to 87.6 after transtendon repair; from 57.8 to 86.9 after conversion and repair) and visual analog scale scores (from 8.6 to 5.4 after transtendon repair; from 9.1 to 5.4 after conversion and repair), with no statistically significant between-group differences. However, subgroup analysis of the Constant scores revealed that full-thickness conversion with subsequent repair led to a significantly greater improvement in postoperative strength than transtendon repair.

Summary

Despite the number of published studies related to PTRCTs, their optimal management continues to be debated. It is likely that different types of PTRCTs have different etiologic factors, leading to different natural histories and successes after nonsurgical or surgical management. In patients with tears smaller than 50%, arthroscopic débridement with or without subacromial decompression can lead to an excellent short-term result. However, the long-term results of using this technique are unclear. Surgical repair usually is considered for patients with a tear larger than 50%, and it has led to excellent clinical results. Although several repair techniques have been described, the published literature is insufficient for determining whether any single technique is superior to the others.

Annotated References

1. Clark JM, Harryman DT II: Tendons, ligaments, and capsule of the rotator cuff: Gross and microscopic anatomy. *J Bone Joint Surg Am* 1992;74(5):713-725.

2. Curtis AS, Burbank KM, Tierney JJ, Scheller AD, Curran AR: The insertional footprint of the rotator cuff: An anatomic study. *Arthroscopy* 2006;22(6):e1.

3. Ruotolo C, Fow JE, Nottage WM: The supraspinatus footprint: An anatomic study of the supraspinatus insertion. *Arthroscopy* 2004;20(3):246-249.

4. Mochizuki T, Sugaya H, Uomizu M, et al: Humeral insertion of the supraspinatus and infraspinatus: New anatomical findings regarding the footprint of the rotator cuff. *J Bone Joint Surg Am* 2008;90(5):962-969.

   A cadaver study described an alternative interpretation of the supraspinatus and infraspinatus tendon insertions. The supraspinatus inserted into the most anterior aspect of the greater tuberosity; in 21% of the specimens, it also inserted into the lesser tuberosity. The infraspinatus curved anteriorly to occupy the lateral aspect of the greater tuberosity.

5. Sano H, Ishii H, Trudel G, Uhthoff HK: Histologic evidence of degeneration at the insertion of 3 rotator cuff tendons: A comparative study with human cadaveric shoulders. *J Shoulder Elbow Surg* 1999;8(6):574-579.

6. Fukuda H: Partial-thickness rotator cuff tears: A modern view on Codman's classic. *J Shoulder Elbow Surg* 2000;9(2):163-168.

7. Lohr JF, Uhthoff HK: The pathogenesis of degenerative rotator cuff tears. *Orthop Trans* 1987;11:237.

8. Sher JS, Uribe JW, Posada A, Murphy BJ, Zlatkin MB: Abnormal findings on magnetic resonance images of asymptomatic shoulders. *J Bone Joint Surg Am* 1995;77(1):10-15.

9. Burkhart SS, Morgan CD, Kibler WB: The disabled throwing shoulder: Spectrum of pathology. Part I: Pathoanatomy and biomechanics. *Arthroscopy* 2003;19(4):404-420.

10. Yamanaka K, Matsumoto T: The joint side tear of the rotator cuff: A follow-up study by arthrography. *Clin Orthop Relat Res* 1994;304:68-73.

11. Mall NA, Kim HM, Keener JD, et al: Symptomatic progression of asymptomatic rotator cuff tears: A prospective study of clinical and sonographic variables. *J Bone Joint Surg Am* 2010;92(16):2623-2633.

    In a prospective evaluation of 195 patients with an asymptomatic rotator cuff tear, 4 of 30 patients with a PTRCT had full-thickness progression with symptoms. No patient progressed while remaining asymptomatic. Level of evidence: III.

12. Maman E, Harris C, White L, Tomlinson G, Shashank M, Boynton E: Outcome of nonoperative treatment of symptomatic rotator cuff tears monitored by magnetic resonance imaging. *J Bone Joint Surg Am* 2009;91(8):1898-1906.

    At a mean 20-month follow-up, 26 of 30 patients (86%) with a PTRCT remained stable as determined by serial MRI. Level of evidence: IV.

13. Lo IK, Denkers MR, More KD, Hollinshead R, Boorman RS: Paper No. 75—Partial thickness rotator cuff tears: Observe or operate? *AAOS 2012 Annual Meeting Proceedings.* CD-ROM, Rosemont, IL, American Acadamy of Orthopaedic Surgeons, 2012, pp 883-884.

    The nonsurgical treatment of PTRCTs was reviewed in 74 patients. The success rate was approximately 50%. Patients with an atraumatic onset involving the nondominant extremity and a tear of less than 50% were most likely to have a successful result. Level of evidence: IV.

14. Teefey SA, Rubin DA, Middleton WD, Hildebolt CF, Leibold RA, Yamaguchi K: Detection and quantification of rotator cuff tears: Comparison of ultrasonographic, magnetic resonance imaging, and arthroscopic findings in seventy-one consecutive cases. *J Bone Joint Surg Am* 2004;86(4):708-716.

15. Teefey SA, Middleton WD, Payne WT, Yamaguchi K: Detection and measurement of rotator cuff tears with sonography: Analysis of diagnostic errors. *AJR Am J Roentgenol* 2005;184(6):1768-1773.

16. de Jesus JO, Parker L, Frangos AJ, Nazarian LN: Accuracy of MRI, MR arthrography, and ultrasound in the diagnosis of rotator cuff tears: A meta-analysis. *AJR Am J Roentgenol* 2009;192(6):1701-1707.

    A meta-analysis of 65 articles evaluating MRI, MRA, and ultrasonography for diagnosing rotator cuff tears found that MRA was significantly more accurate for detecting PTRCTs. Level of evidence: I.

17. Jung JY, Jee WH, Chun HJ, Ahn MI, Kim YS: Magnetic resonance arthrography including ABER view in diagnosing partial-thickness tears of the rotator cuff: Accuracy, and inter- and intra-observer agreements. *Acta Radiol* 2010;51(2):194-201.

    The addition of the abduction–external rotation view increased sensitivity as well as interobserver and intraobserver agreement when MRA was used to detect arthroscopically confirmed PTRCTs. Level of evidence: I.

18. Herold T, Bachthaler M, Hamer OW, et al: Indirect MR arthrography of the shoulder: Use of abduction and external rotation to detect full- and partial-thickness tears of the supraspinatus tendon. *Radiology* 2006;240(1):152-160.

19. Ellman H: Diagnosis and treatment of incomplete rotator cuff tears. *Clin Orthop Relat Res* 1990;254:64-74.

20. Snyder SJ: Arthroscopic classification of rotator cuff lesions and surgical decision making, in *Shoulder Arthroscopy*, ed 2. Philadelphia, PA, Lippincott, Williams & Wilkins, 2003, pp 201-207.

21. Spencer EE Jr, Dunn WR, Wright RW, et al: Interobserver agreement in the classification of rotator cuff tears using magnetic resonance imaging. *Am J Sports Med* 2008;36(1):99-103.

    An evaluation by 10 fellowship-trained orthopaedic shoulder specialists led to high interobserver agreement for distinguishing between FTRCTs and PTRCTs and determining the location of PTRCTs but poor interobserver agreement for determining PTRCT grade. Level of evidence: II.

22. Kuhn JE, Dunn WR, Ma B, et al: Interobserver agreement in the classification of rotator cuff tears. *Am J Sports Med* 2007;35(3):437-441.

    Interobserver agreement by 12 orthopaedic surgeons was high for distinguishing between FTRCTs and PTRCTs and the location of the PTRCT but poor for PTRCT grade when observing videotaped arthroscopic surgery. Level of evidence: II.

23. Weber SC: Arthroscopic debridement and acromioplasty versus mini-open repair in the treatment of significant partial-thickness rotator cuff tears. *Arthroscopy* 1999;15(2):126-131.

24. Mazzocca AD, Rincon LM, O'Connor RW, et al: Intra-articular partial-thickness rotator cuff tears: Analysis of injured and repaired strain behavior. *Am J Sports Med* 2008;36(1):110-116.

    A biomechanical study evaluated the effect on adjacent rotator cuff strain of varying depths and repairs of articular-surface PTRCTs. Rotator cuff strain was significantly increased in tears of 50% or more of tendon thickness and was restored to close to normal after repair.

25. Yang S, Park HS, Flores S, et al: Biomechanical analysis of bursal-sided partial thickness rotator cuff tears. *J Shoulder Elbow Surg* 2009;18(3):379-385.

    A biomechanical study evaluated the effect of increasingly deeper bursal-side PTRCTs on adjacent rotator cuff strain. Strain in the adjacent posterior portion was significantly higher if the tear was at least 60% of tendon thickness.

26. Budoff JE, Rodin D, Ochiai D, Nirschl RP: Arthroscopic rotator cuff debridement without decompression for the treatment of tendinosis. *Arthroscopy* 2005;21(9):1081-1089.

27. Cordasco FA, Backer M, Craig EV, Klein D, Warren RF: The partial-thickness rotator cuff tear: Is acromioplasty without repair sufficient? *Am J Sports Med* 2002;30(2):257-260.

28. Kartus J, Kartus C, Rostgård-Christensen L, Sernert N, Read J, Perko M: Long-term clinical and ultrasound evaluation after arthroscopic acromioplasty in patients with partial rotator cuff tears. *Arthroscopy* 2006;22(1):44-49.

29. Liem D, Alci S, Dedy N, Steinbeck J, Marquardt B, Möllenhoff G: Clinical and structural results of partial supraspinatus tears treated by subacromial decompression without repair. *Knee Surg Sports Traumatol Arthrosc* 2008;16(10):967-972.

    The clinical results of arthroscopic débridement and decompression were evaluated at a mean 50.3-month follow-up of 46 consecutive patients. ASES scores significantly improved, and only 6.5% of the patients had progressed to an FTRCT on ultrasonography. Level of evidence: IV.

30. Park JY, Yoo MJ, Kim MH: Comparison of surgical outcome between bursal and articular partial thickness rotator cuff tears. *Orthopedics* 2003;26(4):387-390.

31. Reynolds SB, Dugas JR, Cain EL, McMichael CS, Andrews JR: Débridement of small partial-thickness rotator cuff tears in elite overhead throwers. *Clin Orthop Relat Res* 2008;466(3):614-621.

    After arthroscopic débridement of a PTRCT, 76% of the elite overhead-throwing athletes were able to return to competitive pitching at a professional level, and 55% were able to return to the same or higher level of competition. Level of evidence: IV.

3: The Rotator Cuff

32. Snyder SJ, Pachelli AF, Del Pizzo W, Friedman MJ, Ferkel RD, Pattee G: Partial thickness rotator cuff tears: Results of arthroscopic treatment. *Arthroscopy* 1991;7(1):1-7.

33. Strauss EJ, Salata MJ, Kercher J, et al: Multimedia article: The arthroscopic management of partial-thickness rotator cuff tears. A systematic review of the literature. *Arthroscopy* 2011;27(4):568-580.

    A systematic review of 16 studies on the arthroscopic management of PTRCTs led to recommendations for surgical treatment. Level of evidence: IV.

34. Gonzalez-Lomas G, Kippe MA, Brown GD, et al: In situ transtendon repair outperforms tear completion and repair for partial articular-sided supraspinatus tendon tears. *J Shoulder Elbow Surg* 2008;17(5):722-728.

    A biomechanical study found that in situ transtendon rotator cuff repair of articular-side PTRCTs led to significantly less gap formation and a higher ultimate failure strength than full-thickness conversion followed by double-row repair.

35. Peters KS, Lam PH, Murrell GA: Repair of partial-thickness rotator cuff tears: A biomechanical analysis of footprint contact pressure and strength in an ovine model. *Arthroscopy* 2010;26(7):877-884.

    A biomechanical study found that transtendon and double-row rotator cuff repair had greater footprint contact pressures than tension-band single-row repair for articular-surface PTRCTs. The ultimate load to failure was higher after a transtendon repair than a double-row or single-row repair.

36. Porat S, Nottage WM, Fouse MN: Repair of partial thickness rotator cuff tears: A retrospective review with minimum two-year follow-up. *J Shoulder Elbow Surg* 2008;17(5):729-731.

    A retrospective study evaluated the success of full-thickness conversion and repair of PTRCTs at a mean 42.4-month follow-up. Thirty of 36 patients had a good to excellent result using UCLA criteria. Level of evidence: IV.

37. Deutsch A: Arthroscopic repair of partial-thickness tears of the rotator cuff. *J Shoulder Elbow Surg* 2007;16(2):193-201.

    A retrospective study evaluated the success of full-thickness conversion and repair of PTRCTs. At a mean 38-month follow-up, there was significant improvement in the ASES score, and 98% of the patients were satisfied. Level of evidence: IV.

38. Kamath G, Galatz LM, Keener JD, Teefey S, Middleton W, Yamaguchi K: Tendon integrity and functional outcome after arthroscopic repair of high-grade partial-thickness supraspinatus tears. *J Bone Joint Surg Am* 2009;91(5):1055-1062.

    Full-thickness conversion and repair of PTRCTs led to a mean ASES score of 82.1 and intact repair on ultrasonography in 88% of the patients. Patients with an intact rotator cuff repair were younger than those with a recurrent tear. Level of evidence: IV.

39. Iyengar JJ, Porat S, Burnett KR, Marrero-Perez L, Hernandez VH, Nottage WM: Magnetic resonance imaging tendon integrity assessment after arthroscopic partial-thickness rotator cuff repair. *Arthroscopy* 2011;27(3):306-313.

    The anatomic results of full-thickness conversion and repair of PTRCTs were evaluated on MRI. In 82% of the patients, there was no evidence of a recurrent FTRCT, but 18% had a persistent defect. Integrity was not correlated with outcome. Level of evidence: IV.

40. Waibl B, Buess E: Partial-thickness articular surface supraspinatus tears: A new transtendon suture technique. *Arthroscopy* 2005;21(3):376-381.

41. Ide J, Maeda S, Takagi K: Arthroscopic transtendon repair of partial-thickness articular-side tears of the rotator cuff: Anatomical and clinical study. *Am J Sports Med* 2005;33(11):1672-1679.

42. Castagna A, Delle Rose G, Conti M, Snyder SJ, Borroni M, Garofalo R: Predictive factors of subtle residual shoulder symptoms after transtendinous arthroscopic cuff repair: A clinical study. *Am J Sports Med* 2009;37(1):103-108.

    At a minimum 2-year follow-up after transtendon repair of a PTRCT, 41% of the 54 patients had some residual symptoms at the extremes of range of motion during activities of daily living or sports, despite excellent shoulder scores. Level of evidence: IV.

43. Castricini R, Panfoli N, Nittoli R, Spurio S, Pirani O: Transtendon arthroscopic repair of partial-thickness, articular surface tears of the supraspinatus: Results at 2 years. *Chir Organi Mov* 2009;93(suppl 1):S49-S54.

    The clinical and anatomic results of 33 patients were reviewed at a mean 33-month follow-up after transtendon repair of a PTRCT. The mean Constant score was 91.6, with no recurrent tears on MRI. Level of evidence: IV.

44. Seo YJ, Yoo YS, Kim DY, Noh KC, Shetty NS, Lee JH: Trans-tendon arthroscopic repair for partial-thickness articular side tears of the rotator cuff. *Knee Surg Sports Traumatol Arthrosc* 2011;19(10):1755-1759.

    A modified transtendon bridging repair technique using medial and lateral anchors led to a mean ASES score of 89, and 22 of 24 patients were satisfied with the procedure. Level of evidence: IV.

45. Tauber M, Koller H, Resch H: Transosseous arthroscopic repair of partial articular-surface supraspinatus tendon tears. *Knee Surg Sports Traumatol Arthrosc* 2008;16(6):608-613.

    The use of an in situ transosseous technique for repair of articular-surface PTRCTs led to a mean UCLA score of 32.8, and 15 of 16 patients were satisfied with the procedure. Level of evidence: IV.

46. Spencer EE Jr: Partial-thickness articular surface rotator cuff tears: An all-inside repair technique. *Clin Orthop Relat Res* 2010;468(6):1514-1520.

A technique for all intra-articular repair of articular-surface PTRCTs was described. At a mean 29-month follow-up, the mean Penn Shoulder Score improved to 92, and 19 of 20 patients were able to return to sports at the same or a higher level. Level of evidence: IV.

47. Castagna A, Gumina S, Borroni M, Delle Rose G, Conti M, Garofalo R: Partial articular-sided supraspinatus tear: A comparison between transtendon repair and tear completion and repair. *American Shoulder and Elbow Surgeons Annual Closed Meeting Proceedings*. White Sulpher Springs, VA, American Shoulder and Elbow Surgeons, 2011, paper 30.

Seventy-four patients with an articular-surface PTRCT were randomly assigned to conversion to an FTRCT and repair or to transtendon repair. Mean Constant and visual analog scale scores improved in both groups of patients, with no significant between-group differences. Patients assigned to conversion had significantly more improvement in strength. Level of evidence: II.

Chapter 15

Surgical Treatment of Full-Thickness Rotator Cuff Tears

Sumant G. Krishnan, MD   Glen H. Rudolph, MD   Raffaele Garofalo, MD

Introduction

Rotator cuff tears represent one of the most common causes of shoulder pain and disability. The spectrum of patients with a rotator cuff lesion ranges from a young elite-level overhead athlete who has a partial-thickness rotator cuff tear to a patient of advanced age who has a massive and irreparable full-thickness tear. One or more tendons may be torn; a tear of the supraspinatus tendon is most common. The prevalence of full-thickness tears was found to increase with age, with an overall prevalence approaching 50% in individuals age 50 years or older.[1]

As the general population ages, orthopaedic surgeons increasingly must treat full-thickness rotator cuff tears. A full-thickness tear of the rotator cuff cannot heal spontaneously. Over time, the tear will reach a steady state or enlarge. In addition, irreversible fatty infiltration and muscle atrophy can occur over time in the affected muscle-tendon units and will compromise the treatment outcome. Surgical repair is indicated if the patient continues to have pain after nonsurgical management. The most popular surgical technique for rotator cuff repair has evolved from open to miniopen to arthroscopic. The primary aim of rotator cuff repair is to restore the anatomy by reinserting the torn tendons on their proximal humeral footprint, thereby improving the patient's pain and function. Unfortunately, not all surgically repaired rotator cuff tears heal. A full

understanding of the biologic and biomechanical factors affecting healing of the surgically repaired rotator cuff has not yet been achieved, and there is no agreement on the most effective methods for repair or postoperative rehabilitation.

Classification

Rotator cuff tears have been classified by etiology, chronicity, size, shape, number of tendons, and topography or trophicity. Because of the great variability in the characteristics of rotator cuff tears, a standard classification does not exist. Several rotator cuff tear classifications are intended to guide treatment decisions. These classifications often describe the tendon tear in a single dimension by measuring the greatest width of the tear or determining the number of torn tendons. A well-informed decision regarding the tear pattern and the preferred repair technique should take into account the three-dimensional information provided by preoperative MRI and subsequent arthroscopy.

A recently proposed geometric classification using coronal (length) and sagittal (width) dimensions of rotator cuff tears can provide guidance for treating a tear and determining the prognosis.[2] A type I tear is crescent shaped (short and wide) and is reparable to the footprint. A type II tear is longitudinal (L or U shaped, long and narrow) and usually is reparable to the footprint, with some side-to-side repair. A type III tear is massive and retracted (long and wide); it is often repaired by margin convergence. A type III tear larger than 2 cm^2 may be partially reparable, but it may require a tendon transfer. A type IV tear occurs with preexisting rotator cuff arthropathy and is associated with loss of the normal acromiohumeral interval and glenohumeral joint space. A type IV tear usually is irreparable and should be treated with arthroplasty.

Associated Lesions

Failure to detect a concomitant shoulder lesion disguised by a rotator cuff tear is a common surgical pitfall. The biceps tendon, glenohumeral joint,

Dr. Krishnan or an immediate family member serves as a board member, owner, officer, or committee member of the American Shoulder and Elbow Surgeons and the Arthroscopy Association of North America; has received royalties from Tornier, TAG Medical, and Ossur; is a member of a speakers' bureau or has made paid presentations on behalf of Tornier; serves as a paid consultant to or is an employee of Tornier and TAG Medical; and has received nonincome support (such as equipment or services), commercially derived honoraria, or other non–research-related funding (such as paid travel) from DePuy Mitek and Tornier. Neither of the following authors nor any immediate family member has received anything of value from or has stock or stock options held in a commercial company or institution related directly or indirectly to the subject of this chapter: Dr. Rudolph and Dr. Garofalo.

3: The Rotator Cuff

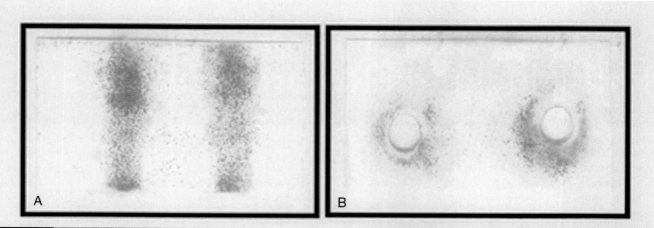

Figure 1 Pressure-sensitive film showing the rotator cuff tendon-bone interface pressure provided by transosseous suture repair (**A**) and suture anchor mattress repair (**B**). (Reproduced with permission from Park MC, Cadet ET, Levine WN, Bigliani LU, Ahmad CS: Tendon-to-bone pressure distributions at a repaired rotator cuff footprint using transosseous suture and suture anchor fixation techniques. *Am J Sports Med* 2005;33:1154-1159.)

acromioclavicular joint, suprascapular nerve, or an os acromiale may be involved in the symptom complex of rotator cuff disease. A favorable outcome requires identifying each lesion during the workup phase and treating it appropriately.

Degenerative glenohumeral joint disease is subjectively described as a pain deep inside the shoulder, sometimes with crepitus or night pain. The diagnosis can be made with plain radiography. The presence of advanced glenohumeral degeneration precludes rotator cuff repair because the postoperative immobilization can lead to worsening of existing arthritis. Acromioclavicular joint arthritis is fairly common among patients with rotator cuff disease. Specific findings include radiographic degenerative changes, tenderness to palpation directly over the acromioclavicular joint, and pain at the joint during cross-arm adduction and/or the active compression test. Open or arthroscopic distal clavicle excision can be done at the time of surgery. An os acromiale is present in approximately 8% of the population and can be identified before surgery on a standard axillary radiograph. Surgical treatment involves reduction and fixation or excision of the unfused fragment. Suprascapular nerve compression can cause shoulder pain and weakness that mimics a full-thickness supraspinatus and/or infraspinatus tear. This condition can occur in conjunction with a tear that involves supraspinatus retraction of at least 2 cm. An electromyography or nerve conduction velocity study should be obtained if a suprascapular nerve lesion is suspected.

Evaluation for an associated symptomatic lesion is crucial to discovering all sources of the patient's pain. A simple injection of 1% lidocaine into an area suspected of being a source of pain can be a powerful tool for diagnosis. This technique requires little time but provides a wealth of information for treatment planning.

Surgical Treatment

The method of repairing a rotator cuff tear should be individually chosen for the patient, with consideration of the size and pattern of the tear as well as the quality and degree of retraction of the tendon. A rotator cuff tear can be successfully treated using an open, an arthroscopically assisted, a miniopen, or an all-arthroscopic technique.[3-5] The goal of all surgical rotator cuff repairs is to obtain secure fixation of tendon to bone at the footprint to allow anatomic healing at the interface. For this purpose, the repair must have high fixation strength, minimal gapping at the time of repair, and continued mechanical stability under cyclic loading.

An open rotator cuff repair using a transosseous suture technique has been considered the gold standard among surgical techniques[6] (**Figure 1**). Regardless of the surgical approach, the coracoacromial arch and the deltoid must be treated with care. The acromion and the coracoacromial ligament in part function to restrain anterosuperior translation of the humeral head. The deltoid is responsible for generating powerful synchronized glenohumeral motion. Deltoid detachment and insufficiency of the coracoacromial arch represent a serious complication of rotator cuff repair that may result in significant disability of the arm. Acromioplasty and subacromial decompression have valid therapeutic roles in rotator cuff surgery. The goal is to reduce pressure and abrasion on the rotator cuff by smoothing the undersurface of the acromion, without disrupting the deltoid origin or destabilizing the coracoacromial arch.

Open Repair

A planned open rotator cuff tear repair should include diagnostic arthroscopy. Arthroscopy enables the surgeon to observe and treat concomitant pathology before the open rotator cuff repair. With a large or massive tear, arthroscopically observed glenohumeral arthritis may be more severe than was suggested by preoperative imaging. As the pathology dictates, the treatment plan can be altered to exclude rotator cuff repair in favor of arthroscopic débridement, subacromial decompression, and biceps tenotomy or tenodesis. Arthroscopic biceps tenotomy or tenodesis can effectively treat the pain and dysfunction caused by an irreparable rotator cuff tear in association with an intact biceps tendon. If the teres minor is atrophic or absent, pseudoparalysis of the shoulder may result. Pseudoparalysis and severe rotator cuff arthropathy are contraindications to isolated arthroscopic biceps tenotomy or tenodesis.[7]

After the diagnostic arthroscopy and before the open rotator cuff repair, the arthroscopic portals should be closed and the shoulder should be reprepared and draped to prevent infection. Skin incisions should be carefully planned to allow for potential revision surgery. Planning is particularly important during an open repair of a large or massive tear. An oblique incision from the posterior edge of the acromioclavicular joint to the anterolateral corner of the acromion, extending 2 to 3 cm distally over the raphe between the anterior and middle deltoid, provides excellent visualization for cuff repair, and it allows anterosuperior access through the same incision for any future reverse shoulder arthroplasty.

A distal clavicle excision and a two-step acromioplasty improve access to the subacromial space without extending the deltoid split. Subacromial bursectomy improves visualization and is facilitated by rotating the arm. The coracohumeral ligament is palpated in external rotation and adduction and is released if it is tight. The rotator cuff is exposed for evaluation, mobilization, and repair. With relatively recent technical advances, arthroscopic rotator cuff repair is largely equivalent to open repair. Single-row, double-row, transosseous, and transosseous-equivalent techniques are discussed here in terms of arthroscopic rotator cuff repair.

Deltoid reattachment to the acromion is a critical component of open rotator cuff repair, and it has specific implications for postoperative rehabilitation. A meticulous and strong repair is essential for avoiding dehiscence during rehabilitation. The longitudinal deltoid split is repaired with nonabsorbable sutures in a simple fashion, and the reattachment to bone often is done using suture around the distal clavicle and through tunnels in the acromion. Overall survivorship (defined as not requiring additional surgery) of 94% or 83% was reported at 5 or 10 years, respectively, after open rotator cuff repair.[8] A repair that did not require surgical intervention within the first 2 years was likely to remain intact at 10 years. Rotator cuff repair survivorship was correlated with the number of tendons repaired.

Miniopen repairs were developed to reduce deltoid morbidity. The results have been similar to those of open repairs.[9] In a randomized study, outcomes at 3-month follow-up were significantly better after miniopen rotator cuff repair than after open repair. However, between-group differences were not significant at 2-year follow-up.[3]

Arthroscopic Repair

Arthroscopic rotator cuff surgery is becoming increasingly popular, but successful and efficient repair requires a methodic stepwise approach. Patient positioning is determined by the surgeon. A modified beach chair position is preferred, with an articulated arm holder used for flexibility in positioning the arm during surgery. Four portals (posterior, posterolateral, anterolateral, and anterosuperior) normally can be used. The three-dimensional evaluation possible with the arthroscope allows the tear pattern to be recognized, and the surgeon can then formulate an appropriate repair technique and configuration. The pattern and size of the tear can best be seen through the lateral portals, and the posterolateral portal may be preferred for viewing the subacromial space and cuff anatomy. A two-step acromioplasty is done first, by removing soft tissues and bony prominences. The coracoacromial ligament may be preserved in a repair of a large or massive tear. A level I study found no benefit to subacromial decompression in association with rotator cuff repair, in terms of functional results.[10] No differences were found between arthroscopic and miniopen repair in terms of range of motion or clinical scores at a mean 24-month follow-up. After miniopen repair there appeared to be a higher rate of complications including revision, arthrofibrosis, and postoperative impingement. The studies of miniopen repair tended to have a relatively long follow-up period, however, possibly accounting for the higher complication rate. In retrospective cohort studies, miniopen repairs led to approximately twice the risk of revision or arthrofibrosis.[9]

Single-Row and Double-Row Repairs

Suture anchors have been used in both open and arthroscopic rotator cuff repairs to reattach the torn tendon to the rotator cuff footprint. For the past two decades, single-row repair has been the standard technique. In the single-row technique, the anchors are placed in a linear fashion close to the medial or the lateral aspect of the footprint, depending on surgeon preference and tendon mobility. The most common mode of failure is suture cutout through the tendon (**Figure 2**). Several strategies have been used to improve tissue grip. The use of a modified Mason-Allen stitch (the Alex stitch) led to a 38% rate of retearing, as observed on ultrasonographic examination at 2-year follow-up.[11] Single-row reconstruction with a modified suture configuration also was able to improve biomechanical properties more than a simple suture repair and had biomechanical results comparable to those of a double-row repair.[12,13] A prospective study compared clinical outcomes when the massive cuff stitch or a simple

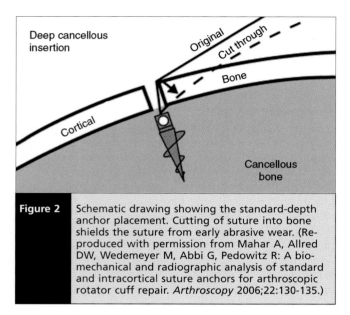

| **Figure 2** | Schematic drawing showing the standard-depth anchor placement. Cutting of suture into bone shields the suture from early abrasive wear. (Reproduced with permission from Mahar A, Allred DW, Wedemeyer M, Abbi G, Pedowitz R: A biomechanical and radiographic analysis of standard and intracortical suture anchors for arthroscopic rotator cuff repair. *Arthroscopy* 2006;22:130-135.) |

stitch was used for arthroscopic repair of a small to medium-size full-thickness rotator cuff tear. No significant difference was found, but the massive cuff stitch was superior to the simple stitch in maintaining repair integrity on ultrasonographic evaluation.[14] The use of multiple sutures per anchor has been promoted for improving integrity in a single-row repair. Triple-loaded sutures were found to be biomechanically superior in a single-row configuration compared with a double-row configuration, but the data have not been supported by a clinical study.[15]

Suture anchors are made from a variety of materials. Claims that any one material is superior to another are not scientifically supported. A randomized prospective study in which full-thickness rotator cuff tears were treated with metal or biodegradable suture anchors did not find between-group functional differences.[16] The angle of anchor insertion influences fixation stability at the suture-tendon interface. In an experimental rotator cuff model, suture anchors placed at 90° to the surface of the footprint provided better soft-tissue fixation than anchors placed at the standard 45° angle.[17] Mechanical failure at the bone-anchor interface can lead to suture anchor loosening, migration, and pullout; this complication has been reported in approximately 0.3% of patients.[18]

There is no clear consensus as to whether single-row or double-row repair of rotator cuff tears is superior. Double-row fixation is more costly, time consuming, and technically difficult when performed arthroscopically. Biomechanical studies found double-row repair to be superior to single-row repair, offering a stronger fixation, better footprint restoration, and decreased gap formation and strain[12,19-22] A bovine study found no biomechanical advantage to single-row or double-row repair, however.[23]

Several recent prospective randomized studies did not find a difference in clinical outcomes and range of motion at short-term follow-up after single-row and double-row repair.[24-30] One study examined postoperative MRI for healing of the cuff to the footprint,[25] and another study found similar rates of retearing.[30] Other studies found a trend suggesting that single-row repair is more likely to lead to recurrence than double-row repair.[26,27]

Tear size may be a determining factor in the choice of technique.[28] At 2-year follow-up, patients had higher outcomes scores after double-row fixation of tears larger than 3 cm.[31] Another study also reported better outcomes after double-row repair of large tears.[32] At a minimum 2-year follow-up after arthroscopic rotator cuff repair, patients with a tear larger than 3 cm had greater clinical strength after double-row anchor repair using a diamond suture configuration than after a single-row suture anchor repair.[33] However, there was no significant MRI-detected difference in repair integrity at 6-month or 24-month follow-up in patients with tears of different sizes. Most published data suggest that double-row fixation may be preferable for a large chronic tear, but single-row fixation is sufficient for a smaller tear (less than 3 cm). Long-term outcomes depend not only on the strength of tendon-to-bone fixation but also the biologic property of the tendon, as shown by the favorable results of patients younger than 40 years who underwent a single-row arthroscopic rotator cuff repair of a full-thickness medium-size or large rotator cuff tear.[34]

Transosseous Repair

Open rotator cuff repair using transosseous sutures has been considered the gold standard technique.[6] In the original transosseous tunnel repair, the suture emerges from the bone tunnel at the most medial aspect of the footprint and then passes through the rotator cuff tendon 1 cm from the free edge. In addition to a greater contact area, the transosseous technique provides higher mean footprint pressures. A finite element model was used to examine stress distribution in simulated supraspinatus tendon repairs with 23 common techniques and suture configurations (single row, double row, and transosseous). Stress concentrations in single-row and double-row repairs were located at the anchor insertion sites. During muscle contraction, the highest stress concentrations were shifted to the bursal surface of the tendon. These data may help explain the retearing pattern in which sutures pull through the tendon, and they support the hypothesis that the weakest part of a suture-anchor repair is at the suture-tendon interface. With transosseous sutures, stress concentration occurs at the bone-tendon interface, with no stress concentrated in the tendon; this pattern suggests that the suture-bone interface is the weakest point in a transosseous repair.[35]

Several attempts have been made to arthroscopically replicate the original open transosseous repair. An anterior cruciate ligament tibial drill guide has been used to create holes in the greater tuberosity. The sutures are passed through the tunnels and subsequently through the rotator cuff using cannulated needles or suture passers.[36] A proposed technique for arthroscopic transosseous rotator cuff repair uses an arthroscopic bone needle to improve the method of suture passage.[37] Dedicated instrumentation for arthroscopic transosseous tunnel and suture placement has been used for several years, with good results.[18] In patients treated with a transosseous anchorless technique using single-use instrumentation, the surgeon was able to arthroscopically create reproducible tunnels for transosseous suture passage with a reliable and successful result.[18]

Transosseous-Equivalent Repair

The suture bridge configuration (known as a transosseous-equivalent repair) was developed to exploit the mechanical properties of a double-row repair while offering the footprint coverage of a transosseous repair. Its favorable pressure properties are attributable to the oblique suture bridge limbs. The suture bridge imparts edge stability by flattening the lateral tendon edge, thereby preventing contact with the acromion-coracoacromial ligament arch, which is believed to lead to failure.[38] The suture-bridging technique and arthroscopic double-row procedures led to comparable patient satisfaction, functional outcomes, and rates of retearing. The only factor that significantly influenced tendon healing was patient age older than 60 years. Two types of retearing were identified: unhealed tendons and medial failures with a healed footprint.[39] In a comparison of the single-row, double-row, and combined double-row and suture bridge (compression double-row) techniques, the combined double-row and suture bridge techniques led to the lowest rate of postoperative retearing; this technique was found to be particularly useful for large or massive tears.[40]

Arthroscopic techniques for rotator cuff repair have advanced significantly in recent years. Transosseous and transosseous-equivalent rotator cuff repair techniques offer low bone-tendon interface motion, excellent footprint restoration, a high number of cycles to failure, and favorable distribution of stress over the repair in biomechanical and clinical evaluation.[35,41-43] Although these techniques are intriguing, there are no clinical studies to show definitive superiority of one technique over another or the best use of each technique.

Summary

Surgical repair of full-thickness rotator cuff tears can now be accomplished by a variety of open and all-arthroscopic techniques. There have been many exciting recent advances, such as arthroscopic transosseous and transosseous-equivalent repairs, but the peer-reviewed literature has not established the definitive superiority of any one technique. Surgeons should be familiar with the strengths and weaknesses of each technique to achieve the best potential outcome for each patient. Ongoing studies are intended to improve the success of these mechanical surgical techniques with respect to healing the repaired rotator cuff.

Annotated References

1. Yamaguchi K, Tetro AM, Blam O, Evanoff BA, Teefey SA, Middleton WD: Natural history of asymptomatic rotator cuff tears: A longitudinal analysis of asymptomatic tears detected sonographically. *J Shoulder Elbow Surg* 2001;10(3):199-203.

2. Davidson J, Burkhart SS: The geometric classification of rotator cuff tears: A system linking tear pattern to treatment and prognosis. *Arthroscopy* 2010;26(3):417-424.

   A useful classification system for rotator cuff tears assigns a prognostic value for each type, after appropriate treatment.

3. Mohtadi NG, Hollinshead RM, Sasyniuk TM, Fletcher JA, Chan DS, Li FX: A randomized clinical trial comparing open to arthroscopic acromioplasty with mini-open rotator cuff repair for full-thickness rotator cuff tears: Disease-specific quality of life outcome at an average 2-year follow-up. *Am J Sports Med* 2008;36(6):1043-1051.

   No difference in long-term outcomes was found after open or miniopen rotator cuff repair. Arthroscopic acromioplasty with a miniopen approach to the rotator cuff led to improved outcome scores at 3-month postoperative follow-up. Level of evidence: I.

4. Zumstein MA, Jost B, Hempel J, Hodler J, Gerber C: The clinical and structural long-term results of open repair of massive tears of the rotator cuff. *J Bone Joint Surg Am* 2008;90(11):2423-2431.

   Patients had improvement 3 to 10 years after massive rotator cuff tears were treated in an open fashion, despite a 57% rate of retearing and an increase in tear size and fatty infiltration.

5. Morse K, Davis AD, Afra R, Kaye EK, Schepsis A, Voloshin I: Arthroscopic versus mini-open rotator cuff repair: A comprehensive review and meta-analysis. *Am J Sports Med* 2008;36(9):1824-1828.

   A meta-analysis compared the results of arthroscopic and miniopen rotator cuff repairs at a minimum 1-year and average 2-year follow-up. There was no statistical difference in functional outcomes or complications.

6. Ramsey ML, Getz CL, Parsons BO: What's new in shoulder and elbow surgery. *J Bone Joint Surg Am* 2009;91(5):1283-1293.

   A review of 2007 and 2008 articles highlighted new and emerging evidence and trends in treating shoulder and elbow disease.

7. Boileau P, Baqué F, Valerio L, Ahrens P, Chuinard C, Trojani C: Isolated arthroscopic biceps tenotomy or te-

3: The Rotator Cuff

nodesis improves symptoms in patients with massive irreparable rotator cuff tears. *J Bone Joint Surg Am* 2007;89(4):747-757.

After isolated biceps tenotomy in selected patients with an irreparable rotator cuff tear, 78% were satisfied with the result and had an overall statistical improvement in Constant score. An intact teres minor was an important factor for success. Level of evidence:III.

8. Millett PJ, Horan MP, Maland KE, Hawkins RJ: Long-term survivorship and outcomes after surgical repair of full-thickness rotator cuff tears. *J Shoulder Elbow Surg* 2011;20(4):591-597.

At 5- or 10-year follow-up after open treatment of rotator cuff tears, survivorship was 94% or 83%, respectively. Survivorship rates and outcomes scores were higher after repair of single-tendon tears than after chronic tears and tears involving the subscapularis. Level of evidence: IV.

9. Nho SJ, Shindle MK, Sherman SL, Freedman KB, Lyman S, MacGillivray JD: Systematic review of arthroscopic rotator cuff repair and mini-open rotator cuff repair. *J Bone Joint Surg Am* 2007;89(suppl 3): 127-136.

A systematic review found no statistically significant differences in functional or clinical outcomes or complication rates after arthroscopic or miniopen rotator cuff repairs at a mean 24-month follow-up. There was a slightly higher percentage of complications after miniopen repair.

10. Milano G, Grasso A, Salvatore M, Zarelli D, Deriu L, Fabbriciani C: Arthroscopic rotator cuff repair with and without subacromial decompression: A prospective randomized study. *Arthroscopy* 2007;23(1):81-88.

In the short term, there was no statistical difference in the outcomes of rotator cuff repair with or without subacromial decompression, with consideration of age, gender, dominance, location, shape, area, retraction, reducibility, and fatty infiltration. Level of evidence: I.

11. Castagna A, Conti M, Markopoulos N, et al: Arthroscopic repair of rotator cuff tear with a modified Mason-Allen stitch: Mid-term clinical and ultrasound outcomes. *Knee Surg Sports Traumatol Arthrosc* 2008; 16(5):497-503.

At a minimum 24-month follow-up of 29 patients treated arthroscopically for an isolated supraspinatus tear with a single anchor and modified Mason-Allen stitch, Constant scores improved significantly, and the retear rate was 38%.

12. Lorbach O, Bachelier F, Vees J, Kohn D, Pape D: Cyclic loading of rotator cuff reconstructions: Single-row repair with modified suture configurations versus double-row repair. *Am J Sports Med* 2008;36(8):1504-1510.

A biomechanical study of single- and double-row suture configurations for rotator cuff repair in a porcine model found that double-row repair with corkscrew anchors had the greatest pull-out strength.

13. Nelson CO, Sileo MJ, Grossman MG, Serra-Hsu F: Single-row modified Mason-Allen versus double-row arthroscopic rotator cuff repair: A biomechanical and surface area comparison. *Arthroscopy* 2008;24(8): 941-948.

A biomechanical study comparing the strength and the contact surface area of a single-row modified Mason-Allen suture configuration and a double-row arthroscopic configuration found no difference in strength. The surface area was better with the double-row technique.

14. Ko SH, Friedman D, Seo DK, Jun HM, Warner JJ: A prospective therapeutic comparison of simple suture repairs to massive cuff stitch repairs for treatment of small- and medium-sized rotator cuff tears. *Arthroscopy* 2009;25(6):583-589, e1-e4.

Clinical outcomes were not significantly different in single row rotator cuff repairs using a massive rotator cuff stitch or a simple stitch. The massive rotator cuff stitch had superior integrity on follow-up ultrasound examination. Level of evidence: III.

15. Barber FA, Herbert MA, Schroeder FA, Aziz-Jacobo J, Mays MM, Rapley JH: Biomechanical advantages of triple-loaded suture anchors compared with double-row rotator cuff repairs. *Arthroscopy* 2010;26(3): 316-323.

A biomechanical study of two single-row and three double-row repair techniques found that a single row of triple-loaded anchors was more resistant to gap formation than any double-row repair. The addition of a ripstop stitch enhanced stretch resistance.

16. Milano G, Grasso A, Salvatore M, Saccomanno MF, Deriu L, Fabbriciani C: Arthroscopic rotator cuff repair with metal and biodegradable suture anchors: A prospective randomized study. *Arthroscopy* 2010; 26(9, suppl):S112-S119.

No difference was found between metal and biodegradable suture anchors when individual patient variables were accounted for. Level of evidence: I.

17. Strauss E, Frank D, Kubiak E, Kummer F, Rokito A: The effect of the angle of suture anchor insertion on fixation failure at the tendon-suture interface after rotator cuff repair: Deadman's angle revisited. *Arthroscopy* 2009;25(6):597-602.

A biomechanical study compared pull-out strength and gap formation in suture anchors inserted at 45° and 90°. Anchors inserted at 90° had better cyclic load to failure and gap formation.

18. Garofalo R, Castagna A, Borroni M, Krishnan SG: Arthroscopic transosseous (anchorless) rotator cuff repair. *Knee Surg Sports Traumatol Arthrosc* 2012; 20(6):1031-1035.

Dedicated single-use instrumentation was used to reliably and reproducibly create bone tunnels and pass sutures through the greater tuberosity for a purely arthroscopic transosseous rotator cuff repair. Preliminary results were reported. Level of evidence: V.

19. Ahmad CS, Kleweno C, Jacir AM, et al: Biomechanical performance of rotator cuff repairs with humeral rotation: A new rotator cuff repair failure model. *Am J Sports Med* 2008;36(5):888-892.

    A biomechanical study compared gap formation in single-row and double-row repairs in neutral, 45° internal, and 45° external rotation. Gapping was less in double-row than single-row repairs. Gapping was greater in internal rotation than in external rotation and was least in neutral.

20. Baums MH, Buchhorn GH, Gilbert F, Spahn G, Schultz W, Klinger HM: Initial load-to-failure and failure analysis in single- and double-row repair techniques for rotator cuff repair. *Arch Orthop Trauma Surg* 2010;130(9):1193-1199.

    A biomechanical study compared single-row repair (Mason-Allen stitches) and double-row repair (single-row repair plus medial horizontal mattress stitches) using polyester or polyblend suture material. The double-row technique was superior with both suture types.

21. Baums MH, Spahn G, Steckel H, Fischer A, Schultz W, Klinger HM: Comparative evaluation of the tendon-bone interface contact pressure in different single- versus double-row suture anchor repair techniques. *Knee Surg Sports Traumatol Arthrosc* 2009;17(12):1466-1472.

    A biomechanical study examined time-zero contact pressures for three single-row and two double-row suture configurations. Contact pressures and footprint coverage were superior with the double-row techniques and the use of arthroscopic Mason-Allen sutures in a single-row construct.

22. Milano G, Grasso A, Zarelli D, Deriu L, Cillo M, Fabbriciani C: Comparison between single-row and double-row rotator cuff repair: A biomechanical study. *Knee Surg Sports Traumatol Arthrosc* 2008;16(1):75-80.

    A biomechanical study compared single-row and double-row rotator cuff repairs with or without tension on the tendon. Single-row repair under tension was significantly inferior to the other repairs in displacement under cyclic loading.

23. Mahar A, Tamborlane J, Oka R, Esch J, Pedowitz RA: Single-row suture anchor repair of the rotator cuff is biomechanically equivalent to double-row repair in a bovine model. *Arthroscopy* 2007;23(12):1265-1270.

    A biomechanical study in a bovine model that compared single-row and double-row repairs found no statistical differences in repair elongation or load to failure.

24. Grasso A, Milano G, Salvatore M, Falcone G, Deriu L, Fabbriciani C: Single-row versus double-row arthroscopic rotator cuff repair: A prospective randomized clinical study. *Arthroscopy* 2009;25(1):4-12.

    A short-term comparison of clinical outcomes after double-row or single-row arthroscopic repair found no statistical differences between the two groups at

25. Burks RT, Crim J, Brown N, Fink B, Greis PE: A prospective randomized clinical trial comparing arthroscopic single- and double-row rotator cuff repair: Magnetic resonance imaging and early clinical evaluation. *Am J Sports Med* 2009;37(4):674-682.

    At 1-year follow-up, a comparison of arthroscopic double-row and single-row rotator cuff repairs found no difference in clinical outcomes or on MRI. One retear occurred in each patient group. Level of evidence: I.

26. Franceschi F, Ruzzini L, Longo UG, et al: Equivalent clinical results of arthroscopic single-row and double-row suture anchor repair for rotator cuff tears: A randomized controlled trial. *Am J Sports Med* 2007;35(8):1254-1260.

    At 2-year follow-up, there were no differences in clinical results or healing rates after single-row or double-row arthroscopic rotator cuff repair. The double-row repairs had greater integrity on MRI. Level of evidence: I.

27. Charousset C, Grimberg J, Duranthon LD, Bellaiche L, Petrover D: Can a double-row anchorage technique improve tendon healing in arthroscopic rotator cuff repair? A prospective, nonrandomized, comparative study of double-row and single-row anchorage techniques with computed tomographic arthrography tendon healing assessment. *Am J Sports Med* 2007;35(8):1247-1253.

    At 6-month follow-up, clinical results and healing (assessed on CT) were compared after double-row or single-row rotator cuff repair. There were no differences, except the double-row repair had superior healing. Level of evidence: II.

28. Sugaya H, Maeda K, Matsuki K, Moriishi J: Repair integrity and functional outcome after arthroscopic double-row rotator cuff repair: A prospective outcome study. *J Bone Joint Surg Am* 2007;89(5):953-960.

    At an average 14-month follow-up, healing of double-row rotator cuff repairs was evaluated using MRI. Retearing rates were 5% for small to medium-sized tears and 40% for large to massive tears. Level of evidence: IV.

29. Aydin N, Kocaoglu B, Guven O: Single-row versus double-row arthroscopic rotator cuff repair in small- to medium-sized tears. *J Shoulder Elbow Surg* 2010;19(5):722-725.

    At a minimum 2-year follow-up, the clinical outcomes of single-row and double-row rotator cuff repairs were compared. All shoulders had functional improvement, with no significant difference in clinical outcomes. Level of evidence: II.

30. Koh KH, Kang KC, Lim TK, Shon MS, Yoo JC: Prospective randomized clinical trial of single- versus double-row suture anchor repair in 2- to 4-cm rotator cuff tears: Clinical and magnetic resonance imaging results. *Arthroscopy* 2011;27(4):453-462.

2 years when individual patient factors were considered. Level of evidence: I.

Clinical and MRI outcomes of large to massive rotator cuff tears were compared after single-row or double-row repair. There were no differences in clinical outcomes or rates of retearing on MRI. Level of evidence: I.

31. Park JY, Lhee SH, Choi JH, Park HK, Yu JW, Seo JB: Comparison of the clinical outcomes of single- and double-row repairs in rotator cuff tears. *Am J Sports Med* 2008;36(7):1310-1316.

   A comparison of clinical outcomes after single-row or double-row rotator cuff repair found no significant differences in scores on three measures at 2-year follow-up. Level of evidence: II.

32. Pennington WT, Gibbons DJ, Bartz BA, et al: Comparative analysis of single-row versus double-row repair of rotator cuff tears. *Arthroscopy* 2010;26(11):1419-1426.

   No clinical difference was found in a comparison of clinical outcomes and MRI-assessed healing after double-row rotator cuff repair or single-row repair using a massive cuff stitch. The healing of similar-size tears was better after double-row repair. Level of evidence: III.

33. Ma HL, Chiang ER, Wu HT, et al: Clinical outcome and imaging of arthroscopic single-row and double-row rotator cuff repair: A prospective randomized trial. *Arthroscopy* 2012;28(1):16-24.

   Clinical outcome, muscle strength, and repair integrity were compared after single-row or double-row rotator cuff repair. At 6-month and 2-year follow-up, the strength of larger tears was significantly better after double-row repair. No other differences were found. Level of evidence: II.

34. Krishnan SG, Harkins DC, Schiffern SC, Pennington SD, Burkhead WZ: Arthroscopic repair of full-thickness tears of the rotator cuff in patients younger than 40 years. *Arthroscopy* 2008;24(3):324-328.

   At a minimum 2-year follow-up, clinical outcomes of rotator cuff repair were evaluated in patients younger than 40 years. Almost all of the tears were traumatic. All of the tears improved, with 90% of the patients returning to their previous level of activity. Level of evidence: IV.

35. Sano H, Yamashita T, Wakabayashi I, Itoi E: Stress distribution in the supraspinatus tendon after tendon repair: Suture anchors versus transosseous suture fixation. *Am J Sports Med* 2007;35(4):542-546.

   A biomechanical study compared stress distribution within the tendon after single-row, double-row, or transosseous repair. The concentrations of stress were significantly higher with suture anchor repair than with transosseous repair.

36. Kim KC, Rhee KJ, Shin HD, Kim YM: Arthroscopic transosseous rotator cuff repair. *Orthopedics* 2008; 31(4):327-330.

   A technique was described for using an anterior cruciate ligament guide to pass transosseous sutures

through the greater tuberosity to repair the rotator cuff. The technique is recommended in the presence of osteoporotic bone that is unable to hold an anchor.

37. Frick H, Haag M, Volz M, Stehle J: Arthroscopic bone needle: A new, safe, and cost-effective technique for rotator cuff repair. *Tech Shoulder Surg* 2010;11: 107-112.

   A technique for arthroscopic use of a bone needle to pass sutures transosseously reduced the cost of surgery by 80%. The mean Constant score normalized for age and sex was 92% at 1-year follow-up.

38. Park MC, Tibone JE, ElAttrache NS, Ahmad CS, Jun BJ, Lee TQ: Part II: Biomechanical assessment for a footprint-restoring transosseous-equivalent rotator cuff repair technique compared with a double-row repair technique. *J Shoulder Elbow Surg* 2007;16(4): 469-476.

   A biomechanical study compared transosseous-equivalent and double-row techniques by measuring stiffness, gap formation, and ultimate load to failure. Stiffness and gap formation were not significantly different. The transosseous-equivalent repair had a greater load to failure.

39. Voigt C, Bosse C, Vosshenrich R, Schulz AP, Lill H: Arthroscopic supraspinatus tendon repair with suture-bridging technique: Functional outcome and magnetic resonance imaging. *Am J Sports Med* 2010;38(5): 983-991.

   Suture bridge treatment of rotator cuff tears led to clinical outcomes and retearing rates similar to those of published double-row repair studies at 4-month, 1-year, and mean 2-year follow-up. Level of evidence: IV.

40. Mihata T, Watanabe C, Fukunishi K, et al: Functional and structural outcomes of single-row versus double-row versus combined double-row and suture-bridge repair for rotator cuff tears. *Am J Sports Med* 2011; 39(10):2091-2098.

   A large study comparing the functional and structural outcomes of three anchor-based techniques for rotator cuff repair found that the combined double-row and suture bridge technique had a significantly lower retearing rate for massive cuff tears compared with single-row and double-row repairs. Level of evidence: III.

41. Zheng N, Harris HW, Andrews JR: Failure analysis of rotator cuff repair: A comparison of three double-row techniques. *J Bone Joint Surg Am* 2008;90(5):1034-1042.

   A biomechanical study of double-row repair using anchors medially with three different techniques for the lateral row found a significantly higher failure rate with the anchor lateral techniques than the Mason-Allen transosseous technique.

42. Frank JB, ElAttrache NS, Dines JS, Blackburn A, Crues J, Tibone JE: Repair site integrity after arthroscopic transosseous-equivalent suture-bridge rotator cuff repair. *Am J Sports Med* 2008;36(8):1496-1503.

Healing after suture bridge rotator cuff repair was evaluated on MRI at a minimum 1-year follow-up. Supraspinatus tears had healed in 89% of patients, supraspinatus-infraspinatus tears had healed in 86%, and massive tears had healed in 100%. Level of evidence: IV.

43. Tocci SL, Tashjian RZ, Leventhal E, Spenciner DB, Green A, Fleming BC: Biomechanical comparison of single-row arthroscopic rotator cuff repair technique versus transosseous repair technique. *J Shoulder Elbow Surg* 2008;17(5):808-814.

A biomechanical study compared arthroscopic single-row repair and Mason-Allen transosseous repair in rotator cuff tears of different sizes. Gapping was greater in massive tears and occurred posteriorly. There were no technique-based differences in gapping.

3: The Rotator Cuff

Chapter 16

Massive Rotator Cuff Tears

Daniel M. Hampton, MD   Ruth A. Delaney, MB BCh, MRCS   Laurence D. Higgins, MD

Introduction

The term massive rotator cuff tear has not been precisely defined, although a variety of definitions and classifications have been proposed. Some are based on a maximum tear diameter of more than 5 cm, and others are based on complete detachment of at least two tendons.[1,2] Because of the variety in definitions, it can be difficult to directly compare studies. A massive tear is caused by an acute injury only occasionally . Most occur as sequelae of chronic rotator cuff tears. An acute-on-chronic massive tear occurs when a traumatic event causes enlargement of a preexisting smaller tear.[3] The prevalence of massive rotator cuff tears ranges from 10% to 40%.[1]

A chronic rotator cuff tear is associated with significant fatty infiltration of the muscles and tendon retraction, both of which make a repair more complicated, and they contribute to making some massive tears irreparable. Not all massive rotator cuff tears are irreparable, and not all irreparable rotator cuff tears are massive. Most patients with a massive rotator cuff tear have significant weakness that contributes to their disability. As a consequence, younger patients experience more disability than older patients. The literature suggests that massive posterosuperior tears (involving the supraspinatus and the infraspinatus) are more common than anterosuperior tears involving the supraspinatus and the subscapularis.[4]

Dr. Higgins or an immediate family member has received nonincome support (such as equipment or services), commercially derived honoraria, or other nonresearch related funding (such as paid travel) from Arthrex, Smith & Nephew, Breg, and DePuy and serves as a board member, owner, officer, or committee member of the American Shoulder and Elbow Surgeons, the Arthroscopy Association of North America, the American Academy of Orthopaedic Surgeons, and the Advocacy for Improvement in Mobility. Neither of the following authors nor any immediate family member has received anything of value from or has stock or stock options held in a commercial company or institution related directly or indirectly to the subject of this chapter: Dr. Hampton and Dr. Delaney.

Biomechanics

The biomechanical function of the rotator cuff is to keep the humeral head centered in the glenoid during movement.[5-7] The stage at which the biomechanics of the normal force couple are altered is not known, however. In a recent cadaver study, the progression of a tear of the entire supraspinatus into the infraspinatus marked the critical stage for significant changes in humeral head kinematics.[8] A tear of the entire supraspinatus without infraspinatus involvement decreased abduction capability at high loads, but humeral head kinematics were not disrupted. These findings suggest that a balanced force couple is maintained in the setting of an isolated supraspinatus tear.

Natural History

The natural history of massive rotator cuff tears has not been well described. Most of our knowledge has been gained by examining the results of nonsurgical treatments, such as pain medication and physical therapy. These results may not reflect the true natural history of massive rotator cuff tears and instead may reflect significant bias because the patients elected not to undergo surgery or had an irreparable tear. Nonetheless, MRI studies found that the size of the tear increased by a mean 3.29 cm during nonsurgical treatment.[2,3] Fatty infiltration significantly increases with Goutallier grade progression of supraspinatus, infraspinatus, and subscapularis involvement. Repairable tears progress to irreparable tears; in one study, 50% of the initially repairable tears progressed to become irreparable as a result of an increase in fatty infiltration and a decrease in the acromiohumeral interval to less than 7 mm. The acromiohumeral interval decreased by a mean of 2.6 mm. In addition, the altered biomechanics of a massive rotator cuff tear led to a radiographic increase in the stage of glenohumeral osteoarthritis. Importantly, several risk factors for progression were identified; the number of ruptured tendons, tear size, and abduction weakness were correlated with increased severity of glenohumeral arthritis, stage of fatty infiltration, and acromiohumeral distance.[3,9]

3: The Rotator Cuff

Clinical Evaluation

Patients usually report pain and weakness. Symptomatic tears often are painful at night and during activities of daily living. Depending on the size of the tear, the patient may have pseudoparalysis, which is defined as an inability to elevate the arm to 90°or higher if the patient has an unrestricted passive range of glenohumeral motion and no neurologic impairment.[10] However, the extent of weakness varies, as does the loss of range of motion. It is important to determine whether the pain reported by the patient is indeed the result of a massive tear. Pain from a cause such as adhesive capsulitis, cervical spine disease, biceps tendon disease, or acromioclavicular arthritis can mimic pain from a rotator cuff tear. Pain associated with a rotator cuff tear typically is located on the anterolateral aspect of the shoulder and often radiates distally toward the deltoid insertion. Pain radiating below the elbow to the hand should raise suspicion of cervical radiculopathy or peripheral nerve compression.

The examination always should begin with an inspection of both shoulders without obstructive clothing. Marked atrophy of the supraspinatus and/or the infraspinatus fossae often is present with a massive tear and often can be easily seen but may be more easily palpated. The active and passive range of motion should be recorded and compared with that of the unaffected side. The differences between passive and active motion can provide important clues as to the functioning of the rotator cuff. It is vital to observe scapular kinematics during active motion. Scapular substitution often is present in a patient with a massive tear and should be noted. Strength testing of the rotator cuff muscles should be performed, and lag signs should be evaluated. Anterosuperior tears tend to cause weakness during internal rotation and painful weakness in elevation. Posterosuperior tears cause weakness during elevation and external rotation.

Several clinical signs portend a poor prognosis for repair. Static anterosuperior subluxation of the humeral head under the skin is a sign of a large anterosuperior tear that cannot be repaired. A tear with dynamic anterosuperior subluxation during resisted abduction also has a poor repair prognosis. Pseudoparalysis and a true drop arm sign indicate severe disease with fatty infiltration of the infraspinatus classified as Goutallier grade 2 or higher.[11,12] A positive hornblower sign indicates that the teres minor has undergone significant fatty infiltration, and repair will not succeed.[13]

In summary, static or dynamic subluxation and chronic substantial lag signs are predictors of an irreparable rotator cuff tear. Although the clinician can measure weakness and correlate it with the disability level, ultimately, the patient must determine whether the current condition is acceptable or must be improved. Further treatment should be pursued only if the patient does not wish to accept the current level of disability or it is possible to halt a highly likely progression of disability.

Table 1

The Hamada Classification of the Acromiohumeral Interval

Grade	Status of the Acromiohumeral Interval
1	Normal (7 to 14 mm)
2	Narrowing
3	Narrowing, with acetabulization of the acromion
4	Narrowing, with acetabulization of the acromion and glenohumeral joint narrowing[a]
5	Narrowing, with acetabulization of the acromion and humeral head collapse

[a] In the Walch classification, 4A = glenohumeral arthritis without subacromial arthritis, and 4B = glenohumeral arthritis with subacromial arthritis.

Imaging

Plain radiographs are the first imaging for a patient with shoulder pain. Radiographs provide information on the status of the glenohumeral joint and the humeral head position, the acromioclavicular joint, and acromial morphology. A true AP view of the shoulder (Grashey view), a scapular Y view (outlet view), and an axillary view are standard for evaluating suspected rotator cuff pathology. On the Grashey view, proximal migration of the humeral head can be observed and quantified.[1]

The acromiohumeral interval is used to quantify the extent of proximal migration.[14] In a healthy shoulder, the normal range is 7 to 14 mm. The acromiohumeral interval was found to be correlated with the size of the rotator cuff tear. The Hamada classification system for the acromiohumeral interval, ranging from grade 1 to grade 5, was modified slightly to divide grade 4 into two subtypes[15,16] (**Table 1**). As the acromiohumeral interval decreases in size (and increases in grade), the extent of fatty infiltration of the rotator cuff muscles increases. A recent review found that in patients who underwent repair of a grade 1 or 2 massive tear, the retearing rate was higher among those with a grade 2 tear. However, none of the repaired tears progressed to grade 3 or higher.[17]

CT or MRI can be useful for precisely identifying the size of the tear, the number of torn tendons, tendon retraction, tissue quality, bony morphology, and fatty infiltration of the muscle bellies. MRI has become the mainstay of soft-tissue evaluation of the shoulder. A rotator cuff tear can be reliably identified and characterized on MRI. If the patient cannot undergo MRI, CT arthrography can be used to obtain good-quality information. CT arthrography was used in developing the initial Goutallier scale for characterizing fatty infiltration of the muscle[18] (**Table 2**). MRI also can be used to assess fatty infiltration; the sagittal T1 sequence is best for evaluating muscle fat content, although the cuts

Table 2

The Goutallier Classification of Fatty Infiltration

Grade	Extent of Fatty Infiltration
0	Normal muscle
1	Some fatty streaks
2	Less fat than muscle
3	Equal amounts of fat and muscle
4	More fat than muscle

must be sufficiently medial for visualizing the muscle belly[19] (**Figure 1**). Severe muscle retraction can cause bunching of the muscle and lead to an underestimation of the extent of fatty infiltration. Recent work has cast doubt on the interobserver and intraobserver reliability of the classification system, however.[20]

The extent of fatty infiltration is an important prognostic indicator for repair. The outcome for a patient with grade 3 or 4 infiltration is likely to be inferior to that of a patient with less fatty infiltration.[12,20] However, a review of 22 patients with grade 3 or 4 infiltration found that some patients had clinical improvement after repair.[21] Despite this finding, most researchers agree that the clinical and radiographic results of surgery are worse with high-grade fatty infiltration. Most studies report consistently superior results in patients whose fatty infiltration is grade 2 or lower.[22,23]

Increased tendon retraction is associated with high grades of fatty infiltration (**Figure 2**). A recent study found that most musculotendinous retraction is from the muscle fibers themselves if the fatty infiltration is grade 3 or lower. Tendon shortening appears to occur only with grade 2 or 3 and higher, and all tendon shortening in grade 3 or 4 appears to come from the tendon. This finding implies that anatomic repair of the tendon, if possible, cannot anatomically restore the muscle-tendon unit in the presence of high-grade fatty infiltration.[24]

Ultrasound is now being used to evaluate the rotator cuff. The advantages of portable shoulder ultrasound are its low cost, noninvasive nature, absence of adverse effects, ability to visualize the rotator cuff dynamically during physiologic motion, and the immediate availability of results. Ultrasound cannot penetrate bone and therefore does not provide much information on large rotator cuff tears if the tendons have retracted medial to the acromion. The accuracy of the evaluation is highly dependent on the experience and the skill of the operator.[25] Recent studies have found a positive predictive value of 96% and a negative predictive value of 95% when the operator was experienced. When tear size was quantified as small (less than 1 cm), medium (1 to 3 cm), or large or massive (more than 3 cm), the size of the larger tears was found to be estimated with greater accuracy.[26]

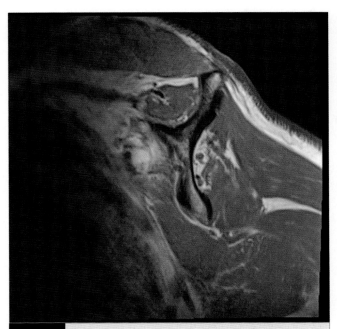

Figure 1   T1-weighted sagittal MRI of the scapular Y, showing significant fatty infiltration of the infraspinatus.

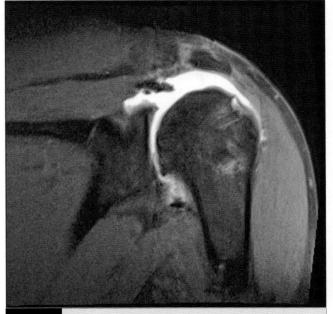

Figure 2   MRI showing substantial retraction of the supraspinatus.

Nonsurgical Treatment

Nonsurgical management may be appropriate for a massive rotator cuff tear in certain circumstances.[3,27] The natural history of massive rotator cuff tears was examined in a retrospective review of 19 consecutive patients, all of whom underwent a standardized

3: The Rotator Cuff

rehabilitation protocol.[3] Nonsurgical treatment was chosen if a patient had low functional demands or refused surgery. At a mean 4-year follow-up, the mean relative Constant score was 83%, the mean Subjective Shoulder Value was 68%, and range of motion was preserved. Glenohumeral arthritis progressed, the acromiohumeral distance decreased, the size of the tendon tear increased, and fatty infiltration increased. Fifty percent of the tears classified as repairable at diagnosis had become irreparable at follow-up. The researchers concluded that moderately symptomatic patients with a massive rotator cuff tear can maintain satisfactory shoulder function after nonsurgical management despite the progression of structural changes. However, they cautioned that a repairable tear may become symptomatic and irreparable. At that point, the surgical treatment options may be limited to technically demanding tendon transfers, open or arthroscopic débridement with limited possibility of success, and reverse total shoulder arthroplasty.

A structured anterior deltoid rehabilitation program was recommended for managing a massive rotator cuff tear in a patient who was medically unable to undergo surgery.[27] A prospective assessment of 17 patients with a massive rotator cuff tear and Goutallier grade 4 fatty infiltration of the supraspinatus and the infraspinatus found improvement in the mean Constant score from 26 to 63 after a structured anterior deltoid rehabilitation program. All components of shoulder motion improved, particularly forward elevation. In most patients, the stabilizing effect of recruiting the anterior deltoid achieved adequate improvement in function and pain. The researchers stated that structured anterior deltoid rehabilitation, in combination with pain medication, should be the first treatment of a massive rotator cuff tear in a patient of advanced age with significant comorbidities.

Débridement and Subacromial Decompression

The goal of surgically relieving pain from a massive, irreparable rotator cuff tear has led to interest in the débridement of massive tears with or without acromioplasty or subacromial decompression. These techniques may not yield functional benefit in terms of strength or range of motion, but they can provide significant pain relief, particularly for a patient with relatively low physical demands. The patient may have secondary functional gains related to decreased pain, especially if other pain generators, such as the biceps tendon, also are treated.[16]

Thirty-one patients (mean age, 70.6 years) underwent arthroscopic débridement of an irreparable rotator cuff tear.[28] Twenty-four of the patients also underwent a biceps tenotomy. To preserve the coracoacromial arch, acromioplasty was not performed. At a mean 47-month follow-up, the mean American Shoulder and Elbow Surgeons Disability Index score had significantly improved from 24.0 to

69.8, and the pain score on visual analog scale had improved from 7.8 to 2.9. The Constant score for the surgically treated shoulder was significantly lower than that for the contralateral shoulder. The result was rated as excellent by 10 patients (32%), good by 7 (22%), average by 9 (29%), and poor by 5 (16%). As with nonsurgical management, radiographic deterioration was evident at follow-up: glenohumeral osteoarthritis had progressed in 10 patients (32%), and the mean acromiohumeral distance had decreased from 8.3 mm to 7.0 mm. Overall, the patients had significant functional improvement despite radiographic progression of degenerative changes.

Anteroinferior partial acromioplasty, as described by Neer,[4] has become an arthroscopic procedure.[4,29] With experience in this procedure, the importance of the coracoacromial arch was discovered, and superior humeral head migration was recognized as a potential complication of acromioplasty in the presence of a massive rotator cuff tear. In a cadaver study of seven shoulders, anterosuperior humeral head translation was measured after the sequential application of an anterosuperior 150-N load in five scenarios: the intact coracoacromial ligament, subperiosteal coracoacromial ligament release, standard acromioplasty, coracoacromial reconstruction, and modified Neer acromioplasty.[30] A significant decrease in anterosuperior migration was found after coracoacromial ligament reconstruction compared with anterior acromioplasty or modified Neer acromioplasty. The researchers deduced that reconstruction of the coracoacromial ligament may provide the necessary stabilizing force in a massive rotator cuff tear to prevent excessive anterosuperior translation and possible humeral head escape from the coracoacromial arch. Only minimal bone should be resected during acromioplasty, and the coracoacromial ligament should be preserved where possible. The researchers also recommended that if the coracoacromial ligament cannot be preserved, anatomic reconstruction of its medial band is warranted. In 16 patients undergoing repair of a massive rotator cuff tear,[31] the coracoacromial ligament was repaired with bone sutures to the acromion. Eight of the 10 patients available for follow-up had a satisfactory result and were able to perform overhead activities, but 2 patients had an unsatisfactory result. Anterosuperior humeral head subluxation did not occur. Although the tears in this study were not irreparable, acromioplasty with coracoacromial ligament preservation or repair was found to maintain some of the passive stabilizing effect of the coracoacromial arch.

In 2002, a procedure was introduced for treating massive, irreparable rotator cuff tears and preserving the coracoacromial ligament. The procedure, described as a tuberoplasty, involves removing exostoses on the humerus and reshaping the greater tuberosity to create a smooth, congruent acromiohumeral articulation. An acromioplasty is not performed. The acromion and the coracoacromial ligament are left intact until a decision is made about the reparability of the cuff; it is vital to

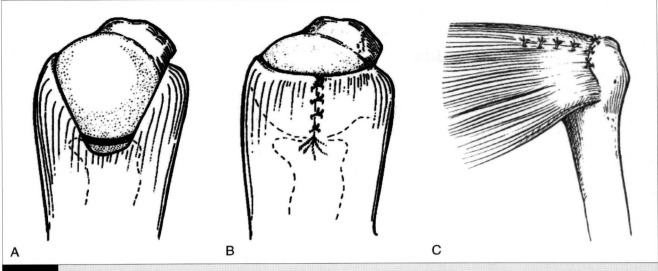

Figure 3 Schematic drawings showing a U-shaped rotator cuff tear (**A**), a partial side-to-side repair (**B**), and the placement of side-to-side sutures and repair of the free margin of the cuff to bone with suture anchors (**C**). During the repair, margin convergence of the tear toward the greater tuberosity increases the cross-sectional area and decreases the length of the tear, thereby decreasing strain. (Reproduced with permission from Burkhart SS: Arthroscopic treatment of massive rotator cuff tears. *Clin Orthop Relat Res* 2001;390:107-118.)

make this determination before the coracoacromial arch is violated. Twenty patients treated with this procedure had disabling preoperative pain and a tear of at least 5 cm involving both the supraspinatus and the infraspinatus; 2 patients also had a partial subscapularis tear. In all patients, rotator cuff repair was abandoned because of excessive retraction and/or poor tissue quality after mobilization. At a minimum 27-month follow-up of 19 patients, the result was excellent in 12 patients, good in 6, and fair in 1. Thirteen patients (68%) were totally pain free, and no patient had night pain after surgery. All patients had residual external rotation weakness. The results clearly showed improvement in pain and function but were inferior to those achieved with acromioplasty and repair of the rotator cuff. The study concluded that in selected patients with a massive, irreparable rotator cuff tear, the importance of the acromion and the coracoacromial ligament cannot be overemphasized, despite their role in the pathogenesis of impingement syndrome.[32]

Débridement of a massive rotator cuff tear and subacromial decompression are inferior to repair of the rotator cuff but may have a role in patients with low physical demands for whom pain relief is the priority and functional goals are limited. The results deteriorate over time, however. A satisfactory result is most likely to be achieved if the patient has an intact posterior rotator cuff before surgery, as indicated by integrity of the deltoid and good external rotation strength.

Partial Repair and Margin Convergence

The term margin convergence describes the side-to-side closure of a massive, U-shaped rotator cuff tear. Most massive rotator cuff tears are not retracted but instead are L shaped with a vertical split from medial to lateral, which assumes a U shape because of the elasticity of the muscle-tendon unit.[33] Repair using a combination of side-to-side tendon-to-tendon sutures and end-on tendon-to-bone sutures was recommended beginning in the 1940s. Mobilization of these tears leads to repair failure because of tension overload at the apex of the tear, but side-to-side closure provides a mechanical advantage because of the biomechanical principle of margin convergence. In margin convergence, the free margin of the tear converges toward the greater tuberosity as side-to-side repair progresses (**Figure 3**). As the margin converges, the strain at the free edge of the cuff is significantly reduced, leaving an almost tension-free converged cuff margin overlying the humeral bone bed for repair. Side-to-side closure of two thirds of a U-shaped tear reduces the strain at the cuff margin to one sixth of the strain at the preconverged cuff margin. The use of this repair lowers the risk of failure of a fixation to bone by anchors or transosseous tunnels. The medial margin of a massive, U-shaped tear should not be sufficiently mobilized from the glenoid and the scapular neck for pulling over to the humeral bone bed; such a mobilization would lead to large tensile forces in the middle of the repaired cuff margin that would predispose the repair to failure.

The principles of margin convergence and force couples must be followed when attempting repair of a massive rotator cuff tear. Partial repair, in which a defect remains in the superior portion of the cuff after margin convergence, can be effective if at least half of the infraspinatus can be repaired to bone. Partial repair is recommended if complete closure of the defect is not possible, but local transfers of rotator cuff tendons

3: The Rotator Cuff

should not be done. In truly nonmobile tears, an interval slide sometimes allows an additional 1 to 2 cm of lateral excursion of the supraspinatus tendon and therefore permits a more complete partial repair.[34] The results of using this technique vary.

Partial repair was compared with no repair, infraspinatus repair, and two-tendon repair in 48 rats 4 weeks after detachment of the infraspinatus and the supraspinatus.[35] Quantitative ambulatory measures (medial-lateral forces, braking, propulsion, and step width) were significantly different in the rats with no repair or infraspinatus repair but were similar in those with infraspinatus or two-tendon repair. Repair of the infraspinatus back to its insertion site without repairing the supraspinatus was found to improve shoulder function to a similar extent as repair of both the infraspinatus and the supraspinatus by restoring the anterior-posterior force couple.

A cadaver study examined whether there was a biomechanical rationale for margin convergence in large, retracted rotator cuff tears. The supraspinatus muscle-tendon unit was removed in 20 cadaver shoulders to create a large retracted rotator cuff tear, and margin convergence was performed in an open fashion by placing simple sutures 5 mm apart beginning at the glenoid rim medially and proceeding laterally. Gap area was measured after each suture placement. Each suture produced statistically significant gap closure amounting to 50% after the first suture, 60% after the second, 67% after the third, and 75% after the fourth suture ($P < 0.05$). Infraspinatus and supraspinatus strain was measured in each specimen in the intact state, after supraspinatus removal, after each convergence suture was placed, and in different positions of rotation and abduction. After suture placement, infraspinatus and subscapularis strain was found to be reduced, as much as 58% at all degrees of rotation at 0° of abduction ($P < 0.05$). As abduction was increased to 60°, the absolute strain values for all positions were reduced but the difference was not statistically significant except in the infraspinatus after the fourth margin convergence suture ($P < 0.05$). Testing also was conducted to calculate glenohumeral joint translation and measure tension in the rotator cuff itself during knot tying and gap closure. There was minimal tension and stress in the rotator cuff during knot tying, although infraspinatus and subscapularis strain increased slightly as the tendons were pulled together. The first margin convergence suture caused the greatest increase in intrinsic rotator cuff tension, with each subsequent suture having a similar but less dramatic effect. Mean humeral head anterior translation with four margin convergence sutures was 4.97 mm.[36] These results supported the hypothesis that margin convergence decreases the size of the tear gap and reduces strain, with minimal effect on glenohumeral translation and intrinsic tendon strain during knot tying.

Tendon Transfers

An irreparable tear can be defined as a tear in which direct tendon-to-bone repair and healing are not possible. Tendon transfers have gained acceptance as a treatment for such tears. Local tendon transposition, distant tendon transfer, and deltoid flap transposition have been proposed as methods of reconstructing the rotator cuff. A portion of the subscapularis and the teres major was used to cover a superior rotator cuff defect with limited success, but the results were not reproducible.[37] More reproducible and long-term success has been achieved by distant tendon transfer in the form of a latissimus dorsi transfer for a massive posterosuperior tear or a pectoralis major transfer for a less common anterosuperior tear.

Latissimus Dorsi Transfer

Latissimus dorsi transfer was proposed in 1988 for reconstructing tears that involve complete loss of the supraspinatus and the infraspinatus.[38] Conversion of the teres major and the latissimus dorsi into external rotators was earlier shown to be effective in children with brachial plexus birth palsy, and reconstruction of a massive rotator cuff tear was considered to be an analogous adult procedure.[39] The latissimus dorsi provides a large, vascularized tendon to close the rotator cuff defect, and the tendon was transferred from its insertion on the humeral shaft to the superolateral humeral head. The transfer of the latissimus dorsi to the superolateral humeral head converts the latissimus dorsi into a humeral head depressor by virtue of its almost-vertical orientation and into an external rotator by virtue of its insertion relative to the humeral head. The technique was used for 14 patients with massive rotator cuff tears, 9 of whom had a severe functional handicap. The rotator cuff could be closed with the aid of the latissimus dorsi in 10 of the patients. Postoperative electromyography in the first 11 patients confirmed normal suprascapular and thoracodorsal nerve function; 1 patient had innervated latissimus dorsi during shoulder flexion, and 3 patients had innervated latissimus dorsi during external rotation. Electromyographic studies suggested that the latissimus dorsi acted mainly by tenodesis to produce external rotation. These patients had promising results at 1-year follow-up, with gains in forward flexion, abduction, and control of external rotation in abduction, as well as a decrease in fatigability of the shoulder when the arm was used between the waist and shoulder levels. The teres major was not transferred with the latissimus dorsi because the teres major often was too bulky to pass under the deltoid, and the teres major tendon was considered to have insufficient amplitude and length.

A later study of 69 shoulders with a massive, irreparable rotator cuff tear showed that the latissimus dorsi transfer had positive long-term results. At mean 53-month follow-up, the average Subjective Shoulder Value had improved from 28% before surgery to 66%. The mean age- and sex-matched Constant-Murley score had improved from 55% to 73% ($P < 0.0001$). The pain score had improved from 6 to 12 of a possible 15 points ($P < 0.0001$). Flexion had increased from 104° to 123°, abduction from 101° to 119°, and external rotation from 22° to 29° ($P < 0.05$). Strength had increased from 0.9 to 1.8 kg ($P < 0.0001$). Thirteen patients had a deficient subscapularis before surgery, as evidenced by a positive lift-off test. These patients did not achieve the improvements in function and pain experienced by those with an intact subscapularis. The researchers concluded that latissimus dorsi transfer durably and substantially improves chronically painful, dysfunctional shoulders with an irreparable rotator cuff tear, especially if the subscapularis is intact. If subscapularis function is deficient, the procedure is of questionable benefit and probably should not be performed.[40]

Preoperative shoulder function and general strength were found to influence the outcome of a latissimus dorsi transfer.[41] In 14 patients who underwent latissimus dorsi transfer for a massive rotator cuff tear, women with poor shoulder function were most likely to have a poor result. The authors reported that the most significant predictors of outcome were preoperative active range of motion and strength in forward flexion and external rotation. Pseudoparalysis cannot be overcome by latissimus dorsi transfer and is considered a contraindication.

The result of 16 patients who underwent latissimus dorsi transfer as a salvage procedure after unsuccessful rotator cuff repair were compared with those of 6 patients who underwent the transfer as a primary procedure for the repair of a massive irreparable rotator cuff, based on a 7-year experience with this technique.[42] Of the 16 patients with a revision transfer, 3 had undergone more than one earlier rotator cuff repair, and 7 had undergone a distal clavicle resection. Patients in the two groups had comparable preoperative modified Constant scores (mean, 37% for patients in the primary group and 36% for those in the revision group). At a mean 25-month follow-up, the relative gain in forward flexion was 60° (range, 30° to 90°) for patients in the primary group and 43° (range, 15° to 75°) for those in the revision group. Six patients in the revision group had 90° of active forward flexion or less, but all patients in the primary group had at least 100° of flexion. Five of the 6 patients in the revision group were found to have deltoid detachment intraoperatively. The modified Constant score improved more than 30% in 6 patients in the primary group, but only 1 patient in the revision group had as much improvement. Poor tendon quality, severe fatty degeneration, and deltoid detachment were predictive of a poor outcome. Poor tendon quality and severe fatty degeneration were equally common among patients in the two groups, but deltoid detachment occurred only in patients undergoing revision surgery (in 7 of 16 patients). The differences in outcome between those with an injured deltoid and those with an intact deltoid were statistically significant, both within the revision group and between the revision and primary groups. Rupture of the transferred latissimus dorsi occurred in 1 of 6 patients in the primary group and 7 of 16 patients in the revision group, at a mean 19 months after surgery (range, 3 to 38 months). The overall 36% incidence of rupture reflected a 17% rate for patients in the primary group and a 44% rate for those in the revision group. Outcomes in the primary group of patients were comparable to those in the original study of latissimus dorsi transfer,[40] but they suggested that latissimus dorsi transfer leads to more limited gains in subjective and objective outcomes when used as a salvage procedure after unsuccessful rotator cuff repair. Almost 20% of the patients in the revision group reported a poor outcome. The researchers believed that deltoid deficiency profoundly affected clinical outcome in patients in the revision group, noting that all patients with deltoid deficiency had an unsuccessful earlier rotator cuff repair. Patient selection is important when latissimus dorsi transfer is used as a salvage procedure because concomitant shoulder pathology and its effect on shoulder function contribute to an inferior outcome. The rotator cuff tear configuration did not appear to influence the outcome. An intact deltoid was considered mandatory for the restoration of shoulder function.[42] Another study also found that deltoid function was linked to the extent of improvement with latissimus dorsi transfer after an unsuccessful rotator cuff repair.[43]

Relatively recent modifications of the latissimus dorsi transfer technique include harvesting of the tendon with a small piece of bone to enable direct transosseous bone-to-bone healing of the transfer, a single-incision technique, and a single-incision technique using a minimally invasive approach that exposes only the humeral tendon insertion and the site of transfer reinsertion.[44-47] Despite the theoretic advantages of these modifications, none of them has led to results superior to those of the original study. The latissimus dorsi tendon transfer can restore shoulder function, but it has not been shown to halt the progression of cuff tear arthropathy.

Pectoralis Major Transfer
A pectoralis major transfer is an option for treating a massive anterosuperior rotator cuff tear. Repair of a chronic subscapularis rupture can be challenging and has not had favorable results. In the initial study, transfer of the pectoralis minor in four patients and transfer of the pectoralis major in one patient after an unsuccessful Bristow procedure led to a good or excellent result.[48] Encouraged by these early results in patients without complete detachment of the subscapularis, the researchers began to use the transfer in patients with a completely absent subscapularis.[49] Pectoralis major and/or pectoralis minor transfer was used in 13 shoulders from 1980 to 1994 for an irreparable subscapularis tear (defined as complete absence of the subscapularis) in patients with anterior glenohumeral instability. At a mean 5-year follow-up, a satisfactory

result was achieved in 10 shoulders and an unsatisfactory result in 3 shoulders, according to the Neer and Foster grading system. All 3 shoulders with an unsatisfactory result had undergone at least two earlier reconstructive procedures. These shoulders had persistent pain, poor strength, and anterior laxity after the tendon transfer. In one patient, failure of the tendon transfer was precipitated by a new trauma. All 10 shoulders with a satisfactory result had active contraction of the transferred muscle and diminished anterior glenohumeral translation. These patients had slight or no pain during activities of daily living or work activities.[49]

Twelve patients (mean age, 65 years) who had an irreparable subscapularis tear were treated with a subcoracoid pectoralis major transfer.[50] The superior half to two thirds of the pectoralis major was used as a substitute for the subscapularis tendon. The pectoralis muscle transfer was routed behind the conjoined tendon (coracobrachialis and short head of the biceps) to the lesser tuberosity to adapt the orientation of the pectoralis to that of the subscapularis (**Figure 4**). At a mean 28-month follow-up, the outcome was excellent in five patients, good in four, and fair in three. The mean Constant score improved from 26.9 to 67.1, and all patients had healing of the transfer on ultrasound.

A study of 30 patients distinguished three groups: in group I, 11 patients (mean age, 37 years) underwent an unsuccessful instability procedure; in group II, 8 patients (mean age, 55 years) who had subscapularis rupture after hemiarthroplasty or total shoulder arthroplasty; and in group III, 11 patients (mean age, 58 years) had a massive rotator cuff tear involving the subscapularis.[51] All patients were treated with split transfer of the sternal head of the pectoralis major passed under the clavicular head. This technique allows the clavicular head to act as a fulcrum for the transferred sternal head when it contracts, and it helps guide the axis of pull of the sternal head of the pectoralis major to be more in line with the vector of the subscapularis. The vector of pull of the transferred pectoralis major remains anterior to the chest wall, in contrast to the vector of the subscapularis, which is posterior to the chest wall. The difference between the vector of the transferred pectoralis major and the vector of the subscapularis in relation to the chest wall is a feature of all pectoralis major transfer techniques (direct, subcoracoid deep to conjoined tendon, and deep to clavicular head). At a minimum 2-year follow-up, pain had improved in 7 of the 11 patients in group I and 7 of the 11 patients in group III, but in only 1 of the 8 patients in group II. Constant scores improved in patients in all groups, but the improvement was least in the patients with subscapularis rupture after shoulder arthroplasty (group II). The tendon transfer failed in 6 of the 8 patients in group II, compared with 3 of the 11 patients in group I and 4 of the 11 in group III. The researchers concluded that the risk of failure is high in a pectoralis major transfer if the patient has an irreparable subscapularis tear after shoulder arthroplasty, particularly with preoperative

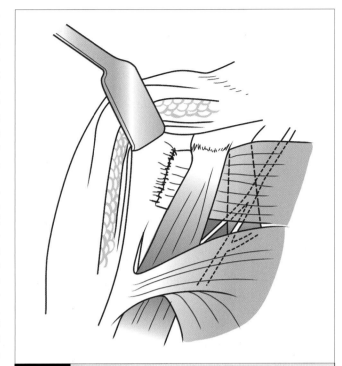

Figure 4 Schematic drawing showing the course of the transferred pectoralis major under the conjoined tendon. (Adapted with permission from Resch H, Povacz P, Ritter E, et al: Transfer of the pectoralis major muscle for the treatment of irreparable rupture of the subscapularis tendon. *J Bone Joint Surg Am* 2000;82[3]:372-382.)

anterior subluxation of the humeral head. Improvement in pain and function can be expected in a patient with isolated subscapularis insufficiency after an unsuccessful stabilization procedure, provided that the glenohumeral joint is concentric. If the shoulder joint is subluxated or not concentric, however, pectoralis tendon transfer is more likely to fail, and an alternative treatment, such as a bone block, transfer of the coracoid, or capsular reconstruction using tendon allograft or autograft, should be considered as a salvage procedure.

Routing the transferred pectoralis major tendon under the conjoined tendon is biomechanically preferable to routing over the conjoined tendon, but there is no evidence that the technically less demanding over-the-tendon technique (**Figure 5**) leads to clinically inferior results.[52,53] In 30 patients (average age, 53 years) with a pectoralis major transfer over the conjoined tendon, the mean relative Constant score improved from 47% before surgery to 70% at 32-month follow-up.[53] The patients with an isolated subscapularis tear or both a subscapularis tear and a repairable supraspinatus tear had a postoperative relative Constant score of 79%. Patients with a subscapularis tear and an irreparable supraspinatus (and infraspinatus) tear had a clearly inferior clinical outcome, as indicated by a 49% relative Constant score at final follow-up. Overall, the results

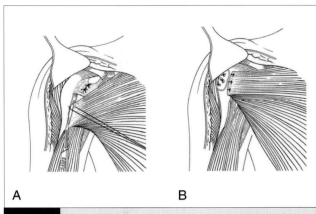

Figure 5 Schematic drawings showing the course of the transferred pectoralis major over the conjoined tendon. **A,** The deltoid muscle is retracted. After mobilization of the subscapularis, an attempt is made to repair the remaining tendon, scar, and fascial tissue to the lesser tuberosity. The pectoralis major tendon is then released completely from its insertion. A reinsertion area for the pectoralis major tendon on the medial aspect of the greater tuberosity is then prepared. **B,** The pectoralis major tendon is transferred to the medial aspect of the greater tuberosity over the conjoined tendon. (Reproduced with permission from Jost B, Puskas GJ, Lustenberger A, Gerber C: Outcome of pectoralis major transfer for the treatment of irreparable subscapularis tears. *J Bone Joint Surg Am* 2003;85[10]:1944-1951.

were comparable to those of patients having an under-the-tendon transfer.[53]

Deltoid Flap Reconstruction
European surgeons have used a deltoid flap to reconstruct posterosuperior tears, with variable results. This technique led to satisfactory medium-term results but poor long-term results in terms of pain relief and improvement in shoulder function: at a mean 13.9-year follow-up, 50% of the deltoid flaps had ruptured and 70% of shoulders had stage 1 or 2 osteoarthritis.[54] No predictive factor for deltoid flap rupture was identified. Another study reported minor functional gains but acceptable pain relief and patient satisfaction after deltoid flap reconstruction.[55] However, ultrasound showed survival of only 16.5% of the deltoid flaps at mid-term follow-up and only 12.5% at long-term follow-up. In neither report did the authors recommend further use of this procedure.

Summary

Massive, irreparable rotator cuff tears remain a clinical challenge. A thorough history and physical examination are vital for accurate diagnosis and understanding of the patient's condition. A variety of imaging modalities can be used, most commonly plain radiography, CT arthrography, and MRI, to help delineate the extent

and severity of the disease. The natural history is not well understood, but some patients do well after nonsurgical treatment with physical therapy and pain management. However, most patients experience increasing pain and disability and require further intervention. In a patient with low physical demands, simple débridement of the tear may provide pain relief, sometimes leading to secondary functional improvement. The results are poorer with a larger tear and deteriorate with time. Partial repair using the margin convergence technique decreases the size of the tear gap and reduces strain, with minimal effect on glenohumeral translation and intrinsic tendon strain. A tendon transfer offers a good result for a patient with a massive, irreparable rotator cuff tear who has intact deltoid function and disabling weakness but not pseudoparalysis. A tendon transfer will not halt the progression of cuff tear arthropathy, however. The treatment modality chosen for a massive, irreparable rotator cuff tear must be tailored to the patient's needs, expectations, and ability to comply with intensive rehabilitation.

Annotated References

1. Bedi A, Dines J, Warren RF, Dines DM: Massive tears of the rotator cuff. *J Bone Joint Surg Am* 2010;92(9): 1894-1908.

   A comprehensive review of massive rotator cuff tears included workup and treatment options.

2. Cofield RH, Parvizi J, Hoffmeyer PJ, Lanzer WL, Ilstrup DM, Rowland CM: Surgical repair of chronic rotator cuff tears: A prospective long-term study. *J Bone Joint Surg Am* 2001;83-A(1):71-77.

3. Zingg PO, Jost B, Sukthankar A, Buhler M, Pfirrmann CW, Gerber C: Clinical and structural outcomes of nonoperative management of massive rotator cuff tears. *J Bone Joint Surg Am* 2007;89(9):1928-1934.

   A retrospective review of 19 patients with a nonsurgically managed massive rotator cuff tear found satisfactory shoulder function despite progression of degenerative structural joint changes and the risk of a repairable tear progressing to an irreparable tear during the 4-year study period. Level of evidence: IV.

4. Harryman DT II, Hettrich CM, Smith KL, Campbell B, Sidles JA, Matsen FA III: A prospective multipractice investigation of patients with full-thickness rotator cuff tears: The importance of comorbidities, practice, and other covariables on self-assessed shoulder function and health status. *J Bone Joint Surg Am* 2003;85-A(4):690-696.

5. Su W-R, Budoff JE, Luo Z-P: The effect of anterosuperior rotator cuff tears on glenohumeral translation. *Arthroscopy* 2009;25(3):282-289.

   A biomechanical study evaluated the effect of an anterosuperior rotator cuff tear in cadaver shoulders. Tears of the superior subscapularis altered mechanics

3: The Rotator Cuff

at low loads, and tears of the entire subscapularis altered mechanics at all loads.

6. Burkhart SS: Fluoroscopic comparison of kinematic patterns in massive rotator cuff tears: A suspension bridge model. *Clin Orthop Relat Res* 1992;284: 144-152.

7. Parsons IM, Apreleva M, Fu FH, Woo SL: The effect of rotator cuff tears on reaction forces at the glenohumeral joint. *J Orthop Res* 2002;20(3):439-446.

8. Oh JH, Jun BJ, McGarry MH, Lee TQ: Does a critical rotator cuff tear stage exist? A biomechanical study of rotator cuff tear progression in human cadaver shoulders. *J Bone Joint Surg Am* 2011;93(22):2100-2109.

   A biomechanical study of cadaver shoulders evaluated the stage at which rotator cuff tears alter kinematics. A tear of the entire supraspinatus tendon was the stage of increasing rotational range of motion and decreasing abduction capability, and progression to the infraspinatus muscle was the critical stage for changes in humeral head kinematics.

9. Gerber C, Wirth SH, Farshad M: Treatment options for massive rotator cuff tears. *J Shoulder Elbow Surg* 2011;20(2, suppl):S20-S29.

   A review of massive rotator cuff tears included nonsurgical treatment, repair, transfers, and arthroplasty.

10. Werner CM, Steinmann PA, Gilbart M, Gerber C: Treatment of painful pseudoparesis due to irreparable rotator cuff dysfunction with the Delta III reverse-ball-and-socket total shoulder prosthesis. *J Bone Joint Surg Am* 2005;87(7):1476-1486.

11. Zumstein MA, Jost B, Hempel J, Hodler J, Gerber C: The clinical and structural long-term results of open repair of massive tears of the rotator cuff. *J Bone Joint Surg Am* 2008;90(11):2423-2431.

    At 10-year follow-up of 23 patients who underwent open repair of a massive rotator cuff tear, 22 patients were satisfied with the outcome, and the retearing rate was associated with preoperative fatty infiltration. Level of evidence: IV.

12. Goutallier D, Postel J-M, Gleyze P, Leguilloux P, Van Driessche S: Influence of cuff muscle fatty degeneration on anatomic and functional outcomes after simple suture of full-thickness tears. *J Shoulder Elbow Surg* 2003;12(6):550-554.

13. Nové-Josserand L, Costa P, Liotard J-P, Safar J-F, Walch G, Zilber S: Results of latissimus dorsi tendon transfer for irreparable cuff tears. *Orthop Traumatol Surg Res* 2009;95(2):108-113.

    A retrospective review of 26 patients after latissimus dorsi transfer found a high satisfaction rate but a variable increase in active external rotation at a mean 34-month follow-up. Level of evidence: IV.

14. Nové-Josserand L, Edwards TB, O'Connor DP, Walch G: The acromiohumeral and coracohumeral in-

tervals are abnormal in rotator cuff tears with muscular fatty degeneration. *Clin Orthop Relat Res* 2005; 433:90-96.

15. Hamada K, Fukuda H, Mikasa M, Kobayashi Y: Roentgenographic findings in massive rotator cuff tears: A long-term observation. *Clin Orthop Relat Res* 1990;254:92-96.

16. Walch G, Edwards TB, Boulahia A, Nové-Josserand L, Neyton L, Szabo I: Arthroscopic tenotomy of the long head of the biceps in the treatment of rotator cuff tears: Clinical and radiographic results of 307 cases. *J Shoulder Elbow Surg* 2005;14(3):238-246.

17. Hamada K, Yamanaka K, Uchiyama Y, Mikasa T, Mikasa M: A radiographic classification of massive rotator cuff tear arthritis. *Clin Orthop Relat Res* 2011; 469(9):2452-2460.

    A retrospective review of 75 patients, 41 of whom were surgically treated, found that those with more acromiohumeral interval narrowing had more muscle fatty degeneration and a higher rate of retearing. Level of evidence: III.

18. Goutallier D, Postel JM, Bernageau J, Lavau L, Voisin MC: Fatty muscle degeneration in cuff ruptures: Pre- and postoperative evaluation by CT scan. *Clin Orthop Relat Res* 1994;304:78-83.

19. Fuchs B, Weishaupt D, Zanetti M, Hodler J, Gerber C: Fatty degeneration of the muscles of the rotator cuff: Assessment by computed tomography versus magnetic resonance imaging. *J Shoulder Elbow Surg* 1999;8(6): 599-605.

20. Lippe J, Spang JT, Leger RR, Arciero RA, Mazzocca AD, Shea KP: Inter-rater agreement of the Goutallier, Patte, and Warner classification scores using preoperative magnetic resonance imaging in patients with rotator cuff tears. *Arthroscopy* 2012;28(2):154-159.

    An MRI review by three board-certified orthopaedic surgeons evaluated the interobserver reliability of three classification schemes. None of the classifications had high interobserver reliability. Level of evidence: III.

21. Burkhart SS, Barth JR, Richards DP, Zlatkin MB, Larsen M: Arthroscopic repair of massive rotator cuff tears with stage 3 and 4 fatty degeneration. *Arthroscopy* 2007;23(4):347-354.

    In a retrospective review of 22 patients with grade 3 or 4 fatty infiltration who underwent repair of a massive rotator cuff tear, all 17 patients with grade 3 infiltration had clinical improvement at a mean 39.3-month follow-up, and 2 of the 5 with grade 4 infiltration had improvement. Level of evidence: IV.

22. Mellado JM, Calmet J, Olona M, et al: Surgically repaired massive rotator cuff tears: MRI of tendon integrity, muscle fatty degeneration, and muscle atrophy correlated with intraoperative and clinical findings. *AJR Am J Roentgenol* 2005;184(5):1456-1463.

23. Yoo JC, Ahn JH, Yang JH, Koh KH, Choi SH, Yoon YC: Correlation of arthroscopic repairability of large to massive rotator cuff tears with preoperative magnetic resonance imaging scans. *Arthroscopy* 2009; 25(6):573-582.

In 51 consecutive patients who underwent arthroscopic repair of a large or a massive tear, those with grade 2 or 3 fatty infiltration had a greater risk of incomplete repair. Level of evidence: II.

24. Meyer DC, Farshad M, Amacker NA, Gerber C, Wieser K: Quantitative analysis of muscle and tendon retraction in chronic rotator cuff tears. *Am J Sports Med* 2012;40(3):606-610.

In an MRI study of 130 shoulders with an intact or a torn supraspinatus (20 or 110 shoulders, respectively), fatty infiltration was graded and retraction of the tendon stump and the musculotendinous junction was measured. In advanced fatty infiltration, a component of shortening arises from the tendon. Level of evidence: III.

25. Iannotti JP, Ciccone J, Buss DD, et al: Accuracy of office-based ultrasonography of the shoulder for the diagnosis of rotator cuff tears. *J Bone Joint Surg Am* 2005;87(6):1305-1311.

26. Al-Shawi A, Badge R, Bunker T: The detection of full thickness rotator cuff tears using ultrasound. *J Bone Joint Surg Br* 2008;90(7):889-892.

An evaluation of the accuracy of portable ultrasonography for detecting rotator cuff tears found that experienced operators were able to most accurately detect large and massive tears.

27. Levy O, Mullett H, Roberts S, Copeland S: The role of anterior deltoid reeducation in patients with massive irreparable degenerative rotator cuff tears. *J Shoulder Elbow Surg* 2008;17(6):863-870.

A prospective assessment of 17 patients with a massive rotator cuff tear treated with an anterior deltoid rehabilitation program found significant clinical improvement at a minimum 9-month follow-up after treatment. Level of evidence: III.

28. Liem D, Lengers N, Dedy N, Poetzl W, Steinbeck J, Marquardt B: Arthroscopic debridement of massive irreparable rotator cuff tears. *Arthroscopy* 2008;24(7): 743-748.

A retrospective review of 31 patients with a massive rotator cuff tear who underwent arthroscopic débridement with or without biceps tenotomy found improvement in clinical scores and no decrease in biceps strength for those with low demands at a mean 47-month follow-up. Level of evidence: IV.

29. Gartsman GM: Arthroscopic acromioplasty for lesions of the rotator cuff. *J Bone Joint Surg Am* 1990;72(2): 169-180.

30. Fagelman M, Sartori M, Freedman KB, Patwardhan AG, Carandang G, Marra G: Biomechanics of coracoacromial arch modification. *J Shoulder Elbow Surg* 2007;16(1):101-106.

A biomechanical study evaluated several coracoacromial arch alterations and found that reconstruction best resisted anterosuperior migration.

31. Flatow EL, Weinstein XA, Duralde CA, et al: Coracoacromial ligament preservation in rotator cuff surgery. *J Shoulder Elbow Surg* 1994;3:573.

32. Fenlin JM Jr, Chase JM, Rushton SA, Frieman BG: Tuberoplasty: Creation of an acromiohumeral articulation—a treatment option for massive, irreparable rotator cuff tears. *J Shoulder Elbow Surg* 2002;11(2): 136-142.

33. Burkhart SS: Arthroscopic treatment of massive rotator cuff tears. *Clin Orthop Relat Res* 2001;390:107-118.

34. Tauro JC: Arthroscopic "interval slide" in the repair of large rotator cuff tears. *Arthroscopy* 1999;15(5): 527-530.

35. Hsu JE, Reuther KE, Sarver JJ, et al : Restoration of anterior-posterior rotator cuff force balance improves shoulder function in a rat model of chronic massive tears. *J Orthop Res* 2011;29(7):1028-1033.

In an in vivo study of rats, creation of a two-tendon tear of the supraspinatus and the infraspinatus was followed by no repair, infraspinatus-only repair, or two-tendon repair. Isolated infraspinatus repair and two-tendon repair restored similar function.

36. Mazzocca AD, Bollier M, Fehsenfeld D, et al: Biomechanical evaluation of margin convergence. *Arthroscopy* 2011;27(3):330-338.

A biomechanical study of 20 shoulders evaluated the effect of margin convergence on retracted rotator cuff tears. There was a significant decrease in rotator cuff strain and gap size after margin convergence in a large retracted tear.

37. Warner JJ: Management of massive irreparable rotator cuff tears: The role of tendon transfer. *Instr Course Lect* 2001;50:63-71.

38. Gerber C, Vinh TS, Hertel R, Hess CW: Latissimus dorsi transfer for the treatment of massive tears of the rotator cuff: A preliminary report. *Clin Orthop Relat Res* 1988;232:51-61.

39. L'Episcopo JB: Tendon transposition in obstetrical paralysis. *Am J Surg* 1934;25:122-125.

40. Gerber C, Maquieira G, Espinosa N: Latissimus dorsi transfer for the treatment of irreparable rotator cuff tears. *J Bone Joint Surg Am* 2006;88(1):113-120.

41. Iannotti JP, Hennigan S, Herzog R, et al: Latissimus dorsi tendon transfer for irreparable posterosuperior rotator cuff tears: Factors affecting outcome. *J Bone Joint Surg Am* 2006;88(2):342-348.

3: The Rotator Cuff

42. Warner JJ, Parsons IM IV: Latissimus dorsi tendon transfer: A comparative analysis of primary and salvage reconstruction of massive, irreparable rotator cuff tears. *J Shoulder Elbow Surg* 2001;10(6):514-521.

43. Birmingham PM, Neviaser RJ: Outcome of latissimus dorsi transfer as a salvage procedure for failed rotator cuff repair with loss of elevation. *J Shoulder Elbow Surg* 2008;17(6):871-874.

    Retrospective review of 18 patients who underwent latissimus dorsi transfer for a massive rotator cuff tear found improved clinical scores and motion at an average 25-month follow-up. Level of evidence: IV.

44. Moursy M, Forstner R, Koller H, Resch H, Tauber M: Latissimus dorsi tendon transfer for irreparable rotator cuff tears: A modified technique to improve tendon transfer integrity. *J Bone Joint Surg Am* 2009;91(8):1924-1931.

    Two latissimus dorsi harvesting techniques were compared: the standard tendon technique and a modification with removal of some bone. At a mean 47-month follow-up, the modified tendon technique led to better clinical scores. Level of evidence: III.

45. Habermeyer P, Magosch P, Rudolph T, Lichtenberg S, Liem D: Transfer of the tendon of latissimus dorsi for the treatment of massive tears of the rotator cuff: A new single-incision technique. *J Bone Joint Surg Br* 2006;88(2):208-212.

46. Gerhardt C, Lehmann L, Lichtenberg S, Magosch P, Habermeyer P: Modified L'Episcopo tendon transfers for irreparable rotator cuff tears: 5-year follow-up. *Clin Orthop Relat Res* 2010;468(6):1572-1577.

    A retrospective review of 20 patients who underwent a modified L'Episcopo tendon transfer for a massive rotator cuff tear found an increase in shoulder function but some progression of rotator cuff arthropathy at 5-year follow-up. Level of evidence: IV.

47. Lehmann LJ, Mauerman E, Strube T, Laibacher K, Scharf HP: Modified minimally invasive latissimus dorsi transfer in the treatment of massive rotator cuff tears: A two-year follow-up of 26 consecutive patients. *Int Orthop* 2010;34(3):377-383.

    A retrospective review of 26 patients who underwent a modified minimally invasive latissimus dorsi transfer for a massive rotator cuff tear found improved clinical scores at a mean 24-month follow-up. Level of evidence: IV.

48. Young DC, Rockwood CA Jr: Complications of a failed Bristow procedure and their management. *J Bone Joint Surg Am* 1991;73(7):969-981.

49. Wirth MA, Rockwood CA Jr: Operative treatment of irreparable rupture of the subscapularis. *J Bone Joint Surg Am* 1997;79(5):722-731.

50. Resch H, Povacz P, Ritter E, Matschi W: Transfer of the pectoralis major muscle for the treatment of irreparable rupture of the subscapularis tendon. *J Bone Joint Surg Am* 2000;82(3):372-382.

51. Elhassan B, Ozbaydar M, Massimini D, Diller D, Higgins L, Warner JJ: Transfer of pectoralis major for the treatment of irreparable tears of subscapularis: Does it work? *J Bone Joint Surg Br* 2008;90(8):1059-1065.

    The outcomes of pectoralis major transfer were evaluated in the setting of an unsuccessful procedure for instability of the shoulder, an unsuccessful shoulder replacement, or a massive rotator cuff tear. Patients who underwent the transfer after an unsuccessful shoulder replacement had the worst outcomes. Level of evidence: III.

52. Resch H, Povacz P, Ritter E, Aschauer E: Pectoralis major muscle transfer for irreparable rupture of the subscapularis and supraspinatus tendon. *Tech Shoulder Elbow Surg* 2002;3:167-173.

53. Jost B, Puskas GJ, Lustenberger A, Gerber C: Outcome of pectoralis major transfer for the treatment of irreparable subscapularis tears. *J Bone Joint Surg Am* 2003; 85(10):1944-1951.

54. Lu XW, Verborgt O, Gazielly DF: Long-term outcomes after deltoid muscular flap transfer for irreparable rotator cuff tears. *J Shoulder Elbow Surg* 2008; 17(5):732-737.

    A retrospective review of long-term outcomes of deltoid muscular flap transfer for a massive rotator cuff tear found satisfactory short- and mid-term results but poor long-term (13.9-year) results. The authors recommended against the procedure. Level of evidence: IV.

55. Glanzmann MC, Goldhahn J, Flury M, Schwyzer HK, Simmen BR: Deltoid flap reconstruction for massive rotator cuff tears: Mid- and long-term functional and structural results. *J Shoulder Elbow Surg* 2010;19(3): 439-445.

    A retrospective review of 31 deltoid flap transfers found that ultrasound-confirmed deltoid flap survival was 16.5% at 53-month follow-up and 12.5% at 175-month follow-up. Deltoid flap survival was correlated with better clinical outcome. The authors did not recommend this procedure. Level of evidence: IV.

3: The Rotator Cuff

Chapter 17

Biologic Augmentation of Rotator Cuff Healing

Kyle A. Caswell, DO   Todd C. Moen, MD   Wayne Z. Burkhead Jr, MD

Introduction

Rotator cuff repair reliably relieves pain in patients with a symptomatic rotator cuff tear, but functional improvement is less predictable. For functional improvement, the repaired tendon must heal to bone. Studies have found a surprisingly high rate of failure of tendon healing, with retears occurring after surgery in 11% to 94% of large and massive rotator cuff tears.[1,2] This high failure rate has led to research into ways to improve tendon healing by using biologic augmentation at the time of surgery. Both open and arthroscopic techniques for rotator cuff repair with biologic augmentation have been described. The biologic augments that have been studied in vivo and in vitro include allograft, extracellular matrices (ECMs), platelet-rich plasma (PRP), growth factors, stem cells, and gene therapy.

Preoperative Evaluation

The preoperative evaluation of a patient who may benefit from augmentation begins with a thorough history and physical examination. The patient's history is critical to identifying risk factors for rotator cuff repair failure, including diabetes, hyperlipidemia, a history of smoking, advanced fatty degeneration of muscle, and advanced age.[3-5] The shoulder girdle should be inspected for atrophy in the supraspinatus and infraspinatus fossae, ruptures of the biceps tendon, and a fixed or dynamic anterosuperior escape of the humeral head from a massive, decompensated rotator cuff tear. The patient may have a lag sign indicative of a massive cuff tear.[6-8] Severe limitation of active motion (especially in external rotation) in a patient with an atrophic rotator cuff may indicate a concomitant suprascapular neuropathy, for which an electrodiagnostic study should be considered before surgical management.[9] Plain radiographs of the shoulder should include at least neutral-rotation AP, axillary, and supraspinatus outlet views. Advanced imaging to detect a massive rotator cuff tear should include MRI with or without intra-articular gadolinium or CT with intra-articular contrast.

Indications and Contraindications

The indications for biologic augmentation of rotator cuff repair remain controversial. Only limited peer-reviewed evidence is available. The current best practice indication for biologic augmentation is a diminished potential for healing because of comorbidity, in an open or arthroscopic repair of a massive rotator cuff tear. Augmentation also may be indicated for revision of an unsuccessful repair. A massive rotator cuff tear has been described as having a diameter greater than 5 cm or involving two or more rotator cuff tendons.[10,11] The ability to repair the musculature in such tears has been correlated with the extent of fibrofatty degeneration of the rotator cuff tendon, as described by Goutallier. In the Goutallier classification, a grade of 2 or lower indicates the presence of more muscle than fat.[12-14] Tear size, tear chronicity, the extent of muscle atrophy, and the amount of fibrofatty degeneration all must be considered in the decision to use biologic augmentation in rotator cuff repairs. Active infection and substantial glenohumeral arthritis are contraindications to the use of tissue augmentation.

Types and Outcomes of Biologic Augmentation

The current clinical biologic augmentation strategies are focused on ECMs and PRP. There are three types of ECMs: allograft, xenograft, and synthetic graft.[15] PRP is a rich source of several growth factors. Some of these factors are derived from platelets, including platelet-derived growth factor, vascular endothelial growth

Dr. Burkhead or an immediate family member has received royalties from Tornier; is a member of a speakers' bureau or has made paid presentations on behalf of Tornier; serves as a paid consultant to or is an employee of Tornier, Wright Medical Technology, Stryker, and Bio2tech I-Flow; and serves as a board member, owner, officer, or committee member of the International Board of Shoulder and Elbow Surgery. Neither of the following authors nor any immediate family member has received anything of value from or owns stock in a commercial company or institution related directly or indirectly to the subject of this chapter: Dr. Caswell and Dr. Moen.

3: The Rotator Cuff

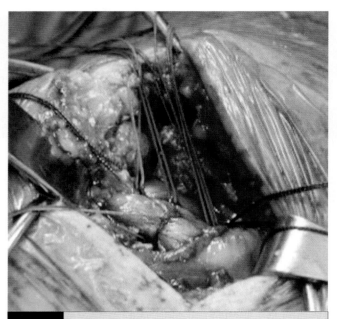

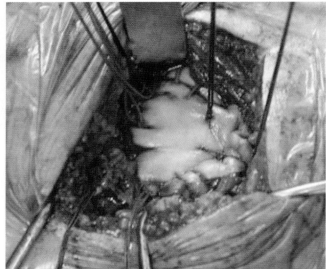

Figure 1 In an open rotator cuff repair, anchoring sutures are placed around the circumference of the cuff repair before augmentation. (Reproduced with permission from Burkhead WZ, Schiffern SC, Krishnan SG: Use of GraftJacket as an augmentation for massive rotator cuff tears. *Semin Arthroplasty* 2007; 18[1]:11-18.)

Figure 2 Biologic augmentation is securely sutured over the previous rotator cuff repair, creating a watertight repair. (Reproduced with permission from Burkhead WZ, Schiffern SC, Krishnan SG: Use of GraftJacket as an augmentation for massive rotator cuff tears. *Semin Arthroplasty* 2007; 18[1]:11-18.)

factor, transforming growth factor–β1, fibroblast growth factor, and epidermal growth factor; others are derived from plasma, including hepatocyte growth factor and insulin-like growth factor–1.[16] Rotator cuff repair with biologic augmentation has been described using both open and arthroscopic techniques[17-20] (**Figures 1 and 2**.)

Porcine Small Intestine Submucosa Xenograft

Several studies of porcine small intestine submucosa xenograft did not find favorable results. In a randomized controlled study of 30 shoulders (30 patients) with a chronic two-tendon rotator cuff tear that was completely reparable with open surgery, 15 patients received porcine small intestine submucosa augmentation, and 15 did not.[21] MRI with intra-articular gadolinium 1 year after the repair revealed rotator cuff healing in four shoulders treated with augmentation compared with nine shoulders not treated with augmentation. Augmentation not only failed to improve healing but also led to a substantially lower median postoperative functional score. Median shoulder and patient satisfaction scores did not differ substantially between patients who were in the treatment group or the control group. On the basis of these results, the researchers did not recommend using porcine small intestine submucosa to augment repair of a massive chronic rotator cuff tear.[21]

Another randomized controlled study assigned patients to be treated with a conventional repair with or without porcine submucosa patch augmentation.[22] The study was abandoned 2 to 4 weeks after surgery because 4 of the 19 patients in the xenograft patch augmentation group had a severe local postoperative reaction requiring surgical irrigation, débridement, and removal of the xenograft patch. The researchers recommended against the use of this xenograft after finding that patients had a retear rate similar to that of the control subjects.[22]

Another prospective study also had poor results after porcine small intestine submucosa xenograft was used to augment a massive rotator cuff repair.[23] Mean scores on the University of California, Los Angeles (UCLA) and American Shoulder and Elbow Surgeons (ASES) scales were better in patients treated with augmentation compared with patients in the control group, but the repairs were partially or completely intact in only 44% of the shoulders on postoperative magnetic resonance arthrography (MRA). Three complications occurred, including one infection and two skin reactions. The researchers recommended against the use of porcine small intestine submucosa as a graft because of the risk of a skin reaction and the poor MRA findings.[23]

A retrospective review of 11 consecutive patients treated with open rotator cuff repair with porcine submucosa augmentation for a large or massive rotator cuff tear found that porcine augmentation did not improve clinical outcomes and was an ineffective reinforcement. Ten patients had MRI-documented recurrence of a large retracted tear at 6-month follow-up. There was no substantial difference between patients' preoperative and postoperative shoulder scores, although five patients had a decline in clinical scores after surgery. The researchers did not recommend the use of interpositional porcine submucosa xenograft for a large or a massive rotator cuff tear.[24]

Porcine Dermal Collagen Xenograft

The use of porcine dermal collagen xenograft was found to improve clinical and radiographic outcomes; however, one study concluded that this graft should not be used to bridge a defect in a rotator cuff repair.[25,26] At 1-year follow-up after a porcine dermal collagen tendon augmentation graft was used to treat a massive rotator cuff tear in 10 consecutive patients, there was statistically significant improvement in mean Constant and pain scores, abduction power, and range of motion in internal rotation, external rotation, and abduction.[25] All patients were able to perform activities of daily living, and all patients except one were satisfied. MRI and ultrasound at an average 4.5-year follow-up revealed an intact graft in eight patients (80%) and graft detachment in two patients. No intraoperative or postoperative complications were noted. The researchers concluded that the use of porcine dermal collagen graft as a biologic augmentation in massive rotator cuff tears is safe and associated with improved clinical outcomes.[25]

Different results were reported in a study of 20 patients, of whom 4 received porcine dermal collagen graft to bridge a residual rotator cuff defect during repair of a massive tear.[26] At 3- to 6-month follow-up, patients who received the graft bridge had signs and symptoms of a recurrent rotator cuff tear, with physical and MRI signs of inflammation and evidence of loss of continuity in the remaining graft material. Two of the four patients subsequently underwent reverse total shoulder replacement. Histologic samples were taken at the time of this surgery, and analysis confirmed necrotic fibrinous material on a background of chronic inflammation, with no sign of an infectious agent. The 16 patients who received a graft to augment a rotator cuff repair had no signs of a similar complication or early failure of the repair at 2-year follow-up. The researchers noted that this graft may have advantages as an augmentation of rotator cuff repair but did not recommend its use to bridge a massive rotator cuff tear.[26]

Human Cadaver Dermal Collagen Allograft

Human dermal collagen allograft augmentation was used in 17 consecutive patients treated with open rotator cuff repair.[17] The primary diagnosis was a primary massive rotator cuff tear in 11 patients and a recurrent massive rotator cuff tear in 6 patients. Pain scores, functional status, and UCLA scores improved substantially after surgery. Two of seven patients who underwent postoperative MRI had a recurrent tear of smaller size. No other complications were observed, such as infection or a sterile inflammatory reaction. The researchers concluded that human dermal collagen allograft augmentation may be effective and safe in primary or revision repair of a massive rotator cuff tear.[17]

Human cadaver dermal collagen allograft also has shown promise in arthroscopy-based studies. In a prospective randomized study of 44 patients treated with arthroscopic repair of a two-tendon rotator cuff tear larger than 3 cm, 22 patients received human dermal collagen matrix augmentation.[27] Statistically significant improvements in ASES and Constant scores were found in the patients treated with augmentation compared with patients in the nonaugmentation group at 24-month follow-up. Gadolinium-enhanced MRI revealed that 85% of the patients who received augmentation (17 of 20 patients) and 40% of those who did not (6 of 15 patients) had an intact rotator cuff at a mean 14.4-month follow-up. The researchers concluded that repair of two-tendon rotator cuff tears with human dermal collagen allograft matrix augmentation is effective and increases the likelihood of complete healing.[27]

Forty-five patients with a massive, irreparable rotator cuff tear were treated with arthroscopic repair and placement of acellular human dermal matrix allograft as a bridging augmentation.[19] Three validated outcome measures (the UCLA, Western Ontario Rotator Cuff, and ASES scales) were used to document clinical outcomes. At a minimum 24-month follow-up, all outcome scores had improved, and the improvement in UCLA scores was statistically significant. The researchers concluded that the procedure is safe, is associated with high patient satisfaction, and avoids the morbidity of tendon transfer or arthroplasty.[19]

A 62-year-old man was treated with a rotator cuff repair augmented with acellular human dermal matrix.[28] Three months later, the patient had mild pain and catching with elevation of the shoulder. MRI showed that the anterior lateral edge of the graft was not attached to bone. An arthroscopic evaluation and repair was performed, with a biopsy of the graft site. Evidence was found that the human acellular dermal matrix had incorporated into the surrounding tissue, aligned with collagen fibers, revascularized with numerous blood vessels, repopulated with host cells, and caused little or no inflammatory response. The researchers concluded that the graft appeared to be suitable for reinforcing the primary repair and acting as a scaffold for remodeling with the host tissue.[28]

Platelet-Rich Plasma

Several studies have investigated the use of PRP during rotator cuff repair. A prospective study randomly assigned 53 patients with a small to massive rotator cuff tear to receive single-row arthroscopic rotator cuff repair alone (27 patients) or with PRP augmentation (26 patients).[29] At 2-year follow-up, MRI found similar rates of retearing in patients with a massive tear (40% of those treated with PRP and 52% of those treated without PRP). At 3-month follow-up, pain level was improved in patients who received PRP, as were shoulder function and strength (as measured by the Simple

Shoulder Test, UCLA, and Constant scales) and strength in external rotation. No difference was found at later time points, and no difference in healing rate on MRI was found at final 2-year follow-up.[15,29]

In a randomized prospective double-blind controlled study, 88 patients with a small to medium-size rotator cuff tear underwent arthroscopic repair with or without autologous platelet-rich fibrin matrix.[30] At 16-month follow-up, no statistically significant between-group difference was found in clinical outcomes or on MRI.

In a randomized study of 79 patients treated with rotator cuff repair with or without platelet-rich fibrin matrix, ultrasound showed no substantial difference in healing 6 or 12 weeks after surgery.[15,31] Two thirds of the patients who received platelet-rich fibrin matrix had an intact repair compared with 80% of those who did not. Between-group outcome scores and strength measurements were similar.[15,31]

Future Approaches to Biologic Augmentation

Mesenchymal Stem Cells

Bone marrow–derived mesenchymal stem cells (MSCs) have been identified as a potential source for biologic augmentation.[32] MSCs may improve the repair of rotator cuff tendon to bone because of their capacity to differentiate into several connective tissue lineages, including those of muscle, bone, ligament, tendon, and cartilage. In a rabbit model, MSCs were found to improve tendon-to-bone healing of the hallucis longus tendon in a calcaneal bone tunnel.[16,33] A comparison of rabbit anterior cruciate ligament reconstruction coated with MSCs or a fibrin glue carrier found that the MSC-treated grafts had large areas of immature fibrocartilage cells at the tendon-bone junction at 2 weeks and by 8 weeks resembled the chondral enthesis of a normal anterior cruciate ligament insertion, with the presence of a mature zone of fibrocartilage blending into adjacent bone and tendon.[34] Biomechanical study at 8 weeks found that the MSC-treated anterior cruciate ligament grafts had a higher failure load and greater stiffness than the fibrin glue–treated grafts.[16,34]

MSCs were used to improve healing at the bone-tendon insertion site during rotator cuff repair in a rat model.[35] One group received 10^6 bone marrow–derived MSCs in a fibrin sealant carrier at the tendon-bone repair site, the second group received a fibrin sealant carrier, and a control group underwent repair only. No between-group difference was found in collagen fiber organization, fibrocartilage formation, or load to failure in histologic and biomechanical studies at 2 and 4 weeks. The researchers concluded that the use of MSCs alone is not sufficient to improve tendon-bone healing in a rotator cuff model because the repair site may lack the molecular or cellular signals needed to induce appropriate differentiation.[35] In humans, connective tissue progenitor cells were harvested from the proximal humerus during arthroscopic rotator cuff re-

pair to serve as a medium with osteogenic potential.[36] These cells have the potential for application at the tendon-bone interface site as an autograft to promote healing.

Growth Factors

Growth factors are a subset of cytokines that promote cell division, maturation, and/or differentiation. These include basic fibroblast growth factor, cartilage oligomatrix protein, connective tissue growth factor, platelet-derived growth factor, transforming growth factor–β, insulin-like growth factor–1, and bone morphogenetic proteins 12, 13, and 14.[37] Research has focused on the use of growth factors in rotator cuff repair models to augment tendon-bone interface healing. The types of growth factors, the timing of application, and delivery methods are being researched.

Gene Therapy

Gene therapy has been identified as an area of biologic augmentation research. Embryonic development studies have identified a marker specific for tendons and ligaments. Scleraxis is a basic helix-loop-helix transcription factor that is expressed in tendons from the early progenitor stage until the formation of mature tendons in chick embryos, mouse embryos, and mouse limb tendons. Tenomodulin is upregulated by scleraxis in tenocytes during chick development, and the loss of tenomodulin expression in gene-targeted mice led to reduced tenocyte density, decreased tenocyte proliferation, and altered tendon ultrastructure.[5,38]

Nanofiber Technology

Nanofiber engineering is of interest because the biologic mimicry of nanofibers makes it an ideal tendon tissue–engineering platform. A polylactide-coglycolide nanofiber-based scaffold was designed for rotator cuff tendon tissue engineering, and the attachment, alignment, gene expression, and matrix elaboration of human rotator cuff fibroblasts were assessed on aligned and unaligned polylactide-coglycolide nanofiber scaffolds.[39] Fibroblasts grown to the aligned fiber scaffolds were more elongated and longitudinally oriented than those on unaligned fibers. The collagen type I fibers had a more organized orientation on the aligned scaffolds. The tensile strength of the aligned scaffolds was greater than that of the unaligned scaffold at all time points. This study showed that nanofiber organization is critical for cell response and scaffold properties. Further research is required to discover whether this type of scaffold can help reestablish the bone-tendon interface in rotator cuff repair.[39]

Summary

Biologic augmentation of rotator cuff repairs is controversial but evolving. Augmentation may be indicated for primary or revision repair of a massive but reparable rotator cuff tear with healing potential. The current clinical biologic augmentation strategies focus on ECMs and PRP. Future biologic augmentation laboratory research will concentrate on the use of MSCs, growth factors, gene therapy, and nanofiber technology to optimize healing after a rotator cuff repair.

Annotated References

1. Lafosse L, Brozska R, Toussaint B, Gobezie R: The outcome and structural integrity of arthroscopic rotator cuff repair with use of the double-row suture anchor technique. *J Bone Joint Surg Am* 2007;89(7): 1533-1541.

   The functional and anatomic results of arthroscopic double-row suture anchor rotator cuff repair were studied using CT or MRA. Level of evidence: IV.

2. Galatz LM, Ball CM, Teefey SA, Middleton WD, Yamaguchi K: The outcome and repair integrity of completely arthroscopically repaired large and massive rotator cuff tears. *J Bone Joint Surg Am* 2004;86(2): 219-224.

3. Nho SJ, Delos D, Yadav H, et al: Biomechanical and biologic augmentation for the treatment of massive rotator cuff tears. *Am J Sports Med* 2010;38(3):619-629.

   The clinical treatment of repair of a massive rotator cuff tear was reviewed, and methods for augmenting the healing of a degenerative rotator cuff tendon were explored.

4. Abboud JA, Kim JS: The effect of hypercholesterolemia on rotator cuff disease. *Clin Orthop Relat Res* 2010;468(6):1493-1497.

   Patients with a rotator cuff tear were more likely to have hypercholesterolemia than control subjects. Level of evidence: II.

5. Kovacevic D, Rodeo SA: Biological augmentation of rotator cuff tendon repair. *Clin Orthop Relat Res* 2008;466(3):622-633.

   This is a review of two studies of rotator cuff repair in sheep using a mixture of osteoinductive factors and bone morphogenetic protein–12, with a detailed review of the current understanding of biologic augmentation of rotator cuff repair healing. Level of evidence:V.

6. Gerber C, Hersche O, Farron A: Isolated rupture of the subscapularis tendon. *J Bone Joint Surg Am* 1996; 78(7):1015-1023.

7. Gerber C, Krushell RJ: Isolated rupture of the tendon of the subscapularis muscle: Clinical features in 16 cases. *J Bone Joint Surg Br* 1991;73(3):389-394.

8. Hertel R, Ballmer FT, Lombert SM, Gerber C: Lag signs in the diagnosis of rotator cuff rupture. *J Shoulder Elbow Surg* 1996;5(4):307-313.

9. Mallon WJ, Wilson RJ, Basamania CJ: The association of suprascapular neuropathy with massive rotator cuff tears: A preliminary report. *J Shoulder Elbow Surg* 2006;15(4):395-398.

10. DeOrio JK, Cofield RH: Results of a second attempt at surgical repair of a failed initial rotator-cuff repair. *J Bone Joint Surg Am* 1984;66(4):563-567.

11. Neer CS II, Craig EV, Fukuda H: Cuff-tear arthropathy. *J Bone Joint Surg Am* 1983;65(9):1232-1244.

12. Goutallier D, Postel JM, Bernageau J, Lavau L, Voisin MC: Fatty muscle degeneration in cuff ruptures: Pre- and postoperative evaluation by CT scan. *Clin Orthop Relat Res* 1994;304:78-83.

13. Fuchs B, Weishaupt D, Zanetti M, Hodler J, Gerber C: Fatty degeneration of the muscles of the rotator cuff: Assessment by computed tomography versus magnetic resonance imaging. *J Shoulder Elbow Surg* 1999;8(6): 599-605.

14. Goutallier D, Postel JM, Gleyze P, Leguilloux P, Van Driessche S: Influence of cuff muscle fatty degeneration on anatomic and functional outcomes after simple suture of full-thickness tears. *J Shoulder Elbow Surg* 2003;12(6):550-554.

15. Montgomery SR, Petrigliano FA, Gamradt SC: Biologic augmentation of rotator cuff repair. *Curr Rev Musculoskelet Med* 2011;4(4):221-230.

    Current research was reviewed pertaining to biologic augmentation of rotator cuff repair using allograft, ECMs, PRP, growth factors, stem cells, and gene therapy. Level of evidence: V.

16. Edwards SL, Lynch TS, Saltzman MD, Terry MA, Nuber GW: Biologic and pharmacologic augmentation of rotator cuff repairs. *J Am Acad Orthop Surg* 2011; 19(10):583-589.

    The basic science of rotator cuff healing was discussed, with a broad overview of current and future biologic and pharmacologic augmentation techniques for rotator cuff repair. Level of evidence: V.

17. Burkhead WZ, Schiffern SC, Krishnan SG: Use of GraftJacket as an augmentation for massive rotator cuff tears. *Semin Arthroplasty* 2007;18(1):11-18.

    A surgical technique for open rotator cuff repair with GraftJacket (Wright Medical Technology) allograft augmentation was reported, with early results. Level of evidence: IV.

18. Labbé MR: Arthroscopic technique for patch augmentation of rotator cuff repairs. *Arthroscopy* 2006; 22(10):e1-e6.

19. Wong I, Burns J, Snyder S: Arthroscopic GraftJacket repair of rotator cuff tears. *J Shoulder Elbow Surg* 2010;19(2, suppl):104-109.

    A surgical technique was presented for arthroscopic

rotator cuff reconstruction using the GraftJacket allograft acellular human dermal matrix, with an update of earlier data. Level of evidence: IV.

20. Seldes RM, Abramchayev I: Arthroscopic insertion of a biologic rotator cuff tissue augmentation after rotator cuff repair. *Arthroscopy* 2006;22(1):113-116.

21. Iannotti JP, Codsi MJ, Kwon YW, Derwin K, Ciccone J, Brems JJ: Porcine small intestine submucosa augmentation of surgical repair of chronic two-tendon rotator cuff tears: A randomized, controlled trial. *J Bone Joint Surg Am* 2006;88(6):1238-1244.

22. Walton JR, Bowman NK, Khatib Y, Linklater J, Murrell GA: Restore orthobiologic implant: Not recommended for augmentation of rotator cuff repairs. *J Bone Joint Surg Am* 2007;89(4):786-791.

    The results of patients who underwent an open rotator cuff repair with xenograft allograft reconstruction were described. Level of evidence: III.

23. Phipatanakul WP, Petersen SA: Porcine small intestine submucosa xenograft augmentation in repair of massive rotator cuff tears. *Am J Orthop (Belle Mead NJ)* 2009;38(11):572-575.

    The results of using porcine small intestine submucosa xenograft to augment the repair of massive rotator cuff tears were described. Level of evidence: IV.

24. Sclamberg SG, Tibone JE, Itamura JM, Kasraeian S: Six-month magnetic resonance imaging follow-up of large and massive rotator cuff repairs reinforced with porcine small intestinal submucosa. *J Shoulder Elbow Surg* 2004;13(5):538-541.

25. Badhe SP, Lawrence TM, Smith FD, Lunn PG: An assessment of porcine dermal xenograft as an augmentation graft in the treatment of extensive rotator cuff tears. *J Shoulder Elbow Surg* 2008;17(1, suppl):35S-39S.

    Clinical, ultrasound, and MRI outcomes of massive rotator cuff repairs using porcine dermal collagen tendon augmentation grafting were analyzed. Level of evidence: IV.

26. Soler JA, Gidwani S, Curtis MJ: Early complications from the use of porcine dermal collagen implants (Permacol) as bridging constructs in the repair of massive rotator cuff tears: A report of 4 cases. *Acta Orthop Belg* 2007;73(4):432-436.

    The clinical, radiographic, and histologic results of repair of a massive rotator cuff tear using a porcine dermal collagen implant in a bridging fashion were described in four patients. Level of evidence: IV.

27. Barber FA, Burns JP, Deutsch A, Labbé MR, Litchfield RB: A prospective, randomized evaluation of acellular human dermal matrix augmentation for arthroscopic rotator cuff repair. *Arthroscopy* 2012;28(1):8-15.

    This study evaluated the safety and effectiveness of arthroscopic acellular human dermal matrix augmentation of large rotator cuff tear repairs. Level of evidence: II.

28. Snyder SJ, Arnoczky SP, Bond JL, Dopirak R: Histologic evaluation of a biopsy specimen obtained 3 months after rotator cuff augmentation with GraftJacket Matrix. *Arthroscopy* 2009;25(3):329-333.

    A biopsy specimen taken from a single rotator cuff augmented 3 months earlier with an acellular human dermal matrix graft was histologically evaluated. Level of evidence: IV.

29. Randelli P, Arrigoni P, Ragone V, Aliprandi A, Cabitza P: Platelet rich plasma in arthroscopic rotator cuff repair: A prospective RCT study, 2-year follow-up. *J Shoulder Elbow Surg* 2011;20(4):518-528.

    A prospective randomized controlled double-blind study reported the results of using autologous PRP in patients undergoing arthroscopic rotator cuff repair. Level of evidence: I.

30. Castricini R, Longo UG, De Benedetto M, et al: Platelet-rich plasma augmentation for arthroscopic rotator cuff repair: A randomized controlled trial. *Am J Sports Med* 2011;39(2):258-265.

    A randomized controlled study investigated the results of autologous platelet-rich fibrin matrix for augmentation of a double-row repair of small- or medium-size rotator cuff tears.

31. Rodeo SA, Delos D, Williams RJ, Adler RS, Pearle A, Warren RF: The effect of platelet-rich fibrin matrix on rotator cuff tendon healing: A prospective, randomized clinical study. *Am J Sports Med* 2012;40(6):1234-1241.

    This randomized controlled trial showed platelet-rich fibrin matrix had no effect on tendon healing, tendon vascularity, manual muscle strength, and clinical rating scales. Level of evidence: II.

32. Caplan AI: Mesenchymal stem cells and gene therapy. *Clin Orthop Relat Res* 2000;379(suppl):S67-S70.

33. Ouyang HW, Goh JC, Lee EH: Use of bone marrow stromal cells for tendon graft-to-bone healing: Histological and immunohistochemical studies in a rabbit model. *Am J Sports Med* 2004;32(2):321-327.

34. Lim JK, Hui J, Li L, Thambyah A, Goh J, Lee EH: Enhancement of tendon graft osteointegration using mesenchymal stem cells in a rabbit model of anterior cruciate ligament reconstruction. *Arthroscopy* 2004; 20(9):899-910.

35. Gulotta LV, Kovacevic D, Packer JD, Deng XH, Rodeo SA: Bone marrow-derived mesenchymal stem cells transduced with scleraxis improve rotator cuff healing in a rat model. *Am J Sports Med* 2011;39(6):1282-1289.

    Bone marrow–derived MSCs were transduced with scleraxis to augment rotator cuff healing at early time points in a rat model. Level of evidence: I.

36. Mazzocca AD, McCarthy MB, Chowaniec DM, Cote MP, Arciero RA, Drissi H: Rapid isolation of human stem cells (connective tissue progenitor cells) from the

proximal humerus during arthroscopic rotator cuff surgery. *Am J Sports Med* 2010;38(7):1438-1447.

A technique was described for arthroscopically obtaining bone marrow aspirate from the proximal humerus and then purifying and concentrating the connective tissue progenitor cells in the operating room. Level of evidence: III.

37. Würgler-Hauri CC, Dourte LM, Baradet TC, Williams GR, Soslowsky LJ: Temporal expression of 8 growth factors in tendon-to-bone healing in a rat supraspinatus model. *J Shoulder Elbow Surg* 2007;16(5, suppl): S198-S203.

The temporal expression of eight different growth factors for tendon-to-bone healing was evaluated in a rat model. Level of evidence: II.

38. Asou Y, Nifuji A, Tsuji K, et al: Coordinated expression of scleraxis and Sox9 genes during embryonic development of tendons and cartilage. *J Orthop Res* 2002;20(4):827-833.

39. Moffat KL, Kwei AS, Spalazzi JP, Doty SB, Levine WN, Lu HH: Novel nanofiber-based scaffold for rotator cuff repair and augmentation. *Tissue Eng Part A* 2009;15(1):115-126.

Bench work efforts were aimed at creating a novel nanofiber-based scaffold for rotator cuff tendon tissue engineering and evaluating the attachment, alignment, gene expression, and matrix elaboration over time of human rotator cuff fibroblasts on aligned and unaligned polylactide-coglycolide nanofiber scaffolds. Level of evidence: II.

3: The Rotator Cuff

Chapter 18

Factors Affecting the Outcome of Rotator Cuff Surgery

Michael E. Angeline, MD   Joshua S. Dines, MD

Introduction

Tears of the rotator cuff are a common cause of disability and pain, and surgical repair of the rotator cuff accounts for approximately 75,000 procedures in the United States each year. All-arthroscopic repairs have good results, with stable functional outcomes after 5 years.[1] Despite the clinical success of rotator cuff repairs, the repair site heals with a fibrovascular scar at the tendon-bone interface. It is important to remember that a rotator cuff repair does not regenerate the native tendon insertion site, which was formed during embryologic development. The construct is mechanically weaker than the normal tendon enthesis and probably is more prone to failure.[2] Recent research supported the belief that patients whose rotator cuff fully heals after a repair tend to have better functional outcomes.[3] There has been much interest in the factors that may affect the outcome of rotator cuff surgery, as well as ways to improve healing rates.

The native rotator cuff tendon-to-bone insertion site functions to minimize stress concentration at the junction between the soft tendinous portion of the enthesis and the hard bony portion. The enthesis is composed of four distinct transition zones: tendon, fibrocartilage, mineralized fibrocartilage, and bone (**Figure 1**). The collagen content differs based on the tissue type.[4] The tendinous portion predominantly is composed of types I and III collagen, and the fibrocartilaginous zone is composed of types I, II, and III collagen. The mineralized fibrocartilage zone contains types I, II, and X collagen. The bone portion of the enthesis is composed of type I collagen.[5,6]

Dr. Dines or an immediate family member has received royalties from Biomet; serves as a paid consultant to Biomimetic and Tornier; and has received research or institutional support from Biomimetic. Neither Dr. Angeline nor any immediate family member has received anything of value from or has stock or stock options held in a commercial company or institution related directly or indirectly to the subject of this chapter.

Biologic Factors

The prevalence of rotator cuff tears in the general population ranges from 5% to 39%.[7] The known risk factors include a history of trauma, injury to the dominant arm, and advancing age. The natural history of symptomatic and asymptomatic rotator cuff tears is suggested by the finding that 39% to 49% of nonsurgically treated tears had increased in size at midrange follow-up.[8] Pain development was found to be associated with an increase in tear size and an increased rate of tear progression.[9] As a rotator cuff tear progresses and becomes more symptomatic, the decision of whether to operate is based on multiple factors. Biologic factors that can affect the outcome of rotator cuff surgery include the patient's age, genetic influences, medical comorbidities, and rotator cuff integrity.

Patient Age

With advancing age, the ability of the rotator cuff tendon to heal is adversely affected by reduced bone quality, tendon cellularity, and vascularity. Several recent case studies examined the outcomes of rotator cuff repair in patients older than 65 years.[10-12] Older patients were found to have improvement in pain, range of motion, and functional status after arthroscopic repair, regardless of whether the study evaluated these patients alone or in comparison with younger patients. These studies suggest that age alone is not associated with poor functional outcomes in older patients. However, most of the studies were at level IV, with only a univariate analysis of age and functional outcomes. In addition, confounding variables may have affected the perceived outcome. For example, the higher physical demands of younger patients may have influenced their perception of the surgical outcome.

In tendon healing, recent research using multivariate analysis found that advanced age was the main biologic limitation at the repair site, even when the biomechanical strength of the repair site was maximized with a double-row repair construct.[13] With advancing age, fatty degeneration of the infraspinatus and tear retraction may become greater and have a further negative influence on anatomic outcomes after a repair. Overall,

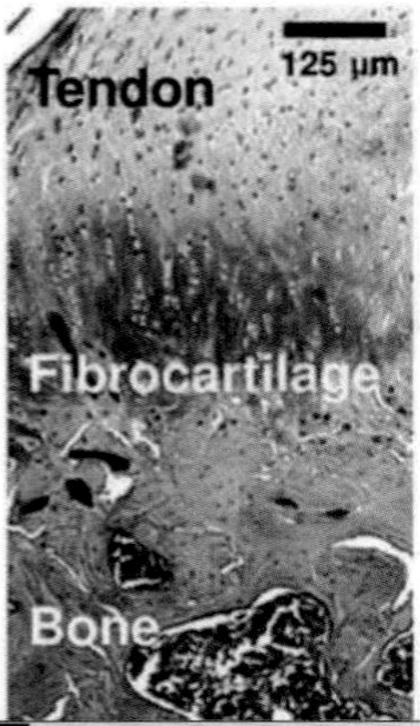

Tissue Region	Cell Type	Major Matrix Component
Tendon	Fibroblasts	Collagen types I, III (Diameter: 40-400 nm)
Nonmineralized Fibrocartilage	Fibrochondrocytes	Collagen types I, II, III
Mineralized Fibrocartilage	Hypertrophic Fibrochondrocytes	Collagen types I, II, X
Bone	Osteoblasts Osteocytes Osteoclasts	Collagen type I (Diameter: 34.5-39.5 nm)

Figure 1 The structure and composition of the direct tendon-to-bone insertion site. (Adapted with permission from Zhang X, Bogdanowicz D, Eriksen C, et al. Biomimetic scaffold design for functional and integrative tendon repair. *J Shoulder Elbow Surg* 2012;21[2]:266–277.)

older patients may have improvement in functional outcome measures after rotator cuff repair, but the repair site has a reduced ability to heal with increasing age.

Genetics

Although no single gene is involved in rotator cuff pathology, the gene pathways are altered in tears and tendinopathies. The resulting changes affect the composition of the rotator cuff tendon in terms of collagen composition, vasculature, and intracellular signaling mechanisms as well as the ability to regenerate the native enthesis after a repair. Within the healing tendon, altered collagen gene expression results in an increase in type III collagen and a decrease in type I collagen, which coincide with a scar-mediated healing pathway. Modulation of the ratio of collagen I to collagen III has the potential for enhancing the structural properties of the healing tendon.

Recently, there has been interest in the levels of expression of the cytokine transforming growth factor–β (TGF-β1, -β2, and -β3), which is believed to influence cellular proliferation, differentiation, and matrix synthesis within the healing tendon. As the adult tendon heals, levels of TGF-β1 and TGF-β2 are elevated, with resultant scar formation and low levels of expressed TGF-β3. Fetal wound healing is known to have higher levels of TGF-β3 expression and a subsequent lack of scar formation.[14]

In a rat supraspinatus repair model, localized delivery of TGF-β3 was found to improve the repair site strength at 4 weeks postoperatively and increase type I collagen expression, reflecting more mature healing.[15] These results are promising, but further research is necessary to establish the optimal dosing and delivery of TGF-β3.

Matrix metalloproteinases (MMPs) and their tissue inhibitors recently have been studied because changes in their dynamic expression patterns were found to regulate remodeling of the extracellular matrix in rotator cuff tears. Loss of the balance between MMPs and their tissue inhibitors results in increased MMP activity, affecting tendon healing through tendon degradation and possible rupture.[16] Localized delivery of an MMP inhibitor in a rat supraspinatus repair model led to significantly greater collagen organization and decreased collagen degradation.[17] These results show that modulating the MMP activity after a rotator cuff repair augments tendon-to-bone healing at the repair site.

Doxycycline, an antibiotic, has MMP inhibitory effects through a pathway independent of its antimicrobial efficacy. The effects of doxycycline on tendon healing were examined in a follow-up study using a rat model.[16] After acute rotator cuff repair, doxycycline-mediated inhibition of MMP activity was associated with improved biomechanical and histologic healing parameters at the tendon-bone interface. Further research is needed to define the exact mechanism of improved tendon healing through MMP inhibition, but doxycycline may become a treatment for improving the outcomes of rotator cuff surgery.

Recent studies also have evaluated the inherited risk of rotator cuff tears or pathology.[18,19] These studies provided evidence of a strong genetic predisposition to rotator cuff disease with increased observed risk among patients' first- and second-degree relatives, and they suggested that individuals having a genetic predisposition may be more affected by age-related tendon degeneration than those without such a predisposition. The role of genetic inheritance patterns on healing of the tendon-bone unit after a repair was not examined, unfortunately. Future research is required to fully identify the predisposing genes responsible for these observations and understand the exact mechanism of genes associated with rotator cuff disease.

Medical Comorbidities

A patient's medical comorbidities can greatly affect tendon healing. Obesity is a worldwide problem associated with a risk of diabetes, vascular disease, and hypercholesterolemia. These disease states result in decreased vascularity and could affect the tendon-to-bone healing response. Two recent retrospective case control studies examined the correlation between obesity and functional outcomes after arthroscopic rotator cuff repair.[20,21] The results were conflicting. One study found a statistically significant correlation between obesity and poor functional outcome, longer hospital stay, and longer surgical time.[20] After controlling for confounding variables, the other study found that body mass index and obesity were not related to outcomes after arthroscopic rotator cuff repair.[21] It is difficult to directly compare these studies because they were based on different outcome measures and follow-up time points as well as the work of different surgeons. At best, the true correlation between obesity and rotator cuff pathology remains unclear.

Diabetes mellitus can affect tendon healing. It was shown that rats with diabetes had poorer biomechanical properties, less fibrocartilage, and less organized collagen at the tendon-bone interface after rotator cuff repair compared with controls.[22] These findings suggest that sustained hyperglycemia can impair rotator cuff tendon-to-bone healing. A recent retrospective study compared patients who had undergone arthroscopic rotator cuff repair, based on whether they had diabetes.[23] Constant scores improved postoperatively in both groups of patients, but improvement was greater in the patients without diabetes, who had better scores for forward flexion, external rotation, activities of daily living, and power components. Patients with diabetes had less forward flexion and external rotation as well as a slightly higher incidence of infection. The findings of basic science and clinical studies on the effects of diabetes on tendon healing should not be construed as precluding these patients from undergoing arthroscopic rotator cuff repair. Patients with diabetes do have improved pain and function postoperatively, although the expected outcomes may not be as good as those of patients without diabetes.

Tendon Integrity

Although the chronicity and the size of a rotator cuff tear are significant, the quality of the rotator cuff musculature, in terms of the extent of atrophy and fatty infiltration, may have an even greater influence on anatomic and functional outcomes after a repair. Research on a sheep chronic rotator cuff tear model showed that the crucial event in the pathogenesis of infraspinatus fatty infiltration is the change in the pennation angle (the angle at which muscle fibers insert into tendon in pennate skeletal muscles).[24] As the pennation angle in-

Table 1

The Goutallier-Bernageau Classification of Fatty Infiltration

Grade	Description
0	Completely normal muscle with no fatty streaking
1	Muscle containing some fatty streaks
2	More muscle than fat
3	As much fat as muscle
4	More fat than muscle

creased, the muscle fibers shortened, and fat was allowed to infiltrate. This factor can result in a poor biologic capacity of the tendon to heal at the insertion site and decreased mechanical properties of the muscle-tendon unit, as has been shown in several clinical studies. Relatively severe preoperative atrophy and fatty infiltration were associated with an increased rate of repair failure, loss of muscle function, and inferior achievable outcomes during the postoperative period.[25-27] The muscle quality and the extent of fatty infiltration of the infraspinatus are more influential than those of the supraspinatus. It is believed that poor infraspinatus function can offset the biomechanics of the glenohumeral joint and lead to a poor patient outcome.[25]

The natural history and the extent of muscle fatty infiltration in rotator cuff tears can be correlated with tear size, location, time to onset, and patient age.[28,29] For example, a large tear in an older patient with a long delay after tendon rupture will result in more severe fatty infiltration. In all tear types, Goutallier grade 2 fatty infiltration was found to occur in the supraspinatus muscle at an average of 4 years after the onset of symptoms[30] (Table 1). The progression was faster in tears that were traumatic or involved more than one tendon. Grade 2 fatty infiltration occurred in the infraspinatus muscle an average of 2.5 years after the onset of symptoms.[28] These fatty changes occurred regardless of whether the tear included an infraspinatus tendon rupture.

With an understanding of the time progression and influencing factors, the clinician should be able to appreciate the extent of atrophy and fatty infiltration before surgery and intervene appropriately (Figure 2). Surgical repair ideally should be attempted before grade 2 fatty infiltration appears, in an effort to avoid poor anatomic and functional results.[25,27] It is important to note that no clinical study has found a postrepair reversal of grade 2 fatty infiltration and the associated structural changes.[23]

3: The Rotator Cuff

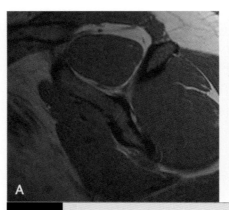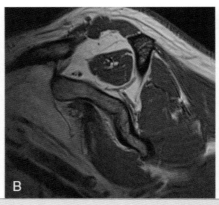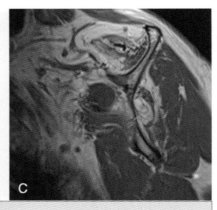

| Figure 2 | Sagittal-view MRI showing fatty infiltration of the supraspinatus muscle: Goutallier grades 0 (**A**), 2 (**B**), and 4 (**C**). |

Social Factors

Social factors including cigarette smoking and a workers' compensation–related claim can have a significant role in the outcome of rotator cuff surgery and are important for the surgeon to recognize. Smoking was found to be more prevalent in patients with a rotator cuff tear than in individuals without a tear, and pain from a rotator cuff disorder is second only to back pain as the most common upper extremity symptom among manual workers.[31,32] Nicotine use was found to negatively affect the amount of collagen deposition and repair at surgical wound sites because its potent vasoconstrictive effects decrease the delivery of oxygen to tissues.[31] These effects were correlated using a rat rotator cuff model, in which nicotine delivery through an implanted osmotic pump was found to affect tendon-to-bone healing by delaying scar degradation and remodeling.[33] Recent research also examined the influence of cigarette smoking on rotator cuff pathology.[31,34] In patients undergoing ultrasound for unilateral atraumatic shoulder pain, a questionnaire revealed a strong association and possible causation between smoking and rotator cuff disease.[31] The findings were independent of age and were both dosage and time dependent. The dosage-dependent relationship involved rotator cuff tear size and the amount of tobacco use; smokers with greater tobacco use had a correspondingly larger and more severe rotator cuff tear.[34]

Patients with a pending workers' compensation claim also were found to have relatively poor outcomes after a rotator cuff repair.[32,35,36] Two recent studies used multivariable analysis and matched case-control analysis to find a negative correlation while controlling for cofounding factors.[32,36] One year after a rotator cuff repair, functional measures were worse for the patients with a compensation claim than for other patients, and a compensation claim had a negative effect on recovery. Although these findings are significant, it is important to recognize that a compensation claim does not pre-clude a patient's receiving surgical management of rotator cuff pathology. Patients with a compensation claim can benefit from surgical intervention and have some improvement on subjective and objective measures.[32]

The potential factors contributing to impairment after a rotator cuff repair in patients with a work-related injury were examined in a recent cross-sectional study.[35] At least one definable explanation for continued impairment was found in half of the patients with reported surgical failure. The reasons were anatomic in nature (missed glenohumeral pathology or fixation failure) or were a consequence of the surgery itself (complex regional pain syndrome or failure of deltoid reattachment in an open repairs). The clinician must look for identifiable causes of surgical failure in a patient with a work-related injury who has a poor outcome.

Physician-Determined Factors

The surgeon can influence the outcome of rotator cuff surgery through decisions involving surgical timing, the surgical procedure, and postsurgical rehabilitation. The decision to operate on a chronic rotator cuff tear should be influenced by the extent of atrophy and fatty infiltration. Surgical repair should be performed before the onset of Goutallier grade 2 fatty infiltration. Fatty degeneration of the infraspinatus muscle has been reported with isolated chronic, degenerative supraspinatus tendon tears.[37] This finding represents a factor that must be considered because muscle quality and extent of fatty infiltration in the infraspinatus can influence the outcome of repair. The surgeon also must be cognizant of surgical timing for an acute rotator cuff tear. Previously, it was believed that a better functional outcome was achieved if an acute rotator cuff tear was repaired within 3 weeks of the time of injury.[38] Two recent retrospective reviews found that patients who underwent a delayed open repair within 3 to 4 months of injury had a satisfactory functional outcome similar to that of patients who underwent an early open re-

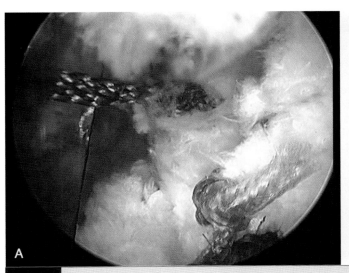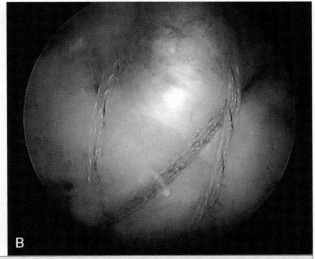

Figure 3   Arthroscopic images showing a single-row (**A**) and a double-row (**B**) rotator cuff repair.

pair.[38] In general, the surgeon can safely delay repair of an acute tear beyond the 3-week window without affecting the functional outcomes.

Surgical Procedures

The surgeon's choice of repair technique can affect the outcome of rotator cuff repair surgery. Concern over a lack of anatomic healing and/or retearing after a repair has led to a persistent debate as to the optimal surgical technique (specifically, single-row, double-row, or transosseous anchorless repair). Current double-row and transosseous repair techniques enhance the biomechanical strength of the repair and increase the surface area of the repaired tendon on the footprint, but their ability to provide superior anatomic and functional outcomes is still controversial (**Figure 3**).

Several recent prospective studies and systematic reviews compared the benefits of single-row and double-row repairs.[39-42] Three recent prospective studies found no significant clinical or anatomic difference between single-row and double-row repair techniques at 1-to 2-year follow-up.[39-41] A recent review found no significant functional difference between the two repair techniques.[43] The muscle strength of the shoulder was found to be greater, however, after double-row repair of a tear larger than 3 cm.[41] In addition, the retearing rate was significantly lower for tears larger than 1 cm after a double-row repair compared with a single-row repair.[42] These studies suggest that there is little difference between single-row and double-row techniques for treating small rotator cuff tears, but patients with a large or a massive tear may benefit from a double-row repair. The surgeon should perform a risk-reward analysis before deciding on the best repair technique. The patient's size, functional demands, and tear characteristics all need to be incorporated into the decision-making process.

Postsurgical Rehabilitation

Stiffness in the shoulder joint before or after surgical repair can occur with any torn rotator cuff tendon. In a rotator cuff model, long periods of immobilization after a repair were found to improve the biomechanical characteristics of the repaired insertion site.[44] Stiffness may be more likely to develop, however. Patients with a full-thickness tear or an acute traumatic tear were observed to have substantially more preoperative stiffness.[45] In a rat rotator cuff model, joint stiffness resulting from immobilization after a repair was transient and, in the long term, was not significantly different from that of nonimmobilized repairs.[46] Furthermore, early passive motion possibly was detrimental to shoulder joint mechanics, resulting in a loss of motion after repair of the supraspinatus tendon in comparison with continuously immobilized shoulders.[44] These findings together highlight the potential beneficial effect of postoperative immobilization for tendon healing. A recent retrospective clinical review supported this concept by finding that 6 weeks of sling immobilization after arthroscopic rotator cuff repair did not affect stiffness or functional outcomes at 1-year follow-up.[47] In addition, there was a trend toward a lower rate of retearing when this conservative postoperative rehabilitation protocol was used. Prospective studies are needed to fully understand the relationship of prolonged postoperative immobilization, stiffness, and tendon healing at the repair site.

3: The Rotator Cuff

Biologic Agents

The challenge in rotator cuff surgery is to stimulate a regenerative rather than a reparative healing pathway. None of the patient or physician-determined factors can enable the healing tendon to regenerate the native tendon-bone interface formed during prenatal development. As a result, the use of biologic agents and cell-based therapies is being examined as potential means of augmenting the repair site and improving tendon healing through a scarless process.

Platelet-Derived Growth Factor

During the early inflammatory phase of tendon healing, platelet-derived growth factor (PDGF) helps direct cell chemotaxis, proliferation, differentiation, and matrix synthesis.[4] The cytokine PDGF basic protein family is composed of two subunits (A and B chains) derived from platelets and other cell types, including smooth muscle. Rotator cuff healing results in reactive scar formation rather than a histologically normal insertion site, and it may be possible to augment the repair site biology by adding PDGF.

Recombinant human PDGF (rhPDGF)-BB is the first exogenous growth factor to be tested in a clinical study of rotator cuff repair. A sheep rotator cuff model was used to examine the effects of rhPDGF-BB on rotator cuff healing.[48] Sutures coated with the growth factor were found to enhance histologic properties after rotator cuff repair but did not improve biomechanical properties compared with standard suture repair. Another sheep rotator cuff repair study examined the effects of an interpositional graft composed of rhPDGF-BB and a type I collagen matrix.[49] Twelve weeks after repair, low- and medium-dosage rhPDGF-BB grafts showed improved biomechanical strength and anatomic appearance compared with control or high-dosage grafts. These studies highlight the importance of growth factor–dependent dosage, timing, and delivery methods. PDGF augmentation holds promise for tendon-to-bone healing, and phase I clinical studies are under way using rhPDGF-BB to augment rotator cuff repairs.

Platelet-Rich Plasma

Many growth factors (cytokines) are upregulated within the cascade of events that leads to natural healing of the tendon-to-bone insertion. Combining and increasing the concentration of these factors has potential for enhancing tenocyte, stem cell, and endothelial cell recruitment and proliferation at the healing interface. Platelet-rich plasma (PRP) has become popular for augmenting tendon healing because it is an autologous concentration of platelets and growth factors including PDGF, vascular endothelial growth factor, TGF-β, fibroblast growth factor–2, and insulinlike growth factor–1. Several recent studies examined the use of PRP

augmentation at the rotator cuff repair site.[50-53] In two cohort studies, PRP application during arthroscopic rotator cuff repair did not improve functional outcome measures compared with those of patients in the control group.[52,53] Another level I randomized study had similar findings at the 6-, 12-, and 24-month postoperative time points.[54] However, pain scores were lower during the first postoperative month, and clinical outcomes were improved 3 months after surgery compared with patients in the control group. These results raise the possibility that PRP may have a positive influence on early tendon healing.

The study results conflicted as to whether PRP augmentation improved the structural integrity of the healing rotator cuff repair site. In contrast, animal and clinical studies of Achilles tendon rupture found that application of PRP enhances healing and functional recovery.[55,56] The effects of PRP may depend on the mechanical loading characteristics of the healing tendon. A recent study also found a difference in the growth factor concentration in three commercially available PRP separation systems.[57] Further research is needed to fully understand the mechanisms by which PRP improves tendon healing and the significance of different growth factor concentrations.

Mesenchymal Stem Cells

As research on regenerative tendon healing has evolved, it has become evident that therapy based on cytokine growth factors alone may not be sufficient for improving the material properties of the tissue. Combining these factors with undifferentiated cells may lead to enhanced tissue healing. Mesenchymal stem cells (MSCs) are distinguished by their unique ability to self-renew and differentiate into cell lines, including adipocytes, tenocytes, and chondrocytes. Currently, autologous stromal cells can be obtained only by isolating them from the bone marrow, but other harvesting techniques are being developed. Cell-based therapy can influence the repair process through a direct local paracrine effect or through anti-inflammatory effects. In a rat rotator cuff model the biomechanical or histologic properties of the tendon attachment site were not enhanced by the addition of bone marrow–derived MSCs alone.[58] A combination of MSCs and other factors may be necessary for augmenting the repair site. The optimal combinations ideally will be based on knowledge of the mechanism and signaling events that lead to the formation of the natural enthesis.

Research involving the use of MSCs and the transcription factor scleraxis has highlighted the potential benefits of combined therapy. Scleraxis was found to play an important role in the developing enthesis and tenogenesis in general, and it remains present during the formation of the tendon proper as well as the tendon-to-bone insertion site. By using bone marrow–derived MSCs transduced with adenoviral-mediated scleraxis in a rat rotator cuff model, a recent study found significantly better biomechanical properties after repair compared with those of controls.[59] The rats treated with adenoviral-mediated scleraxis also had more fibrocartilage, which more closely resembled that of the native tendon-to-bone insertion site. Further research is needed to fully understand the complex signaling events necessary to regenerate the tendon-to-bone insertion site as well as the optimal combination, dosing, and delivery vehicles for biologic augmentation.

Biomimetic Scaffolds

Tissue engineering strategies have evolved to include a biomimetic scaffold that has the potential to achieve functional integration with the host environment. The ideal scaffold design would enable restoration of the histologic and the mechanical properties of the native tendon-to-bone interface. Current research is focused on a biphasic scaffold design composed of polylactide-coglycolide nanofibers and a composite of PLGA nanofibers and hydroxyapatite nanoparticles.[6] The purpose of this biphasic design is to promote the postrepair regeneration of both the nonmineralized and the mineralized fibrocartilaginous regions of the native enthesis. In a rat rotator cuff repair model, the biphasic scaffold was found to stimulate the formation of a continuous noncalcified and calcified matrix region rather than the fibrovascular scarring observed in the control group.

Although biomimetic scaffolding has promise for augmenting and promoting regenerative healing, research is required to gain an in-depth understanding of the signaling mechanisms that lead to the formation of graded structures in the native enthesis.[6] A thorough understanding of developmental biology at the tendon-to-bone insertion site will directly affect future scaffold designs. Growth factors and other signaling molecules may be incorporated into these structures.

Summary

Both patient and physician-derived factors influence the outcome of rotator cuff surgery. The patient factors include age, genetic factors, medical comorbidities, tendon integrity, and social factors. Patient age alone may not influence the functional outcomes of rotator cuff surgery, but age negatively influences anatomic outcomes. There may be a genetic predisposition to rotator cuff disease, and controlling MMP activity or delivering TGF-β3 to the repair site may lead to better tendon healing. Diabetes mellitus is known to negatively affect tendon healing and the outcomes of rotator cuff surgery, but the true correlation between obesity and rotator cuff pathology is unclear. The extent of atrophy and fatty infiltration of the rotator cuff musculature has a significant effect on anatomic and functional outcomes after a repair. Surgery should be performed before Goutallier grade 2 fatty infiltration occurs. Smoking and the presence of a worker's compensation claim were found to negatively affect the outcomes after a rotator cuff repair.

Physician-determined factors that influence the outcomes of rotator cuff surgery include surgical timing, the surgical procedure, and postsurgical rehabilitation. An acute rotator cuff tear can be safely repaired within 3 to 4 months of the injury without negatively affecting the outcome. For a chronic rotator cuff tear, the extent of atrophy and fatty infiltration should be assessed, and the repair should be performed before the onset of Goutallier grade 2 fatty infiltration. A significant difference was found between the single-row and double-row repair techniques in large tears only. Basic science research in a rat model showed that prolonged immobilization can improve the strength of the repair, with only transient stiffness; early passive motion may negatively effect shoulder joint mechanics.

A conservative postsurgical rehabilitation program with six weeks of immobilization was found to have no impact on range of motion or functional outcomes 1 year after surgical repair. A trend toward a reduced retearing rate was noted, based on MRI.

Future directions for augmenting the rotator cuff repair site to improve healing include the use of PDGF, PRP, MSCs, and biomimetic scaffolds. Used alone, PDGF may improve the biomechanical strength and the anatomic appearance of the repaired rotator cuff. In contrast, the use of PRP or MSCs alone may not significantly enhance the biomechanical or histologic properties of the repair site. Further research must establish the optimal combinations of these growth factors (cytokines) as well as the optimal dosing and delivery methods. The use of a biomimetic scaffold to augment regenerative healing has promise, but research is still required.

Annotated References

1. Gulotta LV, Nho SJ, Dodson CC, Adler RS, Altchek DW, MacGillivray JD; HSS Arthroscopic Rotator Cuff Registry: Prospective evaluation of arthroscopic rotator cuff repairs at 5 years: Part I—functional outcomes and radiographic healing rates. *J Shoulder Elbow Surg* 2011;20(6):934-940.

   At 5-year follow-up after arthroscopic rotator cuff repair in 106 patients, functional results remained constant. Healing rates on ultrasound improved over time. Level of evidence: II.

2. Galatz LM, Sandell LJ, Rothermich SY, et al: Characteristics of the rat supraspinatus tendon during tendon-to-bone healing after acute injury. *J Orthop Res* 2006;24(3):541-550.

3. Slabaugh MA, Nho SJ, Grumet RC, et al: Does the literature confirm superior clinical results in radiographically healed rotator cuffs after rotator cuff repair? *Arthroscopy* 2010;26(3):393-403.

   A systematic review examined the correlation between the structural integrity of the rotator cuff after repair and the clinical outcome. Important differences were noted between patients with a healed or an unhealed rotator cuff repair. Level of evidence: IV.

4. Bedi A, Maak T, Walsh C, et al: Cytokines in rotator cuff degeneration and repair. *J Shoulder Elbow Surg* 2012;21(2):218-227.

   The use of cytokines during the healing process after rotator cuff repair is discussed.

5. Galatz L, Rothermich S, VanderPloeg K, Petersen B, Sandell L, Thomopoulos S: Development of the supraspinatus tendon-to-bone insertion: Localized expression of extracellular matrix and growth factor genes. *J Orthop Res* 2007;25(12):1621-1628.

   Using a murine model, the development of the rotator cuff tendon-to-bone insertion site was examined. The rotator cuff was morphologically distinct at 13.5 days postconception, and a shift from TGF-β3 to TGF-β1 expression occurred 2 days later.

6. Zhang X, Bogdanowicz D, Erisken C, Lee NM, Lu HH: Biomimetic scaffold design for functional and integrative tendon repair. *J Shoulder Elbow Surg* 2012; 21(2):266-277.

   A review article examining the current approaches to functional and integrative tendon repair using biomimetic design principles. Level of evidence: Review article.

7. Yamamoto A, Takagishi K, Osawa T, et al: Prevalence and risk factors of a rotator cuff tear in the general population. *J Shoulder Elbow Surg* 2010;19(1):116-120.

   The epidemiology of rotator cuff tears was examined in 683 people (1,366 shoulders). A 20.7% prevalence of full-thickness rotator cuff tears was found. The risk factors involved a history of trauma, the dominant arm, and age. Level of evidence: III.

8. Safran O, Schroeder J, Bloom R, Weil Y, Milgrom C: Natural history of nonoperatively treated symptomatic rotator cuff tears in patients 60 years old or younger. *Am J Sports Med* 2011;39(4):710-714.

   Size change was examined in 61 nonsurgically treated full-thickness rotator cuff tears. At an average 29-month follow-up, half of the tears had increased in size. No correlation was found between tear size and patient age or initial tear size.

9. Mall NA, Kim HM, Keener JD, et al: Symptomatic progression of asymptomatic rotator cuff tears: A prospective study of clinical and sonographic variables. *J Bone Joint Surg Am* 2010;92(16):2623-2633.

   A prospective study of 195 patients with asymptomatic rotator cuff tears found that pain development was associated with an increase in tear size, and larger tears were more likely to develop pain. Level of evidence: III.

10. Verma NN, Bhatia S, Baker CL III, et al: Outcomes of arthroscopic rotator cuff repair in patients aged 70 years or older. *Arthroscopy* 2010;26(10):1273-1280.

Thirty-nine patients age 70 years or older were evaluated after arthroscopic rotator cuff repair. At an average 36.1-month follow-up, American Shoulder and Elbow Surgeons Shoulder Index, Simple Shoulder Test, and visual analog pain scores had significantly improved. Level of evidence: IV.

11. Charousset C, Bellaïche L, Kalra K, Petrover D: Arthroscopic repair of full-thickness rotator cuff tears: Is there tendon healing in patients aged 65 years or older? *Arthroscopy* 2010;26(3):302-309.

    Eighty-eight patients age 65 years or older were evaluated after arthroscopic rotator cuff repair. At an average 41-month follow-up, Constant and Simple Shoulder Test scores had significantly improved. The retear rate was 42% based on a CT arthrogram.

12. Osti L, Papalia R, Del Buono A, Denaro V, Maffulli N: Comparison of arthroscopic rotator cuff repair in healthy patients over and under 65 years of age. *Knee Surg Sports Traumatol Arthrosc* 2010;18(12):1700-1706.

    The outcomes of 28 pairs of matched patients older and younger than 65 years were compared after arthroscopic rotator cuff repair. At an average 27-month follow-up, there were no significant differences in motion or scores on the UCLA Scale or Medical Outcomes Study 36-Item Short Form.

13. Tashjian RZ, Hollins AM, Kim HM, et al: Factors affecting healing rates after arthroscopic double-row rotator cuff repair. *Am J Sports Med* 2010;38(12):2435-2442.

    Forty-eight patients were evaluated at a mean 16-month follow-up after double-row rotator cuff repair. Multivariate regression analysis showed that age was the most important factor influencing tendon healing at the repair site, even with a double-row construct. Level of evidence: IV.

14. Manning CN, Kim HM, Sakiyama-Elbert S, Galatz LM, Havlioglu N, Thomopoulos S: Sustained delivery of transforming growth factor beta three enhances tendon-to-bone healing in a rat model. *J Orthop Res* 2011;29(7):1099-1105.

    In a rat rotator cuff repair model, TGF-β3 was delivered to the repair site using a heparin-fibrin–based delivery system. Sustained delivery of TGF-β3 to the healing tendon-bone insertion led to significant improvement in structural properties at 28 days and material properties at 56 days, compared with controls.

15. Kovacevic D, Fox AJ, Bedi A, et al: Calcium-phosphate matrix with or without TGF-β3 improves tendon-bone healing after rotator cuff repair. *Am J Sports Med* 2011;39(4):811-819.

    In a rat rotator cuff repair model, delivery of TGF-β3 with an injectable calcium-phosphate matrix significantly improved the strength of the repair site at 4 weeks. TGF-β3 delivery also resulted in greater type I rather than type III collagen expression at the healing enthesis.

16. Bedi A, Fox AJ, Kovacevic D, Deng XH, Warren RF, Rodeo SA: Doxycycline-mediated inhibition of matrix metalloproteinases improves healing after rotator cuff repair. *Am J Sports Med* 2010;38(2):308-317.

    Modulation of MMP-13 activity was significantly reduced after oral administration of doxycycline in a rat rotator cuff repair model. The healing enthesis had an increased load to failure at 2 weeks compared with controls.

17. Bedi A, Kovacevic D, Hettrich C, et al: The effect of matrix metalloproteinase inhibition on tendon-to-bone healing in a rotator cuff repair model. *J Shoulder Elbow Surg* 2010;19(3):384-391.

    Local delivery of an MMP inhibitor resulted in reduced collagen degradation at the healing enthesis in a rat rotator cuff repair model. Biomechanical testing revealed no significant differences in stiffness or ultimate load to failure compared with controls.

18. Gwilym SE, Watkins B, Cooper CD, et al: Genetic influences in the progression of tears of the rotator cuff. *J Bone Joint Surg Br* 2009;91(7):915-917.

    The relative risk of full-thickness rotator cuff tears in siblings of patients with a tear was 2.85, compared with control subjects. Full-thickness tears in siblings were significantly more likely to progress over 5 years.

19. Tashjian RZ, Farnham JM, Albright FS, Teerlink CC, Cannon-Albright LA: Evidence for an inherited predisposition contributing to the risk for rotator cuff disease. *J Bone Joint Surg Am* 2009;91(5):1136-1142.

    Patients with diagnosed rotator cuff disease and a known genealogy were analyzed to describe the familial clustering of affected individuals. Significant excess relatedness of patients and elevated risks to both close and distant relatives of patients with rotator cuff disease were observed. Level of evidence: III.

20. Warrender WJ, Brown OL, Abboud JA: Outcomes of arthroscopic rotator cuff repairs in obese patients. *J Shoulder Elbow Surg* 2011;20(6):961-967.

    Retrospective review of 149 patients at 16.3-month follow-up after arthroscopic rotator cuff repair found a significant correlation between obesity and poor functional outcomes, longer surgical times, and longer hospital stay. Level of evidence: III.

21. Namdari S, Baldwin K, Glaser D, Green A: Does obesity affect early outcome of rotator cuff repair? *J Shoulder Elbow Surg* 2010;19(8):1250-1255.

    A retrospective review of 154 patients at a mean 54.8-week follow-up after rotator cuff repair compared preoperative and postoperative scores on the Disabilities of the Arm, Shoulder and Hand questionnaire; the Simple Shoulder Test; and the visual analog scale for pain, function, and quality of life. Obesity and body mass index did not influence early functional outcomes. Level of evidence: III.

22. Bedi A, Fox AJ, Harris PE, et al: Diabetes mellitus impairs tendon-bone healing after rotator cuff repair. *J Shoulder Elbow Surg* 2010;19(7):978-988.

    Diabetes was induced preoperatively in a rat rotator cuff repair model. The sustained hyperglycemia was found to impair both the biomechanical and histomorphometric properties of the healing tendon.

23. Clement ND, Hallett A, MacDonald D, Howie C, McBirnie J: Does diabetes affect outcome after arthroscopic repair of the rotator cuff? *J Bone Joint Surg Br* 2010;92(8):1112-1117.

    The outcomes of arthroscopic rotator cuff repair in 32 patients with diabetes were compared with those of matched control subjects. Patients with diabetes had improvement in pain and function in the short term that was less than that of their counterparts without diabetes.

24. Gerber C, Meyer DC, Frey E, et al: Neer Award 2007: Reversion of structural muscle changes caused by chronic rotator cuff tears using continuous musculotendinous traction. An experimental study in sheep. *J Shoulder Elbow Surg* 2009;18(2):163-171.

    A sheep chronic rotator cuff tear model was used to demonstrate that continuous elongation of the infraspinatus muscle can lead to restoration of normal muscle architecture, partial reversal of muscle atrophy, and arrest of the progression of fatty infiltration.

25. Gladstone JN, Bishop JY, Lo IK, Flatow EL: Fatty infiltration and atrophy of the rotator cuff do not improve after rotator cuff repair and correlate with poor functional outcome. *Am J Sports Med* 2007;35(5):719-728.

    A prospective study of 38 patients found that muscle atrophy and fatty infiltration significantly affected the functional outcome after rotator cuff repair. Tear size significantly influenced repair integrity. Level of evidence: II.

26. Oh JH, Kim SH, Ji HM, Jo KH, Bin SW, Gong HS: Prognostic factors affecting anatomic outcome of rotator cuff repair and correlation with functional outcome. *Arthroscopy* 2009;25(1):30-39.

    Anatomic and functional outcomes after rotator cuff repair were evaluated in 177 patients at an average 29-month follow-up. Multivariate regression analysis showed that tear retraction and fatty degeneration of the infraspinatus were independent determinants of anatomic or functional outcome, but age was not. Level of evidence: IV.

27. Liem D, Lichtenberg S, Magosch P, Habermeyer P: Magnetic resonance imaging of arthroscopic supraspinatus tendon repair. *J Bone Joint Surg Am* 2007;89(8):1770-1776.

    The clinical and structural results of isolated supraspinatus arthroscopic repairs were evaluated in 53 patients at an average 26.4-month follow-up. Relatively great muscular atrophy and fatty infiltration preoperatively were associated with repair failure and an inferior clinical result. Level of evidence: IV.

28. Melis B, Nemoz C, Walch G: Muscle fatty infiltration in rotator cuff tears: Descriptive analysis of

1688 cases. *Orthop Traumatol Surg Res* 2009;95(5): 319-324.

The natural history of fatty infiltration was evaluated in 1,688 patients who underwent surgery for a rotator cuff tear. The mean time to severe fatty infiltration was 5, 4, or 3 years in the supraspinatus, the infraspinatus, or the subscapularis, respectively. Level of evidence: IV.

29. Kim HM, Dahiya N, Teefey SA, Keener JD, Galatz LM, Yamaguchi K: Relationship of tear size and location to fatty degeneration of the rotator cuff. *J Bone Joint Surg Am* 2010;92(4):829-839.

Shoulder ultrasound was performed bilaterally in 262 patients to assess the type of rotator cuff tear and fatty degeneration in the supraspinatus and infraspinatus muscles. Fatty degeneration was found to be closely associated with tear size and location, especially in anterior supraspinatus tendon tears.

30. Goutallier DB, Patte D: L'e ´valuation par le scanner de la trophicite ´ des muscles de la coiffe ayant une rupture tendineuse. *Rev Chir Orthop Reparatrice Appar Mot* 1989;75:126-127.

31. Baumgarten KM, Gerlach D, Galatz LM, et al: Cigarette smoking increases the risk for rotator cuff tears. *Clin Orthop Relat Res* 2010;468(6):1534-1541.

A history of cigarette smoking was obtained in 584 patients who underwent diagnostic shoulder ultrasound for unilateral atraumatic shoulder pain. There was a strong association between smoking and rotator cuff disease, which was both dosage and time dependent. Level of evidence: III.

32. Holtby R, Razmjou H: Impact of work-related compensation claims on surgical outcome of patients with rotator cuff related pathologies: A matched case-control study. *J Shoulder Elbow Surg* 2010;19(3): 452-460.

In 110 patients with a workers' compensation–related injury, there was a significantly higher level of disability before and after rotator cuff surgery in comparison with a historical control group at 1-year follow-up. Level of evidence: III.

33. Galatz LM, Silva MJ, Rothermich SY, Zaegel MA, Havlioglu N, Thomopoulos S: Nicotine delays tendon-to-bone healing in a rat shoulder model. *J Bone Joint Surg Am* 2006;88(9):2027-2034.

34. Carbone S, Gumina S, Arceri V, Campagna V, Fagnani C, Postacchini F: The impact of preoperative smoking habit on rotator cuff tear: Cigarette smoking influences rotator cuff tear sizes. *J Shoulder Elbow Surg* 2012;21(1):56-60.

A correlation was found among cigarette smoking, rotator cuff tears, and tear size by analyzing 408 patients who underwent arthroscopic rotator cuff repair. Tear severity increased with increases in the average number of cigarettes and total lifetime cigarettes smoked.

35. Razmjou H, Lincoln S, Axelrod T, Holtby R: Factors contributing to failure of rotator cuff surgery in persons with work-related injuries. *Physiother Can* 2008; 60(2):125-133.

A cross-sectional study found that of 19 patients with continued impairment after surgical treatment of work-related shoulder injuries, 50% had at least one reason to explain their ongoing symptoms, emotional difficulties, and functional limitations.

36. Henn RF III, Kang L, Tashjian RZ, Green A: Patients with workers' compensation claims have worse outcomes after rotator cuff repair. *J Bone Joint Surg Am* 2008;90(10):2105-2113.

After controlling for confounding factors, 39 patients with a workers' compensation claim were found to have worse outcomes than comparable patients on outcome measures and visual analog shoulder pain, shoulder function, and quality-of-life scales 1 year after repair of a chronic rotator cuff tear. Level of evidence: I.

37. Kim HM, Dahiya N, Teefey SA, et al: Location and initiation of degenerative rotator cuff tears: An analysis of three hundred and sixty shoulders. *J Bone Joint Surg Am* 2010;92(5):1088-1096.

Ultrasound of 360 shoulders showed that degenerative rotator cuff tears most commonly involve a posterior location near the junction of the supraspinatus and infraspinatus. These tears may originate in a region 13 to 17 mm posterior to the biceps tendon.

38. Petersen SA, Murphy TP: The timing of rotator cuff repair for the restoration of function. *J Shoulder Elbow Surg* 2011;20(1):62-68.

Acute, traumatic full-thickness rotator cuff tears in 36 patients were repaired as late as 4 months after injury, with no functional compromise according to American Shoulder and Elbow Surgeons and UCLA scores. Level of evidence: III.

39. Burks RT, Crim J, Brown N, Fink B, Greis PE: A prospective randomized clinical trial comparing arthroscopic single- and double-row rotator cuff repair: Magnetic resonance imaging and early clinical evaluation. *Am J Sports Med* 2009;37(4):674-682.

One year after single-row or double-row rotator cuff repair, there were no differences in measures of postoperative motion or strength. MRI measurements of footprint coverage and the tendon thickness of patients in the two repair groups showed no differences. Level of evidence: I.

40. Grasso A, Milano G, Salvatore M, Falcone G, Deriu L, Fabbriciani C: Single-row versus double-row arthroscopic rotator cuff repair: A prospective randomized clinical study. *Arthroscopy* 2009;25(1):4-12.

The clinical outcomes of arthroscopic rotator cuff repair were compared after single-row or double-row repair. At an average 24.8-month follow-up, no significant between-group clinical differences were noted. Level of evidence: I.

41. Ma HL, Chiang ER, Wu HT, et al: Clinical outcome and imaging of arthroscopic single-row and double-row rotator cuff repair: A prospective randomized trial. *Arthroscopy* 2012;28(1):16-24.

    A randomized study of patients with a rotator cuff tear larger than 3 cm found that double-row fixation resulted in significantly better muscle strength than single-row fixation. There were no between-group differences in cuff integrity at 6-month and 2-year follow-up. Level of evidence: II.

42. Duquin TR, Buyea C, Bisson LJ: Which method of rotator cuff repair leads to the highest rate of structural healing? A systematic review. *Am J Sports Med* 2010; 38(4):835-841.

    A systematic review found that double-row repair leads to significantly lower retearing rates in tears larger than 1 cm compared with single-row methods.

43. Dines JS, Bedi A, ElAttrache NS, Dines DM: Single-row versus double-row rotator cuff repair: Techniques and outcomes. *J Am Acad Orthop Surg* 2010;18(2): 83-93.

    Although a double-row repair provides an improved mechanical environment for the healing enthesis, no clinical difference is noted between either repair technique. Level of evidence: Review article.

44. Peltz CD, Dourte LM, Kuntz AF, et al: The effect of postoperative passive motion on rotator cuff healing in a rat model. *J Bone Joint Surg Am* 2009;91(10):2421-2429.

    Early controlled passive motion had a detrimental effect on shoulder mechanics after surgery in a rat rotator cuff model.

45. Seo SS, Choi JS, An KC, Kim JH, Kim SB: The factors affecting stiffness occurring with rotator cuff tear. *J Shoulder Elbow Surg* 2012;21(3):304-309.

    The type and the direction of the rotator cuff tear and the presence of trauma were found to increase limitation of preoperative joint motion in 119 patients undergoing arthroscopic rotator cuff repair. Level of evidence: IV.

46. Sarver JJ, Peltz CD, Dourte L, Reddy S, Williams GR, Soslowsky LJ: After rotator cuff repair, stiffness—but not the loss in range of motion—increased transiently for immobilized shoulders in a rat model. *J Shoulder Elbow Surg* 2008;17(1, suppl):108S-113S.

    The increase in joint stiffness caused by immobilizing an injured and repaired rat rotator cuff was found to be transient.

47. Parsons BO, Gruson KI, Chen DD, Harrison AK, Gladstone J, Flatow EL: Does slower rehabilitation after arthroscopic rotator cuff repair lead to long-term stiffness? *J Shoulder Elbow Surg* 2010;19(7):1034-1039.

    Sling immobilization for 6 weeks after arthroscopic rotator cuff repair did not result in increased long-term stiffness at 1-year follow-up. MRI showed that conservative rehabilitation after repair may improve the rate of tendon healing. Level of evidence: IV.

48. Uggen C, Dines J, McGarry M, Grande D, Lee T, Limpisvasti O: The effect of recombinant human platelet-derived growth factor BB-coated sutures on rotator cuff healing in a sheep model. *Arthroscopy* 2010;26(11):1456-1462.

    rhPDGF-BB coated sutures produced a more histologically normal tendon insertion site after a repair in a sheep model, but no biomechanical difference was noted compared to controls.

49. Hee CK, Dines JS, Dines DM, et al: Augmentation of a rotator cuff suture repair using rhPDGF-BB and a type I bovine collagen matrix in an ovine model. *Am J Sports Med* 2011;39(8):1630-1639.

    Recombinant human PDGF-BB combined with a type I collagen matrix improved the biomechanical strength and the anatomic appearance of the rotator cuff repair site in an ovine model.

50. Jo CH, Kim JE, Yoon KS, et al: Does platelet-rich plasma accelerate recovery after rotator cuff repair? A prospective cohort study. *Am J Sports Med* 2011; 39(10):2082-2090.

    PRP application in 19 patients during arthroscopic rotator cuff repair did not accelerate recovery clinically or anatomically compared with patients in the control group. This study may have been underpowered, however. Level of evidence: II.

51. Bergeson AG, Tashjian RZ, Greis PE, Crim J, Stoddard GJ, Burks RT: Effects of platelet-rich fibrin matrix on repair integrity of at-risk rotator cuff tears. *Am J Sports Med* 2012;40(2):286-293.

    No difference was found in retearing rates and functional outcomes between 16 patients who had platelet-rich fibrin matrix augmentation of their rotator cuff repair and historical control subjects. Level of evidence: III.

52. Barber FA, Hrnack SA, Snyder SJ, Hapa O: Rotator cuff repair healing influenced by platelet-rich plasma construct augmentation. *Arthroscopy* 2011;27(8): 1029-1035.

    Two matched groups of patients with or without PRP augmentation of their rotator cuff repair were compared at a mean 31-month follow-up. Patients in the PRP group had a lower retearing rate on MRI, but there was no between-group clinical difference aside from Rowe scores. Level of evidence: III.

53. Castricini R, Longo UG, De Benedetto M, et al: Platelet-rich plasma augmentation for arthroscopic rotator cuff repair: A randomized controlled trial. *Am J Sports Med* 2011;39(2):258-265.

    A comparison study found that autologous platelet-rich fibrin matrix augmentation of rotator cuff repairs did not improve functional outcomes at 16-month follow-up. There was no between-group difference in repair integrity based on MRI analysis. Level of evidence: I.

3: The Rotator Cuff

54. Randelli P, Arrigoni P, Ragone V, Aliprandi A, Cabitza P: Platelet rich plasma in arthroscopic rotator cuff repair: A prospective RCT study, 2-year follow-up. *J Shoulder Elbow Surg* 2011;20(4):518-528.

During the first month after rotator cuff repair, autologous PRP augmentation was found to reduce pain. At 3 months after surgery, functional outcomes were significantly higher after PRP augmentation. No difference was noted at 6, 12, or 24 months. Level of evidence: I.

55. Aspenberg P, Virchenko O: Platelet concentrate injection improves Achilles tendon repair in rats. *Acta Orthop Scand* 2004;75(1):93-99.

56. Lyras DN, Kazakos K, Verettas D, et al: The influence of platelet-rich plasma on angiogenesis during the early phase of tendon healing. *Foot Ankle Int* 2009;30(11):1101-1106.

PRP enhanced neovascularization in a rabbit Achilles tendon model during the first 2 weeks of the healing process. The number of newly formed vessels in the PRP-treated rats at 4 weeks was less than that of control rats, and this fact suggests that the healing process was shortened.

57. Castillo TN, Pouliot MA, Kim HJ, Dragoo JL: Comparison of growth factor and platelet concentration from commercial platelet-rich plasma separation systems. *Am J Sports Med* 2011;39(2):266-271.

The three different PRP concentration systems produced differing concentrations of growth factors and white blood cells.

58. Gulotta LV, Kovacevic D, Ehteshami JR, Dagher E, Packer JD, Rodeo SA: Application of bone marrow-derived mesenchymal stem cells in a rotator cuff repair model. *Am J Sports Med* 2009;37(11):2126-2133.

The addition of MSCs to the healing rotator cuff insertion site in a rat model did not improve the structure, composition, or strength of the healing tendon attachment site.

59. Gulotta LV, Kovacevic D, Packer JD, Deng XH, Rodeo SA: Bone marrow-derived mesenchymal stem cells transduced with scleraxis improve rotator cuff healing in a rat model. *Am J Sports Med* 2011;39(6):1282-1289.

MSCs genetically modified with scleraxis were used to augment rotator cuff healing in a rat rotator cuff model. At 4 weeks, fibrocartilage was increased and biomechanical properties were improved at the repair site.

Arthroscopy

SECTION EDITORS:
AUGUSTUS D. MAZZOCCA, MS, MD
MARC SAFRAN, MD

Chapter 19

Arthroscopic Treatment of Subacromial and Acromioclavicular Pathology

Daniel Aaron, MD   Bradford Parsons, MD   Evan Flatow, MD

Introduction

Pathology involving the subacromial space and the acromioclavicular (AC) joint is common, and its symptoms can substantially affect a patient's quality of life. Nonsurgical measures have variable efficacy for treating these conditions, and surgical intervention often is warranted. As techniques and technology have evolved, arthroscopic surgery has become the standard method of surgical management for many of these conditions. The etiology, evaluation, and treatment of the most common conditions affecting the subacromial space and the AC joint are discussed here, with particular attention to arthroscopic technique.

Subacromial Pathology

Anatomy and Etiology

Extrinsic compression or impingement of the rotator cuff is one of the most important proposed mechanisms of rotator cuff disease and tearing. Intrinsic factors also play a critical role. The extent to which mechanical compression of the rotator cuff tendons contributes to symptoms and the development and the progression of tendon pathology is controversial, however.

The anatomy of the subacromial space has been studied with regard to its contribution to the disease

Dr. Parsons or an immediate family member is a member of a speakers' bureau or has made paid presentations on behalf of Zimmer and Arthrex; serves as a paid consultant to or is an employee of Zimmer and Arthrex; and has received research or institutional support from Wyeth. Dr. Flatow or an immediate family member has received royalties from Innomed and Zimmer; is a member of a speakers' bureau or has made paid presentations on behalf of Zimmer; and serves as an unpaid consultant to Zimmer. Neither Dr. Aaron nor any immediate family member has received anything of value from or has stock or stock options held in a commercial company or institution related directly or indirectly to the subject of this chapter.

spectrum of the rotator cuff from subacromial bursitis to impingement syndromes to partial and complete tears of the rotator cuff tendons. Many theories exist concerning the anatomic features of the subacromial space and their relationship to rotator cuff pathology and symptoms.

Neer was the first to describe the anterior acromion as the principal site of impingement on the rotator cuff and the long head of the biceps tendon.[1] Neer noted a ridge of spurs and excrescences on the undersurface of the anterior acromion, with some cadaver specimens having eburnation of the anterior third. These anatomic findings were correlated with intraoperative observations that the supraspinatus, the anterior infraspinatus, and the biceps were the structures most commonly involved in rotator cuff disease, and all of these structures lie anterior to the acromion when the arm is in neutral position. Neer concluded that elevation of the arm in internal or external rotation brought these structures under the anterior acromion, where they were vulnerable to compression, impingement, and, ultimately, mechanical failure.[1] Later anatomic study revealed that the coracoacromial (CA) ligament at the anterior margin of the acromion was stretched by passage of the greater tuberosity beneath it, and the tuberosity and the supraspinatus impinged on the CA ligament and the anterior acromion during flexion and internal rotation.[2] In addition, impingement of the biceps occurred at the CA ligament. Another cadaver study found that the acromiohumeral interval decreased in 60° to 120° of elevation, with contact centered at the supraspinatus insertion. Contact was significantly increased with an anterior-hooked acromion.[3] The association of the anatomy of the anterior acromion and CA ligament with rotator cuff impingement was supported by the finding that flattening of the anterior third of the acromion was necessary to reduce impingement on the rotator cuff.[4]

The use of subacromial decompression in conjunction with rotator cuff repair is controversial, and evidence exists that routine acromioplasty is not needed at the time of routine tendon repair unless spurs are clearly present.[5]

Patient Evaluation

The evaluation of subacromial impingement depends on a focused but thorough patient history and physical examination, with adjunct imaging studies. The typical symptom of impingement is anterolateral shoulder and/or arm pain.[6] Patients often state that particular positions and activities aggravate the pain. Pain may cause difficulty during overhead activities, such as reaching for an object on a high shelf, or activities requiring terminal internal rotation, such as putting on a coat or fastening a brassiere. Lifting objects with an extended arm also frequently causes symptoms.

Physical Examination

As in the physical examination of any shoulder condition, the clinician should begin with a visual assessment of the skin, inspect the contour of the glenohumeral joint and the scapula compared with the contralateral side, and check for the presence of any atrophy or deformity. Passive and active range of motion and rotator cuff strength should be measured. Subacromial impingement can be assessed by performing provocative maneuvers, of which the most commonly used are the Neer and Hawkins tests. The principle of these tests is to decrease the subacromial space and increase contact between the rotator cuff and the bony and ligamentous borders, as validated by several studies. An MRI analysis found that the rotator cuff is in close proximity to the anteroinferior acromion in abduction and internal rotation (the Hawkins sign position) but not in full forward elevation (the Neer sign position).[7] An arthroscopic study found that a positive Neer test is more likely to be related to rotator cuff contact with the glenoid than with the acromion.[8] Another MRI study found that both tests decreased the distance between the supraspinatus insertion and the bony borders of the subacromial space, although the Hawkins test produced more space reduction and rotator cuff contact.[9] A cadaver study also found rotator cuff contact with both tests. The Neer test produced contact with the medial acromion, and the Hawkins test produced contact with the CA ligament. Both tests produced contact between the articular side of the rotator cuff and the anterosuperior glenoid.[10] In clinical practice, both tests are sensitive but not particularly specific.[11]

Imaging

In addition to the patient history and the physical examination, imaging studies should be obtained and assessed. The typical set of shoulder radiographs includes AP views in the normal and scapular planes as well as axillary lateral and outlet or scapula Y views. The normal AP projection offers a view of osteophytes about the AC joint, and the scapular plane AP (true AP, Grashey) view best displays the glenohumeral joint and can show cystic change in the greater tuberosity. The axillary view is best for revealing an os acromiale, and the outlet view is best for acromial morphology. A correlation was observed between impingement and acromiohumeral distance as measured on AP radiographs and coronal plane MRI.[12] Radiographic findings may support a diagnosis of impingement, but they must be correlated with the clinical signs and symptoms.[13]

Nonsurgical Management

A treatment strategy must be developed after shoulder impingement syndrome is diagnosed. The presence or the absence of associated pathology, particularly a rotator cuff tear, is crucial to any treatment plan. If the patient has impingement without full-thickness tearing of the rotator cuff, the treatment algorithm typically begins nonsurgically.

Nonsteroidal Anti-inflammatory Drugs

The use of NSAIDs often is recommended to treat inflammation of the subacromial bursa. These agents can be clinically effective. A molecular basis for their effect was found in the downregulation of inflammatory cytokines and mediating receptors in the subacromial bursa.[14] The detrimental systemic and local effects of NSAIDs make their use controversial. Nonselective NSAIDs (cyclooxygenase [COX] inhibitors) increase the risk of upper gastrointestinal complications, such as ulceration and bleeding. COX-2 inhibitors have decreased the gastrointestinal adverse effect profile but are associated with cardiovascular risk.[15] NSAIDs were shown to inhibit tendon-to-bone healing in an animal model, and this finding raises questions about their use in patients after rotator cuff repair.[16]

Physical Therapy

Physical therapy is a commonly used treatment modality. Compared with patients with subacromial impingement who received nonspecific physical therapy, a significantly lower percentage of patients needed surgical intervention after receiving a specific rehabilitation protocol consisting of stretches, eccentric rotator cuff strengthening, and concentric-eccentric scapular stabilizing exercises.[17]

Subacromial Injections

Subacromial injections often are administered for subacromial impingement syndrome. Corticosteroids are the most commonly injected agent. Corticosteroids also have been shown to downregulate inflammatory cytokines in the subacromial bursa.[14] However, a meta-analysis found only weak support for using corticosteroid injections in treating conditions in the spectrum of rotator cuff disease.[18] Corticosteroid use is contraindicated in certain patients because of the risk of an elevation in blood glucose, and further use is contraindicated in patients who have received multiple injections. A transient decrease in rotator cuff tendon strength and histologic changes were reported after a single administration of methylprednisolone in an animal model.[19]

Nonetheless, corticosteroid injections are a low-risk intervention in most patients, and they may facilitate participation in physical therapy. Newer agents are being investigated that may be clinically effective without the detrimental effects of NSAIDs or corticosteroids. Early results appear promising.[20]

The current American Academy of Orthopaedic Surgeons practice guidelines recommend initial management of subacromial impingement syndrome with physical therapy and NSAIDs but neither support nor refute the use of corticosteroid injections, pulsed electromagnetic fields, iontophoresis, phonophoresis, transcutaneous electrical nerve stimulation, ice, heat, massage, or activity modification.[5]

Surgical Management

If nonsurgical measures are not effective, surgical intervention may be indicated. In the absence of tearing of more than 50% thickness of the rotator cuff, subacromial decompression alone can be effective. This procedure typically consists of removing the subacromial bursa, anterior acromioplasty, and excision of the CA ligament. Flattening of the anterior third of the acromion is adequate to eliminate extrinsic rotator cuff compression.[4] The standard method of decompression is arthroscopic.

Technique

Arthroscopic subacromial decompression (ASD) typically involves the use of two portals. A standard posterior portal is created approximately 2 cm medial and 2 cm distal to the posterolateral corner of the acromion. Palpation of the soft spot of the posterior glenohumeral joint line is recommended to confirm portal placement, although this step can be difficult in a patient with a large deltoid musculature or adipose layer. A No. 11 blade is used to incise the skin. The trocar-cannula assembly is advanced into the subacromial space and can be used to create space for viewing by a sweeping motion along the undersurface of the acromion and the CA ligament. Longitudinal traction on the arm may increase acromiohumeral distance and facilitate entry into the space. The trocar is withdrawn, and the cannula is held in place. When the arthroscope is inserted into the cannula, the camera is aimed superiorly so that the acromion is in view. A standard lateral portal is then created. A spinal needle routinely is used to place this portal so that the anterior acromion and the CA ligament are easily accessible and the angle between the instruments and the acromion will allow an even acromioplasty. The portal is typically located 3 to 4 cm distal to the lateral border of the acromion at the border of the anterior one third and posterior two thirds. It must be kept in mind that the axillary nerve crosses this area 5 to 7 cm distal to the lateral acromial edge. After the portal location has been determined, a transverse portal is created, using a No. 11 blade to incise only 5 mm of skin. A clear plastic cannula is advanced into the space to allow simple insertion and the

removal of instrumentation. A motorized shaver is inserted first to remove bursal tissue and expand the area that can be visualized. Bleeding areas are immediately cauterized. The bursal surface of the rotator cuff is inspected visually and with a probe to rule out tendon tearing. The electrocautery is used to remove all adherent soft tissue from the acromial undersurface. This process begins with a relaxing incision through the deltoid fascia from the cannula entry site directly medial to the acromion edge; the purpose is to improve instrument access to the anterior acromial edge and the CA ligament. The lateral border of the acromion is defined by incising the deltoid fascia until muscle fibers are seen, and the anterior edge is defined by peeling off the CA ligament until none of its fibers remain attached. The ligament is not fully released if there is a large tear of the rotator cuff because the passive stabilizing effect of the arch must be preserved.[5] The remainder of the acromion undersurface can then be exposed. An anterior acromioplasty is performed with a motorized burr. The goal of this step is simply to flatten the anterior surface. After determining how much bony resection will be required, the surgeon resects that thickness at the anterolateral corner. This step-cut technique in effect creates a template for the more medial resection. When the level of resection is even from lateral to medial, the arthroscope is moved to the lateral portal for viewing the acromion in an orthogonal, cutting-block plane. The burr is inserted into the posterior portal, and the acromion is smoothed to the original step-cut. Throughout the procedure, care must be taken to fully define the bony edges but avoid cutting the deltoid muscle. Meticulous hemostasis with the electrocautery and the use of epinephrine in the irrigant solution (1:300,000) are recommended to minimize bleeding, and a low pump pressure (35 torr) is recommended to avoid swelling.

Results

ASD can effectively relieve symptoms originating from impingement syndrome. The results of ASD are superior to those of open decompression. A 1998 review concluded both open and arthroscopic decompression had high success rates that were not significantly different (90.0% and 89.3%, respectively), but the arthroscopic technique allowed earlier rehabilitation because the deltoid was not detached.[21] The importance of the relatively long learning curve of the arthroscopic technique has been largely obviated as it has become more widely used. A recent meta-analysis found that the two techniques had equivalent clinical outcomes, but patients who underwent ASD returned to work more quickly and spent fewer days in the hospital than those who underwent open decompression.[22] Small full-thickness supraspinatus tears did not progress after ASD without tendon repair.[23] There is also evidence that ASD may reduce the risk of future rotator cuff tearing in patients with subacromial impingement; 18% of patients had a rotator cuff tear 15 years after

4: Arthroscopy

ASD (4% had a full-thickness tear), compared with approximately 40% in age-matched historic control patients.[24]

Adjunct to Rotator Cuff Repair

There is debate as to whether ASD performed concurrently with arthroscopic repair of a full-thickness rotator cuff tear leads to an improved outcome. In a study of patients with a full-thickness rotator cuff tear who were treated with repair alone or with repair and ASD, researchers have determined that clinical outcome was correlated with several variables, including patient age, tear pattern, tendon quality and retraction, and repair technique.[25] No correlation was found between concurrent ASD and outcome. In a randomized, prospective study of patients with a full-thickness, single-tendon rotator cuff tear, no significant functional differences were found at 1-year follow-up based on whether the patient's rotator cuff repair included ASD (patients with acromial spurs were excluded).[26] Another study found no significant difference in the clinical outcomes of patients who underwent rotator cuff repair alone or with concurrent ASD, but the reoperation rate was lower in patients who underwent ASD.[27] However, a recent meta-analysis discovered no difference in reoperation rates or functional outcomes.[28] ASD is routinely performed as an adjunct to repair of a full-thickness rotator cuff tear when clear impingement or spurs are noted arthroscopically.

Acromioclavicular Pathology

Etiology

The AC joint may be affected by a degenerative condition, such as osteoarthritis, or a traumatic condition, such as dislocation or separation. Arthritis of the AC joint is common, although almost no motion occurs at the AC joint compared with the sternoclavicular joint. The condition also can develop as a result of inflammatory or crystalline arthropathy, trauma, or joint sepsis.[29] AC arthritis can exist in isolation or in association with another condition affecting the shoulder. Osteolysis of the distal clavicle also leads to pain and tenderness at the AC joint and is believed to be caused by hypervascularization and bone resorption after repeated small subchondral fractures. AC separation typically occurs as a result of trauma.

Anatomy

The AC joint is the articulation between the acromion process of the scapula and the distal end of the clavicle. It is the only connection between the upper extremity and the axial skeleton. It is a diarthrodial joint and contains a fibrocartilaginous disk. The width of the joint space typically is 1 to 3 mm.[30] The joint is stabilized by a complex set of ligamentous and muscular restraints. Anteroposterior translation is primarily limited by the AC ligaments, especially the superior ligament.

Inferior translation is primarily limited by the two coracoclavicular (CC) ligaments, with the conoid being the stronger of the two. The deltotrapezial fascia may also contribute to stability, but its exact role has not been well characterized. The insertions of the stabilizing ligaments are important to understand because resection of the insertion sites can lead to iatrogenic instability, and reconstruction of the ligaments may be more effective if done in anatomic fashion.

An anatomic study of the clavicle and the coracoid in both dry osteologic and fresh cadaver specimens found the average distance from the distal end of the clavicle to the center of the trapezoid tuberosity to be 25.4 (± 3.7) mm in men, and 22.9 (± 3.7) mm in women.[31] The distance to the medial border of the conoid tuberosity was 47.2 (± 4.6) mm and 42.8 (± 5.6) mm in male and female specimens, respectively. Interestingly, the ratio of these distances to overall clavicle length was consistent between the sexes. Specifically, the ratio of the distance to the trapezoid center to overall clavicle length was 0.17 and to the medial border of the conoid tuberosity was 0.31. In the fresh cadaver specimens, the ratio of the distance to the trapezoid to clavicle length was 0.17 and to the conoid center was 0.24.[31]

Patient Evaluation

Patients having pathology of the AC joint frequently experience pain directly over the joint and in the anterolateral neck, the trapezius-supraspinatus region, and the anterolateral deltoid.[6] Physical examination of the AC joint begins with a visual assessment, with attention to prominence of the distal clavicle to detect separation. If separation is suspected, stability of the joint in the anteroposterior and superoinferior planes should be examined. If the AC separation is obvious, reducibility should be assessed by applying a superiorly directed force onto the humerus at the elbow. If no separation is suspected and the pathology is likely to be chronic in nature, the joint should be palpated and tenderness should be noted. Direct tenderness is reported to be 96% to 97% sensitive as a test for AC pathology.[32,33] Also commonly used is the cross-body adduction test, in which pain at the AC joint is elicited by maximally adducting the arm with the shoulder in 90° of elevation. This maneuver has a reported sensitivity of 67%.[33] The O'Brien active compression test also is widely used; the arm is adducted 15° across the body, the shoulder is internally rotated, and the patient actively elevates the arm against resistance. A positive test consists of pain during this maneuver, with substantially less pain when the test is repeated with the shoulder in external rotation. The O'Brien test has reported sensitivity as high as 83%, with 90% specificity.[32,33] In a combined cross-body adduction and O'Brien test, the shoulder is elevated to 90°, the arm is maximally adducted across the body, and the patient actively elevates against resistance with the shoulder in internal rotation.[33] A positive test consists of pain during this maneuver and only slightly less pain with external rotation. The sensitivity of this Bell-van Riet test was reported to be 98%.[33] The sternoclavicular joint should also be examined for tenderness, deformity, and instability.

Imaging of the AC joint begins with standard radiographs. The radiographic views for the AC joint were described as including several AP views: with the beam angled caudad and cephalad by 15°, with the humerus in internal and external rotation, with the arm maximally abducted and in 30° to 35° of cephalad angulation.[30] The most commonly used of these AP radiographs is the so-called Zanca view, in which the beam is angled 15° cephalad (**Figure 1**). A standard AP view often is sufficient (**Figure 2**), but the Zanca view reliably prevents the AC joint from being obscured by the scapular spine and allows detection of erosive changes, osteophyte formation, and joint-space narrowing in the presence of arthritis as well as joint widening and displacement in the setting of trauma.[30,34]

MRI has reported sensitivity of 85% for atraumatic AC joint pain, and it allows ligamentous structures to be seen in patients with AC separation.[32] Nuclear bone scanning also has high accuracy (76%).[32] Ultrasound has been used to detect AC arthritis, but in one study, 65% of the asymptomatic individuals had a positive finding.[35] Intra-articular anesthetic injection is the gold standard for the diagnosis of atraumatic AC joint pathology, although it can be challenging to ensure the anesthetic actually enters the joint.[32]

Management of Acromioclavicular Arthritis and Distal Clavicle Osteolysis

Nonsurgical Management

The management of chronic conditions affecting the AC joint, such as degenerative joint disease and osteolysis, begins nonsurgically with the use of NSAIDs and physical therapy. If these modalities are not effective, intra-articular corticosteroid injections often are used. Recent data suggest that these injections have a low rate of short-term clinical success, but if relief is provided, the benefit is likely to endure.[36] Specifically, only 16 of 58 patients (28%) had adequate relief of pain 1 month after AC joint corticosteroid injection. However, at an average 42-month follow-up, 15 of the 16 patients had relief sufficient to allow them to decline surgery. No complications of corticosteroid injection were noted.[36] Injection of corticosteroid mixed with a local anesthetic can have diagnostic value, and it is a

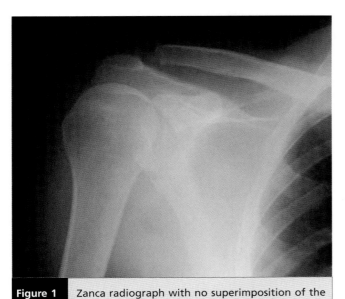

Figure 1 Zanca radiograph with no superimposition of the scapular spine over the AC joint. The even resection of the distal clavicle can be seen.

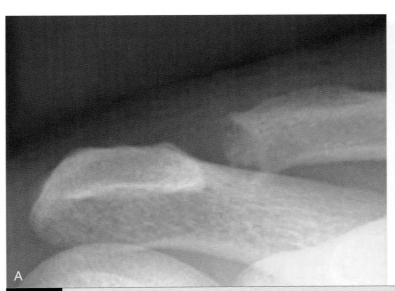
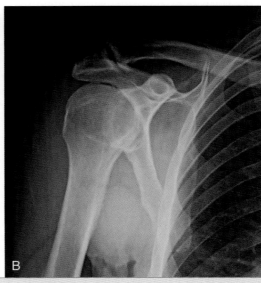

Figure 2 Radiographic appearance of distal clavicle osteolysis (**A**) and osteoarthritis with osteophytes (**B**).

4: Arthroscopy

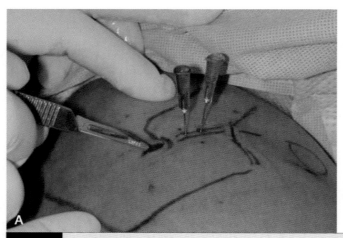 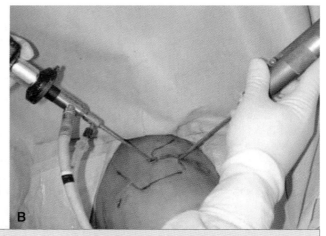

Figure 3 Photographs showing AC joint localization with needles and the creation of the posterior AC portal (**A**) plus instrumentation inserted for a direct arthroscopic approach for distal clavicle resection (**B**).

relatively safe and sometimes effective treatment modality.

Surgical Management

The mainstay surgical treatment of AC joint arthritis or osteolysis is resection of the distal clavicle. Distal clavicle resection (DCR) can be performed open or arthroscopically, although the arthroscopic approach has become the standard. Regardless of the approach, the success of the procedure depends on resecting an adequate amount of distal clavicle bone while avoiding joint destabilization caused by compromise of the supporting ligaments and their bony insertions.

The recommended technique for arthroscopic DCR depends on whether the AC joint pathology is isolated or associated with a condition such as subacromial impingement or rotator cuff tearing. When another condition exists, a bursal approach is used in which ASD is performed first. When the subacromial space is decompressed, the scope is placed in the posterior portal and an additional portal is created at the anterior aspect of the AC joint. The joint is palpated from the outside, and a spinal needle is introduced. The needle should be placed exactly at the midline of the anterior joint line so that the angle of the instruments will provide access for an even resection. When portal placement is confirmed, a No. 11 blade is used to create a 5-mm portal and is inserted completely into the joint until it can be seen through the arthroscope. The portal is expanded with a blunt trocar, and a motorized shaver is inserted. The inferior AC capsule, the intra-articular disk, and other soft tissues are excised. Blood vessels frequently are encountered and are cauterized with the electrocautery. Great care is taken to obtain a complete exposure of the articular surface of the clavicle so that the evenness of the bony resection can be accurately gauged. Although exposure of the superior aspect of the distal clavicle must be obtained, it is important to avoid detaching the superior AC ligament to avoid anteroposte-

rior instability. When all soft tissue is removed, the bony resection is performed with a motorized burr. As with ASD, a step-cut technique is used to ensure an even resection. The burr is used to resect the desired amount of bone at the anterior edge of the clavicle. The burr is then advanced posteriorly, and resection to the level of the step-cut is performed. The surgeon carefully examines the bony contour, with particular attention to the posterior and superior aspects, which often are left incompletely resected. Any undesired remaining bone is removed with the burr. The shaver is then reinserted, and any loose debris is removed. Visualization of the AC joint from the posterior portal sometimes is difficult, and if necessary for this purpose, the posterior aspect of the acromial facet is minimally excised. No more bone should be removed than is necessary to ensure adequate visualization of the joint.

In a patient with isolated AC joint disease, a direct approach is used that can be technically more demanding than the bursal approach but does not violate the bursa and thereby minimizes swelling and bleeding.[37] Furthermore, variability in the orientation of the AC joint can be accommodated because portals are placed according to AC joint anatomy only. In the direct approach, concomitant intra-articular pathology can be ruled out by diagnostic glenohumeral arthroscopy through standard posterior and anterior portals. The exact location and orientation of the AC joint are determined by successful entry into the joint using two or three 22-gauge needles, which then are used to describe the orientation of the AC joint. The joint can be insufflated through these needles to create space, and backflow can confirm intra-articular positioning. A 0.5-cm portal is created at the posterior joint line, and a 2.7-mm arthroscope is inserted (**Figure 3**). The needles in the AC joint are visualized. A spinal needle is used to guide placement of an anterior AC joint portal in the same fashion as for the bursal approach. A 0.5-cm portal is created, a 2.0-mm motorized shaver is inserted,

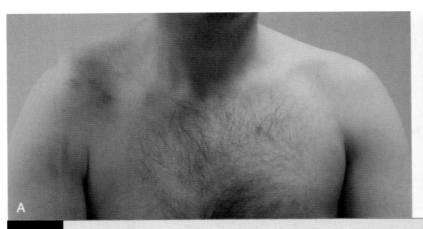
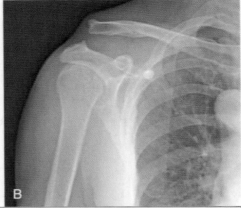

Figure 4 | Photograph (**A**) and Zanca radiograph (**B**) showing the appearance of complete AC joint separation.

and soft tissue is removed. The edges of the AC joint are defined, and a 2.0-mm burr is used to begin the bony resection in step-cut fashion. A standard arthroscope and a larger burr can be used to complete the resection after adequate space has been created. As with the bursal approach, meticulous attention is paid to the depth of resection, the evenness of the joint contour, and the preservation of the superior AC ligament.

In either the bursal or the direct technique, the adequacy of resection can be assessed by inserting an instrument of a known width. Rasps serve this purpose well because they can be used to smooth any remaining rough edges as well as judge the resection. An anatomic study found that the trapezoid insertion lies an average 25.4 mm from the lateral clavicle edge in men and 22.4 mm in women, but a clinical study found that resection of 10 mm can significantly increase anterior translation, even with intact CC and superior and posterior AC ligaments.[31,38] Complete sectioning of the AC capsule significantly increased instability. Therefore, it is recommended that no more than 8 mm of distal clavicle be resected and that the superior capsuloligamentous structures be preserved.

Arthroscopic DCR has favorable results in comparison with open DCR. Several studies found that patients undergoing open or arthroscopic DCR for AC joint arthritis had predictably good pain relief and low rates of complications or reoperation.[39-41] One comparison study found significantly less pain in patients treated with arthroscopic DCR than those treated with open DCR. There was no difference between the two patient groups in amount of resection, surgical time, or functional score.[40] Patients who underwent arthroscopic DCR were found to return to work more quickly, particularly if a direct approach was used.[41] A higher reoperation rate not reaching statistical significance was found when an arthroscopic technique was used.[39] DCR was found to be highly effective for the treatment of osteolysis; 92.6% of patients who underwent arthroscopic DCR for osteolysis of the distal clavicle had a good to excellent result.[42] Treatment for posttraumatic

arthropathy was less consistently successful.[42] Arthroscopic DCR is commonly performed concomitantly with rotator cuff repair in patients with symptomatic AC arthritis in addition to rotator cuff pathology. DCR at the time of rotator cuff repair may be indicated for asymptomatic AC arthritis with inferiorly directed osteophytes; better outcomes at 2-year follow-up and a lower reoperation rate were noted in patients who underwent DCR in addition to rotator cuff repair.[43]

Acromioclavicular Trauma
Mechanism of Injury
Dislocation or separation of the AC joint typically occurs as a result of a direct impact. The direction and the magnitude of the impact force dictate the direction and the severity of joint displacement (**Figure 4**). The most common mechanism is a fall in which ground impact on the superior aspect of the shoulder forces the acromion inferiorly. Injury is more likely and may be more severe if the shoulder is driven into the ground, as might happen in a collision sport.

Classification
AC separations originally were organized into three grades based on the amount of inferior displacement of the acromion relative to the clavicle.[44] Three additional grades subsequently were added, all of which are indications for surgical management.[45] The advent of MRI led to anatomic correlation with the plain radiographic classification, but the relationship may not be consistent.[46]

Anatomic Reconstruction of the Coracoclavicular Ligaments
Most AC separations are managed nonsurgically, but when surgical management is indicated, the trend is to perform an anatomic reconstruction of the CC ligaments. Biomechanical studies found that anatomic reconstruction of both CC ligaments is superior to older techniques in which a single construct was used. In testing of the native CC ligament complex in fresh cadaver

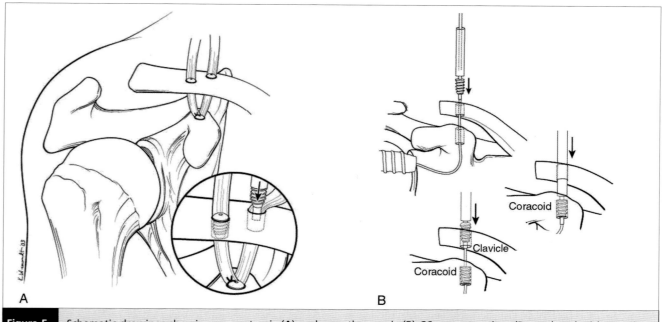

Figure 5 Schematic drawings showing an anatomic (**A**) and an arthroscopic (**B**) CC reconstruction. (Reproduced with permission from Mazzocca AD, Santangelo SA, Johnson ST, Rios CG, Dumonski ML, Arciero RA: A biomechanical evaluation of an anatomic coracoclavicular ligament reconstruction. *Am J Sports Med* 2006;34[2]:236-246.)

specimens, the remaining ligamentous tissue was removed after failure, and an anatomic reconstruction was performed with a semitendinosus graft. Each of the two ends of the graft was passed through a medial or a lateral tunnel in the clavicle, and together they were passed through a single coracoid tunnel. The orientation of the graft ends in the coracoid tunnel re-created the individual specimen's native orientation. The same biomechanical testing was performed on the surgical construct. The absence of significant permanent graft elongation after cyclic loading suggests the ability to withstand early rehabilitation.[47] In a comparison of the biomechanics of anatomic reconstruction with the modified Weaver-Dunn procedure in cadaver specimens, the anatomic reconstruction was achieved with a semitendinosus graft through bone tunnels in the distal clavicle.[48] The tunnel for the conoid ligament was approximately 45 mm medial to the distal end of the clavicle in the posterior half of the shaft. The tunnel for the trapezoid ligament was placed more anteriorly, in the center of the clavicle shaft, and approximately 15 mm lateral to the conoid tunnel (**Figure 5**). The anatomic reconstruction was superior to the modified Weaver-Dunn repair in laxity and both anterior and posterior translation. The authors concluded that anatomic reconstruction is the biomechanically superior procedure and may allow earlier rehabilitation. The biomechanics of anatomic reconstruction depend on the strength of the graft. A recent analysis found that an anatomic reconstruction with the palmaris longus was inadequate and that anatomic reconstruction with the flexor carpi radialis produced a construct superior to that of the modified Weaver-Dunn procedure.[49]

Arthroscopic Coracoclavicular Reconstruction

An early arthroscopic CC reconstruction technique involved arthroscopically guided percutaneous placement of a suture anchor in the coracoid base and percutaneous creation of two bone tunnels in the clavicle. Suture passers were used to pass the suture through the clavicular tunnels, with tying over a titanium plate (**Figure 6**). The anatomic reduction was maintained in 10 of 13 patients, with subluxation in 2 patients and redislocation in 1 patient.[50] Another arthroscopic method involves the use of the TightRope device (Arthrex) to provide nonrigid fixation between the coracoid and the clavicle. Fixation failure was reported in 2 of 12 patients (16.7%) after this procedure, but 11 of 12 patients were satisfied with the results.[51] Significantly greater strength was reported in both vertical and anterior planes when a double-TightRope construct was used for anatomic reconstruction in a cadaver model, compared with native ligaments[52] (**Figures 7 and 8**). The double-TightRope construct also was used clinically in an arthroscopic-assisted anatomic reconstruction.[53] At an average 30-month follow-up, 8 of 23 patients had radiographic evidence of loss of reduction that was not correlated with the clinical outcome. In a study of 10 patients, an all-arthroscopic procedure consisting of DCR and a bone-block transfer of the anterior acromion and the CA ligament to the resected surface (the Chuinard modification of the Weaver-Dunn procedure) was augmented by a four-strand CC ligament reconstruction with heavy braided suture over titanium buttons on the coracoid and clavicular surfaces[54] (**Figure 9**). The rationale for this technique was that the suture construct would maintain reduction

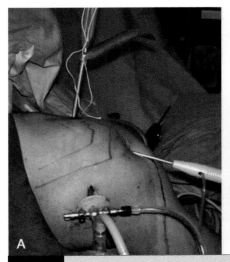
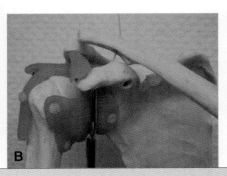
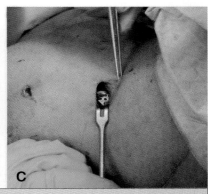

Figure 6 Photographs showing arthroscopic CC reconstruction. **A,** Arthroscopic setup with the camera in the posterior portal and additional instruments in the lateral and anterior portals. **B,** Suture passage shown on a model. **C,** Knot tying over a titanium plate on the clavicle. (Reproduced with permission from Chernchujit B, Tischer T, Imhoff AB: Arthroscopic reconstruction of the acromioclavicular joint disruption: Surgical technique and preliminary results. *Arch Orthop Trauma Surg* 2006;126[9]:575-581.)

4: Arthroscopy

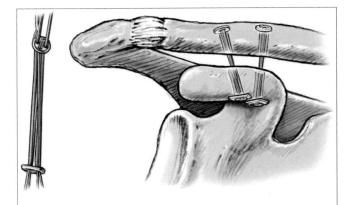

Figure 7 Schematic drawing showing anatomic CC reconstruction using two TightRope devices. (Reproduced with permission from Walz L, Salzmann GM, Fabbro T, Eichhorn S, Imhoff AB: The anatomic reconstruction of acromioclavicular joint dislocations using 2 TightRope devices: A biomechanical study. *Am J Sports Med* 2008;36[12]:2398-2406.)

Some surgeons resect the distal clavicle at the time of CC ligament reconstruction. In situ CC graft forces were found to be increased with sectioning of the AC joint, but no further increase in force is caused by DCR. The increased graft forces remained much lower than their load to failure, and there was no apparent clinical significance.[55]

Os Acromiale

Os acromiale is a condition in which ossification centers in the acromion process of the scapula remain unfused. Often, os acromiale is an incidental radiographic finding, but it causes pain and rotator cuff impingement in some individuals. The incidence of os acromiale is approximately 8%, and it is most common in men and in individuals of African descent.[56]

The acromion consists of the basiacromion, the meta-acromion, the mesoacromion, and the preacromion (**Figure 10**). The entire acromion may fuse as late in life as age 25 years. The posterior, middle, and anterior deltoid fibers attach to the meta-acromion, the mesoacromion, and the preacromion, respectively. The preacromion also is the anchor of the CA ligament.[56]

Evaluation

Any symptoms of os acromiale typically are characteristic of subacromial impingement, including pain with overhead activities. Physical examination may find positive impingement tests, weakness of the rotator cuff, and tenderness to palpation at the site of the nonunion. Os acromiale can be seen, often incidentally, on plain radiographs, CT, MRI, and bone scans[57] (**Figure 11**).

while the bone-block transfer healed, thereby producing a dynamic construct. The bone blocks completely healed in 8 patients and partially healed in 2 patients. No loss of reduction was noted, and all patients were satisfied with the results. Only one patient had not returned to work at 3 months or to preinjury level of sports at the last follow-up.[54] Although this reconstruction method was not anatomic, the two bundles to some extent mimicked the orientation of the CC ligaments, and living biologic tissue was included. Clinical studies of all-arthroscopic anatomic reconstructions with tendon autograft have yet to be published.

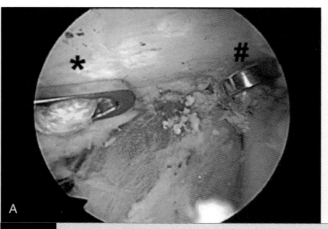

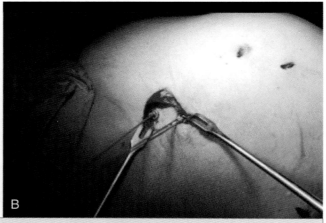

Figure 8 Arthroscopically assisted CC reconstruction using two TightRope devices. **A,** Arthroscopic view from the anterolateral portal. * = posteromedial portal, conoid ligament; # = anterolateral portal, trapezoid ligament. **B,** Photograph showing two clavicle buttons after AC joint reduction and fixation. (Reproduced with permission from Salzmann GM, Walz L, Buchmann S, Glabgly P, Venjakob A, Imhoff AB: Arthroscopically assisted 2-bundle anatomic reduction of acute acromioclavicular joint separations. *Am J Sports Med* 2010;38[6]:1179-1187.)

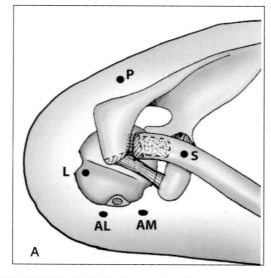

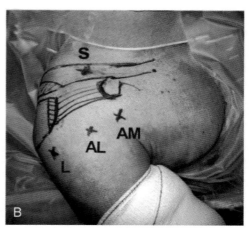

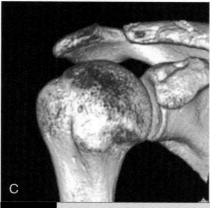

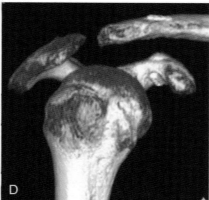

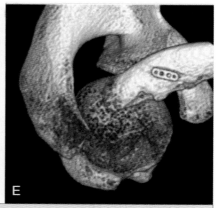

Figure 9 All-arthroscopic Weaver-Dunn-Chuinard repair. Schematic drawing (**A**) and photograph (**B**) showing portal placement. AL = anterolateral, AM = anteromedial, L = lateral, P = posterior, S = superior. Three-dimensional CT reconstruction in the coronal (**C**), sagittal (**D**), and axial (**E**) planes showing button placement on the superior aspect of the lateral clavicle and the inferior aspect of the coracoid. (Reproduced with permission from Boileau P, Old J, Gastaud O, Brassart N, Roussanne Y: All-arthroscopic Weaver-Dunn-Chuinard procedure with double-button fixation for chronic acromioclavicular joint dislocation. *Arthroscopy* 2010;26[2]:149-160.)

Management

The initial treatment of symptoms attributable to os acromiale consists of NSAIDs, physical therapy, and corticosteroid injections.[56] If nonsurgical treatment is unsuccessful, several surgical options are available. Open excision of the distal fragment has had variable results, with most poor outcomes resulting from weakening of the deltoid. Open excision is considered only for a small preacromion fragment.[57] Arthroscopic excision may have a lower rate of deltoid weakening with larger fragments, but no comparison studies have been published.[58] Successful open reduction and internal fixation with cannulated screws or a tension-band construct has been reported, but nonunion rates are high and hardware removal often is required.[58,59]

Os acromiale in the setting of subacromial impingement often is treated with simple acromioplasty that leaves only a thin cortical shell and continues the decompression back to the nonunion site. Extreme care is taken not to violate the deltoid attachment to avoid destabilizing the fragment. DCR is avoided for this reason, but usually it is not necessary because of the AC joint decompression achieved by the aggressive acromioplasty.[57] Eleven of 13 patients had a satisfactory result after ASD for unstable symptomatic os acromiale.[60] However, dynamic impingement is often believed to be refractory to acromioplasty and may be exacerbated by fragment destabilization.[59]

Summary

Arthroscopic management has been found to be safe and effective for many conditions affecting the subacromial space and the AC joint, including subacromial impingement and rotator cuff syndromes, AC joint arthritis, distal clavicle osteolysis, AC joint separation, and os acromiale. The role of arthroscopy is likely to increase as techniques and technology evolve.

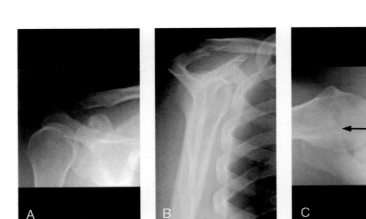

Figure 10 Schematic drawing showing the ossification centers of the acromion. BA = basiacromion, MT = meta-acromion, MS = mesoacromion, PA = preacromion. (Reproduced from Kurtz CA, Humble BJ, Rodosky MW, Sekiya JK: Symptomatic os acromiale. *J Am Acad Orthop Surg* 2006;14[1]:12-19.)

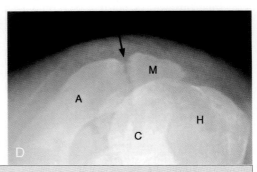

Figure 11 AP (**A**), outlet (**B**), axillary lateral (**C**), and acromion profile (**D**) radiographs of the right shoulder showing an os acromiale *(arrow)* between the meta-acromion and the mesoacromion. A = acromion, C = clavicle, H = humeral head, M = mesoacromion. (Reproduced from Kurtz CA, Humble BJ, Rodosky MW, Sekiya JK: Symptomatic os acromiale. *J Am Acad Orthop Surg* 2006;14[1]:12-19.)

4: Arthroscopy

Annotated References

1. Neer CS II: Anterior acromioplasty for the chronic impingement syndrome in the shoulder: A preliminary report. *J Bone Joint Surg Am* 1972;54(1):41-50.

2. Burns WC II, Whipple TL: Anatomic relationships in the shoulder impingement syndrome. *Clin Orthop Relat Res* 1993;294:96-102.

3. Flatow EL, Soslowsky LJ, Ticker JB, et al: Excursion of the rotator cuff under the acromion: Patterns of subacromial contact. *Am J Sports Med* 1994;22(6): 779-788.

4. Flatow EL, Colman WW, Kelkar R, et al: The effect of anterior acromioplasty on rotator cuff contact: An experimental and computer simulation. *J Shoulder Elbow Surg* 1995;4:S53-S54 7856802

5. Pedowitz RA, Yamaguchi K, Ahmad CS, et al: American Academy of Orthopaedic Surgeons Clinical Practice Guideline on: Optimizing the management of rotator cuff problems. *J Bone Joint Surg Am* 2012;94(2): 163-167.

    The authors discuss issues related to the Clinical Practice Guideline on management of the rotator cuff.

6. Gerber C, Galantay RV, Hersche O: The pattern of pain produced by irritation of the acromioclavicular joint and the subacromial space. *J Shoulder Elbow Surg* 1998;7(4):352-355.

7. Roberts CS, Davila JN, Hushek SG, Tillett ED, Corrigan TM: Magnetic resonance imaging analysis of the subacromial space in the impingement sign positions. *J Shoulder Elbow Surg* 2002;11(6):595-599.

8. Jia X, Ji JH, Pannirselvam V, Petersen SA, McFarland EG: Does a positive Neer impingement sign reflect rotator cuff contact with the acromion? *Clin Orthop Relat Res* 2011;469(3):813-818.

    The high correlation between arthroscopic evaluation of the arm position at which the rotator cuff contacts the superior glenoid and the position of pain in patients with a positive Neer impingement sign suggests that rotator cuff–glenoid contact, not rotator cuff–acromion contact, may be the immediate cause of impingement symptoms.

9. Pappas GP, Blemker SS, Beaulieu CF, McAdams TR, Whalen ST, Gold GE: In vivo anatomy of the Neer and Hawkins sign positions for shoulder impingement. *J Shoulder Elbow Surg* 2006;15(1):40-49.

10. Valadie AL III, Jobe CM, Pink MM, Ekman EF, Jobe FW: Anatomy of provocative tests for impingement syndrome of the shoulder. *J Shoulder Elbow Surg* 2000;9(1):36-46.

11. Park HB, Yokota A, Gill HS, El Rassi G, McFarland EG: Diagnostic accuracy of clinical tests for the different degrees of subacromial impingement syndrome. *J Bone Joint Surg Am* 2005;87(7):1446-1455.

12. Mayerhoefer ME, Breitenseher MJ, Wurnig C, Roposch A: Shoulder impingement: Relationship of clinical symptoms and imaging criteria. *Clin J Sport Med* 2009;19(2):83-89.

    A cross-sectional study of the anatomic relationships and symptoms of impingement syndrome found that the Constant score was correlated with acromiohumeral distance but not with acromial morphology.

13. Harrison AK, Flatow EL: Subacromial impingement syndrome. *J Am Acad Orthop Surg* 2011;19(11): 701-708.

    The pathophysiology and treatment of subacromial impingement syndrome were reviewed.

14. Kim YS, Bigliani LU, Fujisawa M, et al: Stromal cell-derived factor 1 (SDF-1, CXCL12) is increased in subacromial bursitis and downregulated by steroid and nonsteroidal anti-inflammatory agents. *J Orthop Res* 2006;24(8):1756-1764.

15. Labianca R, Sarzi-Puttini P, Zuccaro SM, Cherubino P, Vellucci R, Fornasari D: Adverse effects associated with non-opioid and opioid treatment in patients with chronic pain. *Clin Drug Investig* 2012;32(suppl 1): 53-63.

    The benefits and adverse effect profiles of opioid and nonopioid pain medications were described.

16. Cohen DB, Kawamura S, Ehteshami JR, Rodeo SA: Indomethacin and celecoxib impair rotator cuff tendon-to-bone healing. *Am J Sports Med* 2006;34(3): 362-369.

17. Holmgren T, Björnsson Hallgren H, Öberg B, Adolfsson L, Johansson K: Effect of specific exercise strategy on need for surgery in patients with subacromial impingement syndrome: Randomised controlled study. *BMJ* 2012;344:e787.

    Compared with nonspecific physical rehabilitation, a 12-week course of manual mobilization, eccentric rotator cuff strengthening, and concentric-eccentric strengthening of scapular stabilizers led to decreases in pain and the need for surgery in patients with subacromial impingement after unsuccessful nonsurgical measures. Level of evidence: I.

18. Buchbinder R, Green S, Youd JM: Corticosteroid injections for shoulder pain. *Cochrane Database Syst Rev* 2003;1:CD004016.

19. Mikolyzk DK, Wei AS, Tonino P, et al: Effect of corticosteroids on the biomechanical strength of rat rotator cuff tendon. *J Bone Joint Surg Am* 2009;91(5):1172-1180.

    In rats, a 50%-thickness infraspinatus tear was created. The rats receiving a single injection of methylprednisolone had a transient decrease in biomechanical strength and an increase in fat cells and collagen attenuation.

20. Aaron DL, Bruce BG, Cote M, et al: Abstract: Novel anti-inflammatory agent and CXCR4 inhibitor (AMD 3100) does not impede rotator cuff tendon healing in an animal model. *Annual Meeting Proceedings*. Rosemont, IL, American Academy of Orthopaedic Surgeons, presentation 074. http://www.aaos.org/education/education.asp. Accessed January 2, 2013.

   In a biomechanical comparison of injured rat infraspinatus tendons, no weakening was noted with the administration of an inhibitor of SDF-1α–mediated subacromial bursal inflammation (AMD 3100).

21. Checroun AJ, Dennis MG, Zuckerman JD: Open versus arthroscopic decompression for subacromial impingement: A comprehensive review of the literature from the last 25 years. *Bull Hosp Jt Dis* 1998;57(3): 145-151.

22. Davis AD, Kakar S, Moros C, Kaye EK, Schepsis AA, Voloshin I: Arthroscopic versus open acromioplasty: A meta-analysis. *Am J Sports Med* 2010;38(3):613-618.

   A meta-analysis of studies of open and arthroscopic acromioplasty outcomes found that arthroscopic technique led to faster return to work and fewer inpatient hospital days. No other significant differences were found. Level of evidence: III.

23. Norlin R, Adolfsson L: Small full-thickness tears do well ten to thirteen years after arthroscopic subacromial decompression. *J Shoulder Elbow Surg* 2008; 17(1, suppl):12S-16S.

   In a study of 181 patients who underwent arthroscopic subacromial decompression, those with a small, full-thickness supraspinatus tear had the best results at 10- to 13-year follow-up. The authors concluded that repair of a small, full-thickness supraspinatus tear may be unnecessary and that subacromial decompression may be adequate.

24. Björnsson H, Norlin R, Knutsson A, Adolfsson L: Fewer rotator cuff tears fifteen years after arthroscopic subacromial decompression. *J Shoulder Elbow Surg* 2010;19(1):111-115.

   Rotator cuff integrity was determined by ultrasound in patients who had undergone subacromial decompression 15 years earlier. The prevalence of partial tears was 14% and full tears was 4%, compared with a 40% prevalence of degenerative tears in age-matched historical control subjects. Level of evidence: III.

25. Milano G, Grasso A, Salvatore M, Zarelli D, Deriu L, Fabbriciani C: Arthroscopic rotator cuff repair with and without subacromial decompression: A prospective randomized study. *Arthroscopy* 2007;23(1):81-88.

   A prospective comparison of functional outcomes in patients undergoing rotator cuff repair with or without concurrent subacromial decompression found no significant differences at 2-year follow-up. Level of evidence: I.

26. Gartsman GM, O'Connor DP: Arthroscopic rotator cuff repair with and without arthroscopic subacromial decompression: A prospective, randomized study of one-year outcomes. *J Shoulder Elbow Surg* 2004; 13(4):424-426.

27. MacDonald P, McRae S, Leiter J, Mascarenhas R, Lapner P: Arthroscopic rotator cuff repair with and without acromioplasty in the treatment of full-thickness rotator cuff tears: A multicenter, randomized controlled trial. *J Bone Joint Surg Am* 2011;93(21): 1953-1960.

   A comparison of outcomes after isolated rotator cuff repair or rotator cuff repair with acromioplasty found no differences in outcome scores, but patients who underwent isolated repair had a higher reoperation rate. Level of evidence: I.

28. Chahal J, Mall N, MacDonald PB, et al: The role of subacromial decompression in patients undergoing arthroscopic repair of full-thickness tears of the rotator cuff: A systematic review and meta-analysis. *Arthroscopy* 2012;28(5):720-727.

   A meta-analysis of four level I studies found no differences in outcome after rotator cuff repair alone and with acromioplasty. Level of evidence: I.

29. Noh KC, Chung KJ, Yu HS, Koh SH, Yoo JH: Arthroscopic treatment of septic arthritis of acromioclavicular joint. *Clin Orthop Surg* 2010;2(3):186-190.

   Septic arthritis of the AC joint was successfully treated with arthroscopic débridement and distal clavicle resection in a case report.

30. Zanca P: Shoulder pain: Involvement of the acromioclavicular joint: (Analysis of 1,000 cases). *Am J Roentgenol Radium Ther Nucl Med* 1971;112(3):493-506.

31. Rios CG, Arciero RA, Mazzocca AD: Anatomy of the clavicle and coracoid process for reconstruction of the coracoclavicular ligaments. *Am J Sports Med* 2007; 35(5):811-817.

   In an anatomic description of the distance between the distal clavicle end and the insertion points of the CC ligaments in fresh-frozen cadaver and dry osteologic specimens, the ratios of clavicle length to the distance between the clavicle end and insertion points were found to be consistent in men and women and may serve as a guide to the creation of bone tunnels for anatomic CC reconstruction.

32. Walton J, Mahajan S, Paxinos A, et al: Diagnostic values of tests for acromioclavicular joint pain. *J Bone Joint Surg Am* 2004;86(4):807-812.

33. van Riet RP, Bell SN: Clinical evaluation of acromioclavicular joint pathology: Sensitivity of a new test. *J Shoulder Elbow Surg* 2011;20(1):73-76.

   A new test for AC pathology, consisting of cross-body adduction with elevation against resistance in internal rotation, had a sensitivity of 98%, which was higher than that of four other tests.

34. Mazzocca AD, Spang JT, Rodriguez RR, et al: Biomechanical and radiographic analysis of partial coracoclavicular ligament injuries. *Am J Sports Med* 2008;

4. Arthroscopy

36(7):1397-1402.

The authors studied whether injury to the conoid or trapezoid ligament would result in acromioclavicular joint instability following complete acromioclavicular joint injury.

35. Girish G, Lobo LG, Jacobson JA, Morag Y, Miller B, Jamadar DA: Ultrasound of the shoulder: Asymptomatic findings in men. *AJR Am J Roentgenol* 2011; 197(4):W713-719.

Ultrasound examination of the shoulder found abnormalities in 96% of the asymptomatic subjects, the most common of which were thickening of the subacromial and subdeltoid bursae, AC joint arthritis, and supraspinatus tendinosis.

36. van Riet RP, Goehre T, Bell SN: The long term effect of an intra-articular injection of corticosteroids in the acromioclavicular joint. *J Shoulder Elbow Surg* 2012; 21(3):376-379.

A prospective study of the efficacy of corticosteroid–local anesthetic injection into the AC joint found that the immediate diagnostic value was high; 28% of the patients had pain relief at 1-month follow-up that endured to the final average 42-month follow-up.

37. Flatow EL, Cordasco FA, Bigliani LU: Arthroscopic resection of the outer end of the clavicle from a superior approach: A critical, quantitative, radiographic assessment of bone removal. *Arthroscopy* 1992;8(1):55-64.

38. Beitzel K, Sablan N, Chowaniec DM, et al: Sequential resection of the distal clavicle and its effects on horizontal acromioclavicular joint translation. *Am J Sports Med* 2012;40(3):681-685.

A cadaver biomechanical study of AC joint stability after CC reconstruction and sequential resection of the distal clavicle found significantly greater instability after 10 mm of clavicle resection.

39. Elhassan B, Ozbaydar M, Diller D, Massimini D, Higgins LD, Warner JJ: Open versus arthroscopic acromioclavicular joint resection: A retrospective comparison study. *Arthroscopy* 2009;25(11):1224-1232.

A retrospective comparison of open and arthroscopic distal clavicle resection found no statistically significant difference. Level of evidence: IV.

40. Robertson WJ, Griffith MH, Carroll K, O'Donnell T, Gill TJ: Arthroscopic versus open distal clavicle excision: A comparative assessment at intermediate-term follow-up. *Am J Sports Med* 2011;39(11):2415-2420.

A review of functional and subjective outcomes of open and arthroscopic distal clavicle resection found similar functional scores. Patients who underwent arthroscopic resection had less pain at intermediate-term follow-up. Level of evidence: III.

41. Pensak M, Grumet RC, Slabaugh MA, Bach BR Jr: Open versus arthroscopic distal clavicle resection. *Arthroscopy* 2010;26(5):697-704.

A review of outcome studies of open and arthroscopic distal clavicle resection found better subjective outcomes with arthroscopic procedures, with the direct approach permitting earlier return to athletics. Outcomes were worse in patients with posttraumatic arthrosis than in those with osteoarthritis or osteolysis. Level of evidence: III.

42. Zawadsky M, Marra G, Wiater JM, et al: Osteolysis of the distal clavicle: Long-term results of arthroscopic resection. *Arthroscopy* 2000;16(6):600-605.

43. Kim J, Chung J, Ok H: Asymptomatic acromioclavicular joint arthritis in arthroscopic rotator cuff tendon repair: A prospective randomized comparison study. *Arch Orthop Trauma Surg* 2011;131(3):363-369.

In a randomized prospective comparison of patients with a full-thickness rotator cuff tear and asymptomatic AC joint arthritis with inferior osteophytes, as diagnosed by radiographs, one group underwent isolated rotator cuff repair and the other group underwent rotator cuff repair with distal clavicle resection. Pain and functional scores were lower after distal clavicle resection at 6 and 12 weeks but were higher at 2 years.

44. Tossy JD, Mead NC, Sigmond HM: Acromioclavicular separations: Useful and practical classification for treatment. *Clin Orthop Relat Res* 1963;28:111-119.

45. Rockwood CA, Williams GR, Young DC: *Rockwood and Green's Fractures in Adults*, ed 3. Philadelphia, PA, JB Lippincott, 1991, pp 1181-1239.

46. Barnes CJ, Higgins LD, Major NM, Basamania CJ: Magnetic resonance imaging of the coracoclavicular ligaments: Its role in defining pathoanatomy at the acromioclavicular joint. *J Surg Orthop Adv* 2004; 13(2):69-75.

47. Costic RS, Labriola JE, Rodosky MW, Debski RE: Biomechanical rationale for development of anatomical reconstructions of coracoclavicular ligaments after complete acromioclavicular joint dislocations. *Am J Sports Med* 2004;32(8):1929-1936.

48. Mazzocca AD, Santangelo SA, Johnson ST, Rios CG, Dumonski ML, Arciero RA: A biomechanical evaluation of an anatomical coracoclavicular ligament reconstruction. *Am J Sports Med* 2006;34(2):236-246.

49. Grutter PW, Petersen SA: Anatomical acromioclavicular ligament reconstruction: A biomechanical comparison of reconstructive techniques of the acromioclavicular joint. *Am J Sports Med* 2005;33(11):1723-1728.

50. Chernchujit B, Tischer T, Imhoff AB: Arthroscopic reconstruction of the acromioclavicular joint disruption: Surgical technique and preliminary results. *Arch Orthop Trauma Surg* 2006;126(9):575-581.

51. Thiel E, Mutnal A, Gilot GJ: Surgical outcome following arthroscopic fixation of acromioclavicular joint disruption with the TightRope device. *Orthopedics* 2011;34(7):e267-e274.

A cohort study of high-grade AC separations and one distal clavicle fracture treated with the TightRope device found a 16.67% rate of fixation failure. Patient satisfaction and functional scores were high.

52. Walz L, Salzmann GM, Fabbro T, Eichhorn S, Imhoff AB: The anatomic reconstruction of acromioclavicular joint dislocations using 2 TightRope devices: A biomechanical study. *Am J Sports Med* 2008;36(12):2398-2406.

    A biomechanical cadaver study of anatomic reconstruction of CC ligaments with two TightRope devices found a higher load to failure compared with native ligaments.

53. Salzmann GM, Walz L, Buchmann S, Glabgly P, Venjakob A, Imhoff AB: Arthroscopically assisted 2-bundle anatomical reduction of acute acromioclavicular joint separations. *Am J Sports Med* 2010;38(6):1179-1187.

    Arthroscopically assisted AC joint reduction with two flip-button devices to anatomically reconstruct the CC ligaments found improved pain and functional scores postoperatively, even in patients with radiographic loss of reduction (8 of 23 patients). Level of evidence: IV.

54. Boileau P, Old J, Gastaud O, Brassart N, Roussanne Y: All-arthroscopic Weaver-Dunn-Chuinard procedure with double-button fixation for chronic acromioclavicular joint dislocation. *Arthroscopy* 2010;26(2):149-160.

    Chronic, severe AC separations were treated with an all-arthroscopic Weaver-Dunn-Chuinard procedure augmented with a four-strand suture reconstruction of the CC ligaments. No loss of reduction was seen, all symptoms resolved, and functional outcome scores were high. Level of evidence: IV.

55. Kowalsky MS, Kremenic IJ, Orishimo KF, McHugh MP, Nicholas SJ, Lee SJ: The effect of distal clavicle excision on in situ graft forces in coracoclavicular ligament reconstruction. *Am J Sports Med* 2010;38(11):2313-2319.

    A biomechanical cadaver study assessed in situ graft forces in CC reconstruction, with or without sectioning of the AC ligaments and distal clavicle resection. Higher forces were seen with AC ligament sectioning, but distal clavicle resection did not substantially exacerbate this effect. Although the results were statistically significant, clinical significance could not be established because the increased forces on the graft after AC ligament sectioning and distal clavicle resection remained much lower than load to failure.

56. Kurtz CA, Humble BJ, Rodosky MW, Sekiya JK: Symptomatic os acromiale. *J Am Acad Orthop Surg* 2006;14(1):12-19.

57. Ortiguera CJ, Buss DD: Surgical management of the symptomatic os acromiale. *J Shoulder Elbow Surg* 2002;11(5):521-528.

58. Harris JD, Griesser MJ, Jones GL: Systematic review of the surgical treatment for symptomatic os acromiale. *Int J Shoulder Surg* 2011;5(1):9-16.

    A review of level I through IV evidence of surgical treatment of symptomatic os acromiale found that all evaluated techniques improved outcomes.

59. Warner JJ, Beim GM, Higgins L: The treatment of symptomatic os acromiale. *J Bone Joint Surg Am* 1998;80(9):1320-1326.

60. Wright RW, Heller MA, Quick DC, Buss DD: Arthroscopic decompression for impingement syndrome secondary to an unstable os acromiale. *Arthroscopy* 2000;16(6):595-599.

4. Arthroscopy

Chapter 20

Arthroscopic Rotator Cuff Repair

Charles M. Jobin, MD   Jay D. Keener, MD   Ken Yamaguchi, MD

Introduction

Arthroscopic rotator cuff repair has been widely accepted because of favorable patient outcomes and minimal morbidity when compared with open techniques. The goal of rotator cuff repair is to reduce painful symptoms, obtain tendon-to-bone healing, maximize functional return, and potentially change the natural history of rotator cuff disease. Functional recovery takes many months after repair, and structural healing is highly variable based on many patient- and tear-related factors. Functional outcomes are often improved with healed repairs compared with retorn repairs. Recent studies have highlighted the patient's age, the tear size, and tear chronicity as the most important factors affecting repair integrity. Structural failure of the repair may result in persistent shoulder weakness, but patient satisfaction and clinical outcomes are inconsistently influenced by tendon healing. The optimal repair fixation construct is an area of great interest despite the lack of strong clinical evidence to support the use of one construct over another. A better understanding of the natural history of rotator cuff tears, the strong effect of age on the incidence of rotator cuff disease and the potential for repair healing, and the optimization of repair strategies will help the next generation of surgeons refine the indications for surgical intervention and choose the optimal repair construct for specific patient and tear characteristics.

Epidemiology

Degenerative age-related tears are more common than traumatic tears, although many degenerative tears become symptomatic with acute extension.[1] The pathogenesis of degenerative rotator cuff tears remains debated and probably is a combination of extrinsic mechanical impingement factors and intrinsic biologic factors.[2] A natural history study of 588 patients with

unilateral shoulder pain observed a strong association between tear incidence and patient age.[3] Degenerative rotator cuff tears commonly occur near the junction of the supraspinatus and infraspinatus footprints within the rotator cuff crescent, which is a zone of relative hypovascularity protected by the surrounding rotator cuff cable (**Figure 1**).

Natural History

Rotator cuff disease generally is progressive, and there is little intrinsic ability for spontaneous tendon healing after a tear occurs. Natural history studies have found that painful tears have a tear size progression rate of approximately 50% at 2.5 to 5 years when compared with asymptomatic tears, which progress at a slower rate of 30%.[4,5] Age probably is an important risk factor for tear progression; patients older than 60 years were found to have a 54% rate of tear progression versus 17% in younger patients.[6] Symptomatic tears are associated with supraspinatus atrophy and fatty muscle

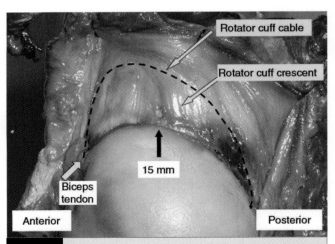

Figure 1 Photograph showing the rotator cuff crescent, a common site of degenerative cuff tearing. The rotator cuff crescent is supported by the suspensory mechanism of the rotator cuff cable. (Adapted with permission from Kim HM, Dahiya N, Teefey SA, et al: Location and initiation of degenerative rotator cuff tears: An analysis of three hundred and sixty shoulders. *J Bone Joint Surg Am* 2010;92[5]:1088-1096.)

Dr. Yamaguchi or an immediate family member has received royalties from Tornier. Neither of the following authors nor any immediate family member has received anything of value from or has stock or stock options held in a commercial company or institution related directly or indirectly to the subject of this chapter: Dr. Jobin and Dr. Keener.

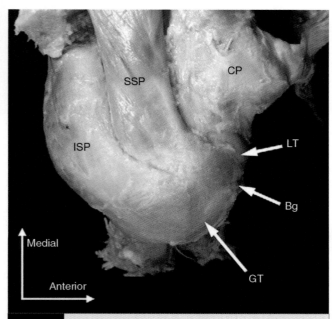

Figure 2 Photograph showing the insertional anatomy of the terminal rotator cuff tendon, with blending of the supraspinatus (SSP) and infraspinatus (ISP) terminal tendons, an anterior vector to the terminal infraspinatus tendon, and a supraspinatus tendon that spans anteriorly to the lesser tuberosity (LT). CP = coracoid process, Bg = biceps groove, GT = greater tuberosity. (Adapted with permission from Mochizuki T, Sugaya H, Uomizu M, et al: Humeral insertion of the supraspinatus and infraspinatus: New anatomical findings regarding the footprint of the rotator cuff. *J Bone Joint Surg Am* 2008;90[5]:962-969.)

changes of Goutallier grade 2 or above.[7] Smoking is also associated with rotator cuff tear progression, with a dosage- and time-dependent relationship to tear size.[8,9]

Extrinsic Versus Intrinsic Factors

Impingement is the most widely described potential extrinsic factor in rotator cuff disease. Repetitive mechanical abrasion of the rotator cuff on the supraspinatus outlet may lead to tearing. The classification of acromial morphology has poor interobserver reliability and has been difficult to correlate with rotator cuff disease. Acromial spurs develop because of ossification within the coracoacromial ligament, and they may signal chronic intrinsic cuff disease. The presence of acromial spurs has been correlated with advancing age and the presence of bursal-side and full-thickness rotator cuff tears.[10,11] Rotator cuff impingement against the acromion during provocative positions was not found in pressure contact studies.[12] Routine acromioplasty during rotator cuff repair did not lead to improved pain or outcome scores in three randomized controlled studies and a meta-analysis.[13-16] The treatment of partial-thickness rotator cuff tears with acromioplasty and débridement does not appear to prevent the progression of tears over time.[17] One study found that the lateral acromial index, a measure of the lateral projection of the acromion relative to the humerus, was correlated with rotator cuff disease and full-thickness tears, but other studies found no such correlation.[10,18] The strong association of rotator cuff disease with age, the frequent presence of bilateral cuff tears, the age-related histologic changes in the rotator cuff, and the frequent absence of an association between trauma and pain onset suggest a primary intrinsic or biologic etiology for most degenerative rotator cuff tears.

Advancements in Understanding Anatomy

Reconstruction of the tendon footprint probably improves healing and anatomic rotator cuff function. Recent anatomic studies of the rotator cuff footprint suggest an important blending of the supraspinatus and infraspinatus terminal tendons with a smaller supraspinatus footprint and a more anterior margin of the infraspinatus footprint[19] (**Figure 2**). Earlier studies separated the footprints of these tendons into two distinct areas with near-equal widths on the greater tuberosity. A more anterior insertion of the supraspinatus was found to include a portion of the lesser tuberosity.[19] The infraspinatus was found to insert as close as 2 mm posterior to the biceps groove at the lateral aspect of the greater tuberosity (**Figure 3**). This finding may explain the infraspinatus fatty muscle changes seen in supraspinatus tears that were previously considered isolated.

Tears of the anterior supraspinatus that involve the anterior rotator cuff cable increasingly are being recognized as at risk for progression and development of fatty changes in the supraspinatus and infraspinatus.[20] Anterior rotator cuff cable tears are located immediately adjacent to the biceps tendon and involve the lateral biceps sling. These tears cause a disruption in the suspensory effect of the rotator cuff cable, allowing greater tension in the thinner crescent area. One study found that proximity of the tear to the biceps tendon was strongly correlated with supraspinatus muscle degenerative changes.[21] Only 11% of tears with an intact anterior supraspinatus tendon had developed supraspinatus muscle degeneration on ultrasound.

Fatty Degeneration of the Rotator Cuff Muscles

The development of muscular fatty changes and muscle atrophy occurs in association with full-thickness rotator cuff tears and is a time-dependent process. Fatty muscle degeneration is generally believed to be irreversible. Goutallier described the association of fatty muscle changes to tear size and tear chronicity.[22] The timing of fatty changes is critically important for surgeons to

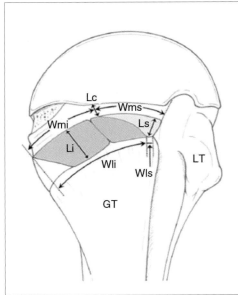

	Average ± standard deviation (mm)
Supraspinatus	
Maximal medial-to-lateral length	6.9 ± 1.4
Anteroposterior width of medial margin	12.6 ± 2.0
Anteroposterior width of lateral margin	1.3 ± 1.4
Infraspinatus	
Maximal medial-to-lateral length	10.2 ± 1.6
Anteroposterior width of medial margin	20.2 ± 6.2
Anteroposterior width of lateral margin	32.7 ± 3.4
Articular capsule	
Medial-to-lateral length at posterior edge of supraspinatus footprint	4.5 ± 0.5

Figure 3 Schematic drawing showing the anatomic dimensions of the rotator cuff footprint, with the average values of the dimensions. The medial-to-lateral dimension of the supraspinatus footprint was found to be narrower than in earlier studies and to stretch across to the lesser tuberosity, sharing significant length with the joint capsule. GT = greater tuberosity, Lc = length of the capsule, Li = length of the infraspinatus footprint, Ls = length of the supraspinatus footprint, LT = lesser tuberosity, Wli = width of the lateral footprint of the infraspinatus, Wls = width of the lateral footprint of the supraspinatus, Wmi = width of medial footprint of the infraspinatus, Wms = width of medial footprint of the supraspinatus. (Adapted with permission from Mochizuki T, Sugaya H, Uomizu M, et al: Humeral insertion of the supraspinatus and infraspinatus: New anatomical findings regarding the footprint of the rotator cuff. *J Bone Joint Surg Am* 2008;90[5]:962-969.)

define the optimal surgical indications. Tendon repair should be attempted before the development of higher grade muscular fatty degeneration, which can affect tendon healing and the clinical results of surgery. This threshold is probably Goutallier grade 2 (equal amounts of fat and muscle); studies have found reduced tendon healing and lower shoulder strength and outcome scores at this stage or higher stages.[23,24]

Studies of the natural history of fatty muscle degeneration suggest that important muscle changes occur more than 2.5 years after the onset of pain. Moderate fatty changes of the supraspinatus were found to occur an average of 3 years after the onset of symptoms, and severe fatty changes and atrophy were present by 5 years.[25] Advanced changes have been found as early as 6 months after an acute supraspinatus rupture. A focused study of infraspinatus fatty changes found moderate fatty changes by 2.5 years and severe changes by 4 years.[26] Retrospective reporting of fatty muscle degeneration has several inherent limitations because the duration of the presence of a tear is unknown, especially in degenerative rotator cuff disease, which may begin as an asymptomatic tear. Fatty degeneration occurs more frequently in the infraspinatus than in the supraspinatus and may occur in the presence of a presumed isolated supraspinatus tear.[27] Infraspinatus degeneration is not well understood but could be related to incorrect anatomic definitions of the cuff footprint insertion, traction on the motor branches of the

suprascapular nerve secondary to tendon retraction, a change in the infraspinatus pennation angle, and disuse atrophy.

Persistent weakness and lower functional scores were observed after repair of rotator cuffs with advanced fatty changes.[22,23] Repairing a torn rotator cuff tendon may limit or slow the progression of fatty muscle changes but does not reverse them.[23] At an average of 2 years after intact repair, the Goutallier stage was found to have increased an average of 0.5 grade.[24] Although the biologic cause of fatty changes remains controversial, the loss of muscular function with advanced muscle changes is a clinical dilemma. In an animal model, a 50% loss of strength, a 68% reduction in active work, and a 35% reduction in tendon excursion were found in chronic rotator cuff tears.[28] Human studies using electrical stimulation found a strong correlation between rotator cuff muscle tension and Goutallier grade. Maximal muscle tension was reduced by 70% with grade 3 fatty changes.[29] Irreversible muscle changes probably affect functional outcomes and strength, even after successful tendon healing.

Biomechanics of Repair Constructs

The biomechanics of rotator cuff repair constructs have been extensively studied in cadaver models. The understanding of optimal pullout strength, tendon-to-bone

4: Arthroscopy

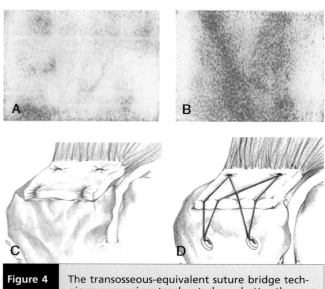

Figure 4 The transosseous-equivalent suture bridge technique pressurizes tendon to bone better than the point fixation of a double-row anchor repair. Suture bridges can be created medial to lateral or anterior to posterior. Pressure-sensitive film recordings (**A** and **B**) and schematic drawings *(bottom row)* showing tendon-to-bone pressurization in the double-row suture-anchor technique (**A** and **C**) and the transosseous-equivalent suture bridge technique (**B** and **D**). (Adapted with permission from Park MC, ElAttrache NS, Tibone JE, Ahmad CS, Jun BJ, Lee TQ: Part I: Footprint contact characteristics for a transosseous-equivalent rotator cuff repair technique compared with a double-row repair technique. *J Shoulder Elbow Surg* 2007;16[4]:461-468.)

pressurization, and tendon-to-bone gapping has advanced, but the clinical translation of these advances is not well understood. The ultimate goal of a repair is biologic healing of tendon to bone before mechanical failure. Biologic healing probably is promoted by minimal motion at the tendon-bone interface, adequate tendon-to-bone pressurization or apposition and, most importantly, favorable biology.

Tissue-grasping suture constructs, such as a modified Mason-Allen stitch, provide optimal tendon fixation but are difficult to perform arthroscopically. Failure of a transosseous repair typically involves suture pullout through bone. Suture anchor constructs typically fail at the suture-tendon interface, with the sutures pulling through the tendon. Double-row repairs appear to be biomechanically superior to most single-row repairs, regardless of suture configuration, ultimate tensile load, and stiffness with cyclic loading.[30,31] Double-row repairs have better fixation strength than single-row or transosseous repairs when exposed to cyclic loading during changes in humeral rotation.[32]

A repair construct that compresses the tendon to bone with a transosseous-equivalent suture bridge has a broader pressurized area than single-row fixation[33] (**Figure 4**). A traditional transosseous repair restores a larger footprint than a single-row repair, and a double-row anchor repair consistently reconstructs most of the native footprint. Biomechanically, transosseous-equivalent repairs have a greater ultimate load strength but similar stiffness under cyclic loading with traditional double-row repairs.[34] Transosseous-equivalent repair constructs also may provide a larger area of pressurized tendon-to-bone contact than double-row repairs.[33] Tuberosity osteopenia or cystic degeneration may preclude secure anchor fixation, and strategies using stronger lateral cortical bone with a suture-bridge technique have been promoted. There is renewed interest in a so-called watertight repair, in which synovial fluid containing degradative enzymes is excluded and healing factors are maintained at the repair site. Transosseous-equivalent constructs had the least articular fluid extravasation in a cadaver model.[35]

Doppler ultrasound was used to find that the primary blood supply for healing comes from the greater tuberosity anchor site and superficial peribursal layer of the rotator cuff.[36] The increased strength and pressurization of rotator cuff repairs may lead to unintended consequences, such as increased rates of medial tendon retearing and reduced vascular supply to the terminal tendon. One study of a double-row suture-bridge construct found that 60% of retears were caused by a failure around the medial row, with loss of continuity to the terminal tendon.[37] These medial retears (**Figure 5**) raise serious concerns because terminal tendon deficiency may preclude revision rotator cuff repair. The cause of these retears is unknown, but some evidence suggests that the vascular supply to the terminal tendon may be compromised with a double-row repair. One study found an immediate 45% reduction in blood flow to the terminal tendon, raising concerns about biologic healing potential with an excessively pressurized repair construct.[38] However, another ultrasound study found an increase in tendon perfusion within the first few months after rotator cuff repair, suggesting that vascularity returns despite repair pressurization.[39]

Factors Influencing Repair Integrity

Numerous factors affect repair integrity, and defining them will help focus research into the most important factors for patient outcomes. Age and its effect on the ability to heal after a repair probably are the most important factors affecting repair integrity, rather than the repair construct itself.[40-46] One study of isolated supraspinatus repairs found a 45% healing rate in patients older than 65 years, compared with an 86% healing rate in younger patients.[40] Another study of patients older than 65 years found a partial or full retear in 25% and 42%, respectively, as confirmed by CT arthrography 6 months after surgery.[45] An ultrasound study 1 and 2 years after surgery found that the average age of patients with a healed repair was 58 years, and the average age of those with a recurrent tear was

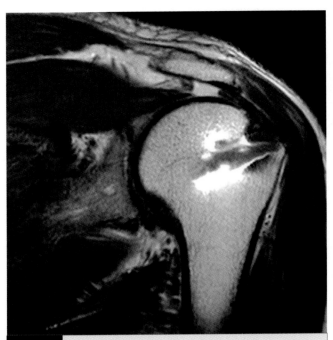

Figure 5 MRI demonstrating medial row retearing after a double-row repair. A tendon deficiency may preclude revision rotator cuff repair. (Adapted with permission from Koh KH, Kang KC, Lim TK, Shon MS, Yoo JC: Prospective randomized clinical trial of single- versus double-row suture anchor repair in 2- to 4-cm rotator cuff tears: Clinical and magnetic resonance imaging results. *Arthroscopy* 2011;27[4]:453-462.)

64 years.[42] This study found that age probably was confounded with tear size and chronicity.

Tear size, tear chronicity, and Goutallier grade are strongly associated with repair failure. Larger tears have lower rates of tendon healing, even with a double-row construct. One study found that 36% of two-tendon tears healed, compared with 67% of single-tendon tears.[43] A systematic review of 1,252 repairs from 23 studies found a strong correlation between tear size and the lack of repair healing.[29] The retear rate for tears smaller than 1 cm was 7% to 17%, compared with 41% to 69% for tears larger than 5 cm. Muscular changes also affect repair structural outcomes. One study found a substantial 40% supraspinatus retear rate in patients with Goutallier grade 2 fatty infiltration compared with 14% to 18% in those with grade 0 or 1 changes.[24] Healing was influenced by age, duration of symptoms, and rotator cuff muscle atrophy.

The repair construct is believed to be an important factor in tendon healing. Some studies of single-row repairs found alarmingly high rates of recurrent tearing. Single-row repairs of large to massive (larger than 3 cm) tears were found to have retear rates ranging from 76% to 94%.[47] Tears with an average size of 2.6 cm had an 88% defect rate on magnetic resonance arthrography (MRA).[48] However, these studies were not sufficiently controlled for adequate comparison.

Most higher level studies have not found that double-row repairs substantially improve repair integrity. A level I randomized controlled study comparing single- and double-row repairs found no statistical difference in rates of recurrent full- or partial-thickness retearing, as observed on MRI.[49] Another level I randomized controlled study found 10% rates of retearing with both constructs, but there was an additional 10% rate of severe tendon thinning in patients treated with a double-row repair.[50] A third level I randomized controlled study found very low, statistically insignificant differences in rates of full-thickness retearing on MRA 2 years after single- and double-row repairs (8% and 4%, respectively).[51] Studies with lower levels of evidence found better structural integrity with a double-row repair construct, but these studies had design weaknesses and should be interpreted with caution. A level II cohort study found better anatomic healing in double-row than in single-row repairs (61% and 40%, respectively) on computed tomographic arthrography, but there was no clinical difference in Constant scores.[52] A level III retrospective cohort study found a significant 25% retear rate after single-row repair versus 10% after double-row repair.[53] Some authors suggested that younger patients with greater rotator cuff strength may benefit from the more robust double-row construct.[29]

Attempts to synthesize the numerous comparison studies of single- and double-row repairs have led to systematic reviews of clinical and structural outcomes. A systematic review of six studies, three of which were level I randomized controlled studies, found inconclusive evidence, although there appeared to be better structural healing and the possibility of functional benefit when a double-row repair was used for tears wider than 3 cm.[54] A review of 23 studies, of which 21 were level IV case studies, concluded that patients with a tear larger than 1 cm had lower retear rates after a double-row repair.[55] The conclusions of these systematic reviews are difficult to interpret because by design they included studies that were subject to bias. Future studies controlling for age, tear size, and muscular changes should better identify the indications for a double-row repair.

Surgical Treatment

Indications and Contraindications
Surgical repair traditionally is indicated for a symptomatic full-thickness or a substantial partial-thickness rotator cuff tear after 3 to 6 months of unsuccessful nonsurgical treatment with nonsteroidal anti-inflammatory drugs, physical therapy, and steroid or local analgesic injections. More urgent surgical repair is indicated in a relatively young patient with a traumatic tear, a patient with an acute tear, or a patient with a substantial acute extension of a chronic tear with an associated decline in function. An acutely torn rotator cuff is most likely

to be successfully repaired within the first 3 weeks of injury.[56]

The indications for rotator cuff surgical intervention are not well defined in the literature. The most common indications for repair were found to be failure of nonsurgical treatment (52%), limitation in activities of daily living (31%), excessive duration of nonsurgical treatment (26%), and a history of nocturnal pain (16%).[57] With a better understanding of the natural history of rotator cuff tears, the indications for surgical intervention are evolving. The presence of a full-thickness rotator cuff tear is not an absolute indication for surgical intervention; nonsurgical treatment may relieve pain, and some such tears are asymptomatic.[3,58] Increasingly, data suggest that rotator cuff tears increase in size over time, become symptomatic with progression, and develop irreversible muscular changes. These considerations justify the argument for early repair of a small or medium-size full-thickness tear or a tear involving the anterior supraspinatus, before the onset of substantial muscle degeneration in a patient younger than 65 years. Surgical intervention for an asymptomatic tear cannot be recommended, but serial evaluation is recommended to monitor symptom development and tear progression.

The contraindications to rotator cuff repair include adequate management by nonsurgical means or the patient's inability to comply with postoperative restrictions and rehabilitation. The relative contraindications include a chronic degenerative tear in a patient older than 65 years, proximal migration of the humeral head as seen on imaging studies, and muscle fatty changes more advanced than Goutallier grade 2, especially if the changes involve more than one rotator cuff muscle. Tear retraction is not a contraindication, but a rotator cuff repair with excessive cuff tension is likely to structurally fail. Attempted repair may be reasonable despite a high likelihood of structural failure because clinical outcomes are good to excellent, even with tendon retearing.[48] In addition, partial repair of a larger or a retracted tear can lead to a good clinical outcome, with the theoretic benefit of restoration of the infraspinatus-subscapularis force couple.

Preoperative Evaluation

Preoperative evaluation includes an assessment of shoulder motion, scapular control, rotator cuff strength, lag signs, and any possibly contributing pathology, such as cervical spine disease, acromioclavicular arthritis, or biceps irritation. Standard radiography, including AP, true AP, axillary, and scapular Y views should be used to assess for glenohumeral arthritis, calcific tendinitis, proximal humeral migration, and anterior subluxation suggestive of a subscapularis tear. Proximal humeral migration is clinically important because it implies the disruption of normal kinematics, which is most often correlated with tearing of the infraspinatus tendon. An acromiohumeral interval of 7 mm or less suggests a large chronic rotator cuff tear

and may imply irreparability.[59] MRI or ultrasound should be used to confirm the presence of a rotator cuff tear. Both MRI and ultrasound are predictive of findings during arthroscopy; show full- and partial-thickness tears with near-equal accuracy; and can quantitate retraction, tear dimensions, and muscle fatty changes.[60] The advantage of MRI is that it shows cartilage, bone, and labrum, thus allowing other pathology to be ruled out. Ultrasound is less expensive, less time consuming, and better tolerated by patients, but it requires a technician experienced in shoulder ultrasound.

Surgical Decision Making

Three general factors influence the success of rotator cuff surgery: biology, surgical technique, and environment. All three can be controlled to some extent by the surgeon. Biology often is predetermined by patient characteristics, including age, tear size, muscle and tendon quality, bone quality, and genetics. Patient selection and surgical indications are the surgeon's best means of controlling biology. Patients younger than 65 years are much more likely to heal than older patients.[40-46] The use of biologics to enhance tendon healing is an area of great interest, but little evidence exists to support clinical use.[61] Extensive research suggests that double-row constructs are mechanically superior to single-row constructs, but they have similar clinical outcomes.[31,32,50,51,58,62,63] Environmental factors, such as the postoperative rehabilitation protocol, patient compliance, patient smoking status, and nonsteroidal anti-inflammatory drug use, probably are important surgeon-influenced variables.

Although only limited clinical evidence suggests superior clinical outcomes after a double-row or an equivalent repair, these repairs are biomechanically stronger, better reestablish the anatomic footprint, and may lead to a higher rate of tendon healing in certain situations. The potential benefits of a double-row repair must be weighed against its disadvantages, which primarily are related to cost and surgical time. Many surgeons selectively use double-row repairs if the healing potential of the patient and the rotator cuff are suboptimal in the hope that the biologic limitations may be overcome by using a superior mechanical construct. This strategy may have limited efficacy. Most partial-thickness tears, small or medium-size full-thickness tears, or acute tears in patients younger than 62 to 65 years have good intrinsic biology and heal with a single- or a double-row repair. Although the use of a double-row repair is often considered if tendon quality is poor, the tear is large or massive, or muscle degeneration is advanced, these conditions often occur in patients who are older and have limited biologic healing capacity. In these patients, a strong repair construct may be of limited value. Further research is needed to refine the indications for the use of specific repair constructs in relation to patient age and tear characteristics.

Surgical Technique

Regional anesthesia is routinely used for rotator cuff repair, supplemented by general endotracheal anesthesia if desired. The risk of reduced cerebral oxygenation may be increased if general anesthesia rather than regional anesthesia is used, with the patient in the beach chair position.[64] Although beach chair positioning is most commonly used, lateral decubitus positioning also is used, based on surgeon experience. Lower extremity sequential compression devices are used for perioperative mechanical prophylaxis against deep vein thrombosis. An articulating arm positioner is useful for controlling the extremity during surgery and allows distraction during subacromial arthroscopy. Subacromial injection of a bupivacaine with epinephrine may aid in hemostasis. Examination under anesthesia can help determine concomitant stiffness or instability.

The posterior viewing portal can be placed in the standard location 2 cm distal and 1 cm medial to the posterolateral acromion. A more lateral portal directly distal to the posterolateral acromion is preferred for visualization of the subacromial space. Surgery begins with a diagnostic arthroscopy in the glenohumeral joint after an anterior portal is established within the rotator cuff interval. The subscapularis; the glenoid labrum; the articular cartilage; and the biceps tendon, sling, and anchor are carefully assessed. Within the subacromial space, one or two lateral portals are established, depending on the tear size. It is important to place all portals sufficiently distal to allow access to the subacromial space despite progressive shoulder swelling. If a lateral portal is used for viewing during tendon mobilization and repair, it is helpful to place an additional lateral working portal as well as an anterior subacromial portal for suture management.

A complete bursectomy is performed so that the torn tendons can be seen. An anterolateral acromioplasty may be necessary if there is evidence of an acromial osteophyte or mechanical impingement characterized by undersurface fraying of the coracoacromial ligament. The boundaries of the rotator cuff are defined, and the edges are débrided back to healthy tendon. The footprint on the greater tuberosity is prepared by removing soft tissue with a shaver, and the greater tuberosity is lightly decorticated to facilitate bleeding. If anchors are to be used, full decortication should be avoided because it could jeopardize fixation.

Tear pattern recognition and assessment of rotator cuff mobility are critical for restoring the tendon footprint. Viewing from the lateral portal helps identify the tear pattern and assess tendon delamination. It is important to define the leading and retracted edges of the tear to avoid unequal tension or malreduction. Sometimes the tear is complex, with delamination and variable degrees of retraction among the different layers. A crescent or C-shaped tear usually can be mobilized to the anatomic footprint without undue tension. An L-, reverse L-, or U-shaped tear may require medial closure with a margin convergence technique.

Full glenoid and acromial side releases of the torn tendons may be needed for adequate mobilization. Tendon releases are aided by the placement of traction sutures to assess tendon mobility and identify sites of further adhesions. For a retracted supraspinatus tear, the anterior rotator cuff interval is released by cutting tissue from the biceps sling to the base of coracoid. More medially, the coracohumeral attachments to the anterior supraspinatus tendon also should be released. The rotator cuff interval slide is a modification of the interval release that preserves the lateral rotator cuff interval tissue to reference the anatomic position for rotator cuff reduction. A superior capsular release between the superior glenoid and the undersurface of the rotator cuff is often helpful. Rarely, a posterior release between the supraspinatus and infraspinatus tendons is needed.

The initial biomechanical strength of a repair is optimized by improving the suture-to-bone and suture-to-tendon fixation, minimizing suture abrasion, improving suture strength, ensuring knot and loop security, and restoring the tendon footprint. Because of technical advances in rotator cuff fixation products, the weakest link in the repair construct is now the suture-tendon interface. The suture usually tears through the tendon when a rotator cuff repair fails. Transosseous repairs most often have failed by suture cutout through bone, but suture anchors have improved the bone fixation site, especially under cyclic loading. Biologic tendon-to-bone healing must occur because mechanical fixation ultimately will fail under cyclic loading.

The numerous repair constructs include transosseous, single-row, double-row, transosseous-equivalent suture-bridge, tension band, mixed suture-bridge with tension band, and other suture-bridge configurations, with many variations (**Figure 6**). All constructs are intended to reduce and fix the tendon to the footprint in an anatomic configuration without excessive tension. If medial-row anchors are used, they are placed just off the articular margin. Care must be taken not to pass the medial sutures too medial because doing so may lateralize the tendon and cause excessive tension on the repair. Medial-row knots can be used, and if a suture-bridge construct is planned, the suture tails are brought out laterally over the tuberosity and secured to compress the terminal tendon to the footprint. The lateral aspect of the greater tuberosity approximately 1 to 2 cm distal to the lateral edge of the footprint is ideal for a lateral-row suture-bridge technique because of the strong cortical bone.

In some procedures, such as revision cuff surgery with tuberosity bone loss, a large tuberosity cyst, or osteoporosis, the tuberosity may be inadequate for suture anchor fixation. A transosseous repair incorporating the lateral tuberosity cortex may offer the only fixation point with reliable strength. Another viable technique is the tension-band construct,[40,65] which transforms rotator cuff tension into compression of the tendon to the bony footprint when the shoulder is in adduction. The tension band technique has had early clinical success,

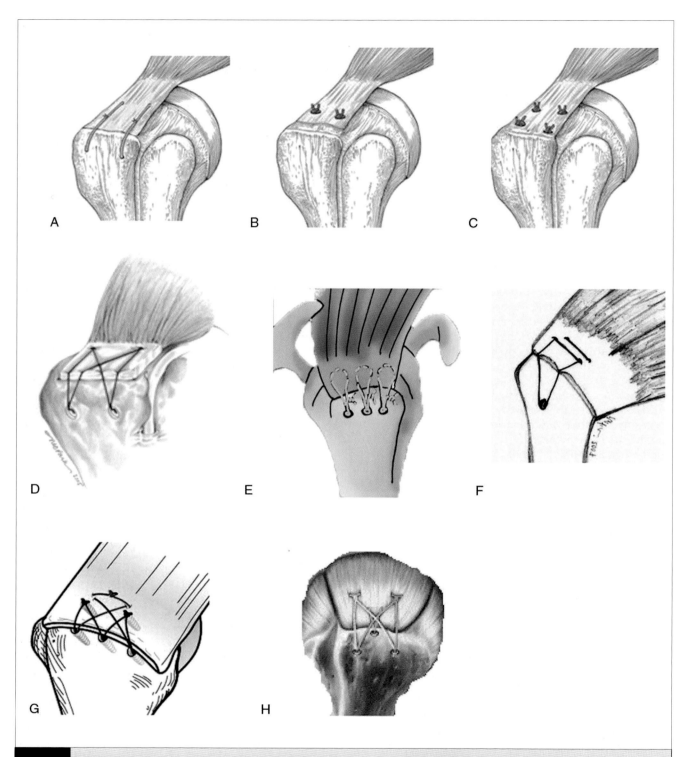

Figure 6   Schematic drawings showing selected rotator cuff repair constructs to highlight the diversity of possible constructs. The unifying principles are point fixation, suture-bridge pressurization, and tension-band compression. **A,** Transosseous. **B,** Single-row. **C,** Double-row. **D,** Transosseous-equivalent suture bridge (two medial-row anchors with lateral suture bridges). **E,** Tension-band (inverted horizontal mattress sutures fixed laterally). **F,** Roman bridge (two medial-row, double-loaded anchors with two anteroposterior suture bridges and a lateral suture bridge). **G,** Diamondback suture-bridge (two medial-row, double-loaded anchors with an anteroposterior suture bridge and a lateral suture bridge to three anchors). **H,** Triple-row (central tension-band repair and transosseous-equivalent suture bridge).

with 70% repair integrity in isolated supraspinatus tears.[40]

Margin convergence or side-to-side repair of the longitudinal aspects of complex tear patterns can be helpful for approximating an otherwise irreparable rotator cuff tear. The key is to recognize the tear pattern and understand that the infraspinatus often retracts in a posteromedial direction, causing a longitudinal split medially in the anterior aspect of the tear. These tears are usually are in the shape of a U, an L, or a reverse L. The marginal convergence repair should be performed medial to lateral before the tendon-to-bone repair because it lateralizes the location for tendon approximation to the footprint, thus reducing tension on the final tendon-to-bone repair construct.

A partial repair should be considered for an otherwise irreparable tear. Partial repairs of large to massive tears have been shown to improve symptoms even if the repair structurally fails.[66] A level III cohort study of massive tears compared 45 complete repairs with 41 partial repairs and found no difference in scores on the the University of California, Los Angeles (UCLA) Shoulder Rating Scale at 2-year follow-up.[67] A case study of 27 patients found good outcomes after partial repair and marginal convergence of irreparable tears measuring 4.2 cm and having a residual defect of 1.2 cm after repair.[68] Scores on the Simple Shoulder Test, Constant, and UCLA Scale substantially improved, but strength was significantly less than in the contralateral shoulder. The etiology of the benefit of a partial repair is unclear. The partial repair may re-create a balanced forced couple and shield the remaining intact cuff from painful tension by redistributing the load, or the benefit may lie in bursectomy, débridement, or another associated procedure.

Postoperative Rehabilitation

Postoperative rehabilitation is crucial to successful recovery, although no high-level evidence supports its use.[69] A well-designed study found no benefit to supervised physical therapy over a home exercise program after rotator cuff repair.[70] Rehabilitation protocols after rotator cuff repair reflect conflicting opinions on immobilization versus early motion. Immobilization may protect the tendon repair from excessive tension and facilitate improvement in structural properties at the repair site, at the expense of early stiffness. Early motion may prevent stiffness and decrease pain, at the cost of increased repair site stress. Delayed rehabilitation protocols typically involve 6 weeks of immobilization with limited passive motion, followed by active-assisted motion, progressing to active motion at 3 months and light resistance exercises at 4 months. Early motion protocols involve passive motion within 2 weeks after surgery, with an early return to active-assisted motion generally within 6 weeks.

The prolonged period of healing after rotator cuff repair is one argument for delaying early motion after surgery. The likelihood that the repair will tear or fail to heal within the first 3 months after surgery indicates that this time period is critical for tendon healing. When repair of tears larger than 3 cm was studied with serial ultrasounds from postoperative day 2 to 2-year follow-up, most of the recurrent tears (78%) occurred within the first 3 months of surgery, and the remaining tears (22%) occuredr 3 to 6 months after surgery.[71] A serial MRI study of medium-size to large rotator cuff repairs found that the structural status of the repair did not change between the 6- and 19-month time points.[72] Another serial ultrasound study found that all intact repairs at 1-year follow-up also were intact at 2-year follow-up.[42]

The mechanobiology of tendon healing has implications for rehabilitation protocols. Rotator cuff tension increases with motions of the glenohumeral joint, such as forward elevation and external rotation. Animal studies found that immobilization enhances tendon-to-bone healing by improving mechanical properties, and it improves histologic properties in comparison with early motion.[73] Complete removal of load was detrimental to tendon healing in a rat model.[74]

Stiffness after rotator cuff repair is associated with open procedures and the development of subdeltoid adhesions. A review of arthroscopic rotator cuff repair found stiffness rates of 0% to 4% with successful return of motion after arthroscopic release if necessary.[75] Stiffness may be an indicator of tendon healing. Patients with shoulder stiffness 6 weeks after surgery had a lower retearing rate versus those with better motion (30% and 64%, respectively).[76]

To allow adequate time for early tendon healing, a delayed physical therapy protocol is recommended for most patients. The shoulder is immobilized with a sling for 6 weeks, but pendulum exercises are allowed after a structurally sound repair. The sling is removed at 6 weeks, and passive range-of-motion exercises are started. At 8 to 10 weeks, active-assisted motion is allowed. Active motion is delayed until 12 weeks, and strengthening is allowed at 4 months.

Clinical Outcomes

The outcomes of rotator cuff repair are good to excellent in most patients. Well-designed studies routinely have found improvements in outcome scores, motion, and pain levels. The typical Disabilities of the Arm, Shoulder and Hand (DASH) questionnaire scores are 10 to 20, Constant scores are 75 to 100, American Shoulder and Elbow Surgeon (ASES) Index scores are 85 to 95, UCLA scores are 28 to 35, and visual analog pain scores are 1 to 3; strength of forward elevation is approximately 13 lb (or 6 kg).[54,55,63,77] Success after a rotator cuff repair does not depend on repair integrity, and improvements in pain, function, and outcome scores are common even with structural failure of the repair. In one study, 94% of patients had a retear, but 72% of these patients had an ASES score greater than 90.[66] Satisfaction and clinical success were not directly associated with repair integrity.[78] A systematic review of 13 studies that investigated the influence of repair integrity on clinical outcome found both a statistical and a clinically relevant association between intact repair and improved strength, but the improvement was not reflected on most outcome measures.[79] This review found statistical improvement in forward elevation strength based on a minimal clinically important difference of more than 5 kg or 20% of the Constant score. Outcome scores rarely reached statistical significance, and there were no clinically significant differences, as evaluated with minimal clinically important difference criteria. In general, this systematic review supports the belief that patient satisfaction and functional scores do not depend on repair integrity, but a healed repair may lead to improved strength.

The long-term clinical outcomes after rotator cuff repair are encouraging, even though the long-term structural integrity of repairs is unknown. A 10-year follow-up study of full-thickness repairs found that clinical outcomes did not deteriorate over time, and increases in the level of patient disability presumably resulted from the concurrent global decrease in activity levels and shoulder demands as the patient aged.[80] A study of 33 single-row repairs at an average 12.5-year follow-up found that 88% of the patients had an excellent or good outcome on the UCLA Shoulder Rating Scale, without loss of motion.[81]

Single- Versus Double-Row Repair

The outcomes are similarly good regardless of whether repairs are with a single- or double-row construct. A level I randomized controlled study of 62 patients with a medium-size to large tear (2 to 4 cm) found no difference in retear rates at 17-month follow-up on MRI; the visual analog scale; or ASES, Constant, or UCLA scores, but surgical times were longer with double-row repair.[49] Another level I randomized controlled study compared single- and double-row repairs in 80 patients followed for 2 years and found no difference in strength, DASH, or Constant scores but did correlate patient age, sex, and preoperative strength with the final outcome.[63] A level I study of 40 patients with an average tear size of 1.8 cm compared single- and double-row repairs on serial MRI and found no differences in structural integrity, strength, or motion or in UCLA, ASES, Constant, Western Ontario Rotator Cuff Index, and Single Assessment Numeric Evaluation scores.[50] A level II cohort study of consecutive patients (average age, 56 years) followed for more than 2 years found no differences between double-row and single-row repairs in terms of ASES and Constant scores, but subgroup analysis of patients with a large to massive tears (larger than 3 cm) found better scores with a double-row repair.[82] A retrospective comparison of massive tears after single- or double-row repairs found that double-row repair was clinically superior at long-term follow-up (more than 5 years).[83] A double-row repair was almost five times more likely to lead to a good or excellent outcome and more improvement on the UCLA Scale,

and patients were more likely to have shoulders that felt close to normal.

Four systematic reviews did not provide significant evidence to support the clinical superiority of double-row over single-row repairs.[54,55,77,84] Based on a single level II study, one review suggested that tears larger than 3 cm may have better ASES and Constant scores after double-row fixation.[54] Another review found that tears larger than 1 cm may benefit from double-row fixation, although only level IV case studies were included, and transosseous repairs were grouped with single-row repairs.[55] Another study found a trend toward functional superiority of double-row repairs.[84] None of the four systematic reviews found a significant difference in the clinical outcomes of single- and double-row repairs.

Complications

With the exception of recurrent tendon tears, complications in arthroscopic rotator cuff repair are uncommon. A review study of almost 3,000 repairs found temporary stiffness in 4%, hardware-related issues in 0.5%, neurovascular injury in 0.2%, deep infection in 0.1%, and a thromboembolic event in 0.1%.[85] Another study found that postoperative stiffness had a 10% occurrence rate, but capsular release was required in only 3% to regain full motion.[75] Delayed recovery of shoulder function has not been well described but occurs frequently after rotator cuff repair. One study found that only 70% of the patients had recovered 6 months after surgery, and the risk factors for delayed recovery included age, preoperative stiffness, and tear size.[86]

Cost Analysis

Rotator cuff repair is a cost-effective treatment when compared with other surgical and medical treatments in terms of quality-adjusted life years. The cost-effectiveness ratio of rotator cuff repair was approximately $3,000 to $13,000 per quality-adjusted life year, depending on the utility measure used. These cost ratios compare favorably to those of total hip arthroplasty, coronary artery bypass graft surgery, and the treatment of hypertension.[87] The cost-effectiveness of open rotator cuff repair is favorable compared with arthroscopic repair because of the greater instrumentation and implant costs of arthroscopic repair. Double-row anchor repairs are more costly than single-row repairs because of greater implant costs and surgical time.[50-53,63,82]

Evidence-Based Strategies

The American Academy of Orthopaedic Surgeons (AAOS) recently published an evidence-based clinical practice guideline for the treatment of rotator cuff disease.[69] Unfortunately, the absence of evidence was the most important finding. Only a few conclusions were stated: exercise and nonsteroidal anti-inflammatory drugs should be used for the treatment of rotator cuff disease other than a full-thickness tear; routine acromioplasty is not required at the time of rotator cuff repair; porcine intestine patches should not be used during rotator cuff repair; and a workers' compensation claim is correlated with a relatively poor outcome of rotator cuff repair.

Summary

Arthroscopic rotator cuff repair requires a risk-reward analysis of the biologic potential for tendon healing as well as environmental factors and surgical techniques. The most important factors influencing tendon healing include the patient's age, the tear size, and tear chronicity. If surgical repair is undertaken, the choice of fixation construct is likely to be less important for a small to medium-size tear or a tear in a younger patient than it is in a larger tear or a tear in an older patient, who may benefit from a double-row fixation. Most patients benefit clinically from arthroscopic rotator cuff repair, even in the absence of full tendon healing. Rotator cuff repair is critically affected by biology more than biomechanics, and a better understanding of the tendon-to-bone healing process is important for optimizing outcomes.

Annotated References

1. Mall NA, Kim HM, Keener JD, et al: Symptomatic progression of asymptomatic rotator cuff tears: A prospective study of clinical and sonographic variables. *J Bone Joint Surg Am* 2010;92(16):2623-2633.

   The development of shoulder pain was associated with an increase in rotator cuff tear size in a prospective study of 195 patients who were asymptomatic. Level of evidence: III.

2. Papadonikolakis A, McKenna M, Warme W, Martin BI, Matsen FA III: Published evidence relevant to the diagnosis of impingement syndrome of the shoulder. *J Bone Joint Surg Am* 2011;93(19):1827-1832.

   A systematic review tested the existence of impingement syndrome in terms of diagnosis, anatomy, pathophysiology, and surgical success and found little high-level evidence. Level of evidence: II.

3. Yamaguchi K, Ditsios K, Middleton WD, Hildebolt CF, Galatz LM, Teefey SA: The demographic and morphological features of rotator cuff disease: A comparison of asymptomatic and symptomatic shoulders. *J Bone Joint Surg Am* 2006;88(8):1699-1704.

4. Yamaguchi K, Tetro AM, Blam O, Evanoff BA, Teefey SA, Middleton WD: Natural history of asymptomatic rotator cuff tears: A longitudinal analysis of asymptomatic tears detected sonographically. *J Shoulder Elbow Surg* 2001;10(3):199-203.

5. Safran O, Schroeder J, Bloom R, Weil Y, Milgrom C: Natural history of nonoperatively treated symptomatic rotator cuff tears in patients 60 years old or younger. *Am J Sports Med* 2011;39(4):710-714.

   A longitudinal ultrasound study of 61 nonsurgically treated full-thickness cuff tears in patents younger than 60 years found an almost-50% progression of tear size at 2.5 years. Level of evidence: IV.

6. Maman E, Harris C, White L, Tomlinson G, Shashank M, Boynton E: Outcome of nonoperative treatment of symptomatic rotator cuff tears monitored by magnetic resonance imaging. *J Bone Joint Surg Am* 2009;91(8):1898-1906.

   Age older than 60 years, a full-thickness tear, and fatty infiltration were the factors associated with progression of a rotator cuff tear on MRI. Level of evidence: IV.

7. Moosmayer S, Tariq R, Stiris MG, Smith HJ: MRI of symptomatic and asymptomatic full-thickness rotator cuff tears: A comparison of findings in 100 subjects. *Acta Orthop* 2010;81(3):361-366.

   A retrospective case-control study found associations between symptoms and rotator cuff tear size greater than 3 cm, significant atrophy, and fatty degeneration of Goutallier grade 2 or higher. The causal relationships are unclear. Level of evidence: III.

8. Baumgarten KM, Gerlach D, Galatz LM, et al: Cigarette smoking increases the risk for rotator cuff tears. *Clin Orthop Relat Res* 2010;468(6):1534-1541.

   A prospective cohort study found that the duration and dosage of cigarette smoking were correlated with an increased risk for rotator cuff tearing. Level of evidence: III.

9. Carbone S, Gumina S, Arceri V, Campagna V, Fagnani C, Postacchini F: The impact of preoperative smoking habit on rotator cuff tear: Cigarette smoking influences rotator cuff tear sizes. *J Shoulder Elbow Surg* 2012;21(1):56-60.

   A cross-sectional survey of rotator cuff repairs found larger tears during arthroscopy among patients who were tobacco smokers compared with those who were not. A dosage and temporal relationship with tobacco use and rotator cuff tear size was seen. Level of evidence: IV.

10. Hamid N, Omid R, Yamaguchi K, Steger-May K, Stobbs G, Keener JD: Relationship of radiographic acromial characteristics and rotator cuff disease: A prospective investigation of clinical, radiographic, and sonographic findings. *J Shoulder Elbow Surg* 2012;21(10):1289-1298.

    The presence of an acromial spur was highly associated with rotator cuff tears in symptomatic and asymptomatic shoulders, but the acromial index had no association with rotator cuff tears. Level of evidence: III.

11. Ogawa K, Yoshida A, Inokuchi W, Naniwa T: Acromial spur: Relationship to aging and morphologic

4: Arthroscopy

changes in the rotator cuff. *J Shoulder Elbow Surg* 2005;14(6):591-598.

12. Lee SB, Itoi E, O'Driscoll SW, An KN: Contact geometry at the undersurface of the acromion with and without a rotator cuff tear. *Arthroscopy* 2001;17(4): 365-372.

13. Chahal J, Mall N, MacDonald PB, et al: The role of subacromial decompression in patients undergoing arthroscopic repair of full-thickness tears of the rotator cuff: A systematic review and meta-analysis. *Arthroscopy* 2012;28(5):720-727.

    A systematic review of four level I studies found no statistically significant difference in subjective outcomes after arthroscopic rotator cuff repair with or without acromioplasty at intermediate follow-up. Level of evidence: I.

14. Gartsman GM, O'Connor DP: Arthroscopic rotator cuff repair with and without arthroscopic subacromial decompression: A prospective, randomized study of one-year outcomes. *J Shoulder Elbow Surg* 2004; 13(4):424-426.

15. Milano G, Grasso A, Salvatore M, Zarelli D, Deriu L, Fabbriciani C: Arthroscopic rotator cuff repair with and without subacromial decompression: A prospective randomized study. *Arthroscopy* 2007;23(1):81-88.

    A randomized controlled study of 80 rotator cuff repairs with or without acromioplasty found no benefit in Constant, DASH, or work-DASH scores at short-term follow-up. Level of evidence: I.

16. MacDonald P, McRae S, Leiter J, Mascarenhas R, Lapner P: Arthroscopic rotator cuff repair with and without acromioplasty in the treatment of full-thickness rotator cuff tears: A multicenter, randomized controlled trial. *J Bone Joint Surg Am* 2011;93(21): 1953-1960.

    A randomized controlled study of 86 rotator cuff repairs with or without acromioplasty found no difference in function and quality of life at 2-year follow-up, except a higher reoperation rate without acromioplasty. There was no structural evaluation of healing. Level of evidence: I.

17. Kartus J, Kartus C, Rostgård-Christensen L, Sernert N, Read J, Perko M: Long-term clinical and ultrasound evaluation after arthroscopic acromioplasty in patients with partial rotator cuff tears. *Arthroscopy* 2006; 22(1):44-49.

18. Torrens C, López JM, Puente I, Cáceres E: The influence of the acromial coverage index in rotator cuff tears. *J Shoulder Elbow Surg* 2007;16(3):347-351.

    A case control study found an increased acromial coverage index among patients with rotator cuff tears compared with normal control subjects. Level of evidence: III.

19. Mochizuki T, Sugaya H, Uomizu M, et al: Humeral insertion of the supraspinatus and infraspinatus: New anatomical findings regarding the footprint of the rotator cuff. *J Bone Joint Surg Am* 2008;90(5):962-969.

    A cadaver anatomic study of 113 shoulders found the supraspinatus tendon footprint to be much smaller than previously believed, and the greater tuberosity was occupied by a substantial amount of the infraspinatus.

20. Kim HM, Dahiya N, Teefey SA, Keener JD, Galatz LM, Yamaguchi K: Relationship of tear size and location to fatty degeneration of the rotator cuff. *J Bone Joint Surg Am* 2010;92(4):829-839.

    A prospective cohort of 262 tears evaluated by ultrasound found that fatty degeneration was closely associated with tear size and loss of integrity of the anterior supraspinatus tendon. Level of evidence: III.

21. Kim HM, Dahiya N, Teefey SA, et al: Location and initiation of degenerative rotator cuff tears: An analysis of three hundred and sixty shoulders. *J Bone Joint Surg Am* 2010;92(5):1088-1096.

    An ultrasound study of 360 rotator cuff tears found that degenerative tears most often involve the junction of the supraspinatus and infraspinatus tendons and may begin 13 to 17 mm posterior to the biceps tendon.

22. Goutallier D, Postel JM, Gleyze P, Leguilloux P, Van Driessche S: Influence of cuff muscle fatty degeneration on anatomic and functional outcomes after simple suture of full-thickness tears. *J Shoulder Elbow Surg* 2003;12(6):550-554.

23. Gladstone JN, Bishop JY, Lo IK, Flatow EL: Fatty infiltration and atrophy of the rotator cuff do not improve after rotator cuff repair and correlate with poor functional outcome. *Am J Sports Med* 2007;35(5): 719-728.

    A MRI cohort study of rotator cuff repairs found that muscle fatty infiltration affected functional outcome, tear size affected repair integrity, and successful repair did not improve muscle degeneration. Muscle degeneration progressed after unsuccessful repair. Level of evidence: II.

24. Liem D, Lichtenberg S, Magosch P, Habermeyer P: Magnetic resonance imaging of arthroscopic supraspinatus tendon repair. *J Bone Joint Surg Am* 2007;89(8): 1770-1776.

    A cohort study found that fatty infiltration could not be reversed by successful rotator cuff repair. Severe preoperative fatty infiltration was associated with tear recurrence, progression of fatty infiltration, and inferior clinical results. Level of evidence: II.

25. Melis B, DeFranco MJ, Chuinard C, Walch G: Natural history of fatty infiltration and atrophy of the supraspinatus muscle in rotator cuff tears. *Clin Orthop Relat Res* 2010;468(6):1498-1505.

    A retrospective case study of 1,688 rotator cuff tears found that moderate supraspinatus fatty infiltration appeared 3 years after the onset of symptoms, and severe infiltration appeared at 5 years. Level of evidence: IV.

26. Melis B, Wall B, Walch G: Natural history of infraspinatus fatty infiltration in rotator cuff tears. *J Shoulder Elbow Surg* 2010;19(5):757-763.

   A retrospective case study of 1,688 rotator cuff tears found that relatively large tears, long duration, and older age were associated with more severe fatty infiltration of the infraspinatus. Grade 2 changes occurred 2.5 years after symptom onset. Level of evidence: IV.

27. Cheung S, Dillon E, Tham SC, et al: The presence of fatty infiltration in the infraspinatus: Its relation with the condition of the supraspinatus tendon. *Arthroscopy* 2011;27(4):463-470.

   This restrospective case series measured rotator cuff tears and MRI Goutallier changes of the supraspinatus and infraspinatus muscles. Increased infraspinatus fatty infiltration was correlated with severity of infraspinatus and supraspinatus tears. Significant infraspinatus fatty infiltration was seen in 18% of those shoulders without and infraspinatus tear. Level of evidence: IV.

28. Meyer DC, Gerber C, Von Rechenberg B, Wirth SH, Farshad M: Amplitude and strength of muscle contraction are reduced in experimental tears of the rotator cuff. *Am J Sports Med* 2011;39(7):1456-1461.

   An animal study created chronic rotator cuff tears in sheep and found loss of muscular strength and contractile amplitude in addition to retraction, fatty infiltration, and atrophy.

29. Gerber C, Schneeberger AG, Hoppeler H, Meyer DC: Correlation of atrophy and fatty infiltration on strength and integrity of rotator cuff repairs: A study in thirteen patients. *J Shoulder Elbow Surg* 2007; 16(6):691-696.

   A case series found that maximal tension of electrically stimulated supraspinatus muscles was strongly correlated with cross-sectional area and inversely with fatty infiltration. One year after successful tendon repair, fatty infiltration had not improved. Level of evidence: IV.

30. Lorbach O, Bachelier F, Vees J, Kohn D, Pape D: Cyclic loading of rotator cuff reconstructions: Single-row repair with modified suture configurations versus double-row repair. *Am J Sports Med* 2008;36(8):1504-1510.

   A biomechanical study found that double-row anchor repairs with modified suture configurations offered the highest failure load and smallest gap formation.

31. Kim DH, Elattrache NS, Tibone JE, et al: Biomechanical comparison of a single-row versus double-row suture anchor technique for rotator cuff repair. *Am J Sports Med* 2006;34(3):407-414.

32. Ahmad CS, Kleweno C, Jacir AM, et al: Biomechanical performance of rotator cuff repairs with humeral rotation: A new rotator cuff repair failure model. *Am J Sports Med* 2008;36(5):888-892.

   A cadaver study found that double-row repairs had better fixation strength than single-row repairs when exposed to cyclic loading and changes in humeral rotation.

33. Park MC, ElAttrache NS, Tibone JE, Ahmad CS, Jun BJ, Lee TQ: Part I: Footprint contact characteristics for a transosseous-equivalent rotator cuff repair technique compared with a double-row repair technique. *J Shoulder Elbow Surg* 2007;16(4):461-468.

   A cadaver rotator cuff repair study found better pressurized contact area and mean pressure with transosseous-equivalent suture-bridge repair when compared with double-row repair.

34. Park MC, Tibone JE, ElAttrache NS, Ahmad CS, Jun BJ, Lee TQ: Part II: Biomechanical assessment for a footprint-restoring transosseous-equivalent rotator cuff repair technique compared with a double-row repair technique. *J Shoulder Elbow Surg* 2007;16(4): 469-476.

   A cadaver biomechanical study found that a transosseous-equivalent suture-bridge repair improved failure loads and restored the footprint better than a double-row repair.

35. Ahmad CS, Vorys GC, Covey A, Levine WN, Gardner TR, Bigliani LU: Rotator cuff repair fluid extravasation characteristics are influenced by repair technique. *J Shoulder Elbow Surg* 2009;18(6):976-981.

   A cadaver study found better fluid extravasation characteristics with double-row suture-bridge repair than with single-row repair.

36. Cadet ER, Adler RS, Gallo RA, et al: Contrast-enhanced ultrasound characterization of the vascularity of the repaired rotator cuff tendon: Short-term and intermediate-term follow-up. *J Shoulder Elbow Surg* 2012;21(5):597-603.

   A Doppler ultrasound study found that peribursal and bone anchor sites were the main conduits of blood flow for the rotator cuff tendon after arthroscopic repair and that flow increased with exercise.

37. Cho NS, Lee BG, Rhee YG: Arthroscopic rotator cuff repair using a suture bridge technique: Is the repair integrity actually maintained? *Am J Sports Med* 2011; 39(10):2108-2116.

   A case study of suture-bridge rotator cuff repairs found a 33% retear rate, with 66% of the retears at the musculotendinous junction. Retearing did not affect the subjective outcomes. Factors affecting healing were age, tear size, and fatty degeneration. Level of evidence: IV.

38. Christoforetti JJ, Krupp RJ, Singleton SB, Kissenberth MJ, Cook C, Hawkins RJ: Arthroscopic suture bridge transosseous equivalent fixation of rotator cuff tendon preserves intratendinous blood flow at the time of initial fixation. *J Shoulder Elbow Surg* 2012;21(4): 523-530.

   An immediate 45% reduction in terminal tendon blood flow was found by intraoperative laser Doppler flowmetry after the lateral row of a transosseous-equivalent repair was tied down.

4. Arthroscopy

39. Funakoshi T, Iwasaki N, Kamishima T, et al: In vivo vascularity alterations in repaired rotator cuffs determined by contrast-enhanced ultrasound. *Am J Sports Med* 2011;39(12):2640-2646.

   A study measured tendon blood flow before and after rotator cuff repair and found increased flow at 1 and 2 months after surgery that decreased at 3 months, with more flow on the bursal side than on the articular tendon side.

40. Boileau P, Brassart N, Watkinson DJ, Carles M, Hatzidakis AM, Krishnan SG: Arthroscopic repair of full-thickness tears of the supraspinatus: Does the tendon really heal? *J Bone Joint Surg Am* 2005;87(6):1229-1240.

41. Keener JD, Wei AS, Kim HM, et al: Revision arthroscopic rotator cuff repair: Repair integrity and clinical outcome. *J Bone Joint Surg Am* 2010;92(3):590-598.

   A retrospective review found reliable outcomes after revision rotator cuff repair. Age and tear size were related to repair integrity, with only 27% of multitendon tears remaining healed. Repair integrity affected abduction strength and the Constant score. Level of evidence: IV.

42. Nho SJ, Adler RS, Tomlinson DP, et al: Arthroscopic rotator cuff repair: Prospective evaluation with sequential ultrasonography. *Am J Sports Med* 2009;37(10):1938-1945.

   A sequential ultrasound study found the integrity of the repair was consistent at 1 and 2 years for 92.5% of patients. Level of evidence: III.

43. Tashjian RZ, Hollins AM, Kim HM, et al: Factors affecting healing rates after arthroscopic double-row rotator cuff repair. *Am J Sports Med* 2010;38(12):2435-2442.

   A case study found that older age and longer follow-up were associated with lower healing rates after double-row rotator cuff repair. Level of evidence: IV.

44. Papadopoulos P, Karataglis D, Boutsiadis A, Fotiadou A, Christoforidis J, Christodoulou A: Functional outcome and structural integrity following mini-open repair of large and massive rotator cuff tears: A 3-5 year follow-up study. *J Shoulder Elbow Surg* 2011;20(1):131-137.

   A case study found that patient age, tear size, and retear size affected the final clinical outcomes. Level of evidence: IV.

45. Charousset C, Bellaïche L, Kalra K, Petrover D: Arthroscopic repair of full-thickness rotator cuff tears: Is there tendon healing in patients aged 65 years or older? *Arthroscopy* 2010;26(3):302-309.

   A case study of rotator cuff repairs in patients older than 65 years found a 42% retear rate despite improved function. These repairs were considered successful. Level of evidence: IV.

46. Kamath G, Galatz LM, Keener JD, Teefey S, Middleton W, Yamaguchi K: Tendon integrity and functional outcome after arthroscopic repair of high-grade partial-thickness supraspinatus tears. *J Bone Joint Surg Am* 2009;91(5):1055-1062.

   A case study found that arthroscopic repair of high-grade partial-thickness rotator cuff tears resulted in a high rate of tendon healing, and patient age was an important factor in tendon healing. Level of evidence: IV.

47. Bishop J, Klepps S, Lo IK, Bird J, Gladstone JN, Flatow EL: Cuff integrity after arthroscopic versus open rotator cuff repair: A prospective study. *J Shoulder Elbow Surg* 2006;15(3):290-299.

48. Meyer M, Klouche S, Rousselin B, Boru B, Bauer T, Hardy P: Does arthroscopic rotator cuff repair actually heal? Anatomic evaluation with magnetic resonance arthrography at minimum 2 years follow-up. *J Shoulder Elbow Surg* 2012;21(4):531-536.

   A retrospective midterm study found good to excellent clinical outcomes after rotator cuff repair but an 88% rate of small or large defects on MRA. There was no correlation between clinical and anatomic outcomes. Level of evidence: IV.

49. Koh KH, Kang KC, Lim TK, Shon MS, Yoo JC: Prospective randomized clinical trial of single- versus double-row suture anchor repair in 2- to 4-cm rotator cuff tears: Clinical and magnetic resonance imaging results. *Arthroscopy* 2011;27(4):453-462.

   A randomized controlled study of 71 patients found similar clinical results and retear rates between double-row and single-row repairs in medium-size to large rotator cuff tears. Level of evidence: I.

50. Burks RT, Crim J, Brown N, Fink B, Greis PE: A prospective randomized clinical trial comparing arthroscopic single- and double-row rotator cuff repair: Magnetic resonance imaging and early clinical evaluation. *Am J Sports Med* 2009;37(4):674-682.

   A randomized controlled study of 40 medium-size tears found no differences in clinical or MRI structural integrity between double- and single-row repairs as late as 1 year after surgery. Level of evidence: I.

51. Franceschi F, Ruzzini L, Longo UG, et al: Equivalent clinical results of arthroscopic single-row and double-row suture anchor repair for rotator cuff tears: A randomized controlled trial. *Am J Sports Med* 2007;35(8):1254-1260.

   A randomized controlled study of 60 patients found no clinical difference between single- and double-row repairs at 2-year follow-up, but there was a trend toward better structural healing in double-row repairs. Level of evidence: I.

52. Charousset C, Grimberg J, Duranthon LD, Bellaiche L, Petrover D: Can a double-row anchorage technique improve tendon healing in arthroscopic rotator cuff repair? A prospective, nonrandomized, comparative study of double-row and single-row anchorage techniques with computed tomographic arthrography ten-

don healing assessment. *Am J Sports Med* 2007;35(8): 1247-1253.

A cohort study of 66 patients found no clinical difference between double- and single-row repairs, but there was better tendon healing on CT arthrography after double-row repair at 6-month follow-up. Level of evidence: II.

53. Sugaya H, Maeda K, Matsuki K, Moriishi J: Functional and structural outcome after arthroscopic full-thickness rotator cuff repair: Single-row versus dual-row fixation. *Arthroscopy* 2005;21(11):1307-1316.

54. Saridakis P, Jones G: Outcomes of single-row and double-row arthroscopic rotator cuff repair: A systematic review. *J Bone Joint Surg Am* 2010;92(3):732-742.

A systematic review of double- and single-row repairs found a trend toward improved structural healing with double-row fixation in large or massive rotator cuff tears.

55. Duquin TR, Buyea C, Bisson LJ: Which method of rotator cuff repair leads to the highest rate of structural healing? A systematic review. *Am J Sports Med* 2010; 38(4):835-841.

A systematic review of 122 repairs from 23 studies, most of which contained level IV evidence, found that double-row repairs led to lower retear rates in tears larger than 1 cm. Level of evidence: IV.

56. Lähteenmäki HE, Virolainen P, Hiltunen A, Heikkilä J, Nelimarkka OI: Results of early operative treatment of rotator cuff tears with acute symptoms. *J Shoulder Elbow Surg* 2006;15(2):148-153.

57. Marx RG, Koulouvaris P, Chu SK, Levy BA: Indications for surgery in clinical outcome studies of rotator cuff repair. *Clin Orthop Relat Res* 2009;467(2): 450-456.

Patient characteristics and indications for surgery were found not to be described in most clinical outcome studies of rotator cuff repair. Level of evidence: III.

58. Dunn W, Kuhn J: Effectiveness of physical therapy in treating atraumatic full thickness rotator cuff tears. *2011 Annual Meeting Proceedings.* Rosemont, IL, American Academy of Orthopaedic Surgeons, 2011, p 703.

This prospective cohort study of atraumatic full thickness rotator cuff tears found more than 90% of the patients elected for nonsurgical treatment after 3 months of physical therapy had significant improvement of ASES, Western Ontario Rotator Cuff, and Single Assessment Numeric Evaluation scores. This low rate of surgical care persisted at 2 years' follow-up, and data collection is ongoing. Level of evidence: II.

59. Nové-Josserand L, Edwards TB, O'Connor DP, Walch G: The acromiohumeral and coracohumeral intervals are abnormal in rotator cuff tears with muscular fatty degeneration. *Clin Orthop Relat Res* 2005;433:90-96.

60. Teefey SA, Rubin DA, Middleton WD, Hildebolt CF, Leibold RA, Yamaguchi K: Detection and quantification of rotator cuff tears: Comparison of ultrasonographic, magnetic resonance imaging, and arthroscopic findings in seventy-one consecutive cases. *J Bone Joint Surg Am* 2004;86(4):708-716.

61. Isaac C, Gharaibeh B, Witt M, Wright VJ, Huard J: Biologic approaches to enhance rotator cuff healing after injury. *J Shoulder Elbow Surg* 2012;21(2):181-190.

A systematic review found a paucity of clinical research into the use of growth factors, stem cell therapy, and tissue-engineering augmentation for rotator cuff healing.

62. Smith CD, Alexander S, Hill AM, et al: A biomechanical comparison of single and double-row fixation in arthroscopic rotator cuff repair. *J Bone Joint Surg Am* 2006;88(11):2425-2431.

63. Grasso A, Milano G, Salvatore M, Falcone G, Deriu L, Fabbriciani C: Single-row versus double-row arthroscopic rotator cuff repair: A prospective randomized clinical study. *Arthroscopy* 2009;25(1):4-12.

A randomized controlled study of 80 patients found no difference between single- and double-row repairs clinically and structurally. Analysis showed that patient age, sex, and baseline strength influenced outcome. Level of evidence: I.

64. Koh J, Levin S, Murphy G: Cerebral oxygenation in the beach chair position: The effect of general anesthesia compared to regional anesthesia. *2012 Annual Meeting Proceedings.* Rosemont, IL, American Academy of Orthopaedic Surgeons, 2012, p 911.

In a prospective study, 60 patients undergoing shoulder surgery in the beach chair position were tested for cerebral desaturation events to avoid neurologic injury. Patients with regional anesthesia and sedation had almost no cerebral desaturation events, unlike patients who had general anesthesia. Level of evidence: II.

65. Millar NL, Wu X, Tantau R, Silverstone E, Murrell GA: Open versus two forms of arthroscopic rotator cuff repair. *Clin Orthop Relat Res* 2009;467(4):966-978.

Arthroscopic knotless repairs had better healing rates compared with knotted or open repairs. The study was not controlled for tear size. Level of evidence: III.

66. Galatz LM, Ball CM, Teefey SA, Middleton WD, Yamaguchi K: The outcome and repair integrity of completely arthroscopically repaired large and massive rotator cuff tears. *J Bone Joint Surg Am* 2004;86(2): 219-224.

67. Iagulli ND, Field LD, Hobgood ER, Ramsey JR, Savoie FH III: Comparison of partial versus complete arthroscopic repair of massive rotator cuff tears. *Am J Sports Med* 2012;40(5):1022-1026.

Retrospective review of 86 patients compared complete and partial repairs of massive rotator cuff

4: Arthroscopy

tears, which had similarly good outcomes. Level of evidence: III.

68. Kim SJ, Lee IS, Kim SH, Lee WY, Chun YM: Arthroscopic partial repair of irreparable large to massive rotator cuff tears. *Arthroscopy* 2012;28(6):761-768.

    A case study of partial repairs of massive rotator cuff tears found satisfactory short-term outcomes. Level of evidence: IV.

69. Pedowitz RA, Yamaguchi K, Ahmad CS, et al; American Academy of Orthopaedic Surgeons: Optimizing the management of rotator cuff problems. *J Am Acad Orthop Surg* 2011;19(6):368-379.

    An AAOS workgroup found a lack of definitive evidence on most rotator cuff issues and made only four moderate-grade recommendations.

70. Büker N, Kitiş A, Akkaya S, Akkaya N: [Comparison of the results of supervised physiotherapy program and home-based exercise program in patients treated with arthroscopic-assisted mini-open rotator cuff repair]. *Eklem Hastalik Cerrahisi* 2011;22(3):134-139.

    No differences except cost were found between a home exercise program and supervised physical therapy in patients' pain, functional status, quality of life, and depression status.

71. Miller BS, Downie BK, Kohen RB, et al: When do rotator cuff repairs fail? Serial ultrasound examination after arthroscopic repair of large and massive rotator cuff tears. *Am J Sports Med* 2011;39(10):2064-2070.

    A serial ultrasound cohort study found that most retears occurred within the first 3 months and were associated with inferior clinical outcomes. Level of evidence: III.

72. Koh KH, Laddha MS, Lim TK, Park JH, Yoo JC: Serial structural and functional assessments of rotator cuff repairs: Do they differ at 6 and 19 months postoperatively? *J Shoulder Elbow Surg* 2012;21(7):859-866.

    A study found that the structural status of a rotator cuff repair could be assessed 6 months after surgery because the integrity of the rotator cuff did not change for as long as 2 years after surgery.

73. Gimbel JA, Van Kleunen JP, Williams GR, Thomopoulos S, Soslowsky LJ: Long durations of immobilization in the rat result in enhanced mechanical properties of the healing supraspinatus tendon insertion site. *J Biomech Eng* 2007;129(3):400-404.

    An animal study found that immobilizing the shoulder improves tendon-to-bone healing by increasing the organization of the collagen and subsequently increasing the mechanical properties.

74. Galatz LM, Charlton N, Das R, Kim HM, Havlioglu N, Thomopoulos S: Complete removal of load is detrimental to rotator cuff healing. *J Shoulder Elbow Surg* 2009;18(5):669-675.

    An animal study found that complete removal of load with pharmacologic paralysis was detrimental to rota-

tor cuff healing, especially when combined with immobilization.

75. Denard PJ, Lädermann A, Burkhart SS: Prevention and management of stiffness after arthroscopic rotator cuff repair: Systematic review and implications for rotator cuff healing. *Arthroscopy* 2011;27(6):842-848.

    A systematic review found that postoperative stiffness resistant to nonsurgical management was uncommon, and arthroscopic capsular release could restore range of motion, if needed. Level of evidence: IV.

76. Parsons BO, Gruson KI, Chen DD, Harrison AK, Gladstone J, Flatow EL: Does slower rehabilitation after arthroscopic rotator cuff repair lead to long-term stiffness? *J Shoulder Elbow Surg* 2010;19(7):1034-1039.

    A retrospective case study found that sling immobilization for 6 weeks after arthroscopic rotator cuff repair did not result in increased long-term stiffness and could improve the rate of tendon healing.

77. Nho SJ, Slabaugh MA, Seroyer ST, et al: Does the literature support double-row suture anchor fixation for arthroscopic rotator cuff repair? A systematic review comparing double-row and single-row suture anchor configuration. *Arthroscopy* 2009;25(11):1319-1328.

    A systematic review found no clinical differences between single- and double-row repairs, but some studies reported that double-row repair might improve tendon healing. Level of evidence: III.

78. Voigt C, Bosse C, Vosshenrich R, Schulz AP, Lill H: Arthroscopic supraspinatus tendon repair with suture-bridging technique: Functional outcome and magnetic resonance imaging. *Am J Sports Med* 2010;38(5):983-991.

    A case study found similar functional outcomes with a suture-bridge technique compared with a double-row repair. Structural failure of the repair was not correlated with clinical failure. Age older than 60 years influenced tendon healing. Level of evidence: IV.

79. Slabaugh MA, Nho SJ, Grumet RC, et al: Does the literature confirm superior clinical results in radiographically healed rotator cuffs after rotator cuff repair? *Arthroscopy* 2010;26(3):393-403.

    A systematic review found increased strength in forward elevation in five of eight studies and improved Constant scores with an intact repair in six of nine studies. These results suggested that repair integrity may improve strength. Level of evidence: IV.

80. Galatz LM, Griggs S, Cameron BD, Iannotti JP: Prospective longitudinal analysis of postoperative shoulder function: A ten-year follow-up study of full-thickness rotator cuff tears. *J Bone Joint Surg Am* 2001;83(7):1052-1056.

81. Marrero LG, Nelman KR, Nottage WM: Long-term follow-up of arthroscopic rotator cuff repair. *Arthroscopy* 2011;27(7):885-888.

Retrospective review found that patients maintained good outcomes 10 years after rotator cuff repair. Level of evidence: IV.

82. Park JY, Lhee SH, Choi JH, Park HK, Yu JW, Seo JB: Comparison of the clinical outcomes of single- and double-row repairs in rotator cuff tears. *Am J Sports Med* 2008;36(7):1310-1316.

    A cohort study comparing double- and single-row repairs found better ASES scores, Constant scores, and strength in patients with a tear larger than 3 cm who were treated with a double-row technique. Level of evidence: II.

83. Denard PJ, Jiwani AZ, Lädermann A, Burkhart SS: Long-term outcome of arthroscopic massive rotator cuff repair: The importance of double-row fixation. *Arthroscopy* 2012;28(7):909-915.

    A retrospective comparative study found double-row repairs of massive rotator cuff tears to have 4.9 times more good or excellent outcomes than single-row repairs at a 5-year minimum follow-up. Level of evidence: III.

84. DeHaan AM, Axelrad TW, Kaye E, Silvestri L, Puskas B, Foster TE: Does double-row rotator cuff repair improve functional outcome of patients compared with single-row technique? A systematic review. *Am J Sports Med* 2012;40(5):1176-1185.

    A systematic review found trends toward higher functional outcomes and a lower retear rate after a double-row repair compared with a single-row repair.

85. Randelli P, Spennacchio P, Ragone V, Arrigoni P, Casella A, Cabitza P: Complications associated with arthroscopic rotator cuff repair: A literature review. *Musculoskelet Surg* 2012;96(1):9-16.

    Rotator cuff repair was found to be a low-risk surgical procedure. Failure of the repair was the most common complication.

86. Manaka T, Ito Y, Matsumoto I, Takaoka K, Nakamura H: Functional recovery period after arthroscopic rotator cuff repair: Is it predictable before surgery? *Clin Orthop Relat Res* 2011;469(6):1660-1666.

    Retrospective review found delayed recovery (more than 6 months) in 28% of patients after rotator cuff repair. Age, shoulder stiffness, and rotator cuff tear size influenced functional recovery time.

87. Vitale MA, Vitale MG, Zivin JG, Braman JP, Bigliani LU, Flatow EL: Rotator cuff repair: An analysis of utility scores and cost-effectiveness. *J Shoulder Elbow Surg* 2007;16(2):181-187.

    A cost-effectiveness study found that rotator cuff repairs compared favorably with other common healthcare interventions.

4: Arthroscopy

Chapter 21

Arthroscopic and Open Treatment of the Proximal Biceps Tendon

Augustus D. Mazzocca, MS, MD   Mark P. Cote, PT, DPT, MSCTR   Knut Beitzel, MA, MD

Introduction

The biceps muscle originates from two proximal tendons: the long head of the biceps tendon (LHBT) and the short head of the biceps tendon. The LHBT is of particular interest because of its intra-articular origin on the supraglenoid tubercle of the glenohumeral joint.[1] The LHBT originates with variable fiber insertions from the superior labrum; most of the fibers arise from the posterior aspect of the superior labrum.[2] The intra-articular portion of the tendon is extrasynovial and has an average length of 34.5 mm (± 4.2 mm). Before entering the intertubercular groove, the tendon is guided by the structures of the pulley system, which consists anteriorly of the superior glenohumeral ligament (SGHL) and the subscapularis tendon and posterolaterally of the coracohumeral ligament and the anterior fibers of the supraspinatus tendon[3] (**Figure 1**). The short head of the biceps tendon originates on the coracoid process of the scapula. In contrast to the origin of the LHBT, the origin of the short head of the biceps tendon is extra-articular.

The biceps muscle crosses both the shoulder and the elbow. The distal biceps acts on the elbow primarily as a forearm supinator and a secondary elbow flexor. The role of the biceps at the shoulder has been the subject of debate.[1,4] The LHBT previously was believed to act as a humeral head depressor, but recent research suggests that this function is unlikely because of the anterior position of the LHBT relative to the glenohumeral joint. Despite debate over the function of the biceps at the shoulder, there is general agreement among surgeons that the proximal LHBT acts as a pain generator.[1,4]

The pathology of the LHBT includes tendinitis and tendon rupture, which are well documented but not fully understood, probably because of the unique anatomic features of the LHBT. The intra-articular portion of the tendon is subject to compression, shearing, and friction forces, whereas the extra-articular distal segment is primarily under the influence of tensional strain. The vascular anatomy of the LHBT also may play a role in the pathogenesis of disorders. The first 3 cm of the intra-articular portion of the tendon, as measured from its insertion on the glenoid, has specific regions of blood supply with significant areas of hypovascularization.[5] These hypovascular regions are correlated with the areas of increased mechanical strain. The combination of specific multidirectional force distributions and the segmental blood supply is believed to be the primary contributor to the intra-articular degenerative processes of the LHBT.

Etiology

Multiple intra-articular lesions of the shoulder joint may generate a secondary lesion of the LHBT, such as bursitis, a rotator cuff tear, a superior labrum anterior to posterior (SLAP) lesion, or an acromioclavicular joint disorder. Primary tendinitis and rupture of the LHBT also have been observed. Rupture almost always occurs near the insertion or at the proximal intertubercular groove. If the rupture is distal to the insertion, the stump can become incarcerated in the joint. Tendinitis of the LHBT has been recognized for more than 50 years but increasingly is reported as an isolated source of shoulder pain or a source of pain in combination with one or more additional disorders. An hourglass biceps is described as a lesion of the biceps tendon complex in which a hypertrophic portion of the intra-articular segment of the LHBT cannot slide during elevation of the arm, resulting in incarceration of the tendon.[6]

Clinical Evaluation

If the tendon is completely ruptured, physical examination may reveal a Popeye deformity, in which hollowness appears proximally and laterally. Patients often describe an onset of pain in the anterior shoulder before

Dr. Mazzocca or an immediate family member serves as a paid consultant to or is an employee of Arthrex and has received research or institutional support from Arthrex and Arthrosurface. Neither of the following authors nor any immediate family member has received anything of value from or has stock or stock options held in a commercial company or institution related directly or indirectly to the subject of this chapter: Dr. Cote and Dr. Beitzel.

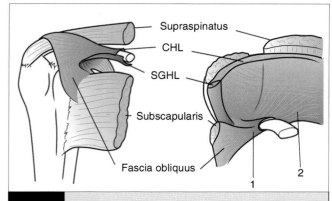

| **Figure 1** | Schematic drawing of the structures of the biceps pulley. 1 = Insertion of the subscapularis tendon, 2 = Insertion of the supraspinatus tendon, CHL = coracohumeral ligament, SGHL = superior glenohumeral ligament. |

rupture, with pain relief after the injury. If the tendon did not rupture, the symptom typically is significant pain with motion, particularly with resisted elbow flexion or forearm supination. Tenderness often is noted at the superior margin of the muscle belly.

The subpectoral biceps tendinitis test can be useful for detecting biceps pathology. The pectoralis tendon is identified by resisted contraction of the upper extremity in a position of adduction and internal rotation. The examiner palpates the biceps in the axilla under the inferior border of the pectoralis tendon. Pain during this maneuver is considered a positive test indicative of biceps pathology. Occasionally, there may be ecchymosis in this area. It is important to examine for associated rotator cuff pathology. The range of motion should be assessed to detect possible incarceration of the biceps tendon stump in the glenohumeral joint (an hourglass biceps). The O'Brien test can be used to identify a SLAP lesion. The Yergason and Speed tests can be used to evaluate pathologies occurring more distally to the tendon (within the sulcus). Clinical tests must be considered as a set because the specificity of each test alone is limited.

The diagnosis often is made clinically but may be supplemented by imaging. Ultrasound is an inexpensive tool for detecting an absence of the LHBT in the bicipital groove or at its insertion. MRI rarely is necessary for diagnosis, but MRI with an intra-articular contrast agent may be the only reliable means of clearly distinguishing between SLAP and pulley lesions. A split of the tendon, as in a type IV SLAP lesion, also can be diagnosed with these methods.

Arthroscopic evaluation may be the only means of objectively proving a diagnosis of tendon instability. Before any surgical procedure, the entire intra-articular length of the LHBT is arthroscopically inspected. The origin of the tendon and the superior labrum is tested with a probe after an additional anterior portal is established to evaluate the biceps tendon anchor for a

SLAP lesion. The tendon is pulled out of the sulcus, and the pulley structures are tested for anterior and posterior stability.

Classification

Multiple classifications of disorders of the LHBT have been proposed, but no consensus exists. The classifications primarily focus on secondary lesions of the shoulder combined with LHBT instability. The lesions of the LHBT can be broadly classified into three groups: isolated tendinitis, tendinitis associated with a SLAP lesion or tendon instability, and tendon instability combined with a high-grade lesion of the stabilizing pulley sling and a rotator cuff tear.

The Habermeyer classification identifies four types of pulley lesions of the LHBT.[7] Type I is a lesion of the SGHL resulting in anterior instability of the LHBT; type II, an SGHL lesion combined with a partial rupture of the anterior portion of the supraspinatus tendon; type III, an SGHL lesion combined with a partial rupture of the cranial portion of the subscapularis tendon; and type IV, a lesion of the anterior supraspinatus tendon combined with a lesion of the cranial portion of the subscapularis tendon. A type IV lesion is believed to result from anteroposterior instability.

The Lafosse arthroscopic classification takes into account the direction and extent of LHBT instability, macroscopic lesions of the LHBT, and concomitant lesions of the subscapularis and/or supraspinatus tendon.[8]

Treatment

Both nonsurgical and surgical treatment schemes have been described, but few objective data exist to determine the best treatment.[4,9] Nonsurgical treatment typically is sufficient for treating a spontaneous rupture. A patient electing nonsurgical care will have a residual cosmetic deformity and may report cramping with strenuous activity. Cramping often resolves but may persist in some patients. Patients generally do well with a home exercise program and rarely have stiffness. Full range of motion, including overhead activity, should be encouraged to allow evaluation for an incarcerated tendon stump.

Some physicians recommend surgical treatment for a physically active patient or a patient who requires unusually great supination strength. A patient who elects surgical treatment often is a manual laborer with a dominant extremity injury. Such patients often report aching pain and spasm with repeated activity. Young athletes and middle-aged patients who do not accept the biceps deformity also may elect surgery. It is preferable to perform the surgery within 3 months of injury.

Several terms are used to delineate locations about the shoulder in reference to tenodesis of the LHBT. The

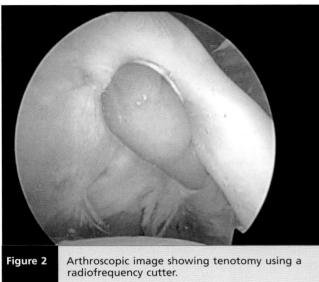

Figure 2 Arthroscopic image showing tenotomy using a radiofrequency cutter.

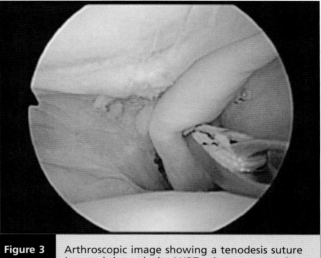

Figure 3 Arthroscopic image showing a tenodesis suture inserted through the LHBT using a penetration instrument.

term proximal often refers to intra-articular arthroscopic tenodesis of the LHBT as part of a rotator cuff repair or extra-articular tenodesis in the groove slightly inferior to the articular margin. The term suprapectoral describes arthroscopic tenodesis of the LHBT below the bicipital groove and above the superior edge of the pectoralis tendon.[10] The term subpectoral describes an open tenodesis of the LHBT underneath the pectoralis tendon through an incision in the axilla.

Arthroscopic Treatment

Tenotomy currently is performed arthroscopically.[1] A standard working portal is used to cut the biceps at the insertion using an arthroscopic scissor or a radiofrequency cutter (**Figure 2**). Damage to the superior labrum should be avoided to retain its function. After detaching the tendon, the surgeon should check that the tendon has slipped into the sulcus. A SLAP lesion in an older adult can be débrided at this time. The available methods for tenodesis of the LHBT can be distinguished by the anatomic regions of fixation of the tendon stump.

Proximal tenodesis almost always is performed arthroscopically. The tendon stump can be fixed with sutures, suture anchors, or tenodesis screws.[11,12] A biomechanical comparison of repair techniques concluded that keyhole tenodesis was substantially stronger than classic interference screw fixation but not stronger than bioabsorbable screw fixation. Keyhole tenodesis failed by tendon splitting and slippage, and interference screw fixation failed exclusively by slippage.[13] Four fixation techniques were compared biomechanically: subpectoral bone tunnel (suture fixation in the bone tunnel), arthroscopic interference screw, subpectoral interference screw, and arthroscopic suture anchor. Bone tunnel fixation had substantially more cyclic displacement than the other three methods, all of which had favorable load-to-failure characteristics.[14]

The advantages of these techniques are the preservation of tendon length and the ability to perform refixation without an additional skin incision. Usually proximal tenodesis is performed before a concomitant procedure, such as rotator cuff repair. A standard posterior portal is used for initial evaluation of the joint and the LHBT. A probe may be used to examine the intertubercular portion of the tendon by pulling the tendon into the joint. A needle is used to pierce the tendon for placement of a shuttle suture, which can be used to shuttle nonabsorbable suture through the tendon. At this point, several methods of fixation may be used. For soft-tissue tenodesis, the tendon is fixed to the rotator cuff interval. Tenodesis also can be done using a suture anchor, such as the 5.5-mm bioabsorbable Corkscrew FT suture anchor (Arthrex) armed with two No. 2 FiberWire (Arthrex) sutures (**Figure 3**), or a biotenodesis screw, such as the 4.5-mm bioabsorbable SwiveLock anchor (Arthrex). In these techniques, the anchor is placed in the entrance of the bicipital groove after decortication with a motorized burr. The suture anchor allows fixation without pulling the tendon out of the anterior portal. For fixation using a tenodesis screw, the tendon stump is pulled out of the anterior portal and loaded into the screw. The tenotomy is done by transecting the tendon proximal to the sutures and close to its origin (**Figure 4**).

In the preferred arthroscopic technique, a tenodesis screw is used for suprapectoral fixation of the tendon stump within the intertubercular groove. A holding suture is placed through the tendon. The tendon then is cut close to its origin, without damaging the superior labral complex. The arthroscope is moved to the subacromial space using the lateral portal. The falciform ligament of the pectoralis tendon is identified, and the biceps tendon is found underneath. The accessory anterior portal is localized with a spinal needle into the rotator cuff interval. The proximal 20 mm of the tendon are removed to eliminate diseased tendon and re-create an anatomic fit. The proximal 15 mm of the remaining tendon stump are whipstitched. (Alternatively, Krakow stitches can be used.) The intertubercular groove is located, and a 2-mm guidewire is inserted. The guidewire is reamed over with a 7- or 8-mm cannulated reamer to a depth of 30 mm. The tendon is pulled out of the accessory anterior portal, and one suture is inserted through the tenodesis screw and tightened. Finally, the screw is inserted into the tunnel, and an arthroscopic knot pusher is used to tie suture over the top of the te-

nodesis screw. The use of a forked tenodesis screw allows direct insertion of the tendon into the hole (**Figure 5**).

Open Treatment

Early surgical techniques for tenodesis involved transferring the tendon to the coracoid process. Because large dissections were necessary with this technique, keyhole tenodesis was devised as an alternative. In this technique, the bicipital groove is exposed through a deltopectoral approach, and a 1-cm hole is burred with a keyhole inferior and sufficiently narrow to contain the tendon. A knot is created in the biceps tendon and delivered into the keyhole. An immediate improvement in cosmesis and supination strength was reported after biceps ruptures were treated using this technique.[15]

The procedure of choice is subpectoral tenodesis using an interference screw. The subpectoral approach is close to the muscle belly of the biceps.[16] Even if initially ruptured, the biceps tendon generally does not retract beyond the point of fixation. Before the tenodesis, arthroscopy is performed to identify any associated pathology and tenotomize and débride the bicipital tendon stump. With the arm abducted and internally rotated, the inferior border of the pectoralis major tendon is palpated. The incision is over the inferior border of the pectoralis tendon to 3 cm below the inferior border on the medial aspect of the arm (**Figure 6, A**). A scalpel is used to cut down through the subcuticular tissue, and an electrocautery is used to control bleeding. A Gelpi or Wheitlaner self-retaining retractor can be used for visualization. The adipose tissue is cleared until the fascia overlying the pectoralis major coracobra-

| Figure 4 | Arthroscopic image showing an intra-articularly fixed LHBT after tenodesis using a Corkscrew FT suture anchor. |

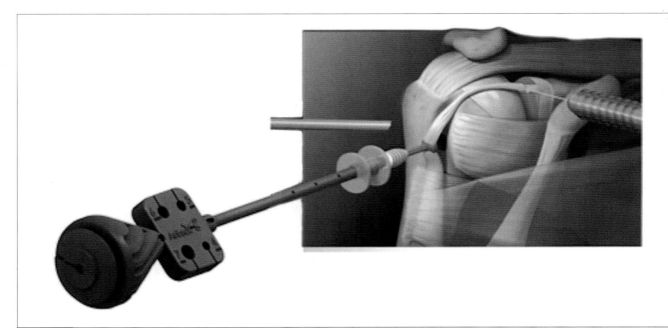

| Figure 5 | Schematic drawing showing arthroscopic suprapectoral tenodesis using a fork-tipped tenodesis screw (SwiveLock, Arthrex) and arthroscopic cannulas. |

4: Arthroscopy

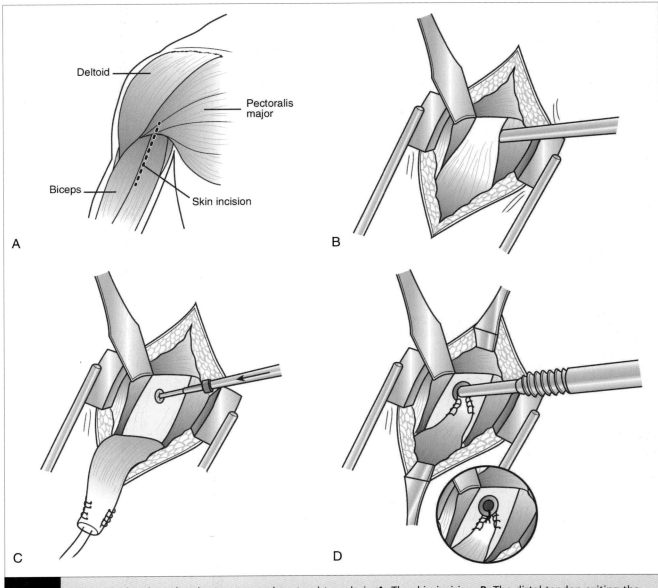

Figure 6   Schematic drawings showing an open subpectoral tenodesis. **A,** The skin incision. **B,** The distal tendon exiting the groove under the pectoralis muscle. **C,** Drilling of the socket for tendon fixation, using a tenodesis screw directly under the retracted tendon of the pectoralis muscle. **D,** Insertion of the interference screw, with the completed subpectoral tenodesis *(inset)*.

chialis and biceps is identified. If these anatomic landmarks are not identified, the dissection could be too lateral. If the cephalic vein can be seen in the deltopectoral groove, the dissection is too proximal and too lateral. When the inferior border of the pectoralis major has been identified, the fascia overlying the coracobrachialis and biceps is incised in a proximal-to-distal manner (**Figure 6, B**). A pointed Hohmann retractor is placed under the pectoralis major and on the proximal humerus to retract the muscle proximally and laterally. A blunt Chandler retractor is placed in the medial aspect of the humerus to retract the coracobrachialis and the short head of the biceps tendon. Vigorous medial retraction should be avoided to prevent injury to the

musculocutaneous nerve. The LHBT musculotendinous junction should be located and then withdrawn from the field. To ensure appropriate tensioning of the LHBT, the proximal portion is resected to leave 20 to 25 mm proximal to the musculotendinous portion of the biceps. One centimeter proximal to the pectoralis major tendon, the periosteum is reflected. A No. 2 nonabsorbable suture, such as FiberWire, is placed onto the tendon, and 12 mm of the tendon is secured to ensure that adequate fixation is maintained and the musculotendinous portion of the biceps will sit underneath the inferior border of the pectoralis major tendon. This step is critical for proper tensioning of the musculotendinous unit as well as cosmesis.

For most patients, an 8-mm cannulated reamer is of adequate size for placing the tendon into the bone tunnel and securing fixation with an 8-mm bioabsorbable interference-fit screw. The calibrated reamer is advanced over the guidepin to the 30-mm mark (**Figure 6, C**). Drilling beyond the posterior cortex of the humerus may increase the risk of complications and is not necessary.

With a wire loop passed through the driver, one limb of the suture is pulled through the screw and the screwdriver handle. The surgeon holds the other limb loosely. The limb that is passed through the driver is pulled tightly until the end of the tendon is securely placed against the tip of the driver. The tip of the driver is placed at the superior aspect of the bone socket and manually inserted until the tendon reaches the base of the tunnel. The bioabsorbable interference screw is placed directly over the top of the tendon until the head of the screw is below the cortex (**Figure 6, D**).

Clinical Results of Surgical Treatment

Studies comparing tenotomy and tenodesis have had varied results, with no technique showing clear clinical superiority.[4,9] Because no surgical procedure can be recommended over others, the choice should be made for each patient individually.[1]

Arthroscopic Treatment

No consensus exists as to whether the LHBT should be treated with tenotomy or tenodesis because both procedures have had good clinical results.[9] Substantial pain reduction and functional improvement occurred after tenotomy, with a 13.3% complication rate.[17] A recent systematic review found comparably favorable results after both tenotomy and tenodesis. The only relevant difference may be that biceps tenotomy led to a higher incidence of cosmetic deformity.[9] Another study had identical results, with 30% of the patients having a cosmetic defect after tenotomy.[18] Cramping and weakness with vigorous activity also has been reported.[1] Tenotomy has been suggested as effective for relief of pain related to LHBT lesions. Tenotomy may be primarily useful for treating older patients or patients having severe comorbidities or other contraindications for tenodesis.

Open Treatment

Good results have been reported for open tenodesis of the LHBT.[4,19,20] Proximal techniques for tenodesis may lead to persistent tenosynovitis and pain.[21] The risk of this complication may be decreased by performing a subpectoral tenodesis.[19,22] No technique has been proved superior to others, and clinical studies are needed to provide evidence for decision making in LHBT surgery.

Summary

Tendinitis and ruptures of the LHBT are well documented but not yet fully understood. Multiple surgical options have been described for treating patients with LHBT-related pain. The results of tenotomy and tenodesis have been variable, with neither technique showing clear clinical superiority. Arthroscopic procedures include simple tenotomy as well as intra-articular and suprapectoral tenodesis. The tendon stump can be fixed using suture anchors or tenodesis screws. An open procedure is preferable for subpectoral tenodesis.

Annotated References

1. Barber A, Field LD, Ryu R: Biceps tendon and superior labrum injuries: Decision-making. *J Bone Joint Surg Am* 2007;89(8):1844-1855.

   Options for the surgical treatment of pathologic biceps conditions include decompression, débridement, tenotomy, and tenodesis. Factors to be considered include patient age, activity and cosmetic expectations, compliance, and associated pathologic entities that can be treated with a tenodesis.

2. Vangsness CT Jr, Jorgenson SS, Watson T, Johnson DL: The origin of the long head of the biceps from the scapula and glenoid labrum: An anatomical study of 100 shoulders. *J Bone Joint Surg Br* 1994;76(6): 951-954.

3. Werner A, Mueller T, Boehm D, Gohlke F: The stabilizing sling for the long head of the biceps tendon in the rotator cuff interval: A histoanatomic study. *Am J Sports Med* 2000;28(1):28-31.

4. Elser F, Braun S, Dewing CB, Giphart JE, Millett PJ: Anatomy, function, injuries, and treatment of the long head of the biceps brachii tendon. *Arthroscopy* 2011; 27(4):581-592.

   Biceps tenotomy and tenodesis were found to be effective for isolated LHBT pathology and combined lesions of the rotator cuff and biceps-labral complex. The function of the LHBT and its role in glenohumeral kinematics are only partially understood because of the difficulty of cadaver and in vivo biomechanical studies.

5. Cheng NM, Pan WR, Vally F, Le Roux CM, Richardson MD: The arterial supply of the long head of biceps tendon: Anatomical study with implications for tendon rupture. *Clin Anat* 2010;23(6):683-692.

   The LHBT was consistently supplied through its osseotendinous and musculotendinous junctions by branches of the thoracoacromial and brachial arteries, respectively, which divided the LHBT into two or three vascular territories, depending on the presence of the mesotenon-derived vascular supply.

6. Ahrens PM, Boileau P: The long head of biceps and associated tendinopathy. *J Bone Joint Surg Br* 2007; 89(8):1001-1009.

Current views on LHBT lesion pathology, diagnosis, and management were described. Surgical management was classified, with details of techniques.

7. Habermeyer P, Magosch P, Pritsch M, Scheibel MT, Lichtenberg S: Anterosuperior impingement of the shoulder as a result of pulley lesions: A prospective arthroscopic study. *J Shoulder Elbow Surg* 2004;13(1): 5-12.

8. Lafosse L, Reiland Y, Baier GP, Toussaint B, Jost B: Anterior and posterior instability of the long head of the biceps tendon in rotator cuff tears: A new classification based on arthroscopic observations. *Arthroscopy* 2007;23(1):73-80.

   The authors assessed 200 patients with rotator cuff tears and reported that the direction of LHBT instability could be arthroscopically observed in 45% of the patients (posterior instability, 19%; anterior instability, 16%; and anteroposterior instability; 10%). The grade of the LHBT lesion became more significant with the increasing size of the tear. The authors used their findings to create a new arthroscopic classification for disorders of the LHBT. Level of evidence: IV.

9. Slenker NR, Lawson K, Ciccotti MG, Dodson CC, Cohen SB: Biceps tenotomy versus tenodesis: Clinical outcomes. *Arthroscopy* 2012;28(4):576-582.

   Tenotomy and tenodesis have comparably favorable results. The only major difference is a higher incidence of cosmetic deformity with biceps tenotomy.

10. Lutton DM, Gruson KI, Harrison AK, Gladstone JN, Flatow EL: Where to tenodese the biceps: Proximal or distal? *Clin Orthop Relat Res* 2011;469(4):1050-1055.

    Arthroscopic suprapectoral biceps tenodesis was described as a new technique for distal tenodesis. A more distal tenodesis location may decrease the incidence of persistent postoperative pain at the bicipital groove, but additional research is needed.

11. Gartsman GM, Hammerman SM: Arthroscopic biceps tenodesis: Operative technique. *Arthroscopy* 2000; 16(5):550-552.

12. Geaney LE, Mazzocca AD: Biceps brachii tendon ruptures: A review of diagnosis and treatment of proximal and distal biceps tendon ruptures. *Phys Sportsmed* 2010;38(2):117-125.

    Surgical repair of distal biceps ruptures was indicated to restore supination strength and endurance. Data suggest increased strength with the cortical button repair, although the best technique has not been determined. Proximal and distal biceps brachii ruptures were reviewed, with a treatment algorithm.

13. Jayamoorthy T, Field JR, Costi JJ, Martin DK, Stanley RM, Hearn TC: Biceps tenodesis: A biomechanical study of fixation methods. *J Shoulder Elbow Surg* 2004;13(2):160-164.

14. Mazzocca AD, Bicos J, Santangelo S, Romeo AA, Arciero RA: The biomechanical evaluation of four fixation techniques for proximal biceps tenodesis. *Arthroscopy* 2005;21(11):1296-1306.

15. Froimson AI, Oh I: Keyhole tenodesis of biceps origin at the shoulder. *Clin Orthop Relat Res* 1975;112: 245-249.

16. Mazzocca AD, Rios CG, Romeo AA, Arciero RA: Subpectoral biceps tenodesis with interference screw fixation. *Arthroscopy* 2005;21(7):896.

17. Gill TJ, McIrvin E, Mair SD, Hawkins RJ: Results of biceps tenotomy for treatment of pathology of the long head of the biceps brachii. *J Shoulder Elbow Surg* 2001;10(3):247-249.

18. Osbahr DC, Diamond AB, Speer KP: The cosmetic appearance of the biceps muscle after long-head tenotomy versus tenodesis. *Arthroscopy* 2002;18(5): 483-487.

19. Mazzocca AD, Cote MP, Arciero CL, Romeo AA, Arciero RA: Clinical outcomes after subpectoral biceps tenodesis with an interference screw. *Am J Sports Med* 2008;36(10):1922-1929.

    At a minimum 1-year follow-up, subpectoral biceps tenodesis with an interference screw was found to be a viable option for patients with symptomatic biceps tendinosis. Anterior shoulder pain and biceps symptoms were resolved, but patients with a coexistent rotator cuff lesion had less favorable outcomes.

20. Millett PJ, Sanders B, Gobezie R, Braun S, Warner JJ: Interference screw vs. suture anchor fixation for open subpectoral biceps tenodesis: Does it matter? *BMC Musculoskelet Disord* 2008;9:121.

    Retrospective review after open subpectoral biceps tenodesis with interference screw fixation or suture anchor fixation found reliable pain relief and improved function at an average 13-month follow-up. There was no statistically significant difference in outcomes. Residual pain may be an issue when suture anchors are used.

21. Friedman DJ, Dunn JC, Higgins LD, Warner JJ: Proximal biceps tendon: Injuries and management. *Sports Med Arthrosc* 2008;16(3):162-169.

    The LHBT is a known pain generator. Numerous pathologic entities may affect this tendon, including tendinitis, partial tearing, and subluxation, and often are associated with rotator cuff tears, especially those involving the subscapularis.

22. Nho SJ, Reiff SN, Verma NN, Slabaugh MA, Mazzocca AD, Romeo AA: Complications associated with subpectoral biceps tenodesis: Low rates of incidence following surgery. *J Shoulder Elbow Surg* 2010;19(5): 764-768.

    In 353 patients treated with an open biceps tenodesis with bioabsorbable interference screw fixation, the 3-year incidence of complications was 2.0%.

Chapter 22

Subscapularis Tears and Subcoracoid Impingement

Richard E. Duey, MD   Stephen S. Burkhart, MD

Anatomy and Function

The subscapularis plays an integral role in glenohumeral kinematics and normal shoulder function. It is the largest and the strongest of the rotator cuff muscles, and it contributes approximately 50% of the total force generated by the rotator cuff.[1] In addition to its function as a dynamic anterior stabilizer of the shoulder joint, the subscapularis is an internal rotator. A recent cadaver study found that the subscapularis is the strongest internal rotator of the glenohumeral joint when the arm is in abduction and forward flexion.[2]

One of the most critical roles of the subscapularis is its contribution to force couples in the coronal and transverse planes[3,4] (**Figure 1**). A cadaver study found that when an anterosuperior rotator cuff tear extends into the upper subscapularis, glenohumeral joint kinematics are substantially altered at higher loads.[5] Higher loads are correlated with the physiologic force transmission exerted by the deltoid in the presence of a massive rotator cuff tear.[6] The alteration in shoulder kinematics probably results from the detachment of the anterior rotator cable, whose anterior attachment points are at the upper border of the subscapularis and the anterior border of the supraspinatus[7] (**Figure 2**). Conversely, glenohumeral kinematics were not altered when an isolated tear of the supraspinatus was simulated and the upper subscapularis was left intact.[5] In the presence of a supraspinatus tear, a substantially higher force must be generated by the subscapularis to maintain stable-fulcrum glenohumeral joint kinematics.[6] The increased force requirements were found to be within the physiologic range of the subscapularis if the anteroposterior dimension of the combined supraspinatus-infraspinatus tear was 7 cm or less. These findings substantiate the importance of the subscapularis in creating balanced force couples in the

shoulder, particularly in the presence of a superior rotator cuff tear.

An understanding of the insertional anatomy of the subscapularis is necessary for the treatment of a subscapularis tear. The footprint of the subscapularis is larger than that of any other rotator cuff tendon.[8] The subscapularis insertion area has been described as trapezoidal; it is widest superiorly and gently tapers as it extends inferiorly.[9,10] The superior-to-inferior footprint length is approximately 25 mm, and the average width is approximately 17 mm superiorly and 3 mm inferiorly. The subscapularis has a muscular attachment along the humeral neck immediately distal to its tendinous insertion, and the entire length of its myotendinous insertion is approximately 40 mm.[10] Approximately 60% of the tendon attaches at the wide superior one third of the footprint.[9,10] This area has been shown to be the strongest attachment point for the subscapularis as well as the point of greatest load transmission.[11] The subscapularis footprint is substantially larger in men than in women, and its length from superior to inferior is significantly correlated with the diameter of the humeral head.[10]

Prevalence and Pathology

Shoulder arthroscopy offers the surgeon an enhanced ability to recognize subscapularis pathology. The description of a subscapularis tear usually includes the location and amount of tendon involvement, whether the tear is partial or full thickness, and whether it is degenerative or traumatic. Most subscapularis tears involve the upper subscapularis insertion and are articular-sided, partial thickness, and degenerative.[12,13] This tear pattern may be caused by subcoracoid stenosis and impingement (the so-called roller-wringer effect).[14] As the subscapularis moves across the coracoid, increased tensile forces on the articular side of the tendon lead to the development of a tensile undersurface fiber failure (TUFF) lesion (**Figure 3**). Subcoracoid impingement can also cause longitudinal splits along the deep surface of the tendon (**Figure 4**).

Recent reports indicate that 27% to 49% of all rotator cuff tears involve the subscapularis.[13,15-17] The

Dr. Duey or an immediate family member serves as a paid consultant to or is an employee of Arthrex. Dr. Burkhart or an immediate family member serves as a board member, owner, officer, or committee member of the Arthroscopy Association of North America; has received royalties from Arthrex; serves as a paid consultant to or is an employee of Arthrex; and has received research or institutional support from Arthrex.

4: Arthroscopy

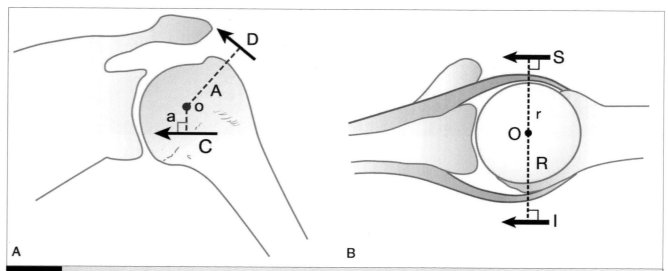

Schematic drawings showing the balanced force couples required to maintain the normal glenohumeral relationship. **A,** In the coronal plane, the combined inferior rotator cuff force (C) is balanced against the deltoid (D). A = moment arm of the deltoid, a = moment arm of the inferior rotator cuff, o = center of rotation. **B,** In the axial plane, the subscapularis (S) is balanced against the infraspinatus and teres minor (I). O = center of rotation, R = moment arm of the infraspinatus and teres minor, r = moment arm of the subscapularis. (Reproduced with permission from Burkhart SS, Lo IKY, Brady PC, Denard PJ: Large and massive rotator cuff tears, in Burkhart SB: *The Cowboy's Companion: A Trail Guide for the Arthroscopic Shoulder Surgeon.* Philadelphia, PA, Lippincott Williams & Wilkins, 2012, pp 129-164.)

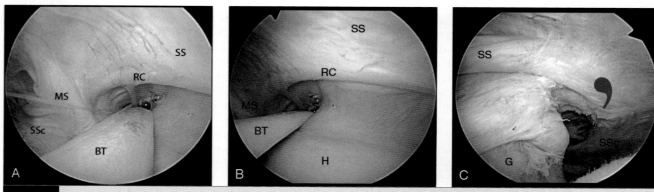

Figure 2 Arthroscopic photographs of a right shoulder as seen from a posterior viewing portal, showing the connection between the subscapularis (SSc) and the supraspinatus (SS) through the medial sling (MS). **A,** The rotator cable (RC) of the rotator cuff merges with the medial sling anteriorly. When the medial sling detaches during a subscapularis tear, the comma sign can be followed to locate the superolateral corner of the subscapularis tendon. **B,** A profile view of the rotator cable (RC) further shows this constant relationship. **C,** In a massive contracted rotator cuff tear, the relationship between the subscapularis and the supraspinatus is maintained, and the comma sign (blue symbol) can be used to identify the superolateral subscapularis tendon. BT = biceps tendon, G = glenoid, H = humerus. (Reproduced with permission from Burkhart SS, Lo IKY, Brady PC, Denard PJ: Subscapularis tendon tears, in Burkhart SB: *The Cowboy's Companion: A Trail Guide for the Arthroscopic Shoulder Surgeon.* Philadelphia, PA, Lippincott Williams & Wilkins, 2012, pp 101-128.)

prevalence of subscapularis tears was found to be almost identical to that of infraspinatus tears.[18] Almost all subscapularis tears occur as part of a massive tear involving two or more rotator cuff tendons.[16-19] However, two relatively recent studies looked solely at isolated subscapularis tendon tears, most of which were the result of traumatic injury.[16,20] The reported mechanisms of injury included forced abduction with external rotation, a fall onto an outstretched upper extremity, severe traction, a direct blow, and heavy lifting. One

study found that most of the isolated tears were full-thickness lesions involving at least the upper one third of the tendinous insertion.[16]

Several studies found a strong correlation between subscapularis tendon tears and pathologic changes involving the long head of the biceps tendon (LHBT).[13,16-22] The reported prevalence of LHBT lesions associated with subscapularis tears ranged from 63% to 85%.[16,18-20,22] Anterior instability of the LHBT almost always occurs in conjunction with a tear of the

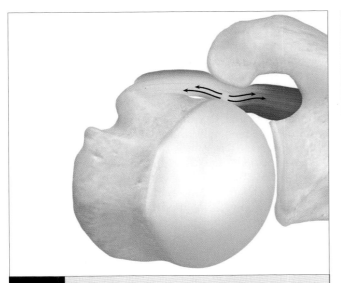

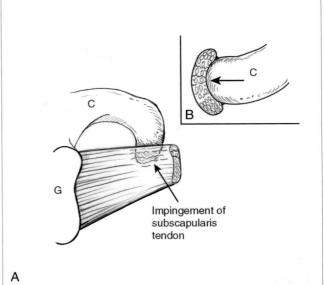

Figure 3 Schematic drawing showing the roller-wringer effect. In a patient with subcoracoid impingement, the prominent coracoid tip indents the superficial surface of the subscapularis tendon, creating tensile forces *(arrows)* on the convex articular surface of the subscapularis tendon and sometimes leading to failure of the subscapularis fibers (a tensile undersurface fiber failure [TUFF] lesion). (Reproduced with permission from Burkhart SS, Lo IKY, Brady PC, Denard PJ Subscapularis tendon tears, in Burkhart SS: *The Cowboy's Companion: A Trail Guide for the Arthroscopic Shoulder Surgeon.* Philadelphia, PA, Lippincott Williams & Wilkins, 2012, pp 101-128.)

Figure 4 Schematic drawings showing subcoracoid impingement. Repetitive compression of the subscapularis tendon fibers by the coracoid tip in the anterior-to-posterior direction causes spreading of the fibers in the superior-to-inferior direction (**A**), with resultant longitudinal splits between subscapularis tendon fiber bundles (**B**). C = coracoid, G = glenoid. (Reproduced with permission from Burkhart SS, Lo IKY, Brady PC, Denard PJ Subscapularis tendon tears, in Burkhart SS: *The Cowboy's Companion: A Trail Guide for the Arthroscopic Shoulder Surgeon.* Philadelphia, PA, Lippincott Williams & Wilkins, 2012, pp 101-128.)

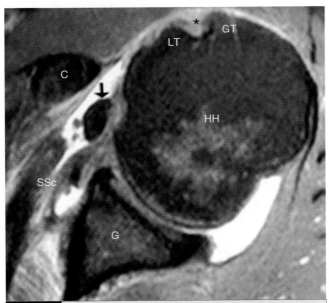

Figure 5 Axial MRI of a left shoulder with a medial dislocation of the long head of the biceps tendon (black arrow) into a split tear of the subscapularis tendon (SSc). The empty biceps groove (*) is seen between the lesser tuberosity (LT) and greater tuberosity (GT). C = coracoid, G = glenoid, HH = humeral head.

subscapularis[13,17,21] (**Figure 5**). The rate of LHBT dislocation also is substantially higher when there is a full-thickness subscapularis tear, particularly if it involves more than one third of the insertion.[13,21]

The strong association between subscapularis tears and LHBT subluxation or dislocation probably results from loss of the stability the subscapularis normally offers the LHBT. The superior insertion of the subscapularis may be the most important restraint keeping the LHBT in place.[23] Anatomic and histologic analysis revealed that the subscapularis forms a buttress that supports the LHBT tendon as it makes its acute turn out of the intertubercular groove before entering the joint.[13,23] The wide uppermost insertion of the subscapularis extends as a distinct tendinous slip over the fovea capitis of the humeral head. This tendinous slip at the widest section of the subscapularis tendon insertion comes into direct contact with the LHBT where it turns over the top of the humeral head. The upper subscapularis insertion directly supports the LHBT, and this tendinous slip serves as a secondary attachment point (in addition to the bone insertion) for the superior glenohumeral ligament and the medial head of the coracohumeral ligament as they spiral to form the medial sling of the biceps and thereby stabilize the LHBT.

4: Arthroscopy

4: Arthroscopy

Clinical Evaluation

Clinical tests can be used to evaluate the integrity and function of the subscapularis. Four tests commonly used for the detection of subscapularis tears were prospectively compared in 50 consecutive patients undergoing shoulder arthroscopy.[24] The exclusion criteria included calcific tendinitis, stiffness, instability, osteoarthritis, and previous surgery. All study patients were examined preoperatively using the lift-off test, internal rotation lag sign, Napoleon test, and belly-off sign. During arthroscopy, subscapularis tears were assessed and graded. The Napoleon test and belly-off sign were most sensitive (88% and 87%, respectively). The belly-off sign was most specific (91%), followed by the lift-off test (79%). The accuracy of the belly-off sign was 90%, and that of the Napoleon test was 74%. The belly-off sign and the Napoleon test were most useful for detecting a partial- or full-thickness tear involving the upper 25% of the subscapularis tendon. The lift-off test and the internal rotation lag sign were more effective if the tear involved more than 50% of the tendinous insertion. Fifteen percent of surgically detected tears were missed on physical examination. This study found a better ability to detect subscapularis tears than previous studies. However, the exclusion of patients with concomitant shoulder pathology, which frequently is encountered in a clinical shoulder practice, probably had a substantial effect on the study outcomes.[24]

In another study, modified lift-off and belly press tests were used to evaluate 17 patients with an arthroscopically treated isolated subscapularis tear.[16] The arthroscopic findings were compared with those of the preoperative physical examination. In the lift-off test, the patient was asked to push on the examiner's hand, and strength was graded. Five patients (29%) were unable to perform the test secondary to pain or stiffness. The lift-off test had a sensitivity of 92% in patients who were able to perform the test. In the modified belly press test, the examiner pushed the patient's elbow, and strength was graded; the sensitivity of the test was 71%. The use of both tests enabled 16 of the 17 subscapularis tears to be identified on physical examination. However, most of these were full-thickness tears involving at least one third of the subscapularis tendon.[16]

Electromyography has been used to evaluate the ability of clinical examination tests to isolate the upper and lower subscapularis muscle-tendon units. In a recent study, electromyographic data were collected on the lift-off, belly press, and bear hug tests.[25] The tests were performed with the arm in various positions, including the ideal position, to determine whether position affected the result. The muscle activity of 28 healthy volunteers was recorded for the upper and lower subscapularis, supraspinatus, infraspinatus, teres major, latissimus dorsi, triceps, and pectoralis major. Each of the three tests was successful in isolating the subscapularis muscle regardless of arm position. There were no significant differences among the tests in their ability to activate the subscapularis. Furthermore, no test preferentially activated the upper or lower subscapularis at different arm positions.[25]

Another study also compared the lift-off, belly press, and bear hug tests using electromyographic data.[26] The bear hug test was performed at 0°, 45°, and 90° of shoulder forward flexion, and muscle activation was monitored in the upper and lower subscapularis, pectoralis major, and latissimus dorsi. The bear hug test at 45° and the belly press test elicited substantially greater activity in the upper and lower subscapularis compared with the pectoralis major and the latissimus dorsi. The lift-off test showed no important difference in activation between the upper and lower subscapularis and the latissimus dorsi. The bear hug test at 45° better isolated the subscapularis than the other two muscles; it also showed 20% greater activation of the upper subscapularis than the lower subscapularis, but this result was not statistically significant. The bear hug test at 90° showed substantially greater activity in the lower subscapularis than in the upper subscapularis, pectoralis major, or latissimus dorsi. Some question remains as to how well the lift-off test isolates the subscapularis, but electromyographic data indicate that it is effectively isolated by both the belly press and bear hug tests. It also appears that the bear hug test causes some preferential activation of the upper and lower subscapularis, depending on shoulder position.[26]

Imaging

Plain radiographs are the initial studies obtained for patients with a suspected rotator cuff tear. Although nonspecific for subscapularis tears, plain radiographs can reveal concomitant pathology, including narrowing of the coracohumeral interval, glenohumeral arthritis, or fracture. Superior migration of the humeral head can also be identified; this condition may result from a long-standing massive rotator cuff tear or an acute injury involving the subscapularis, with loss of the coronal and transverse plane force couples.

MRI, magnetic resonance arthrography, CT arthrography (CTA), and ultrasonography have been used to evaluate the subscapularis. CTA is most commonly used in Europe, and MRI and magnetic resonance arthrography are more commonly used in North America. Ultrasonography is cost-effective, can be used in the clinical setting, and allows dynamic evaluation of the subscapularis. However, its usefulness depends on the expertise of the sonographer. MRI, magnetic resonance arthrography, and CTA are able to detect labral injury, fatty infiltration, and muscle atrophy, but ultrasonography does not have this ability.

One recent study evaluated the accuracy of shoulder ultrasonography in detecting subscapularis tears by comparing its results with findings during arthroscopy.[15] Ninety-six shoulders with rotator cuff pathology underwent ultrasonographic examination by a single radiologist familiar with the technique. The patients subsequently underwent shoulder arthroscopy by a single surgeon. Analysis of the results determined ultrasonography to have a sensitivity of 30% and a specificity of 100% for detecting subscapularis tears. The positive predictive value was 100%, and the negative predictive value was 78%. The false-negative rate was high, but 18 of the 19 false-negative results involved a partial-thickness tear of the subscapularis. Ultrasonography was effective in detecting full-thickness subscapularis tears, with a sensitivity of 86%. None of the tears seen as full thickness on ultrasonograph was found to be a partial-thickness tear during arthroscopy.[15]

A small prospective study of the results of arthroscopic subscapularis repair also examined the effectiveness of CTA in detecting subscapularis tears in 17 patients with an isolated subscapularis lesion.[16] A sensitivity of 94% was reported for CTA. However, 15 of the tears were full-thickness lesions involving at least one third of the tendon insertion.

The accuracy of MRI for detecting subscapularis tears also was recently evaluated.[18] The preoperative MRI studies were interpreted by radiologists and compared with findings at the time of shoulder arthroscopy. MRI had a low sensitivity (36%) but an excellent specificity (100%). The overall accuracy was 69%. Smaller tears of the subscapularis were frequently missed. However, tears involving 50% or more of the tendon insertion were more readily detected; MRI had a sensitivity of 56% and an accuracy of 86%.[18]

A recent study examined the ability of fellowship-trained orthopaedic surgeons to accurately detect subscapularis tears using MRI.[17] Five surgeons prospectively reviewed MRIs of 202 consecutive patients using four specific criteria: in axial images, a tear of the subscapularis tendon off the lesser tuberosity or medial subluxation-dislocation of the LHBT (**Figure 5**); and in sagittal oblique images, a tear from the lesser tuberosity or atrophy of the subscapularis muscle. A subscapularis that met two or more criteria was considered torn. The surgeon evaluated all MRIs before examining the patient or reading the radiologist's report. The presence or absence of a subscapularis tear was determined at the time of shoulder arthroscopy, and a tear was defined as a more-than-10% disruption of the tendinous insertion. This approach had sensitivity of 73%, specificity of 94%, positive predictive value of 90%, negative predictive value of 84%, and accuracy of 86% for detecting subscapularis tears. Neither MRI magnet strength nor the use of intra-articular contrast had an important impact on overall accuracy. However, tears involving more than 50% of the tendinous footprint were more readily identified; the detection rate was higher than 97%. Based on these findings, the systematic use of these criteria may improve a surgeon's ability to preoperatively detect a subscapularis tear on MRI.[17]

These studies show that advanced imaging modalities are most effective in detecting a large, full-thickness tear of the subscapularis; a smaller, partial-thickness tear frequently is not evident. Therefore, a high index of suspicion should be maintained if the clinical findings are consistent with a subscapularis tear.

Treatment

Questions remain as to which subscapularis tears should be treated surgically and which should be treated nonsurgically. An acute, traumatic tear typically is repaired surgically. A small, degenerative tear initially can be treated nonsurgically, particularly if the patient has low demands and is older than approximately 65 years. However, some experts believe that, given the critical role of the subscapularis in shoulder function, most subscapularis tears ultimately lead to substantial disability and should be repaired.[27,28] Even in the presence of substantial fatty infiltration, some experts believe that the subscapularis can and should be repaired for its tenodesis effect, which stabilizes the glenohumeral joint and provides a stable fulcrum for glenohumeral kinematics.[28,29]

A biomechanical rationale has been presented for repairing the subscapularis when the tear is part of an anterosuperior rotator cuff tear.[30] The anterior supraspinatus and superior subscapularis are connected by a comma-shaped arc of tissue called the comma sign.[31] This comma tissue comprises the superior glenohumeral ligament and the medial segment of the coracohumeral ligament where they interdigitate with the superolateral corner of the subscapularis tendon insertion, forming part of the medial sling of the LHBT in the intact rotator cuff. In the presence of a chronic, retracted anterosuperior rotator cuff tear, the comma tissue insertion pulls away from the bone along with the upper subscapularis, and the comma sign becomes the primary means by which to identify the superolateral corner of the subscapularis (**Figure 2**). By preserving the comma tissue and repairing the subscapularis first, the surgeon can bring the anterior portion of the supraspinatus closer to its anatomic footprint.[30] The subsequent repair of the supraspinatus becomes more attainable by decreasing the tension in its muscle-tendon unit. In addition, repair of the subscapularis and the anterior supraspinatus reestablishes the anterior attachment of the rotator cable.

The arthroscopic treatment of subscapularis tears and any associated pathology can be challenging, but evolving techniques and instrumentation are making these repairs easier. The subscapularis can be arthroscopically repaired with the patient in the beach-chair or lateral decubitus position. For a multitendon tear, it is advisable to treat the subscapularis first, before swelling further restricts the already limited subcoracoid space. The anterosuperolateral and anterior portals are the standard working portals. The posterior or lateral portal is used for visualization. Often, tears of the subscapularis can be identified by using a 30° ar-

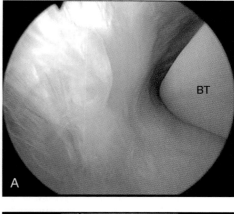

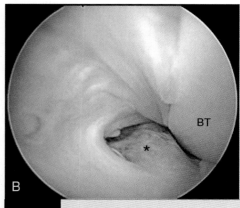

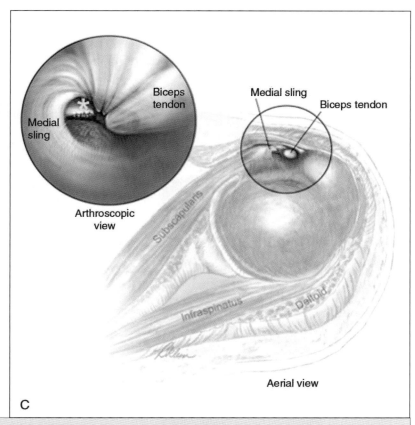

Figure 6 **A,** Arthroscopic photograph of a normal shoulder as seen from a posterior viewing portal with a 70° arthroscope, showing approximately 2 cm of the floor and sidewalls of the bicipital groove. **B,** Arthroscopic photograph of a shoulder with disruption in the medial sidewall, with a bare lesser tuberosity footprint distally. **C,** Schematic drawings of the shoulder in **B,** showing a mid to distal tendon tear of the subscapularis. * = disrupted medial sidewall, BT = biceps tendon. (Reproduced with permission from Burkhart SS, Lo IKY, Brady PC, Denard PJ: Subscapularis tendon tears, in Burkhart SS: *The Cowboy's Companion: A Trail Guide for the Arthroscopic Shoulder Surgeon.* Philadelphia, PA, Lippincott Williams & Wilkins, 2012, pp 101-128.)

throscope in the posterior portal. However, the view of the subscapularis footprint can be substantially improved when a 70° arthroscope is used. Some experts believe that the use of a lateral viewing portal with a 30° arthroscope offers the best view of the subscapularis footprint, but others hold that a posterior viewing portal with a 70° arthroscope provides the best view.[16,27,28]

The 70° arthroscope offers the ability to see 2 cm down the intertubercular groove from a posterior portal.[27] It is essential to inspect the medial sidewall of the intertubercular groove in this manner when evaluating the subscapularis. Doing so may reveal a rent in the sidewall, which usually implies a subtle biceps instability and disruption of the subscapularis. This tear may be obstructed from view by the proximal portion of the medial sling (if it is intact), and looking down the groove with a 70° arthroscope is the only way to identify such a tear (**Figure 6**).

Proper manipulation of the arm also is useful for visualizing the subscapularis. Bringing the arm into forward flexion and internal rotation can be helpful in examining the tendon insertion. With the patient in the lateral decubitus position, applying a so-called posterior lever push not only increases the anterior working space but also improves visualization of the subscapularis insertion.[19,28] This maneuver is performed by stabilizing the patient's elbow while slightly internally rotating the arm with one hand and applying a posteriorly directed force to the proximal humerus with the other hand. The posterior lever push has proved useful for visualization from a posterior portal, particularly with a 70° arthroscope. A similar maneuver with the patient in the beach chair position is much less effective for enhancing visualization of the subscapularis insertion.

A narrowed coracohumeral interval and subscapularis pathology have been significantly correlated.[32,33] Therefore, the subcoracoid space must be dealt with along with a tear of the subscapularis. From an intraarticular viewpoint, it is useful to internally and externally rotate the shoulder and to observe whether the coracoid tip (seen as a rolling bulge at the top of the subscapularis tendon) is compressing and impinging on the subscapularis tendon as the shoulder moves back and forth. This finding is a strong indicator that the coracohumeral interval is substantially narrowed. The

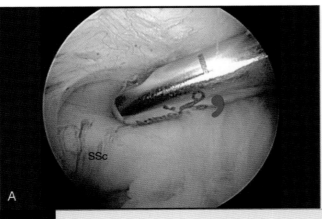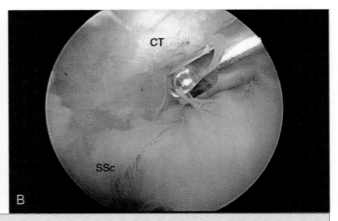

Figure 7 Arthroscopic photographs showing a right shoulder as seen from a posterior viewing portal. **A,** A shaver is used to make a window in the rotator interval medial to the comma tissue *(blue symbol).* **B,** The coracoid tip is located by palpation with the shaver. CT = coracoid tip, SSc = subscapularis tendon. (Reproduced with permission from Burkhart SS, Lo IKY, Brady PC, Denard PJ: Subscapularis tendon tears, in Burkhart SS: *The Cowboy's Companion: A Trail Guide for the Arthroscopic Shoulder Surgeon.* Philadelphia, PA, Lippincott Williams & Wilkins, 2012, pp 101-128.)

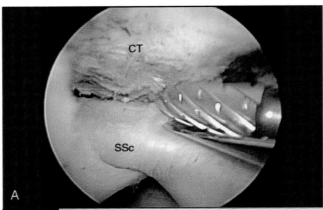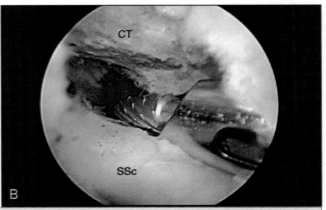

Figure 8 Arthroscopic photographs of a right shoulder as seen from a posterior glenohumeral portal with a 70° arthroscope, showing coracohumeral interval evaluation. **A,** The native coracohumeral interval can be estimated by comparison with the known width of an instrument; here, the width of the interval is less than that of the 5-mm burr. **B,** Coracoplasty has created a coracohumeral interval of at least 7 mm. CT = coracoid tip, SSc = subscapularis tendon. (Reproduced with permission from Burkhart SS, Lo IKY, Brady PC, Denard PJ: Subscapularis tendon tears, in Burkhart SS: *The Cowboy's Companion: A Trail Guide for the Arthroscopic Shoulder Surgeon.* Philadelphia, PA, Lippincott Williams & Wilkins, 2012, pp 101-128.)

coracoid and subcoracoid space can be seen from an intra-articular viewpoint by placing the tip of the arthroscope through a window created in the rotator interval. Care should be taken to preserve the comma tissue during this step (**Figure 7**). A 30° arthroscope initially is used to identify the tip of the coracoid because the use of a 70° arthroscope may be disorienting and cause a drift too far inferiorly. Many surgeons still use a coracohumeral interval of 6 mm or less as an indication for coracoplasty during a subscapularis repair.[22,28,34] The bursa and other soft tissue can be removed from the subcoracoid space by using a combination of electrocautery and shaving. A burr is then used to resect the posterolateral tip of the coracoid in the plane of the conjoined tendon and the subscapularis. The goal is to enlarge the coracohumeral interval

to between 7 and 10 mm[19,28] (**Figure 8**). Coracoplasty also can be done through a subacromial approach, depending on the surgeon's preference. Familiarity with the surrounding anatomy is important during a coracoplasty. Surgery about the posterolateral aspect of the coracoid tip is relatively safe, however, because all major neurovascular structures are located at least 28 mm from the tip of the coracoid.[35]

The effectiveness of arthroscopic coracoplasty recently was examined in a cadaver study of five forequarter shoulder specimens in which an approximately 5- to 10-mm resection of the coracoid tip was made. For each specimen, CT was obtained before and after the procedure and measurements were gathered, including coracoid overlap, coracoid index, and coracohumeral interval. Substantial reductions in subcora-

4: Arthroscopy

coid stenosis were observed after surgery. Partial disruption of the coracoacromial ligament and the conjoined tendon was observed after anatomic dissection. However, limiting the resection of the coracoid to 10 mm or less, depending on the size of the patient, appears to preclude any substantial soft-tissue disruption.[36]

There is a high correlation between LHBT pathology and a subscapularis tendon tear, and often the LHBT must be treated at the same time as a subscapularis tear.[13,16-22] Many surgeons treat the biceps based on its appearance at the time of arthroscopy.[16,20,22] Others routinely perform either a tenodesis or tenotomy of the LHBT during repair of a subscapularis tear, unless the patient is younger than approximately 35 years or is an overhead throwing athlete.[28] The decision to perform a tenodesis rather than tenotomy is based on the patient factors, including age, activity level, concern about cosmesis, and personal preference. Anatomic studies have highlighted the role of the upper subscapularis tendon in stabilizing the LHBT.[13,23] Routinely treating the biceps may, therefore, protect the subscapularis repair. Clinical outcomes were improved after subscapularis repair with LHBT tenotomy or tenodesis, regardless of the appearance of the LHBT at the time of surgery.[37] Two studies found that some patients with a healed subscapularis after arthroscopic repair had an unsatisfactory clinical outcome related to pathology involving the LHBT, although the biceps had a normal appearance at the time of surgery.[16,22] Arthroscopic restabilization of the LHBT in the intertubercular groove was reported to have good short-term results.[38] Instability of the LHBT can recur, however, causing failure of the subscapularis repair. Therefore, most experts prefer to use tenotomy or tenodesis to treat the LHBT in the context of a subscapularis tear.[16,20,22,28,37]

Preparation of the bony footprint is important to a successful repair of the subscapularis. All soft tissue is carefully removed from the bone bed using a combination of a cautery, a shaver, a high-speed burr, and ring curets. The goal is a uniform bleeding bone surface to which the subscapularis can heal and form a strong attachment. In a complete chronic tear, reduced tendon excursion may lead to inadequate apposition of the tendon to the native footprint. If necessary, the footprint can be medialized 5 to 7 mm to improve the contact surface area between the tendon and the bone and to reduce the tension on the repair. A recent study compared two groups of patients after primary arthroscopic repair of a 100% retracted full-thickness subscapularis tear.[39] Patients in one group had a repair to the native footprint, and those in the other group required medialization of the footprint of as much as 7 mm. At a minimum 2-year follow-up, there was no significant between-group difference in functional scores, patient satisfaction, or return to activity.

A chronic tear can leave the subscapularis severely retracted and scarred to adjacent structures. Identifying the tendon margins can be difficult, but the process is facilitated by identification of the comma sign and its attachment to the superolateral corner of the subscapularis tendon insertion[31] (**Figure 2**). A traction stitch then can be placed in the subscapularis tendon, and the meticulous process of releasing the tendon is begun. The posterolateral coracoid is skeletonized, and anterior adhesions between the subscapularis, the conjoined tendon, and the internal deltoid fascia are resected. Care must be taken to avoid straying too far inferior or medial to the conjoined tendon. Often, there are adhesions between the subscapularis and the inferior neck and base of the coracoid process, and a 30° elevator can be extremely useful in releasing these adhesions. The upper subscapular nerve insertion can be as close as 11 mm to the medial aspect of the base of the coracoid. Therefore, it is important to avoid straying medial to the coracoid during this release. A posterior release of the subscapularis from the anterior glenoid neck also should be done. This plane is relatively avascular, and a 15° elevator can be helpful with this portion of the release. Release of the coracohumeral ligament from the base of the coracoid with preservation of the comma tissue can greatly improve tendon excursion. This portion of the release has been called the anterior interval slide in continuity.[40] Release of inferior adhesions between the subscapularis and the axillary nerve and the brachial plexus has been described.[16,41] This step can be dangerous, however, and many surgeons find it unnecessary for gaining adequate tendon excursion before repair.[20,22,28]

Suture anchors usually are placed from inferior to superior along the footprint. In general, one anchor per linear centimeter of torn tendon (in the superior-to-inferior dimension) is used. Sutures can be passed antegrade or retrograde through an anterior or anterosuperolateral portal, depending on the surgeon's preference. Inferior sutures are tied before superior sutures. Superior sutures can be brought medial to the comma tissue over the superior margin of the tendon and tied, thereby using the comma tissue as a rip stop to suture cutout.

Most subscapularis tears are repaired using a single-row technique, and excellent short-term and long-term results have been reported.[16,19,20,22,42,43] However, some surgeons prefer to use a double-row repair if at all possible.[16,28,34,42-44] There is some clinical evidence that improved tendon healing occurs in patients who have double-row repair of a rotator cuff tear.[45] A biomechanical study found that a double-row repair using a suture-bridge technique had substantially higher stiffness and ultimate load for a complete subscapularis tear compared with a single-row repair.[44] Tendon elongation before failure was substantially less in patients with a double-row repair. In fact, the strength of the double-row repair surpassed the predicted loads for everyday activities involving the subscapularis. The use of two accessory anterior portals placed lateral to the conjoined tendon was found to facilitate the use of a suture-bridge technique in the repair of the subscapularis.[34] In this technique, a low anterolateral portal is

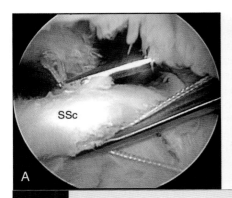
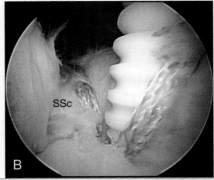
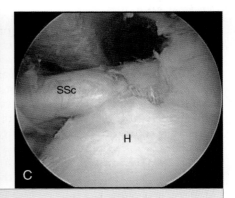

Figure 9 Arthroscopic photographs of a right shoulder as seen from a posterior viewing portal, showing knotless repair of an upper subscapularis tendon tear. **A,** A FiberTape suture is passed antegrade through the upper subscapularis tendon. **B,** The tape is secured to the prepared bone bed with a BioComposite SwiveLock C anchor (Arthrex). **C,** Restoration of the footprint with a low-profile knotless repair. H = humerus, SSc = subscapularis tendon. (Reproduced with permission from Burkhart SS, Lo IKY, Brady PC, Denard PJ: Subscapularis tendon tears, in Burkhart SS: *The Cowboy's Companion: A Trail Guide for the Arthroscopic Shoulder Surgeon.* Philadelphia, PA, Lippincott Williams & Wilkins, 2012, pp 101-128.)

used as a working portal and for the placement of lateral row anchors. An elevator is placed in a low anteromedial portal and is used to retract the conjoined tendon and deltoid muscle to increase the anterior working space.

Tears of the subscapularis typically involve the upper portion of the tendon insertion.[12,13] The use of a double-loaded suture anchor has been described for a double inverted mattress repair of the upper subscapularis.[46] This technique improves the compression of the tendon against the footprint, compared with the use of simple sutures. However, there is a risk of cutout in poor-quality tissue. A knotless technique using a suture tape (FiberTape; Arthrex, Naples, FL) is an option for repairing an upper subscapularis tear.[47] FiberTape is a nonabsorbable 2-mm suture tape with a polyethylene structure similar to that of FiberWire (Arthrex), but it is wider than FiberWire and has stronger failure characteristics than suture when used in degenerative tendon. The FiberTape is placed in the superolateral corner of the subscapularis tendon, and both limbs are brought medial to the comma tissue and secured in the superomedial corner of the footprint using a knotless anchor (**Figure 9**). The wide suture tape provides superior compression of the tendon against the footprint as well as better resistance than suture to tendon cut-through. After the two limbs are secured, the tails can be brought anterior to the comma tissue and secured laterally within a biceps tenodesis construct or with a second knotless suture anchor.[43] This technique provides double-row fixation of an upper subscapularis tear in a relatively straightforward and efficient manner.

After surgery, immobilization in a sling with a small abduction pillow is required. Active elbow motion is allowed. Passive external rotation is limited to 0° with the arm at the side. The use of the sling is discontinued at 6 weeks, and progressive, active-assisted range-of-motion exercises are begun. Strengthening exercises are initiated 12 to 16 weeks after surgery, depending on the size of the tear. A return to full activities requires at least 6 months, depending on the size of the tear.

Results

The overall results of arthroscopic subscapularis repair continue to be promising. Outcome data over the past 5 years have come from several studies. A group of 17 patients with an isolated subscapularis tear (average age at surgery, 47 years) were evaluated at a minimum 2-year follow-up.[16] Thirteen of the tears had resulted from trauma, and all were repaired using arthroscopic techniques. These patients had substantial improvement in pain scores as well as scores on the Constant and University of California, Los Angeles (UCLA) shoulder scales. Substantial gains in active forward flexion, external rotation, and internal rotation were observed, with no postoperative stiffness. Abduction strength also substantially increased. Biceps pathology in nine patients was treated with a biceps tenodesis using a suture anchor construct, but two of these procedures were unsuccessful. No coracoplasty was performed. CTA was used to evaluate the postoperative integrity of the repair; 15 patients had an intact repair, and a partial retear of the upper subscapularis developed in two patients. Overall function tended to be better in patients with an intact repair. There was no postoperative progression of fatty infiltration. Sixteen patients (94%) were satisfied or very satisfied with the results of surgery. The one unsatisfactory outcome was in a patient in whom biceps instability developed after surgery despite a normal-appearing biceps at the time of arthroscopy. Postoperative CTA both confirmed this diagnosis and showed healing of the subscapularis repair.[16]

In a prospective study, 21 patients with an isolated subscapularis tear (average age, 43 years) were treated

4: Arthroscopy

with an arthroscopic repair.[20] The average interval between injury and surgery was 5.8 months. Nineteen of the tears were traumatic in origin, and consequently the surgeon elected not to perform a coracoplasty. The LHBT was treated based on its appearance at the time of surgery; nine tenodeses, one tenotomy, and two recentering procedures were performed. One tenodesis with a suture anchor construct failed after surgery because of a traumatic event. Data were collected at a minimum 2-year follow-up. Patients had substantial improvement in Constant scores, with 19 (90%) having a good or excellent result. One of the remaining two patients was satisfied with the results of surgery, and one was unsatisfied. Postoperative MRI showed an intact repair in 20 patients and no substantial increase in fatty infiltration. One patient with a rerupture of the upper subscapularis had an increase in fatty infiltration. However, the patient was satisfied with the clinical outcome and elected not to undergo revision surgery. Four patients (25%) with an intact repair had atrophy of the upper subscapularis; these patients had a positive postoperative belly press test but a negative lift-off test. The surgically treated shoulders had a substantial decrease in transverse muscle diameter and cross-sectional area of the subscapularis. Subscapularis strength in the contralateral shoulder was measured postoperatively using electronic force measurement plates. A substantial reduction in strength was found in the surgically treated extremity compared with the contralateral side. Investigators observed a trend toward improved functional outcomes and less muscle atrophy in the patients with a shorter time to surgery, but these findings were not clinically significant.[20]

The clinical results of 23 patients who underwent arthroscopic repair of an isolated or combined subscapularis tear were reported.[42] Sixty-one percent of these patients were treated with a biceps tenodesis, and none underwent a coracoplasty. At a minimum 2-year follow-up, the data revealed a substantial improvement in Constant, UCLA, and visual analog pain scale scores. There also was a substantial increase in subjective shoulder function rating scores. Eighty-five percent of patients had a good or very good clinical result. There was a substantial decrease in subscapularis strength in surgically treated shoulders as measured with dynamometric bear hug testing.[42]

In a prospective study of 20 patients (average age, 61.7 years) who underwent arthroscopic treatment of traumatic combined subscapularis tendon tears, 18 (90%) had a good or excellent result.[22] All of the tears involved the subscapularis and the supraspinatus, and seven also involved the infraspinatus. A coracoplasty was required in six patients, all of whom had a coracohumeral interval of less than 6 mm, as seen on MRI and confirmed during arthroscopy. At a minimum 2-year follow-up, patients had significant improvement on the UCLA and Japanese Orthopaedic Association clinical scales. When repair integrity was evaluated postoperatively with MRI, a recurrent tear was found in seven patients (35%), all of whom had improved clinical scores (six reported a good or excellent result, and one a fair result). Patients with an intact repair had a substantially greater improvement in clinical outcome than those with an unsuccessful repair. A positive correlation was found between advanced age, severe tendon retraction, and recurrent tearing. No substantial fatty infiltration was noted postoperatively. This finding and the excellent clinical results were attributed in part to the short time period between injury and surgery. One poor result occurred in a patient who had clinical signs consistent with biceps tendinitis. This patient had a normal-appearing biceps at the time of the index procedure, but second-look arthroscopy revealed a well-healed rotator cuff repair and partial fraying of the biceps. The patient's symptoms resolved after biceps tenotomy.[22]

At a median 5-year follow-up (range, 3 to 7 years) after arthroscopic repair of a subscapularis tear, 40 patients were available, including all patients who underwent a primary subscapularis repair, regardless of concomitant pathology.[19] Biceps tenodesis or tenotomy was routinely performed, and coracoplasty was performed in 17 patients (43%) based on a coracohumeral interval of less than 6 mm at the time of arthroscopy. Visual analog scale, modified UCLA, and modified ASES scores all were substantially improved; 32 patients (80%) had a good or excellent result, 33 patients were able to return to their previous activities, and 35 patients (88%) reported satisfaction with the results of surgery.[19]

The long-term functional outcomes of 79 patients (mean age at surgery, 60.8 years) were retrospectively reviewed after arthroscopic surgery for a subscapularis tear.[41] The tears were both isolated and combined, and 63% were part of a massive rotator cuff tear. Thirty-nine patients (49%) underwent coracoplasty if the coracohumeral interval was less than 6 mm at the time of surgery. The LHBT was routinely treated with a tenodesis or tenotomy. At a minimum 7-year follow-up, UCLA, ASES, and visual analog scale scores all substantially improved postoperatively, and 83% of patients had a good or excellent result. Patients subjectively rated the surgically treated shoulder as having reached 90% of normal function at final follow-up. Ninety-two percent of patients were able to return to their normal activities and were satisfied with the results of surgery.[41]

Summary

The diagnosis and treatment of subscapularis tears and subcoracoid impingement continue to evolve. Arthroscopic shoulder surgery has enabled better recognition and understanding of these clinical entities and has allowed less invasive treatment. Both short- and long-term outcome studies evaluating these techniques have had encouraging results and support their continued use. Further work is needed to better delineate the tenodesis function of the subscapularis as well as the specific role of subcoracoid impingement in subscapularis pathology. Double-row repair techniques may prove clinically advantageous for repairing subscapularis tears, although their use is not always feasible in the presence of severe tendon retraction.

Annotated References

1. Keating JF, Waterworth P, Shaw-Dunn J, Crossan J: The relative strengths of the rotator cuff muscles: A cadaver study. *J Bone Joint Surg Br* 1993;75(1):137-140.

2. Ackland DC, Pandy MG: Moment arms of the shoulder muscles during axial rotation. *J Orthop Res* 2011; 29(5):658-667.

   A biomechanical cadaver study examined the moment arms of muscles that internally or externally rotate the humerus. The subscapularis was found to be the strongest internal rotator of the glenohumeral joint when the shoulder is in abduction or forward flexion.

3. Burkhart SS: Fluoroscopic comparison of kinematic patterns in massive rotator cuff tears: A suspension bridge model. *Clin Orthop Relat Res* 1992;284:144-152.

4. Burkhart SS, Lo IK: Arthroscopic rotator cuff repair. *J Am Acad Orthop Surg* 2006;14(6):333-346.

5. Su WR, Budoff JE, Luo ZP: The effect of anterosuperior rotator cuff tears on glenohumeral translation. *Arthroscopy* 2009;25(3):282-289.

   A cadaver model was used in finding that rotator cuff tears involving both the supraspinatus and the upper subscapularis substantially altered glenohumeral joint kinematics at physiologic loads. When the upper subscapularis tendon was left intact, no alteration in joint kinematics was noted.

6. Hansen ML, Otis JC, Johnson JS, Cordasco FA, Craig EV, Warren RF: Biomechanics of massive rotator cuff tears: Implications for treatment. *J Bone Joint Surg Am* 2008;90(2):316-325.

   When superior rotator cuff tears were created in a cadaver model, increased force transmission was required of the subscapularis for maintaining spheric glenohumeral joint kinematics. These force requirements fell within the physiologic range for the subscapularis with tears as large as 7 cm in the anteroposterior direction.

7. Burkhart SS, Esch JC, Jolson RS: The rotator crescent and rotator cable: An anatomic description of the shoulder's "suspension bridge". *Arthroscopy* 1993; 9(6):611-616.

8. Curtis AS, Burbank KM, Tierney JJ, Scheller AD, Curran AR: The insertional footprint of the rotator cuff: An anatomic study. *Arthroscopy* 2006;22(6):e1, e1.

9. Richards DP, Burkhart SS, Tehrany AM, Wirth MA: The subscapularis footprint: An anatomic description of its insertion site. *Arthroscopy* 2007;23(3):251-254.

   Nineteen cadaver shoulder specimens were used to investigate the insertional anatomy of the subscapularis tendon. The upper 60% of the footprint formed a major attachment point for the tendon and probably plays an important role in load transmission.

10. Ide J, Tokiyoshi A, Hirose J, Mizuta H: An anatomic study of the subscapularis insertion to the humerus: The subscapularis footprint. *Arthroscopy* 2008;24(7): 749-753.

    Forty cadaver shoulders were used to develop a detailed description of the anatomic footprint of the subscapularis tendon and the adjacent bare area. Certain dimensions were substantially larger in specimens from men than in those from women.

11. Halder A, Zobitz ME, Schultz E, An KN: Structural properties of the subscapularis tendon. *J Orthop Res* 2000;18(5):829-834.

12. Sakurai G, Ozaki J, Tomita Y, Kondo T, Tamai S: Incomplete tears of the subscapularis tendon associated with tears of the supraspinatus tendon: Cadaveric and clinical studies. *J Shoulder Elbow Surg* 1998;7(5):510-515.

13. Arai R, Sugaya H, Mochizuki T, Nimura A, Moriishi J, Akita K: Subscapularis tendon tear: An anatomic and clinical investigation. *Arthroscopy* 2008;24(9): 997-1004.

    A clinical investigation established the prevalence of subscapularis tears and their association with biceps pathology. Anatomic dissection showed that the upper portion of the subscapularis insertion functions as an important stabilizer for the LHBT.

14. Lo IK, Burkhart SS: The etiology and assessment of subscapularis tendon tears: A case for subcoracoid impingement, the roller-wringer effect, and TUFF lesions of the subscapularis. *Arthroscopy* 2003;19(10):1142-1150.

15. Singisetti K, Hinsche A: Shoulder ultrasonography versus arthroscopy for the detection of rotator cuff tears: Analysis of errors. *J Orthop Surg (Hong Kong)* 2011; 19(1):76-79.

    The results of ultrasonography of 96 shoulders with rotator cuff symptoms were compared with arthroscopic surgical findings. Ultrasonography had a sensitivity of 30% and a specificity of 100% in the detection of subscapularis tears. Eighteen of the 19 false-negative results involved partial-thickness tears of the upper subscapularis.

16. Lafosse L, Jost B, Reiland Y, Audebert S, Toussaint B, Gobezie R: Structural integrity and clinical outcomes after arthroscopic repair of isolated subscapularis tears. *J Bone Joint Surg Am* 2007;89(6):1184-1193.

    Isolated subscapularis tears were arthroscopically repaired in 17 patients. Most of the tears were traumatic

4: Arthroscopy

and full thickness. Significantly improved short-term clinical outcomes were reported. A retearing rate of 12% was observed on CTA. Sixteen patients were satisfied or very satisfied with the results of surgery. Level of evidence: IV.

17. Adams CR, Brady PC, Koo SS, et al: A systematic approach for diagnosing subscapularis tendon tears with preoperative magnetic resonance imaging scans. *Arthroscopy* 2012;28(11):1592-1600.

   Five orthopaedic surgeons systematically reviewed MRIs for 202 patients, using four specific criteria to determine whether a subscapularis tear was present. This approach led to improved accuracy in recognizing subscapularis tears, compared with previous studies. Level of evidence: III.

18. Adams CR, Schoolfield JD, Burkhart SS: Accuracy of preoperative magnetic resonance imaging in predicting a subscapularis tendon tear based on arthroscopy. *Arthroscopy* 2010;26(11):1427-1433.

   Preoperative shoulder MRI (as interpreted by radiologists) was compared with arthroscopic intraoperative findings. MRI had a sensitivity of 36% and a specificity of 100% for detecting subscapularis lesions. Larger tears were more readily identified using MRI. Level of evidence: III.

19. Adams CR, Schoolfield JD, Burkhart SS: The results of arthroscopic subscapularis tendon repairs. *Arthroscopy* 2008;24(12):1381-1389.

   Retrospective review at a median 5-year follow-up of 40 patients who underwent arthroscopic subscapularis repair found that 80% had a good or excellent clinical outcome and 88% were satisfied with the results of surgery. Level of evidence: IV.

20. Bartl C, Salzmann GM, Seppel G, et al: Subscapularis function and structural integrity after arthroscopic repair of isolated subscapularis tears. *Am J Sports Med* 2011;39(6):1255-1262.

   At a minimum 2-year follow-up of 21 patients who underwent arthroscopic repair of a traumatic isolated subscapularis tear, 19 patients had a good or excellent result. MRI revealed an intact repair in 20 patients. Subscapularis strength was significantly decreased in the surgically treated extremity. Level of evidence: IV.

21. Lafosse L, Reiland Y, Baier GP, Toussaint B, Jost B: Anterior and posterior instability of the long head of the biceps tendon in rotator cuff tears: A new classification based on arthroscopic observations. *Arthroscopy* 2007;23(1):73-80.

   Instability of the LHBT and its association with rotator cuff tearing were evaluated in 200 consecutive patients undergoing arthroscopic rotator cuff repair. Ninety-six percent of patients with anterior instability of the biceps had a concomitant subscapularis tear.

22. Ide J, Tokiyoshi A, Hirose J, Mizuta H: Arthroscopic repair of traumatic combined rotator cuff tears involving the subscapularis tendon. *J Bone Joint Surg Am* 2007;89(11):2378-2388.

Traumatic combined rotator cuff tears that included the subscapularis were arthroscopically repaired in 20 patients. At a minimum 2-year follow-up, 90% reported a good or excellent result. The tear recurrence rate was 35%, based on postoperative MRI. One poor outcome occurred in a patient in whom biceps pathology developed after surgery. Level of evidence: IV.

23. Arai R, Mochizuki T, Yamaguchi K, et al: Functional anatomy of the superior glenohumeral and coracohumeral ligaments and the subscapularis tendon in view of stabilization of the long head of the biceps tendon. *J Shoulder Elbow Surg* 2010;19(1):58-64.

   The importance of the upper subscapularis insertion, superior glenohumeral ligament, and coracohumeral ligament in stabilizing the LHBT was investigated by means of anatomic and histologic analysis. The superior insertion of the subscapularis was found to be the most important restraint preventing dislocation of the LHBT.

24. Bartsch M, Greiner S, Haas NP, Scheibel M: Diagnostic values of clinical tests for subscapularis lesions. *Knee Surg Sports Traumatol Arthrosc* 2010;18(12): 1712-1717.

   Four clinical tests were compared for their ability to accurately detect subscapularis tears in 50 consecutive patients undergoing shoulder arthroscopy. The Napoleon test had the highest sensitivity (88%), and the belly-off sign had the highest specificity (91%). Strict exclusion criteria probably had a substantial effect on the reported outcomes.

25. Pennock AT, Pennington WW, Torry MR, et al: The influence of arm and shoulder position on the bear-hug, belly-press, and lift-off tests: An electromyographic study. *Am J Sports Med* 2011;39(11):2338-2346.

   Electromyographic data were used to analyze the ability of three different physical examination tests to isolate the subscapularis. All three tests were effective for this purpose, and no test appeared superior to the others. None of the tests was able to selectively isolate the upper subscapularis.

26. Chao S, Thomas S, Yucha D, Kelly JD IV, Driban J, Swanik K: An electromyographic assessment of the "bear hug": An examination for the evaluation of the subscapularis muscle. *Arthroscopy* 2008;24(11):1265-1270.

   Electromyographic analysis showed that the bear hug test performed at 45° of shoulder flexion effectively isolates the subscapularis. A 20% increase in activation of the upper subscapularis compared with the lower subscapularis was not significant. At 90° of shoulder flexion, the bear hug test significantly isolated the lower subscapularis compared with the upper subscapularis and other muscles.

27. Koo SS, Burkhart SS: Subscapularis tendon tears: Identifying mid to distal footprint disruptions. *Arthroscopy* 2010;26(8):1130-1134.

   An arthroscopic technique for identifying mid to distal subscapularis tendon tears is described. A 70° arthroscope was used to carefully examine the medial sidewall of the bicipital groove for evidence of occult disruptions of the subscapularis tendon, which can easily be missed.

28. Denard PJ, Lädermann A, Burkhart SS: Arthroscopic management of subscapularis tears. *Sports Med Arthrosc* 2011;19(4):333-341.

    A review of subscapularis anatomy and function is presented along with the means to effectively identify and arthroscopically manage subscapularis pathology. The results of arthroscopic treatment of subscapularis lesions are discussed.

29. Burkhart SS, Tehrany AM: Arthroscopic subscapularis tendon repair: Technique and preliminary results. *Arthroscopy* 2002;18(5):454-463.

30. Ticker JB, Burkhart SS: Why repair the subscapularis? A logical rationale. *Arthroscopy* 2011;27(8):1123-1128.

    Reasons are presented for repairing the subscapularis if it is part of an anterosuperior rotator cuff tear. Maintaining the soft-tissue attachment to the supraspinatus and repairing the subscapularis help reduce the supraspinatus tear, restore the anterior rotator cable attachment, and provide added security to the overall repair.

31. Lo IK, Burkhart SS: The comma sign: An arthroscopic guide to the torn subscapularis tendon. *Arthroscopy* 2003;19(3):334-337.

32. Nové-Josserand L, Edwards TB, O'Connor DP, Walch G: The acromiohumeral and coracohumeral intervals are abnormal in rotator cuff tears with muscular fatty degeneration. *Clin Orthop Relat Res* 2005;433(433):90-96.

33. Richards DP, Burkhart SS, Campbell SE: Relation between narrowed coracohumeral distance and subscapularis tears. *Arthroscopy* 2005;21(10):1223-1228.

34. Park JY, Park JS, Jung JK, Kumar P, Oh KS: Suture-bridge subscapularis tendon repair technique using low anterior portals. *Knee Surg Sports Traumatol Arthrosc* 2011;19(2):303-306.

    Two low-anterior accessory portals were used for the arthroscopic repair of subscapularis tears. The purpose was to facilitate the use of a double-row suture-bridge technique for restoring the anatomic footprint of the subscapularis.

35. Lo IK, Burkhart SS, Parten PM: Surgery about the coracoid: Neurovascular structures at risk. *Arthroscopy* 2004;20(6):591-595.

36. Kleist KD, Freehill MQ, Hamilton L, Buss DD, Fritts H: Computed tomography analysis of the coracoid process and anatomic structures of the shoulder after arthroscopic coracoid decompression: A cadaveric study. *J Shoulder Elbow Surg* 2007;16(2):245-250.

    Arthroscopic coracoplasty was performed on five cadaver specimens. Preoperative and postoperative CT showed substantial changes in the morphology of the coracoid and the subcoracoid space. Resection of 10 mm or less of the coracoid tip appears to prevent undue disruption of the adjacent soft-tissue structures.

37. Edwards TB, Walch G, Sirveaux F, et al: Repair of tears of the subscapularis. *J Bone Joint Surg Am* 2005;87(4):725-730.

38. Bennett WF: Arthroscopic bicipital sheath repair: Two-year follow-up with pulley lesions. *Arthroscopy* 2004;20(9):964-973.

39. Denard PJ, Burkhart SS: Medialization of the subscapularis footprint does not affect functional outcome of arthroscopic repair. *Arthroscopy* 2012;28(11):1608-1614.

    Subscapularis tears involving 100% of the tendinous insertion were retrospectively reviewed. Some patients underwent a repair to the anatomic footprint, and the others had the footprint medialized an average of 5 mm before repair. At a minimum 2-year follow-up, there was no substantial between-group difference in functional outcomes. Level of evidence: III.

40. Lo IK, Burkhart SS: The interval slide in continuity: A method of mobilizing the anterosuperior rotator cuff without disrupting the tear margins. *Arthroscopy* 2004;20(4):435-441.

41. Denard PJ, Jiwani AZ, Lädermann A, Burkhart SS: Long-term outcome of a consecutive series of subscapularis tendon tears repaired arthroscopically. *Arthroscopy* 2012;28(11):1587-1591.

    At a minimum 7-year follow-up of 79 patients who underwent arthroscopic repair of a subscapularis tendon tear, 83% had a good or excellent clinical result, and 92% were satisfied. Both isolated and combined tears were included; 63% involved a massive rotator cuff tear. Level of evidence: IV.

42. Lafosse L, Lanz U, Saintmard B, Campens C: Arthroscopic repair of subscapularis tear: Surgical technique and results. *Orthop Traumatol Surg Res* 2010;96(8, suppl):S99-S108.

    Extensive subscapularis tears were arthroscopically repaired in 23 patients. The surgical technique is described. Short-term follow-up revealed significant improvement in clinical measures. The failure rate was 9%. Level of evidence: IV.

43. Denard PJ, Lädermann A, Burkhart SS: Double-row fixation of upper subscapularis tears with a single suture anchor. *Arthroscopy* 2011;27(8):1142-1149.

    A simplified, efficient technique for double-row fixation of upper subscapularis tears was described. Knotless anchor fixation was used to repair lesions involving as much as 50% of the superior tendon attachment.

44. Wellmann M, Wiebringhaus P, Lodde I, et al: Biomechanical evaluation of a single-row versus double-row repair for complete subscapularis tears. *Knee Surg*

Sports Traumatol Arthrosc 2009;17(12):1477-1484, 48, 4.

A biomechanical cadaver study found that a double-row repair of a simulated subscapularis tear had a substantially higher stiffness and ultimate load to failure than a single-row technique. Tendon elongation before failure was substantially lower with a double-row repair.

45. Charousset C, Grimberg J, Duranthon LD, Bellaiche L, Petrover D: Can a double-row anchorage technique improve tendon healing in arthroscopic rotator cuff repair? A prospective, nonrandomized, comparative study of double-row and single-row anchorage techniques with computed tomographic arthrography tendon healing assessment. *Am J Sports Med* 2007;35(8): 1247-1253.

Two groups of patients underwent arthroscopic repair of a rotator cuff tear using a single-row or double-row technique. No significant difference was noted in short-term clinical outcomes. CTA revealed significantly better tendon healing in those with a double-row repair. Level of evidence: II.

46. Yoo JC, Kim JH, Lee YS, Park JH, Kang HJ: Arthroscopic double mattress repair in incomplete subscapularis tears. *Orthopedics* 2008;31(9):851-854.

A technique for the arthroscopic repair of upper subscapularis tendon tears was described. A double-loaded suture anchor was used in a double, inverted horizontal mattress repair of the torn tendon to its bone footprint.

47. Denard PJ, Burkhart SS: A new method for knotless fixation of an upper subscapularis tear. *Arthroscopy* 2011;27(6):861-866.

A novel technique uses knotless fixation for the repair of subscapularis tears involving as much as 50% of the upper tendinous insertion. This efficient, straightforward technique can be used for most subscapularis tears.

Chapter 23

Arthroscopic Assessment and Treatment of Anterior Glenoid Bone Loss

Frank Martetschläger, MD   Daniel Rios, MD   Robert E. Boykin, MD   Peter J. Millett, MD, MSc

Introduction

Bony deficiency of the anteroinferior glenoid can contribute to recurrent glenohumeral instability.[1] Primary etiologies of this bony deficiency include fracture after an acute shoulder dislocation or bony erosion in patients with chronic anterior instability. The incidence of bony Bankart lesions ranges from 4% to 70% after an acute shoulder dislocation. Men are more likely than women to sustain this injury.[2]

Bony Bankart lesions most often occur between the 2-o'clock and 4-o'clock positions (in a right shoulder) and have been classified into three types according to the percentage of glenoid bone loss. Type I represents a displaced avulsion fracture, and type II represents a malunited avulsion fracture of the anteroinferior glenoid rim. Type III is defined based on the percentage of glenoid erosion; type IIIA represents a less-than-25% bone loss, and type IIIB represents a more-than-25% bone loss.

It is well known that glenoid bone loss is associated with an increased risk of surgical failure after arthroscopic soft-tissue repair.[3] Bony reconstruction is therefore recommended in patients with anteroinferior glenoid bone loss of more than 20%.[3] Although bony reconstruction historically has been performed as an open procedure, in recent years open procedures have been supplanted by advanced arthroscopic procedures.[4-7]

Biomechanics

Numerous biomechanical studies have quantified the critical amount of bone loss that results in recurrent instability even after soft-tissue repair. In a cadaver study, a glenoid width-to-length ratio of less than 21% was found to significantly decrease stability.[8] Another study found that osseous defects resulting in a width-to-length ratio of more than 20% significantly decreased anterior instability.[9] A third cadaver study found that a 50% glenoid width reduction reduced the resistance to humeral dislocation by 30% in comparison with the intact state.[10]

The relationship of the convex humeral head to the concave glenolabral surface, as well as the dynamic pull of the rotator cuff, illustrates the effect of concavity compression on glenohumeral kinematics.[11] Significant glenoid bone loss creates stress risers resulting in pain and further osteolysis. Mean contact pressures were found to be almost doubled in the anteroinferior quadrant, with a concomitant increase in peak pressures, after a 20% loss of glenoid width.[12] Therefore, based on the most recent biomechanical data, repair should be considered if the patient has glenoid bone loss resulting in a 20% to 25% decrease in the width-to-length ratio; the purpose is to prevent recurrent instability as a result of continued osteolysis and a decrease in static stabilization.

Evaluation

History and Physical Examination

A thorough history and physical examination with specific provocative tests are helpful to establish a diagnosis of glenohumeral instability. The number of previous dislocations, the activities that cause apprehension, and

Dr. Martetschläger or an immediate family member has received nonincome support (such as equipment or services), commercially derived honoraria, or other non–research-related funding (such as paid travel) from Arthrex and Steadman Philippon Research Institute. Dr. Millett or an immediate family member has received royalties from Arthrex; serves as a paid consultant to Arthrex; has stock or stock options held in Game Ready and VuMedi; and has received research or institutional support from Arthrex, OrthoRehab, Össur Americas, Siemens Medical Solutions USA, Smith & Nephew, and ConMed Linvatec. Neither of the following authors nor any immediate family member has received anything of value from or owns stock in a commercial company or institution related directly or indirectly to the subject of this article: Dr. Rios and Dr. Boykin.

previous trauma or surgical intervention are particularly useful aspects of the patient history.

The anterior apprehension, relocation, load-and-shift, and anterior-posterior drawer tests can reveal anterior and/or posterior instability after comparison with the contralateral shoulder. It has been shown that the patient's sense of apprehension is much more likely to be diagnostic of instability than the occurrence of pain when these provocative maneuvers are performed.[13] Testing for global, symptomatic ligamentous laxity as well as the sulcus sign (in both 0° and 90° of abduction) is critically important for the diagnosis of multidirectional instability.

The diagnostic usefulness of specific provocative tests such as the load-and-shift, relocation, and anterior-posterior drawer tests is greater when anesthesia is used to eliminate the patient's discomfort and muscle tension.[13] At the time of surgery, the patient should be examined under anesthesia to assess the amount of humeral translation and to evaluate for the presence of crepitus, which may indicate a bony lesion.[14] As always, the findings are compared with the contralateral shoulder. Genetically determined ligamentous laxity should be differentiated from pathologic laxity as the cause of symptoms.

Imaging

The initial radiographic evaluation of all patients with symptomatic instability should include true AP (in internal and external rotation), axillary lateral, scapular Y, and apical oblique views.[15] In addition, the West Point axillary view may be useful to assess for glenoid bone loss, and the Stryker notch view to visualize an associated Hill-Sachs lesion. Bone loss is best evaluated using axial and sagittal CT sequences, and three-dimensional reconstruction may be useful for delineating complex defects. Three-dimensional CT has been shown to accurately predict the need for bone grafting and has been used to create an anatomic glenoid index to measure preoperative glenoid bone loss[16,17] (Figure 1).

Arthroscopic Diagnosis

Diagnostic arthroscopy is the gold standard for confirmation of an osseous glenoid defect found on imaging studies. A view from the rotator interval portal is of particular use in determining the percentage of glenoid bone loss. In most patients with an acute traumatic injury, the osseous fragment is sequestered by the surrounding labroligamentous complex, which also may be injured.[18]

In 2002, a method for the arthroscopic quantification of glenoid bone loss was presented. This method uses the so-called glenoid bare spot as a reference point designating the geometric center of the inferior glenoid[1] (Figure 2). Because the best-fitting circle centered on the bare spot has an average diameter of 24 mm, a measurement taken from the bare spot to the location of bone loss is divided by 24 to represent the approximate percentage of remaining glenoid. For example, a

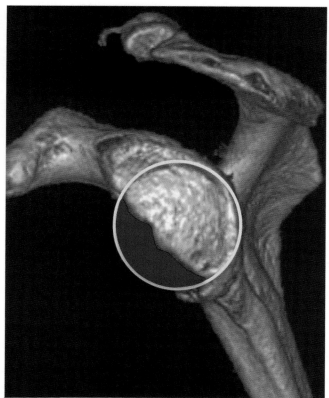

Figure 1   Three-dimensional CT scan of a left shoulder showing anteroinferior bone loss. A normal glenoid would completely fill the circle. The anterior red area represents the amount of bone loss.

calculation of 80% remaining glenoid indicates a 20% glenoid bone loss. This percentage is used to guide surgical management decisions.

Arthroscopic Options for Glenoid Bone Loss

Surgical Indications and Decision-Making

Surgical treatment is recommended for patients with symptomatic instability in the presence of glenoid bone loss.[13] Based on clinical and biomechanical studies, reconstruction of the bony glenoid is recommended if the bony deficiency exceeds 20% to 25% of the inferior glenoid diameter.[3,8,9,12] The threshold for surgical intervention may be decreased for a patient at high risk of recurrent instability, such as a contact athlete.

Reconstruction of the glenoid can be achieved by fixation of the fracture fragment. If the defect is not amenable to primary repair, an autograft or allograft bone block can be used to restore stability. In a patient with attritional glenoid deficiency, a bone graft transfer typically is recommended.[19]

Biomechanical studies have found that a glenoid defect resulting in a 20% glenoid bone loss is amenable to soft-tissue repair that reliably restores stability.[9] Thus,

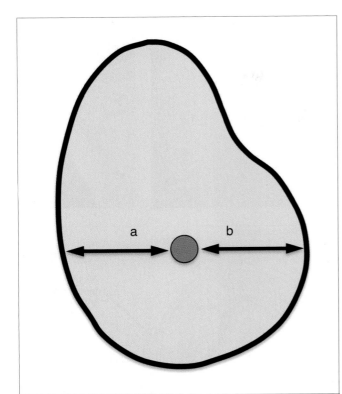

Figure 2 Schematic drawing showing the distance from the glenoid bare spot *(center circle)* to the posterior glenoid rim and the anterior glenoid rim, as measured using a calibrated probe. If the distance (b) from the center to the anterior glenoid rim is less than 50% of the distance (a) from the center to the posterior glenoid rim, the bone loss is at least 25% of the inferior glenoid diameter.

in patients with a glenoid defect of less than 20% of the inferior glenoid diameter, soft-tissue repair (Bankart repair) is recommended. In patients with an engaging Hill-Sachs lesion, the remplissage procedure (first described in 2008) can biomechanically augment stability.[20,21]

In the presence of a bone fragment amenable to repair, arthroscopic internal fixation can be performed using suture anchors or screws.[2,4,5,22,23] The bony Bankart bridge technique, first described in 2009, uses a double row of anchors to secure the bony fragment back to the glenoid rim.[5] For patients with irreparable fragments or attritional deficiency resulting in a defect of greater than 25% of the inferior glenoid diameter, arthroscopic Bristow and Latarjet procedures and osteochondral autograft or allograft procedures have been well described.[21-28]

Arthroscopic Bankart Repair With Remplissage

A standard arthroscopic Bankart repair is performed when, after diagnostic arthroscopy, glenoid bone loss is estimated to be less than 20% of the intact inferior gle-

noid diameter. In addition to the typical portals for an arthroscopic Bankart repair, an accessory portal is placed superolateral to the posterior portal for transtendinous suture anchor placement during remplissage. The glenoid suture anchors can be placed first, with sutures passed through the capsulolabral tissue in a standard manner for anterior and anteroinferior labral repair. To facilitate anchor insertion into the humerus, the sutures are not tied.[20-28]

The bone bed of the Hill-Sachs lesion is prepared with a shaver or angled ring curette through the posterior portal, resulting in mild bleeding without decortication. For visualization, the arthroscope is inserted into the anterosuperolateral portal. Typically, two double-loaded anchors are placed into the defect. A cannula is withdrawn external to the infraspinatus, and the bursa is removed from the subacromial space to allow tying of the sutures. A penetrating grasper is used to pass the sutures through the infraspinatus tendon and posterior capsule both proximal and distal to the initial entry portal and just lateral to the musculotendinous junction. The inferior suture is tied before the superior suture while the arm is in neutral position. The infraspinatus tendon is secured to the humeral defect to complete the standard Bankart repair. Alternatively, the remplissage can be performed before the Bankart repair, and all sutures can be tied at the end of the procedure to balance the anterior and posterior repairs.

Arthroscopic Anchor Repair (The Bony Bankart Bridge Procedure)

The bony Bankart bridge technique uses two-point fixation to compress the bony fragment back to its origin.[5] A high anterosuperior portal and an accessory anteroinferior portal are established, and a 70° arthroscope is introduced to visualize the glenoid neck medial to the fracture site. The labrum and the inferior glenohumeral ligament (IGHL) complex typically are attached to the bony fragment and should be preserved. Instruments are placed through both anterior portals to mobilize the bony fragment as well as the IGHL as a sleeve of continuous tissue inferior to the 6-o'clock position. To enhance bone-to-bone healing, the glenoid neck and the fractured surface of the bony fragment are prepared with a shaver. An elevator is introduced through the anterosuperior portal, and the bony fragment is elevated so that the first anchor can be placed medially on the glenoid neck. This anchor provides the medial fixation point for the bridge. If the fragment is small, only one medial anchor is necessary; it is placed medial to the donor site on the glenoid neck in the midportion of the fracture. If the fragments are relatively large, two medial anchors are placed. Both limbs of the suture are passed through the soft tissues medial to the bony fragment using a 45° curved shuttling device (SutureLasso [Arthrex]) and are shuttled through the anteroinferior cannula. A suture anchor is placed just inferior to the bony fragment on the glenoid rim to secure

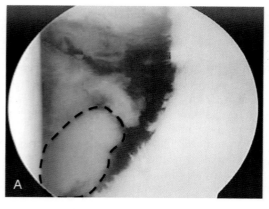
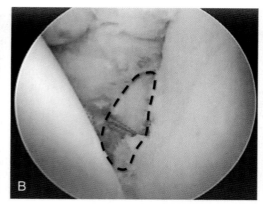
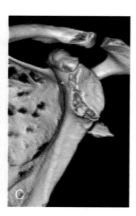

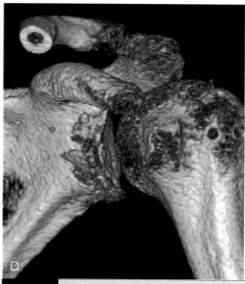
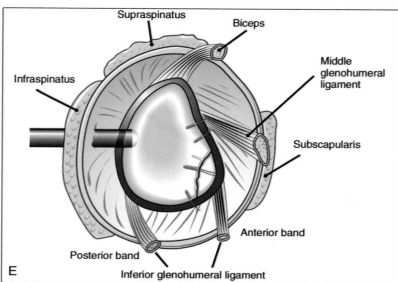

Figure 3 Arthroscopic images of a left shoulder from the posterior, showing a large bony Bankart lesion *(dashed outline)* before **(A)** and after **(B)** refixation of the bony fragment using the Bankart bridge technique. Three-dimensional CT reconstruction of a left shoulder with a large anterior bony Bankart lesion before **(C)** and after **(D)** Bankart bridge repair. **E,** Schematic drawing showing a final bony Bankart bridge repair, with a reduced bony Bankart piece, repaired labrum, and shifted capsule and IGHL complex. (Panel E adapted with permission from Millett PJ, Braun S: The "bony Bankart bridge" procedure: A new arthroscopic technique for reduction and internal fixation of a bony Bankart lesion. *Arthroscopy* 2009;25[1]:102-105.)

the labrum and IGHL complex. The medial suture limb is passed through the IGHL complex, shifting the IGHL complex and labrum superiorly and medially, thereby tightening the axillary pouch. The size of the shift is controlled with a grasper through the anterosuperior portal. The sutures are tied with a sliding-locking Weston knot backed up with two alternating half-hitch knots. Two inferior anchors can be used if a large fragment is present. Appropriate tension for fracture reduction is assessed by determining the optimal position for the lateral fixation anchor on the glenoid face. A drill hole is placed on the glenoid face at the cartilage-fracture margin. The two free limbs of the medial suture anchor are fed into a 3.5-mm knotless anchor (Bio-PushLock [Arthrex]) and tensioned simultaneously as the anchor is inserted into the drill hole. During this process, the bony fragment is compressed back into its donor bed, and an arthroscopic osteosynthesis is achieved. The security of the construct is tested with a probe, and the free limbs are cut flush with the lateral anchor. The superior capsule, labrum, and middle glenohumeral ligament are repaired superiorly to the bony Bankart bridge. Fixing of any torn superior labrum is recommended to provide additional rotational stability. Depending on the size of the bony fragment, one or more bridging techniques can be used to secure the fragment (**Figure 3**).

Arthroscopic Bone Graft Repair

A technique for arthroscopic bone grafting of glenoid defects begins by first establishing an anteroinferior working portal through the rotator cuff interval and an anterosuperior viewing portal behind the biceps tendon.[26] Visualization through the anterosuperior portal

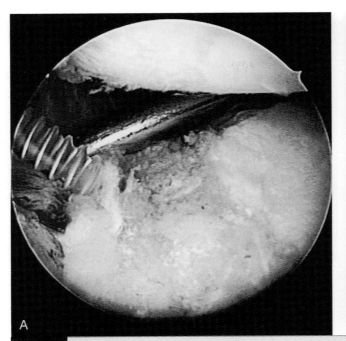
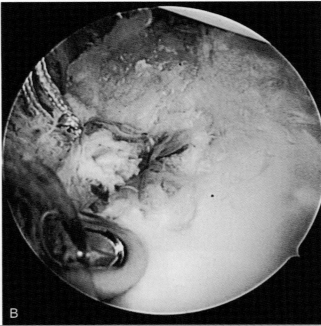

Figure 4 Arthroscopic images showing bone graft reconstruction of a right shoulder using two 2.7- to 3.7-mm Bio-Compression screws **(A)** and final reattachment of the capsuloligamentous complex **(B)**. FasTak suture anchors armed with FiberWire (Arthrex) are placed superiorly and inferiorly to the graft, and horizontal mattress stitches are used. (Reproduced with permission from Scheibel M, Kraus N, Diederichs G, Haas NP: Arthroscopic reconstruction of chronic anteroinferior glenoid defect using an autologous tricortical iliac crest bone grafting technique. Arch Orthop Trauma Surg 2008;128[11]:1295-1300.)

allows for the establishment of an anteroinferior portal through the subscapularis muscle. Two 8.25-mm twist-in cannulas are inserted into the anteroinferior and deep anteroinferior portals, and a 6-mm cannula is used in the posterior portal. A bone graft is harvested from the iliac crest and is shaped using an oscillating saw to approximate the morphology of the anteroinferior glenoid.[29] Through the anteroinferior portal, the capsulolabral complex is mobilized medially beyond the 6-o'clock position, and the glenoid bony surface is débrided with a burr or shaver to create a bleeding bed on which to place the graft. After the cannula is removed from the anterosuperior portal, the graft can be placed intra-articularly using a clamp for insertion. When the graft has been correctly positioned and the graft–joint line relationship has been examined using a hooked probe or Wissinger rod, the graft is temporarily fixed with Kirschner wires. Three Kirschner wires are inserted in line through the anteroinferior and deep anteroinferior portals and percutaneously through the upper third of the subscapularis tendon. The inferior and superior Kirschner wires are overdrilled, and two 2.7- to 3.7-mm cannulated Bio-Compression screws (Arthrex) are inserted for final fixation of the graft. If necessary, the graft is polished to match the native glenoid using a small burr. Finally, the capsuloligamentous tissue is reconstructed using two anchors, one of which is placed superiorly and the other inferiorly to the graft (**Figure 4**).

Arthroscopic Coracoid Transfer

In 2007, an arthroscopic Latarjet procedure was described in which the procedure is divided into five distinct steps: exposure, coracoid preparation, coracoid drilling and osteotomy, coracoid transfer, and bone graft fixation.[25] To achieve appropriate exposure, an anterior capsulectomy is performed with a shaver, and the rotator interval is opened between the superior border of the coracohumeral ligament and the superior part of the subscapularis to allow exposure of the coracoid process. In a right shoulder, the anterior labrum and the middle glenohumeral ligament are resected between the 2-o'clock and 5-o'clock positions, thereby retaining the superior band of the IGHL attachment. The coracohumeral ligament insertion is sectioned next to the coracoid, and the conjoined tendon is mobilized from the deep surface of the deltoid. The bone bed at the anteroinferior glenoid rim (2-o'clock to 6-o'clock) is prepared with a shaver to create a bleeding surface for bony integration.

During the second stage, the coracoid and the axillary nerve (located at the anterior border of the subscapularis) are exposed with the arthroscope in the lateral portal and the anterior portal is used as a working portal. The border of the conjoined tendon is defined medially and laterally from the pectoralis minor, and the brachial plexus is subsequently exposed. A coracoid portal is established as a working portal between the base and the tip of the coracoid process. The arthro-

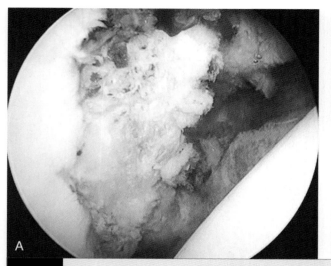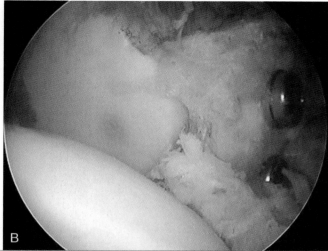

Figure 5   Arthroscopic images showing Latarjet reconstruction of a right shoulder. The coracoid bone graft is fixed to the anterior glenoid rim by two cannulated screws. The correct positioning of the graft is verified from the posterior (**A**) and anterior (**B**) portals. (Reproduced with permission from Agneskirchner JD, Haag M, Lafosse M: Arthroskopischer Korakoidtransfer. *Der Orthopade* 2011;40:41-51.)

scope is inserted through the anterior portal, and the pectoralis minor tendon is sectioned as close as possible to the coracoid process to avoid injuring the plexus, which lies just behind the pectoralis minor. After the tendon is sectioned, the brachial plexus and the axillary neurovascular bundle can be seen. Two vertical drill holes are created 8 mm apart into the inferior half of the coracoid using a 2.9-mm drill and a special drill guide. A suture is passed through the two holes with two long hooks forming a U shape and shuttled out through the coracoid portal. The osteotomy is performed using an osteotome placed 2 to 2.5 cm from the coracoid tip at the junction of the horizontal and vertical parts of the coracoid. The resected coracoid with conjoined tendon is mobilized inferiorly and medially, and the anterior subscapularis is exposed.

During the final stage, the arthroscope is placed in the lateral portal. An anteroinferior portal must be established through the subscapularis tendon by splitting it horizontally. A switching stick inserted through the posterior portal and directed through the subscapularis split works as a lever arm to elevate the upper third of the subscapularis for passage of the graft. Through a cannula, guide screws are placed into the drill holes over the sutures to allow control of the graft during the positioning. The graft is passed through the subscapularis split and placed at the anterior glenoid rim from the 2-o'clock to the 6-o'clock position. With the arthroscope in the anterior portal and the anteroinferior portal used for working, a Kirschner wire is drilled through one of the screws. To avoid distraction of the graft from the glenoid and scapular neck, one screw must be completely inserted before the second screw is placed. Therefore, the guide screw is removed, the wire is overdrilled using a 3.5-mm cannulated drill bit, and a 4.5-mm screw is inserted. The second screw is placed in a similar fashion, and both

screws are tightened under direct visualization. Any step-off at the glenoid-graft interface is corrected using a burr. **Figure 5** shows the final result.

Postoperative Rehabilitation

The rehabilitation protocol should be individualized for the patient. The overall stability of the repair, the size of the treated bony lesion, other concomitant procedures, and the overall health and goals of the patient should be considered. Progression of therapy and return to activity also are determined by these patient-specific factors.

Complications

Multiple authors have reported relatively low complication rates after arthroscopic procedures to address bony glenoid deficiency.[19,22,24,30-32] However, complications such as infection, bleeding, neurovascular damage and anesthetic risks can occur. Because a thin area of bone usually is involved in arthroscopic bony stabilization, hardware complications such as loosening, excessive length with irritation to surrounding structures, and graft resorption can occur.[33]

Arthroscopic bone-grafting procedures can pose a risk of neurovascular injury because of their proximity to neurovascular structures. Cadaver studies have highlighted the advantages of arthroscopically assisted procedures, including optimization of graft position and adequate preparation of the anterior glenoid.[34] These advantages may reduce the risk of early nonunion or late arthritis, both of which are commonly associated with open techniques.

Outcomes

Some experts have concluded that patients with a large bony defect should not undergo arthroscopic soft-tissue stabilization because of its high failure rates.[3,8,35] However, successful outcomes were reported with arthroscopic Bankart repair, even in shoulders with a large (greater than 25%) glenoid defect, as evaluated with three-dimensional CT.[18] At a mean 34-month follow-up of 21 patients who underwent arthroscopic anchor stabilization of a 20% to 30% bony deficiency of the anteroinferior glenoid, 2 of 21 patients (9.5%) had recurrent subluxation, and 1 of 21 (4.8%) had a recurrent dislocation requiring revision.[19] Patients with a bony fragment had an improved outcome compared with those who had attritional bone loss. At 26-month follow-up after an arthroscopic Latarjet procedure, 91% of patients had an excellent clinical outcome score, and 9% had a good score.[32] However, only 35 of the 100 patients were available for clinical review at 26 months. Longer term studies are needed to improve the understanding of performance and patient satisfaction after arthroscopic management of instability with severe bone loss.

The Role of Open Surgery

Advances in arthroscopic techniques have provided surgeons with the ability to perform almost all procedures for instability through an arthroscopic approach. Despite the promising short-term results, however, long-term outcomes for these techniques are not available.[19,22,32,36,37] Many of these techniques require proficiency in advanced arthroscopy. It should be remembered that open techniques provide reliably good results and that the use of a deltopectoral approach generally precludes morbidity.[38-40] Therefore, open surgery remains an important treatment option, particularly if the surgeon lacks the equipment, experience, or technical expertise needed to perform an arthroscopic repair. Conversion to an open procedure may be required during revision surgery, surgery for a soft-tissue deficiency, or surgery with difficult visualization. As arthroscopic techniques continue to evolve, surgeons should carefully consider the indications based on their level of skill as well as the spectrum of pathology in glenohumeral instability.[41]

Summary

Recent improvements in arthroscopic shoulder surgical technique, instrumentation, and implants have allowed minimally invasive management of anterior instability in patients with significant glenoid bone loss. Although these techniques are promising, their true value must be proven by long-term observation. In contrast, open procedures historically have provided good to excellent results. It is therefore important for the surgeon to be proficient in open techniques, especially if a complicated arthroscopic procedure may require conversion to an open procedure. Careful surgical planning is the key to the successful treatment of patients with instability in the presence of glenoid bone loss. The choice of surgical technique should be based on the surgeon's level of experience, the pathology most likely to be encountered, and the patient's comfort throughout the surgical and postsurgical phases.

Annotated References

1. Burkhart SS, Debeer JF, Tehrany AM, Parten PM: Quantifying glenoid bone loss arthroscopically in shoulder instability. *Arthroscopy* 2002;18(5):488-491.

2. Porcellini G, Paladini P, Campi F, Paganelli M: Long-term outcome of acute versus chronic bony Bankart lesions managed arthroscopically. *Am J Sports Med* 2007;35(12):2067-2072.

   A modified Bankart technique was used to repair the capsulolabral complex and fix the avulsed bone fragment with suture anchors in 65 patients. One of the 41 patients with acute injury and 1 of the 24 with chronic injury had a traumatic redislocation. The mean Rowe score increased from 59 to 92 and from 43.5 to 61, respectively (P < 0.001).

3. Burkhart SS, De Beer JF: Traumatic glenohumeral bone defects and their relationship to failure of arthroscopic Bankart repairs: Significance of the inverted-pear glenoid and the humeral engaging Hill-Sachs lesion. *Arthroscopy* 2000;16(7):677-694.

4. Kim KC, Rhee KJ, Shin HD: Arthroscopic three-point double-row repair for acute bony Bankart lesions. *Knee Surg Sports Traumatol Arthrosc* 2009;17(1):102-106.

   An arthroscopic technique for bony Bankart repair was reported to confer effective, firm three-point fixation of the bony Bankart lesion without the suture material crossing the glenoid cavity.

5. Millett PJ, Braun S: The "bony Bankart bridge" procedure: A new arthroscopic technique for reduction and internal fixation of a bony Bankart lesion. *Arthroscopy* 2009;25(1):102-105.

   An easy, reproducible technique for arthroscopic reduction and suture anchor fixation of bony Bankart fragments created a nontilting two-point fixation that compresses the fragment into its bed.

6. Mochizuki Y, Hachisuka H, Kashiwagi K, Oomae H, Yokoya S, Ochi M: Arthroscopic autologous bone graft with arthroscopic Bankart repair for a large bony defect lesion caused by recurrent shoulder dislocation. *Arthroscopy* 2007;23(6):e1-e4.

   An arthroscopic autologous bone graft repair was used for a patient with recurrent dislocation of the shoulder joint and a large bony Bankart lesion. Two bones were harvested from the lateral side of the acromion and transplanted to the large bony defect of the glenoid.

7. Porcellini G, Campi F, Paladini P: Arthroscopic approach to acute bony Bankart lesion. *Arthroscopy* 2002;18(7):764-769.

8. Itoi E, Lee SB, Berglund LJ, Berge LL, An KN: The effect of a glenoid defect on anteroinferior stability of the shoulder after Bankart repair: A cadaveric study. *J Bone Joint Surg Am* 2000;82(1):35-46.

9. Yamamoto N, Itoi E, Abe H, et al: Effect of an anterior glenoid defect on anterior shoulder stability: A cadaveric study. *Am J Sports Med* 2009;37(5):949-954.

    In eight cadaver shoulders, an osseous defect was created stepwise with a 2-mm increment of the defect width. The stability ratio was used to evaluate joint stability. An osseous defect of at least 20% of the glenoid length significantly decreased anterior stability.

10. Gerber C, Nyffeler RW: Classification of glenohumeral joint instability. *Clin Orthop Relat Res* 2002;400:65-76.

11. Lippitt S, Matsen F: Mechanisms of glenohumeral joint stability. *Clin Orthop Relat Res* 1993;291:20-28.

12. Greis PE, Scuderi MG, Mohr A, Bachus KN, Burks RT: Glenohumeral articular contact areas and pressures following labral and osseous injury to the anteroinferior quadrant of the glenoid. *J Shoulder Elbow Surg* 2002;11(5):442-451.

13. Bushnell BD, Creighton RA, Herring MM: Bony instability of the shoulder. *Arthroscopy* 2008;24(9):1061-1073.

    Unrecognized large bony lesions have been identified as a primary cause of recurrent instability or failure of arthroscopic reconstruction for instability, and the diagnosis is difficult. Developments in the diagnosis and treatment of bony instability were reviewed.

14. Matsen FA III, Chebli C, Lippitt S; American Academy of Orthopaedic Surgeons: Principles for the evaluation and management of shoulder instability. *J Bone Joint Surg Am* 2006;88(3):648-659.

15. Bushnell BD, Creighton RA, Herring MM: Hybrid treatment of engaging Hill-Sachs lesions: Arthroscopic capsulolabral repair and limited posterior approach for bone-grafting. *Tech Shoulder Elbow Surg* 2007;8: 194-203.

    A hybrid technique is described in which an engaging Hill-Sachs lesion was treated through arthroscopic capsulolabral repair coupled with an open posterior approach to the humeral head, which involved splitting the posterior deltoid and the infraspinatus muscles.

16. Chuang TY, Adams CR, Burkhart SS: Use of preoperative three-dimensional computed tomography to quantify glenoid bone loss in shoulder instability. *Arthroscopy* 2008;24(4):376-382.

The glenoid index, which is calculated from three-dimensional CT, accurately predicted the need for bone grafting in 24 of 25 patients (96%). Three-dimensional CT can be used for preoperative planning and patient counseling.

17. Nofsinger C, Browning B, Burkhart SS, Pedowitz RA: Objective preoperative measurement of anterior glenoid bone loss: A pilot study of a computer-based method using unilateral 3-dimensional computed tomography. *Arthroscopy* 2011;27(3):322-329.

    A CT-based study confirmed that the normal inferior glenoid surface is a nearly perfect circle with remarkably low variability. A simple, reliable method was described for determining the anatomic glenoid index, used to create an anatomic preoperative description of bone loss.

18. Sugaya H, Moriishi J, Kanisawa I, Tsuchiya A: Arthroscopic osseous Bankart repair for chronic recurrent traumatic anterior glenohumeral instability. *J Bone Joint Surg Am* 2005;87(8):1752-1760.

19. Mologne TS, Provencher MT, Menzel KA, Vachon TA, Dewing CB: Arthroscopic stabilization in patients with an inverted pear glenoid: Results in patients with bone loss of the anterior glenoid. *Am J Sports Med* 2007; 35(8):1276-1283.

    Twenty-one of 23 patients undergoing arthroscopic stabilization surgery were found to have a bony deficiency of 20% to 30% at a mean 34-month follow-up. The procedure can yield a stable shoulder, but outcomes were less predictable with attritional bone loss.

20. Koo SS, Burkhart SS, Ochoa E: Arthroscopic double-pulley remplissage technique for engaging Hill-Sachs lesions in anterior shoulder instability repairs. *Arthroscopy* 2009;25(11):1343-1348.

    A new technique for arthroscopic remplissage was described, in which the eyelets of the two suture anchors were used as pulleys and a double-mattress suture was created.

21. Purchase RJ, Wolf EM, Hobgood ER, Pollock ME, Smalley CC: Hill-Sachs "remplissage": An arthroscopic solution for the engaging Hill-Sachs lesion. *Arthroscopy* 2008;24(6):723-726.

    An arthroscopic technique was described for the treatment of traumatic shoulder instability in patients with glenoid bone loss and a large Hill-Sachs lesion. Capsulotenodesis of the posterior capsule and infraspinatus tendon was used to fill the Hill-Sachs lesion.

22. Sugaya H, Moriishi J, Kanisawa I, Tsuchiya A: Arthroscopic osseous Bankart repair for chronic recurrent traumatic anterior glenohumeral instability: Surgical technique. *J Bone Joint Surg Am* 2006;88(suppl 1 pt 2:)159-169.

23. Zhang J, Jiang C: A new "double-pulley" dual-row technique for arthroscopic fixation of bony Bankart lesion. *Knee Surg Sports Traumatol Arthrosc* 2011; 19(9):1558-1562.

24. Boileau P, Bicknell RT, El Fegoun AB, Chuinard C: Arthroscopic Bristow procedure for anterior instability in shoulders with a stretched or deficient capsule: The "belt-and-suspenders" operative technique and preliminary results. *Arthroscopy* 2007;23(6):593-601.

   A combined arthroscopic Bankart repair was used with a transfer of the coracobiceps tendon to reinforce the deficient anterior capsule in 36 patients. At a minimum 1-year follow-up, 28 patients (78%) were very satisfied, 5 (14%) were satisfied, and 3 (8%) were disappointed.

25. Lafosse L, Lejeune E, Bouchard A, Kakuda C, Gobezie R, Kochhar T: The arthroscopic Latarjet procedure for the treatment of anterior shoulder instability. *Arthroscopy* 2007;23(11):e1-e5.

   The outcomes of 100 patients were reported at 26-month follow-up after an arthroscopic Latarjet procedure. Patient-reported outcome scores were 91% excellent and 9% good. The all-arthroscopic Latarjet technique had excellent results through midterm follow-up, with minimal complications and good graft positioning.

26. Scheibel M, Kraus N, Diederichs G, Haas NP: Arthroscopic reconstruction of chronic anteroinferior glenoid defect using an autologous tricortical iliac crest bone grafting technique. *Arch Orthop Trauma Surg* 2008;128(11):1295-1300.

   An all-arthroscopic reconstruction technique for the anteroinferior glenoid included autologous iliac crest bone grafting using Bio-Compression screws and a capsulolabral repair using suture anchors.

27. Taverna E, Golanò P, Pascale V, Battistella F: An arthroscopic bone graft procedure for treating anterior-inferior glenohumeral instability. *Knee Surg Sports Traumatol Arthrosc* 2008;16(9):872-875.

   An arthroscopic method for treating anteroinferior glenohumeral instability was investigated in a cadaver model. There were six good, two fair, and two poor results.

28. Skendzel JG, Sekiya JK: Arthroscopic glenoid osteochondral allograft reconstruction without subscapularis takedown: Technique and literature review. *Arthroscopy* 2011;27(1):129-135.

   The literature on the surgical treatment of glenoid bone deficiency was reviewed. A novel technique of arthroscopic anteroinferior glenoid reconstruction used glenoid osteochondral allograft without subscapularis takedown.

29. Warner JJ, Gill TJ, O'hollerhan JD, Pathare N, Millett PJ: Anatomical glenoid reconstruction for recurrent anterior glenohumeral instability with glenoid deficiency using an autogenous tricortical iliac crest bone graft. *Am J Sports Med* 2006;34(2):205-212.

30. Lafosse L, Boyle S, Gutierrez-Aramberri M, Shah A, Meller R: Arthroscopic latarjet procedure. *Orthop Clin North Am* 2010;41(3):393-405.

   The value of the arthroscopic Latarjet procedure was described for the treatment of complex shoulder instability. Results were excellent at short- to mid-term follow-up, with minimal complications.

31. Sugaya H, Kon Y, Tsuchiya A: Arthroscopic repair of glenoid fractures using suture anchors. *Arthroscopy* 2005;21(5):635.

32. Lafosse L, Boyle S: Arthroscopic Latarjet procedure. *J Shoulder Elbow Surg* 2010;19(2, suppl):2-12.

   The arthroscopic Latarjet procedure is a valuable tool in the treatment of complex shoulder instability. Introduction of the procedure into practice was described. The procedure was recommended for surgeons with good anatomic knowledge and advanced arthroscopic skills.

33. Tauber M, Resch H, Forstner R, Raffl M, Schauer J: Reasons for failure after surgical repair of anterior shoulder instability. *J Shoulder Elbow Surg* 2004;13(3):279-285.

34. Nourissat G, Nedellec G, O'Sullivan NA, et al: Mini-open arthroscopically assisted Bristow-Latarjet procedure for the treatment of patients with anterior shoulder instability: A cadaver study. *Arthroscopy* 2006;22(10):1113-1118.

35. Kim SH, Ha KI, Cho YB, Ryu BD, Oh I: Arthroscopic anterior stabilization of the shoulder: Two to six-year follow-up. *J Bone Joint Surg Am* 2003;85-A(8):1511-1518.

36. Agneskirchner JD, Haag M, Lafosse L: [Arthroscopic coracoid transfer: Indications, technique and initial results]. *Orthopade* 2011;40(1):41-51.

   The indications, surgical technique, and early results of coracoid transfer related to a completely arthroscopic technique were reviewed.

37. Park MJ, Tjoumakaris FP, Garcia G, Patel A, Kelly JD IV: Arthroscopic remplissage with Bankart repair for the treatment of glenohumeral instability with Hill-Sachs defects. *Arthroscopy* 2011;27(9):1187-1194.

   Twenty patients underwent arthroscopic Bankart repair with remplissage for the treatment of recurrent anterior glenohumeral instability and a large Hill-Sachs defect. At a mean 29-month follow-up, function was restored, pain was diminished, and 85% of the patients were satisfied.

38. Auffarth A, Schauer J, Matis N, Kofler B, Hitzl W, Resch H: The J-bone graft for anatomical glenoid reconstruction in recurrent posttraumatic anterior shoulder dislocation. *Am J Sports Med* 2008;36(4):638-647.

   Long-term results were reported for 47 patients after stabilization with a J-bone graft, which was found to be capable of creating a stable shoulder joint without causing extensive loss of motion. The patients had traumatic glenoid rim fracture after shoulder dislocation. Despite anatomic glenoid reconstruction, some patients had mild to moderate arthropathy.

4: Arthroscopy

39. Hovelius L, Sandström B, Olofsson A, Svensson O, Rahme H: The effect of capsular repair, bone block healing, and position on the results of the Bristow-Latarjet procedure (study III): Long-term follow-up in 319 shoulders. *J Shoulder Elbow Surg* 2012;21(5): 647-660.

   At long-term follow-up of 319 patients after an open Bristow-Latarjet procedure, 837 had a good and consistent result. The rate of recurrence decreased and subjective results improved when a horizontal capsular shift was added to the coracoid transfer.

40. Hovelius L, Vikerfors O, Olofsson A, Svensson O, Rahme H: Bristow-Latarjet and Bankart: A comparative study of shoulder stabilization in 185 shoulders during a seventeen-year follow-up. *J Shoulder Elbow Surg* 2011;20(7):1095-1101.

   Eighty-eight consecutive shoulders underwent Bankart repair, and 97 consecutive shoulders underwent Bristow-Latarjet repair for traumatic anterior recurrent instability. At a mean 17-year follow-up, patients with the Bristow-Latarjet repair had better results than those with Bankart repair done with anchors, in terms of stability and subjective evaluation.

41. Millett PJ, Clavert P, Warner JJ: Open operative treatment for anterior shoulder instability: When and why? *J Bone Joint Surg Am* 2005;87(2):419-432.

Chapter 24

Arthroscopic Treatment of Multidirectional Instability

Brett McCoy, MD   Waqas Munawar Hussain, MD   Michael J. Griesser, MD   Anthony Miniaci, MD

Introduction

Although the understanding of shoulder instability has improved through advances in basic science, clinical research, and imaging, multidirectional instability (MDI) continues to be a difficult clinical diagnosis. This complex condition was first described by Neer and Foster in 1980 and has since been extensively studied.[1] MDI is defined as symptomatic, involuntary instability of the glenohumeral joint in two or more directions (inferior, anterior, and posterior).[2] The mnemonic AMBRI (*a*traumatic, *m*ultidirectional, *b*ilateral, *r*ehabilitation, *i*nferior capsular shift) has been used to describe MDI.[3] However, many inconsistencies in the characterization and the description of MDI have made it difficult to define its prevalence and compare research results.[4]

Despite published results indicating a good or an excellent outcome for more than 80% of patients after nonsurgical treatment including physical therapy,[5] not all patients improve with therapy alone. For these patients, open or arthroscopic surgical stabilization may be indicated.[6] The initial open surgical treatments focused on reducing laxity by decreasing joint volume with capsular retensioning, specifically in the inferior region.[7] Improved arthroscopic techniques and instrumentation and an improved understanding of pathoanatomy have led to the development of minimally invasive surgical methods for treating this complex condition.[8-10]

Pathoanatomy

The glenohumeral articulation allows excellent range of motion in the shoulder. Disruption of the delicate balance between stability and flexibility can predispose an individual to MDI. It is important to understand that laxity is not directly correlated with instability, and to some extent both dynamic and static restraints may be able to compensate for structurally deficient elements. Laxity does play an important role, however, and it can become symptomatic when compensatory mechanisms fail.[11] In contrast to patients with traumatic instability, patients with laxity may have an isolated labrocapsular laxity without a definite labral tear. Nonetheless, patients with chronic instability from MDI can have secondary labral pathology, including tearing, despite the primarily atraumatic nature of the condition.[9,12]

The static stabilizing structures of the shoulder include both bony and ligamentous elements. The shallow concavity of the glenoid acts with the labrum to provide a minor but key contribution to shoulder stability; investigators have observed relatively flat cup surfaces in patients with MDI, compared with normal control patients.[11,13] A very small labrum can contribute to an overall decrease in effective glenoid depth. Glenoid version also can contribute to a propensity for instability.[11] The capsular ligaments, including the superior, middle, and inferior glenohumeral ligaments, have been well characterized; they serve to resist joint translation by reciprocally tightening or loosening, depending on extremity position. An absence or a deficiency of any of these structures can increase the predisposition to instability. Likewise, a defect in the rotator cuff interval has been proposed to increase the amount of inferior translation and may be present in MDI.[2,14] A magnetic resonance arthrography evaluation found that the interval between the subscapularis and the supraspinatus (reflecting the size of the rotator cuff interval) was no greater in patients with MDI than in patients with other types of instability.[15]

Dr. Miniaci or an immediate family member serves as a board member, owner, officer, or committee member of the International Society of Arthroscopy, Knee Surgery, and Orthopaedic Sports Medicine; the American Shoulder and Elbow Surgeons; the Arthroscopy Association of North America; and the American Society for Sports Medicine; has received royalties from Arthrosurface and Zimmer; is a member of a speakers' bureau or has made paid presentations on behalf of Arthrosurface; serves as a paid consultant to or is an employee of Arthrosurface, Smith & Nephew, Stryker, and Zimmer; has stock or stock options held in DePuy, Medtronic, Zimmer, Stryker, and Arthrosurface; and has received noninterest support (such as equipment or services), commercially derived honoraria, or other non–research-related funding (such as paid travel) from Stryker and Arthrosurface. None of the following authors or any immediate family member has received anything of value from or has stock or stock options held in a commercial company or institution related directly or indirectly to the subject of this chapter: Dr. McCoy, Dr. Hussain, and Dr. Griesser.

Dynamic stabilization occurs through musculotendinous elements that are most active in the midarc of the shoulder range of motion, where the capsuloligamentous structures are least effective.[2] The scapulothoracic musculature dynamically alters the position of the shoulder to provide the most appropriate version and inclination of the glenoid for stability.[16] Abnormalities or imbalances in the trapezius, rhomboid, and serratus anterior muscles can affect scapular rotation and ultimately shoulder stability. A study that confirmed the presence of abnormal scapular kinematics in patients with MDI emphasized the importance of incorporating directed stability exercises during rehabilitation.[17] The supraspinatus, infraspinatus, and teres minor vectors increase the contact force between the humeral head and the glenoid through concavity compression.[16] The muscle bellies of the rotator cuff serve as a direct reinforcement or block to prevent abnormal joint motion.[11] Active neuromuscular control and intact proprioceptive feedback mechanisms are necessary for functional dynamic stability of the glenohumeral joint. Differences in rotator cuff function were observed and the electromyography results of patients with MDI were compared with those of normal control patients during pulling, forward punching, elevation, and overhead throwing motions.[18] The irregularities in shoulders with MDI may diminish the ability of the rotator cuff to process and adjust its responses based on small variations in afferent proprioceptive input.

Variations in collagen and elastin may be present in patients with MDI compared with normal control patients. When collagen cross-links, collagen fibril diameter and density, and amino acid and elastin composition were compared, histochemical differences were found in tissue from shoulders with MDI or unidirectional instability compared with normal joints. Capsule from shoulders undergoing revision surgery for MDI differed from tissue harvested from shoulders undergoing primary surgical intervention for MDI. These analyses suggest an underlying connective tissue disorder in this cohort of patients with MDI.[19]

In addition to these factors, the presence of a large, redundant inferior capsule and the accompanying loss of negative intra-articular joint pressure may contribute to MDI. An increase in capsular volume is believed to contribute to a decrease in negative pressure that impairs stability. A cadaver study evaluated intra-articular pressure after capsular shift, before and after venting of the joint. Although the inferior capsular shift decreased joint volume and increased the responsiveness of intra-articular pressure to downward loading, the humeral head dislocated inferiorly in all specimens after venting, even after imbrication.[20] The labrum also is atypical in patients with MDI, and the capsulolabral complex does not have the bumper effect found in normal shoulders.

Clinical Evaluation

The diagnosis of MDI primarily is based on the clinical history and the physical examination. The patient's history may be characterized by nonspecific, activity-related shoulder pain that typically begins before age 30 years. The primary symptom can range from pain to instability. Decreases in athletic performance and strength may be present, with extremity numbness or paresthesias to a lesser extent.[11] Information as to the frequency, reproducibility, and severity of the symptoms as well as inciting or alleviating positions or activities can provide invaluable insight to the extent and the direction of instability. Connective tissue disorders and associated laxity are not uncommon in patients diagnosed with MDI, and both shoulders may be affected. Multidirectional laxity is most prevalent among repetitive overhead athletes, such as swimmers, volleyball players, and gymnasts.[11] Patients with relatively severe symptoms may have instability during more subtle activities, such as overhead lifting, holding objects at the side, or changing position while sleeping.[2,21]

Symptomatic MDI frequently is a result of repetitive microtrauma leading to capsular laxity.[7] Less commonly, a single inciting trauma or event may initiate symptoms. The clinician must maintain heightened awareness to ensure an appropriate diagnosis. MDI can appear as shoulder instability without anatomic injury, in contrast to anterior unilateral instability, which typically appears as anteroinferior capsulolabral damage. MDI always should be considered in patients younger than 40 years who have persistent symptoms despite surgical stabilization.[11]

A patient who is able to voluntarily dislocate the shoulder can selectively control muscle contraction and relaxation to induce repetitive instability.[2] Voluntary dislocation often is associated with an emotional or a psychiatric disorder, and these patients typically have a poor outcome after surgical stabilization.[22] It is important to differentiate patients whose dislocation is related to secondary gain from those who are able to voluntarily induce shoulder dislocation but are careful to avoid provocative maneuvers or positions. These patients often self-protect or autoregulate positional instability, and typically they respond well to surgical stabilization.[11]

The physical examination begins with a visual inspection, with careful observation of any muscular atrophy, scapular asymmetry, or winging. Generalized laxity can be seen as metacarpal hyperextension, thumb-to-wrist opposition, knee and elbow recurvatum, patellar instability, or pes planus (**Figure 1**). The patient may exhibit a sulcus sign, characterized as a gap below the lateral border of the acromion when an inferiorly directed stress is applied to a relaxed adducted shoulder. A sulcus sign seen when the distal extremity is in external rotation (thereby increasing tension on the superior glenohumeral ligament) confirms

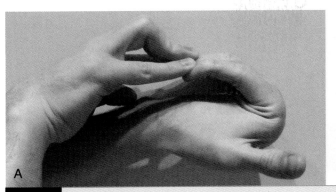
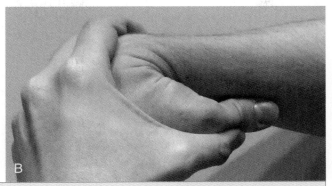

| **Figure 1** | Photographs showing metacarpophalangeal hyperextension (**A**) and thumb-to-wrist opposition (**B**). |

greater laxity related to the superior glenohumeral ligament.

Although the diagnosis of MDI primarily is based on the history and the physical examination, radiographic images should be obtained. The primary purpose is to rule out an anatomic defect or assess for concomitant structural shoulder pathology, such as a Hill-Sachs or a reverse Hill-Sachs lesion or an avulsion of the glenohumeral ligaments. MRI can be obtained to assess the capsular anatomy, the labrum, the rotator cuff, and the biceps. CT is useful for assessing bone quality or defects.[7] In patients who have had unsuccessful earlier surgery for MDI, attention should be focused on the function and the strength of the individual rotator cuff muscles, particularly the subscapularis. Internal rotation strength may be decreased by as much as 30%, resulting in a loss of dynamic stabilization.[21,23]

Nonsurgical and Surgical Treatment Considerations

Determining the appropriate treatment of patients with a diagnosis of MDI requires careful interpretation of both subjective and objective findings. An algorithm to guide clinicians through this process is presented in **Figure 2**. It is important to note that patients whose pain is a key component of the clinical picture may have an etiology unrelated to hyperlaxity. Thus, the painful shoulder in a patient with MDI requires a broad differential diagnosis and a thorough workup. Any asymmetry discovered in the physical examination for instability requires an evaluation for mechanical derangement (for example, a labral or Bankart injury or a SLAP tear), in addition to MDI.

Nonsurgical Treatment

Nonsurgical management is considered the first-line treatment for most patients with MDI. Rehabilitation should treat scapulothoracic dyskinesia and include proprioceptive exercises and rotator cuff strengthening. A study of the nonsurgical management of MDI found that 35 of 39 patients had a good or an excellent result.[5] Subsequent research with long-term follow-up determined that young athletic patients have a relatively poor response to nonsurgical management; 49% of nonsurgically treated patients had a poor result, and 37% required surgery.[24] Shoulder kinematics were found not to return to normal with physical therapy alone, but a combination of therapy and capsular shift had adequately restored normal kinematics at 4-year follow-up.[25] Despite these findings, a minimum 6-month course of physical therapy was recommended before any surgical intervention.[25]

Surgical Treatment

Surgical intervention is reserved for patients with persistent disability despite rehabilitation. The goal of surgery is to treat the pathologic structures, and the focus is on decreasing the capsular volume using capsuloligamentous techniques. It is important to distinguish true MDI from traumatic instability in a patient with systemic hyperlaxity. In Neer's original description of inferior capsular shift, more than half of the patients had an instability episode precipitated by significant trauma.[1] Although the presence of diffuse laxity in the setting of a Bankart repair was found to increase the failure rate, this is a different entity from true MDI.[26] The surgeon should carefully consider whether the patient's condition is a traumatic labral tear rather than true MDI. Relevant patient population data from the literature should be examined when making the diagnosis.

Arthroscopic Treatment Considerations

Historically, open procedures have been used to surgically treat MDI, but laboratory data have shown that open and arthroscopic surgery achieve a comparable amount of volume reduction.[27] In a cadaver model, 1-cm plication stitches decreased capsular volume by 10%, and five plication stitches achieved a volume reduction similar to that of an open shift.[28] A clinical study using the American Shoulder and Elbow Surgeons (ASES) Shoulder Index found a statistically favorable response to arthroscopic compared with open

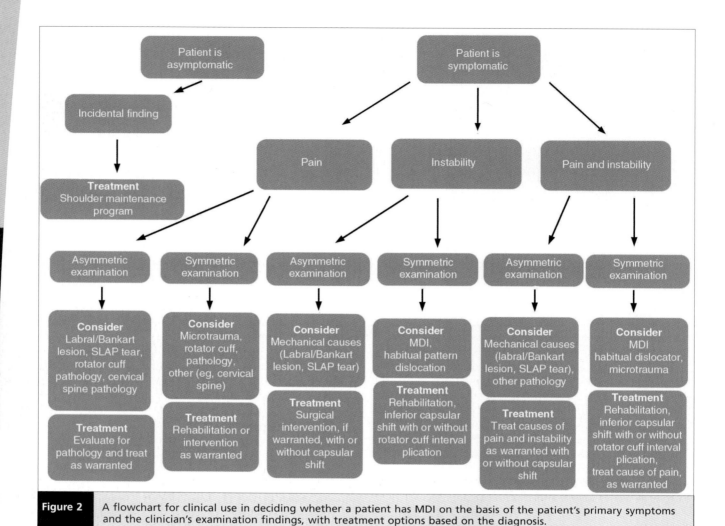

Figure 2 A flowchart for clinical use in deciding whether a patient has MDI on the basis of the patient's primary symptoms and the clinician's examination findings, with treatment options based on the diagnosis.

procedures. Patients with earlier surgery had a relatively low ASES score.[29] A recent systematic review of seven studies comparing open and arthroscopic treatment of MDI found no significant difference in recurrent instability, return to sports, loss of external rotation, or rate of complications. There was a slight trend toward improved return to sports after arthroscopic treatment.[30] This review appropriately excluded patients with a Bankart lesion but contained only level IV studies. The findings are difficult to interpret because of the inherent variation in disease processes and specific mechanisms of treatment. However, the literature suggests that in experienced hands, arthroscopic treatment can achieve the same results as open surgery.

The arthroscopic treatment of MDI involves different techniques, the most common of which involve a capsular plication and/or rotator cuff interval closure. Thermal capsulorrhaphy has fallen out of favor because of reported high rates of failure, chondrolysis, and nerve injury.[31,32] Multiple laboratory studies have evaluated specific techniques for arthroscopic treatment. One study found that capsular plication alone decreased excess motion, but an additional rotator cuff interval closure was necessary to decrease glenohumeral translation.[33] A medial-lateral rotator cuff interval closure more effectively decreased posterior translation than a superior-inferior technique.[34] A comparison of three types of plication stitches found that the simple stitch was comparable to the figure-of 8 and mattress configurations.[35]

Limited clinical data are available on the outcomes of the arthroscopic treatment of MDI. Most of the studies extend only to midterm follow-up, and many of them include patients with a Bankart lesion. A retrospective study of 40 patients at 2- to 5-year follow-up after arthroscopic treatment of MDI found that 91% had satisfactory range of motion, 86% were able to return to sports with minimal or no limitation, and clinical outcome scores were good.[8] In a study of nine young overhead athletes with MDI who were treated with capsular plication and rotator cuff interval closure, seven had a good or an excellent result; seven bxreturned to sports, but three returned at a lower level.[36]

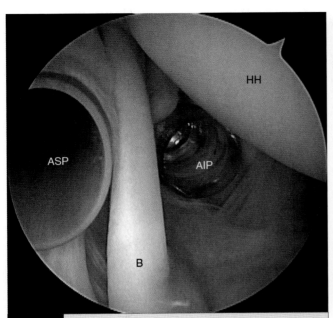

Figure 3 Arthroscopic photograph showing the anterosuperior portal (ASP) used for viewing and the anteroinferior portal (AIP) used for instrumentation. B = biceps, HH = humeral head. (Reproduced from Ryu RKN: Multidirectional instability, in Galatz LM, ed: *Orthopaedic Knowledge Update: Shoulder and Elbow*, ed 3. Rosemont, IL, American Academy of Orthopaedic Surgeons, 2008, pp 303-312.)

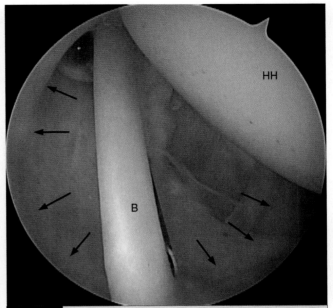

Figure 4 Arthroscopic photograph showing the patulous rotator cuff interval *(arrows)*. B = biceps, HH = humeral head. (Reproduced from Ryu RKN: Multidirectional instability, in Galatz LM, ed: *Orthopaedic Knowledge Update: Shoulder and Elbow*, ed 3. Rosemont, IL, American Academy of Orthopaedic Surgeons, 2008, pp 303-312.)

Arthroscopic Technique

The examination under anesthesia is the first surgical step. All patients with MDI have inferior instability, but it is important to determine whether the primary direction is anterior or posterior. These findings should be compared to those of the contralateral shoulder. After the examination, the patient is positioned in the beach chair or the lateral position.

Establishing the posterior portal in a relatively lateral position is useful for subsequent capsular and labral work. One or two anterior portals should be established in the rotator cuff interval (**Figure 3**). A thorough diagnostic inspection of the shoulder should be conducted, with attention to the patulous nature of the rotator cuff interval and assessment for a Bankart-type labral injury (**Figure 4**). In MDI, the labrum may have some minor changes but should remain attached. Traction on the humerus will lead to a positive drive-through sign, which involves passing the scope from posterosuperior to anteroinferior without obstruction from the glenohumeral joint (**Figure 5**).

Different treatment strategies exist for capsular plication and rotator cuff interval imbrication. It is important to avoid overtightening or axillary nerve injury. The axillary nerve runs approximately 12.4 mm below the 6-o'clock position of the glenoid and can be protected by positioning the arm in abduction, external ro-

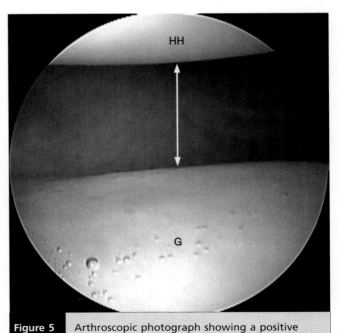

Figure 5 Arthroscopic photograph showing a positive drive-through sign *(arrow)*. G = glenoid, HH = humeral head. (Reproduced from Ryu RKN: Multidirectional instability, in Galatz LM, ed: *Orthopaedic Knowledge Update: Shoulder and Elbow*, ed 3. Rosemont, IL, American Academy of Orthopaedic Surgeons, 2008, pp 303-312.)

4: Arthroscopy

tation, and slight traction.[37,38] Capsular abrasion is performed first and is followed by capsular plication in a sequential pattern that generally begins in the area of primary instability (anterior or posterior, **Figure 6**). It is important to progress from inferior to superior because each plication decreases the volume of the joint and thus inhibits visualization (**Figure 7**). Care must be taken to avoid shifting tissue in a medial to lateral direction because doing so can reduce the rotational motion of the shoulder. After treating the primary direction of instability, the tissue opposite the primary direction of instability is shifted to create a balanced shoulder (**Figure 8**). The centering of the humeral head on the glenoid is checked after sutures are in place, and the shoulder is taken through a range of motion. Sutures may rupture; they also can be removed and retensioned if there are limitations of motion. The sutures can be passed around the capsule and the labrum, or a glenoid suture anchor can be used. The optimal number of sutures, suture configuration, and suture material have not been determined.

The role of rotator cuff interval closure is controversial. Most data supporting rotator interval closure are limited to cadaver studies, and there is minimal high-level clinical evidence. One study suggests no improvement in inferior instability but a decrease in motion.[15] It is important to avoid overtightening and a subsequent loss of external rotation; this can be prevented by positioning the arm in approximately 20° to 30° of external rotation during the repair. The techniques include both medial-lateral and superior-inferior closures.

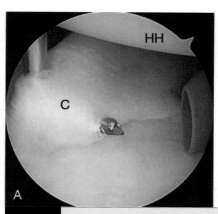

Figure 6 Arthroscopic photograph from the anterosuperior portal, showing careful rasping of the capsule to generate a healing response. G = glenoid, IGHL = inferior glenohumeral ligament, L = labrum. (Reproduced from Ryu RKN: Multidirectional instability, Galatz LM, ed: *Orthopaedic Knowledge Update: Shoulder and Elbow*, ed 3. Rosemont, IL, American Academy of Orthopaedic Surgeons, 2008, pp 303-312.)

Immobilization and Rehabilitation

Immobilization after surgery can be in a neutral position or in a position based on the direction of primary instability. For example, patients with posteroinferior instability can be immobilized in external rotation. Because postoperative stiffness is much less common than residual laxity after surgery for MDI, the recommendation is to proceed slowly with rehabilitation. Sling immobilization is maintained for 6 weeks (or a longer period if the joint remains supple). A gradual return of motion is obtained over a period as long as 6 months.

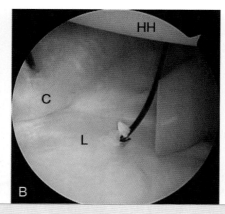
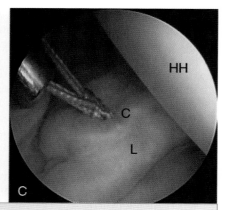

Figure 7 Arthroscopic photographs showing capsular tissue captured with first pass and shifted superiorly before the labrum is engaged (**A**); the suture hook passing through the labrum as the second step, with passage of absorbable suture (**B**); and knot tying on the capsular side of the tissue (**C**). C = capsular tissue, G = glenoid, HH = humeral head, L = labrum, PC = posterior cannula. (Reproduced from Ryu RKN: Multidirectional instability, in Galatz LM, ed: *Orthopaedic Knowledge Update: Shoulder and Elbow*, ed 3. Rosemont, IL, American Academy of Orthopaedic Surgeons, 2008, pp 303-312.)

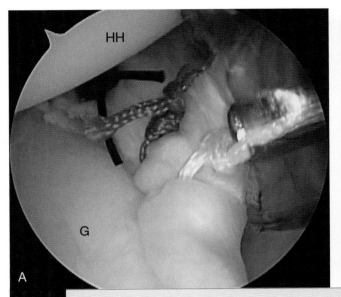
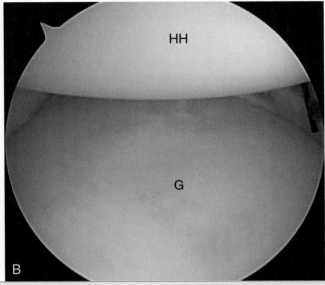

Figure 8 Arthroscopic photographs showing posterior capsular plication after the anteroinferior component was treated (**A**), and the humeral head is balanced and well centered on the glenoid face after multiple plication sutures, as seen from the anterosuperior portal (**B**). G = glenoid, HH = humeral head. (Reproduced from Ryu RKN: Multidirectional instability, in Galatz LM, ed: *Orthopaedic Knowledge Update: Shoulder and Elbow*, ed 3. Rosemont, IL, American Academy of Orthopaedic Surgeons, 2008, pp 303-312.)

Summary

MDI is a difficult clinical entity in terms of both diagnosis and management. It is important to appreciate that true MDI is atraumatic in nature. The first-line treatment is rehabilitation, but some data suggest that certain patients respond poorly to nonsurgical management. The current evidence for surgical intervention is limited, but multiple studies suggest that arthroscopic treatment of MDI can achieve the same goals as open treatment. Continued research is warranted to define specific recommendations regarding surgical technique.

Annotated References

1. Neer CS II, Foster CR: Inferior capsular shift for involuntary inferior and multidirectional instability of the shoulder: A preliminary report. *J Bone Joint Surg Am* 1980;62(6):897-908.

2. Bahu MJ, Trentacosta N, Vorys GC, Covey AS, Ahmad CS: Multidirectional instability: Evaluation and treatment options. *Clin Sports Med* 2008;27(4): 671-689.

   A general review of MDI and treatment options is provided. The initial treatment is with physical therapy, and surgical solutions are appropriate only after unsuccessful nonsurgical treatment.

3. Thomas SC, Matsen FA III: An approach to the repair of avulsion of the glenohumeral ligaments in the management of traumatic anterior glenohumeral instability. *J Bone Joint Surg Am* 1989;71(4):506-513.

4. McFarland EG, Kim TK, Park HB, Neira CA, Gutierrez MI: The effect of variation in definition on the diagnosis of multidirectional instability of the shoulder. *J Bone Joint Surg Am* 2003;(11):2138-2144.

5. Burkhead WZ Jr, Rockwood CA Jr: Treatment of instability of the shoulder with an exercise program. *J Bone Joint Surg Am* 1992;74(6):890-896.

6. Caprise PA Jr, Sekiya JK: Open and arthroscopic treatment of multidirectional instability of the shoulder. *Arthroscopy* 2006;22(10):1126-1131.

7. Cole B: *Surgical Techniques of the Shoulder, Elbow, and Knee in Sports Medicine.* Philadelphia, PA, WB Saunders, 2008.

   A general review of surgical techniques in sports medicine is provided, including open surgical procedures for MDI.

8. Baker CL III, Mascarenhas R, Kline AJ, Chhabra A, Pombo MW, Bradley JP: Arthroscopic treatment of multidirectional shoulder instability in athletes: A retrospective analysis of 2- to 5-year clinical outcomes. *Am J Sports Med* 2009;37(9):1712-1720.

   The mean ASES score was 91.4 at 2- to 5-year follow-up of arthroscopic treatment of MDI in 43 shoulders in athletes age 14 to 39 years. Ninety-one percent of the patients had full or satisfactory range of motion, 98% had full or slightly decreased strength, and 86% had returned to sport with little or no limitation.

9. Alpert JM, Verma N, Wysocki R, Yanke AB, Romeo AA: Arthroscopic treatment of multidirectional shoulder instability with minimum 270 degrees labral re-

pair: Minimum 2-year follow-up. *Arthroscopy* 2008; 24(6):704-711.

At a mean 56-month follow-up of 13 patients (mean age, 27.2 years) after arthroscopic stabilization for MDI and a labral tear of at least 270°, 85% had a good result on physical examination and measures including ASES.

10. ElAttrache NS: *Surgical Techniques in Sports Medicine.* Philadelphia, PA, Lippincott, Williams & Wilkins, 2007.

Surgical techniques in sports medicine are reviewed, with a technique for arthroscopic surgical stabilization of MDI.

11. Gaskill TR, Taylor DC, Millett PJ: Management of multidirectional instability of the shoulder. *J Am Acad Orthop Surg* 2011;19(12):758-767.

The definition, diagnosis, physical examination, physical therapy, and arthroscopic stabilization of MDI are reviewed.

12. Werner AW, Lichtenberg S, Schmitz H, Nikolic A, Habermeyer P: Arthroscopic findings in atraumatic shoulder instability. *Arthroscopy* 2004;20(3):268-272.

13. Kim SH, Noh KC, Park JS, Ryu BD, Oh I: Loss of chondrolabral containment of the glenohumeral joint in atraumatic posteroinferior multidirectional instability. *J Bone Joint Surg Am* 2005;87(1):92-98.

14. Schenk TJ, Brems JJ: Multidirectional instability of the shoulder: Pathophysiology, diagnosis, and management. *J Am Acad Orthop Surg* 1998;6(1):65-72.

15. Provencher MT, Dewing CB, Bell SJ, et al: An analysis of the rotator interval in patients with anterior, posterior, and multidirectional shoulder instability. *Arthroscopy* 2008;24(8):921-929.

The magnetic resonance arthrograms of patients with an anteriorly, posteriorly, or multidirectionally unstable shoulder were compared with those of control the subjects. The distance between the supraspinatus and the subscapularis was well preserved in all instability patterns. The long head of the biceps tendon assumes a more anterior position relative to the supraspinatus in posterior instability, compared with the anteriorly unstable or stable shoulder.

16. Lippitt S, Matsen F: Mechanisms of glenohumeral joint stability. *Clin Orthop Relat Res* 1993;291:20-28.

17. Ogston JB, Ludewig PM: Differences in 3-dimensional shoulder kinematics between persons with multidirectional instability and asymptomatic controls. *Am J Sports Med* 2007;35(8):1361-1370.

Patients with MDI had abnormal scapular kinematics in upward rotation, abduction, and internal rotation in comparison with control subjects. This finding highlights the importance of scapular stability and positioning exercises during MDI rehabilitation.

18. Illyés A, Kiss RM: Electromyographic analysis in patients with multidirectional shoulder instability during pull, forward punch, elevation and overhead throw. *Knee Surg Sports Traumatol Arthrosc* 2007;15(5): 624-631.

An electromyelography study compared patients with MDI and control subjects. Centralization of the glenohumeral joint is attempted by increasing rotator cuff musculature activation in patients with MDI, but there is an increased time difference in the peak activity of these muscle groups.

19. Rodeo SA, Suzuki K, Yamauchi M, Bhargava M, Warren RF: Analysis of collagen and elastic fibers in shoulder capsule in patients with shoulder instability. *Am J Sports Med* 1998;26(5):634-643.

20. Yamamoto N, Itoi E, Tuoheti Y, et al: The effect of the inferior capsular shift on shoulder intra-articular pressure: A cadaveric study. *Am J Sports Med* 2006;34(6): 939-944.

21. Forsythe B, Ghodadra N, Romeo AA, Provencher MT: Management of the failed posterior/multidirectional instability patient. *Sports Med Arthrosc* 2010;18(3): 149-161.

Presentation, physical examination findings, and radiographic analysis are described for patients after unsuccessful surgery for posterior instability or MDI, with options for a revision surgical solution.

22. Rowe CR, Pierce DS, Clark JG: Voluntary dislocation of the shoulder: A preliminary report on a clinical, electromyographic, and psychiatric study of twenty-six patients. *J Bone Joint Surg Am* 1973;55(3):445-460.

23. Warner JJ, Micheli LJ, Arslanian LE, Kennedy J, Kennedy R: Patterns of flexibility, laxity, and strength in normal shoulders and shoulders with instability and impingement. *Am J Sports Med* 1990;18(4):366-375.

24. Misamore GW, Sallay PI, Didelot W: A longitudinal study of patients with multidirectional instability of the shoulder with seven- to ten-year follow-up. *J Shoulder Elbow Surg* 2005;14(5):466-470.

25. Nyiri P, Illyés A, Kiss R, Kiss J: Intermediate biomechanical analysis of the effect of physiotherapy only compared with capsular shift and physiotherapy in multidirectional shoulder instability. *J Shoulder Elbow Surg* 2010;19(6):802-813.

A comparison of 32 patients with MDI treated only with physical therapy, 19 patients with MDI treated with capsular shift and physical therapy, and 50 healthy control subjects found that the alterations in kinematic parameters could be returned to normal with physical therapy alone but could be restored for at least 4 years with capsular shift and physical therapy.

26. Chechik O, Maman E, Dolkart O, Khashan M, Shabtai L, Mozes G: Arthroscopic rotator interval closure in shoulder instability repair: A retrospective

study. *J Shoulder Elbow Surg* 2010;19(7):1056-1062.

In a retrospective review of patients with recurrent instability after arthroscopic Bankart repair, with or without arthroscopic rotator cuff interval closure, systemic joint hyperlaxity was associated with recurrent instability. Patients with arthroscopic rotator cuff interval closure had a more limited range of motion, with 75% having a good or an excellent functional result.

27. Sekiya JK, Willobee JA, Miller MD, Hickman AJ, Willobee A: Arthroscopic multi-pleated capsular plication compared with open inferior capsular shift for reduction of shoulder volume in a cadaveric model. *Arthroscopy* 2007;23(11):1145-1151.

In seven fresh-frozen cadaver shoulders, arthroscopic plication resulted in a 58% mean volume decrease. Open inferior capsular shift resulted in a mean volume decrease of 45%. This study showed that the arthroscopic method could be as effective as the open method.

28. Ponce BA, Rosenzweig SD, Thompson KJ, Tokish J: Sequential volume reduction with capsular plications: Relationship between cumulative size of plications and volumetric reduction for multidirectional instability of the shoulder. *Am J Sports Med* 2011;39(3):526-531.

In 12 fresh-frozen cadaver shoulders, a 1-cm plication stitch resulted in a 10% volume reduction. Five plication stitches resulted in a 49% to 52% reduction, which is similar to the result in an open lateral-based capsular shift.

29. Yeargan SA III, Briggs KK, Horan MP, Black AK, Hawkins RJ: Determinants of patient satisfaction following surgery for multidirectional instability. *Orthopedics* 2008;31(7):647.

A review of 50 shoulders in 46 patients after stabilization surgery for MDI found that subjective variables, such as symptoms and motion, had the greatest correlation with patient satisfaction.

30. Jacobson ME, Riggenbach M, Wooldridge AN, Bishop JY: Open capsular shift and arthroscopic capsular plication for treatment of multidirectional instability. *Arthroscopy* 2012;28(7):1010-1017.

A systematic review of seven studies with 197 patients found that arthroscopic capsular plication yielded results comparable to those of open capsular shift in terms of recurrent instability, return to sport, external rotation loss, and overall complications.

31. D'Alessandro DF, Bradley JP, Fleischli JE, Connor PM: Prospective evaluation of thermal capsulorrhaphy for shoulder instability: Indications and results, two- to five-year follow-up. *Am J Sports Med* 2004;32(1):21-33.

32. Hawkins RJ, Krishnan SG, Karas SG, Noonan TJ, Horan MP: Electrothermal arthroscopic shoulder capsulorrhaphy: A minimum 2-year follow-up. *Am J Sports Med* 2007;35(9):1484-1488.

At 2-year follow up, 37 of 85 thermal capsulorrhaphies had failed, and almost 60% had failed in patients with posterior, multidirectional, or anteroposterior instability. Augmenting these procedures with capsular plication and/or rotator cuff interval closure is recommended to improve results.

33. Shafer BL, Mihata T, McGarry MH, Tibone JE, Lee TQ: Effects of capsular plication and rotator interval closure in simulated multidirectional shoulder instability. *J Bone Joint Surg Am* 2008;90(1):136-144.

Seven cadaver shoulders received anterior plication, posterior plication, and rotator cuff interval closure. Capsular plication alone resulted in reduced range of motion in the intact state, but reduction of glenohumeral translation required the addition of rotator cuff interval closure.

34. Farber AJ, ElAttrache NS, Tibone JE, McGarry MH, Lee TQ: Biomechanical analysis comparing a traditional superior-inferior arthroscopic rotator interval closure with a novel medial-lateral technique in a cadaveric multidirectional instability model. *Am J Sports Med* 2009;37(6):1178-1185.

Eight match-paired cadaver shoulders underwent either superior-inferior or medial-lateral rotator cuff interval closure. Medial-lateral closure more closely restored range of motion to the intact state and significantly reduced posterior translation with the shoulder in an abducted, externally rotated position.

35. Nho SJ, Frank RM, Van Thiel GS, et al: A biomechanical analysis of shoulder stabilization: Posteroinferior glenohumeral capsular plication. *Am J Sports Med* 2010;38(7):1413-1419.

Twenty-one fresh-frozen cadaver shoulders underwent capsulolabral plication with a simple stitch, a horizontal mattress, or a figure-of-8 configuration. All three configurations were effective in plication, but the simple stitch may be preferred because of technical ease.

36. Voigt C, Schulz AP, Lill H: Arthroscopic treatment of multidirectional glenohumeral instability in young overhead athletes. *Open Orthop J* 2009;3:107-114.

Ten shoulders in nine young overhead athletes were treated with arthroscopic anteroposterior capsular plication and rotator cuff interval closure after unsuccessful nonsurgical treatment of MDI. Seven of the nine patients were able to return to their previous level of sport, but three returned at a lower level.

37. Uno A, Bain GI, Mehta JA: Arthroscopic relationship of the axillary nerve to the shoulder joint capsule: An anatomic study. *J Shoulder Elbow Surg* 1999;8(3):226-230.

38. Price MR, Tillett ED, Acland RD, Nettleton GS: Determining the relationship of the axillary nerve to the shoulder joint capsule from an arthroscopic perspective. *J Bone Joint Surg Am* 2004;(10):2135-2142.

4: Arthroscopy

Chapter 25

Superior Labrum Anterior to Posterior Lesions

James R. Andrews, MD   Brett Shore, MD

4: Arthroscopy

Introduction

Before the advent of shoulder arthroscopy, the etiology of shoulder dysfunction in the overhead athlete was believed to relate to external impingement of the undersurface of the acromion on the bursal side of the rotator cuff.[1] The primary treatment was open acromioplasty, which had poor results in overhead athletes; the failure rate was 50%, and only 22% returned to the preinjury level of play.[2] In 1985, lesions of the superior labrum associated with the long head of the biceps were first reported in high-level overhead athletes.[3] Fraying and detachment of the labrum were found, sometimes associated with tearing of the biceps tendon. These athletes also commonly had undersurface tearing of the rotator cuff. The proposed mechanism of this constellation of findings was attrition secondary to repetitive tension overloading on the rotator cuff and the biceps-labrum complex. In 1990, the name superior labrum anterior posterior (SLAP) was applied to these lesions, and they were defined as starting posterior to the biceps anchor and extending anteriorly to involve the biceps anchor.[4] Four types of lesions were included in the initial Snyder classification, which later was expanded to include all identifiable pathology of the superior labrum. Several more recent studies examined the pathogenesis, presentation, and treatment of SLAP lesions, thus improving understanding of these injuries and their management.

Dr. Andrews or an immediate family member has received royalties from Biomet Sports Medicine; serves as a paid consultant to or is an employee of Biomet Sports Medicine, Bauerfiend, Theralase, MiMedx, and Physiotherapy Associates; has stock or stock options held in Patient Connection and Connective Orthopaedics; and serves as a board member, owner, officer, or committee member of FastHealth, the American Orthopaedic Society for Sports Medicine, and Physiotherapy Associates. Neither Dr. Shore nor any immediate family member has received anything of value from or has stock or stock options held in a commercial company or institution related directly or indirectly to the subject of this chapter.

Classification

The original four types of SLAP lesions have been expanded to 10 types, although the original classification is still most widely used[4-6] (**Figure 1**). The interobserver reliability of this classification system has been inconsistent, although at least one study found good interobserver reliability among experienced surgeons.[7,8] A type I lesion is degenerative fraying of the inner margin of the superior labrum, without detachment of the labrum or the biceps anchor. Type I is the most common type of SLAP lesion; often it is asymptomatic and typically is found incidentally in middle-aged patients. A type II SLAP lesion is detachment of the superior labrum at the biceps insertion; this is the most com-

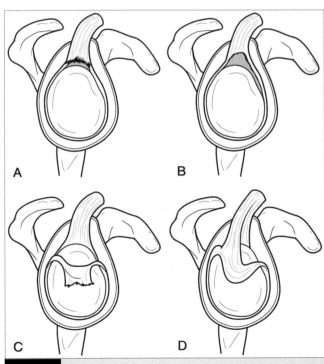

Figure 1 Schematic drawings showing the Snyder classification of SLAP lesions: types I (**A**), II (**B**), III (**C**), and IV (**D**).

mon, clinically important type. Type II SLAP tears can be subcategorized as anterior, predominately posterior, or combined anterior and posterior (in relation to the biceps anchor) (**Figure 2**). Throwing athletes most commonly have posterior extension of the lesion. A type III SLAP lesion is characterized by a bucket-handle tear of the superior labrum, with displacement into the joint and an intact biceps anchor. A type IV SLAP lesion is a bucket-handle tear that extends into the biceps tendon, resulting in the appearance of a split tendon; part of the biceps anchor may still be attached to the superior glenoid. The additional Gartsman and Ryu types of SLAP lesions involve an associated instability lesion, such as a

Bankart lesion, a posterior labral lesion, middle glenohumeral ligament involvement, or a 360° labral lesion (**Table 1**).

Anatomy and Biomechanics

The glenoid labrum is a fibrocartilaginous ring that surrounds and deepens the glenoid. The labrum also serves as the attachment point for the glenohumeral ligaments and the biceps tendon. The superior labrum can be meniscoid in appearance and attached to the glenoid peripherally, or it can be firmly attached to the glenoid

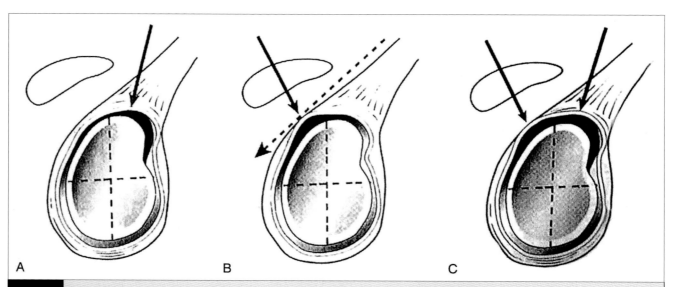

| Figure 2 | Schematic drawings showing the anterior (**A**), posterior (**B**), and combined anterior and posterior (**C**) subtypes of the Snyder type II SLAP lesion. Solid arrows = primary location of the tear (anterior, posterior, or combined anterior and posterior), dashed vertical and horizontal lines = glenoid quadrants, dashed arrow = orientation of the force producing a posterior SLAP tear (**B**). (Reproduced with permission from Morgan CD, Burkhart SS, Palmeri M, Gillespie M: Type II SLAP lesions: Three subtypes and their relationships to superior instability and rotator cuff tears. *Arthroscopy* 1998;14[6]:553-565.) |

Table 1

The Classification of SLAP lesions

Type	Description
I	Fraying of superior labrum
II	Detachment of biceps anchor and superior labrum
III	Bucket-handle tear of superior labrum with intact biceps anchor
IV	Bucket-handle tear of superior labrum extending into the biceps tendon
V	Extension of Bankart lesion to include detachment of the biceps anchor
VI	Anterior or posterior labral flap with type II biceps lesion
VII	Biceps anchor detachment extending into the middle glenohumeral ligament
VIII	Type II with posterior labral extension
IX	Type II with 360° labral detachment
X	Type II with posteroinferior labral detachment

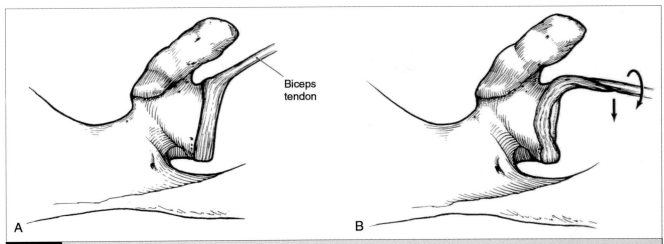

Figure 3 Schematic drawings showing a superior view of the resting position of the biceps anchor (**A**) and vertical force (*arrows*) transmitted to the posterosuperior labrum with abduction and external rotation (**B**). (Reproduced with permission from Burkhart SS, Morgan CD: The peel-back mechanism: Its role in producing and extending posterior type II SLAP lesions and its effect on SLAP repair rehabilitation. *Arthroscopy* 1998;14[6]:637-640.)

both centrally and peripherally. The long head of the biceps attaches to the posterosuperior labrum and the supraglenoid tubercle, which lies 5 mm medial to the superior glenoid rim. Approximately 40% to 60% of the biceps tendon fibers attach to the supraglenoid tubercle, with the remainder attaching directly to the labrum. The primary site of attachment of the biceps to the labrum varies; in most individuals, it attaches purely or primarily posterior, with some anterior component, but it also can be primarily anterior. The blood supply to the labrum comes through capsular and periosteal vessels that branch from the suprascapular, posterior humeral circumflex, and circumflex scapular arteries. The peripheral labrum has the greatest concentration of vessels, the central portion of the labrum is relatively avascular, and the superior labrum has the least robust blood supply.

The biceps tendon serves as a humeral head depressor and a secondary restraint to glenohumeral translation, particularly in abduction and external rotation.[9] A SLAP tear reduces resistance to external rotation force in the abducted and externally rotated position. Simulated SLAP lesions were found to increase anteroinferior translation, increasing tension on the inferior glenohumeral ligament complex.[10] The biceps was found to have a greater stabilizing effect as glenohumeral stability decreased.[11]

The peel-back sign results from the effect of the throwing position on the superior labrum and the biceps anchor[12] (**Figure 3**). The throwing position of maximal abduction and external rotation forces the biceps tendon into a relatively posterior and vertically oriented position, twisting the posterosuperior labrum in the process. This motion is effectively resisted by the biceps anchor in an intact shoulder, but in the presence of a type II SLAP lesion, the labrum rotates medially over the glenoid and onto the posterior scapular neck.

Repair of a type II SLAP lesion restores stability to the superior labrum and eliminates the peel-back sign.

Pathogenesis

The proposed mechanisms for the etiology of the SLAP lesion include repetitive overhead activity, traction, and compression, all of which have been evaluated in cadaver models. A single traumatic event is responsible for a SLAP lesion in patients who have not had an extended period of symptoms, and repetitive overhead activity is the cause specifically in throwing athletes. In a cadaver study, direct compression or impaction resulted in a SLAP lesion, particularly when the arm was flexed forward.[13] Another study found that traction with inferior subluxation consistently produced a SLAP lesion.[14]

The cause of type II SLAP lesions in overhead athletes is complex and controversial. In one proposal, glenohumeral internal rotation deficit (GIRD) accompanied by posterior capsular contracture leads to posterosuperior migration of the humeral head with abduction and external rotation and subsequently to increased shear and torsional forces at the biceps anchor.[12,15] Although evidence of this peel-back mechanism was observed during arthroscopic examination of the shoulder, there is little direct evidence that symptomatic GIRD with an associated posterior capsular contracture is a prerequisite for the development of a SLAP lesion. The peel-back mechanism may be the norm in overhead athletes who have increased external rotation, commonly with decreased internal rotation, in the throwing shoulder (**Figure 4**). It may be this hyperexternal rotation that puts abnormal stresses on the biceps anchor, independent of posterior capsular contracture. Internal impingement occurs when the posterosuperior rotator cuff is pinched between the greater

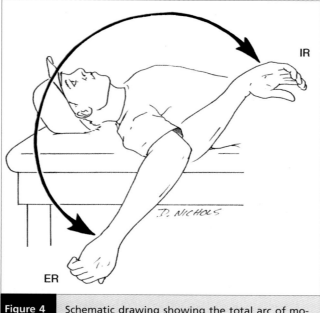

Figure 4 Schematic drawing showing the total arc of motion concept, in which external rotation (ER) + internal rotation (IR) = total motion. (Reproduced with permission from Wilk KE, Meister K, Andrews JR: Current concepts in the rehabilitation of the overhead throwing athlete. *Am J Sports Med* 2002;30[1]:136-151.)

tuberosity and the posterosuperior glenoid labrum at 90° abduction and 90° external rotation.[16] This impingement is repeated thousands of times in the late cocking phase of throwing, and it may cause a SLAP lesion.

Although each of these etiologies is plausible for type II SLAP lesions in overhead athletes, the so-called weed-pulling hypothesis probably provides an adequate explanation for a SLAP lesion in most patients.[17] The weed-pulling hypothesis suggests that SLAP tears are created by repetitively alternating forces during late cocking, which creates a posterior force on the biceps-labral complex, and deceleration–follow-through, which creates an anterior force. The result is the characteristic SLAP lesion in throwing athletes.

Clinical Evaluation

Patients with a symptomatic SLAP lesion broadly fall into two groups: overhead athletes, most of whom are baseball pitchers (although some are baseball position players, swimmers, tennis players, javelin throwers, or volleyball players), and people who have undergone an acute traumatic event causing traction or compression. SLAP lesions also develop in military personnel because of the rigorous and repetitive nature of their training. Military personnel who underwent shoulder arthroscopy were found to have a 22% incidence of SLAP lesions, 69% of which were type II.[18]

An accurate and thorough history of symptoms is critical to patient evaluation for a SLAP lesion. An overhead athlete may describe a vague onset of symptoms of somewhat unclear duration, without a clear inciting event. It is important to elicit the nature of the overhead activity, including changes in velocity, mechanics, stamina, and pain. The symptoms of internal impingement often are similar to those of a SLAP lesion, including vague pain and so-called dead arm syndrome with hard throwing. Dead arm syndrome recently was redefined as an inability to throw with preinjury velocity and control because of pain and unease in the throwing shoulder.[19] Mechanical symptoms such as locking, catching, or popping may be present, especially with rotational shoulder motions.

The physical examination for a suspected SLAP lesion should include evaluation for scapular dysfunction or pathologic shoulder motion (such as GIRD or crepitus) as well as provocative tests for shoulder pathology. Muscular atrophy should be evaluated; atrophy of the infraspinatus suggests a spinoglenoid notch ganglion cyst, which has been associated with SLAP lesions. In the absence of other pathology, a patient with a SLAP lesion should have normal rotator cuff strength and active shoulder motion (in a throwing athlete, defined as a less-than-25° difference between the dominant and nondominant arms). The examination for shoulder instability is critical for detecting associated labral pathology; the anterior apprehension-relocation and posterior load-and-shift tests should be included. The O'Brien active compression, biceps load II, forced shoulder abduction and elbow flexion, dynamic labral shear, crank, and resisted supination external rotation tests also have been described for detecting a SLAP lesion[20-25] (**Figure 5**).

An evaluation of several well-described and new tests found that the dynamic labral shear test was the most accurate single test, and the dynamic labral shear and O'Brien tests were the most useful combination for detecting a SLAP lesion.[26] A recent meta-analysis of studies that evaluated the clinical usefulness of provocative tests for SLAP lesions found that the active compression, crank, and Speed tests were the most sensitive and specific, and the anterior slide test was significantly less accurate.[27] A case-control study found that the biceps load II test was the most accurate in identifying a SLAP-only lesion, and the O'Brien, dynamic labral shear, Speed, and labral tension tests did not accurately identify SLAP lesions.[28] However, there was objection that the dynamic labral shear test was incorrectly performed in this study. The test is correctly performed with the patient supine and the shoulder off the side of the table, with the scapula supported but the humerus free. The shoulder is brought into 90° abduction, and the elbow is flexed to 90°. The shoulder is externally rotated to its natural limit, the elbow is dropped back to its natural limit of horizontal abduction, and the shoulder is passively elevated while horizontal abduction and external rotation are maintained. A positive

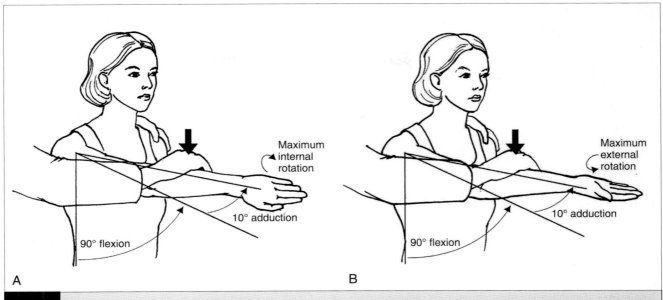

Figure 5 Schematic drawings showing the O'Brien active compression test. A downward force is resisted while the flexed and adducted shoulder is rotated internally (**A**) or externally (**B**). The reduction of symptoms in external rotation is a positive test. (Reproduced with permission fr om Parentis MA, Jobe CM, Pink MM, Jobe FW: An anatomic evaluation of the active compression test. *J Shoulder Elbow Surg* 2004;13[4]:410-416.)

test reproduces the patient's pain when the shoulder is moved through the arc of motion (usually 90° to 120°); a painful click may be felt. The active compression test is performed with downward pressure on a patient's arm while the shoulder is flexed to 90°, the elbow is extended, the arm is slightly adducted (at 10° to 15°), and the hand is first in maximal pronation and then in supination. The test is positive if the pain from the test in pronation is reduced or eliminated in supination. The Speed test is performed with downward pressure on the arm while the shoulder is flexed to 60° and the elbow is extended. The test is positive if the pain is localized to the bicipital groove. The crank test is performed with the shoulder elevated to 160° and an axial load applied while the humerus is internally and externally rotated. The test is positive with pain in external rotation, and clicking or catching also may occur. The biceps load II test is performed with the patient supine, the shoulder abducted to 120°, the elbow flexed to 90°, and the forearm supinated. The shoulder is maximally externally rotated, and the patient flexes the elbow against resistance. In a positive test, the patient's pain is reproduced.

Several tests should be used in combination with a thorough history, although their overall reliability is highly variable. Positive test results are suggestive rather than diagnostic of a SLAP lesion.

Imaging

The initial imaging studies are plain radiographs (the AP, scapular AP, axillary, and outlet views), which are not specific for SLAP lesions but can help identify other shoulder pathology. MRI is the study of choice for identifying SLAP lesions as well as concomitant labral, chondral, and rotator cuff pathology. Although the benefit of magnetic resonance arthrography (MRA) for identifying labral pathology has been extensively debated, it is quite useful for identifying subtle lesions of the labrum when intra-articular contrast is added. The abduction and external rotation view accentuates both superior and anterior labral pathology and is useful because of the anatomic variability of the superior labrum.[29] External rotation of the shoulder was found to improve the sensitivity and specificity of MRA for identifying SLAP lesions.[30] MRA findings consistent with a SLAP lesion include increased signal in the superior labrum with T2-weighting and the appearance of contrast between the glenoid and the superior labrum on coronal MRA (**Figure 6**). Identification of an anterosuperior labral tear on axial MRI or MRA also suggests a SLAP lesion. MRI is useful for identifying suprascapular and spinoglenoid cysts that may be associated with a SLAP lesion.

MRI for identifying SLAP lesions has a reported sensitivity of 67% to 98% and a specificity of 63% to 100%.[31-35] A side-by-side comparison using a 3-tesla magnet found that MRA had greater sensitivity than conventional MRI (83% versus 98%).[36] CT arthrography was found to be accurate and have good interobserver reliability for identifying SLAP lesions, comparable that of MRA for labral pathology.[37,38] Despite the advances in shoulder imaging, accurate diagnosis of a SLAP lesion also requires the patient history and examination findings.

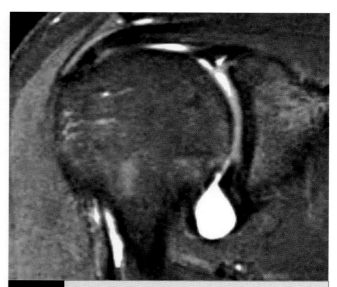

Figure 6 T2-weighted coronal magnetic resonance arthrogram showing dye tracking between the superior labrum and the glenoid. (Reproduced from Keener JD, Brophy RH: Superior labral tears of the shoulder: Pathogenesis, evaluation and treatment. *J Am Acad Orthop Surg* 2009;17[10]:627-637.)

Management

Nonsurgical Treatment

The nonsurgical treatment of a SLAP lesion consists of rest from the inciting activity, anti-inflammatory drugs, posterior capsular stretching, and strengthening of the rotator cuff and scapular stabilizers. A four-phase protocol is used for rehabilitation in athletes with a shoulder condition such as a SLAP tear, rotator cuff pathology, tendinitis, GIRD, or internal impingement.[39] The goals in the acute phase are to reduce pain, decrease inflammation, restore normal motion (especially internal rotation and horizontal adduction), and restore muscle strength and proprioception. The intermediate phase focuses on progressively increasing strength, improving flexibility, and facilitating neuromuscular control. In the advanced strengthening phase, aggressive strengthening drills, functional drills, and plyometrics are used. The final phase is the return-to-throwing (or other overhead sport) phase; it includes an interval throwing program or another sport-specific progression until pain-free athletic participation is achieved. In one study, nonsurgical treatment was successful in 19 of 39 patients (49%), but the remaining patients required surgery after unsuccessful nonsurgical treatment.[40] Before surgical intervention is considered, the athlete should attempt to regain full motion nonsurgically, especially in internal rotation.

Surgical Treatment

Surgical treatment of a SLAP lesion generally is performed arthroscopically. Several techniques can be chosen, depending on the type of lesion, activity level of the patient, and associated pathology. The indications for surgical treatment generally include 3 months of unsuccessful nonsurgical treatment, although early surgical intervention can be considered for a high-level overhead athlete, particularly in the off-season. For an in-season athlete who can perform despite the pain associated with a SLAP lesion, surgical treatment can be delayed until the season ends. The treatment of SLAP lesions in patients who are not high-level athletes has been heavily debated, and questions remain as to which patients can benefit from surgery and which procedure should be used. Surgical treatment of a SLAP lesion is recommended if nonsurgical treatment has been unsuccessful, the patient's symptoms and examination findings are correlated with those of a SLAP lesion, and the biceps anchor is unstable on arthroscopy. Biceps tenodesis is favored over repair in patients older than 40 years who have a symptomatic SLAP lesion.

The choice of surgical treatment depends on the type of SLAP lesion, as determined using the original four-type Snyder classification. Other classification types essentially consist of a SLAP lesion plus an instability lesion, which generally is surgically treated as it would be in the absence of extension into the superior labrum. The recommendation is to repair the SLAP lesion concomitant with the instability procedure. A type I SLAP lesion can be treated with gentle débridement back to a stable base, but in the absence of symptoms may not require surgical treatment. A type II SLAP lesion by definition destabilizes the biceps anchor. Reattachment of the biceps-labrum complex to the superior glenoid generally is required, but primary biceps tenodesis can be used in revision surgery or for a patient who is older than 40 years or relatively inactive. A type III SLAP lesion can be treated with débridement of the bucket-handle labrum and repair of any unstable labral rim. In addition, the middle glenohumeral ligament should be repaired if it is attached to the bucket-handle labrum. The choice of surgical treatment of a type IV lesion depends on the severity of the injury to the biceps tendon. With minimal biceps involvement, débridement of the biceps plus labral repair is appropriate, but the treatment of choice for a severely injured biceps is open or arthroscopic primary biceps tenodesis.

Surgical Technique

Many techniques of SLAP repair have been described; the technique preferred by this chapter's authors is described here (**Figures 7** and **8**). Beach chair or lateral decubitus positioning of the patient can be used for arthroscopy. The posterior portal should be established in standard fashion. It can be helpful to establish a very medial portal (near the glenoid) if a Bankart lesion is also present; a more lateral portal is helpful for a SLAP lesion with substantial posterior extension. An anterior

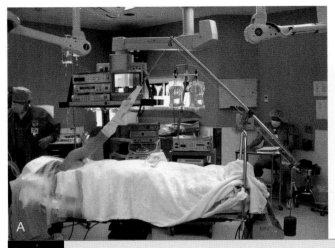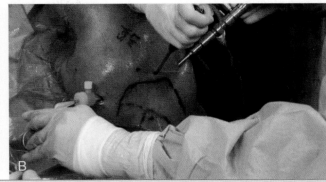

Figure 7 Photographs showing repair of a SLAP lesion. **A,** The lateral decubitus patient position is preferred for an all-arthroscopic procedure, but the beach chair position also can be used. **B,** The position of the anterior portal (green cannula), the posterior viewing portal, and an accessory portal for anchor placement (not always necessary) are shown.

portal is established in the rotator cuff interval, and diagnostic arthroscopy is performed to identify any concomitant pathology. Additional portals are used for anchor placement, depending on the nature of the SLAP lesion, including an accessory lateral portal (approximately 1 cm from the anterolateral corner of the acromion), the portal of Wilmington (approximately 1 cm anterolateral to the posterolateral corner of the acromion) and the Neviaser portal, which can be used for suture passage. It is rarely necessary to establish all of these portals. A cannula should be used only in the anterior portal, not through the rotator cuff.[41] Any portal through the rotator cuff should be made with a No. 11 blade oriented in line with the fibers of the rotator cuff to minimize iatrogenic pathology.

The SLAP lesion should be probed and classified to determine the appropriate surgical treatment. Determining the stability of the biceps anchor is critical. The labrum should be freed from the glenoid, essentially completing the tear. The next step is the preparation of a bleeding bony bed for healing, as in any labral repair. This step typically is done from the anterior portal. Good control of the shaver, commonly used on the reverse setting, is important to avoid the tendency to skive during preparation on the glenoid face. The next step is anchor placement at the articular margin; the use of suture tacks has largely been abandoned because of reports of synovitis and articular damage.[42,43] Standard 3.0-mm biocomposite suture anchors are preferred, although knotless techniques were found to be an acceptable alternative.[44] One anchor should be placed anterior to the biceps anchor, using a spinal needle to identify the appropriate angle of approach from the accessory lateral portal (45° from the center of the glenoid). This portal usually can be used to place one anchor posterior to the biceps, but the portal of Wilmington should be used if the SLAP lesion has substan-

tial posterior extension. It is important to avoid compromising the anchor placement or the orientation to save a portal. Suture passage can be accomplished using a suture retrieval device that passes through a spinal needle, a rigid retrograde suture-passing device, a curved suture loop, or a suture-retrieving instrument. The suture configuration can be a simple loop, in which only one suture limb is passed around the superior labrum, or a mattress stitch, in which both limbs are passed. Biomechanical data suggest that one mattress suture has a higher load to failure than one simple suture, one double-loaded anchor provides a load to failure equivalent to that of two single-loaded anchors, and two posterior anchors are equivalent to one anterior and one posterior anchor (on a posteriorly directed vector simulating the peel-back mechanism).[45-47] Surgical treatment of any paralabral cyst can be performed concomitantly and usually arthroscopically.[48] A paralabral cyst may resolve without direct decompression through repair of the SLAP lesion, but direct decompression is preferred if there is substantial muscle atrophy.[49]

Postoperative Care

The choice of a specific rehabilitation protocol after SLAP lesion repair depends on the nature of the repair (a slower progression is required for a relatively extensive tear) as well as any additional pathology identified during surgery.[50] The first 6 weeks of the postoperative period are focused on regaining range of motion and dynamic stability of the shoulder, and the next 6 weeks are devoted to strengthening and regaining proprioception.

Rehabilitation can be fairly aggressive after a simple débridement procedure, but repair of a type II SLAP lesion requires a more gradual, structured protocol. For the first 4 weeks, the allowable range of motion is be-

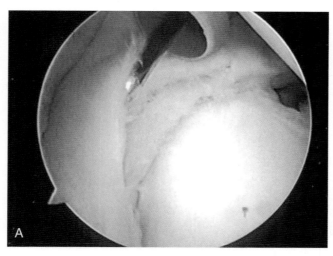

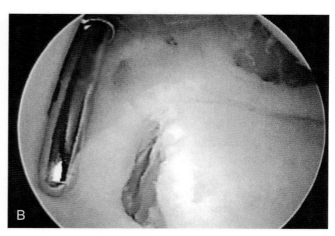

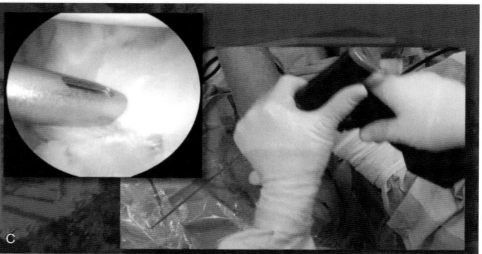

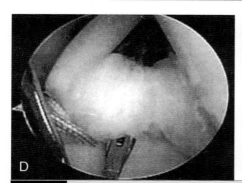

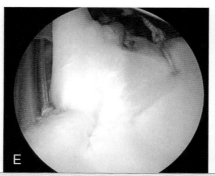

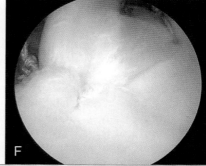

Figure 8 Photograph and arthroscopic images showing repair of a SLAP lesion. **A,** Biceps anchor involvement in the lesion. **B,** The labrum is elevated from the glenoid, and a shaver is used to prepare the superior glenoid rim by removing soft tissue and leaving a bleeding bony bed. **C,** Anchors are placed at the superior glenoid margin, most commonly just anterior and posterior to the biceps tendon, through the standard portals or an accessory posterior portal. **D,** A retrograde suture passer is used to grasp one limb of the paired suture for a simple configuration or both limbs for a mattress configuration. **E,** The suture is tied down, with care to keep the suture away from the glenoid face. **F,** The completed SLAP repair.

low 90° of elevation; internal rotation is allowed to a greater extent than external rotation. Full motion is to be obtained by 8 weeks after surgery, with throwing motion by 12 weeks. Isometric strengthening is initiated immediately after surgery to promote dynamic stabilization, but weight-bearing exercises are avoided until 7 weeks have passed, and biceps strengthening is initiated after 12 weeks.

Rehabilitation after a type IV lesion repair is similar to that for a type II lesion, with additional emphasis on management of the biceps tendon. If the biceps was released, active biceps exercises begin at 6 weeks. If a tenodesis was performed, it is advisable to begin active biceps exercises after 12 weeks.

Outcomes

Most reports of SLAP lesion outcomes have focused on type II lesions. At 1-year follow-up, 78% of the patients who underwent simple débridement of a SLAP lesion had an excellent result, but at 2-year follow-up, only 63% had an excellent result, and only 44% had returned to sports.[51]

The results of a SLAP lesion repair depend on the method of fixation. The use of bioabsorbable tacks has led to relatively poor outcomes, particularly as related to night pain, the expected level of postoperative activity, and return to sports.[41,52] Arthroscopic repair of a SLAP lesion was found to eliminate the peel-back sign, with a 97% rate of good or excellent results.[53] At 1-year follow-up, 44 of 53 pitchers (87%) had returned to play. The results were worse in patients with an undersurface rotator cuff tear, all of whom had a substantial internal rotation deficit. A study of 23 elite overhead athletes found relatively poor return-to-play results in patients who had an undersurface rotator cuff tear.[54] At a mean 38-month follow-up, 22 patients (96%) had a good to excellent American Shoulder and Elbow Index score. However, only 12 patients (52%) had a good to excellent score on the Kerlan-Jobe Orthopaedic Clinic measure,[55] and 13 (57%) had returned to play. A recent prospective study of 47 patients found that 40 (87%) had a good to excellent result at an average 2.7-year follow-up, with better patient-reported outcomes and a higher return-to-play rate in patients with an acute traumatic event than in those with an atraumatic etiology.[56] At an average 3.5-year follow-up, overhead athletes had an overall satisfaction rate of 93%, a perceived rate of return to preinjury performance of 84%, and average American Shoulder and Elbow Surgeons and Kerlan-Jobe Orthopaedic Clinic scores of 87.9 and 73.6, respectively.[57] This study confirmed the Kerlan-Jobe score as the superior measure for assessing outcomes in throwing athletes.

An 87% overall rate of good to excellent results was found in a study of patients with an average age of 39.7 years.[58] Sixty-five percent of patients with a workers' compensation claim had good to excellent results versus 95% of patients with no claim, and there was a trend toward worse results that did not reach statistical significance in patients older than 40 years. Similarly, another study found no significant difference in outcomes after SLAP repair based on age younger or older than 40 years.[59] Good results were reported for concomitant SLAP and rotator cuff repairs in older patients (mean age, 57 years).[60] A study of patients age 45 to 60 years found débridement of type II SLAP lesions to be superior to repair in combination with rotator cuff repair.[61] Data are limited on revision SLAP repair, but in one small study, revision repair had significantly worse results in 12 patients than primary repair in historical control patients, particularly in patients who were overhead athletes or had a workers' compensation claim.[62]

Primary biceps tenodesis recently has been proposed as a reasonable alternative for treating a SLAP lesion, particularly in patients who are older or not involved in overhead sports. A comparison of results in primary arthroscopic tenodesis and SLAP repair found significantly better Constant scores, satisfaction, and return to play after tenodesis. The patients treated with tenodesis were significantly older than those treated with repair (average age, 52 and 37 years, respectively), and extrapolation of the data to a younger patient population is problematic.[63]

Complications

The most common complication of SLAP repair is postoperative stiffness with decreased range of motion, which can be minimized with adequate postoperative physical therapy. Additional reported complications include night pain with penetration of the rotator cuff, synovitis, and chondral damage related to loose bodies and metallic anchors.[52,64-66] Isolated suprascapular nerve injury has been reported.[67,68]

Summary

SLAP lesions are commonly found in two distinct populations: patients who have had a single traumatic event and those who participate in overhead sports. The classic type II SLAP lesion is found in the dominant arm of a male overhead athlete younger than 40 years. The pathogenesis of SLAP lesions in overhead athletes is controversial. The clinical evaluation for a SLAP lesion is somewhat unreliable; an accurate diagnosis is dependent on high-quality imaging (3-tesla MRA) and can be confirmed arthroscopically. Nonsurgical treatment sometimes is effective, but surgical repair is the standard for overhead athletes. Surgical repair of a SLAP lesion has good results with respect to pain and overall shoulder function, but return to high-level athletic activity is less predictable. Major complications are uncommon with modern repair techniques. Structured rehabilitation based on the extent of the injury and the nature of the repair is important to a successful outcome.

Annotated References

1. Neer CS II: Anterior acromioplasty for the chronic impingement syndrome in the shoulder: A preliminary report. *J Bone Joint Surg Am* 1972;54(1):41-50.

4: Arthroscopy

2. Tibone JE, Jobe FW, Kerlan RK, et al: Shoulder impingement syndrome in athletes treated by an anterior acromioplasty. *Clin Orthop Relat Res* 1985;188:134-140.

3. Andrews JR, Carson WG Jr, McLeod WD: Glenoid labrum tears related to the long head of the biceps. *Am J Sports Med* 1985;13(5):337-341.

4. Snyder SJ, Karzel RP, Del Pizzo W, Ferkel RD, Friedman MJ: SLAP lesions of the shoulder. *Arthroscopy* 1990;6(4):274-279.

5. Maffet MW, Gartsman GM, Moseley B: Superior labrum-biceps tendon complex lesions of the shoulder. *Am J Sports Med* 1995;23(1):93-98.

6. Powell SE, Nord KD, Ryu RK: The diagnosis, classification and treatment of SLAP lesions. *Oper Tech Sports Med* 2004;12:99-110.

7. Gobezie R, Zurakowski D, Lavery K, Millett PJ, Cole BJ, Warner JJ: Analysis of interobserver and intraobserver variability in the diagnosis and treatment of SLAP tears using the Snyder classification. *Am J Sports Med* 2008;36(7):1373-1379.

   This is a cohort study in which 22 video vignettes of shoulder arthroscopy were sent to members of the Arthroscopy Association of North America, the American Shoulder and Elbow Surgeons, and the American Orthopaedic Society for Sports Medicine. They were asked to review the images, classify the SLAP lesions, and recommend treatment; a total of 73 members returned analyses. Surgeons had the most difficulty differentiating between type III and type IV lesions and between type II lesions and normal shoulders; additionally, the treatment of type III lesions was most variable. Overall, moderate interobserver agreement was found with respect to the Snyder classification, which improved significantly when the diagnoses were analyzed based on treatment desision. Level of evidence: II.

8. Jia X, Yokota A, McCarty EC, et al: Reproducibility and reliability of the Snyder classification of superior labral anterior posterior lesions among shoulder surgeons. *Am J Sports Med* 2011;39(5):986-991.

9. Kumar VP, Satku K, Balasubramaniam P: The role of the long head of biceps brachii in the stabilization of the head of the humerus. *Clin Orthop Relat Res* 1989;244:172-175.

10. Pagnani MJ, Deng XH, Warren RF, Torzilli PA, Altchek DW: Effect of lesions of the superior portion of the glenoid labrum on glenohumeral translation. *J Bone Joint Surg Am* 1995;77(7):1003-1010.

11. Warner JJ, McMahon PJ: The role of the long head of the biceps brachii in superior stability of the glenohumeral joint. *J Bone Joint Surg Am* 1995;77(3):366-372.

12. Burkhart SS, Morgan CD: The peel-back mechanism: Its role in producing and extending posterior type II SLAP lesions and its effect on SLAP repair rehabilitation. *Arthroscopy* 1998;14(6):637-640.

13. Clavert P, Bonnomet F, Kempf JF, Boutemy P, Braun M, Kahn JL: Contribution to the study of the pathogenesis of type II superior labrum anterior-posterior lesions: A cadaveric model of a fall on the outstretched hand. *J Shoulder Elbow Surg* 2004;13(1):45-50.

14. Bey MJ, Elders GJ, Huston LJ, Kuhn JE, Blasier RB, Soslowsky LJ: The mechanism of creation of superior labrum, anterior, and posterior lesions in a dynamic biomechanical model of the shoulder: The role of inferior subluxation. *J Shoulder Elbow Surg* 1998;7(4):397-401.

15. Burkhart SS, Morgan CD, Kibler WB: The disabled throwing shoulder: Spectrum of pathology. Part I: Pathoanatomy and biomechanics. *Arthroscopy* 2003;19(4):404-420.

16. Walch G, Boileau P, Noel E, Donell ST: Impingement of the deep surface of the supraspinatus tendon on the posterosuperior glenoid rim: An arthroscopic study. *J Shoulder Elbow Surg* 1992;1(5):238-245.

17. Jazrawi LM, McCluskey GM III, Andrews JR: Superior labral anterior and posterior lesions and internal impingement in the overhead athlete. *Instr Course Lect* 2003;52:43-63.

18. Kampa RJ, Clasper J: Incidence of SLAP lesions in a military population. *J R Army Med Corps* 2005;151(3):171-175.

19. Burkhart SS, Morgan CD, Kibler WB: Shoulder injuries in overhead athletes: The "dead arm" revisited. *Clin Sports Med* 2000;19(1):125-158.

20. O'Brien SJ, Pagnani MJ, Fealy S, McGlynn SR, Wilson JB: The active compression test: A new and effective test for diagnosing labral tears and acromioclavicular joint abnormality. *Am J Sports Med* 1998;26(5):610-613.

21. Kim SH, Ha KI, Ahn JH, Kim SH, Choi HJ: Biceps load test II: A clinical test for SLAP lesions of the shoulder. *Arthroscopy* 2001;17(2):160-164.

22. Nakagawa S, Yoneda M, Hayashida K, Obata M, Fukushima S, Miyazaki Y: Forced shoulder abduction and elbow flexion test: A new simple clinical test to detect superior labral injury in the throwing shoulder. *Arthroscopy* 2005;21(11):1290-1295.

23. Liu SH, Henry MH, Nuccion SL: A prospective evaluation of a new physical examination in predicting glenoid labral tears. *Am J Sports Med* 1996;24(6):721-725.

24. Myers TH, Zemanovic JR, Andrews JR: The resisted supination external rotation test: A new test for the diagnosis of superior labral anterior posterior lesions. *Am J Sports Med* 2005;33(9):1315-1320.

25. Cheung EV, O'Driscoll SW: Abstract: The dynamic labral shear test for superior labral anterior posterior tears of the shoulder. *74th Annual Meeting Proceedings.* Rosemont, IL, American Academy of Orthopaedic Surgeons, 2007, p 574.

    The authors assess the dynamic labral shear test in the diagnosis of SLAP tears in 105 shoulders.

26. Ben Kibler W, Sciascia AD, Hester P, Dome D, Jacobs C: Clinical utility of traditional and new tests in the diagnosis of biceps tendon injuries and superior labrum anterior and posterior lesions in the shoulder. *Am J Sports Med* 2009;37(9):1840-1847.

    In a cohort study of 325 consecutive patients who underwent six commonly described clinical tests and two new tests (uppercut and dynamic labral shear), clinical findings were correlated with findings at surgery. The uppercut test was the most accurate for biceps disease, and the dynamic labral shear test as the most accurate single test for SLAP lesions.

27. Meserve BB, Cleland JA, Boucher TR: A meta-analysis examining clinical test utility for assessing superior labral anterior posterior lesions. *Am J Sports Med* 2009;37(11):2252-2258.

    Six of 198 studies met the inclusion criteria for a meta-analysis of clinical tests for the diagnosis of SLAP lesions. The accuracy of the anterior slide test was poor. The recommendation was to use the active compression test first, the crank test second, and the Speed test third when a SLAP lesion is suspected.

28. Cook C, Beaty S, Kissenberth MJ, Siffri P, Pill SG, Hawkins RJ: Diagnostic accuracy of five orthopedic clinical tests for diagnosis of superior labrum anterior posterior (SLAP) lesions. *J Shoulder Elbow Surg* 2012;21(1):13-22.

    A case control study of 87 patients with shoulder pathology evaluated the clinical accuracy and usefulness of five commonly described tests for the diagnosis of SLAP lesions. Only the biceps load II test had clinical usefulness for identifying isolated SLAP lesions, and none of the tests were accurate in isolation. Level of evidence: III.

29. Borrero CG, Casagranda BU, Towers JD, Bradley JP: Magnetic resonance appearance of posterosuperior labral peel back during humeral abduction and external rotation. *Skeletal Radiol* 2010;39(1):19-26.

    A retrospective review of patients younger than 40 years found MRI sensitivity of 73%, specificity of 100%, positive predictive value of 100%, and negative predictive value of 78% for the presence of a peel-back lesion.

30. Jung JY, Ha DH, Lee SM, Blacksin MF, Kim KA, Kim JW: Displaceability of SLAP lesion on shoulder MR arthrography with external rotation position. *Skeletal Radiol* 2011;40(8):1047-1055.

    MRA in neutral and external rotation of 210 patients who underwent shoulder arthroscopy found sensitivity improved from 64.4% (neutral) to 78.5% (external rotation), accuracy improved from 71% to 81.9%, and specificity constant at 93.6%.

31. Connell DA, Potter HG, Wickiewicz TL, Altchek DW, Warren RF: Noncontrast magnetic resonance imaging of superior labral lesions: 102 cases confirmed at arthroscopic surgery. *Am J Sports Med* 1999;27(2):208-213.

32. Bencardino JT, Beltran J, Rosenberg ZS, et al: Superior labrum anterior-posterior lesions: Diagnosis with MR arthrography of the shoulder. *Radiology* 2000;214(1):267-271.

33. Jee WH, McCauley TR, Katz LD, Matheny JM, Ruwe PA, Daigneault JP: Superior labral anterior posterior (SLAP) lesions of the glenoid labrum: Reliability and accuracy of MR arthrography for diagnosis. *Radiology* 2001;218(1):127-132.

34. Tung GA, Entzian D, Green A, Brody JM: High-field and low-field MR imaging of superior glenoid labral tears and associated tendon injuries. *AJR Am J Roentgenol* 2000;174(4):1107-1114.

35. Pandya NK, Colton A, Webner D, Sennett B, Huffman GR: Physical examination and magnetic resonance imaging in the diagnosis of superior labrum anterior-posterior lesions of the shoulder: A sensitivity analysis. *Arthroscopy* 2008;24(3):311-317.

    Fifty-one consecutive patients with a SLAP lesion confirmed arthroscopically and no shoulder instability were evaluated with MRI or MRA and physical examination. Test sensitivities were active compression, 90%; dynamic shear, 80%; and Jobe relocation, 76%. MRI sensitivity was 67% (surgeon) and 53% (radiologist); MRA sensitivity was 72% (surgeon) and 50% (radiologist). Level of evidence: II.

36. Magee T: 3-T MRI of the shoulder: Is MR arthrography necessary? *AJR Am J Roentgenol* 2009;192(1):86-92.

    In 150 consecutive patients younger than 50 years, MRA was more sensitive than MRI for detecting partial-thickness rotator cuff tears, SLAP lesions, and anterior labral tears.

37. Kim YJ, Choi JA, Oh JH, Hwang SI, Hong SH, Kang HS: Superior labral anteroposterior tears: Accuracy and interobserver reliability of multidetector CT arthrography for diagnosis. *Radiology* 2011;260(1):207-215.

    A review of 161 CT arthrograms for the detection of SLAP lesions found sensitivity of 94.3% to 97%, specificity of 72.6% to 76.7%, and accuracy of 86.3%, with good interobserver agreement ($\kappa = 0.72$).

38. Oh JH, Kim JY, Choi JA, Kim WS: Effectiveness of multidetector computed tomography arthrography for

4: Arthroscopy

the diagnosis of shoulder pathology: Comparison with magnetic resonance imaging with arthroscopic correlation. *J Shoulder Elbow Surg* 2010;19(1):14-20.

Similar sensitivity, specificity and interobserver agreement were found for CT arthrography and MRA in the diagnosis of labral pathology and full-thickness rotator cuff tears, but MRA was better at identifying partial-thickness rotator cuff tears. Level of evidence: I.

39. Wilk KE, Obma P, Simpson CD, Cain EL, Dugas JR, Andrews JR: Shoulder injuries in the overhead athlete. *J Orthop Sports Phys Ther* 2009;39(2):38-54.

Shoulder anatomy, pathology, biomechanics, and rehabilitation of the overhead athlete were reviewed. Level of evidence: V.

40. Edwards SL, Lee JA, Bell JE, et al: Nonoperative treatment of superior labrum anterior posterior tears: Improvements in pain, function, and quality of life. *Am J Sports Med* 2010;38(7):1456-1461.

Nineteen patients who were nonsurgically treated for a documented SLAP lesion had overall improvement on functional outcomes measures at a minimum 1-year follow-up, with 71% of the athletes returning to their earlier sports levels.

41. O'Brien SJ, Allen AA, Coleman SH, Drakos MC: The trans-rotator cuff approach to SLAP lesions: Technical aspects for repair and a clinical follow-up of 31 patients at a minimum of 2 years. *Arthroscopy* 2002; 18(4):372-377.

42. Freehill MQ, Harms DJ, Huber SM, Atlihan D, Buss DD: Poly-L-lactic acid tack synovitis after arthroscopic stabilization of the shoulder. *Am J Sports Med* 2003; 31(5):643-647.

43. Sassmannshausen G, Sukay M, Mair SD: Broken or dislodged poly-L-lactic acid bioabsorbable tacks in patients after SLAP lesion surgery. *Arthroscopy* 2006; 22(6):615-619.

44. Oh JH, Lee HK, Kim JY, Kim SH, Gong HS: Clinical and radiologic outcomes of arthroscopic glenoid labrum repair with the BioKnotless suture anchor. *Am J Sports Med* 2009;37(12):2340-2348.

A study of 97 patients with a labral tear repaired with the BioKnotless suture anchor found overall good results, with significant improvements in functional outcomes scores and a return to normal recreation and sport in 81.1% of the patients with anterior instability and 83.3% of those with a SLAP lesion. Level of evidence: IV.

45. Domb BG, Ehteshami JR, Shindle MK, et al: Biomechanical comparison of 3 suture anchor configurations for repair of type II SLAP lesions. *Arthroscopy* 2007; 23(2):135-140.

A biomechanical cadaver study evaluated the load to failure of three suture configurations used for SLAP repair. The single anchor with mattress suture through the biceps anchor was the strongest configuration, fol-lowed by two anchors with simple sutures anterior and posterior to the anchor. A simple suture anterior to the anchor was the weakest configuration.

46. Baldini T, Snyder RL, Peacher G, Bach J, McCarty E: Strength of single- versus double-anchor repair of type II SLAP lesions: A cadaveric study. *Arthroscopy* 2009;25(11):1257-1260.

A biomechanical study found that using two single-loaded anchors is biomechanically equivalent to using a single double-loaded anchor with respect to mean load to failure in SLAP repair.

47. Morgan RJ, Kuremsky MA, Peindl RD, Fleischli JE: A biomechanical comparison of two suture anchor configurations for the repair of type II SLAP lesions subjected to a peel-back mechanism of failure. *Arthroscopy* 2008;24(4):383-388.

A biomechanical study found an equivalent load to failure in two suture configurations for SLAP repair (two anchors placed posterior to the biceps anchor, one anchor placed anterior and one placed posterior to the biceps anchor).

48. Westerheide KJ, Dopirak RM, Karzel RP, Snyder SJ: Suprascapular nerve palsy secondary to spinoglenoid cysts: Results of arthroscopic treatment. *Arthroscopy* 2006;22(7):721-727.

49. Youm T, Matthews PV, ElAttrache NS: Treatment of patients with spinoglenoid cysts associated with superior labral tears without cyst aspiration, debridement, or excision. *Arthroscopy* 2006;22(5):548-552.

50. Wilk KE, Reinold MM, Dugas JR, Arrigo CA, Moser MW, Andrews JR: Current concepts in the recognition and treatment of superior labral (SLAP) lesions. *J Orthop Sports Phys Ther* 2005;35(5):273-291.

51. Cordasco FA, Steinmann S, Flatow EL, Bigliani LU: Arthroscopic treatment of glenoid labral tears. *Am J Sports Med* 1993;21(3):425-430, discussion 430-431.

52. Cohen DB, Coleman S, Drakos MC, et al: Outcomes of isolated type II SLAP lesions treated with arthroscopic fixation using a bioabsorbable tack. *Arthroscopy* 2006;22(2):136-142.

53. Morgan CD, Burkhart SS, Palmeri M, Gillespie M: Type II SLAP lesions: Three subtypes and their relationships to superior instability and rotator cuff tears. *Arthroscopy* 1998;14(6):553-565.

54. Neri BR, ElAttrache NS, Owsley KC, Mohr K, Yocum LA: Outcome of type II superior labral anterior posterior repairs in elite overhead athletes: Effect of concomitant partial-thickness rotator cuff tears. *Am J Sports Med* 2011;39(1):114-120.

A cohort study evaluated the results of SLAP repair in overhead athletes using two outcomes measures. The Kerlan-Jobe score was more strongly correlated with return to play than the American Shoulder and Elbow Index score. Level of evidence: III.

55. Alberta FG, ElAttrache NS, Bissell S, et al: The development and validation of a functional assessment tool for the upper extremity in the overhead athlete. *Am J Sports Med* 2010;38(5):903-911.

In a cross-sectional study, 282 competitive overhead athletes completing the new Kerlan-Jobe Orthopaedic Clinic questionnaire were self-stratified into three injury categories: playing without pain, playing with pain, or not playing as a result of pain. The new score correctly stratified patients by injury category and had excellent responsiveness after treatment of injury.

56. Brockmeier SF, Voos JE, Williams RJ III, Altchek DW, Cordasco FA, Allen AA; Hospital for Special Surgery Sports Medicine and Shoulder Service: Outcomes after arthroscopic repair of type-II SLAP lesions. *J Bone Joint Surg Am* 2009;91(7):1595-1603.

A prospective study of 47 patients who underwent repair of a type II SLAP lesion found good overall scores on outcomes measures and high patient satisfaction at a minimum 2-year follow-up. Patient satisfaction and return-to-play rates were higher in patients who had discrete trauma. Level of evidence: IV.

57. Neuman BJ, Boisvert CB, Reiter B, Lawson K, Ciccotti MG, Cohen SB: Results of arthroscopic repair of type II superior labral anterior posterior lesions in overhead athletes: Assessment of return to preinjury playing level and satisfaction. *Am J Sports Med* 2011;39(9):1883-1888.

A review found overall good results and high patient satisfaction in 30 overhead athletes who underwent SLAP repair, at an average 3.5-year follow-up. Functional outcomes scores and overall satisfaction were relatively low. Level of evidence: IV.

58. Denard PJ, Lädermann A, Burkhart SS: Long-term outcome after arthroscopic repair of type II SLAP lesions: Results according to age and workers' compensation status. *Arthroscopy* 2012;28(4):451-457.

A review of long-term outcomes of isolated type II SLAP repairs found a good to excellent result in 87%, with significantly poorer results in patients with a worker's compensation claim. Level of evidence: IV.

59. Alpert JM, Wuerz TH, O'Donnell TF, Carroll KM, Brucker NN, Gill TJ: The effect of age on the outcomes of arthroscopic repair of type II superior labral anterior and posterior lesions. *Am J Sports Med* 2010;38(11):2299-2303.

A review of 52 patients at a minimum 2-year follow-up after type II SLAP repair found no significant difference in outcomes scores or patient satisfaction stratified by age (age 40 years or younger versus older than 40 years). Level of evidence: III.

60. Forsythe B, Guss D, Anthony SG, Martin SD: Concomitant arthroscopic SLAP and rotator cuff repair. *J Bone Joint Surg Am* 2010;92(6):1362-1369.

A retrospective study compared the results of rotator cuff repair with or without concomitant SLAP repair in older patients. Functional outcomes scores were comparable. Level of evidence: III.

61. Abbot AE, Li X, Busconi BD: Arthroscopic treatment of concomitant superior labral anterior posterior (SLAP) lesions and rotator cuff tears in patients over the age of 45 years. *Am J Sports Med* 2009;37(7):1358-1362.

In a cohort study of patients older than 45 years who had a rotator cuff tear and a type II SLAP lesion, all patients had a rotator cuff repair and were randomly assigned to débridement or SLAP lesion repair. The patients who underwent débridement had better outcomes scores, improved function, and better motion that those with SLAP repair. Level of evidence: II.

62. Park S, Glousman RE: Outcomes of revision arthroscopic type II superior labral anterior posterior repairs. *Am J Sports Med* 2011;39(6):1290-1294.

At a mean follow-up of 50.5 months, 12 patients (mean age, 32.6 years) who underwent an isolated revision SLAP repair had overall worse results than with a primary repair. The worst results were in patients with a workers' compensation claim and overhead athletes. Level of evidence: IV.

63. Boileau P, Parratte S, Chuinard C, Roussanne Y, Shia D, Bicknell R: Arthroscopic treatment of isolated type II SLAP lesions: Biceps tenodesis as an alternative to reinsertion. *Am J Sports Med* 2009;37(5):929-936.

Poorer results were found in 10 patients (mean age, 37 years) who had a SLAP repair than in 15 patients (mean age, 52 years) who had an arthroscopic biceps tenodesis. The significant age difference between the groups makes it difficult to draw any definitive conclusions. Level of evidence: III.

64. Edwards DJ, Hoy G, Saies AD, Hayes MG: Adverse reactions to an absorbable shoulder fixation device. *J Shoulder Elbow Surg* 1994;3(4):230-233.

65. Burkart A, Imhoff AB, Roscher E: Foreign-body reaction to the bioabsorbable Suretac device. *Arthroscopy* 2000;16(1):91-95.

66. Kaar TK, Schenck RC Jr, Wirth MA, Rockwood CA Jr: Complications of metallic suture anchors in shoulder surgery: A report of 8 cases. *Arthroscopy* 2001;17(1):31-37.

67. Yoo JC, Lee YS, Ahn JH, Park JH, Kang HJ, Koh KH: Isolated suprascapular nerve injury below the spinoglenoid notch after SLAP repair. *J Shoulder Elbow Surg* 2009;18(4):e27-e29.

An isolated suprascapular nerve injury occurred after arthroscopic SLAP repair.

68. Kim SH, Koh YG, Sung CH, Moon HK, Park YS: Iatrogenic suprascapular nerve injury after repair of type II SLAP lesion. *Arthroscopy* 2010;26(7):1005-1008.

A suprascapular nerve injury at the spinoglenoid notch was caused by improper insertion of a suture anchor during a type II SLAP repair.

4: Arthroscopy

Chapter 26

Arthroscopic Treatment of the Arthritic Shoulder

Emilie V. Cheung, MD   Marc Safran, MD   John Costouros, MD

4: Arthroscopy

Introduction

The management of a painful arthritic shoulder in a young or active patient poses a treatment dilemma for the orthopaedic surgeon. The definition of "young" must be based on both chronologic and physiologic age in the context of activity demands. The primary goals of treatment are pain relief and functional improvement. Nonsurgical treatment may not provide satisfactory pain relief, and patients may become frustrated by their functional decline during activities of daily living and recreational pursuits. Total shoulder arthroplasty offers the most favorable and predictable results, but the long-term success of shoulder arthroplasty is relatively unpredictable in young patients. The risk of complications, including glenoid component loosening and glenoid erosion that leads to a need for revision surgery, should be taken into account when shoulder arthroplasty is being considered for a young or active patient.

At a minimum 15-year follow-up after total shoulder arthroplasty or hemiarthroplasty in 78 arthritic shoulders in patients age 50 years or younger, the estimated survival rate (defined as being free of revision surgery) at 20 years was 84% for total shoulder arthro-

plasty and 75% for hemiarthroplasty.[1] There was marked long-term pain relief and improvement in motion after shoulder arthroplasty. However, the use of the Neer clinical rating system indicated that almost half of the patients had an unsatisfactory result, usually because of limitations in motion. The researchers concluded that great care must be exercised and alternative methods of treatment must be considered before shoulder joint arthroplasty is offered to patients age 50 years or younger. The reasons for revision surgery after total shoulder arthroplasty include infection, glenoid loosening, and rotator cuff tearing. Painful glenoid erosion is a leading reason for revision surgery after hemiarthroplasty.

The findings were similar in a report of revision rates after 1,285 consecutive shoulder arthroplasties (455 hemiarthroplasties and 830 total shoulder arthroplasties) performed to treat primary osteoarthritis, rheumatoid arthritis, or osteonecrosis.[2] Traumatic injuries were excluded from the study. There were no statistically significant between-group differences in demographic factors or diagnoses. The difference in surgical revision rates was statistically significant at an average 42-month follow-up, at 4.2% for those treated with hemiarthroplasty and 1.9% for those treated with total shoulder arthroplasty. The primary reasons for revision were symptomatic glenoid wear in those treated with hemiarthroplasty and glenoid component loosening in those treated with total shoulder arthroplasty.

These study findings suggest that other treatments should be actively considered for young patients before prosthetic replacement is considered. The options include arthroscopic débridement, the removal of loose bodies, chondroplasty, capsular release, and the treatment of associated pathology that may be contributing to pain. The well-described benefits of arthroscopy compared with open reconstruction include smaller incisions, shorter surgical time, less bleeding and postoperative pain, lower rates of infection, an outpatient surgical setting, and faster overall recovery.

The Outerbridge classification, although originally used to describe chondral and osteochondral lesions of the patella, has been used clinically to describe chondral and osteochondral lesions in other joints, including the shoulder. An Outerbridge grade I lesion is charac-

Dr. Cheung or an immediate family member serves as a board member, owner, officer, or committee member of the American Academy of Orthopaedic Surgeons. Dr. Safran or an immediate family member has received royalties from Stryker; serves as a paid consultant to Cool Systems and Arthrocare; serves as an unpaid consultant to Cool Systems, Cradle Medical, Ferring Pharmaceuticals, Biomimedica, and Eleven Blade Solutions; has stock or stock options held in Cool Systems, Cradle Medical, Biomimedica, and Eleven Blade Solutions; has received research or institutional support from Ferring Pharmaceuticals and Smith & Nephew; and serves as a board member, owner, officer, or committee member of the American Orthopaedic Society for Sports Medicine; the International Society of Arthroscopy, Knee Surgery, and Orthopaedic Sports Medicine; and the International Society for Hip Arthroscopy. Neither Dr. Costouros nor any immediate family member has received anything of value from or has stock or stock options held in a commercial company or institution related directly or indirectly to the subject of this chapter.

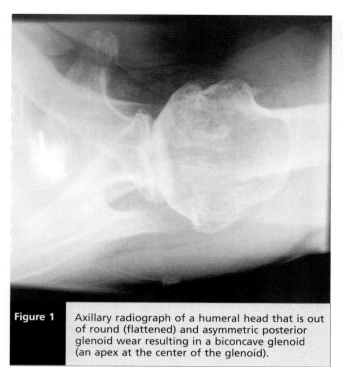

Figure 1 Axillary radiograph of a humeral head that is out of round (flattened) and asymmetric posterior glenoid wear resulting in a biconcave glenoid (an apex at the center of the glenoid).

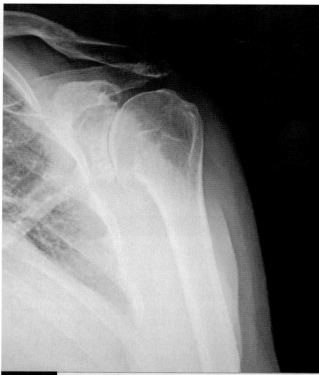

Figure 2 AP radiograph of the shoulder showing osteoarthritic changes, including joint space narrowing, inferior humeral osteophyte formation, subchondral cyst formation, and subchondral sclerosis.

terized by softening of the articular surface, grade II by fissuring of the hyaline articular cartilage, grade III by fibrillation of cartilage, and grade IV by exposed subchondral bone.[3] Chondromalacia with grade III or IV lesions is treated at the time of shoulder arthroscopy with débridement of the articular surface to create a smoother bearing surface and remove loose chondral flaps that may be causing mechanical pain.

Clinical Evaluation

Radiographic studies should include a true AP or Grashey view of the shoulder. In the Grashey view, the positioning is perpendicular to the scapular plane rather than to the plane of the body. The x-ray beam is angled approximately 40° laterally to obtain a proper view of the glenohumeral joint space. An axillary view of the shoulder is used to evaluate for eccentric glenoid wear and the presence of glenohumeral subluxation[4] (**Figure 1**). The radiographic changes of osteoarthritis include joint space narrowing, inferior humeral osteophyte formation, subchondral cyst formation, and subchondral sclerosis (**Figure 2**).

The Samilson-Prieto radiologic classification system has been used to describe the extent of shoulder arthropathy.[5] Mild arthrosis by definition includes inferior humeral head and/or glenoid exostosis less than 3 mm in height. Moderate arthrosis includes inferior humeral head and/or glenoid exostosis measuring 3 mm to 7 mm, with slight glenohumeral irregularity. Severe arthrosis includes inferior humeral head and/or glenoid exostosis more than 7 mm in height, with gle-

nohumeral joint space narrowing and sclerosis. Loose bodies also may be seen on radiographs. MRI is useful in identifying rotator cuff tears, labral or biceps pathology, and focal chondral lesions.

Arthritis often does not occur in isolation. The coexistent shoulder pathology may include subacromial impingement, rotator cuff tearing, acromioclavicular joint arthritis, long head biceps tendinopathy, capsular contracture, labral tearing, and suprascapular neuropathy. A detailed and comprehensive physical examination can guide the surgeon in identifying potential pain generators in the shoulder, in addition to advanced osteoarthritis. These sources of shoulder pain can be treated at the time of surgery despite the presence of osteoarthritis.

Surgical Contraindications and Indications

The surgical contraindications for arthroscopic débridement, such as an active infection or a medical comorbidity that precludes the use of general anesthesia, are similar to those for any surgical procedure. Lack of medical fitness to undergo general anesthesia is a relative contraindication because shoulder arthroscopic débridement can be done using regional anesthesia (interscalene block).

The indications for arthroscopic débridement include lack of improvement after at least 3 months of nonsurgical treatment. Nonsurgical treatment includes physical therapy for maintaining range of motion, NSAIDs, and intra-articular injection of corticosteroid. Patients with Milwaukee shoulder syndrome had pain relief at 6-month follow-up after simple closed needle irrigation of the shoulder followed by cortisone injection.[6]

Arthroscopic débridement often is included in the treatment algorithm of shoulder arthritis for a young, active patient who is not a candidate for arthroplasty or is unwilling to adhere to postoperative restrictions, thus increasing the risk of early implant failure. The best candidates for surgery may be patients who are physiologically young (younger than 60 years) and have a diagnosis of osteoarthritis, mild loss in range of motion, and concentric wear of the glenohumeral joint. Total shoulder arthroplasty often is not recommended for patients who participate in contact sports or have an occupation requiring heavy manual labor or lifting. These patients may be better served with a less invasive procedure, such as arthroscopic débridement. Shoulder arthroscopy has been shown to be a safe procedure with a low complication rate.[7,8] However, it is generally accepted that arthroscopic treatment of shoulder arthritis is a temporizing procedure and is not definitive. Those who undergo arthroscopic débridement often required shoulder arthroplasty several years later.

Surgical Technique

The surgical technique for arthroscopic débridement includes a complete diagnostic arthroscopy of the glenohumeral joint and the subacromial space (**Figures 3** and **4**). The use of regional anesthesia (an interscalene blockade) facilitates working in a contracted joint and is effective for postoperative pain control. The glenohumeral joint space is extremely narrowed as an effect of advanced osteoarthritis as well as capsular contracture. To avoid inadvertent chondral injury by the trocar in a tight shoulder, traction can be applied to the humeral head while the arthroscope is introduced into the glenohumeral joint. Another helpful technique is to introduce the trochar more superiorly than is usual when entering the joint, near the superior aspect of the humeral head at the joint line. Alternatively, a disposable plastic cannula can be used to enter the joint initially and replaced by the metallic cannula over a switching stick. A standard anterior working portal in the rotator cuff interval is created using an outside-in technique.

Coexistent lesions that may be causing shoulder pain may need to be treated at the time of surgery. Loose osteochondral fragments are removed. A motorized shaver is used to débride osteochondral lesions, and unstable flaps are débrided to a stable base with a shaver, a curette, and/or a rongeur. Outerbridge grade III articular cartilage is débrided to smooth tapering margins.

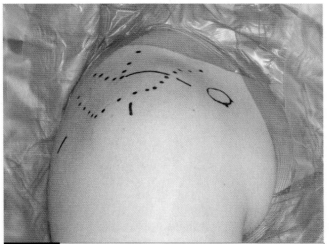

Figure 3 Photograph showing the standard setup for beach chair positioning of a patient undergoing arthroscopy of the right shoulder. The bony landmarks are marked, including the scapular spine and the clavicle *(dotted lines)*, the acromioclavicular joint *(long solid line)*, and the coracoid *(circle)*. The standard posterior, lateral, and anterior portal locations are marked *(short solid lines)*.

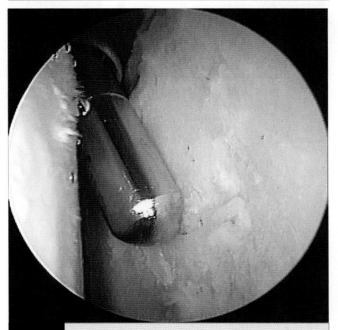

Figure 4 Intraoperative photograph showing the glenohumeral joint as seen through the standard posterior viewing portal in a left shoulder. Severe degenerative joint disease has affected the humeral head and the glenoid articular surfaces.

Large inferior humeral head osteophytes can cause mechanical symptoms, such as locking and crepitus. The surgeon can choose to shave down large inferior osteophytes from the humeral head using a motorized

4: Arthroscopy

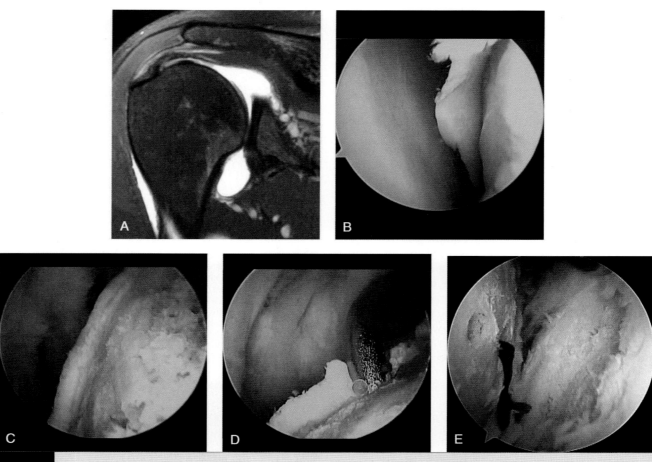

Figure 5   An isolated full-thickness chondral lesion of the humeral head. **A,** Preoperative MRI. Intraoperative photographs showing the lesion with a flap of articular cartilage at its edge (**B**), the lesion after débridement with a curette (**C**), and the microfracture awl penetrating the subchondral bone (**D**). **E,** Intraoperative photograph (of a different patient) showing blood leaking out of a hole in the bone made by the awl after microfracture of the humeral head.

burr. The use of an accessory anteroinferior working portal and devices that are curved allow easier access to the inferior humeral head. In addition, adjusting the rotation of the humeral head during surgery can facilitate the removal of inferior osteophytes. Although surgical removal of this potential mechanical block can improve motion of an arthritic shoulder, ultimately the capsular release is more important for improving motion. The risk of injury to the axillary nerve must be considered during débridement of osteophytes near the axillary pouch.[9]

Microfracture (drilling of intact subchondral bone) may be performed for focal lesions. The purpose is to cause an influx of pluripotent mesenchymal cells into the bleeding bed of subchondral bone, leading to fibrocartilage deposition and filling of the articular defect. After the cartilage defect is prepared to a stable rim, the zone of calcified cartilage is removed at the base of the lesion with a curette. Microfracture can be considered for a full-thickness cartilage defect of the humerus or glenoid, using criteria similar to those for the knee (for example, size less than 8 cm²). A microfracture awl is

used to penetrate the subchondral bone to a depth of 2 mm, with 2-mm spacing between the bony penetrations[10] (**Figure 5**). The clinical indications for microfracture and its results in the shoulder remain under investigation.

Arthroscopic glenoidplasty with osteocapsular arthroplasty has been described as an effective technique for patients with osteoarthritis of the shoulder for whom prosthetic replacement is considered unsuitable.[11] A nonconcentric glenohumeral joint is treated by correcting the articular contour of the misshapen glenoid, which in a patient with osteoarthritis characteristically has posterior wear. The procedure is analogous to eccentric reaming in open shoulder surgery. An arthroscopic burr and rasp are used to contour the anterior glenoid or smooth the osteochondral ridge in a biconcave glenoid. The glenoid is converted to a concentric concave shape, leading to improvement in pain and motion. It may be necessary to create multiple portals to gain access to large osteophytes around the humeral head. Arthroscopic synovectomy and capsular release can be performed, if indicated, to restore the position of the humeral head and theoretically to in-

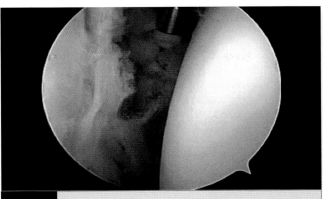

Figure 6 Intraoperative photograph from a posterior viewing portal showing arthroscopic capsular release of the anterior capsule using a radiofrequency device.

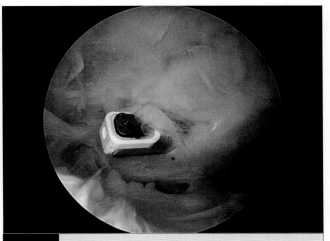

Figure 7 Intraoperative photograph showing the subacromial space from the posterior portal of a right shoulder. Bursectomy has been performed with a radiofrequency probe and an arthroscopic shaver. The coracoclavicular ligament (the shiny structure) remains intact, and the intact rotator cuff is seen in the lower part of the arthroscopic field.

crease the joint contact surface area. Arthroscopic synovectomy and capsular release is a technically challenging procedure, however, and should be reserved for the experienced shoulder arthroscopist.

Approximately 30% of patients undergoing arthroscopic débridement of shoulder osteoarthritis have capsular contractures.[12,13] Arthroscopic débridement alone cannot restore motion in these patients. Capsular release is recommended if the patient has lost significant motion, and it may help reestablish a concentric joint. A flat humeral head will not rotate, even after capsular release, and the preoperative evaluation should include careful inspection of the radiographs to be sure the humeral head is still round and the joint is concentric. Some surgeons believe that capsular releases reduce the contact pressures and thereby reduce pain.

The capsular release can be performed using a radiofrequency device or a handheld biting instrument. A standard anterior working portal is created using an outside-in technique through the rotator cuff interval. The rotator cuff interval capsule and the coracohumeral ligament are incised 1 cm lateral to the glenoid rim using the radiofrequency device. The thick capsular tissue within the rotator interval is completely released, and the middle glenohumeral ligament is released (**Figure 6**). The exposure of rotator cuff interval tissue may be facilitated by external rotation of the arm in adduction. Care should be taken to preserve the subscapularis tendon and the medial aspect of the biceps sling to prevent destabilizing the biceps tendon. The thick capsule covering the subscapularis should be released to the anterior inferior capsular pouch. The subscapularis and the capsule can be differentiated by their appearance: the subscapularis tendon fibers are oriented transversely, and the capsule has an amorphous appearance.

The posterior capsular release can be done by working through the posterior portal while viewing through the anterior portal or an accessory transcuff portal.[14]

The posterior capsule and associated glenohumeral ligament generally are less robust than the anterior capsular structures. Internal rotation during the release may be helpful for visualizing the posterior capsule.

Release of the inferior capsule should be performed with the arm in adduction to minimize the risk of injury to the axillary nerve, which often is in close proximity to the inferior glenoid. Rather than risk radiofrequency or direct mechanical injury to the axillary nerve, some surgeons prefer to complete the inferior release with manual manipulation, by placing the arm in maximal forward elevation while stabilizing the scapula.

The subacromial space is entered to perform a subacromial decompression, and a distal clavicle resection can be performed if clinically indicated (**Figure 7**). The subacromial bursectomy may be critical to the success of arthroscopic débridement of the shoulder for glenohumeral arthritis. A radiofrequency device is used for ablation of the subacromial bursa. Care is taken to preserve the coracoacromial ligament, especially in the context of a massive rotator cuff tear, reduce the risk of humeral head anterosuperior escape, especially if an arthroplasty eventually may be required.

The shoulder is gently manipulated with the patient under anesthesia. Special care should be taken in a patient with osteoporotic bone, who may be predisposed to iatrogenic fracture. It is helpful to use one hand to stabilize the scapula and the other hand to grasp the humeral shaft as close to the axilla as possible. This technique helps to shorten the lever arm during manipulation and reduce the risk of fracture. The manipulation leads to disruption of the inferior capsular fibers, which remain at the 6-o'clock position. Manipulation is performed in forward flexion, abduction, external rotation at the side, internal rotation at the side, external rotation in abduction, and internal rotation in abduction, and the achieved motion is recorded.

Postoperative Rehabilitation

A sling is used for comfort only after surgery, and the patient is encouraged to move the arm actively and passively. The patient should begin physical therapy immediately after surgery for aggressive passive and active range-of-motion exercises to maintain the motion achieved during surgery and prevent the development of adhesions. The patient should be taught to obtain forward elevation in the scapular plane, external rotation at the side, external rotation in abduction, and internal rotation. Exercises performed in the supine position limit scapulothoracic motion and help isolate the glenohumeral joint. The patient should perform these exercises not only during supervised physical therapy but also several times daily in a home program. Cryotherapy is routinely useful for controlling postoperative swelling and pain. The use of anti-inflammatory medications also may be helpful during the postoperative period. Strengthening exercises generally are incorporated as postoperative range of motion improves and pain subsides.

Results

The arthroscopic management of early shoulder arthritis was found to be effective in most studies with a relatively short term follow-up.[15] In one study, 25 patients with early shoulder arthritis (defined as arthritis without severe radiographic changes) were treated with arthroscopic débridement, the removal of loose bodies, and subacromial bursectomy.[16] At an average 34-month follow-up, 80% of patients had a good or excellent result. The minimum duration of pain relief was 8 months. The authors did not recommend this procedure for shoulders with a loss of glenohumeral joint space on the axillary radiograph or a loss of concentricity in the joint; however, data were not provided to support their recommendation.

Surgical procedures for coexistent pathology may be beneficial for patients with early osteoarthritis without obvious radiographic evidence. For example, all 21 patients with grade IV osteochondral lesions had improved pain and function after arthroscopic acromioplasty.[17] Other studies reported similarly favorable results when arthroscopic débridement was combined with arthroscopic bursectomy, labral débridement, or débridement of partial-thickness rotator cuff tears.[13,16,18]

Arthroscopic management of patients with isolated, focal grade IV chondral lesions of the glenohumeral joint (with no radiographic evidence of arthritis) was found to be effective.[12] Significant pain relief continuing at least 28 months was documented in 88% of patients. The addition of concomitant procedures, such as acromioplasty, distal clavicle resection, labral débridement, or labral repair, did not have a negative impact on the functional results. Osteochondral lesions larger than 2 cm^2 were associated with return of pain and failure of the procedure. The authors recommended arthroscopic capsular release for patients with a loss of passive shoulder motion.

In a prospective study, 19 patients with severe degenerative arthritis of the shoulder had arthroscopic débridement, the removal of loose bodies, and subacromial bursectomy.[19] The average follow-up was 24 months (range, 12 to 50 months). All patients had complete joint space loss and large osteophytes, and they had been referred for total shoulder arthroplasty. No osteophyte excision, glenoidplasty, acromioplasty, or other bony procedure was performed, and no capsulotomy or capsulectomy was added. After surgery, 16 patients (82%) were classified as having a good to excellent result. The maximal pain relief occurred at 3 months, the maximal functional improvement occurred at 6 months, and patient satisfaction reached a plateau at 6 months. The results were maintained in 78% of the patients at 2- to 4-year follow-up. One patient underwent arthroplasty at 1 year, and one patient underwent revision arthroscopic débridement at 3 years.

A study of arthroscopic débridement without subacromial bursectomy in 19 patients found that the results had appeared to deteriorate at longer-term follow-up (4 years).[20] Thirteen patients (68%) were satisfied with their pain relief, although function and motion were unchanged relative to presurgical levels. Three patients (16%) underwent hemiarthroplasty within the follow-up interval.

The outcomes of arthroscopic management were reported for 20 shoulders in 19 patients younger than 55 years with Outerbridge grade II to IV changes.[21] In addition to arthroscopic débridement, 9 of the patients had concomitant subacromial decompression, and 4 others had subacromial bursectomy without acromioplasty; 13 patients had subacromial bursectomy. At a minimum 12-month follow-up (average, 20 months; range, 12 to 33 months), the survivorship rate was 85%; three patients had undergone shoulder arthroplasty. The outcomes scores were similar for patients with a grade II or III chondral injury and those with grade IV changes. Patients with unipolar lesions (glenoid or humeral head) had a better outcome than those with chondral loss on both sides of the joint. The average postarthroscopy score on the American Shoulder and Elbow Surgeons Shoulder Index was 75, and nine patients (five of whom had grade IV changes) had a score greater than 80.

Only one study appears to have specifically investigated arthroscopic capsular release with débridement in patients with severe glenohumeral arthritis.[22] The treatment of glenohumeral osteoarthritis with débridement and capsular release in eight patients led to improvement in pain and functional outcome scores at short-term follow-up. Capsular release to gain motion is most beneficial in patients with osteoarthritis who have concentric wear. In patients with posterior wear, a biconcave glenoid and a flat humeral head with osteophytes are unlikely to gain motion with a capsular release, and pain may increase. Although osteophyte excision has not been extensively studied, early reports suggest that it may improve the outcomes of arthroscopic débridement.[9]

The results of arthroscopic glenoidplasty with osteocapsular arthroplasty were encouraging in 14 patients with severe arthritis with biconcave glenoid surfaces.[11] There was consistent relief of impingement and rest pain at average 3-year follow-up. The favorable prognostic indicators were impingement pain at the end points of motion, large humeral osteophytes, posterior glenoid erosion, humeral head subluxation, and large loose bodies, all of which were structurally treated at the time of surgery. The negative predictors were pain in the mid-arc of motion, pain with glenohumeral compression during humeral rotation, and a concentric glenohumeral joint. Although this procedure is technically difficult, in experienced hands it may be effective for well-selected patients.

Favorable pain relief and recovery of shoulder function were reported for 55 of 71 patients at an average follow-up of slightly more than 2 years.[23] Twenty of the patients had undergone earlier surgery. The patients were rated from 0 to 4 on the Samilson-Prieto radiographic scale, and all had Outerbridge grade II to IV lesions. These patients were self-selected in that they chose the arthroscopic option; they were "not considered to be candidates for arthroplasty based on the degree of disease on radiography, the patient's age or activity level, and/or the patient's desire to avoid arthroplasty."[23] The surgery was performed by one of four surgeons and included a variety of concomitant procedures: capsular release (44 patients), biceps tenodesis or tenotomy (14 patients), microfracture (11 patients), loose body or osteophyte removal (12 patients), and subacromial decompression (28 patients). Because data on the concomitant procedures were not studied, their effect is not clear. Sixteen patients (22%) underwent total shoulder arthroplasty at an average 10 months after arthroscopy. The other 55 patients had not required arthroplasty at an average 27-month follow-up (range, 12 to 90 months). In patients who underwent total shoulder arthroplasty, the mean joint space width was 1.5 mm, and the mean Samilson-Prieto grade was 2.4. The patients who did not undergo total shoulder arthroplasty had a mean joint space width of 2.6 mm and a mean Samilson-Prieto grade of 1.9.

Microfracture of the shoulder is an emerging area in the treatment of focal chondral lesions of the humerus and the glenoid and is largely based on techniques derived from the knee. Microfracture was used to treat full-thickness lesions of the shoulder in 30 patients with a mean age of 43 years.[10] At minimum 2-year follow-up, 19% of the procedures were considered unsuccessful, and these patients required another shoulder surgery at a mean 47-month follow-up. The remaining patients reported improvement in pain and function. The procedure was most effective for relatively small lesions and lesions affecting the humerus only.

Summary

Arthroscopic débridement and capsular release are effective for treating an osteoarthritic shoulder in a young, active patient. Concomitant shoulder pathology, such as rotator cuff disease, impingement syndrome, biceps and labral pathology, and acromioclavicular arthritis, should be treated at the time of surgery. Encouraging results with regard to pain relief and restoration of function have been reported at short-term follow-up, even in patients with severe glenohumeral arthritis. The benefits of capsular release, osteophyte excision, and microfracture remain under investigation. Although arthroscopic débridement is not a substitute for joint arthroplasty, it provides a treatment alternative for some patients and may delay the need for prosthetic replacement.

Annotated References

1. Sperling JW, Cofield RH, Rowland CM: Minimum fifteen-year follow-up of Neer hemiarthroplasty and total shoulder arthroplasty in patients aged fifty years or younger. *J Shoulder Elbow Surg* 2004;13(6): 604-613.

2. Yian EH, Navarro RA, Funahashi T, et al: Hemiarthroplasty and total shoulder arthroplasty (TSA) revision rates: Analysis of 1,311 elective shoulder replacements in a community setting. American Shoulder and Elbow Surgeons Specialty Day, February 2011. http://www.ases-assn.org. Accessed September 20, 2012.

3. Outerbridge RE, Dunlop JA: The problem of chondromalacia patellae. *Clin Orthop Relat Res* 1975;110: 177-196.

4. Gerber C, Costouros JG, Sukthankar A, Fucentese SF: Static posterior humeral head subluxation and total shoulder arthroplasty. *J Shoulder Elbow Surg* 2009; 18(4):505-510.

   Static posterior subluxation of the humeral head often is associated with glenohumeral arthritis. This condition can be corrected in most shoulders undergoing total shoulder arthroplasty, but recentering is not correlated with glenoid version or its correction.

5. Samilson RL, Prieto V: Dislocation arthropathy of the shoulder. *J Bone Joint Surg Am* 1983;65(4):456-460.

4: Arthroscopy

6. Epis O, Caporali R, Scirè CA, Bruschi E, Bonacci E, Montecucco C: Efficacy of tidal irrigation in Milwaukee shoulder syndrome. *J Rheumatol* 2007;34(7): 1545-1550.

Ten patients with Milwaukee shoulder syndrome underwent ultrasound examination, tidal irrigation, and instillation of methylprednisolone and tranexamic acid. This minimally invasive procedure led to a significant improvement in pain and active motion. Patients with recent-onset disease recovered completely.

7. Bigliani LU, Flatow EL, Deliz ED: Complications of shoulder arthroscopy. *Orthop Rev* 1991;20(9): 743-751.

8. Small NC: Complications in arthroscopic surgery of the knee and shoulder. *Orthopedics* 1993;16(9): 985-988.

9. Millett PJ, Gaskill TR: Arthroscopic management of glenohumeral arthrosis: Humeral osteoplasty, capsular release, and arthroscopic axillary nerve release as a joint-preserving approach. *Arthroscopy* 2011;27(9): 1296-1303.

A technique for arthroscopic management of glenohumeral arthrosis in young, high-demand patients combines traditional glenohumeral débridement and capsular release with inferior humeral osteoplasty and arthroscopic transcapsular axillary nerve decompression. Symptom relief may be greater than with débridement alone.

10. Millett PJ, Huffard BH, Horan MP, Hawkins RJ, Steadman JR: Outcomes of full-thickness articular cartilage injuries of the shoulder treated with microfracture. *Arthroscopy* 2009;25(8):856-863.

In 30 patients, microfracture in glenohumeral joints with full-thickness chondral lesions led to significant improvement in ability to work, activities of daily living, and sports activity. The greatest improvement occurred with relatively small humeral lesions; the poorest was with bipolar lesions.

11. Kelly EW, Steinmann SP, O'Driscoll SW: Arthroscopic glenoidplasty and osteocapsular arthroplasty for advanced glenohumeral osteoarthritis. *67th Annual Meeting Proceedings*. Rosemont, IL, American Academy of Orthopaedic Surgeons, 1999.

12. Cameron BD, Galatz LM, Ramsey ML, Williams GR, Iannotti JP: Non-prosthetic management of grade IV osteochondral lesions of the glenohumeral joint. *J Shoulder Elbow Surg* 2002;11(1):25-32.

13. Ogilvie-Harris DJ, Wiley AM: Arthroscopic surgery of the shoulder: A general appraisal. *J Bone Joint Surg Br* 1986;68(2):201-207.

14. Costouros JG, Clavert P, Warner JJ: Trans-cuff portal for arthroscopic posterior capsulorrhaphy. *Arthroscopy* 2006;22(10):e1-e5.

15. Elser F, Braun S, Dewing CB, Millett PJ: Glenohumeral joint preservation: Current options for managing articular cartilage lesions in young, active patients. *Arthroscopy* 2010;26(5):685-696.

Shoulder joint preservation techniques are reviewed, with a guide to surgical decision making and summaries of the current treatments for focal chondral defects and more massive structural osteochondral defects (microfracture, osteoarticular transplantation, autologous chondrocyte implantation, bulk allograft reconstruction, and biologic resurfacing).

16. Weinstein DM, Bucchieri JS, Pollock RG, Flatow EL, Bigliani LU: Arthroscopic debridement of the shoulder for osteoarthritis. *Arthroscopy* 2000;16(5):471-476.

17. Ellowitz AS, Rosas R, Rodosky MW, Buss DD: The benefit of arthroscopic decompression for impingement in patients found to have unsuspected glenohumeral osteoarthritis. *64th Annual Meeting Final Program*. Rosemont, IL, American Academy of Orthopaedic Surgeons, 1997, p 206.

18. Ogilvie-Harris DJ: Arthroscopy and arthroscopic surgery of the shoulder. *Semin Orthop* 1987;2:246-258.

19. Safran MR, Wolde-Tsadik G: Prospective outcome study of arthroscopic debridement for the treatment of grade IV glenohumeral arthritis. *Annual Meeting Proceedings*. Rosemont, IL, American Academy of Orthopaedic Surgeons, 2002, p 659.

20. Feldmann DD, Orwin JF: Efficacy of arthroscopic debridement for treatment of glenohumeral arthritis. *Transactions of the 19th Open Meeting*. Rosemont, IL, American Shoulder and Elbow Surgeons, 2003, p. 30.

21. Kerr BJ, McCarty EC: Outcome of arthroscopic débridement is worse for patients with glenohumeral arthritis of both sides of the joint. *Clin Orthop Relat Res* 2008;466(3):634-638.

Arthroscopic glenohumeral débridement in 19 patients (20 shoulders) younger than 55 years with Outerbridge grade II to IV articular cartilage changes was found to be effective for managing symptoms and delaying the need for prosthetic replacement.

22. Richards DP, Burkhart SS: Arthroscopic debridement and capsular release for glenohumeral osteoarthritis. *Arthroscopy* 2007;23(9):1019-1022.

Range of motion and pain were improved by using electrocautery to release the rotator cuff interval, the anterior capsule, the posterior capsule, and the axillary recess. A reduction in joint contact pressures is believed to be the primary mechanism for pain relief after capsular release.

23. Van Thiel GS, Sheehan S, Frank RM, et al: Retrospective analysis of arthroscopic management of glenohumeral degenerative disease. *Arthroscopy* 2010;26(11): 1451-1455.

A retrospective review of 71 shoulders after arthroscopic débridement for degenerative joint disease suggested that patients with residual joint space and an absence of large osteophytes can avoid arthroplasty at short-term follow-up and have increased function with decreased pain. Significant risk factors include the presence of grade IV bipolar disease, large osteophytes, and joint space of less than 2 mm.

4: Arthroscopy

Arthritis and Arthroplasty

SECTION EDITOR:
T. BRADLEY EDWARDS, MD

Chapter 27

Proximal Humeral Anatomy and Prosthetic Reconstruction

Christopher R. Chuinard, MD, MPH

Introduction

The history of proximal humeral arthroplasty dates from 1893, when French surgeon Jules Emile Pean performed a two-stage procedure (resection followed by staged implantation) on a patient with extensive tuberculosis osteomyelitis.[1] The implant was crafted by a dentist, had a platinum shaft, and was more like a modern reverse prosthesis than a nonconstrained design. The prosthesis performed admirably for a short time but eventually failed because of recurrent infection. Pean had been inspired by Themistocles Gluck, a German surgeon who designed several proximal humeral replacements, including one with modular ivory heads.[1] Both surgeons were prescient in their approaches but not in their execution. Modern arthroplasty has little use for noble metals and ivory resurfacing, but it has benefited from more than a century of development. Prostheses have evolved into approximations of native humeral anatomy as well as designs that do not resemble anything in nature.

Humeral Anatomy

The goal of an unconstrained primary arthroplasty is to re-create normal, patient-specific humeral anatomy. To reproducibly and reliably accomplish this goal, the surgeon must have an understanding of normal humeral anatomy, glenoid anatomy, and glenohumeral kinematics. The primary consideration for glenohumeral arthroplasty is the humerus itself. It is important to understand the relationship between the articular surface and the axis of motion. Because the normative shape of

the humeral head may be lost during arthroplasty, the surgeon must understand relationships between humeral size, shape, and radius of curvature for accurate reproduction of the anatomy.

Humeral Head Size and Shape

Although multiple cadaver studies have provided some average values for humeral head size and shape, the reported norms vary. The articular surface of the humeral head approximates one third of a sphere, but it becomes slightly ellipsoid at the periphery, averaging 2 mm less in the axial plane than in the coronal plane.[2-6] Because of this relationship, there is a fairly constant ratio between humeral head diameter and thickness; this implies that there is a single head height for each radius.[2-8] The average thickness of the humeral head radius of curvature is 24 mm in men and 19 mm in women. The average humeral head diameter is 2 mm greater in both dimensions in men than in women.[4,8,9] Studies reported an average humeral head diameter of 43.4 mm or 44.5 mm at the anatomic neck.[2-4] Across studies, there is a fairly consistent 70% to 80% ratio of humeral head radius to humeral head height. The between-study variations may have to do with differing methodologies[4-11] (Figure 1).

The use of a large prosthetic head was found to constrain the first and last 20° of abduction, leading to proximal humeral migration, loss of external rotation, and more posterior translation. Using a smaller head led to an inferior migration.[10] An increase in humeral head height to 5 mm above normal will significantly reduce motion, and a reduction of an equal amount can decrease joint excursion by 24°.[7] A displacement of 5 mm, corresponding to 20% of the radius of the humeral head, altered the lever arm of the rotator cuff by 20%.[12]

Humeral Neck-Shaft Angle

The angle between the center line of the humeral head and the axis of the humeral canal is the neck-shaft angle (Figure 2). Reported values range from 129.6° to 137.0°, with a weighted average of 134.4°.[2-5,13] A study of 2,058 cadaver humeri found that 78% of the humeri fell between 130° and 140°, with 135° the most com-

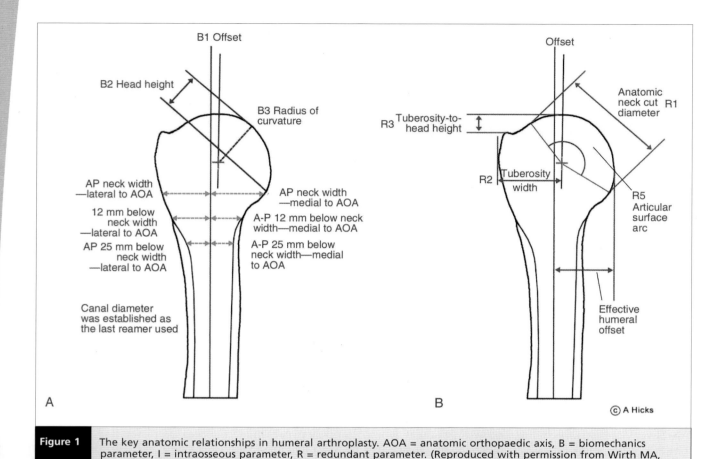

Figure 1 The key anatomic relationships in humeral arthroplasty. AOA = anatomic orthopaedic axis, B = biomechanics parameter, I = intraosseous parameter, R = redundant parameter. (Reproduced with permission from Wirth MA, Ondrla J, Southworth C, Kaar K, Anderson BC, Rockwood CA III: Replicating proximal humeral articular geometry with a third-generation implant: A radiographic study in cadaveric shoulders. *J Shoulder Elbow Surg* 2007;16[suppl3]:S111-S116.)

mon measurement and a mean of 134.7° (range, 115° to 148°).[14] The clinical relevance is that an extreme varus or valgus angle can make prosthetic reconstruction challenging unless an adaptable prosthesis is used. However, variations in cutting technique allowed appropriate reconstruction of the articular surface with a fixed-angle prosthesis. For a varus neck-shaft angle, the humeral osteotomy should begin at the superolateral point; for a valgus neck-shaft angle the osteotomy should begin from the inferomedial point [14] (**Figure 3**). Because alterations of the neck-shaft angle during prosthetic reconstruction could lead to a change in the length of the abductor muscles, thereby shifting the center of rotation and leading to impingement or rotator cuff dysfunction, the surgeon must mate the prosthesis with the line of the humeral head resection and restore the appropriate articular surface arc to the humerus.[14-16]

Humeral Head Offset

It is important to consider the offset of the center of rotation of the humeral head from the axis of the humeral shaft in both the transverse and the coronal planes. Because the center of rotation of the humeral head is not coincident with the axis of the humeral shaft (the so-

called orthopaedic axis), small variations in position can lead to large alterations in glenohumeral kinematics. The orthopaedic axis represents the central reaming axis of the humerus; the actual center of rotation of the humeral head lies an average 2.1 mm posterior (ranges 2 to 4 mm in the axial plane) and 6.6 mm medial (ranges 6 to 9 mm in the coronal plane) to the humeral axis, thus creating a combined center of rotation that is posteromedial to the longitudinal axis of the humeral canal[2,5,8,13,16-19] (**Figure 4**).

Humeral Head Retroversion

Humeral head retroversion or retrotorsion is the angle between the epicondylar axis of the distal humerus and the central axis of the humeral head. Reported values range from 17.9° (± 13.7°) to 21.4° (± 3.3°). Humeral head retroversion may be more affected than other parameters by patient age, sex, and ethnicity, and it can vary between sides in the same individual.[2,20-23] A correlation may exist between the position of the bicipital groove and the equator of the humeral head; the bicipital groove lies an average of 8 to 9 mm from the equator, allowing it to be used as an additional landmark for humeral retroversion.[5,20-22] When CT was used to

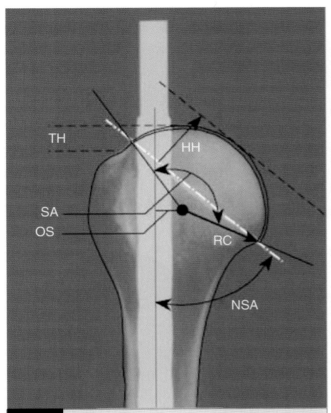

Figure 2 True AP radiograph showing the coronal anatomic parameters of the proximal humerus. Black dot = center of rotation, dashed white line = base of articular surface, vertical black line = center line of reamed canal, HH = humeral head height, NSA = neck-shaft angle, OS = medial offset, RC = radius of curvature. TH = tuberosity-to-head height. (Adapted with permission from Pearl ML: Proximal humeral anatomy in shoulder arthroplasty: Implications for prosthetic design and surgical technique. *J Shoulder Elbow Surg* 2005;14[Suppl 1]:S99-S104.)

and visualizing the insertion of the rotator cuff before performing the humeral osteotomy[17] (**Figure 5**).

Humeral Shaft Morphology

In the past 10 years, increasing attention has been given to the proximal humeral shaft and metaphyseal morphology. Three morphotypes of the proximal humerus were identified: low offset, standard, and high offset[5] (**Figure 6**). These terms refer to the relative amount of offset of the head to the humeral shaft in the metaphyseal segment. Decreasing the offset may make the insertion of a straight stem more difficult. Curved stems, so-called finless stems, and reduced-geometry stems were developed based on improved understanding of this anatomy. As more attention was directed to creating adaptable prostheses, the limitations of some press-fit designs became apparent. Some press-fit stems displaced the center of rotation superiorly and laterally by 12 mm and 8 mm, respectively, leading to rotator cuff dysfunction.[26,27] Elevation of the prosthetic humeral head by as little as 5 mm can decrease the moment arms of the rotator cuff musculature and can even change their vectors when the arm is adducted.[28-30] The greater tuberosity–to–humeral head height averages 6 mm; if the humerus is too high, the inferior capsule will be overly tight with the arm in abduction, and the rotator cuff will be under excessive tension with the arm in adduction[4,31] (**Figure 1**).

Prosthesis Design Considerations

First-, Second-, and Third-Generation Humeral Implants

Modern shoulder arthroplasty began with Charles Neer's monobloc design in 1951.[32] This system offered five stem diameters and one humeral head size. The stem resembled a modern fracture stem, with fenestrations to allow bony growth. Neer's early success with this implant led to the 1974 introduction of an implant that borrowed from successful hip arthroplasty, with a cemented stem, two humeral head options, and a polyethylene glenoid component. The second generation of shoulder arthroplasty was launched by the introduction of modularity between the humeral head and shaft to allow a more anatomic reconstruction. This system facilitated more anatomic placement of the humeral head relative to the tuberosities and the rotator cuff, allowing easier soft-tissue tensioning by providing different head heights and variable offset between the shaft and the head.[33] However, many second-generation stems had a gap between the head and the collar of the stem: a smaller head size and a corresponding loss of articular surface arc led to premature contact between the nonarticular portions of the humerus and glenoid.[26,27] The step-off between the collar of the stem and the humeral head with a second-generation implant made it easy to overstuff the joint or position the humeral head in an overly superior position relative to the greater tu-

determine retroversion in 120 cadavers, an average of 17.6° of retroversion was measured from the transepicondylar axis, and an average of 28.8° was measured from the forearm axis.[24] A three-dimensional laser analysis of the articular surface yielded an average retroversion of 18.6°, with articular geometry approximating a centroid.[20] Another study found that retroversion could be reliably measured based on the lateral margin of the lesser tuberosity and arrived at an average of 48°.[25] The researchers measured 185 dry bone specimens with a special jig to determine that the lesser tuberosity was a more reliable reference point than the bicipital groove or the transepicondylar line. Many humeral systems for arthroplasty reconstruction reference retroversion based on the axis of the forearm. When relying on a humeral cutting guide that uses the forearm for reference, the surgeon should account for natural variation by considering the 10° to 15° carrying angle

5: Arthritis and Arthroplasty

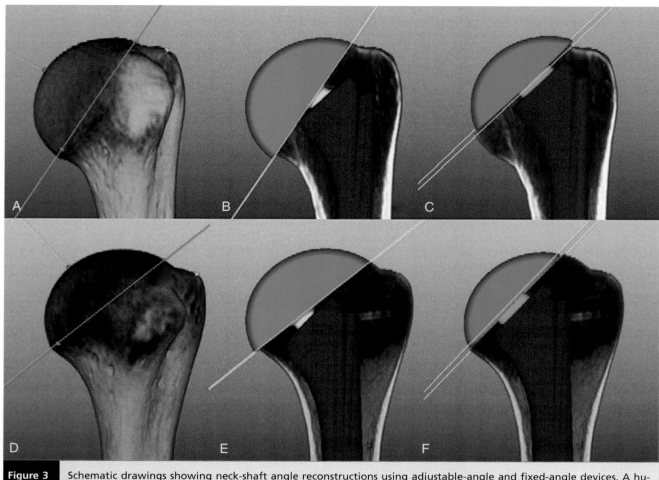

Figure 3 Schematic drawings showing neck-shaft angle reconstructions using adjustable-angle and fixed-angle devices. A humerus with a varus neck-shaft angle (**A**) can be treated with an adjustable-angle device and a humeral osteotomy at the anatomic neck (**B**) or a fixed-angle prosthesis and a 135° osteotomy with a modified cut from the superolateral point of the neck plane (**C**). A humerus with a valgus neck-shaft angle (**D**) can be treated with an adjustable-angle device and a humeral osteotomy at the anatomic neck (**E**) or a fixed-angle prosthesis and a 135° osteotomy with a modified cut from the superolateral point of the neck plane (**F**). Green line = anatomic neck (defining the native neck-shaft angle), yellow line = prosthetic neck and neck-shaft angle. Blue area = fixed-angle prosthetic neck, green area = prosthetic humeral head, red area = prosthetic body, yellow area = variable-angle prosthetic neck. (Reproduced with permission from Jeong J, Bryan J, Iannotti JP: Effect of a variable prosthetic neck-shaft angle and the surgical technique on replication of normal humeral anatomy. *J Bone Joint Surg Am* 2009;91[8]:1932-1941.)

berosity.[16] Usually, soft-tissue tensioning is easiest to judge when the humeral head rests on the cut surface, but implants with a step-off between the stem and the head made this step challenging. Most second-generation implants have a preset neck-shaft angle that necessitates a cut using a specific osteotomy guide. Cementing these implants may improve the ability to accurately reproduce the anatomy, but they can be unforgiving when press fit.

The modern adaptable shoulder prosthesis is based on anatomic norms.[2,3] These third-generation stems have multiple areas of adjustment to account for variation in neck-shaft angle as well as more anatomic head sizes and variable offset. Compared with a second-generation implant, the anatomic implant more accurately restored glenohumeral motion and minimize eccentric loading of the glenoid. Furthermore, the second-generation implant produced eight times the joint reactive force at the superior aspect of the glenoid.[34] Further evolution of implant adaptability has allowed near-normalization of the center of rotation in prosthetic reconstruction of the proximal humerus.[35] With a third-generation implant, the surgeon can perform an anatomic osteotomy of the humeral head and be confident that the prosthesis will reproduce the anatomy. The prosthesis can be adapted to the patient, rather than the patient adapted to the prosthesis. Cementation of the stem can provide an additional degree of freedom in third- as well as second-generation implants.

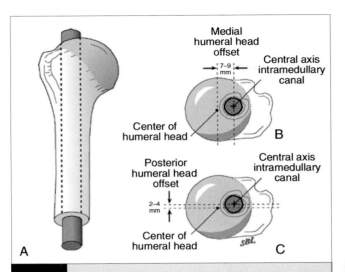

Figure 4 Schematic drawings showing the humeral head offset. **A,** The central axis of the intramedullary canal. **B,** The humeral head offset in the coronal plane (approximately 7 to 9 mm medial to the central axis of the intramedullary canal). **C,** The humeral head offset in the axial plane (2 to 4 mm posterior to the central axis of the intramedullary canal). (Reproduced with permission from Iannotti JP, Lippitt SB, Williams GR Jr: Variation in neck-shaft angle: Influence in prosthetic design. *Am J Orthop (Belle Mead NJ)* 2007;36[12, suppl 1]:9-14.)

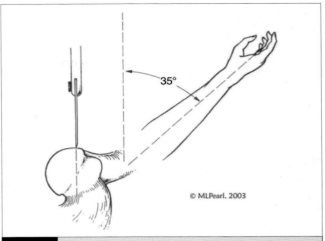

Figure 5 Schematic drawing showing a humeral osteotomy made in excessive retroversion. With a standard osteotomy at 35° of retroversion, anatomic reconstruction is difficult, and there is a risk of violating the rotator cuff. (Reproduced with permission from Pearl ML: Proximal humeral anatomy in shoulder arthroplasty: Implications for prosthetic design and surgical technique. *J Shoulder Elbow Surg* 2005;14[1 suppl 1]:S99-S104.)

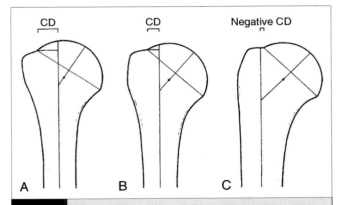

Figure 6 Schematic drawings showing proximal humeral morphology and the types of offset of the articular surface relative the proximal metaphysis: high offset (**A**), standard (**B**), and low offset (**C**). CD = critical distance or greater tuberosity offset, defined as the distance between the medial insertion of the supraspinatus and the longitudinal axis of the humeral shaft; as the CD decreases, insertion of a straight-stemmed prosthesis becomes more difficult. Angled lines = humeral head inclination angle relative to the shaft, dot = geometric center of rotation, vertical line = longitudinal axis of the humeral shaft. (Adapted with permission from Hertel R, Knothe U, Ballmer FT: Geometry of the proximal humerus and implications for prosthetic design. *J Shoulder Elbow Surg* 2002;11[4]:331-338.)

Long-, Short-, and No-Stem Humeral Implants and Humeral Resurfacing

In recent years, increasing attention has been directed to the shaft portion of the humeral implant. The concepts of hip arthroplasty have been extended to shoulder arthroplasty. Many of the original concepts of humeral implants were based on those of femoral implants. Resurfacing shoulder arthroplasty also was adapted from the hip precedent and has been used for several years. The resurfacing should remove only the remaining cartilage and underlying subchondral bone, with the intent of easily reproducing the offset, the radius of curvature, the diameter, and the head height of the proximal humerus while preserving proximal humeral bone stock and avoiding stem-associated complications.[36-38]

Advocates of resurfacing believe that this bone-preserving operation may be preferable to total or stemmed hemiarthroplasty in young, active patients.[36-42] Conversion to a stemmed implant or an arthrodesis is thought to be easy. In a study of 36 patients younger than 55 years who underwent a resurfacing hemiarthroplasty, there was no short-term implant loosening or glenoid wear, and 35 patients reported high satisfaction.[38] If a stem is not used, re-creating the instant center of rotation may be easier because the position of the articular surface is not dictated by the humeral canal. In total shoulder arthroplasty, however, the approach to the glenoid is challenging if the humerus is not resected (**Figure 7, A**). Caution should be exercised if there is insufficient bone stock, osteopenic bone, significant osteonecrosis, or proximal humeral deformity. In some patients with a focal cartilaginous

5: Arthritis and Arthroplasty

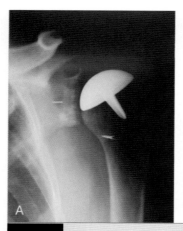
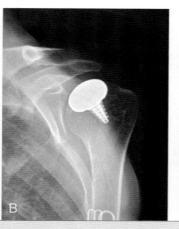
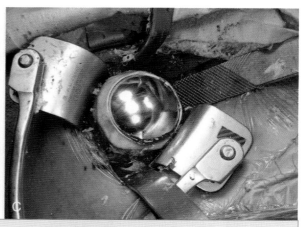

Figure 7 **A,** Grashey radiograph showing a resurfacing total shoulder arthroplasty. Grashey radiograph (**B**) and intraoperative photograph of the same patient (**C**) showing a focal resurfacing to treat osteonecrosis.

defect or osteonecrosis, it may be necessary to resurface the isolated pathologic area[43] (**Figure 7, B**).

Current stem designs focus on metaphyseal fixation of the humeral stem. These designs derive their press fit from the proximal metaphyseal bone rather than more distal cortical bone. In Europe, research is being conducted on stemless implants that have purchase in the metaphysis below the resection plane. Stemless designs are not resurfacing implants; instead, the surgeon makes an anatomic head cut, and the device is centered on the cut, thus eliminating the concerns of offset and allowing the surgeon to re-create the native center of rotation independent of the axis of the humeral shaft. With fixation in the metaphyseal region, there is no stem to force the device into varus or incorrect version. Recent studies have reported good short-term clinical success, even with distorted proximal humeral anatomy, after anatomic humeral reconstruction and glenoid replacement with a bone-conserving device that allowed traditional glenoid exposure.[44-46] The use of a stemless implant may not be preferable in patients with osteoporotic bone, many of whom are older women.[46,47]

The advantages of a design with a relatively long stem are the larger bone-implant interface to distribute the forces and the larger surface area to resist rotational or torsional loads, which lead to good long-term stability. The disadvantages include stem-related complications, such as intraoperative or postoperative periprosthetic fracture, alterations in kinematics, and difficult revision. The advantages of a stemless device include the preservation of proximal bone, which may be an advantage for later revision or repair of a rotator cuff tear. Because the humeral head is resected in the same fashion as in a primary arthroplasty, access to the glenoid is facilitated. Stemless implants have less metal and therefore may be less stiff, share more load across the bone, and have better long-term survivability.[44]

Humeral resurfacing may be necessary if hemiarthroplasty is indicated. A relatively young patient, a patient with distorted proximal humeral anatomy (as with fracture sequelae), or a patient with a pristine concentric glenoid may be an ideal candidate for resurfacing rather than stemmed hemiarthroplasty or traditional total shoulder arthroplasty.[38] Because the proximal humerus is reamed or milled to accommodate a metallic shell that restores a smooth, spherical articular surface, advocates claim that the resurfacing procedure can easily re-create the anatomic instant center of rotation of the humerus. However, the joint can be easily overstuffed, and care must be taken to ensure that the guidepin is perpendicular to the plane of the anatomic neck before humeral preparation.[39,40,43] The same soft-tissue releases as in a total shoulder arthroplasty should be performed to ensure adequate exposure of the humerus during preparation, but good long-term satisfaction and survivorship are possible.[41,42,48]

The short-stemmed implant represents a compromise between conventional and stemless or resurfacing stem designs. A shorter stem can provide the rotational control and excellent stability of a traditional stemmed design but obtains its press-fit biologic fixation in the metaphysis of the proximal humerus. Long-term follow-up may reveal that the short stem provides less stress shielding, with accompanying proximal humeral osteolysis or resorption, because the forces are concentrated adjacent to the humeral head rather than distally to the humeral shaft. Although the short-stemmed implant may be subject to the same long-term issues as a longer-stemmed device, near-term data are promising. Furthermore, the shorter-stemmed implant holds promise for bone-conserving arthroplasty, which may be important in revision surgery or the treatment of future pathology such as rotator cuff disease.

Bony (Anatomic) and Soft-Tissue Balancing

For proper postarthroplasty functioning, the reconstruction must restore the anatomy, and the muscle forces must be appropriately balanced. Most often, soft-tissue balancing involves releasing excessively tight tissues from the anterior aspect of the joint to allow appropriate alignment, stability, and range of motion. Less commonly, it may be necessary to plicate redundant soft tissues in the posterior aspect of the joint. Humeral head size fell within eight fixed combinations in 85% of the population; therefore, the implant size can be selected to provide the ideal amounts of range of motion, stability, and translation. Implant head height or thickness can be varied to alter the relative soft-tissue tension.[4,18,49]

The concept of bony balancing implies that the humeral anatomy will be reconstructed to essentially the native dimensions, or, at a minimum, those determined by the humeral head resection.[3] Under the assumption that humeral head thickness is related to the diameter of the anatomic neck or the resection plane, the resection will predetermine the humeral head thickness.[2] Therefore, when the osteophytes are removed, the anatomic neck identified, and the resection is performed, the critical steps have been completed and what remains is primarily a matter of covering the resection.

The subsequent restoration of the bony anatomy should restore normal glenohumeral kinematics. Overstuffing can occur with a proper cut if the stem is placed in a varus position or if the stem is placed correctly but the head cut is inadequate.[16,28-30] In either case, the head should be centered on the metaphysis; this task is made easier by using a modern adaptable implant, which can minimize the difference between bone and soft-tissue balancing. The superior aspect of the head should sit 5 to 10 mm above the summit of the greater tuberosity.[4,7,8,31] The offset of the humeral shaft necessitates the use of an offset head more often than a centered head.[2,3,5] If the particular system lacks a centered option, the surgeon must choose the appropriate direction for overhang; with a lesser tuberosity osteotomy, an anterior overhang may mate well with the area reconstituted by the osteotomy. Alternatively, a cemented stem can be used, as is more commonly done in Europe than in the United States. A cemented stem allows the surgeon to float the humeral implant into the ideal location for reconstructing the articular geometry.

If the soft tissues appear symmetrically tight, the humeral head may be too large or the resection may be inadequate.[49] Attention should be directed to the capsule, ensuring that the soft-tissue releases have been adequate. To correct excessive posterior translation, the humeral head size can be increased at the expense of range of motion (external rotation); more posterior offset can be placed; or posterior plication sutures can be placed in the capsule or through the humerus (as in repair of a posterior humeral avulsion of the glenohumeral ligament).[48,49] After soft-tissue reconstruction, the arm should allow 40° of external rotation in the adducted position; the head should translate 50% of the width of the glenoid with a posteriorly directed force; and there should be 60° of internal rotation with the arm in the abducted position.[50] (This is the so-called 40-50-60 rule.)

Cemented and Cementless Fixation

Fixation is a relative term because bone is a dynamic, living structure. Immediately after surgery, the bone-implant interface is different from the interface at 2-year follow-up. As the surgical trauma is replaced by a zone of healing, the thinner the transition zone is, the better the force is distributed to the surrounding bone. The surgeon must create an environment that supports appropriate force transmission between the implant and the bone so that the component does not loosen over time, leading to pain or prosthetic failure. Until material science creates an implant that replicates the stiffness of the native tissues, there will be a relative mismatch between the implant and the bone. This mismatch in stiffness leads to micromotion and eventual loosening of the implant.[51] The prosthetic design and interface should be loaded in compression to distribute the forces as evenly as possible in an attempt to keep micromotion to less than 70 microns. Minimizing the load across the interface for the first 6 to 12 weeks may encourage maturation of the healing zone but is not practical. Therefore, it is important to distribute the forces as evenly as possible to minimize shear and maximize compression. To achieve even force distribution, the implant must register appropriately with the native glenoid or the glenoid component, articulating with as much rotational kinematics as possible and minimizing rolling or gliding.[52]

A cementless prosthesis is designed to achieve initial fixation through a macroscopic interlock between the surface of the prosthesis and the bone. It is essential to minimize the shear forces that occur if the implant pistons within the canal or convert them to compressive force at the bone-implant interface. Impaction bone grafting may enhance the metaphyseal fit and prevent the stem from moving into varus.[53] Ideally, the forces should be transmitted through the implant to the bone, resulting in minimal shear stresses at the bone-prosthesis interface and transmitting the load to the bone in series rather than in parallel or by load sharing.[54] The next phase allows bone ingrowth or ongrowth at the interstices of the prosthesis to lock it in place. This is a dynamic process because bone is constantly turning over.[51] Some prosthetic designs have fared better than others, and recent radiographic concerns have been raised that a collared or distally press-fit implant may stress shield proximally, leading to bone resorption along the medial calcar.[55] Proximal humeral bone loss results in more micromotion and ultimately to prosthetic loosening.[56] Metaphyseal press fit was more efficacious than distal stem press fit, and this design trend has continued in the evolution of smaller tapered stems.[57]

The practical concerns and considerations related to press-fit designs have to do with the relative ease of implantation rather than the stability of the initial press fit. Large fins can force the stem into a varus position, may not always align with the cut, or may force the stem into poor inclination or version. Smaller cylindrical bodies have been replaced by those with a more proximal wedge shape to prevent settling within the bone; a tight metaphyseal fit can be augmented by impaction grafting along the medial calcar.[53,57] On the other hand, a cemented stem can float in the cement mantle, allowing the surgeon to place it precisely over the cut surface to accurately re-create the resected anatomy and center of rotation. Published loosening rates with unconstrained shoulder arthroplasty range from 0% with a bony ingrowth model or 1.5% in a cemented application to 10.0% with a limited-ingrowth monoblock stem, and some studies suggest that certain cemented stem designs may outperform cementless applications.[52,58-61] It is important to recognize that there will be variation based on the suitability of the stem for the specific application; for example, the results are poor if a stem designed for a cemented application is used as a press-fit stem or vice versa. A study of 1,584 primary arthroplasties identified risk factors for humeral component failure, including male sex, relatively young age, a metal-backed glenoid, and posttraumatic arthropathy.[58] Improved rotational micromotion was found with a proximal cemented stem compared with a press-fit stem, and there was no advantage to full cementation.[62] Therefore, in a patient without a fracture, it may be preferable to proximally apply cement only to the metaphyseal portion of the stem before implantation. A level I study that compared cemented and noncemented implantation of a specific stem found better outcomes in terms of range of motion, strength, and quality of life when the cemented application was used.[63]

Soft-Tissue Considerations

The subscapularis is critical for successful function after a shoulder arthroplasty. A rotator cuff tear or a subscapularis deficiency was identified in 72% of painful shoulder arthroplasties, and subscapularis deficiency was implicated in poor long-term outcomes.[64-66] Recent studies of a transosseous repair found a 25% rate of subscapularis deficiency.[67] Concern over the integrity of subscapularis repair has led to the development of alternative approaches to tenotomy.[68] The variations range from a periosteal sleeve elevation to several types of lesser tuberosity osteotomy, in which the tendon and the capsule usually are taken together to preserve blood supply (**Figure 8**). Biomechanically, a superior load to failure was found with a lesser tuberosity osteotomy and a double-row repair, although more recent studies found little difference in repair strength with osteotomy or tenotomy.[66,69-73] Of 45 patients, 41 had a negative lift-off test, and all 45 had a negative belly-press test result after routine tenotomy and repair.[74] Excellent bone-to-bone healing and excellent clinical results were

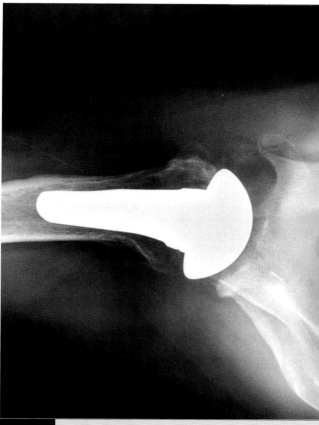

Figure 8 Axillary radiograph showing a fibrous union after a lesser tuberosity osteotomy. The patient had no deficit.

reported after a lesser tuberosity osteotomy; nonetheless, 44% of the patients had fatty infiltration of the muscle belly.[65,66] Better function of the subscapularis was found in patients who underwent osteotomy compared with a historical cohort of patients who underwent tenotomy.[75] Ultimately, surgeon preference may dictate the approach to the subscapularis and its repair.

A report of a subscapularis-sparing approach through the rotator cuff interval noted the advantage of immediate full activity without limitation. This approach is technically demanding and requires specialized instruments, and it may not be suitable for patients with a stiff shoulder, a large inferior osteophyte, or a large deltoid.[76] In the 22 studied patients, the concerns were "nonanatomic humeral head osteotomies in 6, residual inferior humeral neck osteophytes in 8, and the humeral head prosthesis undersized in 5."[76]

Future Directions

Concern remains about glenoid wear or glenoid implant prosthetic loosening, and research continues for prosthetic reconstruction that provides as much pain relief as a total shoulder arthroplasty while requiring less surgical time, difficulty, and expense. The creation

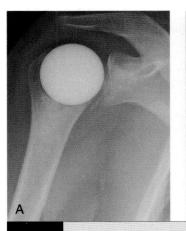
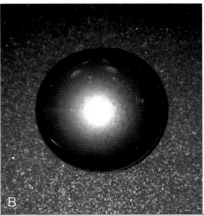
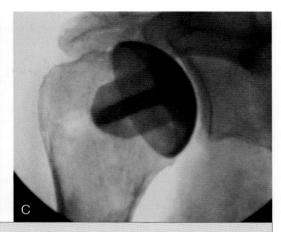

Figure 9 Two pyrolytic carbon implants commercially available in Europe. Grashey radiograph (**A**) and photograph (**B**) showing the so-called snooker ball implant (Tornier); Grashey radiograph (**C**) showing a resurfacing arthroplasty implant (Integra). (Panel A, Courtesy of Gilles Walch, MD; panel C, courtesy of Integra.)

of a humeral implant that is less stiff and provides improved wear characteristics over current materials is desirable. No hard-on-hard bearings are commercially available for shoulder arthroplasty, but research is being done for suitable applications.[77] Composite materials may be better suited to the humerus rather than ceramic or metal-on-metal applications. With a modulus of elasticity of 29.4 GPa, pyrolytic carbon may be a future option for shoulder arthroplasty because it is closer to the modulus of cortical bone (23 GPa) and may exhibit better wear characteristics against cartilage, making it ideal for consideration in a hemiarthroplasty.[78] Pyrolytic carbon has been used in mechanical heart valves since the 1960s and for small-joint arthroplasty since 1979; in Europe, several hundred pyrolytic carbon humeral arthroplasties have been performed[79] (**Figure 9**).

Summary

Modern unconstrained shoulder arthroplasty attempts reconstruction of the native proximal humeral anatomy, thereby relieving pain and restoring normal glenohumeral kinematics. The evolution of prosthesis design has led to modular implants that adapt to patient anatomy while minimizing surgical trauma and improving long-term implant survivability.[80] However, improved prosthesis design is not a substitute for rigorous surgical technique. Soft-tissue considerations still are of paramount importance for providing long-term stability and functionality after reconstruction. Material science may provide compounds with biomechanical properties similar to those of the host bone and thereby increase device longevity.

Annotated References

1. Bankes MJ, Emery RJ: Pioneers of shoulder replacement: Themistocles Gluck and Jules Emile Péan. *J Shoulder Elbow Surg* 1995;4(4):259-262.

2. Boileau P, Walch G: The three-dimensional geometry of the proximal humerus: Implications for surgical technique and prosthetic design. *J Bone Joint Surg Br* 1997;79(5):857-865.

3. Walch G, Boileau P: Prosthetic adaptability: A new concept for shoulder arthroplasty. *J Shoulder Elbow Surg* 1999;8(5):443-451.

4. Iannotti JP, Gabriel JP, Schneck SL, Evans BG, Misra S: The normal glenohumeral relationships: An anatomical study of one hundred and forty shoulders. *J Bone Joint Surg Am* 1992;74(4):491-500.

5. Hertel R, Knothe U, Ballmer FT: Geometry of the proximal humerus and implications for prosthetic design. *J Shoulder Elbow Surg* 2002;11(4):331-338.

6. Pearl ML: Proximal humeral anatomy in shoulder arthroplasty: Implications for prosthetic design and surgical technique. *J Shoulder Elbow Surg* 2005;14 (1 Suppl S):99S-104S.

7. Pearl ML, Volk AG: Coronal plane geometry of the proximal humerus relevant to prosthetic arthroplasty. *J Shoulder Elbow Surg* 1996;5(4):320-326.

8. Robertson DD, Yuan J, Bigliani LU, Flatow EL, Yamaguchi K: Three-dimensional analysis of the proximal part of the humerus: Relevance to arthroplasty. *J Bone Joint Surg Am* 2000;82(11):1594-1602.

5: Arthritis and Arthroplasty

9. Wataru S, Kazuomi S, Yoshikazu N, Hiroaki I, Takaharu Y, Hideki Y: Three-dimensional morphological analysis of humeral heads: A study in cadavers. *Acta Orthop* 2005;76(3):392-396.

10. Vaesel MT, Olsen BS, Søjbjerg JO, Helmig P, Sneppen O: Humeral head size in shoulder arthroplasty: A kinematic study. *J Shoulder Elbow Surg* 1997;6(6):549-555.

11. Wirth MA, Ondrla J, Southworth C, Kaar K, Anderson BC, Rockwood CA III: Replicating proximal humeral articular geometry with a third-generation implant: A radiographic study in cadaveric shoulders. *J Shoulder Elbow Surg* 2007;16(Suppl 3):S111-S116.

    Radiographic measurements confirmed that a third-generation arthroplasty can accurately reproduce the native anatomy of the humerus.

12. Fischer LP, Carret JP, Gonon GP, Dimnet J: Etude cinématique des mouvements de l'articulation scapulo-humérale (articulatio humeri). *Rev Chir Orthop Reparatrice Appar Mot* 1977;63(Suppl 2):108-115.

13. Roche C, Angibaud L, Flurin PH, Wright T, Fulkerson E, Zuckerman J: Anatomic validation of an "anatomic" shoulder system. *Bull Hosp Jt Dis* 2006; 63(3-4):93-97.

14. Jeong J, Bryan J, Iannotti JP: Effect of a variable prosthetic neck-shaft angle and the surgical technique on replication of normal humeral anatomy. *J Bone Joint Surg Am* 2009;91(8):1932-1941.

    Both fixed-angle and variable-angle prostheses have the ability to replicate native anatomy, but humeral head height may need to be adjusted when a fixed-angle device is used, and care must be taken not to alter the available surface arc.

15. Takase K, Yamamoto K, Imakiire A, Burkhead WZ Jr: The radiographic study in the relationship of the glenohumeral joint. *J Orthop Res* 2004;22(2):298-305.

16. Iannotti JP, Spencer EE, Winter U, Deffenbaugh D, Williams G: Prosthetic positioning in total shoulder arthroplasty. *J Shoulder Elbow Surg* 2005;14(1, Suppl S):111S-121S.

17. Pearl ML, Volk AG: Retroversion of the proximal humerus in relationship to prosthetic replacement arthroplasty. *J Shoulder Elbow Surg* 1995;4(4):286-289.

18. Pearl ML, Kurutz S, Postacchini R: Geometric variables in anatomic replacement of the proximal humerus: How much prosthetic geometry is necessary? *J Shoulder Elbow Surg* 2009;18(3):366-370.

    A computer algorithm was used to conclude that increased geometric variability in a prosthesis allowed for closer approximation of normal anatomy.

19. Iannotti JP, Lippitt SB, Williams GR Jr: Variation in neck-shaft angle: Influence in prosthetic design. *Am J Orthop (Belle Mead NJ)* 2007;36(12, Suppl 1):9-14.

    Introducing variability in the neck-shaft angle of the prosthesis was thought to allow more accurate reproduction of the instant center of rotation.

20. Harrold F, Wigderowitz C: A three-dimensional analysis of humeral head retroversion. *J Shoulder Elbow Surg* 2012;21(5):612-617.

    The anterior cartilage–metaphyseal junction may not accurately reproduce true retroversion when used as the reference for humeral resection.

21. Tillett E, Smith M, Fulcher M, Shanklin J: Anatomic determination of humeral head retroversion: The relationship of the central axis of the humeral head to the bicipital groove. *J Shoulder Elbow Surg* 1993;2(5): 255-256.

22. Doyle AJ, Burks RT: Comparison of humeral head retroversion with the humeral axis/biceps groove relationship: A study in live subjects and cadavers. *J Shoulder Elbow Surg* 1998;7(5):453-457.

23. Edelson G: Variations in the retroversion of the humeral head. *J Shoulder Elbow Surg* 1999;8(2): 142-145.

24. Hernigou P, Duparc F, Hernigou A: Determining humeral retroversion with computed tomography. *J Bone Joint Surg Am* 2002;84(10):1753-1762.

25. Hromádka R, Kubena AA, Pokorný D, Popelka S, Jahoda D, Sosna A: Lesser tuberosity is more reliable than bicipital groove when determining orientation of humeral head in primary shoulder arthroplasty. *Surg Radiol Anat* 2010;32(1):31-37.

    Based on a study of 185 humeri, the lesser tuberosity was believed to be a more reliable landmark for retroversion because the bicipital groove is variable along its length.

26. Pearl ML, Kurutz S: Geometric analysis of commonly used prosthetic systems for proximal humeral replacement. *J Bone Joint Surg Am* 1999;81(5):660-671.

27. Pearl ML, Kurutz S, Robertson DD, Yamaguchi K: Geometric analysis of selected press fit prosthetic systems for proximal humeral replacement. *J Orthop Res* 2002;20(2):192-197.

28. Nyffeler RW, Sheikh R, Jacob HA, Gerber C: Influence of humeral prosthesis height on biomechanics of glenohumeral abduction: An in vitro study. *J Bone Joint Surg Am* 2004;86(3):575-580.

29. Favre P, Moor B, Snedeker JG, Gerber C: Influence of component positioning on impingement in conventional total shoulder arthroplasty. *Clin Biomech (Bristol, Avon)* 2008;23(2):175-183.

    Component position had an effect on impingement through the arc of motion. One factor under the surgeon's control is the position of the implant along the resection line.

30. Williams GR Jr, Wong KL, Pepe MD, et al: The effect of articular malposition after total shoulder arthroplasty on glenohumeral translations, range of motion, and subacromial impingement. *J Shoulder Elbow Surg* 2001;10(5):399-409.

31. Takase K, Imakiire A, Burkhead WZ Jr: Radiographic study of the anatomic relationships of the greater tuberosity. *J Shoulder Elbow Surg* 2002;11(6):557-561.

32. Neer CS II: Articular replacement for the humeral head. *J Bone Joint Surg Am* 1955;37-A(2):215-228.

33. Fenlin JM Jr, Vaccaro A, Andreychik D, Lin S: Modular total shoulder: Early experience and impressions. *Semin Arthroplasty* 1990;1(2):102-111.

34. Büchler P, Farron A: Benefits of an anatomical reconstruction of the humeral head during shoulder arthroplasty: A finite element analysis. *Clin Biomech (Bristol, Avon)* 2004;19(1):16-23.

35. Irlenbusch U, End S, Kilic M: Differences in reconstruction of the anatomy with modern adjustable compared to second-generation shoulder prosthesis. *Int Orthop* 2011;35(5):705-711.

    The variation in proximal humeral geometry supports the use of a prosthesis that can be adapted to patient anatomy. Modern prostheses more closely approximated the native humeral anatomy compared with second-generation implants.

36. Hammond G, Tibone JE, McGarry MH, Jun BJ, Lee TQ: Biomechanical comparison of anatomic humeral head resurfacing and hemiarthroplasty in functional glenohumeral positions. *J Bone Joint Surg Am* 2012;94(1):68-76.

    Humeral resurfacing may more accurately re-create the geometric center of rotation than hemiarthroplasty.

37. Jensen KL: Humeral resurfacing arthroplasty: Rationale, indications, technique, and results. *Am J Orthop (Belle Mead NJ)* 2007;36(12, Suppl 1):4-8.

    Guidelines for humeral resurfacing arthroplasty were provided in this report.

38. Bailie DS, Llinas PJ, Ellenbecker TS: Cementless humeral resurfacing arthroplasty in active patients less than fifty-five years of age. *J Bone Joint Surg Am* 2008;90(1):110-117.

    These data supported the use of resurfacing for arthritis in the young patient. Level of evidence: IV.

39. Thomas SR, Sforza G, Levy O, Copeland SA: Geometrical analysis of Copeland surface replacement shoulder arthroplasty in relation to normal anatomy. *J Shoulder Elbow Surg* 2005;14(2):186-192.

40. Thomas SR, Wilson AJ, Chambler A, Harding I, Thomas M: Outcome of Copeland surface replacement shoulder arthroplasty. *J Shoulder Elbow Surg* 2005;14(5):485-491.

41. Pritchett JW: Long-term results and patient satisfaction after shoulder resurfacing. *J Shoulder Elbow Surg* 2011;20(5):771-777.

    The author reported that shoulder resurfacing had 96% survivorship and 95% patient satisfaction at 20-year follow-up.

42. Burgess DL, McGrath MS, Bonutti PM, Marker DR, Delanois RE, Mont MA: Shoulder resurfacing. *J Bone Joint Surg Am* 2009;91(5):1228-1238.

    The history, indications, technique, and advantages of resurfacing arthroplasty of the shoulder were thoroughly reviewed. Longer-term data will be necessary to determine whether resurfacing is preferable to total shoulder arthroplasty, but initial data are promising. This procedure may be the preferred option for younger patients.

43. Scalise J, Miniaci A, Iannotti J: Resurfacing arthroplasty of the humerus: Indications, surgical technique, and clinical results. *Tech Shoulder Elbow Surg* 2007;8:152-160.

    Techniques for shoulder resurfacing were reported, with particular attention given to surgical technique.

44. Huguet D, DeClercq G, Rio B, Teissier J, Zipoli B; TESS Group: Results of a new stemless shoulder prosthesis: Radiologic proof of maintained fixation and stability after a minimum of three years' follow-up. *J Shoulder Elbow Surg* 2010;19(6):847-852.

    In early results, the use of a stemless device was equivalent to that of stemmed implants.

45. Collin P, McGourbey G, Boileau P, Walch G: Complications of the Simpliciti stemless prosthesis, in Walch G, Boileau P, Molé D, Favard L, Lévigne C, Sirveaux F, eds: *Shoulder Concepts 2012: Complications in Shoulder Arthroplasty*. Montpellier, France, Sauramps Medical, 2012, pp 57-61.

    The combined experience from three shoulder centers in France was reported for 23 patients. The results were similar to those of standard arthroplasty, but caution may be needed in patients with poor bone quality.

46. Tauber M, Habermeyer P, Magosch P: Is a stemless prosthesis better? in Walch G, Boileau P, Molé D, Favard L, Lévigne C, Sirveaux F, eds: *Shoulder Concepts 2012: Complications in Shoulder Arthroplasty*. Montpellier, France, Sauramps Medical, 2012, pp 49-56.

    The results from a single institution and a multicenter study in France were reported at 3- to 5-year follow-up after the use of a stemless design. The results were similar to those of traditional third- and fourth-generation shoulder arthroplasty prosthesis. The complication rate was 9.8% to 12.1%.

47. Barvencik F, Gebauer M, Beil FT, et al: Age- and sex-related changes of humeral head microarchitecture: Histomorphometric analysis of 60 human specimens. *J Orthop Res* 2010;28(1):18-26.

    Regions of less dense bone in the proximal humerus were identified in humeri harvested at autopsy.

5: Arthritis and Arthroplasty

48. Williams G, Iannotti J: Unconstrained prosthetic arthroplasty for glenohumeral arthritis with an intact or repairable rotator cuff: Indications, techniques, and results, in Iannotti J, Williams G, eds: *Disorders of the Shoulder*, ed 2. Philadelphia, PA, Lippincott, Williams, & Wilkins, 2007, pp 713-715.

    The authors summarized the history, indications, results, and complications of shoulder arthroplasty.

49. Harryman DT, Sidles JA, Harris SL, Lippitt SB, Matsen FA III: The effect of articular conformity and the size of the humeral head component on laxity and motion after glenohumeral arthroplasty: A study in cadavera. *J Bone Joint Surg Am* 1995;77(4):555-563.

50. Matsen F, Clinton J, Rockwood C, Wirth M, Lippitt S: *The Shoulder*, ed. 4. Philadelphia, PA, Saunders, 2009, pp 1093-1096.

    The authors summarized the conventional theoretical and technical aspects of shoulder arthroplasty.

51. Jobe CM, Phipatanakul WP, Bowsher JG: *Revision and Complex Shoulder Arthroplasty*. Philadelphia PA, Wolters Kluwer/Lippincott, Williams & Wilkins, 2010, pp 83-94.

    The biomechanics of prosthetic fixation were clearly discussed, providing insight into possible modes of failure.

52. Cofield R: Loosening of cemented and uncemented humeral stems, in Walch G, Boileau P, Molé D, Favard L, Lévigne C, Sirveaux F, eds: *Shoulder Concepts 2012: Complications in Shoulder Arthroplasty*. Montpellier, France, Sauramps Medical, 2012, pp 23-27.

    The Mayo experience of cemented and cementless shoulder arthroplasty was concisely described. Cemented stems may have better survivability.

53. Boorman RS, Hacker S, Lippitt SB, Matsen FA: A conservative broaching and impaction grafting technique for humeral component placement and fixation in shoulder arthroplasty: The procrustean method. *Tech Shoulder Elbow Surg* 2001;2:172-173.

54. Orr TE, Carter DR: Stress analyses of joint arthroplasty in the proximal humerus. *J Orthop Res* 1985; 3(3):360-371.

55. Edwards B: Can a short-stem avoid the potential complications of the longer stems? The Aequalis Ascend experience, in Walch G, Boileau P, Molé D, Favard L, Lévigne C, Sirveaux F, eds: *Shoulder Concepts 2012: Complications in Shoulder Arthroplasty*. Montpellier, France, Sauramps Medical, 2012, pp 147-149.

    The author's experience with a short-stem humeral prosthesis was described. A near-term improvement in calcar resorption was reported.

56. Cuff D, Levy JC, Gutiérrez S, Frankle MA: Torsional stability of modular and non-modular reverse shoulder humeral components in a proximal humeral bone loss model. *J Shoulder Elbow Surg* 2011;20(4):646-651.

    Rotational stability with humeral stems in a reverse

model was studied. Monoblock stems performed best, especially when the proximal humerus was intact.

57. Matsen FA III, Iannotti JP, Rockwood CA Jr: Humeral fixation by press-fitting of a tapered metaphyseal stem: A prospective radiographic study. *J Bone Joint Surg Am* 2003;85(2):304-308.

58. Cil A, Veillette CJ, Sanchez-Sotelo J, Sperling JW, Schleck CD, Cofield RH: Survivorship of the humeral component in shoulder arthroplasty. *J Shoulder Elbow Surg* 2010;19(1):143-150.

    The least amount of radiolucency was seen around cemented components, but all maintained good survivability.

59. Gonzalez JF, Alami GB, Baque F, Walch G, Boileau P: Complications of unconstrained shoulder prostheses. *J Shoulder Elbow Surg* 2011;20(4):666-682.

    This meta-analysis of unconstrained shoulder arthroplasty reported excellent survivability, with a trend toward better results with cemented rather than cementless implants.

60. Sperling JW, Cofield RH, O'Driscoll SW, Torchia ME, Rowland CM: Radiographic assessment of ingrowth total shoulder arthroplasty. *J Shoulder Elbow Surg* 2000;9(6):507-513.

61. Throckmorton TW, Zarkadas PC, Sperling JW, Cofield RH: Radiographic stability of ingrowth humeral stems in total shoulder arthroplasty. *Clin Orthop Relat Res* 2010;468(8):2122-2128.

    A press-fit design that included porous coating circumferentially around the metaphysis performed much better than earlier implants that had ingrowth surface only on the undersurface of the collar. No loosening was reported at short-term to midterm follow-up.

62. Harris TE, Jobe CM, Dai QG: Fixation of proximal humeral prostheses and rotational micromotion. *J Shoulder Elbow Surg* 2000;9(3):205-210.

63. Litchfield RB, McKee MD, Balyk R, et al: Cemented versus uncemented fixation of humeral components in total shoulder arthroplasty for osteoarthritis of the shoulder: A prospective, randomized, double-blind clinical trial—A JOINTs Canada Project. *J Shoulder Elbow Surg* 2011;20(4):529-536.

    Cementation of a humeral arthroplasty implant had better results than cementless fixation. The stem originally was designed for cemented use. Level of evidence: I.

64. Sperling JW, Potter HG, Craig EV, Flatow E, Warren RF: Magnetic resonance imaging of painful shoulder arthroplasty. *J Shoulder Elbow Surg* 2002;11(4): 315-321.

65. Gerber C, Yian EH, Pfirrmann CA, Zumstein MA, Werner CM: Subscapularis muscle function and structure after total shoulder replacement with lesser tuberosity osteotomy and repair. *J Bone Joint Surg Am* 2005;87(8):1739-1745.

66. Gerber C, Pennington SD, Yian EH, Pfirrmann CA, Werner CM, Zumstein MA: Lesser tuberosity osteotomy for total shoulder arthroplasty: Surgical technique. *J Bone Joint Surg Am* 2006;88(Suppl 1, Pt 2): 170-177.

67. Liem D, Kleeschulte K, Dedy N, Schulte TL, Steinbeck J, Marquardt B: Subscapularis function after transosseous repair in shoulder arthroplasty: Transosseous subscapularis repair in shoulder arthroplasty. *J Shoulder Elbow Surg* 2012;21(10):1322-1327.

   A 25% rate of subscapularis dysfunction was reported after a transosseous repair.

68. Armstrong A, Lashgari C, Teefey S, Menendez J, Yamaguchi K, Galatz LM: Ultrasound evaluation and clinical correlation of subscapularis repair after total shoulder arthroplasty. *J Shoulder Elbow Surg* 2006; 15(5):541-548.

69. Krishnan SG, Stewart DG, Reineck JR, Lin KC, Buzzell JE, Burkhead WZ: Subscapularis repair after shoulder arthroplasty: Biomechanical and clinical validation of a novel technique. *J Shoulder Elbow Surg* 2009;18(2):184-192, discussion 197-198.

   A sound reconstruction technique was described for lesser tuberosity osteotomy repair.

70. Van Thiel GS, Wang VM, Wang F-C, et al: Biomechanical similarities among subscapularis repairs after shoulder arthroplasty. *J Shoulder Elbow Surg* 2010; 19(5):657-663.

   No difference was found among multiple types of subscapularis repairs, including osteotomy.

71. Van den Berghe GR, Nguyen B, Patil S, et al : A biomechanical evaluation of three surgical techniques for subscapularis repair. *J Shoulder Elbow Surg* 2008; 17(1):156-161.

   Tendon-to-bone repair was not as strong as bone-to-bone repair for an osteotomy or tendon-to-tendon repair.

72. Giuseffi SA, Wongtriratanachai P, Omae H, et al: Biomechanical comparison of lesser tuberosity osteotomy versus subscapularis tenotomy in total shoulder arthroplasty. *J Shoulder Elbow Surg* 2012;21(8): 1087-1095.

   Little difference was found in a comparison of tendon-to-tendon and osteotomy repairs.

73. Ahmad CS, Wing D, Gardner TR, Levine WN, Bigliani LU: Biomechanical evaluation of subscapularis repair used during shoulder arthroplasty. *J Shoulder Elbow Surg* 2007;16(Suppl 3):S59-S64.

Transosseous tunnels altered the anatomy and were less strong than tendon-to-tendon repairs or combined constructs.

74. Caplan JL, Whitfield B, Neviaser RJ: Subscapularis function after primary tendon to tendon repair in patients after replacement arthroplasty of the shoulder. *J Shoulder Elbow Surg* 2009;18(2):193-197-198.

   Excellent results were reported after traditional subscapularis tenotomy and repair.

75. Qureshi S, Hsiao A, Klug RA, Lee E, Braman J, Flatow EL: Subscapularis function after total shoulder replacement: Results with lesser tuberosity osteotomy. *J Shoulder Elbow Surg* 2008;17(1):68-72.

   Excellent results were reported after a lesser tuberosity osteotomy technique was used for total shoulder arthroplasty.

76. Lafosse L, Schnaser E, Haag M, Gobezie R: Primary total shoulder arthroplasty performed entirely thru the rotator interval: Technique and minimum two-year outcomes. *J Shoulder Elbow Surg* 2009;18(6): 864-873.

   Good results were reported after the use of a subscapularis-sparing approach to the shoulder joint. The surgery is technically demanding.

77. Williams GR Jr, Iannotti JP: Alternative bearing surfaces—do we need them? *Am J Orthop (Belle Mead NJ)* 2007;36(12, Suppl 1):15-17.

   The risks and benefits of metal-on-metal, ceramic-on-ceramic, and ceramic-on-polyethylene bearings in the shoulder were described, as was cross-linking of the polyethylene.

78. Cook SD, Thomas KA, Kester MA: Wear characteristics of the canine acetabulum against different femoral prostheses. *J Bone Joint Surg Br* 1989;71(2):189-197.

79. Stanley J, Klawitter J, More R: Joint replacement technology, in Revell P, ed: *Joint Replacement Technologies.* Boca Raton, FL, CRC Press, 2008, pp 631-656.

   The material properties, manufacturing, and clinical use of pyrolytic carbon for joint arthroplasty were described.

80. Buzzell JE, Lutton DM, Shyr Y, Neviaser RJ, Lee DH: Reliability and accuracy of templating the proximal humeral component for shoulder arthroplasty. *J Shoulder Elbow Surg* 2009;18(5):728-733.

   Preoperative templating was found to approximate surgical reconstruction with a modern prosthesis.

5: Arthritis and Arthroplasty

Chapter 28

Glenoid Anatomy and Prosthetic Reconstruction

Patric Raiss, MD   T. Bradley Edwards, MD   Gilles Walch, MD

Introduction

Hemiarthroplasty of the proximal humerus is a standard procedure for treating degenerative pathologies of the glenohumeral joint, and it can lead to good results. However, resurfacing of the glenoid bone has many advantages. Total shoulder arthroplasty has been described as superior for pain relief, functional outcome, and patient satisfaction compared with hemiarthroplasty.[1] The major concern in total shoulder arthroplasty is loosening of the glenoid component, which has been frequently observed at mid- and long-term follow-up.[2-5] Therefore, some surgeons avoid implanting a glenoid component, especially in relatively young patients with a high level of activity and a long life expectancy.[6] The outcomes have varied with the use of different fixation concepts (cemented or uncemented) and glenoid component designs (keeled or pegged, flat-back or convex-back).

Glenoid Anatomy

Knowledge of the anatomy of the glenoid is crucial for every shoulder surgeon, especially when total shoulder arthroplasty is being considered. The surgeon needs to know the version, inclination, height, width, and shape of the patient's glenoid.[7] A surgical plan can be formulated using this information.

The glenoid cavity is covered with cartilage, with the thinnest part in the center. The thickness of the cartilage increases from the center to the periphery. The cartilage terminates at the glenoid labrum, which consists of strong fibrocartilage. The morphology of the glenoid surface can be described as the shape of a pear or an inverted comma. The supraglenoid tubercle with its insertion of the long head of the biceps tendon is the superiormost point of the glenoid, and the infraglenoid tubercle with its insertion of the long head of the triceps tendon is the inferiormost point. Multiple studies have analyzed the average dimensions of the glenoid surface in nonarthritic shoulders, with slightly differing results.[8-11] Mean glenoid height measured from superior to inferior was found to range from 35 to 39 mm, and mean glenoid width to range from 23 to 29 mm.[8-11] An analysis of the articulating surface area and the volume of the glenoid vault found a mean surface area of 8.7 cm^2 and a volume of 11.9 cm^3.[10] Glenoid version is routinely measured on CT using different methods.[12] A mean retroversion of 7.4° was found in 75% of analyzed shoulders, and an anteversion of 2° to 10° was found in 25%.[13] A mean retroversion of 1.2° was found in 344 human scapulas.[8]

Neither Dr. Raiss nor any immediate family member has received anything of value from or owns stock in a commercial company or institution related directly or indirectly to the subject of this article. Dr. Edwards or an immediate family member has received royalties from Tornier and Orthohelix; is a member of a speakers' bureau or has made paid presentations on behalf of Tornier; serves as a paid consultant to Kinamed and Tornier; serves as an unpaid consultant to Gulf Coast Surgical Services; has received research support from Tornier; has received nonincome support (such as equipment or services), commercially derived honoraria, or other non–research-related funding (such as paid travel) from Tornier; and serves as a board member, owner, officer, or committee member of the American Shoulder and Elbow Surgeons. Dr. Walch or an immediate family member has received royalties from Tornier, and has received nonincome support (such as equipment or services), commercially derived honoraria, or other non–research-related funding (such as paid travel) from Tornier.

Prosthetic Considerations

Glenoid components can be fixed with or without the use of bone cement. Several implant designs and fixation concepts are available.

Uncemented Glenoid Components

Higher rates of revision surgery and complications have been reported with the use of uncemented glenoid components than with cemented components. A prospective, double-blinded randomized study compared the results of using an uncemented metal-back bone ingrowth glenoid component with the results of using a cemented keeled flat-back component (each in 20 shoulders).[2] The rate of radiolucent lines around the

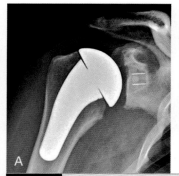

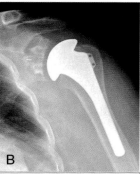

Figure 2 Immediate postoperative AP radiographs of a total shoulder replacement in which an uncemented stem is combined with a cemented keeled glenoid component (**A**) or a cemented pegged glenoid component (**B**).

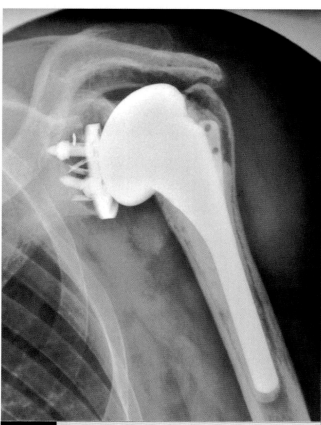

Figure 1 AP radiograph showing a total shoulder replacement 14 years after implantation of a cemented stem with an uncemented metal-back glenoid component. Proximal migration of the humerus and gross loosening of the glenoid component with breakage of one screw and wear of the polyethylene inlay can be seen.

components was significantly higher in the shoulders with a cemented component (85% versus 25%, *P*<0.01), but loosening was found in 4 shoulders with an uncemented component (20%) and three implant revisions were required (**Figure 1**). No loosening was detected in the shoulders with a cemented component. In 2005, the results of 147 consecutive shoulder arthroplasties were reported at a mean 7.5-year follow-up.[14] In 11% of shoulders, the metal-back glenoid component had been removed because of clinical failure, and an additional 8% of shoulders had asymptomatic broken hardware evident on radiographs. Multiple investigations have recently confirmed the high complication rates with the use of different metal-back designs.[15-17] The most common complication apparently is loosening of the component, followed by severe polyethylene wear or dissociation of the polyethylene from the metal portion of the implant. Only one study described excellent mid- and long-term results.[18] In this study, 35 arthroplasties in 35 patients were performed between 1996 and 2005 using a metal-back glenoid component consisting of a titanium alloy shell coated with porous titanium and hydroxyapatite and secured by two

6.5-mm screws. The indication for the use of this type of glenoid component is unclear. The researchers found neither loosening nor complications at a mean 6-year follow-up. Further mid- and long-term studies of new uncemented glenoid implants are necessary to confirm these findings.

Cemented Glenoid Components

The results of using cemented all-polyethylene glenoid components have been well documented. The phenomenon of radiolucent lines around cemented glenoid implants is common, with reported rates of 0% to 96%.[19] Although the radiolucent lines often are visible on immediate postoperative radiographs, their presence is not always predictive of component loosening or clinical symptoms.

The two predominant types of cemented glenoid components are keeled and pegged (**Figure 2**). An analysis of immediate postoperative radiographs of 328 total shoulder arthroplasties found significantly higher rates of radiolucent lines when a keeled component was used.[19] These data were supported by two prospective randomized studies that found significantly more radiolucent lines around keeled components than around pegged components at 2-year follow-up.[20,21] A biomechanical study found that the maximal tensile edge displacement was significantly less in pegged than in keeled components.[22] However, another study found no difference in the occurrence of radiolucent lines at a mean 4-year follow-up of 50 patients with a keeled component and 50 with a pegged component.[23]

The long-term results of using cemented keeled glenoid components have been well documented. Implant survival recently was reported in 972 all-polyethylene cemented glenoid components, with revision as the end point.[24] The overall survival rate was 95% at 10 years and 92% at 15 years; at 15 years, the survival rate for the Cofield 1 prosthesis (Smith & Nephew) was 87%, and the rate for the Neer 2 prosthesis (Smith & Nephew) was 94%. The Cofield 2 prosthesis (Smith & Nephew) also had good survival, at 99% after 5 years and 94% after 10 years. Two multicenter studies of implant survival with a flat-back or a convex-back glenoid component had comparable results.[3,4] In patients with osteoarthritis but without a rotator cuff tear or preoperative instability, 263 total shoulder replacements with a cemented flat-back keeled glenoid were evaluated clinically and radiographically at a mean 10-year follow-up (range, 5 to 20 years).[3] Rates of implant survival with glenoid component revision as the end point were 94.5% at 10 years and 79.4% at 15 years. The results were less promising when radiographic loosening was defined as the end point; the survival rates were 80.3% at 10 years and only 33.6% at 15 years. The same investigators analyzed 333 total shoulder arthroplasties with a convex-back cemented glenoid component and reported survival rates of 99.7% at 5 years and 98.3% at 10 years, with revision of the glenoid component as the end point. With radiologic loosening of the glenoid component as the end point, implant survival was 99.7% at 5 years but only 51.5% at 10 years. In both studies, significant associations were found between radiographic loosening and clinical deterioration in pain level, activity level, and shoulder motion.

A recent study of 518 cemented total shoulder arthroplasties with a convex-back or flat-back keeled glenoid component analyzed patterns of loosening of the glenoid component at a mean 8.6-year follow-up (range, 5 to 18 years).[25] The three predominant mechanisms of failure were medial subsidence (in 7.9%), superior tilting (in 10%), and posterior tilting (in 6.4%). Medial subsidence of the glenoid component was associated with excessive reaming during glenoid preparation and complete removal of the subchondral bone (P <0.001). The risk factors for superior tilting were an inferior position of the glenoid component, a superiorly oriented position of the glenoid component on the immediate postoperative radiographs, and superior migration of the humeral head (P<0.05). The risk factors for posterior tilting were preoperative posterior subluxation of the humeral head and excessive reaming during glenoid preparation, with complete removal of the subchondral bone (P<0.01). The overall rate of radiographic loosening was 32%, and the authors concluded that protection of the subchondral bone is important for the long-term survival of the glenoid component.[25]

Despite the promise shown by pegged glenoid components in comparative studies, few mid- to long-term data exist on these implants. The published study with the longest follow-up period (mean, 5 years) reported that the pegged all-polyethylene Cofield 2 implant had a survival rate similar to that of keeled implants, with revision as the end point.[24] This prosthesis differs from most current pegged implants in that it has three in-line pegs, rather than four or five pegs in a nonlinear configuration. Longer follow-up is needed to better elucidate any advantages of a pegged implant design over a keeled design.

Partially Cemented All-Polyethylene Components

Implant design has evolved during the past decade to include variations in component morphology, the number and location of fixation pegs, and the fixation method. The anchor-pegged glenoid implant (Anchor Peg Glenoid, DePuy; Cortiloc, Tornier) is a minimally cemented all-polyethylene design in which the finned central peg is impacted into the center drill hole without cement and the small peripheral pegs are conventionally cemented. Although the mechanism by which cancellous bone grows into the central peg is not understood, good results have been reported.[26-28] More than 33,000 shoulder replacements have been performed with this type of glenoid implant,[28] but only three studies with limited numbers of patients have been published. At a mean 43-month follow-up, a CT-based study of 35 patients treated with this implant found bone ingrowth around the central uncemented peg in a mean 4.5 of the 6 fins in 32 implants (91%) and no bone ingrowth in 3 implants (9%).[27] Another study used radiographs under fluoroscopic control and detected bone formation around the fins of the anchor peg in 15 of 20 patients at a minimum 5-year follow-up.[26] Radiolucency or osteolysis was detected around the central peg in the remaining 5 patients. Another study of this type of implant radiographically followed 44 shoulders for a mean of 3 years.[28] When the system devised by Lazarus et al was used to analyze cementing and seating of the glenoid components, 86% were scored as "better cementing" and "better seating."[19] Osteolysis around the central peg was found in 7%, and 68% had adequate bone growth around the fins of the central peg. A gross loosening was detected in one implant.

Another hybrid glenoid component (Comprehensive Shoulder System, Biomet) also has cemented peripheral pegs, with an uncemented porous-coated titanium central peg for bone ingrowth. No results of its use have been published.

Flat-Back Versus Convex-Back Components

The back side of the glenoid can be flat or curved. Convex-back implants attempt to match the shape of the back of the implant to the concave surface of the patient's glenoid. Hemispherical reamers usually are available for glenoid preparation in a convex-back system. A flat reamer is used in bone preparation for a flat-back component. One disadvantage of flat-back components, in comparison with convex-back components, is that in general they require more extensive bone removal during reaming because the convexity of the native glenoid must be reamed to a flat surface to match the shape of the back of the implant. Biomechanically, convex-back components were found to resist micromotion better than flat-back components.[22] However, clinical investigations have not shown either component to be superior.

The use of a flat-back component has been shown to

lead to more radiolucent lines in the short term, but this difference is mitigated at longer term follow-up.[29,30] A prospective study of 66 arthroplasties found a significant difference at 2-year follow-up between the mean Molé radiolucent line scores of the flat-back components (4.2 points) and the convex-back components (3.2 points).[31,32] At 10-year follow-up of the same patients, 56 arthroplasties had survived, but the mean radiolucent line score had increased to 9.8 points for the flat-back components and 8.3 points for the convex-back components.[33] This 10-year difference was not statistically significant, but the authors found that at 10-year follow-up patients younger than 60 years at the time of arthroplasty had a significantly higher radiolucent line score ($P<0.03$), there were more radiolucent lines if the shoulder was dominant ($P<0.017$), and the presence of radiolucent lines on immediate postoperative radiographs significantly predicted the progression of radiolucent lines ($P<0.018$). This study is the only available clinical comparison of the results of flat-back and convex-back glenoid components.

Prosthetic Mismatch

The term prosthetic mismatch describes the difference in the radius of curvature between the glenoid and humeral components. The osseous radial glenohumeral mismatch can range from 8 to 9 mm, whereas the cartilaginous radial glenohumeral mismatch can be as small as 0.1 mm.[34] In total shoulder replacement, the range of mismatch depends on the implant and ultimately is selected by the surgeon. A complete conformity between the humeral and glenoid components increases the contact area of the components and therefore decreases the contact pressure.[35] In a conforming system, however, the contact area between the components is markedly reduced as the humeral head translates on the glenoid and increased forces are transmitted to the rim of the glenoid component.[36] This rim loading may increase the risk of glenoid component loosening.[37] Conversely, increasing glenohumeral mismatch reduces the contact area between the head and the glenoid components, resulting in increased contact pressure that can accelerate polyethylene wear and increase glenohumeral instability.[34-36] Most investigators recommend some mismatch of the components to avoid excessive loading of the glenoid rim.[34,35] Only one clinical study has analyzed the influence of the mismatch on the formation of radiolucent lines around cemented glenoid components.[34] In 319 shoulders treated with the Aequalis total shoulder arthroplasty system (Tornier), all patients had the same diagnosis of primary glenohumeral osteoarthritis, and a cemented keeled glenoid component was used.[34] The patients were assigned to one of four glenohumeral mismatch groups: group 1, 0 to 4 mm; group 2, 4.5 to 5.5 mm; group 3, 6 to 7 mm; and group 4, more than 7 mm. At a mean 4.5-year follow-up, lower mean Molé et al radiolucent line scores were found in groups 3 and 4 (3.8 and 3.7 points, respectively) than in groups 1 and 2

(6.4 and 5.8 points, respectively). The authors concluded that a glenohumeral mismatch between 6 and 10 mm most favorably influences the development of radiolucent lines.[34]

Technical Considerations

Glenoid Preparation Technique

Adequate exposure of the glenoid surface is critical for preparation of the native glenoid during component implantation. Many techniques for glenoid exposure and preparation have been described. The preferred technique of the senior author is described here.

A humeral head retractor is inserted into the joint after the tenotomy of the subscapularis tendon. After a release of the medial and inferior glenohumeral ligaments, the humeral head is retracted posteriorly to expose the anterior glenoid rim. The subscapularis tendon is placed into the subscapularis recess on the anterior scapula and held with an anterior glenoid rim retractor. The long head of the biceps tendon is released from its insertion on the supraglenoid tubercle and tenodesis of the upper border of the pectoralis major tendon is performed using nonabsorbable suture. The glenoid labrum and capsule are released starting just anteroinferior to the coracoid and terminating at the 5 o'clock or 7 o'clock position (in a right or left shoulder, respectively). The inferior capsule and lateral extent of the triceps tendon is released around to the 8 o'clock or 4 o'clock position (in a right or left shoulder, respectively). This inferior release is the key step for adequate glenoid exposure and implant insertion (**Figure 3**). The humeral head is dislocated anteriorly and resected. When the preparation of the humerus is complete, the proximal humerus is retracted posteriorly to expose the glenoid. Any residual cartilage can be removed from the glenoid using a curette. Glenoid osteophytes can be observed and removed. The center of the glenoid surface is marked using electrocautery. If a cannulated system is being used, the central guidewire can be inserted; a center hole can be drilled if a noncannulated system has been selected. A motorized reamer is used to prepare the surface of the glenoid. To protect the subchondral bone, which is important for implant longevity, minimal reaming is performed.[4,24] If a pegged component is being used, the remaining peg holes can be drilled. If a keeled component is being used, the impaction technique is recommended.[31] This technique involves minimal bone removal and uses a keel punch to impact the bone. It has been shown that this technique leads to significantly better radiolucent line scores around keeled glenoid components in comparison with a traditional curettage technique.[31] The implant can be fixed as recommended by the prosthesis manufacturer.

Cementing Technique

After glenoid preparation, the keel slot or the peg holes are irrigated by pulsatile lavage to remove blood and

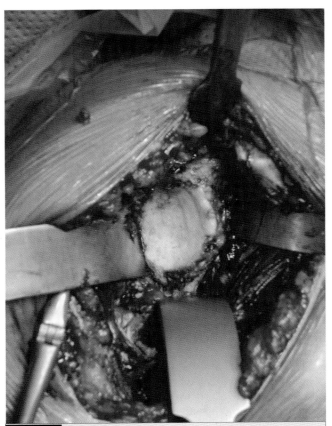

Figure 3 Photograph showing the exposure of a right glenoid after a deltopectoral approach was used. A Lambotte retractor is placed in the posterior part of the glenoid, and a Link retractor is placed in the anterior part. One Hohmann retractor is placed superoinferiorly at the glenoid.

debris from the cancellous bone. The benefits of pulsatile lavage irrigation are well established in hip arthroplasty, although similar efficacy has not been proved in shoulder arthroplasty. The glenoid bone should be dried after irrigation. A comparison of three methods of drying the glenoid before keeled implant cementation (the use of thrombin-soaked gel foam, compressed gas lavage, or saline-solution lavage followed by simple sponge use) on immediate postoperative radiographs did not find a statistically significant difference in radiolucent lines around the glenoid component, based on the drying method.[38] In the weep-hole technique for drying the glenoid vault, a hole is drilled into the coracoid process to connect it to the glenoid vault, and continuous suction is performed over this hole during implant cementation.[39] A clinical study found significantly improved cement mantles and fewer radiolucent lines around keeled and pegged glenoid components when the weep-hole technique was used.[39] A CT-based in vitro study found significantly deeper cement penetration into the glenoid vault when the weep-hole technique was used, in comparison with a standard technique.[40] A potential problem with this technique is that the drill

hole might weaken the coracoid process, leading to fracture.

Many types of cement are available, including slow- or fast-curing low-, medium-, or high-viscosity cements that may contain an antibiotic. The cement can be manually mixed in a bowl or can be mixed using a vacuum centrifuge to reduce porosity. No data are available comparing the outcomes of using different types of cement for glenoid component implantation.

Multiple techniques have been described for inserting the cement into the glenoid vault directly or with a syringe. In vitro syringe application was found to result in better cement penetration than manual application, and cement penetration was deeper in one patient with osteoporosis.[41] This finding was confirmed in a study that found a strong negative correlation between local bone mineral density in the glenoid vault and cement penetration.[29] Pressurization is a well-established method for improving cement penetration in hip and knee arthroplasty. A few studies have been published on this technique in total shoulder arthroplasty. The occurrence of radiolucent lines around all-polyethylene glenoid components was compared based on whether a "free-hand packing technique" or a "new instrumented pressurization technique" was used.[30] The incidence and thickness of radiolucent lines around the glenoid component were significantly greater on immediate postoperative radiographs after treatment with the free-hand technique ($P<0.05$). Pegged glenoid components had significantly fewer radiolucent lines than keeled components ($P<0.05$). When a 60-mL syringe was used in combination with a pressurizer sponge for cement application into the peg holes, 90% of the 69 shoulders had no radiolucent lines on immediate postoperative radiographs.[42] A size-matched pegged component used in combination with cement pressurization and the study authors' surgical technique was found to lead to a low incidence of radiolucent lines. Longer term follow-up data are not yet available. More recently, a silicone pressurization device with a slot for a keeled component or a hole for a pegged component was introduced.[43] This device can easily be attached to a cement gun. In an in vitro study, the use of this device led to more homogenous and deeper cement penetration into the glenoid bone, in comparison with a conventional cementing technique. After pressurization of cement, the authors recommend holding the component in place until the cement polymerizes and removing any cement extrusion to avoid foreign bodies in the joint, which could induce third-body polyethylene wear.

Future Directions

Glenoid loosening is the weak link in total shoulder arthroplasty. This factor is especially problematic for relatively young patients who have a longer life expectancy as well as a higher activity level than most older patients.[6,44] So-called alternative bearing surfaces have been introduced for the purpose of avoiding conventional glenoid component implantation.

Biologic Resurfacing

One possibility for resurfacing the glenoid without implanting a conventional component is to use a soft-tissue graft. The principle is to create a smooth biologic glenoid surface and thereby to reduce mechanical friction between the prosthetic humeral component and the glenoid.[45] Graft materials including meniscal allograft, joint capsule, fascia lata autograft, Achilles tendon allograft, and extracellular matrix products have been described.[45-48] Thirty-six shoulders in patients with multiple diagnoses were treated with biologic glenoid resurfacing combined with humeral head replacement.[48] The anterior capsule was used in 7 shoulders, autogenous fascia lata in 11 shoulders, and Achilles tendon allograft in 18 shoulders.[48] At 2- to 15-year follow-up, the mean overall score on the American Shoulder and Elbow Surgeons Pain and Disability Index had improved to 91 points from 39 points before surgery. According to the Neer criteria, 50% of the patients were very satisfied with the result of surgery, 36% were satisfied, and 14% were not satisfied. All shoulders had a postoperative decrease in joint space, but there was no progression at 5 years. The patients in whom allograft was used had better results for glenohumeral mobility and radiographic glenoid erosion than those in whom autograft was used. Four additional procedures had been performed; one was a débridement related to wound infection, and three were conversions to total shoulder arthroplasty. In all patients who underwent conversion to total shoulder arthroplasty, the anterior capsule had been initially used for glenoid resurfacing. The authors recommended an Achilles tendon allograft for biologic resurfacing of the glenoid.

Contrary results were reported when hemiarthroplasty was combined with biologic resurfacing of the glenoid.[49] Thirteen patients (mean age, 34 years) underwent glenoid resurfacing with an Achilles tendon allograft in 11 patients, fascia lata autograft in 1 patient, or anterior capsule autograft in 1 patient. Only 1 patient was satisfied 3 years after the procedure. The remaining 12 patients underwent revision surgery. A total shoulder replacement was required in 10 patients because of severe shoulder pain and joint space narrowing. In 2 patients, an infection was treated with débridement and a resection arthroplasty. The authors concluded that the graft material used in these patients was not durable and that biologic resurfacing of the glenoid should be pursued with caution.

In another study, 30 shoulders were treated using a metallic humeral head replacement and a meniscal allograft for resurfacing the glenoid.[47] Although there were significant improvements in all clinical outcome measures, 17% of the shoulders had required revision surgery at 1-year follow-up. Two patients underwent conversion to a total shoulder replacement, and a third

patient underwent graft removal with retention of the hemiarthroplasty. An infection requiring removal of all implants developed in one patient, and another patient underwent an arthroscopic débridement procedure.

Arthroscopic resurfacing of the glenoid using a patch without replacement of the humerus led to satisfaction with the result in 75% of patients at 3- to 6-year follow-up.[50] All scores on the Constant and American Shoulder and Elbow Surgeons measures were greatly improved. However, 25% of the patients underwent revision to a hemiarthroplasty. These inconsistent results led to the conclusion that biologic resurfacing may be a viable option for degenerative pathology of the shoulder joint in a young adult, but it should be used with caution. Prospective studies are needed to compare the results of techniques including biologic resurfacing, hemiarthroplasty, and total shoulder replacement.

The Ream-and-Run Procedure

Although hemiarthroplasty leads to inferior functional outcomes and less pain relief than total shoulder arthroplasty, it is a viable option for treating degenerative pathologies of the shoulder joint.[1] Especially in a relatively young patient, glenoid component loosening is a concern. In shoulders with eccentric glenoid wear, the outcomes of hemiarthroplasty have been inferior in comparison with shoulders in which the humeral head is centered in the glenoid.[51] The so-called ream-and-run procedure was introduced as a means of correcting the biconcavity of eccentric glenoid wear without the use of a glenoid component.[36,52] During this procedure, the glenoid is prepared with a large-diameter reamer, and a humeral head 2 mm smaller than the diameter of curvature of the glenoid reamer is chosen.[36] Although it has been shown that the intrinsic stability of the reamed glenoid can be restored and that a fibrocartilaginous surface is created on the reamed surface, few data are available as to the clinical and radiologic outcome of this type of procedure.[52-54] There was a significant improvement in shoulder function at a mean 2.7-year follow-up of 35 shoulders; pain relief after surgery was described in 32 shoulders, with no change in 1 shoulder and more pain in 2 shoulders.[52] One patient with pain and stiffness after the procedure underwent revision surgery with rereaming of the glenoid and a capsular release. Progressive medial erosion was radiographically detected in 11.4% of the shoulders, and recurrent posterior wear was detected in 17.1%.

Inset Glenoid Components

In an inset glenoid component technique, the prosthesis is inset into the bone, in comparison with the onset technique used with a conventional glenoid component. The glenoid surface is reamed to a depth of 2 to 3 mm to create a circumferential cortical rim around the implant.[55] The inset component was introduced for resurfacing glenoids with severe eccentric erosion. In a case study of seven patients, significant improvements in function and pain relief were found at a mean 4.3-year follow-up, with no signs of radiologic loosening of the components.[55] Although mechanical testing and finite element analysis showed that the inset implant had favorable results when compared with a conventional implant, it must be recognized that reaming through the cortex of the native glenoid prevents preservation of the subchondral bone, which is critical to the longevity of cemented keeled glenoid components.[56]

Summary

Significant improvement in function and pain relief can be expected after total shoulder replacement. The results appear to be superior to those of hemiarthroplasty. The glenoid component seems to be the weak point in total shoulder arthroplasty, however. High rates of loosening have been described with cemented keeled components, and no long-term data (more than 5 years) are available for pegged implants. Uncemented glenoid components had high rates of failure in the past, and many have had to be abandoned. Further investigation is necessary to analyze the long-term results of using the newer glenoid implant concepts and designs and to identify the ideal treatment for the glenoid side of the shoulder.

Annotated References

1. Radnay CS, Setter KJ, Chambers L, Levine WN, Bigliani LU, Ahmad CS: Total shoulder replacement compared with humeral head replacement for the treatment of primary glenohumeral osteoarthritis: A systematic review. *J Shoulder Elbow Surg* 2007;16(4): 396-402.

   The results of hemiarthroplasty and total shoulder arthroplasty are systematically reviewed.

2. Boileau P, Avidor C, Krishnan SG, Walch G, Kempf JF, Molé D: Cemented polyethylene versus uncemented metal-backed glenoid components in total shoulder arthroplasty: A prospective, double-blind, randomized study. *J Shoulder Elbow Surg* 2002;11(4): 351-359.

3. Young A, Walch G, Boileau P, et al: A multicentre study of the long-term results of using a flat-back polyethylene glenoid component in shoulder replacement for primary osteoarthritis. *J Bone Joint Surg Br* 2011; 93(2):210-216.

   A multicenter study examined the long-term results of cemented glenoid implantation. Level of evidence: IV.

4. Walch G, Young AA, Melis B, Gazielly D, Loew M, Boileau P: Results of a convex-back cemented keeled glenoid component in primary osteoarthritis: Multicenter study with a follow-up greater than 5 years. *J Shoulder Elbow Surg* 2011;20(3):385-394.

   A multicenter study examined the mid- and long-term results of cemented convex-back glenoid implantation. Level of evidence: IV.

5. Kasten P, Pape G, Raiss P, et al: Mid-term survivorship analysis of a shoulder replacement with a keeled glenoid and a modern cementing technique. *J Bone Joint Surg Br* 2010;92(3):387-392.

   The midterm results of cemented keeled glenoid implantation are reported. Level of evidence: IV.

6. Burroughs PL, Gearen PF, Petty WR, Wright TW: Shoulder arthroplasty in the young patient. *J Arthroplasty* 2003;18(6):792-798.

7. Schrumpf M, Maak T, Hammoud S, Craig EV: The glenoid in total shoulder arthroplasty. *Curr Rev Musculoskelet Med* 2011;4(4):191-199.

   The options for glenoid replacement are presented.

8. Churchill RS, Brems JJ, Kotschi H: Glenoid size, inclination, and version: An anatomic study. *J Shoulder Elbow Surg* 2001;10(4):327-332.

9. Mallon WJ, Brown HR, Vogler JB III, Martinez S: Radiographic and geometric anatomy of the scapula. *Clin Orthop Relat Res* 1992;277(277):142-154.

10. Kwon YW, Powell KA, Yum JK, Brems JJ, Iannotti JP: Use of three-dimensional computed tomography for the analysis of the glenoid anatomy. *J Shoulder Elbow Surg* 2005;14(1):85-90.

11. Iannotti JP, Gabriel JP, Schneck SL, Evans BG, Misra S: The normal glenohumeral relationships: An anatomical study of one hundred and forty shoulders. *J Bone Joint Surg Am* 1992;74(4):491-500.

12. Rouleau DM, Kidder JF, Pons-Villanueva J, Dynamidis S, Defranco M, Walch G: Glenoid version: How to measure it? Validity of different methods in two-dimensional computed tomography scans. *J Shoulder Elbow Surg* 2010;19(8):1230-1237.

   The validity of two-dimensional CT for evaluating glenoid version is examined. Level of evidence: IV.

13. Saha AK: The classic: Mechanism of shoulder movements and a plea for the recognition of "zero position" of glenohumeral joint. *Clin Orthop Relat Res* 1983; 173:3-10.

14. Martin SD, Zurakowski D, Thornhill TS: Uncemented glenoid component in total shoulder arthroplasty: Survivorship and outcomes. *J Bone Joint Surg Am* 2005; 87(6):1284-1292.

15. Fucentese SF, Costouros JG, Kühnel SP, Gerber C: Total shoulder arthroplasty with an uncemented soft-metal-backed glenoid component. *J Shoulder Elbow Surg* 2010;19(4):624-631.

   The use of a new uncemented glenoid component led to high failure rates. Level of evidence: IV.

5: Arthritis and Arthroplasty

16. Groh GI: Survival and radiographic analysis of a glenoid component with a cementless fluted central peg. *J Shoulder Elbow Surg* 2010;19(8):1265-1268.

    The short-term results of using the anchor-peg glenoid implant are presented. Level of evidence: IV.

17. Taunton MJ, McIntosh AL, Sperling JW, Cofield RH: Total shoulder arthroplasty with a metal-backed, bone-ingrowth glenoid component: Medium to long-term results. *J Bone Joint Surg Am* 2008;90(10):2180-2188.

    The mid- and long-term results of using uncemented glenoid components were found to be unsatisfactory. Level of evidence: IV.

18. Castagna A, Randelli M, Garofalo R, Maradei L, Giardella A, Borroni M: Mid-term results of a metal-backed glenoid component in total shoulder replacement. *J Bone Joint Surg Br* 2010;92(10):1410-1415.

    The use of an uncemented glenoid component design led to excellent midterm results. Level of evidence: IV.

19. Lazarus MD, Jensen KL, Southworth C, Matsen FA III: The radiographic evaluation of keeled and pegged glenoid component insertion. *J Bone Joint Surg Am* 2002;84(7):1174-1182.

20. Gartsman GM, Elkousy HA, Warnock KM, Edwards TB, O'Connor DP: Radiographic comparison of pegged and keeled glenoid components. *J Shoulder Elbow Surg* 2005;14(3):252-257.

21. Edwards TB, Labriola JE, Stanley RJ, O'Connor DP, Elkousy HA, Gartsman GM: Radiographic comparison of pegged and keeled glenoid components using modern cementing techniques: A prospective randomized study. *J Shoulder Elbow Surg* 2010;19(2):251-257.

    The short-term results of using a cemented pegged glenoid component were superior to those of using a keeled glenoid component. Level of evidence: I.

22. Anglin C, Wyss UP, Pichora DR: Mechanical testing of shoulder prostheses and recommendations for glenoid design. *J Shoulder Elbow Surg* 2000;9(4):323-331.

23. Throckmorton TW, Zarkadas PC, Sperling JW, Cofield RH: Pegged versus keeled glenoid components in total shoulder arthroplasty. *J Shoulder Elbow Surg* 2010;19(5):726-733.

    No difference was found in the development of radiolucent lines after a cemented pegged or keeled glenoid component was used. Level of evidence: IV.

24. Fox TJ, Cil A, Sperling JW, Sanchez-Sotelo J, Schleck CD, Cofield RH: Survival of the glenoid component in shoulder arthroplasty. *J Shoulder Elbow Surg* 2009; 18(6):859-863.

    The survival of different glenoid components is compared. Level of evidence: IV.

25. Walch G, Young AA, Boileau P, Loew M, Gazielly D, Molé D: Patterns of loosening of polyethylene keeled glenoid components after shoulder arthroplasty for primary osteoarthritis: Results of a multicenter study with more than five years of follow-up. *J Bone Joint Surg Am* 2012;94(2):145-150.

    Patterns of loosening are described at mid- and long-term follow-up after implantation of cemented keeled glenoid components. Level of evidence: IV.

26. Churchill RS, Zellmer C, Zimmers HJ, Ruggero R: Clinical and radiographic analysis of a partially cemented glenoid implant: Five-year minimum follow-up. *J Shoulder Elbow Surg* 2010;19(7):1091-1097.

    The 5-year results of the use of anchor-pegged glenoid components is presented. Level of evidence: IV.

27. Arnold RM, High RR, Grosshans KT, Walker CW, Fehringer EV: Bone presence between the central peg's radial fins of a partially cemented pegged all poly glenoid component suggest few radiolucencies. *J Shoulder Elbow Surg* 2011;20(2):315-321.

    Anchor-pegged glenoid components are analyzed. Level of evidence: IV.

28. Wirth MA, Loredo R, Garcia G, Rockwood CA Jr, Southworth C, Iannotti JP: Total shoulder arthroplasty with an all-polyethylene pegged bone-ingrowth glenoid component: A clinical and radiographic outcome study. *J Bone Joint Surg Am* 2012;94(3):260-267.

    The short- and mid-term results of using anchor-pegged glenoid components are presented. Level of evidence: IV.

29. Raiss P, Pape G, Kleinschmidt K, et al: Bone cement penetration pattern and primary stability testing in keeled and pegged glenoid components. *J Shoulder Elbow Surg* 2011;20(5):723-731.

    A CT examination of cement mantles and biomechanical testing of primary stability in cemented glenoid components is presented.

30. Klepps S, Chiang AS, Miller S, Jiang CY, Hazrati Y, Flatow EL: Incidence of early radiolucent glenoid lines in patients having total shoulder replacements. *Clin Orthop Relat Res* 2005;435(435):118-125.

31. Szabo I, Buscayret F, Edwards TB, et al: Radiographic comparison of two glenoid preparation techniques in total shoulder arthroplasty. *Clin Orthop Relat Res* 2005;431:104-110.

    Glenoid preparation technique influences implant survival and the occurrence of radiolucent lines when a cemented keeled glenoid component is used. Level of evidence: IV.

32. Molé D, Roche O, Riand N, Levigne C, Walch G: Results in osteoarthritis and rheumatoid arthritis, in Walch G, Boileau P, eds: *Shoulder Arthroplasty.* New York, NY, Springer, 1998.

33. Collin P, Tay AK, Melis B, Boileau P, Walch G: A ten-year radiologic comparison of two-all polyethylene glenoid component designs: A prospective trial. *J Shoulder Elbow Surg* 2011;20(8):1217-1223.

Cemented keeled flat-back and convex-back glenoid components are prospectively compared. Level of evidence: II.

34. Walch G, Edwards TB, Boulahia A, Boileau P, Molé D, Adeleine P: The influence of glenohumeral prosthetic mismatch on glenoid radiolucent lines: Results of a multicenter study. *J Bone Joint Surg Am* 2002;84(12):2186-2191.

35. Terrier A, Büchler P, Farron A: Influence of glenohumeral conformity on glenoid stresses after total shoulder arthroplasty. *J Shoulder Elbow Surg* 2006;15(4):515-520.

36. Matsen FA III, Bicknell RT, Lippitt SB: Shoulder arthroplasty: The socket perspective. *J Shoulder Elbow Surg* 2007;16(5, suppl):S241-S247.

An overview of hemiarthroplasty, total shoulder arthroplasty, and the ream-and-run procedure is presented.

37. Collins D, Tencer A, Sidles J, Matsen F III: Edge displacement and deformation of glenoid components in response to eccentric loading: The effect of preparation of the glenoid bone. *J Bone Joint Surg Am* 1992;74(4):501-507.

38. Edwards TB, Sabonghy EP, Elkousy H, et al: Glenoid component insertion in total shoulder arthroplasty: comparison of three techniques for drying the glenoid before cementation. *J Shoulder Elbow Surg* 2007;16(3, suppl):S107-S110.

Drying methods before cementation of glenoid components are compared. Level of evidence: I.

39. Gross RM, High R, Apker K, Haggstrom J, Fehringer JA, Stephan J: Vacuum assist glenoid fixation: Does this technique lead to a more durable glenoid component? *J Shoulder Elbow Surg* 2011;20(7):1050-1060.

The results of using the weep-hole technique for cementation of glenoid components are presented. Level of evidence: IV.

40. Hasan SA, Cox WK, Syed M, Suva LJ: Microcomputed tomography assessment of glenoid component cementation techniques in total shoulder arthroplasty. *J Orthop Res* 2010;28(5):559-564.

The standard and weep-hole techniques for cementation of glenoid components are compared.

41. Nyffeler RW, Meyer D, Sheikh R, Koller BJ, Gerber C: The effect of cementing technique on structural fixation of pegged glenoid components in total shoulder arthroplasty. *J Shoulder Elbow Surg* 2006;15(1):106-111.

42. Barwood S, Setter KJ, Blaine TA, Bigliani LU: The incidence of early radiolucencies about a pegged glenoid component using cement pressurization. *J Shoulder Elbow Surg* 2008;17(5):703-708.

Fewer radiolucent lines developed when cement pressurization of glenoid components was used. Level of evidence: IV.

43. Raiss P, Sowa B, Bruckner T, et al: Pressurisation leads to better cement penetration into the glenoid bone: A cadaveric study. *J Bone Joint Surg Br* 2012;94(5):671-677.

Cement mantle thickness and homogeneity are analyzed after insertion of a cemented pegged or keeled glenoid component using the standard technique or a cement restrictor.

44. Raiss P, Aldinger PR, Kasten P, Rickert M, Loew M: Total shoulder replacement in young and middle-aged patients with glenohumeral osteoarthritis. *J Bone Joint Surg Br* 2008;90(6):764-769.

The clinical results of young patients who underwent cemented total shoulder replacement are presented. Level of evidence: IV.

45. Burkhead WZ Jr, Krishnan SG, Lin KC: Biologic resurfacing of the arthritic glenohumeral joint: Historical review and current applications. *J Shoulder Elbow Surg* 2007;16(5, suppl):S248-S253.

Options and outcomes of biologic resurfacing of the glenoid are reviewed.

46. Creighton RA, Cole BJ, Nicholson GP, Romeo AA, Lorenz EP: Effect of lateral meniscus allograft on shoulder articular contact areas and pressures. *J Shoulder Elbow Surg* 2007;16(3):367-372.

Biomechanical testing of pressures and contacts after meniscus allograft on the glenoid are described.

47. Nicholson GP, Goldstein JL, Romeo AA, et al: Lateral meniscus allograft biologic glenoid arthroplasty in total shoulder arthroplasty for young shoulders with degenerative joint disease. *J Shoulder Elbow Surg* 2007;16(5, suppl):S261-S266.

Clinical results are described after glenoid resurfacing using meniscal allografts. Level of evidence: IV.

48. Krishnan SG, Nowinski RJ, Harrison D, Burkhead WZ: Humeral hemiarthroplasty with biologic resurfacing of the glenoid for glenohumeral arthritis: Two to fifteen-year outcomes. *J Bone Joint Surg Am* 2007;89(4):727-734.

Short- to long-term results are reported after biologic resurfacing of the glenoid. Level of evidence: IV.

49. Elhassan B, Ozbaydar M, Diller D, Higgins LD, Warner JJ: Soft-tissue resurfacing of the glenoid in the treatment of glenohumeral arthritis in active patients less than fifty years old. *J Bone Joint Surg Am* 2009;91(2):419-424.

Results are reported for biologic resurfacing of the glenoid in young patients. Level of evidence: IV.

5: Arthritis and Arthroplasty

50. Savoie FH III, Brislin KJ, Argo D: Arthroscopic glenoid resurfacing as a surgical treatment for glenohumeral arthritis in the young patient: Midterm results. *Arthroscopy* 2009;25(8):864-871.

    The midterm results are reported after arthroscopic resurfacing of the glenoid. Level of evidence: IV.

51. Hettrich CM, Weldon E III, Boorman RS, Parsons IM IV, Matsen FA III: Preoperative factors associated with improvements in shoulder function after humeral hemiarthroplasty. *J Bone Joint Surg Am* 2004;86(7): 1446-1451.

52. Lynch JR, Franta AK, Montgomery WH Jr, Lenters TR, Mounce D, Matsen FA III: Self-assessed outcome at two to four years after shoulder hemiarthroplasty with concentric glenoid reaming. *J Bone Joint Surg Am* 2007;89(6):1284-1292.

    The clinical outcomes of the ream-and-run procedure are reported. Level of evidence: IV.

53. Matsen FA III, Clark JM, Titelman RM, et al: Healing of reamed glenoid bone articulating with a metal humeral hemiarthroplasty: A canine model. *J Orthop Res* 2005;23(1):18-26.

54. Weldon EJ III, Boorman RS, Smith KL, Matsen FA III: Optimizing the glenoid contribution to the stability of a humeral hemiarthroplasty without a prosthetic glenoid. *J Bone Joint Surg Am* 2004;86(9):2022-2029.

55. Gunther SB, Lynch TL: Total shoulder replacement surgery with custom glenoid implants for severe bone deficiency. *J Shoulder Elbow Surg* 2012;21(5):675-684.

    The short-term results of a glenoid inset implant for bone deficiency are reported. Level of evidence: IV.

56. Gunther SB, Lynch TL, O'Farrell D, Calyore C, Rodenhouse A: Finite element analysis and physiologic testing of a novel, inset glenoid fixation technique. *J Shoulder Elbow Surg* 2012;21(6):795-803.

    Biomechanical testing and finite element analysis of inlay and onlay glenoid components are reported.

Chapter 29

Hemiarthroplasty and Reverse Shoulder Arthroplasty for Acute Proximal Humeral Fractures

Pascal Boileau, MD   Daniel Grant Schwartz, MD   Tjarco D. Alta, MD

Introduction

Proximal humeral fractures account for approximately 5% of all fractures. In patients older than approximately 70 years, however, proximal humeral fractures are the third most common fractures (exceeded in incidence only by hip and distal radius fracture).[1] Only three- and four-part displaced proximal humeral fractures customarily are treated with arthroplasty. The infrequent use of arthroplasty, combined with low interobserver and intraobserver agreement regarding surgeon treatment algorithms, contribute to the difficulty of managing proximal humeral fractures for even the most experienced surgeon.[2] Success requires a clear understanding of the indications, treatment options, prosthetic design rationales, and technical considerations related to tuberosity repair and prosthesis placement.

In 1953, Neer first described hemiarthroplasty for proximal humeral fractures; his "satisfactory but imperfect" results included a 90% rate of patients with an excellent or satisfactory result when prosthetic replacement was used for displaced three- and four-part fractures.[3,4] No subsequent study was able to replicate Neer's results.[5,6] During the intervening decades, an understanding of metallurgy, an ability to create anatomic shoulder prostheses, and technical comprehension of tuberosity repair and prosthetic placement have improved the ability to restore the native anatomy with arthroplasty.

Dr. Boileau or an immediate family member has received royalties from Tornier; serves as a paid consultant to or is an employee of Smith & Nephew and DePuy; and serves as a board member, owner, officer, or committee member of the European Society for Surgery of the Shoulder and the Elbow. Dr. Alta or an immediate family member has received nonincome support (such as equipment or services), commercially derived honoraria, or other non–research-related funding (such as paid travel) from Tornier. Neither Dr. Schwartz nor any immediate family member has received anything of value from or has stock or stock options held in a commercial company or institution related directly or indirectly to the subject of this chapter.

Reverse shoulder arthroplasty has become increasingly popular for treating proximal humeral fractures in patients older than 70 years, but the concept is not new. Grammont performed 22 reverse shoulder arthroplasties between 1989 and 1993 in patients with proximal humeral fractures or fracture sequelae.[7] Multiple reports have shown that reverse shoulder arthroplasty is a crucial tool in the arsenal of the orthopaedic surgeon.

Fracture Classification

In 1934, Codman classified proximal humeral fractures by whether the anatomic fragment was in the greater tuberosity, the lesser tuberosity, the surgical neck, or the humeral head.[8] Neer expanded on this concept to suggest that an anatomic fragment must be displaced at least 1 cm or angulated 45° to be considered part of a so-called displaced fracture.[9] Therefore, a four-part fracture would involve the humeral head displaced and/or angulated from the diaphysis, with both the greater and lesser tuberosities displaced and/or angulated. The more parts to the fracture, the more likely it is to involve compromise to the vascular supply of the humeral head.

The AO-ASIF fracture classification system is not commonly used in clinical practice but is based on both comminution and the potential for disruption of the blood supply to the humeral head.[10] A type A fracture is entirely extra-articular and has one fracture line. A type B fracture also is entirely extra-articular but has two fracture lines. A type C fracture is intra-articular and is subclassified, in order of increasing severity, as a C1 fracture, indicating slight displacement, to a C3 fracture-dislocation, which carries the greatest risk for humeral head ischemia. The Hertel binary-based classification and the so-called LEGO classification also are not used in clinical practice.[11]

5: Arthritis and Arthroplasty

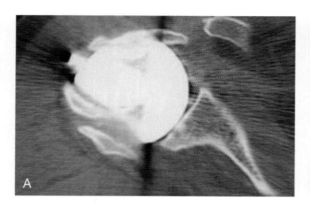
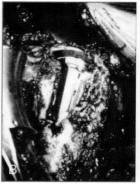
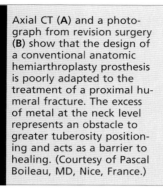

Figure 1 Axial CT (**A**) and a photograph from revision surgery (**B**) show that the design of a conventional anatomic hemiarthroplasty prosthesis is poorly adapted to the treatment of a proximal humeral fracture. The excess of metal at the neck level represents an obstacle to greater tuberosity positioning and acts as a barrier to healing. (Courtesy of Pascal Boileau, MD, Nice, France.)

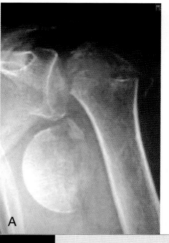
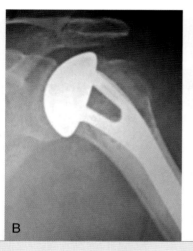
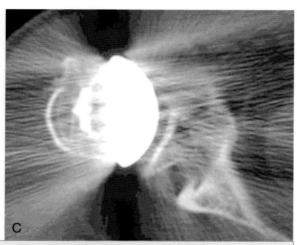

Figure 2 Proximal humeral reconstruction after a four-part fracture-dislocation, using a fracture-specific implant. **A,** Preoperative AP radiograph showing that the humeral head fragment is located in the axillary fold, disconnected from all capsular attachments, and devascularized. **B,** Postoperative AP radiograph showing anatomic tuberosity reconstruction around a fracture-specific stem. **C,** Axial CT showing accurate positioning of the tuberosities and cancellous bone harvested from the head fragment and used as a bone graft to promote tuberosity healing around the fracture stem. (Courtesy of Pascal Boileau, MD, Nice, France.)

Indications and Contraindications for Arthroplasty

Hemiarthroplasty classically has been indicated for severe fracture patterns, including fracture-dislocations, certain three- and four-part fractures, humeral head–splitting fractures, and fractures involving more than 40% of the articular surface.[7,12-14] A valgus-impacted four-part fracture is relatively unlikely to lead to osteonecrosis of the humeral head, and some surgeons may treat it less aggressively than fractures in other patterns.[15] A conserved medial soft-tissue hinge, a metaphyseal fragment longer than 8 mm, and periosteal integrity may explain the relatively low risk of osteonecrosis in a valgus-impacted four-part fracture.[11] Patient age is somewhat controversial as an indication for hemiarthroplasty; some surgeons restrict hemiarthroplasty to patients older than 70 years, but others perform hemiarthroplasty for patients who are as young as 55 years, or even younger in some situations.[2,14,16] A discerning surgeon closely examines the physiologic age of the patient, including any coexisting medical conditions, and discusses all risks and benefits with the patient before the treatment decision is made.

Reverse shoulder arthroplasty can be an alternative to hemiarthroplasty in a patient older than 70 years who has low functional demands.[17] Poor tuberosity bone stock, as a result of a comminuted fracture or osteoporosis, might preclude union with the shaft and the prosthesis, and this concern favors the choice of reverse shoulder arthroplasty. Preexisting rotator cuff arthropathy and massive rotator cuff rupture are additional indications for reverse shoulder arthroplasty.

Hemiarthroplasty and reverse shoulder arthroplasty are contraindicated if a patient has an active infection or is too medically unstable to tolerate surgery. Although there is no absolute minimum age for hemiarthroplasty or reverse shoulder arthroplasty, open reduction and internal fixation should be attempted for a relatively young patient with a heavily comminuted fracture. The surgeon should not choose hemiarthroplasty unless a patient is able to participate in a structured rehabilitation program because physical therapy is fundamental to obtaining a good result. Reverse

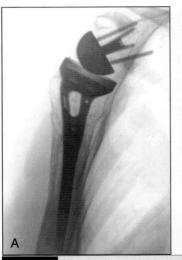
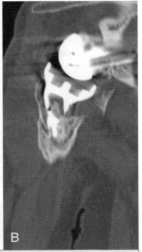

Figure 3 A fracture-specific implant 3 months after reverse shoulder arthroplasty. Tuberosity consolidation and union of the bone graft can be seen through the fracture stem window on an AP radiograph (**A**) and CT (**B**). (Courtesy of Pascal Boileau, MD, Nice, France.)

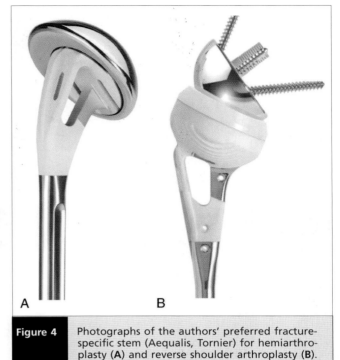

Figure 4 Photographs of the authors' preferred fracture-specific stem (Aequalis, Tornier) for hemiarthroplasty (**A**) and reverse shoulder arthroplasty (**B**). (Courtesy of Pascal Boileau, MD, Nice, France.)

shoulder arthroplasty should not be performed in patients with an axillary nerve palsy or insufficient glenoid bone stock to support a baseplate.

The Role of the External Rotator Cuff Muscles

In general, the surgeon should consider a displaced three- or four-part fracture of the proximal humerus as a massive rotator cuff tear that requires repair. The fractured tuberosities are displaced by medial traction of the rotator cuff muscles and tendons; the greater tuberosity is pulled posteromedially by the supraspinatus, the infraspinatus, and the teres minor, and the lesser tuberosity is pulled anteromedially by the subscapularis. The tuberosities must heal to the humeral shaft and to each other for proper rotator cuff function. Greater tuberosity migration, malunion, or nonunion was found to be the major cause of poor outcomes after hemiarthroplasty to treat fracture.[5] Greater tuberosity positioning and healing are the keys to success. Because the shoulder is unfavorably balanced toward muscles of internal rotation (the pectoralis major, subscapularis, latissimus dorsi, and teres major muscles), loss of the greater tuberosity with its attached muscles (the infraspinatus and teres minor muscles) leaves the shoulder with no true external rotators. The surgeon must focus great attention on securely fixing the greater tuberosity; otherwise, the natural predominance of internal rotation in the shoulder could become even stronger in the face of tuberosity malunion or nonunion.

Greater tuberosity fixation and healing are important in reverse shoulder arthroplasty. Although reverse shoulder arthroplasty may allow restoration of active forward elevation in a rotator cuff–deficient shoulder, the absence of external rotator cuff muscles because of displacement or an improperly healed greater tuberosity leads to the absence of active external rotation. Active external rotation is of paramount importance for the patient's ability to control the position of the arm in space and perform activities of daily living (such as shaving, brushing teeth, combing hair, shaking a hand, opening a door, and using a spoon).[18] In the absence of external rotator muscles in greater tuberosity malunion or nonunion, there is no muscle to counteract the weight of the forearm during elevation or abduction, and the upper limb swings toward the trunk when attempting to elevate or abduct.

Repair of the tuberosities often is overlooked during reverse shoulder arthroplasty after trauma, but this omission predictably leads to a loss of external rotation. One recent study comparing the results of reverse shoulder arthroplasty and hemiarthroplasty found better Constant shoulder scores, abduction, and forward flexion after reverse shoulder arthroplasty but better external rotation after hemiarthroplasty.[19] This result was predictable, however, because the tuberosities were reinserted in only one patient. To maximize the ability to perform activities of daily living involving external rotation, tuberosity repair should be attempted for every patient. The surgeon must understand that, from a functional standpoint, positioning and healing of the greater tuberosity is crucial regardless of whether hemiarthroplasty or reverse shoulder arthroplasty is used.

5: Arthritis and Arthroplasty

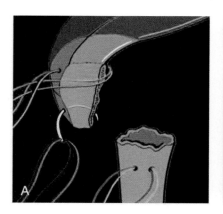
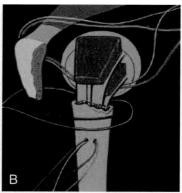
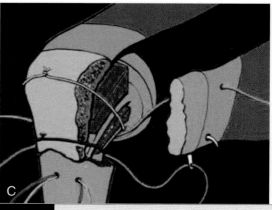
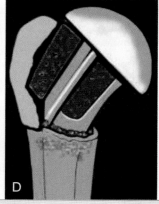
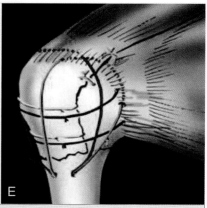

Figure 5 Schematic drawings showing a tuberosity repair. Six sutures are used, including four horizontal cerclages and two vertical tension band sutures. **A,** Two sutures are placed in the teres minor, two in the infraspinatus, and two in the humeral shaft. **B,** The four horizontal sutures are placed around the prosthetic neck. **C,** The greater tuberosity is primarily fixed with two horizontal cerclage sutures passed medial to the prosthetic neck. The lesser tuberosity is repaired with two additional horizontal cerclage sutures, and two vertical tension band sutures neutralize the construct. **D,** The fracture stem prosthesis with bone graft within the window. **E,** The final construct with the cerclage and tension band sutures tied. (Courtesy of Pascal Boileau, MD, Nice, France.)

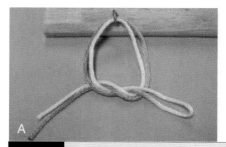
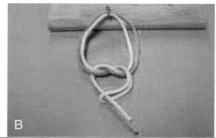
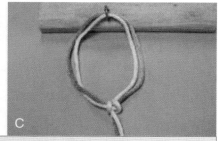

Figure 6 The double-suture Nice knot is used for the fixation of the tuberosities around the prosthesis with cerclage sutures. A square knot is created (**A**), the two free strands are introduced into the loop (**B**), and the knot is created and tightened by pulling on both strands (**C**). Three half-hitch knots are added to definitively lock the knot (Courtesy of Pascal Boileau, MD, Nice, France.).

Prosthesis Design Considerations

Advances in third-generation anatomic shoulder prostheses help to re-create the normal anatomy of the proximal humerus in patients with osteoarthritis.[6] However, conventional anatomic humeral prostheses can be too bulky to allow anatomic reduction of the tuberosities, and they allow only minimal contact between the tuberosities and the diaphysis. Because of the volume of metal around the neck, the probability of bony union is low, and the risk of tuberosity migration and malunion is high (**Figure 1**).

Accurate surgical placement of the tuberosities and their ability to remain nondisplaced have been correlated with improved clinical results.[5,20,21] Prosthesis stems that can aid in this process have been recently de-

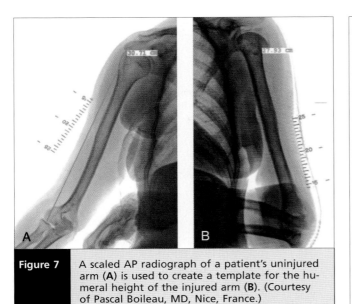

Figure 7 A scaled AP radiograph of a patient's uninjured arm (**A**) is used to create a template for the humeral height of the injured arm (**B**). (Courtesy of Pascal Boileau, MD, Nice, France.)

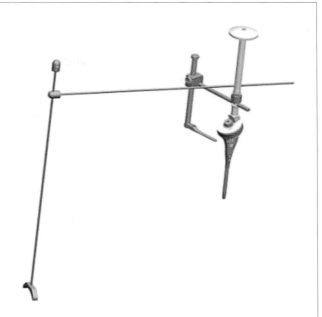

Figure 8 Photograph showing the Fracture-Jig (Tornier), which allows accurate control of the version and the height of the prosthesis during fracture reconstruction. (Courtesy of Pascal Boileau, MD, Nice, France.)

veloped. A low-profile prosthesis with relatively little metal allows unaltered tuberosities to be reduced anatomically, with more space available for bone grafting to further promote healing (**Figure 2**). One low-profile stem incorporates a window into the metaphysis to allow placement of additional bone graft, which could facilitate union between the tuberosity fragments.[16] On some prostheses, the metal around the metaphysis is roughened to increase bony stability by ingrowth into a rough hydroxyapatite-coated surface or a porous tantalum microsurface. Cerclage sutures are placed around the neck of the prosthesis, but these may tear if they come into contact with a roughened metal surface. The use of a smooth medial prosthetic neck can avoid this problem.[6] With a lower profile fracture-dedicated implant, tuberosity migration and nonunion were reduced by 50%.[21]

Fracture-specific reverse shoulder arthroplasty stems also are being developed. A hybrid implant with a smooth diaphysis allows cementation, and its roughened hydroxyapatite-coated proximal portion (with a window for bone grafting) promotes tuberosity consolidation[7] (**Figure 3**). The use of low-profile implants for both hemiarthroplasty and reverse shoulder arthroplasty is recommended to allow bone grafting and maximize the likelihood of tuberosity healing (**Figure 4**).

Fracture-Specific Stems

Hemiarthroplasty
In a recent study of 61 patients, postoperative Constant scores significantly improved if the greater tuberosity healed in an anatomic position (*P* = 0.0004), and the type of implant influenced both anatomic and functional outcomes. At a mean 45-month follow-up, the greater tuberosity was healed in an anatomic position

in 26 of 30 patients (87%) with a fracture-specific stem and was healed at a mean 81-month follow-up in 14 of 31 patients (45%) with a conventional stem (*P* < 0.0001). Active forward elevation, active external rotation, and Constant scores were significantly better with a fracture-specific stem (136°, 34°, and 68, respectively) than with a conventional stem (113°, 23°, and 58, respectively; *P* < 0.0001). Regardless of the type of implant used, women and patients older than 75 years had significantly lower functional results and higher rates of tuberosity complication (*P* < 0.0001).[22]

Reverse Shoulder Arthroplasty
In a prospective multicenter cohort study, 75 consecutive patients (76 shoulders) with a displaced proximal humeral fracture were treated using a fracture-specific reverse shoulder arthroplasty stem.[23] At a minimum 1-year follow-up of 49 patients (50 shoulders), the mean active mobility measurements were 131° (range, 40° to 170°) for anterior elevation, 24° (range, 0° to 50°) for external rotation, and 5 points (range, 0 to 10 points) for internal rotation. The mean score on a 10-point visual analog scale for pain was 1 (range, 0 to 5 points). The mean Constant score was 64 (range, 31 to 91 points) and 93% (range, 45% to 142%) when adjusted for age and gender. The mean subjective shoulder value was 70% (range, 50% to 90%). No complications were recorded, and no patient required further surgery. Forty-three shoulders (86%) had complete radiographic greater tuberosity healing. Five shoulders had

5: Arthritis and Arthroplasty

Table 1

Studies Reporting Functional Results After Reverse Shoulder Arthroplasty

Study (Year)	Number of Patients	Mean Patient Age, in Years	Mean Follow-up, in Months (Range)	Mean Active External Rotation
Tuberosity Resection				
Cazeneuve and Cristofari[44] (2006)	30	75		
Cazeneuve et al[45] (2008)	25 of 36	75	72	
Cazeneuve and Cristofari[43] (2009), Cazeneuve and Cristofari[46] (2010), Cazeneuve and Cristofari[47] (2011)	30 of 41	75	78 (12 to 168)	
Gallinet et al[19] (2009)	16	74	12 (6 to 18)	98°
Klein and Juschka[48] (2008)	20	75	33 (24 to 52)	122°
Tuberosity Reattachment				
Bufquin et al[42] (2007)	40	78	22 (6 to 58)	97°
Sirveaux et al[49] (2006)	20		79	107°
Levy and Badman[50] (2011)	7	86	14 (12 to 23)	117°
Reitman and Kerzhner[51] (2011)	13	70	28 (8 to 46)	125°
Lenarz et al[52] (2011)	30	77	23 (12 to 36)	138°
Tisher et al[53] (2008)	1	79	33	150°
Tuberosity Reattachement With Fracture Prosthesis				
Alta et al[23] (2012)	50	80	18 (12 to 39)	131°

early postoperative tuberosity migration, which healed in that position in two shoulders, led to nonunion and osteolysis in two shoulders, and led to osteolysis in one shoulder. Two shoulders had late tuberosity migration: one shoulder had a nonunion of the greater tuberosity with osteolysis, and the other had osteolysis alone. No glenoid or humeral loosening was observed.

Regardless of patient age, tuberosity healing can be achieved by reattachment and bone grafting around a specific reverse fracture prosthesis. The use of a fracture-specific implant may encourage a reliable atmosphere for tuberosity healing.

Technical Considerations

Tuberosity Bone Grafting and Fixation

Because the healing of the tuberosities strongly affects clinical outcome, the technique for fixation should fa-cilitate anatomic reduction and stable fixation.[5,20,21,24,25] The ideal construct uses six sutures—four horizontal cerclage sutures and two vertical tension band sutures—which securely fix the tuberosities to one another as well as the prosthesis and the diaphysis and thereby maximizes interfragmentary stability[26] (**Figure 5**). Two sutures are placed in the teres minor, and two are placed in the infraspinatus. Two vertical sutures are placed in the humeral shaft, with one strand for the subscapularis and the supraspinatus and the other strand for the supraspinatus and the infraspinatus. The greater tuberosity is primarily fixed with two cerclage sutures passed medial to the prosthetic neck. The lesser tuberosity also is repaired with two cerclage sutures, with one strand each from the infraspinatus and teres minor cerclage sutures. The same technique is used for tuberosity repair with a reverse prosthesis.[17,26]

The Nice knot is a sliding knot that is self-stabilizing (nonslipping) and strong (because it uses a doubled su-

Table 1

Studies Reporting Functional Results After Reverse Shoulder Arthroplasty (continued)

Mean Active External Rotation	Mean Constant Score (Range)	Mean Age- and Sex-Adjusted Constant Score	Complications
	59		12 (40%): 7 proximal humeral bone lysis, 2 instability, 1 infection, 1 glenoid loosening, and 1 humeral loosening
	59		1 instability, 1 infection, 2 acute respiratory distress syndrome, 1 glenoid loosening, and 6 proximal humeral bone lysis
	53		4 (13%): 2 acute respiratory distress syndrome, 1 infection, 1 dislocation, and 18 (60%) progressive radiolucent lines, scapular notching, spur formation
9°	53 (34 to 76)		1 deep and 1 superficial infection, 1 acute respiratory distress syndrome, and 5 humeral-side radiolucent lines without loosening
25°	67 (47 to 98)		1 dislocation and 2 early infections
8°	44 (16 to 69)	66% (25% to 97%)	11 (28%): 1 glenoid and 1 acromial fracture, 1 dislocation, 1 deltoid rupture, 5 transitory nerve palsy, and 3 acute respiratory distress syndrome
10°	55 (31 to 73)	81% (45% to 106%)	
19°			1 tuberosity nonunion and acromion fracture and 1 nonbridging heterotopic bone formation
	67 (45 to 77)		2 postinjury axillary nerve palsies, 1 postinjury radial nerve palsy, and 1 postoperative wound hematoma
27°			1 patient with complex regional pain syndrome, deep venous thrombosis, and tuberosity resorption
0°	61	88%	
24°	64 (31 to 91)	93% (45% to 142%)	1 hematoma and 1 pulmonary embolism

ture) as well as easy to tie and tighten (**Figure 6**). This novel fixation technique has been successfully used for the past 7 years to fix fractured tuberosities around a hemiarthroplasty or a reverse shoulder arthroplasty.[27]

Prosthetic Positioning

Several methods have been proposed for determining the need for restoring humeral length after arthroplasty for fracture. The principle of restoring the native anatomy is a constant, regardless of whether the method is to restore the gothic arch between the lateral edge of the scapula and the medial humerus or to measure the distance from the superior edge of the pectoralis major to the superior aspect of the humeral head (mean, 5.5 cm).[28-30] Scaled radiographs of the injured and uninjured arms allow templating of the appropriate humeral height and humeral head size (**Figure 7**). With the help of a jig, it is easy to determine how much of the stem must remain out of the diaphysis to restore anatomic humeral length

and, in turn, facilitate tuberosity repair (**Figure 8**). The Fracture-Jig (Tornier) also is helpful for restoring retroversion, based on alignment with the forearm.

Results

Recent studies have confirmed a benefit to arthroplasty for traumatic fractures but still find the satisfactory but imperfect results Neer noted decades ago.[4,9] A randomized controlled study of patients with a displaced four-part proximal humeral fracture found that patients treated with hemiarthroplasty had a significantly higher quality of life and lower pain scores than those treated nonsurgically.[31] This study underscores the importance of surgical treatment for some patients in preference to so-called benign neglect. A current study is further investigating this finding.[32] Decreased postoperative pain but imperfect range of motion are common findings in

5: Arthritis and Arthroplasty

published reports.[33-39] In one study, 30 of 57 patients had an unsatisfactory result, and 11 of these patients were in moderate to severe pain or required revision.[35] The Norwegian Arthroplasty Register found an 8% revision rate for hemiarthroplasty within the first 10 years, and the rates for relatively young patients were even higher.[40] A nonrandomized study found similar functional results in patients with fracture after osteosynthesis or hemiarthroplasty, despite an older average age in the patients who underwent hemiarthroplasty.[41] Another study found poorer results after hemiarthroplasty than after open reduction and internal fixation.[25] These findings may illustrate the importance of patient selection and surgeon experience in determining results. Despite the imperfect results, hemiarthroplasty has a definite place in the hands of an experienced orthopaedic surgeon.

Reverse shoulder arthroplasty is a newer technique than hemiarthroplasty but has not been proved significantly better for treating patients with fracture. A review of 43 patients who received a reverse prosthesis for a three- or four-part fracture found that the functional results were similar to those of hemiarthroplasty.[42] Another study found slightly better results after reverse shoulder arthroplasty than after hemiarthroplasty, except for lower external rotation scores. Glenoid notching occurred frequently, however.[19] Glenoid notching was found in more than 70% of the postoperative radiographs after reverse shoulder arthroplasty.[43] **Table 1** summarizes the results of reverse shoulder arthroplasty for the treatment of proximal humeral fractures.[19,23,42-53]

Summary

Controversy remains regarding the optimal treatment of proximal humeral fractures. It can be difficult for the surgeon to determine whether a patient is best treated nonsurgically or with open reduction and internal fixation, hemiarthroplasty, or reverse shoulder arthroplasty. There is no consensus among surgeons as to appropriate management.[2] Ongoing investigations will be helpful for determining which fracture patterns may have a poor outcome,[54,55] but clinical studies are needed to establish the use of hemiarthroplasty and reverse shoulder arthroplasty in this context.

Annotated References

1. Baron JA, Barrett JA, Karagas MR: The epidemiology of peripheral fractures. *Bone* 1996;18(3, suppl):209S-213S.

2. Petit CJ, Millett PJ, Endres NK, Diller D, Harris MB, Warner JJ: Management of proximal humeral fractures: Surgeons don't agree. *J Shoulder Elbow Surg* 2010;19(3):446-451.

Interobserver and intraobserver reliability were evaluated in proximal humeral fracture treatment. The moderate interobserver reliability improved when fewer surgical choices were presented. Intraobserver reliability was low. Level of evidence: IV.

3. Neer CS, Brown TH Jr, McLaughlin HL: Fracture of the neck of the humerus with dislocation of the head fragment. *Am J Surg* 1953;85(3):252-258.

4. Neer CS II: Displaced proximal humeral fractures: II. Treatment of three-part and four-part displacement. *J Bone Joint Surg Am* 1970;52(6):1090-1103.

5. Boileau P, Krishnan SG, Tinsi L, Walch G, Coste JS, Molé D: Tuberosity malposition and migration: Reasons for poor outcomes after hemiarthroplasty for displaced fractures of the proximal humerus. *J Shoulder Elbow Surg* 2002;11(5):401-412.

6. Boileau P, Sinnerton RJ, Chuinard C, Walch G: Arthroplasty of the shoulder. *J Bone Joint Surg Br* 2006; 88(5):562-575.

7. Sirveaux F, Roche O, Molé D: Shoulder arthroplasty for acute proximal humerus fracture. *Orthop Traumatol Surg Res* 2010;96(6):683-694.

This is an excellent review of current concepts in arthroplasty for acute fractures, including hemiarthroplasty and reverse shoulder arthroplasty.

8. Codman E: *The Shoulder: Rupture of the Supraspinatus Tendon and Other Lesions in or About the Subacromial Bursa*. Boston, MA, Thomas Todd, 1934.

9. Neer CS II: Displaced proximal humeral fractures: I. Classification and evaluation. *J Bone Joint Surg Am* 1970;52(6):1077-1089.

10. Müller ME: *Manual of Internal Fixation: Techniques Recommended by the AO-ASIF Group*, 3rd ed. Berlin, Germany, Springer, 1991, pp 118-125.

11. Hertel R, Hempfing A, Stiehler M, Leunig M: Predictors of humeral head ischemia after intracapsular fracture of the proximal humerus. *J Shoulder Elbow Surg* 2004;13(4):427-433.

12. Cadet ER, Ahmad CS: Hemiarthroplasty for three- and four-part proximal humerus fractures. *J Am Acad Orthop Surg* 2012;20(1):17-27.

Treatment algorithms, techniques, and results related to hemiarthroplasty are reviewed.

13. Nho SJ, Brophy RH, Barker JU, Cornell CN, MacGillivray JD: Management of proximal humeral fractures based on current literature. *J Bone Joint Surg Am* 2007;89(suppl 3):44-58.

The management options for proximal humeral fractures are discussed based on a review of the current literature.

14. Voos JE, Dines JS, Dines DM: Arthroplasty for fractures of the proximal part of the humerus. *J Bone Joint Surg Am* 2010;92(6):1560-1567.

    The rationale, surgical technique, rehabilitation, and outcomes of arthroplasty for fractures of the proximal humerus are discussed.

15. Iannotti JP, Ramsey ML, Williams GR Jr, Warner JJ: Nonprosthetic management of proximal humeral fractures. *Instr Course Lect* 2004;53:403-416.

16. Boileau P, Pennington SD, Alami G: Proximal humeral fractures in younger patients: Fixation techniques and arthroplasty. *J Shoulder Elbow Surg* 2011;20(2, suppl):S47-S60.

    This excellent review is focused on the difficulties of treating younger patients with a proximal humeral fracture, with surgical tips.

17. Sirveaux F, Navez G, Roche O, Mole D, Williams MD: Reverse prosthesis for proximal humerus fracture: Technique and results. *Tech Shoulder Elbow Surg* 2008;9:15-22.

    The indications, contraindications, and technique for a reverse shoulder arthroplasty are discussed with respect to a proximal humeral fracture.

18. Boileau P, Rumian AP, Zumstein MA: Reversed shoulder arthroplasty with modified L'Episcopo for combined loss of active elevation and external rotation. *J Shoulder Elbow Surg* 2010;19(2, suppl):20-30.

    The technique, outcomes, and rationale for latissimus dorsi and teres major transfer during reverse shoulder arthroplasty are described for patients with no active external rotation. The importance of external rotation in activities of daily living is highlighted. Level of evidence: IV.

19. Gallinet D, Clappaz P, Garbuio P, Tropet Y, Obert L: Three or four parts complex proximal humerus fractures: Hemiarthroplasty versus reverse prosthesis. A comparative study of 40 cases. *Orthop Traumatol Surg Res* 2009;95(1):48-55.

    The 16 patients who received a reverse prosthesis had higher postoperative Constant scores and better forward flexion and abduction than the 17 who underwent hemiarthroplasty. However, both internal and external rotation were poorer in those with a reverse prosthesis. Level of evidence: IV.

20. Kralinger F, Schwaiger R, Wambacher M, et al: Outcome after primary hemiarthroplasty for fracture of the head of the humerus: A retrospective multicentre study of 167 patients. *J Bone Joint Surg Br* 2004;86(2):217-219.

21. Loew M, Heitkemper S, Parsch D, Schneider S, Rickert M: Influence of the design of the prosthesis on the outcome after hemiarthroplasty of the shoulder in displaced fractures of the head of the humerus. *J Bone Joint Surg Br* 2006;88(3):345-350.

22. Boileau P, Winter M, Cikes A, et al: Can surgeons predict what makes a good hemiarthroplasty for fracture? in Boileau P, ed: *Shoulder Concepts 2012: Arthroscopy, Arthroplasty, and Fractures.* Paris, France, Sauramps Medical, 2012, pp 329-344.

    In a study of 61 patients, postoperative Constant scores significantly improved if the greater tuberosity healed in an anatomic position. The type of implant influenced both anatomic and functional outcomes. Regardless of the type of implant, women and patients older than 75 years had significantly lower functional results and higher rates of tuberosity complication.

23. Alta T, Decroocq L, Moineau G, et al: Reverse shoulder arthroplasty for the treatment of proximal humeral fractures in the elderly: Results with a minimum one-year follow-up. Saint Genis Laval, France, *24th Congress Scientific Program.* European Society for Surgery of the Shoulder and the Elbow, 2012, paper OP16. http://secec.com. Accessed September 10, 2012.

    Seventy-five consecutive patients (76 shoulders) with a displaced proximal humeral fracture were treated using a fracture-specific reverse shoulder arthroplasty stem. At a minimum 1-year follow-up of 49 patients (50 shoulders), the mean active mobility measurements were 131° for anterior elevation and 24° for external rotation. The mean score on a 10-point visual analog scale for pain was 1, and the mean Constant score was 64. Forty-three shoulders (86%) had complete radiographic greater tuberosity healing.

24. Mighell MA, Kolm GP, Collinge CA, Frankle MA: Outcomes of hemiarthroplasty for fractures of the proximal humerus. *J Shoulder Elbow Surg* 2003;12(6):569-577.

25. Solberg BD, Moon CN, Franco DP, Paiement GD: Surgical treatment of three and four-part proximal humeral fractures. *J Bone Joint Surg Am* 2009;91(7):1689-1697.

    A retrospective study of 122 consecutive patients with proximal humeral fractures found that patients who received locked plating had higher postoperative Constant scores than those who had hemiarthroplasty. Level of evidence: III.

26. Boileau P, Walch G, Krishnan SG: Tuberosity osteosynthesis and hemiarthroplasty for four-part fractures of the proximal humerus. *Tech Shoulder Elbow Surg* 2000;1:96-109.

27. Boileau P, Rumian AP: A non-slipping and secure fixation of bone fragments and soft tissues usable in open and arthroscopic surgery, in Boileau P, ed: *Shoulder Concepts 2010: Arthroscopy and Arthroplasty.* Paris, France, Sauramps Medical, 2010, pp. 245-251.

    The technique for using a novel double-limbed suture was described for both soft-tissue and bony fixation in open or arthroscopic surgery.

28. Krishnan SG, Bennion PW, Reineck JR, Burkhead WZ: Hemiarthroplasty for proximal humeral fracture: Restoration of the Gothic arch. *Orthop Clin North Am* 2008;39(4):441-450, vi.

5: Arthritis and Arthroplasty

A technique is described for establishing anatomic humeral length with hemiarthroplasty for proximal humeral fractures. The alignment of the lateral border of the scapula with the medial calcar of the humerus was found to be helpful.

29. Murachovsky J, Ikemoto RY, Nascimento LG, Fujiki EN, Milani C, Warner JJ: Pectoralis major tendon reference (PMT): A new method for accurate restoration of humeral length with hemiarthroplasty for fracture. *J Shoulder Elbow Surg* 2006;15(6):675-678.

30. Torrens C, Corrales M, Melendo E, Solano A, Rodríguez-Baeza A, Cáceres E: The pectoralis major tendon as a reference for restoring humeral length and retroversion with hemiarthroplasty for fracture. *J Shoulder Elbow Surg* 2008;17(6):947-950.

   CT was used to measure the distance between the superior border of the tendon and the apex of the humeral head.

31. Olerud P, Ahrengart L, Ponzer S, Saving J, Tidermark J: Hemiarthroplasty versus nonoperative treatment of displaced 4-part proximal humeral fractures in elderly patients: A randomized controlled trial. *J Shoulder Elbow Surg* 2011;20(7):1025-1033.

   A randomized controlled study compared health-related quality of life in patients with a four-part proximal humeral fracture treated nonsurgically or with hemiarthroplasty. Those treated with hemiarthroplasty had higher quality-of-life scores and less pain. Level of evidence: I.

32. Den Hartog D, Van Lieshout EM, Tuinebreijer WE, et al: Primary hemiarthroplasty versus conservative treatment for comminuted fractures of the proximal humerus in the elderly (ProCon): A multicenter randomized controlled trial. *BMC Musculoskelet Disord* 2010;11:97.

   This is the protocol for an ongoing level I randomized controlled study to detect differences between nonsurgical management and hemiarthroplasty.

33. Kontakis G, Koutras C, Tosounidis T, Giannoudis P: Early management of proximal humeral fractures with hemiarthroplasty: A systematic review. *J Bone Joint Surg Br* 2008;90(11):1407-1413.

   This systematic review examined the results and the complications of hemiarthroplasty for proximal humeral fractures. In 808 patients from 16 studies, the postoperative mean active anterior elevation was 105.7°, mean abduction was 92.4°, and the mean Constant score was 56.63.

34. Grönhagen CM, Abbaszadegan H, Révay SA, Adolphson PY: Medium-term results after primary hemiarthroplasty for comminute proximal humerus fractures: A study of 46 patients followed up for an average of 4.4 years. *J Shoulder Elbow Surg* 2007;16(6):766-773.

   A retrospective study evaluated the midterm functional and radiographic results of hemiarthroplasty for fracture. The mean Constant score was 42, with near-universal relief of pain. Radiographic examination found that 24 of the 46 prostheses had superiorly migrated. Level of evidence: IV.

35. Antuña SA, Sperling JW, Cofield RH: Shoulder hemiarthroplasty for acute fractures of the proximal humerus: A minimum five-year follow-up. *J Shoulder Elbow Surg* 2008;17(2):202-209.

   A retrospective study evaluated long-term outcomes of hemiarthroplasty for acute fractures. The average external rotation was 30°, and average forward elevation was 100°, with 16% of the patients reporting moderate to severe pain. Level of evidence: IV.

36. Fallatah S, Dervin GF, Brunet JA, Conway AF, Hrushowy H: Functional outcome after proximal humeral fractures treated with hemiarthroplasty. *Can J Surg* 2008;51(5):361-365.

   A retrospective study of 45 patients after hemiarthroplasty for proximal humeral fracture found that mean active elevation was 87°, mean abduction was 63°, 15% of the patients reported severe pain, and 25% were unable to sleep on the affected extremity.

37. Greiner SH, Kääb MJ, Kröning I, Scheibel M, Perka C: Reconstruction of humeral length and centering of the prosthetic head in hemiarthroplasty for proximal humeral fractures. *J Shoulder Elbow Surg* 2008;17(5):709-714.

   The study focused on whether using the pectoralis major tendon reference to determine the length of the humerus after hemiarthroplasty led to better results. The overall mean postoperative Constant score was 47.7, but it was higher in patients for whom the pectoralis major tendon was used to reference humeral height.

38. Padua R, Bondì R, Ceccarelli E, Campi A, Padua L: Health-related quality of life and subjective outcome after shoulder replacement for proximal humeral fractures. *J Shoulder Elbow Surg* 2008;17(2):261-264.

   Patient-relevant quality-of-life measures were assessed after hemiarthroplasty for proximal humeral fracture. Scores were lower in the patients compared with healthy control subjects.

39. Pavlopoulos DA, Badras LS, Georgiou CS, Skretas EF, Malizos KN: Hemiarthroplasty for three- and four-part displaced fractures of the proximal humerus in patients over 65 years of age. *Acta Orthop Belg* 2007;73(3):306-314.

   A prospective case study followed patients with three- or four-part fracture treated with hemiarthroplasty. No patients had complete recovery of strength and full range of motion. Of the 50 patients, 34 were able to resume all activities of daily living.

40. Fevang BT, Lie SA, Havelin LI, Skredderstuen A, Furnes O: Risk factors for revision after shoulder arthroplasty: 1,825 shoulder arthroplasties from the Norwegian Arthroplasty Register. *Acta Orthop* 2009; 80(1):83-91.

   In a review of 1,825 arthroplasties performed in Norway during a 12-year period, Kaplan-Meier failure curves and a Cox regression revealed revision rates of approximately 8%, with higher rates for younger patients.

41. Bastian JD, Hertel R: Osteosynthesis and hemiarthroplasty of fractures of the proximal humerus: Outcomes in a consecutive case series. *J Shoulder Elbow Surg* 2009;18(2):216-219.

   A prospective nonrandomized comparison study found that osteosynthesis and hemiarthroplasty had similar functional results. The average Constant score was 77 points for patients treated with osteosynthesis and 70 points for those treated with hemiarthroplasty. Level of evidence: II.

42. Bufquin T, Hersan A, Hubert L, Massin P: Reverse shoulder arthroplasty for the treatment of three- and four-part fractures of the proximal humerus in the elderly: A prospective review of 43 cases with a short-term follow-up. *J Bone Joint Surg Br* 2007;89(4):516-520.

   A prospective review of 43 patients with three- or four-part fractures who were treated with reverse shoulder arthroplasty found a mean active anterior elevation of 97° and a mean active external rotation in abduction of 30°. The Constant score improved to a mean of 44.

43. Cazeneuve JF, Cristofari DJ: Delta III reverse shoulder arthroplasty: Radiological outcome for acute complex fractures of the proximal humerus in elderly patients. *Orthop Traumatol Surg Res* 2009;95(5):325-329.

   A retrospective review of radiographic results after reverse shoulder arthroplasty for fracture of the proximal humerus found unsatisfactory images, notching, radiolucent lines, or inferior spurring for 70% of the patients.

44. Cazeneuve JF, Cristofari DJ: Grammont reversed prosthesis for acute complex fracture of the proximal humerus in an elderly population with 5 to 12 year follow-up. *Rev Chir Orthop Reparatrice Appar Mot* 2006;92(6):543-548.

45. Cazeneuve JF, Hassan Y, Kermad F, Brunel A: Delta III reverse-ball-and-socket total shoulder prosthesis for acute complex fractures of the proximal humerus in elderly population. *Eur J Orthop Surg Traumatol* 2008;18:81-86.

   A Grammont style prosthesis was used to treat 25 consecutive patients with three- or four-part fractures or fracture-dislocations. The results were good with respect to pain, activity, strength, anterior elevation, and abduction but poor for internal and external rotation.

46. Cazeneuve JF, Cristofari DJ: The reverse shoulder prosthesis in the treatment of fractures of the proximal humerus in the elderly. *J Bone Joint Surg Br* 2010;92(4):535-539.

   The clinical and radiologic outcomes of 36 patients with a proximal humeral fracture were reported at a mean 6.6-year follow-up. The mean Constant score was 53, in contrast to 58.5 at an earlier mean 6-year follow-up (range, 1 to 12 years). The reduction in Constant score and the further development of scapular notching was of concern.

47. Cazeneuve JF, Cristofari DJ: Long term functional outcome following reverse shoulder arthroplasty in the elderly. *Orthop Traumatol Surg Res* 2011;97(6):583-589.

   Thirty-five patients had improvement in function with limitations in rotation after receiving a reverse prosthesis for a complex proximal humerus fracture. Scapular notching was present in 20 patients, with associated decreased function and abnormal humeral radiographic images.

48. Klein M, Juschka M, Hinkenjann B, Scherger B, Ostermann PA: Treatment of comminuted fractures of the proximal humerus in elderly patients with the Delta III reverse shoulder prosthesis. *J Orthop Trauma* 2008;22(10):698-704.

   Twenty patients (mean age, 74.85 years) were followed for 33.3 months after receiving a reverse shoulder prosthesis. The average range of motion in abduction was 112.5° (± 38.2°) and in anterior elevation was 122.7° (± 32.84°). The mean Constant Score was 67.85° (± 13.56°). The good functional outcomes and the short intervention times, with no need for a sufficient rotator cuff for implementation purposes, suggested that the Delta III reverse shoulder prosthesis is a useful treatment option for older patients with a comminuted fracture of the proximal humerus.

49. Sirveaux F, Navez G, Favard L, Boileau P, Walch G, Molé D: The multi-centre study, in Walch G, Boileau P, Molé D, eds: *Reverse Shoulder Arthroplasty: Clinical Results, Complications, Revision.* Montpellier, France, Sauramps Medical, 2006, pp 73-80.

50. Levy JC, Badman B: Reverse shoulder prosthesis for acute four-part fracture: Tuberosity fixation using a horseshoe graft. *J Orthop Trauma* 2011;25(5):318-324.

   This technical article described the use of a horseshoe graft technique to increase the possibility of tuberosity repair in patients receiving a reverse prosthesis for fracture. Six of seven patients had healing with good functional results.

51. Reitman RD, Kerzhner E: Reverse shoulder arthoplasty as treatment for comminuted proximal humeral fractures in elderly patients. *Am J Orthop (Belle Mead NJ)* 2011;40(9):458-461.

   At short-term follow-up of 13 patients after reverse shoulder arthroplasty for a proximal humeral fracture, the mean Constant score was 67, and no recurrent instability occurred. Three nerve palsies were reported, but no revisions were required.

52. Lenarz C, Shishani Y, McCrum C, Nowinski RJ, Edwards TB, Gobezie R: Is reverse shoulder arthroplasty appropriate for the treatment of fractures in the older patient? Early observations. *Clin Orthop Relat Res* 2011;469(12):3324-3331.

At short-term follow-up after the use of reverse shoulder arthroplasty for a proximal humeral fractures, functional scores had improved, and the complication rate compared favorably with those of other treatment alternatives.

53. Tischer T, Rose T, Imhoff AB: The reverse shoulder prosthesis for primary and secondary treatment of proximal humeral fractures: A case report. *Arch Orthop Trauma Surg* 2008;128(9):973-978.

An older woman required bilateral reverse shoulder arthroplasty for bilateral proximal humerus fractures. Her functional and radiographic outcomes were reported.

54. Lee CW, Shin SJ: Prognostic factors for unstable proximal humeral fractures treated with locking-plate fixation. *J Shoulder Elbow Surg* 2009;18(1):83-88.

Forty-five unstable proximal humeral fractures were analyzed to determine risk factors for loss of reduction. Lack of comorbidities and restoration of the medial metaphysis predicted a good result from osteosynthesis.

55. Solberg BD, Moon CN, Franco DP, Paiement GD: Locked plating of 3- and 4-part proximal humerus fractures in older patients: The effect of initial fracture pattern on outcome. *J Orthop Trauma* 2009;23(2): 113-119.

Worse clinical outcomes and radiographic results were found in 24 patients with initial varus displacement of the humeral head than in 46 patients with initial valgus displacement.

Chapter 30

Arthroplasty for Sequelae of Proximal Humeral Fractures

Armodios M. Hatzidakis, MD   Benjamin W. Sears, MD

Introduction

Proximal humeral fractures are relatively common, accounting for approximately 185,000 emergency department visits annually in the United States.[1] Although most of these fractures are successfully treated nonsurgically, significant functional impairment can occur in the presence of osseous deformity, nonunion, or osteonecrosis and collapse resulting from the injury.[2-4] The delayed complications of proximal humeral fractures range from isolated tuberosity malunion or nonunion, which often can be managed with arthroscopic or open reduction and internal fixation, to a complex articular surface incongruency, which often leads to destruction of the articular surface and early-onset arthritis.[4,5] In patients with significant deformity of the proximal humeral anatomy or articular surface destruction, prosthetic arthroplasty may be the only reliable means of restoring a functional joint and providing pain relief.

Prosthetic arthroplasty for the management of the sequelae of proximal humeral fractures can be challenging because of injury complexity, rotator cuff insufficiency, bone loss, scarring, and distortion of the osseous anatomy. The decisions related to arthroplasty are even more challenging because patients with symptomatic proximal humeral fracture sequelae often are relatively young and active. Surgical treatment of such a patient can be difficult and have a less predictable outcome than for a patient with primary osteoarthritis.[3,6]

Dr. Hatzidakis or an immediate family member is a member of a speakers' bureau or has made paid presentations on behalf of Tornier; serves as a paid consultant to or is an employee of Tornier; has received research or institutional support from Tornier; and has stock or stock options held in Tornier. Neither Dr. Sears nor any immediate family member has received anything of value from or has stock or stock options held in a commercial company or institution related directly or indirectly to the subject of this chapter.

Fracture Sequelae Classification

The Boileau classification of proximal humeral fracture sequelae is based on a radiographic evaluation of 71 patients treated with nonconstrained (anatomic) arthroplasty.[2] The delayed fracture complications are classified into four types (**Figure 1**). Type I refers to a fracture sequela associated with impaction and humeral head collapse or necrosis, and type II refers to locked anterior or posterior proximal humeral dislocation or fracture-dislocation. Types I and II are categorized as intracapsular and have predictably good results after nonconstrained arthroplasty. Fractures that proceed to surgical neck nonunion are type III, and those with a severe tuberosity malunion and gross proximal humeral deformity are type IV. Types III and IV are categorized as extracapsular and have less predictable outcomes after anatomic arthroplasty. An assessment of the need for greater tuberosity osteotomy or fixation during arthroplasty is a critical component of the classification system. Greater tuberosity nonunion or associated greater tuberosity osteotomy is consistently associated with poor results after nonconstrained shoulder arthroplasty.[2-4,7,8]

The Boileau classification is useful for surgical planning. Intracapsular sequelae (types I and II) are associated with minimal distortion of the proximal humeral anatomy and maintenance of the tuberosity-diaphysis continuity. Predictable, satisfactory results can generally be achieved with nonconstrained arthroplasty without tuberosity osteotomy (**Figure 2**). In these patients, a near-anatomic relationship of the greater tuberosity to the humeral head can be restored without the need for osteotomy. Using a modular, adaptable third-generation humeral prosthesis facilitates the restoration of this relationship.

Extracapsular sequelae (types III and IV) are associated with severe distortion of proximal humeral anatomy and/or a disruption of the tuberosity-diaphysis continuity. In these patients, an unconstrained prosthesis has less predictable long-term results, primarily because of the difficulty or the impossibility of achieving greater tuberosity healing in a near-anatomic position with respect to the humeral prosthesis. Therefore, primary fixation with bone graft (for a type III nonunion)

Intracapsular impacted fracture sequelae	Type 1 Cephalic collapse or necrosis	Type II Locked dislocation or fracture-dislocation

Slight distortion of anatomy
Tuberosity-diaphysis continuity

▼

Greater tuberosity osteotomy
not needed

▼

Good, predictable results using
unconstrained prosthesis

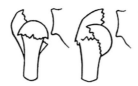

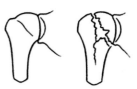

Extracapsular disimpacted fracture sequelae	Type III Surgical neck nonunion	Type IV Severe tuberosity malunion

Severe distortion of anatomy
Tuberosity-diaphysis discontinuity

▼

Greater tuberosity
osteotomy needed

▼

Poor, unpredictable results
using unconstrained prosthesis

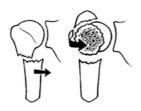

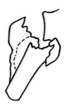

Figure 1 The Boileau classification of proximal humeral fracture sequelae. (Adapted with permission from Boileau P, Chuinard C, Le Huec JC, Walch G, Trojani C: Proximal humerus fracture sequelae: Impact of a new radiographic classification on arthroplasty. *Clin Orthop Relat Res* 2006;442:121-130.)

or a semiconstrained (reverse) prosthesis should be considered.

Indications and Contraindications to Arthroplasty

Prosthetic shoulder arthroplasty should be considered for a patient with symptomatic fracture sequelae, pain, and loss of function. The contraindications for arthroplasty include the presence of active infection, a severe neurologic injury, a comorbidity precluding a surgical procedure, or extremely poor bone quality preventing adequate prosthetic fixation. The options include using an unconstrained shoulder prosthesis (hemiarthroplasty, humeral head resurfacing, and total shoulder arthroplasty) and the use of a semiconstrained prosthesis (reverse total shoulder arthroplasty).

Hemiarthroplasty, Total Shoulder Arthroplasty, and Humeral Head Resurfacing

Hemiarthroplasty remains the treatment of choice if the fracture sequela involves minor tuberosity malunion or nonunion and the deformity of proximal humeral anatomy is minimal, as seen in type I or II fractures and some type III sequelae.[3,4] Advancements in prosthesis design (such as modularity and head eccentricity) have improved the ability of the implant to adapt to altered osseous anatomy. Total shoulder arthroplasty often is

unnecessary because the patient has minimal arthritic changes to the glenoid, even if there are significant degenerative changes to the humeral head. However, degenerative changes in the glenoid are best seen at the time of surgery, and sometimes resurfacing the glenoid results in the most predictable pain relief, return to function, and avoidance of revision (**Figure 2**).

Anatomic prostheses include those with a humeral stem as well as resurfacing prostheses. Although stemmed implants have traditionally been preferred, their adaptability is limited by the intramedullary component. A resurfacing prosthesis is not constrained by the required connection to the humeral shaft, and this characteristic may allow increased adaptability in severe malunion, especially in relation to the neck-shaft angle. Good outcomes based on Constant shoulder scores were recently reported in 28 patients undergoing resurfacing arthroplasty for type I or II proximal humeral fracture sequelae, with only one reported complication. Resurfacing arthroplasty was found to be a viable prosthetic option for patients with posttraumatic osteoarthritis, provided the patient had adequate bone stock and relative preservation of humeral head sphericity[9] (**Figure 3**). In patients with humeral head collapse or severely distorted anatomy, humeral head resurfacing may not be ideal because the implant must be adequately fixed to the epiphyseal surface and may not sufficiently adapt to the osseous anatomy.

5: Arthritis and Arthroplasty

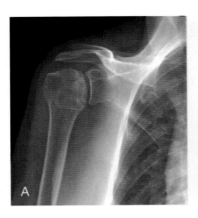
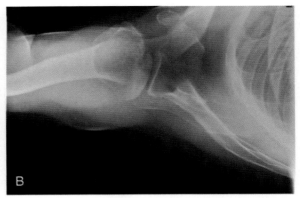

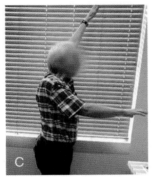
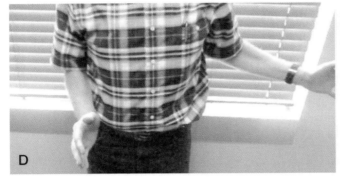
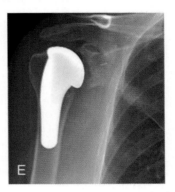

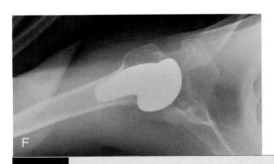
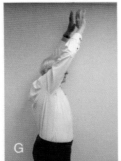
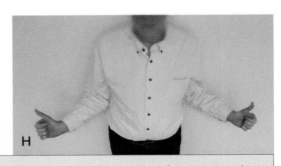

Figure 2 A 66-year-old man had osteonecrosis and humeral head collapse (type I sequele) after healing of an intracapsular proximal humeral fracture. Significant glenoid articular wear was observed during surgery, and glenoid resurfacing was performed. The patient had excellent function with minimal pain at 1-year follow-up. **A,** Preoperative AP radiograph shows osteonecrosis and humeral head collapse. **B,** Preoperative axillary radiograph showing collapse of the articular surface and mild distortion of the tuberosities. Preoperative photographs showing active forward flexion (**C**) and active external rotation (**D**). AP (**E**) and axillary (**F**) radiographs 1 year after total shoulder arthroplasty showing near-anatomic reconstruction of the tuberosity–humeral head relationship. Photographs obtained 1 year after total shoulder arthroplasty showing active forward flexion (**G**) and active external rotation (**H**).

Reverse Shoulder Arthroplasty

Reverse shoulder arthroplasty is most commonly used to treat fracture sequelae in patients older than 70 years or in patients with severe tuberosity malunion, nonunion, and/or rotator cuff deficiency.[10,11] Reverse shoulder arthroplasty greatly reduces the reliance on tuberosity positioning or rotator cuff function for glenohumeral motor power and stability, and it is the treatment of choice for patients who have low physical demands, severe tuberosity malunion, or distortion of the proximal humeral anatomy (type IV sequelae), or

sequelae with concurrent rotator cuff deficiency.[3,10] Reverse shoulder arthroplasty has resulted in good pain relief and postoperative elevation in patients older than 70 years who have intracapsular (type I or II) sequelae.[4,12] Reverse arthroplasty also can be used as a salvage procedure after failed hemiarthroplasty to treat fracture sequelae and should be considered as a primary treatment option in patients who have type I sequelae with a poor-quality or an irreparable rotator cuff (**Figure 4**). Patients with chronic anterior instability who undergo reverse arthroplasty may experience

5: Arthritis and Arthroplasty

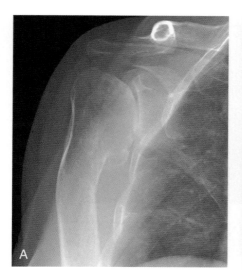

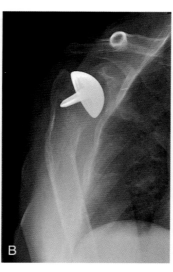

Figure 3 Severe malunion of the surgical neck of the proximal humerus or proximal humeral diaphysis may preclude stemmed humeral prosthetic replacement without humeral osteotomy. The use of a resurfacing humeral component, as in this 72-year-old man, may obviate the need for proximal humeral osteotomy, with or without placement of a glenoid component. **A,** Preoperative AP radiograph showing a proximal humeral malunion with severe osteoarthritis of the glenohumeral joint. **B,** AP radiograph showing total shoulder arthroplasty using a resurfacing humeral component.

improved joint stability.[10] Two studies reported good outcomes for use of reverse arthroplasty in patients with proximal humeral nonunion (type III sequela).[13,14] However, when compared with successful treatment using an unconstrained implant, treatment with reverse arthroplasty generally is associated with more extensive permanent activity restrictions and diminished active shoulder rotation.

Relative contraindications for reverse arthroplasty include patient age and level of function. Reverse arthroplasty should be used cautiously for patients younger than 70 years, regardless of the type of proximal humeral fracture sequelae. However, reverse arthroplasty is the only satisfactory treatment option for many patients with severe tuberosity nonunion or malunion.

Results

In a recent study, 55 patients with proximal humeral sequelae underwent arthroplasty with an anatomic prosthesis for type I or II sequelae or reverse total shoulder arthroplasty for type III or IV sequelae.[13] The 36 patients with the anatomic prosthesis were followed for an average of 24 months, and the 19 patients with a reverse prosthesis were followed for an average of 19.3 months. Patients in both groups had significant postoperative improvement in pain and function, although the extent of improvement relative to sequelae type was not reported. The mean Constant score increased from 19 to 68 points in patients with an anatomic prosthesis and from 9 to 47.5 points in patients with a reverse prosthesis.

Several studies specifically examined the treatment of patients with chronic dislocation (type II sequela) using an anatomic prosthesis. A retrospective review of 11 patients with fixed anterior glenohumeral dislocation treated with a nonconstrained arthroplasty reported significant improvement in pain and function

scores.[15] However, 4 patients (36%) had postoperative anterior instability, and definite radiographic loosening of the glenoid component developed in 2 of these 4 patients. Another study found that pain and function significantly improved in 12 patients with chronic posterior glenohumeral dislocation treated with nonconstrained shoulder arthroplasty; however, 3 patients (25%) required revision surgery for instability or component loosening.[16] Ultimately, anatomic shoulder arthroplasty for patients with a fixed shoulder dislocation reliably reduces pain and improves shoulder function but may be associated with residual instability and component loosening. The outcomes of arthroplasty for chronic posterior glenohumeral dislocation generally are better than the outcomes of arthroplasty for anterior dislocation.

The indications for reverse shoulder arthroplasty have broadened substantially during the past decade. Although this procedure primarily is reserved for patients who are older than 70 years and have low demands, its use as a salvage procedure in patients with fracture sequelae has allowed for the management of previously untreatable glenohumeral disorders. Several recent studies examined the role of reverse arthroplasty in proximal humeral fracture sequelae. When reverse arthroplasty was used to treat proximal humeral nonunion in 18 patients, there was significant improvement in motion, including rotation, as well as subjective shoulder scores.[14] However, 5 patients had postoperative complications, including infection in 2, nerve palsy in 1, and prosthetic dislocation that required revision to a larger glenosphere in 2. The researchers concluded that reverse arthroplasty improves function in patients with symptomatic proximal humeral nonunion that is not amenable to anatomic arthroplasty, albeit with a high complication rate. In another study, 16 patients with proximal humeral malunions were treated with reverse shoulder arthroplasty for severe pain or functional limitations, without an osteotomy of the

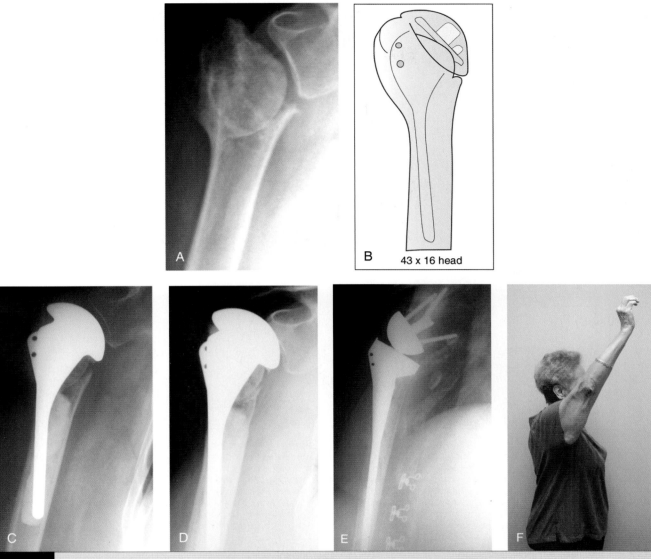

Figure 4 A 67-year-old woman had a painful, dysfunctional shoulder with type I fracture sequelae. Because the acromio-humeral interval was normal and the rotator cuff was intact, she was treated with a third-generation hemiarthro-plasty. During surgery, the superior rotator cuff was observed to be thin and required repair. Initially, the humeral head was properly centered on the glenoid, but within 1 year, it eccentrically migrated superiorly and posteriorly, leading to a poor functional result. The patient had chronic pain and dysfunction that did not respond to nonsurgical care. Revision to a long-stem reverse total shoulder prosthesis resulted in improvement in comfort and function. **A,** Prehemiarthroplasty AP radiograph showing type I fracture sequelae with a nearly anatomically aligned greater tuberosity. **B,** Patient-specific prehemiarthroplasty template showing a near-anatomic reconstruction of the greater tuberosity–humeral head relationship. **C,** Posthemiarthroplasty AP radiograph showing an adequate hemiarthroplasty position. **D,** AP radiograph obtained 1 year after hemiarthroplasty showing the superiorly migrated humeral head. **E,** AP radiograph showing revision to a long-stem reverse total shoulder arthroplasty. **F,** Photograph showing active forward flexion after the reverse shoulder arthroplasty.

malunited tuberosities or remaining proximal humerus.[17] At 2-year follow-up, pain and function scores (including rotation) improved significantly on the American Shoulder and Elbow Surgeons score, the visual analog scale, and the Simple Shoulder Test, with no major complications. The researchers concluded that reverse arthroplasty for severe proximal humeral malunion yields satisfactory outcomes.

Technical Considerations

Placement of Humeral Prosthesis Without Greater Tuberosity Osteotomy
If the proximal humerus is amenable to prosthesis placement without a tuberosity osteotomy (as in types I and II sequelae), the glenohumeral joint is exposed us-

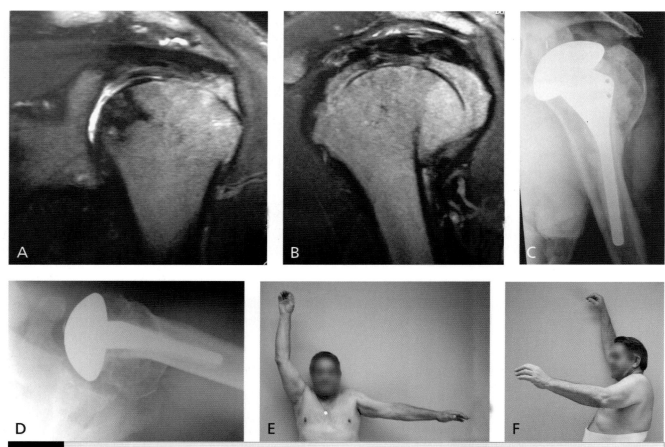

Figure 5 A 63-year-old man with a healed proximal humeral malunion had posterior displacement of the greater tuberosity. An anatomic humeral implant was chosen to achieve adequate reconstruction without osteotomy of the greater tuberosity. At 1-year follow-up, the patient had improved pain relief but persistently limited elevation. **A,** Coronal MRI showing a healed proximal humeral fracture with possible type I sequelae. **B,** Sagittal oblique MRI shows the posteriorly healed greater tuberosity. **C,** AP radiograph 1 year after total shoulder arthroplasty showing satisfactory implant position. **D,** Axillary radiograph obtained 1 year after total shoulder arthroplasty shows anterior subluxation of the humerus on the glenoid. **E,** Photograph showing limited active abduction. **F,** Photograph obtained 1 year after total shoulder arthroplasty shows limited active forward flexion.

ing a deltopectoral approach. Although it is important to maintain the healed position of the greater tuberosity, a lesser tuberosity osteotomy can be performed to gain access to the joint and manage the subscapularis.[18] The subacromial, subdeltoid, and subcoracoid spaces should be cleared of scar tissue and mobilized to allow maximal exposure of the glenohumeral joint.

When access has been gained, the humeral head, rotator cuff, and glenoid surfaces are assessed. A humeral head cut should be planned with the goal of restoring natural glenohumeral anatomy (with the superior aspect of the implant resting 5 mm above the greater tuberosity), while preserving tuberosity integrity. In some patients with advanced necrosis (type I sequela), the humeral head may be collapsed to the point that no cut is required. If a stemmed implant is selected, the stem should be thin and the implant should be cemented to allow an increased offset. Resurfacing arthroplasty can be used to avoid humeral stem placement if a severe distortion of the neck-shaft angle is encountered.

Osteotomy of a Greater Tuberosity Malunion

Although arthroplasty of a greater tuberosity malunion has been shown to have significantly worse results with osteotomy than without osteotomy, the options for maintaining tuberosity integrity sometimes are limited because of tuberosity displacement, patient age, level of function, or the extent of degenerative changes.[3,4,7,8] The relative indications for tuberosity osteotomy include more than 1 cm of posterior displacement or an inability to adequately place the prosthesis because of altered anatomy.[19] Anatomic reconstruction with more relatively severe greater tuberosity malunion may result in less predictable return of shoulder function (**Figure 5**).

When a greater tuberosity osteotomy is required, the osteotomy should be made obliquely to allow as much contact area as possible for subsequent union. The insertion of the rotator cuff on the tuberosity should be protected, and the rotator cuff should be mobilized to optimize excursion. If possible, the distal periosteal

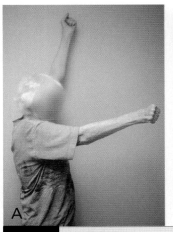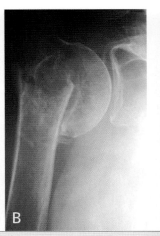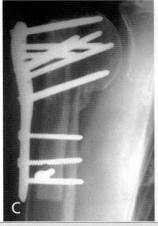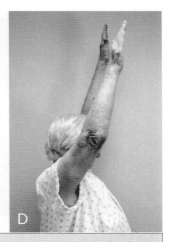

Figure 6 A 72-year-old woman with type III sequela and a surgical neck nonunion. She was treated with open takedown of the nonunion, reduction, and internal fixation with an intramedullary allograft bone peg and locked plate and screws. At 2-year follow-up, the fracture had healed, and active function had improved. **A,** Preoperative photograph shows limited active forward flexion. **B,** AP radiograph showing type III fracture sequelae (surgical neck nonunion). **C,** AP radiograph obtained 1 year after surgery shows healed proximal humerus with locked plating. **D,** Photograph shows improved forward flexion.

connection to the tuberosity should be elevated but not severed, so the soft-tissue attachment and the blood supply to the osseous fragment are maintained. After prosthetic placement, bone graft from the humeral head should be placed along the proximal aspect of the implant and the tuberosity undersurface to augment healing. Finally, the tuberosities are secured around the implant using heavy, nonabsorbable cerclage sutures. Depending on the intraoperative range of motion, a limited program of passive shoulder range of motion can be initiated for the first 6 weeks after surgery to minimize stiffness and optimize healing of the greater tuberosity and subscapularis.

Arthroplasty for Proximal Humeral Nonunion
Open reduction and internal fixation, with or without bone grafting, is the first-line treatment of type III sequelae without advanced degenerative changes[3] (**Figure 6**). For patients with advanced arthritis or limited healing capability (poor bone quality or cavitation of the humeral head), humeral head replacement with an anatomic or a reverse prosthesis may lead to the best outcome.[13,14] Regardless of the type of prosthesis (anatomic or reverse), fixation and healing of the tuberosities to the humeral implant are critical for function, including active rotation after reverse arthroplasty.

A deltopectoral approach typically is used. The long head of the biceps tendon can be used as a guide to the rotator cuff interval. If possible, the lesser tuberosity should be left in continuity with the greater tuberosity, and the subscapularis is mobilized using a peel-down or a tenotomy to gain access to the joint. The humeral head cut should be made with great caution to preserve the viability of the greater tuberosity. After shaft preparation, the final humeral stem is skewered through the ring-shaped greater and lesser tuberosity fragment and cemented in the humeral diaphysis. The proximal fragment is grafted to the humeral shaft and the implant, and the subscapularis is repaired. Depending on the intraoperative range of motion, a limited program of passive shoulder range of motion can be initiated for the first 6 weeks after surgery.

Management of Chronic Locked Dislocations
Prosthetic replacement may be required for a patient who has a chronic glenohumeral dislocation (type II sequela) extending beyond 6 months after the index injury or involving a humeral defect of more than 40% of the articular surface.[15,16] For a posteriorly directed chronic dislocation, hemiarthroplasty or resurfacing arthroplasty is the treatment of choice (**Figure 7**). Posterior capsular plication can be considered if the posterior capsule is excessively patulous and stability is not achieved by restoring the architecture of the humeral head alone.

Patients with an anterior fracture-dislocation are at increased risk for instability compared with those with a posteriorly directed dislocation.[15] Bone graft may be necessary to augment a glenoid deficiency if the humerus is unstable or if the glenoid component is unsupported. The options for glenoid bone augmentation include using an osteotomized humeral head, an iliac crest autograft, coracoid transfer, or a distal tibial allograft. If there is concern for stability or if the rotator cuff is irreparable, reverse arthroplasty may be considered.

Future Directions
The indications and the techniques for treating proximal humeral fracture sequelae with anatomic or reverse shoulder arthroplasty continue to be advanced and refined. Healing of the greater tuberosity is a critical fac-

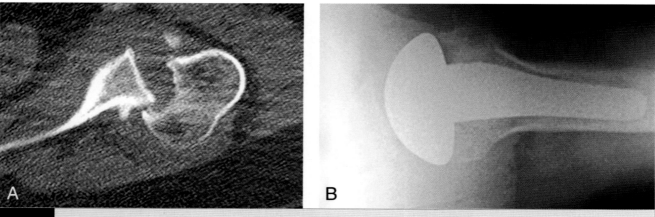

Figure 7 A 30-year-old man with type II fracture sequelae had a locked posterior fracture-dislocation and significant humeral bone loss. Anatomic hemiarthroplasty restored the anatomic location of the shoulder joint. **A**, Axial CT showing a locked posterior fracture dislocation with a large reverse Hill-Sachs lesion. **B**, Postoperative axillary lateral radiograph showing anatomic reconstruction of the humeral head with a well-located glenohumeral joint.

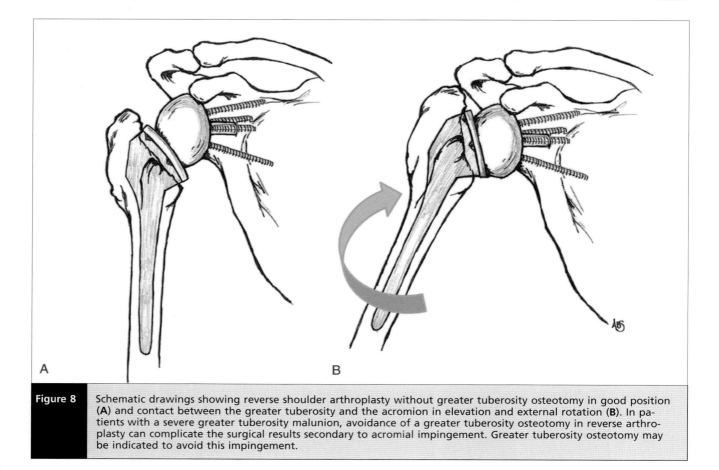

Figure 8 Schematic drawings showing reverse shoulder arthroplasty without greater tuberosity osteotomy in good position (**A**) and contact between the greater tuberosity and the acromion in elevation and external rotation (**B**). In patients with a severe greater tuberosity malunion, avoidance of a greater tuberosity osteotomy in reverse arthroplasty can complicate the surgical results secondary to acromial impingement. Greater tuberosity osteotomy may be indicated to avoid this impingement.

tor in determining functional results after anatomic or reverse shoulder arthroplasty for treating an acute fracture or fracture sequelae. New fracture stem designs for anatomic and reverse prostheses may have potential for improving the healing of the greater tuberosity with acute fractures and sequelae.[20]

Greater tuberosity osteotomy for proximal humeral malunion with reference to anatomic arthroplasty has been discussed in detail in the current literature. Greater tuberosity osteotomy also may be required in reverse arthroplasty for proximal humeral malunion. The greater tuberosity often is displaced superiorly, laterally, and posteriorly in relation to the humeral shaft. Placement of a reverse humeral stem without greater tuberosity osteotomy sometimes leads to impingement of the malunited greater tuberosity with the acromion in abduction or with the acromion and/or the glenoid in external rotation. The impingement may result in decreased range of motion and instability (**Figure 8**). This factor may contribute to the less satisfactory outcomes of reverse shoulder arthroplasty for fracture sequelae when compared with the outcomes of reverse shoulder arthroplasty for rotator cuff tear arthropathy.

Summary

Sequelae after proximal humeral fractures can cause significant pain and functional limitations, commonly leading to prosthetic replacement. Planning appropriate surgical management for these sequelae requires careful evaluation of the proximal humeral anatomy distortion and determination of the need for a greater tuberosity osteotomy. In general, patients who require arthroplasty with greater tuberosity osteotomy have worse functional outcomes than patients whose normal greater tuberosity–humeral head relationship can be restored without osteotomy. Patients with humeral head impaction or necrosis (type I), or chronic dislocation (type II) do not require greater tuberosity osteotomy and can be treated with an anatomic arthroplasty. Patients with proximal humeral nonunion (type III) often can be treated with bone graft and internal fixation, although recent studies have found good outcomes after reverse shoulder arthroplasty in some of these patients. Patients with severe anatomic distortion and tuberosity malunion (type IV) or irreparable rotator cuff deficiency are most reliably treated with reverse shoulder arthroplasty.

Annotated References

1. Kim SH, Szabo RM, Marder RA: Epidemiology of humerus fractures in the United States: Nationwide emergency department sample, 2008. *Arthritis Care Res (Hoboken)* 2012;64(3):407-414.

   An analysis of the 2008 Nationwide Emergency Department Sample revealed 370,000 US emergency room visits resulting from humeral fractures. More than 490,000 annual emergency room visits resulting from humeral fractures are projected to occur by 2030. Level of evidence: IV.

2. Boileau P, Trojani C, Walch G, Krishnan SG, Romeo A, Sinnerton R: Shoulder arthroplasty for the treatment of the sequelae of fractures of the proximal humerus. *J Shoulder Elbow Surg* 2001;10(4):299-308.

3. Boileau P, Chuinard C, Le Huec JC, Walch G, Trojani C: Proximal humerus fracture sequelae: Impact of a new radiographic classification on arthroplasty. *Clin Orthop Relat Res* 2006(442):121-130.

4. Cheung EV, Sperling JW: Management of proximal humeral nonunions and malunions. *Orthop Clin North Am* 2008;39(4):475-482, vii.

   The results of corrective osteotomy, osteosynthesis with bone grafting, and arthroplasty are reviewed for patients with nonunion or malunion of the proximal humerus.

5. Martinez AA, Calvo A, Domingo J, Cuenca J, Herrera A: Arthroscopic treatment for malunions of the proximal humeral greater tuberosity. *Int Orthop* 2010; 34(8):1207-1211.

   Eight patients with malunion of the greater tuberosity were treated with arthroscopic acromioplasty, tuberoplasty of the greater tuberosity, and repair of the rotator cuff. One patient had an excellent result, six had a good result, and one had a poor result on the UCLA Shoulder Rating Scale.

6. Norris TR, Green A, McGuigan FX: Late prosthetic shoulder arthroplasty for displaced proximal humerus fractures. *J Shoulder Elbow Surg* 1995;4(4):271-280.

7. Antuña SA, Sperling JW, Sánchez-Sotelo J, Cofield RH: Shoulder arthroplasty for proximal humeral malunions: Long-term results. *J Shoulder Elbow Surg* 2002;11(2):122-129.

8. Mansat P, Guity MR, Bellumore Y, Mansat M: Shoulder arthroplasty for late sequelae of proximal humeral fractures. *J Shoulder Elbow Surg* 2004;13(3):305-312.

9. Pape G, Zeifang F, Bruckner T, Raiss P, Rickert M, Loew M: Humeral surface replacement for the sequelae of fractures of the proximal humerus. *J Bone Joint Surg Br* 2010;92(10):1403-1409.

   Surface replacement arthroplasty in 28 shoulders resulted in good outcomes in shoulders with types I, II, and III proximal humeral fracture sequelae. The advantages of surface replacement include improved implant position, the preservation of bone stock, and the avoidance of periprosthetic fracture.

10. Neyton L, Garaud P, Boileau P: Results of reverse shoulder arthroplasty in proximal humerus fracture sequelae, in Walch G, Boileau P, Mole D, Favard L, Levigne C, Sirveaux F, eds: *Reverse Shoulder Arthroplasty*. Montpellier, France, Sauramps Medical, 2006.

11. Stechel A, Fuhrmann U, Irlenbusch L, Rott O, Irlenbusch U: Reversed shoulder arthroplasty in cuff tear arthritis, fracture sequelae, and revision arthroplasty. *Acta Orthop* 2010;81(3):367-372.

    At a mean 4-year follow-up of 59 patients, reverse shoulder arthroplasty for severe arthropathy (rotator cuff tear, fracture sequelae, or revision) was suitable for restoring function and attaining pain relief, but reverse shoulder arthroplasty should be reserved for patients in whom conventional methods were unsuccessful.

12. Martin TG, Iannotti JP: Reverse total shoulder arthroplasty for acute fractures and failed management after

proximal humeral fractures. *Orthop Clin North Am* 2008;39(4):451-457, vi.

Reverse shoulder arthroplasty was used for conditions involving insufficient rotator cuff function and proximal humeral malunion after unsuccessful hemiarthroplasty.

13. Kılıç M, Berth A, Blatter G, et al: Anatomic and reverse shoulder prostheses in fracture sequelae of the humeral head. *Acta Orthop Traumatol Turc* 2010; 44(6):417-425.

    In 55 patients with fracture sequelae who underwent anatomic total shoulder arthroplasty (for type I or II) or reverse total shoulder arthroplasty (for type III or IV), there was significant improvement in pain and function.

14. Martinez AA, Bejarano C, Carbonel I, Iglesias D, Gil-Alvaroba J, Herrera A: The treatment of proximal humerus nonunions in older patients with the reverse shoulder arthroplasty. *Injury* 2012.

    Eighteen patients with proximal humeral atrophic nonunion were followed for 28 months after reverse shoulder arthroplasty. Two postoperative dislocations occurred, and one patient developed transient axillary neurapraxia. Average active motion including rotation significantly improved in all patients.

15. Matsoukis J, Tabib W, Guiffault P, et al: Primary unconstrained shoulder arthroplasty in patients with a fixed anterior glenohumeral dislocation. *J Bone Joint Surg Am* 2006;88(3):547-552.

16. Sperling JW, Pring M, Antuna SA, Cofield RH: Shoulder arthroplasty for locked posterior dislocation of the shoulder. *J Shoulder Elbow Surg* 2004;13(5):522-527.

17. Willis M, Min W, Brooks JP, et al: Proximal humeral malunion treated with reverse shoulder arthroplasty. *J Shoulder Elbow Surg* 2012;21(4):507-513.

    Sixteen patients underwent reverse shoulder arthroplasty for proximal humeral malunion. Active motion including rotation significantly improved, and no major complications were reported. Reverse shoulder arthroplasty was indicated for treating severe fracture sequelae.

18. Scalise JJ, Ciccone J, Iannotti JP: Clinical, radiographic, and ultrasonographic comparison of subscapularis tenotomy and lesser tuberosity osteotomy for total shoulder arthroplasty. *J Bone Joint Surg Am* 2010; 92(7):1627-1634.

    Arthroplasty in 35 shoulders was performed with a standard subscapularis tenotomy or a lesser tuberosity osteotomy to release the subscapularis. The lesser tuberosity osteotomy resulted in higher outcome scores, a lower rate of tendon tears, and healing of the osteotomy. Level of evidence: III.

19. Tauber M, Resch H: Prosthetic arthroplasty for delayed complications of proximal humerus fracture, in Cofield RH and Sperling JW, eds: *Revision and Complex Shoulder Arthroplasty*. Philadelphia, PA, Lippincott Williams & Wilkins, 2010.

20. Krishnan SG, Reineck JR, Bennion PD, Feher L, Burkhead WZ Jr: Shoulder arthroplasty for fracture: Does a fracture-specific stem make a difference? *Clin Orthop Relat Res* 2011;469(12):3317-3323.

    A retrospective review of 170 proximal humeral fractures treated with hemiarthroplasty found that the use of a fracture-specific stem resulted in better function and tuberosity healing than the use of a standard stem. Level of evidence: IV.

Chapter 31

Reverse Shoulder Arthroplasty for Chronic Shoulder Pathology

Randall J. Otto, MD   Phillip T. Nigro, MD   Mark A. Frankle, MD

Introduction

Reverse shoulder arthroplasty (RSA) is one of numerous advances in shoulder arthroplasty over the past half-century for the treatment of end-stage shoulder disease. Anatomic total shoulder arthroplasty (TSA) has good results and is durable for the treatment of glenohumeral osteoarthritis with a balanced soft-tissue envelope. However, patients with arthritis and unbalanced soft tissues who are treated with TSA may have failure of the glenoid component caused by uneven forces. RSA was developed to improve the outcomes of patients with a rotator cuff–deficient shoulder. The early failures of constrained devices led Grammont to develop a nonanatomic semiconstrained device.[1] This device initially led to improved function and decreased pain.[2] Over time, the design has been modified and has evolved into the current reverse shoulder prostheses.

Design Rationale

The purpose of the reverse shoulder prosthesis is to provide a stable glenohumeral fulcrum.[1] The reversed articulation blocks superior migration of the humerus, and the superiorly directed translational forces of the

Dr. Otto or an immediate family member is a member of a speakers' bureau or has made paid presentations on behalf of DJ Orthopaedics. Dr. Nigro or an immediate family member is a member of a speakers' bureau or has made paid presentations on behalf of DJ Orthopaedics. Dr. Frankle or an immediate family member has received royalties from DJ Orthopaedics; is a member of a speakers' bureau or has made paid presentations on behalf of DJ Orthopaedics; serves as a paid consultant to DJ Orthopaedics; serves as an unpaid consultant to DePuy; has received research or institutional support from DJ Orthopaedics, EBI, Eli Lilly, and Encore Medical; has received nonincome support (such as equipment or services), commercially derived honoraria, or other non–research-related funding (such as paid travel) from DJ Orthopaedics, EBI, Eli Lilly, and Encore Medical; and serves as a board member, owner, officer, or committee member of the American Shoulder and Elbow Surgeons, American Academy of Orthopaedic Surgeons, and Florida Medical Association.

deltoid are converted into rotational moments. When the glenohumeral articulation is reestablished, the remaining rotator cuff muscles and periscapular musculature are able to restore humerus-trunk motion in conjunction with the deltoid.

Grammont designed the reverse prosthesis with a humeral component in extreme valgus (155°) and a hemisphere directly centered on the fixation and the bony glenoid surface (**Figure 1**). This valgus humeral component was designed to tension the deltoid by lengthening the arm and to provide compression between the humeral socket and the glenosphere, thus stabilizing the articulation. In addition, medializing the center of rotation of the hemisphere could enhance the recruitment of deltoid muscle fibers, thereby allowing for a more efficient deltoid lever arm.[3] It was postulated that locating a humeral center of rotation as close as possible to the glenoid bone surface would decrease baseplate loosening.

Despite clinical improvements resulting from the use of the Grammont device, several mechanical problems emerged, including a substantial reduction in the impingement-free range of motion of the glenohumeral joint and a significant alteration in the proximal humeral lateral and inferior offset.[4,5] These deviations from the structural anatomic shoulder and the subsequent change in mechanics led to unforeseen complications including prosthetic abutment of bone and soft tissue and loss of the appearance of the shoulder form with the alteration in shoulder function. Numerous clinical and biomechanical studies have aimed at improving the prosthetic design and surgical technique of RSA.

Indications and Contraindications

Indications

The indications for RSA have continued to expand as it has become more widely used for treating patients with severe shoulder pathology. Originally, RSA was used for patients with glenohumeral arthritis in the setting of rotator cuff deficiency. More recently, RSA has been successfully used for patients who have severe rotator cuff deficiency without glenohumeral arthritis; osteoar-

5: Arthritis and Arthroplasty

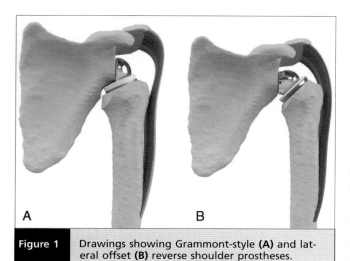

Figure 1 Drawings showing Grammont-style **(A)** and lateral offset **(B)** reverse shoulder prostheses.

thritis, an intact rotator cuff, and glenohumeral instability; rheumatoid arthritis; a three- or four-part proximal humeral fracture; or a fracture malunion. RSA also is successfully used for patients needing reconstruction after tumor resection and for patients who have undergone an unsuccessful hemiarthroplasty for fracture or rotator cuff tear arthropathy, TSA, or earlier RSA.

RSA is considered if the patient reports pain more severe than 5 on a 10-point scale and/or has significant impairment in shoulder function. Often patients have clinical or radiographic pseudoparesis of the shoulder caused by lack of a stable fulcrum, most commonly in the anterosuperior direction. Although not required, residual posterior and anterior rotator cuff repair during surgery can aid in regaining rotational motion after RSA. The less common indications for RSA include a musculoskeletal tumor or a deep shoulder infection. A one- or two-stage procedure can be chosen.[6] Future study is needed to refine and expand the indications for RSA.

Contraindications

Adequate deltoid muscle function is required for elevating the arm after RSA. Thus, RSA is absolutely contraindicated if the patient has a nonfunctioning deltoid, probably as a result of neurologic injury, deltoid avulsion, extensive intramuscular scarring, or other neuromuscular injury. If the middle deltoid muscle belly is insufficient, it is unlikely the muscle will provide adequate function after RSA. RSA has been successful in the treatment of infectious processes with a single- or two-stage procedure. In the setting of an active gross infection, however, an antibiotic spacer is the treatment of choice.

RSA usually has not been recommended for patients younger than 70 years because of concern about implant durability. This factor may become less important as implant designs and surgical techniques advance. RSA was found to be durable and have good results at midterm follow-up.[7-9] The considerations in a younger

patient include the severity of the clinical condition, pain, reduction of shoulder function, and advanced pathology as well as the patient's willingness to accept that the implant may not be sufficiently durable. In a patient who has relatively limited pathology (for example, a massive rotator cuff tear without arthritis), clinical severity plays an important role in predicting satisfaction. It is difficult to anticipate the extent of postoperative clinical improvement if the patient has a relatively good preoperative range of motion. Hence, integrating a patient's symptoms and pathology is critical for deciding on the appropriate treatment.

In the past, glenoid erosion was considered a strong contraindication to RSA. Recent studies have found that RSA can be successful in patients with a glenoid deficiency, and the RSA technique has been modified to expand its use in treating moderate or severe glenoid erosion.[10] However, very severe glenoid deficiency precludes implant fixation and remains a contraindication to RSA.

The general contraindications to joint arthroplasty apply to patients being considered for RSA. These contraindications include severe medical illness, inability to tolerate surgery, the presence of a metal allergy, and an inability to follow postoperative restrictions. In addition, the surgeon must be aware of the learning curve required for RSA in the treatment of advanced pathology. As with any new technology, the surgeon's level of experience affects outcomes and complication rates.[11]

Changing Prosthetic Designs

The clinical limitations of the Grammont reverse-shoulder devices led to the development of devices that maintained the reversed articulation while minimizing the distortion of humeral offset and maximizing the impingement-free range of motion of the glenohumeral joint. The current designs were developed to reduce the incidence of notching, lack of rotational function, instability, and glenoid-side failure. The changes have included the use of glenospheres placed eccentric to the surface of the glenoid and humeral components placed in less valgus than the original design. Current prosthetic designs offer spheres with a center of rotation offset from the glenoid surface. These spheres are larger than those of the original design and have a center of rotation as much as 10 mm lateral or 4 mm inferior to the surface of the glenoid.[12,13] Many current designs also have a more anatomic neck-shaft angle; in several designs, the neck-shaft angle is 135°.

Scapular Notching

Maximizing the impingement-free range of motion is critical not only for patient function but also for implant survivability, implant stability, and relief of unexplained pain. One consequence of decreasing the impingement-free range of motion is abutment of the scapular neck with the inferior aspect of the humeral socket when physiologic adduction is attempted (Figure 2). The adduction deficit leads to the radiographic appearance of a notch. Polyethylene wear and glenoid loosening are of concern with notching. The presence of a notch and its size have a negative effect on outcome scores and can cause glenoid component loosening.[14,15] Reduction in impingement-free range of motion increases the likelihood of prosthetic abutment with soft tissue or bone, leading to pain or levering out of the implant.

With a Grammont-style implant, maximal restoration of glenohumeral motion is prevented by the limited ability to adequately balance the soft tissues and provide a sufficient range of impingement-free motion. The surgical technique can be altered to avoid the adduction deficit. When a virtual simulation computer model was used to evaluate factors contributing to scapular notching, an adduction deficit was found to be best avoided by a varus humeral neck-shaft angle (130°).[4,5] The most important factor for maximizing the impingement-free range of motion was the use of a glenosphere with a center of rotation lateral to the gle-noid surface. Clinical studies have confirmed this conclusion; the risk of scapular notching is almost eliminated if a glenosphere with lateral offset is used.[7,16-20] One modification of the Grammont device uses an autogenous bone graft between the glenoid and the baseplate to increase the lateral offset.[13] Scapular notching was observed in 19% of patients; this rate is lower than with the use of a standard medialized RSA implant.

Lack of External Rotation Improvement

The Grammont-style device repeatedly was found to improve function and provide pain relief, but the improvement in external rotation has been unreliable.[21-24] Grammont speculated that RSA could improve external rotation by allowing posterior deltoid recruitment, but few biomechanical data exist to support this theory.[25] Loss of external rotation strength might be explained by the altered anatomy seen in rotator cuff tear arthropathy, which can decrease the efficiency of contraction of the remaining rotator cuff. In addition, medializing the center of rotation causes slackening of the remaining rotator cuff muscles and prevents sufficient muscle contraction (Figure 3). Some evidence suggests that patients who do not have improvement in external rotation are less satisfied with their function.[22]

RSA implant designs with a lateral center of rotation allow more consistent external rotation improvement than the Grammont prosthesis.[12] In patients with rotator cuff deficiency, the proximally migrated humerus may prevent the intact rotator cuff muscles from functioning properly. Positioning the humerus in a more anatomic position restores joint stability and tensions the remaining rotator cuff muscles, leading to an improvement in external rotation. Several clinical studies confirmed that restoring the lateral offset of the humerus improves postoperative external rotation in patients with different pathologic conditions.[7,16-20] However, patients who have an absent or atrophic teres minor before surgery will not gain in external rotation, and they may require a latissimus dorsi transfer for improvement of external rotation.

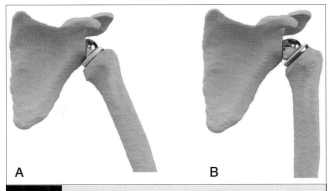
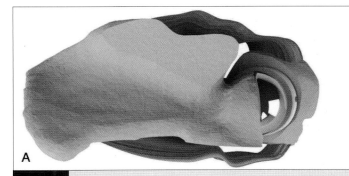

Figure 2 Drawings showing a Grammont-style prosthesis (A) in a shoulder with an adduction deficit with abutment of the inferior humeral socket on the scapular neck and a lateral offset prosthesis (B) without abutment of the inferior humeral socket on the scapular neck.

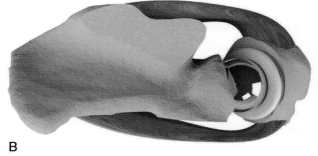

Figure 3 Drawings showing slackening of the remaining rotator cuff external rotators with a medial offset device (A) and tensioning of the remaining rotator cuff external rotators with a lateral offset device (B).

5: Arthritis and Arthroplasty

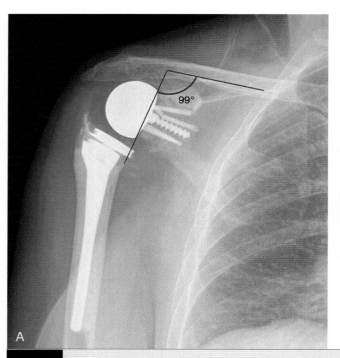
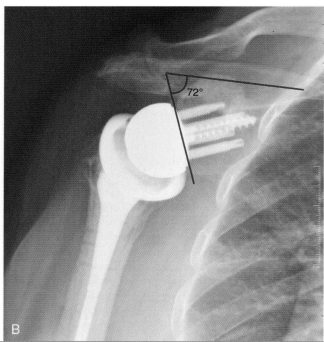

Figure 4   Grashey radiographs showing superior glenosphere tilt with **(A)** and without **(B)** baseplate failure.

Instability

Instability after RSA remains a concern. Rates of dislocation as high as 30% have been reported with the use of the Grammont design. The factors contributing to instability include glenosphere diameter, humeral socket constraint, soft-tissue tensioning, impingement, erroneous version of the prosthesis, and deltoid dysfunction.

Several researchers have suggested that the stability of the glenohumeral joint is improved by restoring muscle tension and thus increasing compression on the humerus.[7,16-20] The stability of the glenohumeral joint is compromised with medialization of the humerus and subsequent slackening of the remaining rotator cuff muscles. Medialization of the humerus can turn the deltoid into a distracting force if there is glenoid bone loss and thereby can increase the possibility of dislocation.[26] An alternative method of improving stability with these implants is to lengthen the humerus and use a valgus humeral socket.[21] However, this method adds to the risk of acromial fracture, brachial plexopathy, deltoid overtensioning, and loss of motion. Increasing the glenoid-tuberosity distance by lateralizing the humerus is another method of improving stability by increasing the compressive forces across the glenohumeral joint.

Several prosthetic design factors including socket depth, glenosphere size, and compression forces were evaluated for their relation to instability.[27] The most important parameter for improving stability was increased compression forces across the joint, followed by increased humeral socket depth. The remaining rotator cuff muscle tension is restored by lateralizing the humerus, thus increasing the compression across the joint. Studies have found that lateralizing the humerus increases joint reactive forces.[27,28]

The initial management of a dislocation after RSA involves closed reduction followed by a period of sling immobilization. Open revision surgery is indicated if closed reduction is not possible or if instability recurs after closed reduction. Adequate inferior release of tissue around the implant should be performed to remove soft tissue that can impinge on the prosthesis and cause it to lever out. Soft-tissue tension should be assessed. A thicker polyethylene socket can be chosen to increase the lateral offset and tension. A more constrained socket or a larger glenosphere can be chosen to help improve stability. If these measures are not successful, the version and placement of the components should be considered as the cause of instability.

Baseplate Failure

Failure of the attachment of the glenoid component to the bony glenoid has been reported by many authors.[2,12,20,29-33] All reverse components designed since 1985 are intended to allow bony ingrowth on the glenoid side. If ingrowth does not occur, the attachment is with fibrous tissue and is less durable. Factors that lead to failure to achieve ingrowth might include the design of the prosthesis, glenoid bone deficiency, and malpositioning of the component. Grammont's theory that centering the sphere over the fixation and the glenoid bone would eliminate the risk of glenoid failure has not been uniformly confirmed. As many as 50% of glenoid components failed in some early studies of patients who

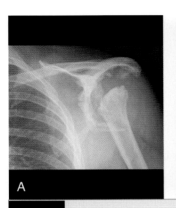 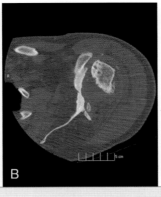 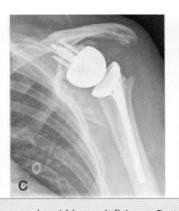 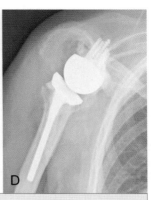

Figure 5 Grashey radiograph **(A)** and axillary CT **(B)** showing severe glenoid bone deficiency. Postoperative Grashey radiographs showing treatment with the use of the alternate center line for adequate fixation **(C)** and the use of glenoid bone grafting and a large glenosphere **(D)**.

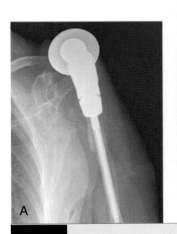 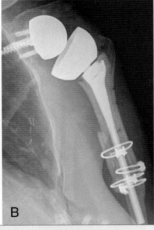

Figure 6 Grashey radiographs showing a failed shoulder hemiarthroplasty with bone loss **(A)** and the use of a prosthesis-allograft composite to treat proximal humeral bone loss **(B)**.

had rheumatoid arthritis or in whom scapular notching developed.[29,30] Other early devices also had high rates of mechanical failure.

In the original report of a device with an ovoid sphere and a center of rotation 10 mm from the glenoid surface, the glenoid component failure rate was almost 12%.[12] A 15° inferior tilt of the glenosphere resulted in the most uniform compressive forces and the least micromotion at the bone-baseplate interface when a glenosphere with a lateral center of rotation was used.[34] This finding suggests a reduced risk of baseplate failure. Another study by the same researchers confirmed the earlier study and provided additional evidence that a glenosphere centered over the glenoid bony surface (the original Grammont design) has optimal force at a bone-baseplate interface with an inferior vertical tilt, compared with a baseplate perpendicular to the bony surface.[5] The most unstable components were superiorly tilted (**Figure 4**). This pattern was different if ec-

centric inferior glenospheres were selected, with inferior tilt providing the least stable mechanical environment.

A biomechanical analysis of baseplate constructs using locked 5.0-mm and unlocked 3.5-mm screw combinations found that baseplates fixed with 5.0-mm locked screws had better fixation and less micromotion.[35] A subsequent clinical study of a modified design using 5.0-mm locked screws and inferior tilt found that glenoid failure was reduced to 0.4% at a minimum 2-year follow-up.[19]

When current implantation techniques are used, Grammont-style devices with locking-screw fixation have comparably low baseplate loosening rates, ranging from 0 to 5% in patients who underwent primary RSA[15,21,24] and from 0 to 8% in those who underwent RSA for rheumatoid arthritis or revision.[9,21,36] Modern techniques allow durable glenoid implant fixation with both Grammont-style and lateral offset devices. The glenoid fixation remains stable in the setting of decreased glenoid bone quality from patient disease or earlier arthroplasty.

Technical Considerations

Glenosphere Positioning
The incidence of scapular notching has been reduced through improved implant design. In addition, surgical technique has been altered to change the position of the glenosphere in an attempt to avoid inferior scapular neck impingement when the arm is at the side.[37] A biomechanical evaluation analyzed four different glenoid component positions to assess their influence on range of motion and mechanical impingement.[3] Placing the glenosphere beyond the inferior rim of the glenoid and tilting the component 15° were found to significantly reduce mechanical impingement. The importance of inferior glenosphere placement for avoiding impingement was subsequently validated clinically.[14]

5: Arthritis and Arthroplasty

Table 1

Studies of Reverse Shoulder Arthroplasty for Rotator Cuff Deficiency

Study	Number of Patients	Pathology (Number of Patients)	Average Follow-up	Preoperative/ Postoperative Range of Motion Forward Flexion
Devices With Medial Center of Rotation				
Boulahia et al[2] (2002)	16	Rotator cuff tear arthropathy	35 months	70°/138°
Sirveaux et al [33] (2004)	77	Rotator cuff tear arthropathy	44 months	73°/138°
Vanhove and Beugnies[45] (2004)	24	Rotator cuff tear arthropathy	31 months	–
Seebauer et al[32] (2005)	57	Rotator cuff tear arthropathy	18.2 months	–/145°
Guery et al[15] (2006)	57	Rotator cuff tear (48) Rheumatoid arthritis (6) Fracture (2) Revision (1)	69.6 months	–
Wall et al[23] (2007)	191	Various	39.9 months	86°/137°
Gerber et al[44] (2007)	10	Massive rotator cuff tear (received latissimus dorsi transfer)	18 months	94°/139°
Simovitch et al[22] (2007)	77	Rotator cuff tear arthropathy	44 months	65/115°
		No notching (43)	47 months	–/127°
		Notching (34)	42 months	–/110°
Favard et al[8] (2011)	148	Rotator cuff tear arthropathy	7.8 years	69/129
Melis et al[9] (2011)	68	Uncemented (34)	9.6 years	–/123°
		Cemented (34)	9.6 years	–132°
Devices With Lateral Center of Rotation				
Frankle et al[12] (2005)	60	Rotator cuff tear arthropathy	33 months	55°/105.1°
Cuff et al[19] (2008)	96	Rotator cuff deficiency (70) Rotator cuff deficiency with arthroplasty (23) Proximal humeral nonunion (30)	27.5 months	63.5°/118°
Mulieri et al[7] (2010)	60	Rotator cuff tear without arthritis	52 months	53°/134°
Klein et al[10] (2010)	143	Rotator cuff deficiency: Normal glenoid (87) Glenoid erosion (56)	30.9 months	67/140

[a] Measured using the Constant Shoulder Score or American Shoulder and Elbow Surgeons (ASES) Index.

Another biomechanical study used a computer simulation to determine the factors that can minimize the risk of an adduction deficit and subsequent impingement.[4] The second most important factor in avoiding

Table 1

Studies of Reverse Shoulder Arthroplasty for Rotator Cuff Deficiency (continued)

Abduction	External Rotation	Preoperative/Postoperative Outcome Scores[a]	Complications (Number)
–	6°/3°	31/85 (Constant)	Traumatic glenoid loosening (1), scapular notching (10), dislocation (1), postoperative phlebitis (1), postoperative hematoma (1)
–	3.5°/11.2°	22.6/65.6 (Constant)	Glenoid loosening (5), dissociation of glenoid component (7), device failure (3), scapular notching (49), infection (1)
–	–	–/60 (Constant)	Device failure (1), glenoid notching (12)
–/140°	–	–/67 (Constant)	Glenosphere loosening (1), polyethylene wear (1), deep infection (2), reflex sympathetic dystrophy (1), scapular notching (13)
–	–	–/>30 (Constant) (Survival: 88% at 72 months, 58% at 120 months)	Infection (3), dislocation (3), glenoid loosening (3)
–	8°/6°	23/60 (Constant)	Dislocation (15), infection (8), glenoid fracture (1), humeral fracture (1), symptomatic hardware (1), musculocutaneous nerve palsy (1), radial nerve palsy (1), glenosphere loosening (1), glenoid base loosening (1)
87°/145°	12°/19°	34/70 (Constant)	Infection (1), hematoma (1)
63/111°	–	38/78 (Constant)	None reported
–/118°	15°/17°	–/83-Constant)	–
–/102°	34°/31°	–/61 (Constant)	–
–	5/11°	24/62 (Constant)	22% complication rate
–	–/7°	–/53 (Constant)	Instability (4), humeral fracture (2), acromial fracture (1)
–	–/11°	–/60 (Constant)	
41.4°/101.8°	12°/41.1°	34.3/68.2 (ASES)	Scapular fracture (1), acromial fracture (2), hardware failure (1), infection (2), humeral dissociation (1), base plate failure (8)
61°/109.5°	13.4°/28.2°	30/77.6 (ASES)	Dislocation (2), traumatic dislocation (2), traumatic acromial fracture (1), infection (2), hematoma (1), glenoid loosening (1)
49°/125°	27°/51°	33/75 (ASES)	Proximal humerus fracture (1), failed baseplate (4), broken center screw (1), deep infection (1), hematoma (1), acromial fracture (2), scapular body fracture (1), dislocation (1)
65/126	19.8/49	39.1/79.1 (ASES)	Acromial fracture (2), humeral fracture (1), infection (2)

[a] Measured using the Constant Shoulder Score or American Shoulder and Elbow Surgeons (ASES) Index.

inferior scapular impingement was found to be inferior placement of the glenosphere, and the most important factor was the use of a varus (130°) humeral neck-shaft angle.

Table 2

Studies of Reverse Shoulder Arthroplasty for Proximal Humeral Fracture

Study	Number of Patients	Average Follow-up	Postoperative Range of Motion Forward Flexion
Bufquin et al[48] (2007)	43	22 months	97
Klein et al[53] (2008)	20	33 months	122°
Gallinet et al[54] (2009)	16	12 months	98°
Cazeneuve and Cristofari[55] (2010)	36	6.6 years	–
Lenarz et al[56] (2011)	30	23 months	139°

[a] Measured using the Constant Shoulder Score or American Shoulder and Elbow Surgeons (ASES) Index.

Table 3

Studies of Reverse Shoulder Arthroplasty for Rheumatoid Arthritis

Study (Year)	Number of Patients	Average Follow-up	Preoperative/Postoperative Range of Motion Forward Flexion
Rittmiester et al[29] (2001)	7	54 months	–
Young et al[36] (2011)	18	3.8 years	78/139
Holcomb et al[46] (2010)	21	36 months	52°/126°

[a] Measured using the Constant Shoulder Score or American Shoulder and Elbow Surgeons (ASES) Index.

Glenoid Bone Deficiency

In a normal shoulder, the glenoid center line is perpendicular to the glenoid surface and in approximately 10° of retroversion. The center line serves as a pillar of bone under which the humeral head rests, and this relationship is maintained throughout the range of motion with a coupling of glenohumeral and scapulothoracic motion. This relationship is disrupted by unbalanced forces in a rotator cuff–deficient shoulder, leading to mechanical alteration and pathologic glenoid wear patterns in as many as 36% of patients who undergo RSA.[38] Depending on the pathology, these wear patterns occur in a spectrum ranging from no wear to superior, anterior, posterior, and global wear. It is important to recognize the wear pattern for purposes of preoperative planning.

The glenoid component ideally is placed along the glenoid center line, where 2.5 to 3.5 cm of bone is accessible for fixation placement in a normally shaped glenoid. If the glenoid has substantial or eccentric wear, this placement is not always feasible. The use of an alternate glenoid center line has been proposed, in which the line is aimed at the dense bone where the scapular spine meets the scapular body.[38] This line is not always perpendicular to the remaining glenoid surface. The implantation of the glenoid component along this line allows the surgeon to achieve adequate bony fixation in the scapular body–scapular spine junction.

A review of nine patients who underwent Grammont-style RSA with glenoid bone grafting for severe bone loss found good pain relief but low functional outcome scores at a minimum 2-year follow-up.

Table 2

Studies of Reverse Shoulder Arthroplasty for Proximal Humeral Fracture (continued)

Postoperative Range of Motion

Abduction	External Rotation	Postoperative Outcome Scores[a]	Complications
86	30	44 (Constant)	Nerve injury (5), reflex sympathetic dystrophy (3), dislocation (1), glenoid fracture (1), acromial fracture (1), deltoid anterior interval dehiscence (1)
113	25°	68 (ASES) 68 (Constant)	Recurrent dislocation (1), infection (2)
–	9°	53 (Constant)	Deep infection (1), superficial infection (1), reflex sympathetic dystrophy (1)
–	–	53 (Constant)	Reflex sympathetic dystrophy (2), infection (1), dislocation (4), baseplate loosening (1)
–	27°	78 (ASES)	Complex regional pain syndrome, deep vein thrombosis, and tuberosity resorption (1)

[a] Measured using the Constant Shoulder Score or American Shoulder and Elbow Surgeons (ASES) Index.

Table 3

Studies of Reverse Shoulder Arthroplasty for Rheumatoid Arthritis (continued)

Preoperative/Postoperative Range of Motion

Abduction	External Rotation	Preoperative/Postoperative Outcome Scores[a]	Complications
–	–	17/63 (Constant)	Revision (3), glenoid loosening (2), failed acromial open reduction and internal fixation (1)
–	17/46	22/64.9 (Constant)	Acromial fracture (1), scapular spine fracture (1), coracoid fracture (1), greater tuberosity avulsion (2), transient axillary nerve palsy (1)
55°/116°	19°/33°	28/82 (ASES)	Periprosthetic glenoid fracture (1), infection (2), scapular spine fracture (1), intraoperative glenoid fracture (1), radiographic baseplate loosening (1)

[a] Measured using the Constant Shoulder Score or American Shoulder and Elbow Surgeons (ASES) Index.

Six of the patients had radiographic evidence of scapular notching.[39] RSA using a lateral offset device was compared in 56 patients with an acquired glenoid bone defect and 87 patients with normal glenoid morphology.[10] A bone graft was used in 22 of the 56 patients with an abnormal glenoid, and the alternate glenoid center line was used for glenoid fixation in all 56 patients (**Figure 5**). A larger glenosphere was used in the patients with an abnormal glenoid, and a glenosphere with an extended hood was used to impact the graft in the patients with a bone graft. Significant improvements were reported in range of motion and functional outcomes, with no differences between the patients with a normal glenoid and those with an abnormal glenoid. One patient was dissatisfied with the result, and there were five complications (two acromial fractures, two infections, and one periprosthetic fracture). These results show that a glenoid bone defect is not a contraindication to RSA if the surgical technique is altered.

Humeral Bone Loss

The use of RSA in the setting of proximal humeral bone loss was found to improve function and relieve pain.[16] However, proximal humeral bone deficiency resulted in high rates of instability, early prosthetic loosening, and rotational weakness.[16] The use of a proximal humeral allograft in conjunction with RSA improved results in patients with severe proximal humeral deficiency[16,18] (**Figure 6**). The allograft also provides rotational stability for the humeral stem component. This factor is especially important with modular humeral components, which have a greater risk of mechanical failure than nonmodular humeral components when used in patients with proximal humeral bone

5: Arthritis and Arthroplasty

Table 4

Studies of Revision Reverse Shoulder Arthroplasty

Study (Year)	Number of Patients	Procedure and/or Pathology (Number of Patients)	Average Follow-up	Preoperative/ Postoperative Range of Motion Forward Flexion
Devices with Medial Center of Rotation				
Werner et al[24] (2005)	58	Primary rotator cuff tear arthroplasty (17) Revision arthroplasty (41)	38 months	42°/100°
Boileau et al[21] (2006)	45	Primary rotator cuff tear arthroplasty (17) Revision after hemiarthroplasty (19) Revision for fracture sequelae (7)	40 months	55°/121°
Melis et al[57] (2012)	37	Conversion of total shoulder arthroplasty to reverse shoulder arthroplasty	47 months	68/121
Lateral center of rotation devices				
Levy et al[17] (2007)	19	Revision of hemiarthroplasty	35 months	49.7°/76.1°
Werner et al[24] (2005)	29	Revision of hemiarthroplasty	35 months	38.1°/72.7°
Cuff et al[19] (2008)	96	Rotator cuff deficiency (70) Rotator cuff deficiency with arthroplasty (23) Proximal humeral nonunion (3)	27.5 months	63.5°/118°
Holcomb et al[58] (2009)	14	Reverse shoulder arthroplasty	33 months	51/118
Chacon et al[18] (2009)	25	Revision of hemiarthroplasty with allograft	30 months	33/82
Walker et al[59] (2012)	22	Revision of failed total shoulder arthroplasty	40 months	50/130

loss.[40] The allograft restores the natural contour of the proximal humerus, maintains the height of the prosthesis-bone construct, and resists subsidence of the humeral implant, thereby helping to optimize deltoid tension. The allograft lateralizes the line of pull of the deltoid muscles, increasing the resultant force of the deltoid as a pulley.

Latissimus Dorsi Tendon Transfer

Patients who undergo RSA are less satisfied with their outcome if they do not have improvement in active external rotation, which is necessary for many activities of daily living.[22,41] Even with prosthetic design changes to lateralize the humerus for the purpose of restoring

Table 4

Studies of Revision Reverse Shoulder Arthroplasty (continued)

		Preoperative/ Postoperative Range of Motion		
Abduction	**External Rotation**	**Preoperative/ Postoperative Outcome Scores[a]**	**Complications**	
43°/90°	17°/12°	18/56 (Constant)	Overall (50%), reoperation (33%) Hematoma (12), dislocation (5), infection (1), nerve lesion (1), glenoid loosening (3), humeral stem loosening (1), scapular fracture (4), polyethylene dissociation (1)	
	7°/11°	17/58 (Constant)	Dislocation (3), deep infection (3), aseptic humeral loosening (1), periprosthetic humeral fracture (2), intraoperative glenoid fracture (1), wound hematoma (1), acromial fracture (2), axillary nerve palsy (1)	
		24/55 (Constant)	Glenoid loosening (3), instability (3), humeral subsidence (2), infection (2), hematoma (1)	
Lateral center of rotation devices				
42.2°/77.2°		29.1/61.2 (ASES)	Failed polyethylene (2), periprosthetic humeral fracture (1), humeral loosening (2), periprosthetic scapular fracture (2), base plate loosening (2), infection (1), hematoma (1)	
34.1°/70.4°	11.2°/17.6°	22.3/52.1 (ASES)	Periprosthetic fracture (1), polyethylene fracture (4), polyethylene dissociation (1), dislocation (4), infection (1), failed baseplate/broken screws (1), humeral stem loosening (1), radial nerve palsy (1)	
61°/109.5°	13.4°/28.2°	30/77.6 (ASES)	Dislocation (2), traumatic dislocation (2), traumatic acromial fracture (1), infection (2), hematoma (1), glenoid loosening (1)	
38/112	8°/22°	23/70 (ASES)	Glenoid failure (1), dislocation (1), hematoma (1)	
40/82	10°/18°	32/69 (ASES)	Recurrent instability (1), acromial fracture (1), allograft fracture (1), allograft and polyethylene fracture (1)	
45/100	12.5/49.5	38.5/67.5 (ASES)	Scapula fracture (1), acromial fracture (1), dislocation (1), glenoid loosening (1), glenoid and humeral loosening (1)	

external rotation and strength, an absence or atrophy of the teres minor means that a patient will not have improvement in external rotation. The patient will have the hornblower's sign and an external rotation lag when the arm is at the side. The use of a modified latissimus dorsi–teres major tendon transfer has been proposed in conjunction with RSA in these patients to restore active elevation and external rotation, thereby improving patient function and satisfaction.[40-44]

Seventeen patients with a massive rotator cuff tear and an absent teres minor underwent RSA combined with latissimus dorsi–teres major tendon transfer and had significant improvement in functional outcomes, range of motion, and ability to perform activities of

5: Arthritis and Arthroplasty

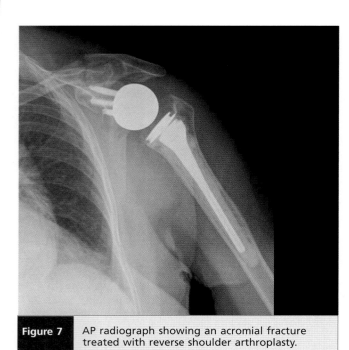

Figure 7 AP radiograph showing an acromial fracture treated with reverse shoulder arthroplasty.

daily living.[43] Similarly, 12 shoulders in 11 patients with pseudoparesis of active elevation and external rotation were treated with RSA and latissimus dorsi transfer, with significant improvement in functional outcomes, range of motion, and ability to perform activities of daily living.[44]

The decision to perform a latissimus dorsi–teres major tendon transfer should be made only after the subscapularis tendon has been repaired. If the soft tissues limit passive external rotation to no more than 45°, the gains may not warrant the morbidity associated with the tendon transfer.

Results

High complication rates were described in the initial reports of RSA used to treat patients with a rotator cuff deficiency. Nonetheless, RSA has proved to be a durable treatment, even after the earlier designs were used. Refinements in implant technology and improved surgical techniques may lead to findings of greater implant durability in future studies. Specific study results are outlined in **Tables 1, 2, 3,** and **4.**

Complications

RSA has been a powerful tool for the treatment of end-stage shoulder pathology, but several complications are associated with its nonanatomic design.

Infection

Rates of infection after RSA have ranged from 1% to 12%.[12,29,45] Infection may result from direct inoculation during surgery, postoperative seeding of hematoma, hematogenous spread, or reactivation of indolent organisms after multiple shoulder surgeries. The infection rate after RSA is higher than it is after conventional shoulder arthroplasty, possibly because of the greater subacromial dead space, the older patient population, or the use of RSA in revision procedures. Hematoma formation may be associated with deep infection, especially if there is persistent drainage.

Patients with rheumatoid arthritis are at a relatively high risk of infection after RSA as well as other joint arthroplasty procedures. A prospective study found a 9.5% infection rate in 21 patients with rheumatoid arthritis.[46] Revision surgery also increases the rate of infection after RSA. Infection rates as high as 6.7% have been documented after RSA was used for revision of hemiarthroplasty or conventional TSA.[9,15-17,21]

Efforts to prevent infection should involve meticulous sterile technique and the use of preoperative antibiotics. An acute infection (of less than 6 weeks' duration) can be treated with débridement, antibiotics, and polyethylene exchange. A chronic infection can be treated with a one- or two-stage revision procedure, with concurrent intravenous antibiotics. The decision to perform a one-stage procedure should be based on the adequacy of the initial débridement.[6]

Acromial Fractures and Intraoperative Fractures

Acromial fracture after RSA can be detrimental to the results (**Figure 7**). The patient may have acetabularization of the acromion, causing thinning of the bone. The increased tension on the deltoid with inferior placement of the glenosphere can contribute to the likelihood of acromial fracture after RSA. A review of 527 patients identified a 3% incidence of acromial fracture.[47] Other studies documented an incidence of acromial fracture ranging from 0 to 4.4%.[46,48-50] The surgeon should suspect an acromial fracture if the patient does not have pain relief, has an acute change in pain and function during the early postoperative period, or has a slow progression of rehabilitation. Acromial fracture may be visible on a plain radiograph but often is more reliably visible on CT. An initial period of immobilization is indicated.

An intraoperative glenoid fracture may occur during reaming.[33,46,48] Unless care is taken to start the reamer before it comes into contact with the glenoid bone, excessive torque may result. Decreased glenoid bone quality also may create a predisposition toward fracture. Stable fracture fixation can be achieved before placing the baseplate or by using screws placed through the baseplate. In a device with a central screw, redirecting the screw into a different bone may allow stable fixation. If adequate fixation is not achieved by redirecting the screw, a two-stage glenoid reconstruction may be necessary.

Intraoperative humeral fracture can result from excessive torque on the humerus or the use of a press-fit implant. If the bone is osteopenic, care must be taken to avoid excessive humeral rotation during exposure. Because fracture also can occur during humeral canal reaming, the use of hand reamers is preferred. Fractures should be stabilized with cerclage wire, with or without a plate, before humeral component placement. The use of a long-stemmed component can be considered.

Neurologic Injury

Neurologic dysfunction, often transient in nature, has been reported after RSA in 1% to 4% of patients. Intraoperative stretching of the brachial plexus, especially during glenoid exposure, combined with lengthening of the arm to tension the deltoid, may place patients at risk for injury. In 191 patients treated with RSA, one musculocutaneous and one radial nerve palsy appeared in separate patients.[23] One transient axillary nerve palsy was found after RSA in 16 patients with rheumatoid arthritis.[36] Numerous other studies also have documented infrequent nerve injury after RSA. The incidence of subclinical nerve injury may be relatively high, however. A 57% incidence of intraoperative nerve alerts was described during anatomic shoulder arthroplasty and hemiarthroplasty.[51] Nine of 19 patients had electromyographic changes 4 weeks after RSA.[52] Patients who underwent RSA had 10.9 times the risk of acute postoperative nerve injury compared with patients who underwent total shoulder arthroplasty. Most of these lesions involved the axillary nerve, and eight of nine injuries resolved completely within 6 months.

Miscellaneous

Relatively uncommon complications reported after RSA include humeral loosening, periprosthetic fracture, glenosphere dissociation, polyethylene dissociation, and polyethylene fracture.

Future Directions

RSA is a relatively new treatment of rotator cuff deficiency arising from one of several etiologies. The available follow-up data are limited to midterm results. Future studies will need to determine the long-term durability of the available RSA designs as well as the durability of RSA in relatively young, active patients. A focus on improving implant design and surgical technique is likely to expand the current indications for RSA.

Annotated References

1. Grammont PM, Baulot E: Delta shoulder prosthesis for rotator cuff rupture. *Orthopedics* 1993;16(1):65-68.

2. Boulahia A, Edwards TB, Walch G, Baratta RV: Early results of a reverse design prosthesis in the treatment of arthritis of the shoulder in elderly patients with a large rotator cuff tear. *Orthopedics* 2002;25(2):129-133.

3. Nyffeler RW, Werner CM, Gerber C: Biomechanical relevance of glenoid component positioning in the reverse Delta III total shoulder prosthesis. *J Shoulder Elbow Surg* 2005;14(5):524-528.

4. Gutiérrez S, Comiskey CA IV, Luo Z-P, Pupello DR, Frankle MA: Range of impingement-free abduction and adduction deficit after reverse shoulder arthroplasty: Hierarchy of surgical and implant-design-related factors. *J Bone Joint Surg Am* 2008;90(12):2606-2615.

   A virtual computer model of RSA was used to evaluate five surgical and implant-related factors and their effect on abduction-adduction. A lateral center of rotation resulted in the largest impingement-free abduction motion, followed by an inferior glenosphere placement, an inferior glenosphere tilt, a varus humeral neck-shaft angle, and glenosphere size.

5. Gutiérrez S, Levy JC, Lee WE III, Keller TS, Maitland ME: Center of rotation affects abduction range of motion of reverse shoulder arthroplasty. *Clin Orthop Relat Res* 2007;458:78-82.

   The effects of glenosphere center of rotation on abduction motion in RSA were biomechanically evaluated using an electronic goniometer and digital video analysis of a model. There is a positive lineal correlation between glenosphere offset and abduction range of motion.

6. Cuff DJ, Virani NA, Levy J, et al: The treatment of deep shoulder infection and glenohumeral instability with debridement, reverse shoulder arthroplasty and postoperative antibiotics. *J Bone Joint Surg Br* 2008;90(3):336-342.

   Deep shoulder infection was treated in 21 patients (22 shoulders) using débridement, RSA, and antibiotics. At a mean 43-month follow-up, there was no evidence of recurrent infection, and patients had improvement in range of motion and in all measured outcomes. Outcomes of single-stage and two-stage procedures did not differ. Level of evidence: IV.

7. Mulieri P, Dunning P, Klein S, Pupello D, Frankle M: Reverse shoulder arthroplasty for the treatment of irreparable rotator cuff tear without glenohumeral arthritis. *J Bone Joint Surg Am* 2010;92(15):2544-2556.

   Irreparable cuff tear without arthritis was treated with RSA in 69 patients (72 shoulders). At a minimum 2-year follow-up, 60 shoulders had significant improvement in range of motion in all planes and improved pain and function scores. Level of evidence: IV.

8. Favard L, Levigne C, Nerot C, Gerber C, De Wilde L, Mole D: Reverse prostheses in arthropathies with cuff tear: Are survivorship and function maintained over time? *Clin Orthop Relat Res* 2011;469(9):2469-2475.

   In 464 patients at a minimum 2-year follow-up after RSA and 148 patients at a minimum 5-year follow-up, there were 107 complications. Survivorship at 10 years was 89% with revision as an end point and was 72% with a Constant score lower than 30 as the end point. Despite the low 10-year revision rate, radiographic and outcome deterioration occurred over time. Caution is warranted when RSA is considered for younger patients. Level of evidence: IV.

9. Melis B, DeFranco M, Lädermann A, et al: An evaluation of the radiological changes around the Grammont reverse geometry shoulder arthroplasty after eight to 12 years. *J Bone Joint Surg Br* 2011;93(9):1240-1246.

A multicenter study with a mean 9.6-year follow-up evaluated radiographic changes in 68 RSAs. Scapular notching was observed in 88% of patients and was associated with a superolateral approach. Glenoid lucency was observed in 16% of patients. Stem subsidence was more common after cemented than uncemented RSA. Stress shielding and tuberosity resorption were more common in uncemented components.

10. Klein SM, Dunning P, Mulieri P, Pupello D, Downes K, Frankle MA: Effects of acquired glenoid bone defects on surgical technique and clinical outcomes in reverse shoulder arthroplasty. *J Bone Joint Surg Am* 2010;92(5):1144-1154.

Acquired glenoid bone defects treated with RSA in 56 patients were compared with normal glenoids in 87 patients to detect any difference in clinical outcome. At 2-year follow-up, there were no graft failures or resorption; five complications and one unsatisfactory result occurred. Level of evidence: IV.

11. Kempton LB, Ankerson E, Wiater JM: A complication-based learning curve from 200 reverse shoulder arthroplasties. *Clin Orthop Relat Res* 2011;469(9):2496-2504.

In 200 consecutive RSAs performed by one surgeon, shoulder-related complications occurred in 23.1% of the first 40 patients and 6.5% of the remaining 160 patients. After revision surgery, the local complication rate was 17.5%, compared with 7.9% after primary surgery. Level of evidence: IV.

12. Frankle M, Siegal S, Pupello D, Saleem A, Mighell M, Vasey M: The Reverse Shoulder Prosthesis for glenohumeral arthritis associated with severe rotator cuff deficiency: A minimum two-year follow-up study of sixty patients. *J Bone Joint Surg Am* 2005;87(8):1697-1705.

13. Boileau P, Moineau G, Roussanne Y, O'Shea K: Bony increased-offset reversed shoulder arthroplasty: Minimizing scapular impingement while maximizing glenoid fixation. *Clin Orthop Relat Res* 2011;469(9):2558-2567.

In a prospective study, 42 patients with rotator cuff deficiency were treated with bony increased-offset RSA to reduce notching and prosthetic instability. At a mean 28-month follow-up, the graft was completely incorporated in 98% of patients, with no graft resorption, glenoid failure, or prosthetic instability. Level of evidence: IV.

14. Simovitch RW, Zumstein MA, Lohri E, Helmy N, Gerber C: Predictors of scapular notching in patients managed with the Delta III reverse total shoulder replacement. *J Bone Joint Surg Am* 2007;89(3):588-600.

In 76 patients (77 shoulders) treated with RSA, inferior notching occurred in 44%, posterior notching in 30%, and anterior notching in 8%. Inferior notching was associated with significantly poorer clinical outcome and can be avoided with optimal positioning of the glenosphere. Level of evidence: II.

15. Guery J, Favard L, Sirveaux F, Oudet D, Mole D, Walch G: Reverse total shoulder arthroplasty: Survivorship analysis of eighty replacements followed for five to ten years. *J Bone Joint Surg Am* 2006;88(8):1742-1747.

16. Levy J, Frankle M, Mighell M, Pupello D: The use of the reverse shoulder prosthesis for the treatment of failed hemiarthroplasty for proximal humeral fracture. *J Bone Joint Surg Am* 2007;89(2):292-300.

In 29 patients, revision to an RSA was required after unsuccessful hemiarthroplasty for proximal humeral fracture. Pain and function scores improved. Forward elevation improved from 38° to 73°, and abduction improved from 34° to 70°. The complication rate was 28%. Level of evidence: IV.

17. Levy JC, Virani N, Pupello D, Frankle M: Use of the reverse shoulder prosthesis for the treatment of failed hemiarthroplasty in patients with glenohumeral arthritis and rotator cuff deficiency. *J Bone Joint Surg Br* 2007;89(2):189-195.

In 18 patients (19 shoulders) who underwent RSA after unsuccessful hemiarthroplasty with rotator cuff deficiency and joint arthritis, pain and functional outcomes significantly improved. Mean flexion improved by 26°, and abduction improved by 35°. The complication rate was 32%, mostly associated with severe glenoid or proximal humeral bone loss. Level of evidence: IV.

18. Chacon A, Virani N, Shannon R, Levy JC, Pupello D, Frankle M: Revision arthroplasty with use of a reverse shoulder prosthesis-allograft composite. *J Bone Joint Surg Am* 2009;91(1):119-127.

In 25 patients with mean proximal humeral bone loss of 53.6 mm (range, 34.5 to 150.3 mm) who were treated using a revision prosthesis–allograft composite, pain and function scores were significantly improved at a minimum 2-year follow-up. Forward elevation, abduction, and internal rotation significantly improved. Nineteen patients had a good or excellent result, 5 had a satisfactory result, and 1 reported an unsatisfactory result. Level of evidence: IV.

19. Cuff D, Pupello D, Virani N, Levy J, Frankle M: Reverse shoulder arthroplasty for the treatment of rotator cuff deficiency. *J Bone Joint Surg Am* 2008;90(6):1244-1251.

In 112 patients (114 shoulders) treated with RSA for rotator cuff deficiency, pain and function scores had significantly improved at a minimum 2-year follow-up.

Blinded range-of-motion analysis showed significantly improved motion in all planes, including external rotation. Fifty-five percent of patients had an excellent result, 27% had a good result, 12% had a satisfactory result, and 6% had an unsatisfactory result. Level of evidence: IV.

20. Valenti P, Sauzières P, Katz D, Kalouche I, Kilinc AS: Do less medialized reverse shoulder prostheses increase motion and reduce notching? *Clin Orthop Relat Res* 2011;469(9):2550-2557.

    In 76 patients treated with a lateral offset RSA for pseudoparalytic shoulder with rotator cuff deficiency, Constant scores had improved from 24 to 59 at a minimum 24-month follow-up. Active elevation improved by 61°, external rotation at the side improved by 15°, and external rotation with 90° of abduction improved by 30°. Level of evidence: IV.

21. Boileau P, Watkinson D, Hatzidakis AM, Hovorka I: Neer Award 2005: The Grammont reverse shoulder prosthesis: Results in cuff tear arthritis, fracture sequelae, and revision arthroplasty. *J Shoulder Elbow Surg* 2006;15(5):527-540.

22. Simovitch RW, Helmy N, Zumstein MA, Gerber C: Impact of fatty infiltration of the teres minor muscle on the outcome of reverse total shoulder arthroplasty. *J Bone Joint Surg Am* 2007;89(5):934-939.

    In 42 patients treated with RSA for rotator cuff deficiency or cuff tear arthropathy, Goutallier stage 3 or 4 fatty infiltration led to significantly lower Constant scores and Subjective Shoulder Value (SSV) scores, as well as significantly less external rotation and a lower score for extremity positioning. Level of evidence: II.

23. Wall B, Nové-Josserand L, O'Connor DP, Edwards TB, Walch G: Reverse total shoulder arthroplasty: A review of results according to etiology. *J Bone Joint Surg Am* 2007;89(7):1476-1485.

    Outcome based on etiology was evaluated in 232 patients (240 shoulders) at a minimum 2-year follow-up after RSA. The results were good for several pathologies, but patients who underwent revision arthroplasty or had posttraumatic arthritis had less improvement and higher complication rates. Level of evidence: II.

24. Werner CM, Steinmann PA, Gilbart M, Gerber C: Treatment of painful pseudoparesis due to irreparable rotator cuff dysfunction with the Delta III reverse-ball-and-socket total shoulder prosthesis. *J Bone Joint Surg Am* 2005;87(7):1476-1486.

25. Boileau P, Watkinson DJ, Hatzidakis AM, Balg F: Grammont reverse prosthesis: Design, rationale, and biomechanics. *J Shoulder Elbow Surg* 2005;14(1, Suppl S):147S-161S.

26. Norris TR, Kelly JD, Humphrey CS: Management of glenoid bone defects in revision shoulder arthroplasty: A new application of the reverse total shoulder prosthesis. *Tech Shoulder Elbow Surg* 2007;8:37-46.

    A technique is described for a single-stage reconstruction for RSA using iliac crest bone graft for glenoid bone defects.

27. Gutiérrez S, Keller TS, Levy JC, Lee WE III, Luo Z-P: Hierarchy of stability factors in reverse shoulder arthroplasty. *Clin Orthop Relat Res* 2008;466(3):670-676.

    A biomechanical study assessed the hierarchy of stability factors by evaluating the force required to dislocate the humerosocket from the glenosphere in eight commercially available reverse shoulder prostheses. The most important factor was joint compressive force, followed by socket depth and glenosphere size.

28. Terrier A, Reist A, Merlini F, Farron A: Simulated joint and muscle forces in reversed and anatomic shoulder prostheses. *J Bone Joint Surg Br* 2008;90(6):751-756.

    A finite element model was used to compare joint forces in reversed and anatomic prostheses. With the reversed prosthesis, abduction was possible without rotator cuff muscles and required 20% less deltoid force to achieve. The mechanical advantage of RSA in cuff deficiency was thus confirmed.

29. Rittmeister M, Kerschbaumer F: Grammont reverse total shoulder arthroplasty in patients with rheumatoid arthritis and nonreconstructible rotator cuff lesions. *J Shoulder Elbow Surg* 2001;10(1):17-22.

30. Delloye C, Joris D, Colette A, Eudier A, Dubuc JE: [Mechanical complications of total shoulder inverted prosthesis]. *Rev Chir Orthop Reparatrice Appar Mot* 2002;88(4):410-414.

31. Frankle MA, Siegal S, Pupello DR, Gutierrez S, Griewe M, Mighell M: Coronal plane tilt angle affects risk of catastrophic failure in patients treated with a reverse shoulder prosthesis. *J Shoulder Elbow Surg* 2007;16:e46.

    Coronal tilt was evaluated in 262 patients treated with RSA to determine whether there was a correlation between tilt angle and baseplate fixation failure. Patients with a superior-tilted baseplate were at a greater risk of catastrophic mechanical failure.

32. Seebauer L, Walter W, Keyl W: Reverse total shoulder arthroplasty for the treatment of defect arthropathy. *Oper Orthop Traumatol* 2005;17(1):1-24.

33. Sirveaux F, Favard L, Oudet D, Huquet D, Walch G, Molé D: Grammont inverted total shoulder arthroplasty in the treatment of glenohumeral osteoarthritis with massive rupture of the cuff: Results of a multicentre study of 80 shoulders. *J Bone Joint Surg Br* 2004;86(3):388-395.

34. Gutiérrez S, Walker M, Willis M, Pupello DR, Frankle MA: Effects of tilt and glenosphere eccentricity on baseplate/bone interface forces in a computational model, validated by a mechanical model, of reverse shoulder arthroplasty. *J Shoulder Elbow Surg* 2011;20(5):732-739.

5: Arthritis and Arthroplasty

The forces at the bone-baseplate interface in concentric and eccentric glenospheres, as well as the effect of tilt on these forces, were biomechanically evaluated. For lateralized and concentric glenospheres, inferior tilt provided the most even distribution of forces, and a superior tilt provided the most uneven distribution. For eccentric glenospheres, an inferior tilt provided a more uneven distribution of forces than a neutral tilt.

35. Harman M, Frankle M, Vasey M, Banks S: Initial glenoid component fixation in "reverse" total shoulder arthroplasty: A biomechanical evaluation. *J Shoulder Elbow Surg* 2005;14(1, Suppl S):162S-167S.

36. Young AA, Smith MM, Bacle G, Moraga C, Walch G: Early results of reverse shoulder arthroplasty in patients with rheumatoid arthritis. *J Bone Joint Surg Am* 2011;93(20):1915-1923.

    Sixteen patients (18 shoulders) with rheumatoid arthritis and rotator cuff deficiency were treated with RSA and followed for a mean 3.8 years. Patients had significant improvement in functional outcome scores and range of motion. Scapular notching was observed in 10 of 18 shoulders. There was no component loosening or revision. Level of evidence: IV.

37. Lévigne C, Boileau P, Favard L, et al: Scapular notching in reverse shoulder arthroplasty. *J Shoulder Elbow Surg* 2008;17(6):925-935.

    At an average 47-month follow-up (range, 24 to 120 months), notching occurred in 62% of 326 consecutive patients (337 shoulders) treated with RSA and was more common with preoperative cuff tear arthropathy, grade 3 or 4 fatty infiltration of the infraspinatus, narrowed acromiohumeral distance, and superiorly oriented glenoids. Glenosphere placement influences notching; superior positioning and superior tilting should be avoided.

38. Frankle MA, Teramoto A, Luo Z-P, Levy JC, Pupello D: Glenoid morphology in reverse shoulder arthroplasty: Classification and surgical implications. *J Shoulder Elbow Surg* 2009;18(6):874-885.

    The morphology of 216 glenoids was evaluated with CT, and the effect on possible glenoid component fixation was determined. The subjects were graded on the presence of an abnormality, with subclassification based on location of erosions. The standard centerline was significantly shorter in abnormal glenoids, and the peripheral screw placement area was reduced by 42%.

39. Neyton L, Boileau P, Nové-Josserand L, Edwards TB, Walch G: Glenoid bone grafting with a reverse design prosthesis. *J Shoulder Elbow Surg* 2007;16(3, Suppl): S71-S78.

    Nine patients treated with RSA required glenoid bone grafting for bone loss. Most patients were satisfied and had pain relief despite low Constant scores. There was no glenoid component loosening or graft failure at a minimum 2-year follow-up, but six patients had inferior notching. Level of evidence: IV.

40. Cuff D, Levy JC, Gutiérrez S, Frankle MA: Torsional stability of modular and non-modular reverse shoulder humeral components in a proximal humeral bone loss model. *J Shoulder Elbow Surg* 2011;20(4):646-651.

    Modular and nonmodular reverse humeral stem designs were evaluated biomechanically in the setting of proximal humeral bone loss compared with the intact humerus. The proximal bone loss constructs had significantly greater rotational micromotion. Two of 12 intact humerus constructs failed testing, and 5 of 12 bone loss constructs failed; all 7 were modular humeral designs.

41. Boileau P, Chuinard C, Roussanne Y, Bicknell RT, Rochet N, Trojani C: Reverse shoulder arthroplasty combined with a modified latissimus dorsi and teres major tendon transfer for shoulder pseudoparalysis associated with dropping arm. *Clin Orthop Relat Res* 2008;466(3):584-593.

    Eleven consecutive patients with combined loss of active elevation and external rotation were treated with RSA and latissimus dorsi–teres major tendon transfer. Mean active elevation improved from 70° to 148°, and external rotation improved from −18 to 18°. All patients had improvement in Constant scores, subjective assessment, and activities of daily living. Level of evidence: IV.

42. Boileau P, Chuinard C, Roussanne Y, Neyton L, Trojani C: Modified latissimus dorsi and teres major transfer through a single delto-pectoral approach for external rotation deficit of the shoulder: As an isolated procedure or with a reverse arthroplasty. *J Shoulder Elbow Surg* 2007;16(6):671-682.

    Fifteen consecutive patients underwent latissimus dorsi–teres major tendon transfer through a deltopectoral incision (eight were combined with RSA). The mean active elevation improved by 34.7°, and the mean active external rotation improved by 28°. Constant and SSV scores improved, with 14 of 15 patients satisfied or very satisfied with the result.

43. Boileau P, Rumian AP, Zumstein MA: Reversed shoulder arthroplasty with modified L'Episcopo for combined loss of active elevation and external rotation. *J Shoulder Elbow Surg* 2010;19(2, Suppl)20-30.

    Seventeen consecutive patients underwent RSA combined with latissimus dorsi–teres major tendon transfer for loss of active elevation and external rotation. Mean elevation improved from 74° to 149°, and mean external rotation improved from −21° to 13°. Patient satisfaction, Constant scores, SSV scores, and activities of daily living all improved. Level of evidence: IV.

44. Gerber C, Pennington SD, Lingenfelter EJ, Sukthankar A: Reverse Delta-III total shoulder replacement combined with latissimus dorsi transfer: A preliminary report. *J Bone Joint Surg Am* 2007;89(5):940-947.

    Eleven patients (12 shoulders) underwent RSA combined with latissimus dorsi transfer for loss of active elevation and external rotation. Mean elevation improved from 94° to 139°. External rotation improved only from 12° to 19°, but functional external rotation improved on Constant scores. SSV scores and activities of daily living also significantly improved. Level of evidence: IV.

45. Vanhove B, Beugnies A: Grammont's reverse shoulder prosthesis for rotator cuff arthropathy: A retrospective study of 32 cases. *Acta Orthop Belg* 2004;70(3):219-225.

46. Holcomb JO, Hebert DJ, Mighell MA, et al: Reverse shoulder arthroplasty in patients with rheumatoid arthritis. *J Shoulder Elbow Surg* 2010;19(7):1076-1084.

    RSA was performed in 21 patients with rheumatoid arthritis. Outcome scores, pain, and range of motion improved postoperatively. Severe glenoid erosion occurred in 10 shoulders, 5 of which required structural grafting. Reoperation was required for infection in 2 patients and periprosthetic fracture in 1 patient. Level of evidence: IV.

47. Molé D, Favard L: [Excentered scapulohumeral osteoarthritis]. *Rev Chir Orthop Reparatrice Appar Mot* 2007;93(6, Suppl):37-94.

    A fracture of the acromion occurred in 16 of 527 patients who underwent RSA (3%). The risk factors included a deltopectoral approach and high tension of the deltoid caused by excessive lateralization and humeral lengthening. Level of evidence: IV.

48. Bufquin T, Hersan A, Hubert L, Massin P: Reverse shoulder arthroplasty for the treatment of three- and four-part fractures of the proximal humerus in the elderly: A prospective review of 43 cases with a short-term follow-up. *J Bone Joint Surg Br* 2007;89(4):516-520.

    The 43 patients treated with RSA for proximal humerus fracture had good range of motion and functional scores despite tuberosity healing in only 58%. There was a 28% complication rate. Level of evidence: IV.

49. Walch G, Mottier F, Wall B, Boileau P, Molé D, Favard L: Acromial insufficiency in reverse shoulder arthroplasties. *J Shoulder Elbow Surg* 2009;18(3):495-502.

    Of 457 patients treated with RSA, 41 had preoperative acromial insufficiencies that were not found to contraindicate RSA. Patients with postoperative scapular spine fracture had a worse outcome. Level of evidence: III.

50. Crosby LA, Hamilton A, Twiss T: Scapula fractures after reverse total shoulder arthroplasty: Classification and treatment. *Clin Orthop Relat Res* 2011;469(9):2544-2549.

    Forty of 400 patients had acromial fracture after RSA. The authors proposed a classification and recommended treatment. Because a scapular spine fracture (type III) is likely to have a relatively poor result, open reduction and internal fixation is recommended. Level of evidence: II.

51. Nagda SH, Rogers KJ, Sestokas AK, et al: Neer Award 2005: Peripheral nerve function during shoulder arthroplasty using intraoperative nerve monitoring. *J Shoulder Elbow Surg* 2007;16(3, Suppl):S2-S8.

    Continuous intraoperative monitoring of the brachial plexus was done in 30 consecutive patients undergoing shoulder arthroplasty. Seventeen (57%) patients had episodes of nerve dysfunction during surgery. Of the 7 patients whose intraoperative nerve dysfunction did not return to normal with repositioning, 4 had electromyographic abnormalities at 4 weeks.

52. Lädermann A, Lübbeke A, Mélis B, et al: Prevalence of neurologic lesions after total shoulder arthroplasty. *J Bone Joint Surg Am* 2011;93(14):1288-1293.

    The correlation of neurologic injury with lengthening of the arm after RSA was evaluated in a comparison of 19 patients treated with RSA with 23 patients treated with anatomic TSA. Postoperative electromyography showed evidence of neurologic lesions in 9 of 19 patients with RSA and 1 of 23 patients with TSA, although the lesions usually were transient. The mean lengthening of the arm in patients with RSA was 2.7 cm (± 1.8 cm).

53. Klein M, Juschka M, Hinkenjann B, Scherger B, Ostermann PA: Treatment of comminuted fractures of the proximal humerus in elderly patients with the Delta III reverse shoulder prosthesis. *J Orthop Trauma* 2008;22(10):698-704.

    Twenty patients treated with RSA for acute proximal humeral fracture were evaluated based on clinical and radiographic outcome. Good outcomes were attainable at a mean 33-month follow-up. Level of evidence: IV.

54. Gallinet D, Clappaz P, Garbuio P, Tropet Y, Obert L: Three or four parts complex proximal humerus fractures: Hemiarthroplasty versus reverse prosthesis. A comparative study of 40 cases. *Orthop Traumatol Surg Res* 2009;95(1):48-55.

    Twenty-one patients treated with hemiarthroplasty for proximal humeral fracture were compared with 19 patients treated with RSA. Elevation and abduction range of motion and Constant scores were better after RSA, and internal and external rotation were better after hemiarthroplasty. There were 3 abnormal tuberosity fixations with hemiarthroplasty, and 15 of 19 patients had notching with RSA. Level of evidence: IV.

55. Cazeneuve JF, Cristofari DJ: The reverse shoulder prosthesis in the treatment of fractures of the proximal humerus in the elderly. *J Bone Joint Surg Br* 2010;92(4):535-539.

    In 36 patients with proximal humeral fracture treated with RSA and followed for a mean 6.6 years, Constant scores declined with longer follow-up, and 63% had radiographic evidence of notching, with development over time. One patient had aseptic loosening at 12-year follow-up. Level of evidence: IV.

56. Lenarz C, Shishani Y, McCrum C, Nowinski RJ, Edwards TB, Gobezie R: Is reverse shoulder arthroplasty appropriate for the treatment of fractures in the older patient? Early observations. *Clin Orthop Relat Res* 2011;469(12):3324-3331.

    In 30 patients treated with RSA for three- or four-part proximal humeral fracture (mean age, 77 years), there were significant improvements in pain and function

5: Arthritis and Arthroplasty

scores and range of motion at a minimum 12-month follow-up. Three complications were noted. Level of evidence: IV.

57. Melis B, Bonnevialle N, Neyton L, et al: Glenoid loosening and failure in anatomical total shoulder arthroplasty: Is revision with a reverse shoulder arthroplasty a reliable option? *J Shoulder Elbow Surg* 2012;21(3): 342-349.

Thirty-seven patients underwent revision to RSA after unsuccessful TSA. Mean forward elevation improved from 68° to 120°. Constant scores improved from 24 to 55. Three patients had postoperative glenoid baseplate loosening, and 3 had instability. Level of evidence: IV.

58. Holcomb JO, Cuff D, Petersen SA, Pupello DR, Frankle MA: Revision reverse shoulder arthroplasty for glenoid baseplate failure after primary reverse shoulder arthroplasty. *J Shoulder Elbow Surg* 2009;18(5):717-723.

Revision RSA was performed in 14 patients for glenoid baseplate failure after primary RSA. Range-of-motion and American Shoulder and Elbow Surgeons Index scores improved postoperatively, and there were no differences between prefailure and postrevision outcome data. Revision RSA was found to restore pain relief and function to levels obtained after the index RSA. Two patients underwent a second revision RSA because of baseplate failure and dislocation. Level of evidence: IV.

59. Walker M, Willis MP, Brooks JP, Pupello D, Mulieri PJ, Frankle MA: The use of the reverse shoulder arthroplasty for treatment of failed total shoulder arthroplasty. *J Shoulder Elbow Surg* 2012;21(4):514-522.

Twenty-two patients treated with RSA for unsuccessful TSA were followed for a minimum of 2 years. There were significant improvements in scores on the American Shoulder and Elbow Surgeons Index, Simple Shoulder Test, and visual analog scale as well as range of motion in all planes. Fourteen patients reported an excellent result, 3 a good result, 3 a satisfactory result, and 2 an unsatisfactory result. The overall complication rate was 22.7%. Level of evidence: IV.

Chapter 32

Complications of Reverse Shoulder Arthroplasty

Stephanie Muh, MD   Reuben Gobezie, MD

Introduction

Long-term projections show that the demand for all types of shoulder arthroplasty will continue to increase.[1] As the indications for reverse shoulder arthroplasty (RSA) have expanded, the number of associated complications also has grown. Overall complication rates of 11% to 50% have been reported after RSA.[2-5] These rates are higher than those for conventional primary total shoulder arthroplasty and are still higher after revision RSA.[4,6,7] The complications specifically associated with RSA are related to the nonanatomic design of the prosthesis, its use in patients who have abnormal morphology, and the surgeon's level of experience with RSA. Higher complication and mortality rates were found to occur if the surgeon performs a relatively small number of arthroplasties.[8,9] The complications associated with RSA include joint infection, neurologic injury, instability, scapular notching, fracture, and baseplate failure.

Intraoperative Complications

Neurologic Injury

The reported incidence of neurologic injury after RSA ranges from 1% to 10%, but the injury often resolves spontaneously.[2,10-13] During RSA, moving the center of rotation more medially and distally lengthens the involved arm and tensions the brachial plexus.[14,15] The symptoms vary from transitory pain to persistent dysesthesia and may include a catastrophic loss of shoulder function, particularly in a patient with a lesion of the axillary nerve.

Dr. Gobezie or an immediate family member has received royalties from Arthrex; serves as a paid consultant to or is an employee of Arthrex and Tornier; and has received research or institutional support from Arthrex and Tornier. Neither Dr. Muh nor any immediate family member has received anything of value from or has stock or stock options held in a commercial company or institution related directly or indirectly to the subject of this chapter.

A cadaver study found that nerve damage was related to the amount of strain.[14] An 8% lengthening of the nerve was critical for initiating blood flow arrest in the sciatic nerve, and complete arrest of blood flow occurred at 15% of strain. The brachial plexus sustained a large strain after RSA (as much as 19.3%). This finding suggests that lengthening caused by RSA may be a factor leading to brachial plexus injury in some patients.

A combination of intraoperative traction, limb manipulation, and lengthening of the arm necessitated by the nonanatomic design of the prosthesis contributes to the risk of neurologic injury. In a prospective study of 19 patients with primary RSA, 9 patients had subclinical electromyographic changes primarily involving the axillary nerve.[16] Compared with anatomic total shoulder arthroplasty, RSA led to an increased relative risk of 10.9 for postoperative nerve injury. The treated arm was lengthened a mean of 2.7 cm in RSA. However, eight of the nine nerve lesions spontaneously resolved within 6 months. A prospective study of intraoperative nerve injury in shoulder arthroplasty found a 56.7% incidence of nerve dysfunction or so-called nerve alerts during surgery.[17] Most of these nerve alerts (76.7%) returned to baseline after the arm was repositioned into a neutral position from extreme external rotation, extension, abduction, or adduction for glenoid preparation. The researchers concluded that extreme arm positions and the use of retractors should be minimized.

Intraoperative Fracture

Intraoperative glenoid fracture is a rare but devastating complication related to reaming and initial implant fixation. The common causes of glenoid fracture include a failure to start the reamer before making contact with the glenoid bone and reaming of the glenoid beyond the subchondral bone, thus causing the reamer to catch the underreamed subchondral bone. Small fractures of the peripheral rim often can be ignored because they have no effect on stable fixation of the glenosphere. However, larger glenoid fractures that extend to the central portion are more problematic. Stable fixation of the glenoid, by augmented baseplate fixation or grafting, must be achieved before inserting the glenosphere. If a central screw baseplate design is used, the screw can be repositioned within the glenoid to achieve a similar outcome. If sufficient stability cannot be achieved, the RSA may need to be converted to a hemiarthroplasty.

Iatrogenic humeral fracture is the most common humeral complication. Patients often have osteopenia that places them at risk for fracture. The risk can be minimized by limiting the amount of torque placed on the humerus and maintaining awareness of humeral position during preparation, especially during reaming of the humeral canal when the arm is in an extended, adducted, and externally rotated position. A fracture at the humeral diaphysis should be reduced, and a long-stem humeral prosthesis can be placed. The radial nerve should be identified when a plate and cerclage wires are used for fracture reduction and fixation.

Postoperative Complications

Infection

Infection can be a devastating complication of RSA. A delay in diagnosis can lead to chronic pain, instability, poor functional motion, sepsis, or the need for extensive revision surgery. The reported rate of infection after conventional total shoulder arthroplasty is approximately 0.7%, but infection rates associated with RSA range from 1% to 15%.[3,5,11,18-21] Infection usually is related to a breach in sterile technique, postoperative hematoma formation, prolonged surgical time, or revision surgery. Not surprisingly, patients with a comorbidity, such as diabetes, inflammatory arthropathy, or another immunosuppressive disorder, are at an increased risk for infection. Patients undergoing revision surgery also are at increased risk for infection.

The diagnosis of infection in shoulder arthroplasty is challenging. The indolent nature of common shoulder pathogens leads to symptoms that usually are nonspecific in nature. Pain is the primary complaint. *Propionibacterium acnes*, *Staphylococcus epidermidis*, and *Staphylococcus aureus* are the most common sources of infection related to shoulder surgery.[22] *P acnes* is an increasingly common cause of infection after shoulder arthroplasty.[23,24] This gram-positive, aerotolerant, non–spore-forming, anaerobic bacillus commonly is found in moist areas (such as the axilla) of healthy skin and the sebaceous glands. Successful diagnosis and treatment of *P acnes* infection remains a challenge because of its low virulence. A patient with *P acnes* infection may report chronic nonspecific complaints, and laboratory values often are normal. Standard laboratory tests, such as C-reactive protein (CRP) level, erythrocyte sedimentation rate (ESR), and white blood cell counts, are routinely done but often are nondiagnostic for periprosthetic infection.

In a retrospective review of 19 shoulder arthroplasties with confirmed periprosthetic infection, the optimized ESR cutoff (26 mm/h) for detecting shoulder arthroplasty infection was found to have a sensitivity of 32% and specificity of 93%.[25] The optimized cutoff level for CRP (7 mg/L) had a sensitivity of 63% and specificity of 73%. The researchers concluded that ESR and CRP level had poor sensitivity for the diagnosis of shoulder implant infection.

Newer biochemical markers, including interleukin-6, tumor necrosis factor–α, and procalcitonin-C, are being investigated as diagnostic tools. A sonication technique for the diagnosis of prosthetic shoulder infection was described as having better sensitivity and similar specificity compared with traditional intraoperative tissue culturing.[26] Adding to the difficulty of diagnosis is the relatively long incubation period needed to culture the organism; the average time for culture was reported to be 13.3 days (range, 4 to 21 days).[27]

Perioperative infection prevention is critical. Perioperative antibiotics should be prophylactically administered within 1 hour of incision. A chlorhexidine scrub was found to be the most effective means of eliminating coagulase-negative *Staphylococcus* and *Propionibacterium* from the shoulder region.[28] Long surgical time also has been identified as a risk factor for infection.[24] The use of antibiotic-loaded bone cement recently was found to reduce the rate of deep infection in primary RSA compared with cement without antibiotics.[29] Some evidence suggests that hematoma formation in the dead space associated with RSA is a risk factor for infection.[30] Therefore, it is important to avoid postoperative hematoma formation by meticulous intraoperative hemostasis and the postoperative placement of a drain.

The management of postoperative infection after RSA is similar to that after other total joint arthroplasty procedures. Several authors have noted that early administration of organism-specific antibiotics plays an important role in eradicating infection.[31] The current surgical treatment options include irrigation and débridement, antibiotic suppression, one- or two-stage revision surgery, resection arthroplasty, and arthrodesis.[32,33] Acute infection (of less than 6 weeks' duration) can be successfully treated with aggressive débridement, intravenous antibiotics, and polyethylene exchange; or with a single-stage reimplantation.[31,34,35] The best treatment of a chronic infection (of more than 3 months' duration) is controversial. The evidence is conflicting regarding the efficacy of one-stage and two-stage revision procedures for eradicating chronic infection.[31,33-35] Most experience has been with two-stage revision, in keeping with recommendations found in the lower extremity arthroplasty literature. The most reproducible results in terms of functional outcomes and infection eradication were found with a two-stage revision consisting of aggressive débridement, prosthesis removal, and the placement of a polymethyl methacrylate spacer, followed by 6 weeks of intravenous antibiotics and reimplantation.[32,36] Resection arthroplasty has been used for patients who are unable to undergo surgical reimplantation or have been unsuccessfully treated with every other option. Resection arthroplasty provides reasonable pain relief but limits postoperative function.

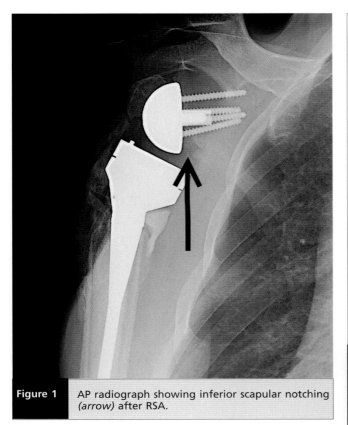

Figure 1 AP radiograph showing inferior scapular notching *(arrow)* after RSA.

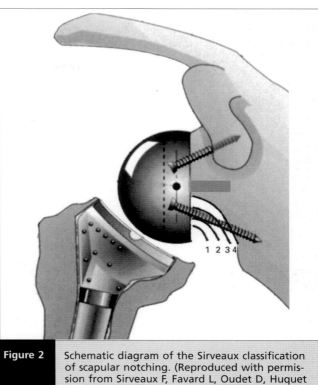

Figure 2 Schematic diagram of the Sirveaux classification of scapular notching. (Reproduced with permission from Sirveaux F, Favard L, Oudet D, Huquet D, Walch G, Molé D: Grammont inverted total shoulder arthroplasty in the treatment of glenohumeral osteoarthritis with massive rupture of the cuff: Results of a multicentre study of 80 shoulders. *J Bone Joint Surg Br* 2004;86[3]:388-395.)

Scapular Notching

Scapular notching, first described in 1997, is a radiographic finding associated only with RSA (**Figure 1**). Scapular notching occurs when the medial edge of the humeral socket impinges on the inferior border of the glenoid. The incidence of scapular notching varies with the implant design. The incidence with the traditional Grammont-style RSA implant ranges from 19% to 96%.[3-5,11,13,37-39] A more recent RSA implant with a relatively lateral center of rotation appears to have a decreased incidence of scapular notching, with a range of 0% to 16%.[18,37,40] Other factors, such as surgical approach, glenosphere positioning, native scapular anatomy (scapular neck length, glenoid erosion, and scapular neck angle), prosthesis neck angle, and patient activity level, also have been implicated in the development of scapular notching.[39,41,42] A biomechanical study of factors that cause impingement on the inferior scapular neck found that a relatively varus humeral component neck-shaft angle, inferior position of the glenosphere, and large glenosphere center-of-rotation offset were important in decreasing impingement.[43]

The diagnosis of scapular notching is made radiographically with a true AP (Grashey) view of the shoulder. Notching usually occurs 6 weeks to 14 months after surgery. In the Sirveaux classification, a grade I notch is limited to the inferior scapular pillar, a grade II notch is in contact with the inferior screw of the baseplate, a grade III notch extends beyond the inferior screw, and a grade IV notch extends under the baseplate and approaches the central peg[44] (**Figure 2**). Inferomedial scapular osteophytes commonly accompany scapular notching (**Figure 3**).

Controversy exists regarding the importance of scapular notching and whether it progresses over time. Scapular notching at a mean 4.5 months after surgery had stabilized at a mean 18 months after surgery.[42] The incidence of notch progression was 48% at 1 year after surgery, 60% at 2 years, and 68% at 3 years, and the incidence of grade III and IV notches increased over time.[38]

The implications of scapular notching also have been debated. Several studies found that scapular notching was not correlated with scores on the Constant-Murley pain scale or with active forward flexion.[4,5,39,41] A negative correlation was found between scapular notching and the Constant-Murley score, the Subjective Shoulder Value, active forward flexion, and abduction.[2,38,42,44] Although the long-term implications of scapular notching are not well understood, most experts agree that surgical techniques should avoid notching, usually by placing the glenosphere as far inferior as possible. Designs incorporating a more lateral center of rotation and new designs such as the BIO-RSA (Tornier) have been introduced as a way to lateralize the glenoid component and avoid

5: Arthritis and Arthroplasty

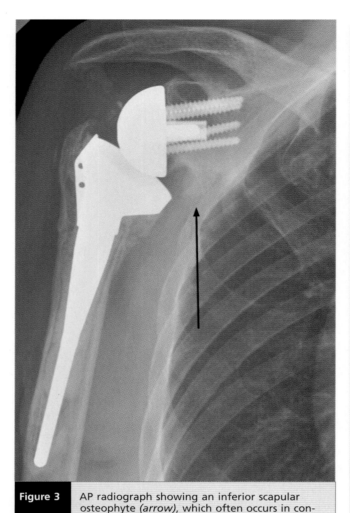

Figure 3   AP radiograph showing an inferior scapular osteophyte *(arrow)*, which often occurs in conjunction with scapular notching.

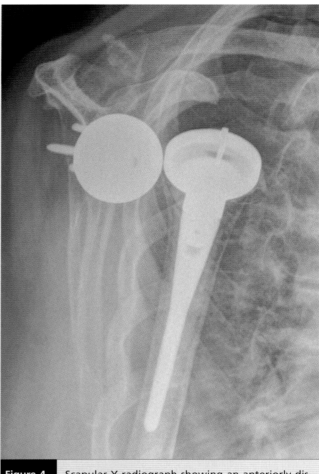

Figure 4   Scapular Y radiograph showing an anteriorly dislocated reverse shoulder prosthesis.

notching. In the novel BIO-RSA technique, lateralization is reproduced by placing an autogenous bone graft from the patient's humeral head on a baseplate designed with a relatively long central post. When the bone graft has healed, the center of rotation is maintained at the glenoid bone–prosthesis interface.[10]

Instability

Dislocation remains one of the most common complications after RSA, with rates ranging from 1% to 31%.[4-6,11,13,15,19,20] Multiple factors contribute to instability, including soft-tissue tension, mechanical impingement, prosthesis version, proximal bone loss, prosthesis height, and axillary nerve dysfunction. Patients who had RSA secondary to fracture sequelae have a higher rate of instability than those undergoing RSA for primary rotator cuff tear arthropathy, massive rotator cuff tear with pseudoparalysis, acute fracture, or instability arthropathy.[6] Adequate soft-tissue tension is critical for stability. If the patient lacks a functioning rotator cuff, appropriate lengthening of the deltoid is paramount and allows increased compression forces across the prosthesis to maintain stability. If the deltoid is not appropriately tensioned, the risk of dislocation is increased.[15] Surgical techniques such as minimizing humeral bone resection, positioning the glenosphere with an inferior tilt, and eccentric placement of the glenosphere allow the surgeon to gain stability by lowering the humerus relative to the glenoid and thus to increase deltoid tension. A prosthesis design with a more valgus head-neck angle, a larger glenosphere diameter, a lateral offset, or a thicker polyethylene insert also can be used to achieve appropriate soft-tissue tension. Mechanical impingement, in which the humeral component levers off the inferior aspect of the scapular neck, is a less common cause of instability that often is related to a too-superior placement of the glenoid component. Another possible risk factor for instability is related to the status of the subscapularis tendon. Some recent studies found that patients with subscapularis insufficiency at the time of surgery had a higher rate of instability than those with a repairable subscapularis tendon, but another study found that subscapularis incompetency did not significantly affect the risk of dislocation.[6,45,46]

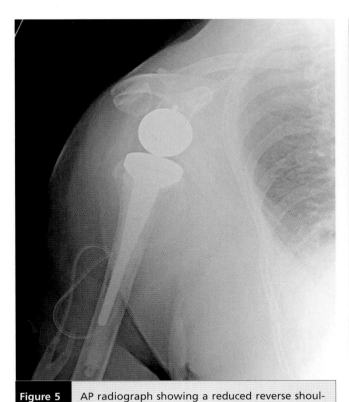

Figure 5 | AP radiograph showing a reduced reverse shoulder prosthesis.

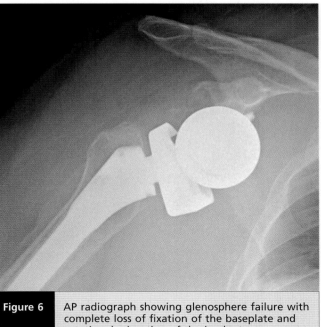

Figure 6 | AP radiograph showing glenosphere failure with complete loss of fixation of the baseplate and rotational migration of the implant.

Most dislocations occur after a combination of extension, adduction, and internal rotation, as in a hand-behind-the-back position. The direction of dislocation is anterior (**Figures 4** and **5**). In most patients, the dislocated prosthesis can be treated with closed reduction. After the prosthesis is reduced, the shoulder should be examined under fluoroscopy to determine whether mechanical impingement is the cause of instability. If closed reduction of the prosthesis is not possible, the shoulder must be reduced with open measures. An early dislocation (within the first 3 months of surgery) usually results from a technical error and cannot be treated with closed reduction alone. During revision surgery, the surgeon should evaluate for appropriate version, soft-tissue impingement, and appropriate tension of the deltoid. Any of these variables should be corrected if it is causing the instability. A late dislocation (more than 1 year after surgery) usually can be treated with closed reduction and a period of immobilization.[47]

Glenoid Baseplate Failure

Glenoid baseplate or component failure occurred after many early RSAs (**Figures 6** and **7**).[18,21] In the early RSA designs, a glenosphere with a laterally offset center of rotation created excessive torque and shear forces at the junction of the baseplate and the glenoid bone. Innovations and implant design changes have decreased the rate of glenoid baseplate failure.[20,21] The Grammont reverse prosthesis medialized the center of rotation, which led to more concentric forces and reduced the torque at the prosthesis-bone junction. This design allowed stable fixation of the glenoid baseplate; implant survivorship was reported to be 84% at 10-year follow-up.[48]

The minimal implant pore size for achieving bony ingrowth is 150 μ.[49] Lack of bone ingrowth onto the baseplate is associated with baseplate failure. Inferior tilt and the use of locking screws minimize forces at the baseplate-bone interface and thereby reduce the rate of failure, regardless of prosthesis design.[50] Newer devices with a lateral eccentric center of rotation use 5.0-mm peripheral locking screws, with a resulting decrease in the risk of mechanical baseplate failure.[20] The reported rate of glenoid loosening is low with modern reverse prosthesis designs that incorporate locking technology in the baseplate. However, every effort should be made to optimally fix the glenosphere at the inferior border of the glenoid and onto good bone stock.

Acromial Stress Fracture

Acromial stress fracture is another complication uniquely associated with RSA. This fracture has received little attention as an RSA complication, but interest recently has increased. The reported incidence of acromial fractures after RSA is 0.8% to 6.9%.[3,5,15,18,20,37,51] Acromial stress fracture often appears within 1 year after surgery and may not be associated with a traumatic event[5,18,51] (**Figure 8**). It is common for a patient to do well after surgery but have a sudden onset of pain or loss of function with no history of trauma. A 4.4% rate of acromial stress fracture was reported in a retrospective review of 45 patients; the researchers believed that overtensioning of the deltoid

5: Arthritis and Arthroplasty

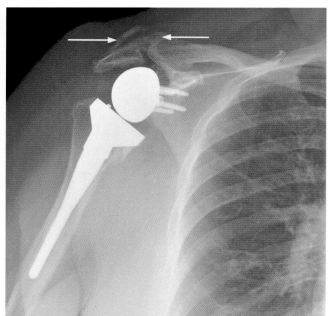

Figure 8 AP radiograph showing acromial fracture *(arrows)* with inferior tilting after reverse shoulder arthroplasty.

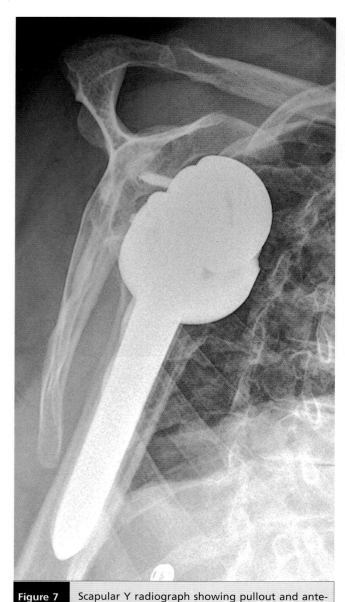

Figure 7 Scapular Y radiograph showing pullout and anterior migration and rotation of the entire glenosphere.

might lead to acromial fracture in patients with severe osteoporosis or eroded acromial bone, as occurs with severe rotator cuff arthropathy.[21] A 0.8% rate was reported in a study of 457 patients.[51]

The treatment of acromial stress fracture is controversial. The outcome was satisfactory when minimally displaced fractures were treated nonsurgically with a period of immobilization.[15,18,20] In a study of 457 patients who underwent RSA, 4 patients had a postoperative acromial fracture. Three fractures were treated nonsurgically, and one was treated with an open reduction with tension band, which eventually failed and required hardware removal.[51] A persistent nonunion developed in two patients, and two patients healed with nonsurgical treatment but had an inferior acromial tilt

of at least 40°. The four patients with postoperative acromial fracture had a worse result in terms of Constant score, active elevation, and subjective satisfaction compared with other patients in the study. The optimal treatment could not be determined, but 6 weeks of nonsurgical treatment with an abduction splint was recommended to limit pain and acromial tilt. A high degree of suspicion was recommended whenever rehabilitation after RSA progresses slowly, is painful, or suddenly deteriorates within the first postoperative year.[51]

Summary and Future Directions

Despite its higher complication rates in comparison with primary total shoulder arthroplasty, RSA has been shown to restore function and improve pain relief in appropriate patients. To minimize the risk of complications in RSA, the surgeon must be familiar with shoulder anatomy, the surgical exposure, and the complications related to the procedure. Complication rates will continue to decrease as surgeons become more experienced in the procedure. The midterm results of RSA are promising, but the long-term outcomes and complication rates remain unknown. The long-term results will clarify the clinical consequences of scapular notching. The long-term survivorship of RSA also is of concern; Constant scores, radiographic results, and survivorship were found to have deteriorated 6 to 8 years after RSA.[48] The increase in the need for RSA revision surgery and its higher complication rates also need to be examined.

Annotated References

1. Day JS, Lau E, Ong KL, Williams GR, Ramsey ML, Kurtz SM: Prevalence and projections of total shoulder and elbow arthroplasty in the United States to 2015. *J Shoulder Elbow Surg* 2010;19(8):1115-1120.

   Trends and projections of procedure volume for shoulder and elbow arthroplasty in the United States were examined. The number of procedures is expected to increase 192% to 322% by 2015.

2. Cazeneuve JF, Cristofari DJ: The reverse shoulder prosthesis in the treatment of fractures of the proximal humerus in the elderly. *J Bone Joint Surg Br* 2010; 92(4):535-539.

   The clinical and radiographic outcomes of RSA were reported for 36 fractures at a mean 6.6-year follow-up. Mean Constant scores decreased with longer follow-up and progressive scapular notching.

3. Naveed MA, Kitson J, Bunker TD: The Delta III reverse shoulder replacement for cuff tear arthropathy: A single-centre study of 50 consecutive procedures. *J Bone Joint Surg Br* 2011;93(1):57-61.

   Active forward elevation, American Shoulder and Elbow Surgeons Disability Index scores, and Oxford scores were improved at a mean 39-month follow-up after 50 RSAs for rotator cuff tear arthropathy.

4. Wall B, Nové-Josserand L, O'Connor DP, Edwards TB, Walch G: Reverse total shoulder arthroplasty: A review of results according to etiology. *J Bone Joint Surg Am* 2007;89(7):1476-1485.

   A review of 91 RSAs by etiology found that patients with primary rotator cuff tear arthropathy, rotator cuff tear with primary arthritis, or a massive rotator cuff tear had best outcomes. Level of evidence: II.

5. Werner CM, Steinmann PA, Gilbart M, Gerber C: Treatment of painful pseudoparesis due to irreparable rotator cuff dysfunction with the Delta III reverse-ball-and-socket total shoulder prosthesis. *J Bone Joint Surg Am* 2005;87(7):1476-1486.

6. Trappey GJ IV, O'Connor DP, Edwards TB: What are the instability and infection rates after reverse shoulder arthroplasty? *Clin Orthop Relat Res* 2011;469(9): 2505-2511.

   A prospective review of 284 RSAs found a 5% instability rate after primary RSA and an 8% rate after revision surgery. Patients with a repairable subscapularis tendon had a 1% rate of instability. Rates of infection were higher after revision than primary RSA. Level of evidence: III.

7. Zumstein MA, Pinedo M, Old J, Boileau P: Problems, complications, reoperations, and revisions in reverse total shoulder arthroplasty: A systematic review. *J Shoulder Elbow Surg* 2011;20(1):146-157.

   A review of studies on postoperative complications after RSA found global rates of 44%, 24%, 3.5%, and 10%, respectively, for notching, glenoid lucent lines, or hematoma formation without clinical significance; complications; reoperations; and revision procedures. Instability and infection were the most common causes of revision.

8. Walch G, Bacle G, Lädermann A, Nové-Josserand L, Smithers CJ: Do the indications, results, and complications of reverse shoulder arthroplasty change with surgeon's experience? *J Shoulder Elbow Surg* 2012; 21(11):1470-1477.

   Two consecutive series of 240 RSAs were compared. The rates of revision surgery and complications were found to decrease with increased surgeon experience. Changes were noted in patient selection and clinical results but not in rates of notching. Level of evidence: IV.

9. Lyman S, Jones EC, Bach PB, Peterson MG, Marx RG: The association between hospital volume and total shoulder arthroplasty outcomes. *Clin Orthop Relat Res* 2005;432:132-137.

10. Boileau P, Moineau G, Roussanne Y, O'Shea K: Bony increased-offset reversed shoulder arthroplasty: Minimizing scapular impingement while maximizing glenoid fixation. *Clin Orthop Relat Res* 2011;469(9): 2558-2567.

    A prospective review of 42 patients who underwent RSA using an autologous humeral head graft found an early 98% rate of complete graft incorporation, improved clinical function, and a 19% incidence of scapular notching. Level of evidence: IV.

11. Boileau P, Watkinson D, Hatzidakis AM, Hovorka I: The Grammont reverse shoulder prosthesis: Results in cuff tear arthritis, fracture sequelae, and revision arthroplasty. *J Shoulder Elbow Surg* 2006;15(5): 527-540.

12. Wierks C, Skolasky RL, Ji JH, McFarland EG: Reverse total shoulder replacement: Intraoperative and early postoperative complications. *Clin Orthop Relat Res* 2009;467(1):225-234.

    Complications were compared after the first and second groups of 10 RSAs. Intraoperative complications were found to decrease after the first 10 procedures, but there was no significant difference in postoperative complications. Level of evidence: II.

13. Valenti P, Sauzières P, Katz D, Kalouche I, Kilinc AS: Do less medialized reverse shoulder prostheses increase motion and reduce notching? *Clin Orthop Relat Res* 2011;469(9):2550-2557.

    A retrospective review of 76 RSAs using a lateralized center-of-rotation glenosphere found a 0% incidence of scapular notching or glenoid loosening and improved forward flexion, external rotation, and Constant scores. Level of evidence: IV.

14. Van Hoof T, Gomes GT, Audenaert E, Verstraete K, Kerckaert I, D'Herde K: 3D computerized model for measuring strain and displacement of the brachial plexus following placement of reverse shoulder pros-

5: Arthritis and Arthroplasty

thesis. *Anat Rec (Hoboken)* 2008;291(9):1173-1185.

Three-dimensional reconstruction of the cadaver brachial plexus and changes in strain and displacement after RSA showed 15% and 19% increases in strain in the lateral and medial roots of the median nerve, respectively, and a 10% decrease in the length of the axillary nerve.

15. Lädermann A, Williams MD, Melis B, Hoffmeyer P, Walch G: Objective evaluation of lengthening in reverse shoulder arthroplasty. *J Shoulder Elbow Surg* 2009;18(4):588-595.

A radiographic review of 58 RSAs found an average 2 mm of humeral lengthening and 23 mm of arm lengthening. Humeral and arm lengthening occurred less often in patients with postoperative instability. Level of evidence: III.

16. Lädermann A, Lübbeke A, Mélis B, et al: Prevalence of neurologic lesions after total shoulder arthroplasty. *J Bone Joint Surg Am* 2011;93(14):1288-1293.

A comparison of the incidence of neurologic lesions in 19 RSAs and 23 total shoulder arthroplasties found a 10.9 higher relative risk of acute postoperative nerve injury after RSA, with a mean lengthening of 2.7 cm. Nerve lesions usually were transient.

17. Nagda SH, Rogers KJ, Sestokas AK, et al: Peripheral nerve function during shoulder arthroplasty using intraoperative nerve monitoring. *J Shoulder Elbow Surg* 2007;16(3, suppl):S2-S8.

A 56.7% incidence of nerve alerts during shoulder arthroplasty was reported; most returned to baseline after retractors were removed and the arm was repositioned to neutral. Extreme arm positions and retractors should be used for the minimal time necessary.

18. Frankle M, Siegal S, Pupello D, Saleem A, Mighell M, Vasey M: The reverse shoulder prosthesis for glenohumeral arthritis associated with severe rotator cuff deficiency: A minimum two-year follow-up study of sixty patients. *J Bone Joint Surg Am* 2005;87(8):1697-1705.

19. De Wilde L, Sys G, Julien Y, Van Ovost E, Poffyn B, Trouilloud P: The reversed Delta shoulder prosthesis in reconstruction of the proximal humerus after tumour resection. *Acta Orthop Belg* 2003;69(6):495-500.

20. Cuff D, Pupello D, Virani N, Levy J, Frankle M: Reverse shoulder arthroplasty for the treatment of rotator cuff deficiency. *J Bone Joint Surg Am* 2008;90(6):1244-1251.

In 96 RSAs with a lateralized center of rotation, the overall complication rate was 6.25%, with improved postoperative abduction, forward flexion, and external rotation. There was no evidence of scapular notching at a mean 27.5-month follow-up. Level of evidence: IV.

21. Boileau P, Watkinson DJ, Hatzidakis AM, Balg F: Grammont reverse prosthesis: Design, rationale, and biomechanics. *J Shoulder Elbow Surg* 2005;14(1, suppl):147S-161S.

22. Topolski MS, Chin PY, Sperling JW, Cofield RH: Revision shoulder arthroplasty with positive intraoperative cultures: The value of preoperative studies and intraoperative histology. *J Shoulder Elbow Surg* 2006;15(4):402-406.

23. Dodson CC, Craig EV, Cordasco FA, et al: *Propionibacterium acnes* infection after shoulder arthroplasty: A diagnostic challenge. *J Shoulder Elbow Surg* 2010;19(2):303-307.

Eleven patients were diagnosed with *P acnes* infection after shoulder arthroplasty. The diagnosis was difficult because of indolent clinical symptoms, resistance to broad-spectrum antibiotics, and the need to keep cultures at least 2 weeks. Level of evidence: IV.

24. Kanafani ZA, Sexton DJ, Pien BC, Varkey J, Basmania C, Kaye KS: Postoperative joint infections due to Propionibacterium species: A case-control study. *Clin Infect Dis* 2009;49(7):1083-1085.

P acnes that occurred a mean 210 days after shoulder arthroplasty was diagnosed in 40 patients. Only 23% of cases occurred within 1 month of surgery. A history of earlier surgery and male sex were independent risk factors.

25. Piper KE, Fernandez-Sampedro M, Steckelberg KE, et al: C-reactive protein, erythrocyte sedimentation rate and orthopedic implant infection. *PLoS One* 2010;5(2):e9358.

CRP level and ESR were analyzed in patients who underwent hip, knee, or shoulder arthroplasty. CRP level and ESR were found to have poor sensitivity for the diagnosis of shoulder infection. Sensitivity and specificity for detecting shoulder infection were 23% and 93%, respectively.

26. Piper KE, Jacobson MJ, Cofield RH, et al: Microbiologic diagnosis of prosthetic shoulder infection by use of implant sonication. *J Clin Microbiol* 2009;47(6):1878-1884.

The accuracy of sonicate fluid for detecting prosthetic shoulder infection in revision or resection shoulder arthroplasty was studied. Sonicate fluid was 66.7% sensitive and periprosthetic tissue culture was 54.5% sensitive for detecting prosthetic shoulder infection in revision or resection shoulder arthroplasty.

27. Lutz MF, Berthelot P, Fresard A, et al: Arthroplastic and osteosynthetic infections due to Propionibacterium acnes: A retrospective study of 52 cases, 1995-2002. *Eur J Clin Microbiol Infect Dis* 2005;24(11):739-744.

28. Saltzman MD, Nuber GW, Gryzlo SM, Marecek GS, Koh JL: Efficacy of surgical preparation solutions in shoulder surgery. *J Bone Joint Surg Am* 2009;91(8):1949-1953.

A prospective study comparing three surgical preparation solutions (ChloraPrep, DuraPrep, and povidone-iodine scrub) found ChloraPrep to be the most effective for eliminating bacteria before surgery. Level of evidence: I.

29. Nowinski RJ, Gillespie RJ, Shishani Y, Cohen B, Walch G, Gobezie R: Antibiotic-loaded bone cement reduces deep infection rates for primary reverse total shoulder arthroplasty: A retrospective, cohort study of 501 shoulders. *J Shoulder Elbow Surg* 2012;21(3): 324-328.

A retrospective study compared the incidence of deep infection after RSA in patients treated with antibiotic-loaded cement or plain cement. No deep infections developed in patients with antibiotic-loaded cement, compared with 3% in those with plain cement. Level of evidence: III.

30. Cheung EV, Sperling JW, Cofield RH: Infection associated with hematoma formation after shoulder arthroplasty. *Clin Orthop Relat Res* 2008;466(6):1363-1367.

Hematoma formation required reoperation after 12 of 4,147 shoulder arthroplasties. Six of nine patients had positive cultures, and two eventually had a resection arthroplasty. Hematoma formation is often associated with a positive intraoperative culture. Level of evidence: IV.

31. Weber P, Utzschneider S, Sadoghi P, Andress HJ, Jansson V, Müller PE: Management of the infected shoulder prosthesis: A retrospective analysis and review of the literature. *Int Orthop* 2011;35(3):365-373.

In a retrospective review of 10 patients treated for an infected shoulder prosthesis, a two-stage exchange yielded only slightly better results than resection arthroplasty. Level of evidence: IV.

32. Sabesan VJ, Ho JC, Kovacevic D, Iannotti JP: Two-stage reimplantation for treating prosthetic shoulder infections. *Clin Orthop Relat Res* 2011;469(9):2538-2543.

A retrospective review found that two-stage reimplantation for prosthetic shoulder infection led to improved shoulder function and pain. There was a 35% incidence of complications, including five dislocations and one reinfection. Level of evidence: IV.

33. Grosso MJ, Sabesan VJ, Ho JC, Ricchetti ET, Iannotti JP: Reinfection rates after 1-stage revision shoulder arthroplasty for patients with unexpected positive intraoperative cultures. *J Shoulder Elbow Surg* 2012; 21(6):754-758.

Infection recurred in 5.9% of 17 patients who underwent a one-stage revision without prolonged antibiotic therapy after unsuccessful shoulder arthroplasty and a positive intraoperative culture. Infection recurred in 5.9%. Level of evidence: IV.

34. Beekman PD, Katusic D, Berghs BM, Karelse A, De Wilde L: One-stage revision for patients with a chronically infected reverse total shoulder replacement. *J Bone Joint Surg Br* 2010;92(6):817-822.

Ten of 11 patients who underwent a one-stage revision of infected shoulder arthroplasty were considered free of infection at a median 24-month follow-up. The mean postoperative score gain on the Constant-Murley Scale was 10.

35. Coste JS, Reig S, Trojani C, Berg M, Walch G, Boileau P: The management of infection in arthroplasty of the shoulder. *J Bone Joint Surg Br* 2004;86(1):65-69.

36. Sperling JW, Kozak TK, Hanssen AD, Cofield RH: Infection after shoulder arthroplasty. *Clin Orthop Relat Res* 2001;382:206-216.

37. Mulieri P, Dunning P, Klein S, Pupello D, Frankle M: Reverse shoulder arthroplasty for the treatment of irreparable rotator cuff tear without glenohumeral arthritis. *J Bone Joint Surg Am* 2010;92(15):2544-2556.

A retrospective review found that American Shoulder and Elbow Surgeons Disability Index scores, Simple Shoulder Test scores, visual analog scale scores, active forward flexion, abduction, internal rotation, and external rotation improved after RSA in 72 shoulders with an irreparable rotator cuff tear. Level of evidence: IV.

38. Lévigne C, Garret J, Boileau P, Alami G, Favard L, Walch G: Scapular notching in reverse shoulder arthroplasty: Is it important to avoid it and how? *Clin Orthop Relat Res* 2011;469(9):2512-2520.

A retrospective review found that notching occurred in 68% of 448 patients after RSA and increased with longer follow-up time. Notching was associated with decreased strength and forward elevation but not with pain or the Constant-Murley score. Level of evidence: IV.

39. Boileau P, Gonzalez JF, Chuinard C, Bicknell R, Walch G: Reverse total shoulder arthroplasty after failed rotator cuff surgery. *J Shoulder Elbow Surg* 2009;18(4):600-606.

A retrospective review of RSA in 42 patients after unsuccessful rotator cuff surgery found that patients with poor preoperative motion were able to restore active elevation. Patients with maintained preoperative motion (more than 90°) risked loss of motion and lower satisfaction.

40. Kempton LB, Balasubramaniam M, Ankerson E, Wiater JM: A radiographic analysis of the effects of prosthesis design on scapular notching following reverse total shoulder arthroplasty. *J Shoulder Elbow Surg* 2011;20(4):571-576.

A comparison of two prosthesis designs found that patients having the prosthesis with a lateralized center of rotation had a lower incidence of notching compared with those having the prosthesis with no center of rotation. Level of evidence: III.

41. Lévigne C, Boileau P, Favard L, et al: Scapular notching in reverse shoulder arthroplasty. *J Shoulder Elbow Surg* 2008;17(6):925-935.

A retrospective review of 337 shoulders with a 62% incidence of notching after RSA found that the highest incidence of notching was in those with rotator cuff tear arthropathy. The rate was higher if an anterosuperior approach was used rather than a deltopectoral approach.

5: Arthritis and Arthroplasty

42. Simovitch RW, Zumstein MA, Lohri E, Helmy N, Gerber C: Predictors of scapular notching in patients managed with the Delta III reverse total shoulder replacement. *J Bone Joint Surg Am* 2007;89(3):588-600.

The angle between the glenosphere and the scapular neck and the height of glenosphere implantation were highly correlated with the development of scapular notching. Patients with notching had a relatively poor clinical outcome. Level of evidence: II.

43. Gutiérrez S, Levy JC, Frankle MA, et al: Evaluation of abduction range of motion and avoidance of inferior scapular impingement in a reverse shoulder model. *J Shoulder Elbow Surg* 2008;17(4):608-615.

A biomechanical study found that the glenosphere center of rotation offset had the greatest effect on range of motion. The neck-shaft angle had the greatest effect on scapular notching.

44. Sirveaux F, Favard L, Oudet D, Huquet D, Walch G, Molé D: Grammont inverted total shoulder arthroplasty in the treatment of glenohumeral osteoarthritis with massive rupture of the cuff: Results of a multicentre study of 80 shoulders. *J Bone Joint Surg Br* 2004;86(3):388-395.

45. Edwards TB, Williams MD, Labriola JE, Elkousy HA, Gartsman GM, O'Connor DP: Subscapularis insufficiency and the risk of shoulder dislocation after reverse shoulder arthroplasty. *J Shoulder Elbow Surg* 2009; 18(6):892-896.

The incidence of dislocation was compared in patients with a repairable or irreparable subscapularis. An irreparable subscapularis tendon was found to be a significant risk factor for postoperative dislocation. Level of evidence: IV.

46. Clark JC, Ritchie J, Song FS, et al: Complication rates, dislocation, pain, and postoperative range of motion after reverse shoulder arthroplasty in patients with and without repair of the subscapularis. *J Shoulder Elbow Surg* 2012;21(1):36-41.

No correlation was found between subscapularis repair and post-RSA complications, dislocation, pain, or motion. Level of evidence: III.

47. Gerber C, Pennington SD, Nyffeler RW: Reverse total shoulder arthroplasty. *J Am Acad Orthop Surg* 2009; 17(5):284-295.

The design rationale, indications, and the technique for RSA are reviewed, and clinical experience and common complications are discussed.

48. Guery J, Favard L, Sirveaux F, Oudet D, Mole D, Walch G: Reverse total shoulder arthroplasty: Survivorship analysis of eighty replacements followed for five to ten years. *J Bone Joint Surg Am* 2006;88(8): 1742-1747.

49. Jasty M, Bragdon C, Burke D, O'Connor D, Lowenstein J, Harris WH: In vivo skeletal responses to porous-surfaced implants subjected to small induced motions. *J Bone Joint Surg Am* 1997;79(5):707-714.

50. Gutiérrez S, Keller TS, Levy JC, Lee WE III, Luo ZP: Hierarchy of stability factors in reverse shoulder arthroplasty. *Clin Orthop Relat Res* 2008;466(3): 670-676.

A biomechanical study concluded that compressive forces generated by muscles are the most important factor in maintaining stability after RSA.

51. Walch G, Mottier F, Wall B, Boileau P, Molé D, Favard L: Acromial insufficiency in reverse shoulder arthroplasties. *J Shoulder Elbow Surg* 2009;18(3): 495-502.

In 457 patients with RSA, preoperative acromial lesions had no effect on range of motion, Constant score, or subjective results. Those with postoperative acromial fracture had inferior functional and subjective results. Level of evidence: III.

Section 6

Trauma and Fractures

SECTION EDITOR:
ANAND M. MURTHI, MD

Chapter 33

Proximal Humeral Fractures

John-Erik Bell, MD, MS

Introduction

Proximal humeral fracture is the third most common extremity fragility fracture in individuals older than 65 years, behind hip and distal radius fractures. Although these fractures most frequently occur in older adults as a consequence of low-energy trauma, as in a fall, they also occur in younger patients as a result of higher energy trauma. Most proximal humeral fractures are nondisplaced or minimally displaced, and usually they are treated nonsurgically. Nonsurgical treatment of a minimally displaced fracture leads to a predictably good outcome. The options for managing a displaced fracture include nonsurgical treatment, percutaneous pinning, open reduction and internal fixation, and primary arthroplasty. The management of displaced fractures can be difficult, controversial, and fraught with complications. The aging of the US population and the widespread osteoporosis associated with aging mean that rates of proximal humeral fracture probably will increase, as will those of other fragility fractures. Proximal humeral fractures are likely to impose a significant and increasing burden on the healthcare system.

Anatomy and Classification

Codman first described the epiphyseal lines of the proximal humerus in 1934; he divided the proximal humerus into four anatomic fragments: the articular segment, the greater tuberosity, the lesser tuberosity, and the humeral shaft.[1] Neer built his widely adopted classification system on parts he defined as angulation of 45° or displacement of 1 cm of any of the four fragments described by Codman.[2] Displacement of one of the parts is determined by its musculotendinous attachments. The supraspinatus and infraspinatus pull the greater tuberosity posteriorly and superiorly. The subscapularis pulls the lesser tuberosity anteriorly and medially. The pectoralis major and deltoid pull the humeral shaft proximally and medially, producing apex anterior angulation.

Neither Dr. Bell nor any immediate family member has received anything of value from or has stock or stock options held in a commercial company or institution related directly or indirectly to the subject of this chapter.

It is important to understand the vascularity of the proximal humerus because the risk of osteonecrosis is higher in some fracture patterns than in others, and this risk influences both the surgical indications and the prognosis. Originally the anterior circulation was believed to provide the dominant blood supply of the humeral head. The anterolateral branch of the anterior circumflex humeral artery enters bone at the junction of the intertubercular groove and the greater tuberosity proximally after ascending along the lateral aspect of the long head of the biceps, and it becomes the arcuate artery as it assumes an intraosseous course.[3] The importance of the posterior circulation recently has been emphasized.[4,5] The posterior humeral circumflex artery was found to contribute 64% of the articular segment blood supply; this finding helps to explain why not all fractures with complete disruption of the anterior circulation go on to osteonecrosis.

The Neer system is straightforward and relatively easy to apply, but does not directly take into account the vascularity of the proximal humerus, and it has mediocre interobserver and intraobserver reliability. The AO-ASIF classification system is based on both the fracture complexity and the extent of disruption of the humeral head blood supply. The three basic types are divided into a total of 27 groups and subgroups.[6] This classification system is comprehensive and correlated with outcomes and osteonecrosis, but it is very complex and has worse interobserver and intraobserver reliability than the Neer system.

The valgus-impacted fracture pattern was not part of the original Neer classification, but it was included in the updated 2002 Neer classification system.[7] In this three- or four-part fracture pattern, the head position relative to the shaft is in valgus and impacted onto the shaft (**Figure 1**). The greater tuberosity usually is displaced superiorly relative to the head. It is important to recognize this pattern because the blood supply usually is preserved, in contrast to most displaced three- and four-part fracture patterns. Rates of osteonecrosis are lower in valgus-impacted four-part fractures than in displaced four-part fractures and fracture-dislocations presumably because of preservation of the medial hinge blood supply.[8,9]

The intimate anatomic relationship between nerves and fractured structures in the proximal humerus leads to a high rate of neurologic injury in these fractures. The rate of electromyography-documented axillary

6: Trauma and Fractures

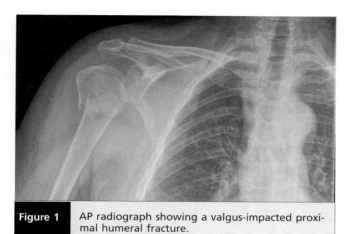

Figure 1 AP radiograph showing a valgus-impacted proximal humeral fracture.

nerve abnormality is 58%, and the rate of suprascapular nerve abnormality is as high as 48%.[10] Injury of the axillary artery has been reported as a complication of proximal humeral fracture, most commonly with fracture-dislocation.

Evaluation and Imaging

The patient history should include any preexisting shoulder symptoms that could indicate rotator cuff pathology, arthritis, or preinjury instability. The history also should include the mechanism of injury, any systemic comorbidities that might affect the safety of surgery or anesthesia, and the patient's social situation. The evaluation should include a thorough neurovascular examination, inspection of the skin, evaluation for associated injuries, and appropriate radiographs. The neurovascular examination should include the radial, median, ulnar, musculocutaneous (and lateral antebrachial cutaneous sensation), axillary, and suprascapular nerves. For the axillary nerve, deltoid muscle contraction and intact lateral shoulder sensation should be confirmed. The vascular examination always is important and is even more important with dislocation of the glenohumeral joint. Doppler or angiogram imaging may be included if there is a question of vascular injury.

The standard shoulder trauma radiographs include the true AP, scapular Y, and axillary views. Additional radiographs to evaluate for specific pathology include internal-external rotation views for occult surgical neck or greater tuberosity fracture, the West Point axillary view for anterior glenoid rim fracture, and the Stryker notch view for a Hill-Sachs lesion. These specialized views have been largely supplanted by the ready availability of CT, which usually provides much more detailed information for surgical decision making and planning.

Decision Making and Nonsurgical Treatment

The characteristics of the patient as well as the fracture must be considered in determining the best treatment course. The patient's comorbidities, activity level, hand dominance, age, and ability to comply with postoperative restrictions and instructions are important considerations. Fracture characteristics including bone quality, fracture pattern and displacement, humeral head vascularity, and neurologic status also should factor into the decision-making process.

The risk of osteonecrosis of the humeral head increases with fracture complexity.[11] Predictors of vascular disruption and subsequent osteonecrosis include length of the metaphyseal head extension (less than 8 mm), fracture type, and integrity of the medial hinge. The risk of osteonecrosis is increased in anatomic neck fractures, four-part displaced fractures, and all three-part fractures unless there is no fracture between the tuberosities. A longer metaphyseal extension is believed to be correlated with preservation of the posteromedial blood supply through the posterior humeral circumflex artery.[12]

Nondisplaced and minimally displaced fractures should be treated nonsurgically. This treatment is not controversial and is widely accepted as the standard of care. Most patients, even those with a stable fracture, are treated with 2 to 4 weeks of sling immobilization. Early physical therapy is recommended and is associated with an improved outcome in stable fractures. Usually, gentle range-of-motion exercises are safe, beginning with pendulums and pulleys and progressing over the first few weeks to passive range of motion.[13] At 6 weeks, active-assisted and active range-of-motion exercises usually can begin, provided that radiographs show no further displacement and there is evidence of early healing. Patients typically have a good result. High radiographic union rates, good functional outcomes, low complication rates, and minimal differences between the injured and contralateral sides on validated outcome scales have been reported.[14,15]

Fracture-dislocation can be treated in some patients with closed reduction and subsequent nonsurgical treatment. Prereduction radiographs should be scrutinized, however, because occult surgical neck fractures can become displaced during the reduction maneuver, potentially changing a nonoperative fracture to a difficult surgical case (**Figure 2**). A dislocation with nondisplaced fracture lines may require general anesthesia with fluoroscopic imaging to minimize the amount of force required and avoid displacement.

The surgical indications are more controversial for a displaced three- or four-part proximal humeral fracture. Recent prospective randomized studies have investigated these fracture patterns. Open reduction and internal fixation with a locking plate was compared with nonsurgical treatment of displaced three-part fractures; no statistically significant difference in outcome was found, but 30% of the patients treated with open re-

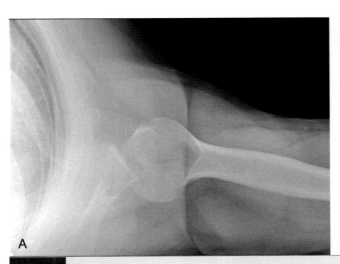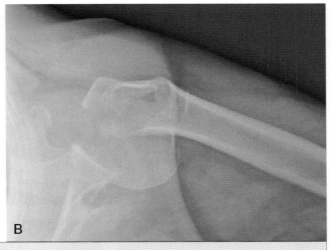

Figure 2 **A,** Axillary radiograph showing a posterior fracture-dislocation with an engaging reverse Hill-Sachs lesion. A nondisplaced crack extends into the surgical neck. **B,** After an attempted closed reduction, the fracture has become displaced.

duction and internal fixation required additional surgery.[16] These researchers conducted another prospective randomized controlled study to compare hemiarthroplasty and nonsurgical treatment of displaced four-part fractures. The patients treated with hemiarthroplasty had significant improvement in pain and quality of life, but there was no between-group difference in range of motion.[17] A systematic review published in 2004 found inadequate evidence to identify a consensus treatment of four-part fractures.[18]

Because no definitive evidence supports a surgical or nonsurgical treatment strategy for displaced proximal humeral fractures, the treatment often is determined by the experience and preference of the surgeon. There are significant regional variations in the proportion of fractures treated surgically or nonsurgically.[19,20]

Surgical Treatment

Surgical treatment of proximal humeral fractures typically is done with the patient in the beach-chair or supine position. General or regional anesthesia or a combination is used. The fluoroscopy machine is parallel to the table to allow orthogonal views of the shoulder without the need to move the arm significantly. The standard deltopectoral approach and the deltoid-splitting (anterolateral) approach are most commonly used. The deltopectoral approach is extensile and utilitarian for both fracture fixation and arthroplasty, although reaching the lateral and posterior aspects of the proximal humerus can be difficult. The anterolateral deltoid-splitting approach provides excellent exposure of the lateral humerus and greater tuberosity for fracture fixation, but it places the axillary nerve at increased risk and is not extensile.[21]

Percutaneous pinning is a good option for a surgical neck fracture or a valgus-impacted fracture with an intact medial hinge. Significant medial calcar communion

is a relative contraindication to pinning. The advantages of percutaneous pinning include preservation of fracture hematoma and a minimal need for incision, soft-tissue stripping, and permanent hardware, as well as a relatively low risk of osteonecrosis. The disadvantages include technical difficulty, the need for hardware removal, and an inability to initiate early range-of-motion exercises because of less secure fixation and pin prominence. Figure 3 illustrates the steps in percutaneous pinning. A small, 1-cm incision is made in the deltopectoral line, and a hemostat or Cobb elevator is inserted to elevate the head to the correct position. The head is pinned to the shaft using 2.8-mm terminally threaded pins. The greater tuberosity is reduced percutaneously with a hemostat and pinned to the head with 1.25-mm cannulated screw guidewires, which are overdrilled for 4.0-mm cannulated screw placement. The pins typically are removed at 3 to 4 weeks, and range-of-motion exercises then can be initiated. The results of percutaneous pinning generally are good.[22-25] In 27 patients with a two-, three-, or four-part fracture, percutaneous pinning led to a mean pain score of 1.4 on a 10-point visual analog pain scale, an American Shoulder and Elbow Surgeons (ASES) Shoulder Index score of 83.4, and a Constant Shoulder Score of 73.9 at an average 35-month follow-up.[26]

Open reduction and internal fixation has become an increasingly popular method of treatment since the introduction of locking-plate technology approximately 10 years ago. In addition to the locking plate, many other methods of open reduction and internal fixation have been described, including suture or wire, plate and screw, cannulated screw, and intramedullary fixation. The optimal fixation construct depends on both the fracture pattern and bone quality. Bone quality usually is poor, especially in the head. Frequently the best fixation method for the tuberosities avoids the tuberosity bone entirely and consists of suture fixation in the ro-

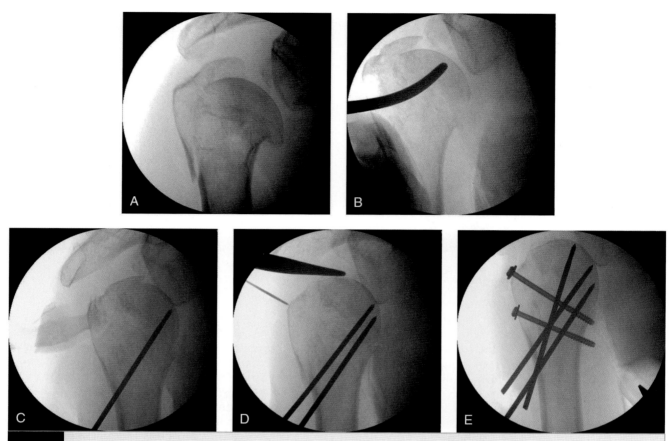

Figure 3   AP fluoroscopic images showing the technique for percutaneous pinning of a valgus-impacted three-part proximal humeral fracture. **A,** The humeral head is valgus impacted, and the greater tuberosity is elevated. **B,** A percutaneously placed hemostat is used to disimpact and elevate the head out of valgus. **C,** The head position is secured relative to the shaft using 2.8-mm terminally threaded pins. **D,** The percutaneous hemostat is used to reduce the greater tuberosity, which is provisionally fixed with guidewires for 4.0-mm cannulated screws. **E,** The cannulated screws with washers are advanced over guidewires to complete the construct.

tator cuff tendon insertion. If significant metaphyseal comminution is present, a fixed-angle construct (a blade plate or locking plate) or intramedullary fixation is preferred to prevent failure into varus.

Locking plates initially were shown to be biomechanically superior to the existing fixation constructs including T plates and buttress plates. The key feature of the proximal humeral locking plate is that the screws are directed toward the humeral head but are locked in different orientations, thereby increasing the pullout strength of the entire construct.[27-29] Locking-plate technology offers an option for open reduction and internal fixation in osteoporotic bone, for which arthroplasty or nonsurgical treatment had been the only other options. Locking-plate technology also offers a desirable option for young patients with relatively good bone stock who have a highly unstable high-energy fracture or a head-splitting fracture (**Figure 4**).

Although the use of locking plates has become popular and has allowed open reduction and internal fixation where it had not previously been possible, the associated rates of complications and reoperation are high. Most of the reported complications are related to hardware and technique, and they underscore the difficulty of treating these fractures, even for experienced surgeons. Many recent studies have documented the high complication and reoperation rates.[19,30-35] A large multicenter study of 187 patients reported a 34% complication rate when proximal humeral locking plates were used; 19% of the patients required a second, unplanned surgery within 12 months of the index procedure.[30] The complications include hardware penetration, varus collapse caused by loss of fixation, malunion, nonunion, infection, neurologic injury, adhesive capsulitis, and osteonecrosis, which often results in late hardware penetration as the humeral head collapses but the locked screws do not (**Figure 5**).

Attention to several specific points can minimize the risk of fixation-related complications. The most commonly reported early complication is screw penetration of the humeral head. This complication can best be avoided by measuring carefully, subtracting 5 mm from the measured length of each screw, and checking orthogonal images of all screws before leaving the operat-

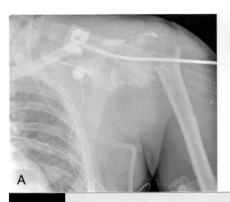 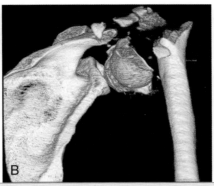 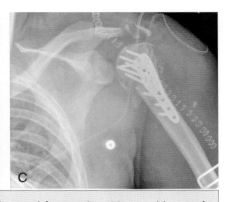

Figure 4   **A,** AP radiograph showing a high-energy comminuted four-part proximal humeral fracture in a 28-year-old man after a motor vehicle crash. **B,** Three-dimensional CT reconstruction showing intra-articular humeral head splitting. **C,** Postoperative AP radiograph showing open reduction and internal fixation with a locking proximal humerus plate.

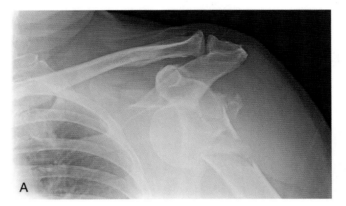

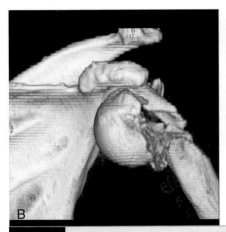 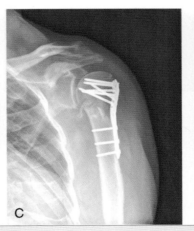 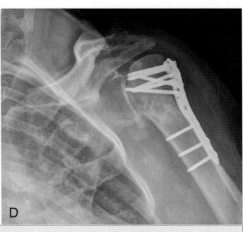

Figure 5   AP radiograph **(A)** and three-dimensional CT reconstruction **(B)** showing fracture-dislocation of the proximal humerus in a 45-year-old man. **C,** Postoperative AP radiograph showing open reduction and internal fixation with a locking proximal humerus plate. **D,** AP radiograph 1 year after surgery showing osteonecrosis causing pain and crepitus. The humeral head has collapsed. Because the screws are locking, they did not back out as the head collapsed and remained fixed, eventually penetrating past the subchondral bone into the glenohumeral joint.

ing room. Supplemental heavy suture fixation first through the rotator cuff bone-tendon junction and then through the plate can help prevent failure of tuberosity fixation or varus collapse. Most proximal humeral locking plates are designed to accommodate suture fix-

ation through the proximal aspect. Salvage of failed proximal humeral open reduction and internal fixation is technically challenging. For some complications, such as osteonecrosis, chronic rotator cuff insufficiency, or tuberosity nonunion, conversion to arthroplasty may

6: Trauma and Fractures

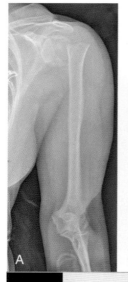
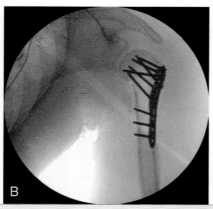
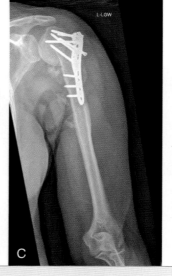
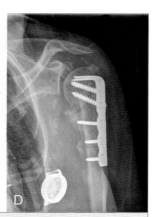

Figure 6 **A,** AP radiograph showing a displaced two-part proximal humeral fracture in a 60-year-old woman. **B,** AP fluoroscopic image showing initial treatment with a locking proximal humerus plate. **C,** AP radiograph showing varus collapse 6 weeks after surgery. **D,** AP radiograph showing revision to a 90° blade plate, which led to painless bony union.

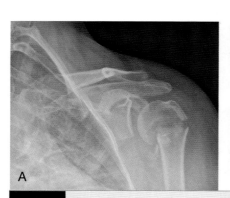
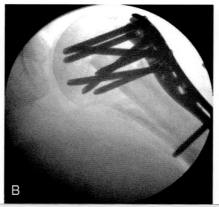
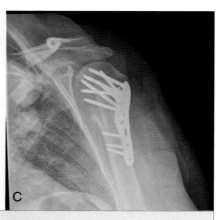

Figure 7 **A,** AP radiograph taken 4 weeks after a surgical neck two-part proximal humeral fracture in a 60-year-old patient with rheumatoid arthritis. The initial fracture treatment was nonsurgical, but the patient elected open reduction and internal fixation after progressive varus angulation and resorption at the fracture margins. AP fluoroscopic image (**B**) and AP radiograph (**C**) showing a standard proximal humeral locking plate applied with intramedullary fibular allograft strut for additional medial support against varus collapse.

be the best option. For fixation failure caused by a technical factor, revision to blade plate fixation is a reasonable option because often there is sufficient residual bone stock in the head to allow a successful revision (**Figure 6**).

Augmentation of internal fixation constructs with intramedullary allograft has received recent attention since it was first described in 2008.[36] Clinical results and recent biomechanical data have confirmed that intramedullary fibular strut augmentation of locking-plate fixation improves both maximal load to failure and initial construct stiffness.[36-38] This technique is most useful in fracture patterns with varus angulation

and loss of medial support, and it has been shown to prevent varus collapse (**Figure 7**).

Primary shoulder arthroplasty is an option for three-part, four-part, and head-splitting fractures. The decision to perform arthroplasty rather than open reduction and internal fixation depends not only on the fracture pattern but also on patient characteristics including age, activity level, and expectations. (**Figure 8**). The traditional standard has been hemiarthroplasty, but the reverse total shoulder prosthesis has become increasingly popular for managing these fractures, particularly in patients older than 70 years who have relatively low physical demands. The outcome of primary

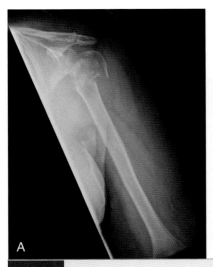
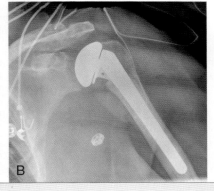
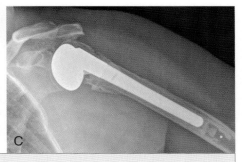

| Figure 8 | AP radiographs showing a displaced four-part proximal humeral fracture in an active 62-year-old woman before (A) and after (B) hemiarthroplasty. In (B), the tuberosity is in the appropriate position relative to the head. C, AP radiograph at 4-year follow-up, showing that the tuberosities are well healed. The patient had active forward elevation of 150° without pain. |

hemiarthroplasty is better than that of secondary arthroplasty after a proximal humeral fracture.[39] The most important factor in the outcome of hemiarthroplasty for fracture is the appropriate positioning and healing of the tuberosities.[40,41] Improper tuberosity position leads to poor postoperative strength and range of motion.[42] The ideal construct for tuberosity repair should consist of both horizontally and vertically oriented heavy sutures placed directly through the bone-tendon junction of the rotator cuff and through the prosthesis, if possible. The medial circumferential cerclage suture is biomechanically important for the stability of the repair construct.[43]

The indications for reverse shoulder arthroplasty continue to be refined and in recent years have included acute proximal humeral fractures in patients older than 70 years and with relatively low demands. Several recent studies have evaluated the outcome of reverse shoulder arthroplasty as the primary treatment of proximal humeral fracture. In the short term, the reverse arthroplasty predictably relieves pain and improves function.[44,45] In contrast to hemiarthroplasty, reverse shoulder arthroplasty can result in improved pain and function even if tuberosity healing does not occur. Nonetheless, tuberosity reconstruction is recommended with reverse arthroplasty for fracture to maximize external rotation function. A direct comparison of the outcomes of reverse shoulder arthroplasty and hemiarthroplasty found better abduction and overhead elevation with reverse arthroplasty but better internal and external rotation with hemiarthroplasty.[46] However, recent studies have documented mild deterioration in function and the development of lucent lines around the glenoid component at midterm follow-up.[47,48] Patients reported increasing pain, loss of strength, and deterioration of the Constant score between the 1-year

and mean 6.6-year follow-up. Only 58% of the patients were satisfied or very satisfied. The complication rate was 23%, and the reoperation rate was 17%.[48] Although early results have been promising, this study highlights the need for studies with longer term results before reverse shoulder arthroplasty for acute fractures of the proximal humerus can be widely recommended.

Summary

Proximal humeral fractures are common, and incidence in the United States is likely to increase based on changing demographics. An understanding of the anatomy and vascularity of the proximal humerus is necessary to accurately classify these fractures and formulate an appropriate treatment plan. Each of the many treatment options has distinct indications and complications, some of which can be significant. There is consensus that nondisplaced and minimally displaced fractures should be treated nonsurgically, but no consensus exists on whether surgery improves outcomes significantly for displaced fractures or on the best surgical treatment for a given fracture pattern. More level I studies are needed to provide this evidence.

Annotated References

1. Codman E: *The Shoulder: Rupture of the Supraspinatus Tendon and Other Lesions in or About the Subacromial Bursa.* Brooklyn, NY, G Miller, 1934.

2. Neer CS II: Displaced proximal humeral fractures: Part I. Classification and evaluation. 1970. *Clin Orthop Relat Res* 2006;442:77-82.

3. Laing PG: The arterial supply of the adult humerus. *J Bone Joint Surg Am* 1956;38-A(5):1105-1116.

4. Hettrich CM, Boraiah S, Dyke JP, Neviaser A, Helfet DL, Lorich DG: Quantitative assessment of the vascularity of the proximal part of the humerus. *J Bone Joint Surg Am* 2010;92(4):943-948.

    A cadaver study evaluated the vascularity of the humeral head using gadolinium and polymer injections. The posterior circumflex humeral artery was found to contribute 64% and the anterior humeral circumflex artery to contribute 36%.

5. Brooks CH, Revell WJ, Heatley FW: Vascularity of the humeral head after proximal humeral fractures: An anatomical cadaver study. *J Bone Joint Surg Br* 1993;75(1):132-136.

6. Marsh JL, Slongo TF, Agel J, et al: Fracture and dislocation classification compendium - 2007: Orthopaedic Trauma Association classification, database and outcomes committee. *J Orthop Trauma* 2007;21(10, suppl):S1-S133.

7. Neer CS II: Four-segment classification of proximal humeral fractures: Purpose and reliable use. *J Shoulder Elbow Surg* 2002;11(4):389-400.

8. Jakob RP, Miniaci A, Anson PS, Jaberg H, Osterwalder A, Ganz R: Four-part valgus impacted fractures of the proximal humerus. *J Bone Joint Surg Br* 1991;73(2):295-298.

9. DeFranco MJ, Brems JJ, Williams GR Jr, Iannotti JP: Evaluation and management of valgus impacted four-part proximal humerus fractures. *Clin Orthop Relat Res* 2006;442:109-114.

10. Visser CP, Coene LN, Brand R, Tavy DL: Nerve lesions in proximal humeral fractures. *J Shoulder Elbow Surg* 2001;10(5):421-427.

11. Lee CK, Hansen HR: Post-traumatic avascular necrosis of the humeral head in displaced proximal humeral fractures. *J Trauma* 1981;21(9):788-791.

12. Hertel R, Hempfing A, Stiehler M, Leunig M: Predictors of humeral head ischemia after intracapsular fracture of the proximal humerus. *J Shoulder Elbow Surg* 2004;13(4):427-433.

13. Koval KJ, Gallagher MA, Marsicano JG, Cuomo F, McShinawy A, Zuckerman JD: Functional outcome after minimally displaced fractures of the proximal part of the humerus. *J Bone Joint Surg Am* 1997;79(2):203-207.

14. Iyengar JJ, Devcic Z, Sproul RC, Feeley BT: Nonoperative treatment of proximal humerus fractures: A systematic review. *J Orthop Trauma* 2011;25(10):612-617.

    A systematic review of nonsurgically treated proximal humeral fractures found a 98% rate of radiographic union and a predictably good Constant score averaging 74. The complication rate was 13%, with varus malunion the most common.

15. Hanson B, Neidenbach P, de Boer P, Stengel D: Functional outcomes after nonoperative management of fractures of the proximal humerus. *J Shoulder Elbow Surg* 2009;18(4):612-621.

    A prospective case study followed 124 patients for 1 year after a nonsurgically treated proximal humeral fracture. The difference between the injured and normal shoulders on the Constant and Disabilities of the Arm, Shoulder and Hand questionnaire scores was only 8.2 and 10.2, respectively.

16. Olerud P, Ahrengart L, Ponzer S, Saving J, Tidermark J: Internal fixation versus nonoperative treatment of displaced 3-part proximal humeral fractures in elderly patients: A randomized controlled trial. *J Shoulder Elbow Surg* 2011;20(5):747-755.

    A comparison of locking-plate and nonsurgical treatment of displaced three-part fractures found a trend toward better outcomes in patients treated with a locking plate, but there was no statistically significant between-group difference in pain or function. The surgically treated patients had a 30% reoperation rate. Level of evidence: I.

17. Olerud P, Ahrengart L, Ponzer S, Saving J, Tidermark J: Hemiarthroplasty versus nonoperative treatment of displaced 4-part proximal humeral fractures in elderly patients: A randomized controlled trial. *J Shoulder Elbow Surg* 2011;20(7):1025-1033.

    A comparison of hemiarthroplasty and nonsurgical treatment of displaced four-part proximal humeral fractures found that pain relief was significantly better in patients treated with hemiarthroplasty; there was no between-group difference in range of motion. Level of evidence: I.

18. Bhandari M, Matthys G, McKee MD; Evidence-Based Orthopaedic Trauma Working Group: Four part fractures of the proximal humerus. *J Orthop Trauma* 2004;18(2):126-127.

19. Bell J-E, Leung BC, Spratt KF, et al: Trends and variation in incidence, surgical treatment, and repeat surgery of proximal humeral fractures in the elderly. *J Bone Joint Surg Am* 2011;93(2):121-131.

    Using Medicare data, this study found a 25.6% increase in surgically managed proximal humeral fractures from 1999 to 2005, with significant regional variation in the proportion of fractures treated surgically and increasing rates of reoperation.

20. Sporer SM, Weinstein JN, Koval KJ: The geographic incidence and treatment variation of common fractures of elderly patients. *J Am Acad Orthop Surg* 2006;14(4):246-255.

21. Nicandri GT, Trumble TE, Warme WJ: Lessons learned from a case of proximal humeral locked plating gone awry. *J Orthop Trauma* 2009;23(8):607-611.

A case report documented entrapment of the axillary nerve between the plate and the humerus during open reduction and internal fixation using the direct lateral approach.

22. Herscovici D Jr, Saunders DT, Johnson MP, Sanders R, DiPasquale T: Percutaneous fixation of proximal humeral fractures. *Clin Orthop Relat Res* 2000; 375(375):97-104.

23. Jaberg H, Warner JJ, Jakob RP: Percutaneous stabilization of unstable fractures of the humerus. *J Bone Joint Surg Am* 1992;74(4):508-515.

24. Resch H, Povacz P, Fröhlich R, Wambacher M: Percutaneous fixation of three- and four-part fractures of the proximal humerus. *J Bone Joint Surg Br* 1997; 79(2):295-300.

25. Magovern B, Ramsey ML: Percutaneous fixation of proximal humerus fractures. *Orthop Clin North Am* 2008;39(4):405-416, v.

    Indications, techniques, and outcomes are reviewed for percutaneous pinning of proximal humeral fractures.

26. Keener JD, Parsons BO, Flatow EL, Rogers K, Williams GR, Galatz LM: Outcomes after percutaneous reduction and fixation of proximal humeral fractures. *J Shoulder Elbow Surg* 2007;16(3):330-338.

    A case study reviewed proximal humeral fractures reduced and treated percutaneously in 35 patients. At an average 35-month follow-up, all fractures had healed and ASES and Constant scores were 83.4 and 73.9, respectively, with a mean visual analog pain score of only 1.4.

27. Liew AS, Johnson JA, Patterson SD, King GJ, Chess DG: Effect of screw placement on fixation in the humeral head. *J Shoulder Elbow Surg* 2000;9(5):423-426.

28. Weinstein DM, Bratton DR, Ciccone WJ II, Elias JJ: Locking plates improve torsional resistance in the stabilization of three-part proximal humeral fractures. *J Shoulder Elbow Surg* 2006;15(2):239-243.

29. Hessmann MH, Hansen WS, Krummenauer F, Pol TF, Rommens PM: Locked plate fixation and intramedullary nailing for proximal humerus fractures: A biomechanical evaluation. *J Trauma* 2005;58(6):1194-1201.

30. Südkamp N, Bayer J, Hepp P, et al: Open reduction and internal fixation of proximal humeral fractures with use of the locking proximal humerus plate: Results of a prospective, multicenter, observational study. *J Bone Joint Surg Am* 2009;91(6):1320-1328.

    In a prospective observational study of 187 proximal humeral fractures treated with locking plates, the average Constant score was 85% of that of the contralateral shoulder at 1-year follow-up. There was a 34% complication rate with a 19% reoperation rate.

31. Brunner F, Sommer C, Bahrs C, et al: Open reduction and internal fixation of proximal humerus fractures using a proximal humeral locked plate: A prospective multicenter analysis. *J Orthop Trauma* 2009;23(3): 163-172.

    At 1-year follow-up of 157 patients treated with a proximal humeral locking plate, good functional outcomes were reported. The average Constant score was 72 (87% of the contralateral side score), but with a 35% complication rate.

32. Ricchetti ET, Warrender WJ, Abboud JA: Use of locking plates in the treatment of proximal humerus fractures. *J Shoulder Elbow Surg* 2010;19(2, suppl):66-75.

    In 54 patients with a proximal humeral fracture treated with a locking plate who were followed for a minimum of 6 months, overall good results were reflected in an average ASES score of 70.8, but with a 20.4% complication rate.

33. Röderer G, Erhardt J, Kuster M, et al: Second generation locked plating of proximal humerus fractures: A prospective multicentre observational study. *Int Orthop* 2011;35(3):425-432.

    In a multicenter prospective study of 131 patients who underwent locked plating of proximal humeral fractures through a deltopectoral or direct lateral approach, the complications included screw perforation (15%) and displacement after open reduction and internal fixation (8%).

34. Röderer G, Erhardt J, Graf M, Kinzl L, Gebhard F: Clinical results for minimally invasive locked plating of proximal humerus fractures. *J Orthop Trauma* 2010;24(7):400-406.

    In a prospective study of 13 patients treated with a locking plate, three fractures had not healed at a minimum 6-month follow-up. The general complication rate was 21%, and the implant-related complication rate was 17%.

35. Ong C, Bechtel C, Walsh M, Zuckerman JD, Egol KA: Three- and four-part fractures have poorer function than one-part proximal humerus fractures. *Clin Orthop Relat Res* 2011;469(12):3292-3299.

    Outcomes were compared for patients with a two-part fracture treated nonsurgically and patients with a three- or four-part fracture treated with a locking plate. The patients with a locking plate had inferior outcomes, as shown by Medical Outcomes Study 36-Item Short Form and ASES scores, with more complications. Range of motion was similar between groups.

36. Gardner MJ, Boraiah S, Helfet DL, Lorich DG: Indirect medial reduction and strut support of proximal humerus fractures using an endosteal implant. *J Orthop Trauma* 2008;22(3):195-200.

    The steps were outlined for using a fibular allograft in the endosteal canal to support fixation of proximal humerus locking plate constructs.

6: Trauma and Fractures

37. Osterhoff G, Baumgartner D, Favre P, et al: Medial support by fibula bone graft in angular stable plate fixation of proximal humeral fractures: An in vitro study with synthetic bone. *J Shoulder Elbow Surg* 2011; 20(5):740-746.

    A synthetic bone study compared the biomechanics of locking-plate fixation with those of locking plate fixation with intramedullary fibular allograft. Treatment with allograft was found to decrease migration and increase stiffness.

38. Bae J-H, Oh J-K, Chon C-S, Oh CW, Hwang JH, Yoon YC: The biomechanical performance of locking plate fixation with intramedullary fibular strut graft augmentation in the treatment of unstable fractures of the proximal humerus. *J Bone Joint Surg Br* 2011; 93(7):937-941.

    A biomechanical study compared two-part surgical neck fractures in cadavers treated with a proximal humeral locking plate or a locking plate with intramedullary fibular strut graft. Maximum load to failure and stiffness were greater and displacement was less for those with fibular strut graft combined with a locking plate.

39. Bosch U, Skutek M, Fremerey RW, Tscherne H: Outcome after primary and secondary hemiarthroplasty in elderly patients with fractures of the proximal humerus. *J Shoulder Elbow Surg* 1998;7(5):479-484.

40. Kralinger F, Schwaiger R, Wambacher M, et al: Outcome after primary hemiarthroplasty for fracture of the head of the humerus: A retrospective multicentre study of 167 patients. *J Bone Joint Surg Br* 2004; 86(2):217-219.

41. Boileau P, Krishnan SG, Tinsi L, Walch G, Coste JS, Molé D: Tuberosity malposition and migration: Reasons for poor outcomes after hemiarthroplasty for displaced fractures of the proximal humerus. *J Shoulder Elbow Surg* 2002;11(5):401-412.

42. Frankle MA, Greenwald DP, Markee BA, Ondrovic LE, Lee WE III: Biomechanical effects of malposition of tuberosity fragments on the humeral prosthetic reconstruction for four-part proximal humerus fractures. *J Shoulder Elbow Surg* 2001;10(4):321-326.

43. Frankle MA, Ondrovic LE, Markee BA, Harris ML, Lee WE III: Stability of tuberosity reattachment in proximal humeral hemiarthroplasty. *J Shoulder Elbow Surg* 2002;11(5):413-420.

44. Lenarz C, Shishani Y, McCrum C, Nowinski RJ, Edwards TB, Gobezie R: Is reverse shoulder arthroplasty appropriate for the treatment of fractures in the older patient? Early observations. *Clin Orthop Relat Res* 2011;469(12):3324-3331.

    At 12-month follow-up, 30 patients who underwent primary reverse shoulder arthroplasty for acute three- or four-part proximal humeral fracture had a mean ASES score of 78, a mean active forward elevation of 139°, and a visual analog scale pain score of only 1.1. The complication rate was 10%.

45. Bufquin T, Hersan A, Hubert L, Massin P: Reverse shoulder arthroplasty for the treatment of three- and four-part fractures of the proximal humerus in the elderly: A prospective review of 43 cases with a short-term follow-up. *J Bone Joint Surg Br* 2007;89(4):516-520.

    A case study of 43 patients who underwent reverse shoulder arthroplasty for proximal humeral fracture reported satisfactory clinical outcomes despite tuberosity migration at a mean 22-month follow-up.

46. Gallinet D, Clappaz P, Garbuio P, Tropet Y, Obert L: Three or four parts complex proximal humerus fractures: Hemiarthroplasty versus reverse prosthesis. A comparative study of 40 cases. *Orthop Traumatol Surg Res* 2009;95(1):48-55.

    This study is the only direct comparison of reverse shoulder arthroplasty and hemiarthroplasty for three- and four-part proximal humeral fractures. Forty patients were studied. Patients treated with reverse shoulder arthroplasty had greater active forward elevation, and those treated with hemiarthroplasty had greater active external rotation. Their scores on the Disabilities of the Arm, Shoulder and Hand questionnaire scores were equivalent.

47. Cazeneuve JF, Cristofari D-J: The reverse shoulder prosthesis in the treatment of fractures of the proximal humerus in the elderly. *J Bone Joint Surg Br* 2010; 92(4):535-539.

    A case study of reverse shoulder arthroplasty for proximal humerus fractures found radiographic glenoid loosening in 23 of 36 patients (63%) at a mean 6.6-year follow-up, with advancing scapular notching and decreasing Constant scores compared with short-term outcomes.

48. Cazeneuve J-F, Cristofari D-J: Long term functional outcome following reverse shoulder arthroplasty in the elderly. *Orthop Traumatol Surg Res* 2011;97(6):583-589.

    When 36 reverse shoulder arthroplasties were followed for a mean 6.6 years, a 63% incidence of radiographic glenoid loosening was found, with progressive notching and gradual deterioration of Constant scores over time.

Chapter 34

Treatment of Severe Acute Proximal Humeral Fractures

Mark J. Jo, MD   Michael J. Gardner, MD

Introduction

Most proximal humeral fractures are minimally displaced and stable, and they can be successfully treated without surgery. The indications for surgical treatment are not well defined. The main goal of treatment is a pain-free shoulder that functions to the patient's satisfaction. Patient factors need to be strongly considered when the best course of treatment is being determined, with the emphasis on the patient's physiologic age, not chronologic age. In the past, chronologic age was used as a definitive indication for treatment. Patients older than 65 years often were referred to as elderly and were assumed to lead sedentary or relatively inactive lives. The patient population is rapidly changing, however. Patients in their 60s and 70s are leading more active lifestyles, and chronologic age has become a broad variable.

Treatment decision making should be guided by the needs and expectations of the individual patient. A patient with limited function or cognitive limitations may tolerate a painless nonunion and a stiff shoulder, but a physiologically young and active patient would expect a well-united shoulder with a greater functional range of motion. Most patients with proximal humeral fractures fall between these two extremes, but they tend to be relatively old and less active, and they may do well with some malunion, decreased range of motion, and decreased function. The quantifiable risks of surgical treatment, such as those associated with general or regional anesthesia, surgical dissection, and fixation failure, must be weighed against the patient's functional demands, preinjury activity level, and mental status. Whether the fracture is in the dominant or the nondominant upper extremity also must be considered.

Dr. Gardner or an immediate family member serves as a paid consultant to or is an employee of Synthes, DGIMed, Amgen, Stryker, and RTI Biologics; has received research or institutional support from Synthes and Amgen; and serves as a board member, owner, officer, or committee member of the Orthopaedic Trauma Association. Neither Dr. Jo nor any immediate family member has received anything of value from or has stock or stock options held in a commercial company or institution related directly or indirectly to the subject of this chapter.

Epidemiology and Mechanisms of Injury

Proximal humeral fractures represent approximately 5% of all fractures; approximately 80,000 occur annually in the United States.[1] As the osteoporosis epidemic continues, the prevalence of proximal humeral fragility fractures is increasing. Like most fractures, proximal humeral fractures occur in a bimodal distribution among relatively young and old patients (patients in their 20s and 30s as well as patients older than 65 years). Proximal humeral fractures occur more frequently in women than in men.

Most proximal humeral fractures occur in patients of advanced age as a result of a low-energy mechanism, such as a fall from a standing height. Such a fracture should be considered truly pathologic, and a workup for osteoporosis should be initiated. The position of the arm at the moment of impact (adducted at the side or abducted and flexed, landing on an outstretched hand) determines the specific fracture pattern (varus or valgus). In younger patients, the typical mechanisms of proximal humeral fracture include high-energy accidents, such as a motor vehicle crash or a fall from a height.

Clinical Evaluation

Physical Examination

The physical examination should include an overall general assessment of the patient, including Advance Trauma Life Support protocols if a high-energy mechanism of injury occurred. A mental status examination may be indicated to rule out potential concomitant cerebral trauma in an older patient after a fall. A full examination of the skin around the shoulder should be performed, paying particular attention to any lacerations in the axilla that might indicate an open fracture. Gentle palpation to assess tenderness and crepitus may help delineate additional injured structures, such as the clavicle, scapula, elbow, and wrist. A careful, complete vascular and neurologic examination of the distal extremity should be performed.

In fracture patterns that involve the surgical neck, the anatomic proximity of the axillary nerve makes it

6: Trauma and Fractures

particularly vulnerable to injury from contusion or entrapment at the fracture site. Accurate assessment of axillary nerve motor function in a patient with an acute injury is difficult, but often it is possible to visualize firing of the deltoid muscle, particularly the anterior head, without active elevation. Axillary nerve sensation over the lateral shoulder girdle should be assessed.

The rotator cuff frequently is ruptured in a displaced proximal humeral fracture. A large tear in a healthy tendon may occur in younger patients, and an acute-on-chronic tear more frequently occurs in older patients. A recent MRI study of 76 patients with a nonsurgically treated acute proximal humeral fracture revealed 22 rotator cuff tears, 4 of which were full-thickness tears.[2] Assessment of rotator cuff function and integrity in an acutely fractured proximal humerus is difficult, but suspicion should be maintained as the fracture heals and rehabilitation progresses to active motion exercises.

Imaging

Appropriate, high-quality imaging is critical for accurately assessing a proximal humeral fracture and devising a treatment plan. A true scapular AP view is angled approximately 30° from the midline and profiles the glenohumeral joint. An internal rotation view can better visualize the tuberosities; this view may be useful for an isolated tuberosity fracture but typically is not necessary for an acute fracture that involves the proximal humeral metaphysis. A scapular Y view can provide additional information on sagittal plane displacement and fracture site contact. The axillary view is difficult to obtain, but it is important for ruling out associated dislocation of the glenohumeral joint and can provide information about neck displacement as well as the integrity and position of the lesser tuberosity. The axillary view requires abduction of the patient's arm, which can be painful with an acute fracture. However, most patients can tolerate 30° of abduction, which often is sufficient for a useful axillary view. A Velpeau axillary view may be obtained in lieu of a true axillary view.

CT is not required to fully assess most proximal humeral fractures but can be helpful in a high-energy injury in which the fracture lines are unpredictable and difficult to visualize because of displacement or comminution. If a clear profile of the fracture is not otherwise available, CT should be obtained to better understand the fracture and help guide treatment decision making. Three-dimensional CT has increased in popularity but adds significant expense and rarely affects the treatment plan.

The rotator cuff is vitally important for the functional outcome of patients with a proximal humeral fracture. MRI can be used to evaluate the rotator cuff before surgery, or the rotator cuff can be evaluated under direct visualization during surgery. Ultrasonography can be used after surgery, when metal implants would distort MRI. Some experts use MRI for fracture

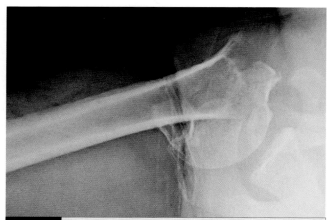

Figure 1 Axillary radiograph showing a reduced glenohumeral joint with anterior angulation of the proximal humeral fracture and a minimally displaced lesser tuberosity fracture. The amount of bony contact between the humeral head fragment and humeral shaft can be seen. The axillary view can provide critical information about the status of the glenohumeral joint, tuberosity displacement, and angulation and translation of the metaphyseal fracture.

patterns correlated with rotator cuff injury, such as a fracture with greater tuberosity displacement of more than 5 mm, a three- or four-part fracture, or an AO type 11B or 11C fracture.[3,4]

Nonsurgical Treatment

Indications

Multiple factors must be considered when determining the feasibility of nonsurgical treatment of a specific patient. The fracture pattern variables should be analyzed in terms of the two main consequences of fracture fragment displacement: the risk of nonunion and the effect of malunion on functional outcomes. Fractures that progress to nonunion clearly have a negative effect on function. Fractures with minimal bony contact, most commonly at the surgical neck level, are at increased risk for nonunion. The typical anterior angulation and translation of the humeral shaft often are best assessed using the axillary view (**Figure 1**). Radiographs should be interpreted given the patient's position because the supine position allows gravity to accentuate the deformity. Many moderately displaced fractures have a propensity to heal given the metaphyseal nature of the region and the relatively redundant blood supply. However, a malunion can lead to functional deficits. Greater tuberosity malunion can lead to shortening of the rotator cuff lever arm as well as impingement on the acromion during abduction and external rotation, thus limiting range of motion. Similarly, varus malunion can lead to impingement and limited shoulder motion. The precise amount of displacement that causes motion limitations is not clear. It is not advisable to adhere strictly to the traditional Neer thresholds of 1 cm and 45° of greater tuberosity displacement because they are not accurate for the prediction of stability and function. With displacement this extensive, a concomitant rotator cuff tear should be sought.

Aside from the functional effects of a fracture healing in its position at the time of the injury, fracture instability must be considered. The propensity for further displacement with nonsurgical treatment can be difficult to predict, but certain fracture features can shift the overall pattern toward greater instability. Displacement at the anatomic neck or the surgical neck, particularly with decreasing bony contact, creates a relatively unstable environment. Varus angulation in the proximal humerus typically is more unstable than valgus angulation. Comminution or displacement along the medial column (the calcar region) also predisposes the fracture to further displacement.

Treatment

When nonsurgical treatment is chosen based on fracture stability, the shoulder should be mobilized as soon as possible.[5] The use of a well-fitting sling for several days generally is sufficient for controlling pain and subsequently allowing early pendulum exercises. Whenever possible, passive exercises supervised by a physical therapist should be initiated within 14 days of injury to minimize adhesion formation and stiffness. Active-assisted exercises typically are initiated 4 to 6 weeks after injury. Strengthening exercises with a focus on the deltoid and periscapular muscles are begun when there is radiographic evidence of fracture healing.

If nonsurgical treatment is used for an unstable fracture because the patient has limited functional requirements or dementia, immobilization for 2 to 4 weeks should be considered to facilitate early fracture consolidation. The goal is to avoid further fracture displacement and thereby minimize the risk of nonunion.

Assessing stability or the risk of future displacement with early rehabilitation is difficult. Many factors must be considered, including the fracture variables and patient motivation. Fractures deemed to be stable may become displaced, requiring the treatment plan to be altered. For this reason, early and frequent radiographic follow-up is necessary if nonsurgical treatment is chosen.

Some patients may benefit from closed reduction of the fracture. Closed reduction can improve fracture alignment and bony contact, leading to improved healing and functional outcome.[6] A closed reduction can be done in the clinical setting, particularly if the patient is a poor surgical candidate or has moderate to severe fracture displacement but prefers to avoid surgery.

Surgical Treatment

The goal of surgical fixation is to achieve reduction and secure the reduction in a position that ensures reliable healing and maximizes function. Successful treatment depends on bone quality, humeral head viability, and the ability to maintain the reduction until healing can occur. Bone quality is patient dependent, can be evaluated preoperatively, and should be taken into consideration when planning treatment.[7] Poor bone stock may necessitate the use of mechanical augments, such as a fibular strut graft or biologic augmentation with an osteobiologic agent. The viability of the humeral head is based on its blood supply. Plain radiographs or CT can help determine whether the fracture is comminuted or markedly displaced. Humeral head blood flow can be predicted by observing the fracture pattern about the medial calcar region. Fractures with less than 8 mm of metaphyseal head extension and a disrupted medial hinge were more prone to humeral head ischemia.[8] A humeral head-splitting fracture formerly was considered to be dysvascular, but an improved understanding of outcomes and the availability of minifragment implants allow such a fracture to be considered for open reduction and internal fixation, particularly in a younger patient.

The Surgical Setup

The deltopectoral approach traditionally has been most widely used for the surgical fixation of proximal humeral fractures because it is extensile and allows visualization of the humeral shaft as well as the glenohumeral joint. Because this approach is anterior, the subscapularis, biceps tendon, and lesser tuberosity are easily accessible. Using the internervous plane between the deltoid and pectoral muscles minimizes the risk of neurologic injury, although the surgeon must be careful because the musculocutaneous and axillary nerves can be injured by vigorous retraction under the conjoined tendon or retractor misplacement under the deltoid. The anterior approach has an increased risk of injury to the cephalic vein or, more importantly, the anterior humeral circumflex artery, which provides a critical blood supply to the humeral head.[9] Injury to the anterior humeral circumflex artery can lead to osteonecrosis or nonunion. Extensive soft-tissue dissection may be necessary to gain access to the fracture and can strip the bone of its vascular supply. The most significant disadvantage of the deltopectoral approach is the limited access to the greater tuberosity and the lateral aspect of the humeral head, which is used as the footprint for most modern locking plates. Sutures typically are placed in the rotator cuff to allow internal rotation of the proximal fragment and improve access to the lateral humerus.

The anterolateral acromial approach was developed to eliminate some of the difficulties of using the deltopectoral approach.[10,11] Because this approach is on the lateral side of the shoulder, the axillary nerve is at risk. Anatomic studies have shown that the location of the anterior branch of the axillary nerve can be reliably located approximately 65 mm from the edge of the acromion.[10] This location should be measured and marked on the patient before incision. The anterolateral acromial approach usually requires a longitudinal incision beginning at the anterolateral corner of the acromion and extending approximately 12 to 15 cm distally (**Figure 2**). A shoulder strap incision that follows the skin tension lines also has been used and may be more cosmetically acceptable.[12-15] The deeper dissection exploits the avascular plane between the anterior and middle heads of the deltoid muscle. Blunt dissection is extended through the raphe. The axillary nerve is palpated and protected as the dissection is extended proximally and distally to the neurovascular bundle, creating both a proximal and a distal window through the fracture, whcih can be reduced and stabilized.

The anterolateral acromial approach allows direct visualization of the footprint for plate placement and improves access to the tuberosity fragments. The surgical plane is in line with the trajectory for the plate placement and locking screw. This approach allows access to the fracture lines as well as access for improved manipulation and reduction maneuvers for the fracture fragments. If the predominant fracture deformity is medialization of the humeral shaft, the plate can be used as an indirect reduction tool (**Figure 3**). The approach can be extended superiorly to gain access to the subacromial space for supraspinatus and infraspinatus visualization and access, which may reveal rotator cuff tearing that requires repair. The minimally invasive nature of the anterolateral acromial approach reduces the amount of soft-tissue disruption. Its main disadvantage is that the axillary nerve can be put at risk. The nerve must be correctly identified, carefully dissected, and meticulously protected during the entire procedure. The anterolateral acromial approach is not extensile and can limit access to the anterior surface of the humerus unless undue tension is placed on the axillary nerve.

Both the deltopectoral and the anterolateral acromial approaches can be used to successfully treat proximal humeral fractures. The fracture characteristics, the anticipated reduction techniques, and the surgeon's experience should be weighed to select the optimal ap-

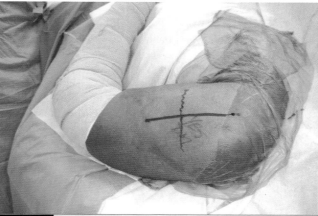

Figure 2 Photograph showing the skin incision for the anterolateral acromial approach, marked from the anterolateral corner of the acromion distally along the axis of the humeral shaft. The approximate position of the axillary nerve is marked at 65 mm from the palpable edge of the acromion. (Reproduced with permission from Gardner MJ: Open reduction and internal fixation of fractures of the proximal humerus: The anterolateral acromial approach, in Levine WN, Cadet ER, Ahmad CS, eds: *Shoulder and Elbow Trauma*. London, England, JP Medical Publishers, 2012, pp 51-60.)

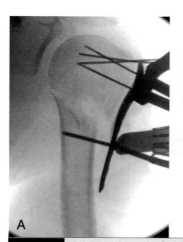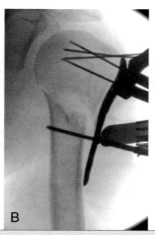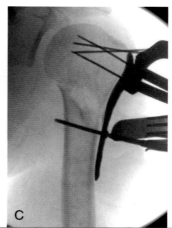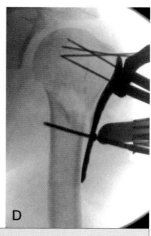

Figure 3 Fluoroscopic images showing the use of a plate as an indirect reduction tool through an anterolateral acromial approach. **A,** A well-placed proximal humeral plate, with residual medial displacement of the humeral shaft. **B** and **C,** The plate is used as a reduction device. As the screw is placed into the diaphysis and tightened, the humeral shaft is lateralized to the plate to achieve an anatomic reduction. **D,** A well-reduced proximal humerus. The reduction screw usually is long enough to facilitate the reduction. A shorter screw can be substituted after the humeral shaft is secured to the plate through the remaining holes. (Reproduced with permission from Gardner MJ: Open reduction and internal fixation of fractures of the proximal humerus: The anterolateral acromial approach, in Levine WN, Cadet ER, Ahmad CS, eds: *Shoulder and Elbow Trauma*. London, England, JP Medical Publishers, 2012, pp 51-60.)

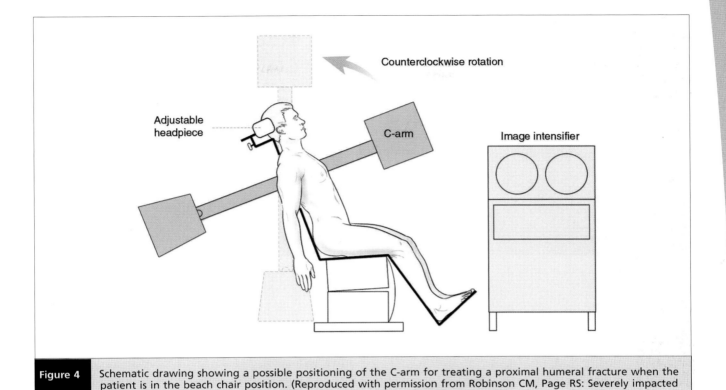

Figure 4 Schematic drawing showing a possible positioning of the C-arm for treating a proximal humeral fracture when the patient is in the beach chair position. (Reproduced with permission from Robinson CM, Page RS: Severely impacted valgus proximal humeral fractures. *J Bone Joint Surg Am* 2004;86[suppl 1]:143-155.)

proach. Because the deltopectoral approach is extensile, it may be better suited for arthroplasty or treatment of a severe malunion or nonunion. Arthroplasty performed through an anterior approach is more likely to be reproducible because much of the technique and instrumentation was developed for this approach. Access to the anterior humerus also is better through a deltopectoral approach when the lesser tuberosity is retracted medially more than 1 cm or access to the subscapularis tendon is required. The anterolateral acromial approach also can be used in treating a nonunion or a malunion, but access can be limited by the need to protect the axillary nerve from excessive traction. Arthroplasty can be performed through an anterolateral acromial approach if the surgeon is comfortable with this technique.

The deltopectoral or the anterolateral acromial approach can be used with the patient in a supine or beach chair position. If the beach chair position is used, fluoroscopy can be done lateral to the patient, on the opposite side of the patient, or from the head of the patient (**Figure 4**). Using a table with a specialized cutout behind the shoulder area can improve intraoperative imaging. The supine position is recommended; the patient is brought to the edge of the table, and the injured extremity is placed on a radiolucent support. It is critical to ensure that the bed rails are radiolucent or are not obstructing the AP view and that standard arm boards are not used. The C-arm is at the patient's head and can be moved to obtain AP and axillary views

(**Figure 5**). Regardless of technique, fluoroscopic images should be obtained before final preparation and draping to ensure that adequate images are obtained and identify any leads or wires that compromise the images.

Closed Reduction and Percutaneous Fixation

Closed reduction of the fracture is performed under fluoroscopic imaging. Manual traction can be used alone or with percutaneous reduction techniques, such as the insertion of elevators or other surgical instruments through stab incisions. After reduction is achieved, the fracture is secured using Kirschner wires or percutaneously placed screws.[16-19] The percutaneous technique is advantageous because it minimizes soft-tissue disruption and stripping from the humerus and surrounding soft tissues. Extensive surgical dissection can lead to postoperative scarring, osteonecrosis, and nonunion of the humeral head.[18] One or two Kirschner wires are placed in the lateral shaft below the insertion of the deltoid: one wire is placed in the anterior cortex, and, if needed, a second wire is placed from the greater tuberosity toward the medial calcar.[16] Anatomic studies have defined the optimal location of the pins[19,20] (**Figure 6**). To avoid injury to the anterior branch of the axillary nerve, the lateral pins should start at a distance of at least two humeral head diameters distal to the superiormost aspect of the humerus. Care should be taken to avoid the cephalic vein and the biceps tendon, which can be injured by the anterior pin. The wire in the

6: Trauma and Fractures

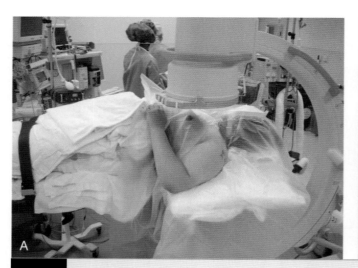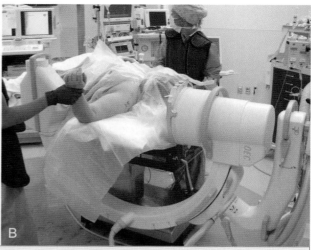

| Figure 5 | Photographs showing the patient in the supine position (**A**) and brought to the edge of the table with a radiolucent support for the arm (**B**) to obtain unencumbered AP and axillary radiographs. (Reproduced with permission from Gardner MJ: Open reduction and internal fixation of fractures of the proximal humerus: The anterolateral acromial approach, in Levine WN, Cadet ER, Ahmad CS, eds: *Shoulder and Elbow Trauma.* London, England, JP Medical Publishers, 2012, pp 51-60.) |

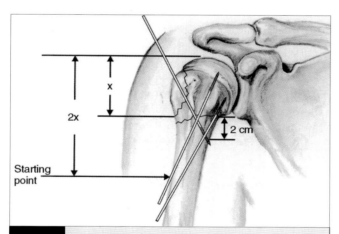

| Figure 6 | Schematic drawing showing the placement of lateral and greater tuberosity pins. The starting point for the proximal lateral pin should be at or distal to a point twice the distance from the superior aspect of the humeral head to the inferiormost margin of the humeral head. The greater tuberosity pins should engage the cortex of the humeral neck 20 mm from the inferiormost aspect of the humeral head. (Reproduced with permission from Rowles DJ, McGrory JE: Percutaneous pinning of the proximal part of the humerus: An anatomic study. *J Bone Joint Surg Am* 2001;83[11]:1695-1699.) |

greater tuberosity should penetrate the medial calcar region at least 2 cm distal to the inferior margin of the humeral head to avoid injury to the axillary nerve and the posterior circumflex artery. Although the percutaneous technique has been described for two-, three-, and four-part proximal humeral fractures, the outcome is poor if fixation of the greater tuberosity fails.[19] As with other minimally invasive techniques involving in-

direct reduction, percutaneous fixation can be technically challenging, and a mini-open technique should be considered for reduction and wire placement.

Suture Fixation

Suture fixation of a proximal humeral fracture eliminates some of the risks associated with a plate construct or arthroplasty. Transosseous suture techniques can decrease soft-tissue disruption and scarring and help preserve the vascular supply to the humeral head. The suture or wire technique was described by Neer for treating three-part fractures but has not been widely used.[21] Several recent studies have reported on this technique, however. In a study of 28 two- and three-part greater tuberosity or surgical neck proximal humeral fractures treated with a suture technique, 78% of the patients had an excellent result, and 11% had a satisfactory result.[22] At final follow-up in 165 two-, three-, and four-part fractures treated with a transosseous suture technique, the mean adjusted Constant score was 94%, compared with the unaffected shoulder[23,24] (Figure 7).

Plate Fixation

Techniques and indications for the surgical fixation of proximal humeral fractures have evolved over the years. Many of the early difficulties resulted from poor screw purchase in the humeral head. Many patients with a proximal humeral fracture frequently have poor bone quality in the metaphysis and the humeral head, and the surgery often led to screw cutout and collapse of the humeral head. Because of the high rate of fixation failure in complex fractures, arthroplasty was the recommended treatment for a three- or four-part fracture.[21] The development of angular stable locking-

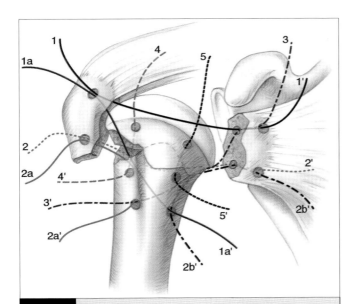

Figure 7 Schematic drawing showing surgical technique for suture-only fixation of a displaced four-part proximal humeral fracture. The suture strands are placed in the numbered order through the designated drill holes. ' = the suture end. Suture 1 fixes the greater tuberosity and the humeral shaft; 1a and 2, the greater tuberosity and the lesser tuberosity; 2a, the greater tuberosity and the humeral shaft; 3, the humeral shaft and the lesser tuberosity; 4 and 5, the humeral head and the humeral shaft. (Reproduced with permission from Dimakopoulos P, Panagopoulos A, Kasimatis G: Transosseous suture fixation of proximal humeral fractures: Surgical technique. *J Bone Joint Surg Am* 2009;91 [suppl 2]:8-21.)

screw technology and the availability of site-specific implants have helped reduce the risk of fixation failure. The fixed angle provides better fixation of the humeral head, and the trajectories and the number of screw options help to maximize fixation in the humeral head. Surgical fixation with plates and screws offers a more rigid construct than other modes of fixation but may require more soft-tissue dissection to adequately reduce and position the implant. The amount of soft-tissue disruption can be minimized by using the anterolateral acromial approach and an implant system designed for a minimally invasive technique. Although this newer technology has helped overcome some of the difficulties of treating proximal humeral fractures, it is not without complications.[25,26] Screw penetration of the humeral head and implant failure still can occur.

An accurate reduction is crucial for providing adequate mechanical stability, healing, and function of the shoulder.[6,27-29] After the medial calcar is properly reduced, placing an inferomedial screw is important for maintaining the reduction.[29] In a fracture that is displaced into varus, an overreduction into valgus may be preferable to improve the bony contact and prevent the fracture from falling back into varus. The position of the plate determines the trajectory and the position of the screw used for this purpose and the screws in the humeral head. Caution is required; although a site-specific plate is designed to fit the proximal humerus, the anatomy of individual patients varies. The plate must be placed sufficiently inferior to avoid impingement when the arm is abducted. The trajectory of the humeral head and the inferomedial screws should be checked to ensure that the fixation is maximized and the joint is not at risk for intra-articular penetration. The plate also must be placed posterior to the bicipital groove to preserve the blood supply to the humeral head. The reduction and the eventual healing of the tuberosities can greatly affect function and the outcome of the surgery. Nonabsorbable sutures should be placed in the tuberosity fragments and secured to one another and/or to the plate itself.

Augmentation

Some fractures may require structural or biologic augmentation or both. Although a proper reduction is the most important factor in the mechanical stability of a construct, the presence of osteoporosis, soft metaphyseal bone, or cancellous bone of the humeral head may limit bone-to-bone contact, even with an anatomic reduction. In many fractures, the bone fragments are impacted at the time of injury. Reduction requires disimpaction of the fragments, and large voids may remain after an adequate reduction. Autograft, allograft, cement, or bone substitutes can be used to fill the voids and provide structure or biologic support to the fracture.[30,31] Endosteal strut allografts may be useful in treating a comminuted posteromedial calcar or nonunion, or with revision surgery. Fibular strut allografts or femoral head allografts can be used to provide stability or strengthen the bone for screw purchase.[32]

Intramedullary Nail Fixation

Intramedullary nail fixation is an option for stabilizing a proximal humeral fracture. Newer nail designs have integrated interlocking screws that create an angular-stable implant. The advantage of intramedullary nail fixation is preservation of the soft-tissue envelope and the blood supply of the humerus. Earlier surgical techniques used the greater tuberosity as the entry site, with the risk of injury to the rotator cuff complex or postoperative shoulder pain. Some of these difficulties can be avoided by meticulous dissection and repair of the rotator cuff and by using a medial articular entry portal away from the footprint of the rotator cuff tendons.[33,34] The main indication for intramedullary nail fixation of a proximal humeral fracture has been a two-part fracture involving the surgical neck, but intramedullary nailing supplemented with suture fixation also has been used to treat three- and four-part fractures.[35-40] A humeral nail is excellent for use in proximal humeral fractures with metaphyseal or diaphyseal extension.

External Fixation

External fixation can be used to treat a proximal humeral fracture.[41-43] Like other minimally invasive techniques, external fixation minimizes soft-tissue stripping and blood loss. However, external fixation has several disadvantages. Anatomic structures are at risk during pin placement, and pin sites can become infected or loosen with time. The external frame can be cumbersome and is cosmetically unacceptable for some patients. External fixation may be useful in situations such as polytrauma, in which the patient cannot undergo a lengthy procedure or has significant soft-tissue injuries. Two- and three-part fractures have been treated with this technique with good results.[41-43] As with the percutaneous techniques described previously, the reduction is assisted by using an indirect technique or a mini-open approach, after which the pins are placed in the fragments and externally secured with bars and clamps

Evidence-Based Outcomes

Data from the US Medicare database indicate that the incidence of proximal humeral fractures in patients at least 65 years of age did not change from 1999 to 2005, but the use of surgical management increased by 25%.[1] The great variation in rates of surgical management among US geographic regions suggests a lack of consensus on the indications for open reduction and internal fixation for these injuries. Recent high-level evidence has begun to shed light on this debate.

The choice of surgical fixation or arthroplasty for a specific patient and fracture pattern depends on many factors and has evolved over time, particularly after the development of locking implants. Few studies have directly compared the procedures, and no randomized studies have been conducted. A recent retrospective review compared patients older than 55 years who had a three- or four-part fracture treated with a locking plate (38 patients) or hemiarthroplasty (48 patients).[27] In patients with a three-part fracture, treatment with a locking plate led to a better outcome than treatment with hemiarthroplasty (Constant score, 72 or 60, respectively; $P < 0.001$). The trend was similar for four-part fractures (Constant score, 65 or 60; $P = 0.19$). However, patients with a varus-extension pattern had a greater risk of complications, reduction loss, and poor outcomes than did other patients.[26] The use of acute reverse total shoulder arthroplasty for treating physiologically old patients with a severely displaced and comminuted proximal humeral fracture and a rotator cuff deficiency has increased.[44] It is important to recognize that tuberosity fixation is as crucial in arthroplasty as in internal fixation procedures.

In 53 patients older than 60 years who had a displaced proximal humeral fracture treated with locked plating, the complication rate was 36%, with a 43% incidence of screw cutout.[45] This study did not control for reduction accuracy, which is known to be critical for success with locked plating.[30] Another option for treating proximal humeral fractures is polyaxial locked plating. Despite the theoretic advantage of having more options for screw placement, a recent randomized study found no differences in functional outcomes based on whether polyaxial or standard locking screws were used.[46]

Intramedullary nailing remains the treatment of choice for several proximal humeral fracture patterns. A recent prospective randomized study of 51 patients with a two-part proximal humeral fracture found that at 1-year follow-up, patients treated with locking plates had better functional status than those treated with intramedullary nailing. Complication rates were higher in those treated with a plate, however.[36] At 3 years, there were no between-group differences in function. Patients in both groups had significantly improved function between 1-year and 3-year follow-up. In a retrospective study, 38 patients with a two-part fracture treated with an angular-stable nail through an articular entry point had reliable fracture healing, a favorable outcome, and minimal shoulder pain.[35]

Nonsurgical treatment still is a viable option for many patients, although the ideal indications remain somewhat unclear. In a study of 70 consecutive patients age 60 to 85 years with a nonsurgically treated displaced or nondisplaced fracture, those with a displaced fracture had a poor functional outcome (Constant score, 59); those with a nondisplaced fracture fared better (Constant score, 74), and those with a four-part fracture had the worst function (Constant score, 34).[47] Eighteen patients with low physical demands who had a displaced three- or four-part fracture had relatively poor function after nonsurgical treatment (mean Constant score, 61) at an average 39-month follow-up.[48] These studies were not corroborated by a recent randomized comparison of surgical and nonsurgical treatment in 50 patients older than 60 years who had a displaced three- or four-part fracture.[6] The nonsurgically treated patients underwent a closed reduction of the metaphysis and early physical therapy. One year after injury, no between-group differences in functional outcome were reported.

Summary

Proximal humeral fractures are challenging to treat, but careful consideration of the patient's expectations and prudent application of the chosen treatment can lead to a successful outcome. The optimal treatment of a proximal humeral fracture has not been fully elucidated. The introduction of new techniques and technology has spurred a significant shift in treatment trends, even before an opportunity for consistent improvements in patient outcomes existed. Studies have clearly shown that most proximal humeral fractures can be successfully treated without surgery. Surgical management should be reserved for the few patients who are at high risk of nonunion or who may require a higher level of function than can be provided by nonsurgical treatment. Individual patient factors are most important in determining whether surgery is appropriate. As the population ages and life expectancies increase, patients increasingly are more active later in life and may have different expectations of the outcome after a proximal humeral fracture than earlier generations. A variety of surgical options are available, and the selection should be made based on applicability to the fracture and the surgeon's experience.

Annotated References

1. Bell JE, Leung BC, Spratt KF, et al: Trends and variation in incidence, surgical treatment, and repeat surgery of proximal humeral fractures in the elderly. *J Bone Joint Surg Am* 2011;93(2):121-131.

   An analysis of Medicare data on treatment trends for proximal humeral fractures over 5 years found that the incidence of proximal humeral fractures was unchanged, but the rate of surgical treatment increased significantly.

2. Fjalestad T, Hole MO, Blücher J, Hovden IA, Stiris MG, Strømsøe K: Rotator cuff tears in proximal humeral fractures: An MRI cohort study in 76 patients. *Arch Orthop Trauma Surg* 2010;130(5):575-581.

3. Gallo RA, Sciulli R, Daffner RH, Altman DT, Altman GT: Defining the relationship between rotator cuff injury and proximal humerus fractures. *Clin Orthop Relat Res* 2007;458:70-77.

   An analysis of radiographic and MRI characteristics of proximal humeral fractures revealed that greater severity of rotator cuff injury was correlated with a higher AO or Neer classification and with 5 mm or more displacement of the greater tuberosity. Level of evidence: II.

4. Gallo RA, Altman DT, Altman GT: Assessment of rotator cuff tendons after proximal humerus fractures: Is preoperative imaging necessary? *J Trauma* 2009;66(3):951-953.

   The usefulness of MRI for proximal humeral fractures was reviewed, and a treatment algorithm was proposed. One- and two-part fractures associated with less than 5 mm of greater tuberosity displacement were found not to warrant MRI. MRI may be useful for two-part fractures with more than 5 mm of greater tuberosity displacement as well as three- and four-part fractures.

5. Lefevre-Colau MM, Babinet A, Fayad F, et al: Immediate mobilization compared with conventional immobilization for the impacted nonoperatively treated proximal humeral fracture: A randomized controlled trial. *J Bone Joint Surg Am* 2007;89(12):2582-2590.

   Patients with a proximal humeral fracture were randomly assigned to mobilization earlier than a few days or at 3 weeks. Early mobilization led to improved outcomes and no complications. Level of evidence: I.

6. Fjalestad T, Hole MO, Hovden IA, Blücher J, Strømsøe K: Surgical treatment with an angular stable plate for complex displaced proximal humeral fractures in elderly patients: A randomized controlled trial. *J Orthop Trauma* 2012;26(2):98-106.

   A comparison study of the surgical and nonsurgical treatment of older patients with a proximal humeral fracture found no difference in functional outcome at 1-year follow-up. Level of evidence: I.

7. Tingart MJ, Apreleva M, von Stechow D, Zurakowski D, Warner JJ: The cortical thickness of the proximal humeral diaphysis predicts bone mineral density of the proximal humerus. *J Bone Joint Surg Br* 2003;85(4):611-617.

8. Hertel R, Hempfing A, Stiehler M, Leunig M: Predictors of humeral head ischemia after intracapsular fracture of the proximal humerus. *J Shoulder Elbow Surg* 2004;13(4):427-433.

9. Gardner MJ, Voos JE, Wanich T, Helfet DL, Lorich DG: Vascular implications of minimally invasive plating of proximal humerus fractures. *J Orthop Trauma* 2006;20(9):602-607.

10. Gardner MJ, Griffith MH, Dines JS, Briggs SM, Weiland AJ, Lorich DG: The extended anterolateral acromial approach allows minimally invasive access to the proximal humerus. *Clin Orthop Relat Res* 2005;434:123-129.

11. Gardner MJ, Boraiah S, Helfet DL, Lorich DG: The anterolateral acromial approach for fractures of the proximal humerus. *J Orthop Trauma* 2008;22(2):132-137.

    Fifty-two patients with a proximal humeral fracture were treated using a minimally invasive anterolateral approach, which led to a good functional outcome and no axillary nerve injuries.

12. Robinson CM, Murray IR: The extended deltoid-splitting approach to the proximal humerus: Variations and extensions. *J Bone Joint Surg Br* 2011;93(3):387-392.

    Variations and extensions of the anterolateral surgical approach for the surgical treatment of proximal humeral fractures were presented, with a description of the indications and approaches used in 386 patients during a 12-year period.

13. Robinson CM, Khan L, Akhtar A, Whittaker R: The extended deltoid-splitting approach to the proximal humerus. *J Orthop Trauma* 2007;21(9):657-662.

    Experience with an extended deltoid-splitting approach for the treatment of proximal humeral fractures was presented. During a 9-year period, 226 patients underwent surgical fixation using this approach, with no major complications.

14. Robinson CM, Page RS: Severely impacted valgus proximal humeral fractures: Results of operative treatment. *J Bone Joint Surg Am* 2003;85-A(9):1647-1655.

15. Robinson CM, Page RS: Severely impacted valgus proximal humeral fractures. *J Bone Joint Surg Am* 2004;86-A(Suppl 1, Pt 2):143-155.

16. Jaberg H, Warner JJ, Jakob RP: Percutaneous stabilization of unstable fractures of the humerus. *J Bone Joint Surg Am* 1992;74(4):508-515.

17. Resch H, Povacz P, Fröhlich R, Wambacher M: Percutaneous fixation of three- and four-part fractures of the proximal humerus. *J Bone Joint Surg Br* 1997; 79(2):295-300.

18. Keener JD, Parsons BO, Flatow EL, Rogers K, Williams GR, Galatz LM: Outcomes after percutaneous reduction and fixation of proximal humeral fractures. *J Shoulder Elbow Surg* 2007;16(3):330-338.

    A cohort study revealed that in selected patients, percutaneous fixation led to reliable union and good clinical outcome.

19. Rowles DJ, McGrory JE: Percutaneous pinning of the proximal part of the humerus: An anatomic study. *J Bone Joint Surg Am* 2001;83(11):1695-1699.

20. Kamineni S, Ankem H, Sanghavi S: Anatomical considerations for percutaneous proximal humeral fracture fixation. *Injury* 2004;35(11):1133-1136.

21. Neer CS II: Displaced proximal humeral fractures: II. Treatment of three-part and four-part displacement. *J Bone Joint Surg Am* 1970;52(6):1090-1103.

22. Park MC, Murthi AM, Roth NS, Blaine TA, Levine WN, Bigliani LU: Two-part and three-part fractures of the proximal humerus treated with suture fixation. *J Orthop Trauma* 2003;17(5):319-325.

23. Dimakopoulos P, Panagopoulos A, Kasimatis G: Transosseous suture fixation of proximal humeral fractures. *J Bone Joint Surg Am* 2007;89(8):1700-1709.

    In a large study of selected patients treated with a transosseous suture fixation technique, radiographic and clinical outcomes were favorable at 5-year follow-up.

24. Dimakopoulos P, Panagopoulos A, Kasimatis G: Transosseous suture fixation of proximal humeral fractures: Surgical technique. *J Bone Joint Surg Am* 2009;91(Suppl 2, Pt 1):8-21.

    Experience with transosseous suture fixation in 165 patients over an 11-year period was presented. The mean Constant score was 94%. Level of evidence: IV.

25. Egol KA, Ong CC, Walsh M, Jazrawi LM, Tejwani NC, Zuckerman JD: Early complications in proximal humerus fractures (OTA Types 11) treated with locked plates. *J Orthop Trauma* 2008;22(3):159-164.

    A retrospective analysis over a 3-year period revealed that locked plating of the proximal humerus had a very good union rate but a large number of complications, most of which were screw penetration of the humeral head.

26. Solberg BD, Moon CN, Franco DP, Paiement GD: Locked plating of 3- and 4-part proximal humerus fractures in older patients: The effect of initial fracture pattern on outcome. *J Orthop Trauma* 2009;23(2): 113-119.

    A retrospective analysis of older patients with a three- or a four-part fracture treated with locked plating revealed that varus angulation of the fracture was associated with relatively poor outcomes and an increased rate of complications. Valgus fractures with an intact metaphysis had the best outcomes.

27. Solberg BD, Moon CN, Franco DP, Paiement GD: Surgical treatment of three and four-part proximal humeral fractures. *J Bone Joint Surg Am* 2009;91(7): 1689-1697.

    A retrospective analysis of older patients with a three- or four-part fracture found that internal fixation led to better outcomes than hemiarthroplasty, especially in three-part fractures, but was associated with a higher complication rate.

28. Olerud P, Ahrengart L, Ponzer S, Saving J, Tidermark J: Internal fixation versus nonoperative treatment of displaced 3-part proximal humeral fractures in elderly patients: A randomized controlled trial. *J Shoulder Elbow Surg* 2011;20(5):747-755.

    Older patients with a moderately displaced three-part fracture proximal humeral fracture were randomly assigned to be treated nonsurgically or with locking plate fixation. Surgery had a slight short-term benefit, but no significant long-term difference was reported between the two groups.

29. Gardner MJ, Weil Y, Barker JU, Kelly BT, Helfet DL, Lorich DG: The importance of medial support in locked plating of proximal humerus fractures. *J Orthop Trauma* 2007;21(3):185-191.

    A retrospective study of proximal humeral fractures treated with locked plating revealed the importance of the inferomedial calcar region to the mechanical stability of the fracture reduction.

30. Robinson CM, Wylie JR, Ray AG, et al: Proximal humeral fractures with a severe varus deformity treated by fixation with a locking plate. *J Bone Joint Surg Br* 2010;92(5):672-678.

    Patients with varus displacement were successfully treated with anatomic reduction, locked plating, and structural allograft.

31. Gerber C, Werner CM, Vienne P: Internal fixation of complex fractures of the proximal humerus. *J Bone Joint Surg Br* 2004;86(6):848-855.

32. Gardner MJ, Boraiah S, Helfet DL, Lorich DG: Indirect medial reduction and strut support of proxi-

mal humerus fractures using an endosteal implant. *J Orthop Trauma* 2008;22(3):195-200.

Fibula strut allograft was used to improve the stability of a locking plate construct for a proximal humeral fracture.

33. Mittlmeier TW, Stedtfeld HW, Ewert A, Beck M, Frosch B, Gradl G: Stabilization of proximal humeral fractures with an angular and sliding stable antegrade locking nail (Targon PH). *J Bone Joint Surg Am* 2003; 85(suppl 4):136-146.

34. Park JY, Pandher DS, Chun JY, Md ST: Antegrade humeral nailing through the rotator cuff interval: A new entry portal. *J Orthop Trauma* 2008;22(6):419-425.

An alternative starting portal for intramedullary nail fixation of proximal humeral fractures was used to avoid some of the complications associated with the classic starting point.

35. Hatzidakis AM, Shevlin MJ, Fenton DL, Curran-Everett D, Nowinski RJ, Fehringer EV: Angular-stable locked intramedullary nailing of two-part surgical neck fractures of the proximal part of the humerus: A multicenter retrospective observational study. *J Bone Joint Surg Am* 2011;93(23):2172-2179.

Patients with a two-part surgical neck fracture were successfully treated using an articular starting portal. Patients had reliable healing and good functional outcomes with minimal postoperative shoulder pain.

36. Zhu Y, Lu Y, Shen J, Zhang J, Jiang C: Locking intramedullary nails and locking plates in the treatment of two-part proximal humeral surgical neck fractures: A prospective randomized trial with a minimum of three years of follow-up. *J Bone Joint Surg Am* 2011; 93(2):159-168.

Locked plating and intramedullary nail fixation were compared in randomly assigned patients with two-part surgical neck fractures. Between-group functional scores were similar at 3 years. Patients treated with intramedullary nailing had fewer complications. Those treated with plating had a better 1-year outcome. Level of evidence: I.

37. Park JY, Kim JH, Lhee SH, Lee SJ: The importance of inferomedial support in the hot air balloon technique for treatment of 3-part proximal humeral fractures. *J Shoulder Elbow Surg* 2012;21(9):1152-1159.

A study of 43 patients over a 12-year period analyzed the importance of medial calcar support in three-part proximal humeral fractures treated with intramedullary nail and suture fixation. Reduction of the medial calcar and the use of an inferomedial screw improved stability and clinical outcomes.

38. Konrad G, Audigé L, Lambert S, Hertel R, Südkamp NP: Similar outcomes for nail versus plate fixation of three-part proximal humeral fractures. *Clin Orthop Relat Res* 2012;470(2):602-609.

Intramedullary nail and locking plate fixation were compared in 211 patients treated for a three-part

proximal humeral fracture. Outcome scores were similar at 1-year follow-up.

39. Koike Y, Komatsuda T, Sato K: Internal fixation of proximal humeral fractures with a Polarus humeral nail. *J Orthop Traumatol* 2008;9(3):135-139.

Intramedullary nail fixation was used to treat 54 patients with a three-part proximal humeral fracture. No major complications were reported, and 79% of the patients had a satisfactory to excellent result.

40. Adedapo AO, Ikpeme JO: The results of internal fixation of three- and four-part proximal humeral fractures with the Polarus nail. *Injury* 2001;32(2): 115-121.

41. Ebraheim NA, Patil V, Husain A: Mini-external fixation of two- and three-part proximal humerus fractures. *Acta Orthop Belg* 2007;73(4):437-442.

External fixation was used to treat two-part and three-part proximal humeral fractures, with good results. The minimally invasive procedure was suggested for patients with polytrauma.

42. Martin C, Guillen M, Lopez G: Treatment of 2- and 3-part fractures of the proximal humerus using external fixation: A retrospective evaluation of 62 patients. *Acta Orthop* 2006;77(2):275-278.

43. Zhang J, Ebraheim N, Lause GE: Surgical treatment of proximal humeral fracture with external fixator. *J Shoulder Elbow Surg* 2012;21(7):882-886.

External fixation was used to treat 32 patients with a proximal humeral fracture. The result was good to excellent in 81% of the patients. Level of evidence: IV.

44. Cazeneuve JF, Cristofari DJ: The reverse shoulder prosthesis in the treatment of fractures of the proximal humerus in the elderly. *J Bone Joint Surg Br* 2010; 92(4):535-539.

At 6-year follow-up of 36 proximal humeral fractures treated with reverse shoulder arthroplasty, a drop in Constant score was reported as well as increased evidence of glenoid component loosening and scapular notching compared with previously reported data.

45. Owsley KC, Gorczyca JT: Fracture displacement and screw cutout after open reduction and locked plate fixation of proximal humeral fractures [corrected]. *J Bone Joint Surg Am* 2008;90(2):233-240.

A retrospective analysis revealed that locked plating led to a high rate of complications, most of which involved screw cutout, in older patients with a three- or four-part fracture.

46. Voigt C, Geisler A, Hepp P, Schulz AP, Lill H: Are polyaxially locked screws advantageous in the plate osteosynthesis of proximal humeral fractures in the elderly? A prospective randomized clinical observational study. *J Orthop Trauma* 2011;25(10):596-602.

Polyaxial and nonpolyaxial locked screw-plate constructs were compared for treating proximal humeral

6: Trauma and Fractures

fractures in older patients. No clinically significant difference was reported in functional outcomes.

47. Torrens C, Corrales M, Vilà G, Santana F, Cáceres E: Functional and quality-of-life results of displaced and nondisplaced proximal humeral fractures treated conservatively. *J Orthop Trauma* 2011;25(10):581-587.

    Nonsurgical treatment led to good pain relief but decreased function in older patients. Quality-of-life perception was unchanged.

48. Yüksel HY, Yimaz S, Akşahin E, Celebi L, Muratli HH, Biçimoğlu A: The results of nonoperative treatment for three- and four-part fractures of the proximal humerus in low-demand patients. *J Orthop Trauma* 2011;25(10):588-595.

    Eighteen patients older than 65 years were nonsurgically treated for a proximal humeral fracture. Functional outcomes were satisfactory and not well correlated with radiographic appearance.

6: Trauma and Fractures

Chapter 35

Sequelae of Proximal Humeral Fractures

Robert Z. Tashjian, MD

Introduction

Proximal humeral fractures account for approximately 5% of all fractures, and they are among the most commonly treated musculoskeletal injuries. Most of these injuries are minimally displaced and can be treated nonsurgically to achieve almost complete healing, a near-normal range of motion, and an excellent functional outcome.[1] Nonetheless, residual complications, including osteonecrosis, malunion, nonunion, degenerative arthritis, and stiffness, can ensue after nonsurgical or surgical care of proximal humeral fractures.

Osteonecrosis

Osteonecrosis of the humeral head results from a loss of circulation that leads to bone cell death. Initially, the bone of the avascular area attempts to repair itself with necrotic bone resorption and new bone deposition. Subchondral fracture may develop, leading to articular surface collapse and glenohumeral arthritis.[2] The etiology of proximal humeral osteonecrosis can be atraumatic, as in corticosteroid or alcohol use or sickle cell disease, or traumatic, as with a proximal humeral fracture. Posttraumatic osteonecrosis can occur after nonsurgical or surgical care of a proximal humeral fracture. The risk of osteonecrosis primarily is determined by the severity of the fracture.[3] Overall rates of osteonecrosis in large groups have been reported as 2% after nonsurgical treatment and 8% after surgical treatment.[1,4] Studies of three- and four-part fractures reported osteonecrosis rates of 28% after nonsurgical treatment and 35% after surgical treatment.[3,5] These studies indicate a greater risk of osteonecrosis after a severe injury compared with the overall risk.

Posttraumatic osteonecrosis most often is associated with clinical disability, although the level of disability has improved over time from the dismal results once

Neither Dr. Tashjian nor any immediate family member has received anything of value from or has stock or stock options held in a commercial company or institution related directly or indirectly to the subject of this chapter.

expected for patients with posttraumatic osteonecrosis In 25 patients with partial or complete collapse of the humeral head as a result of posttraumatic osteonecrosis, the clinical outcome depended on the extent of humeral head collapse and malunion of the fracture fragments.[6] Another study similarly found that the presence or absence of a malunion was one of the major predictors of outcomes in patients with posttraumatic osteonecrosis after a four-part fracture.[7] Although many patients with osteonecrosis without substantial collapse or malunion have a reasonable clinical result, severe collapse and malunion often require reconstruction with hemiarthroplasty or reverse total shoulder arthroplasty, depending on the residual malposition of the greater tuberosity.[8] In the absence of substantial humeral head collapse or malunion, a more limited surgical procedure, such as arthroscopic débridement or open or arthroscopic core decompression, can be considered for a patient with persistent symptoms secondary to osteonecrosis.[9-12]

Evaluation and Classification

The initial symptom of osteonecrosis of the proximal humerus typically is a deep, poorly localized shoulder pain similar to that of early glenohumeral arthrosis. The pain often radiates to the elbow and is exacerbated by overuse. The typical location of the osteonecrotic lesion is superomedial, and abduction and forward flexion may elicit symptoms as the diseased portion of the humeral head contacts the glenoid surface. Some patients are relatively asymptomatic.

Standard shoulder radiographs and MRI are the main imaging diagnostic tools. The shoulder radiographs should include true AP views in internal and external rotation as well as an axillary lateral view. Radiographic changes typically occur during later stages of the disease, but early changes can be detected on MRI. Bone scanning is inadequate as a diagnostic tool for osteonecrosis of the shoulder.

Staging is extremely important because it dictates the treatment and predicts the outcome. The most commonly used classification is the Cruess system, which is a modification of the Ficat-Arlet classification of osteonecrosis of the hip.[13] The classification primarily is

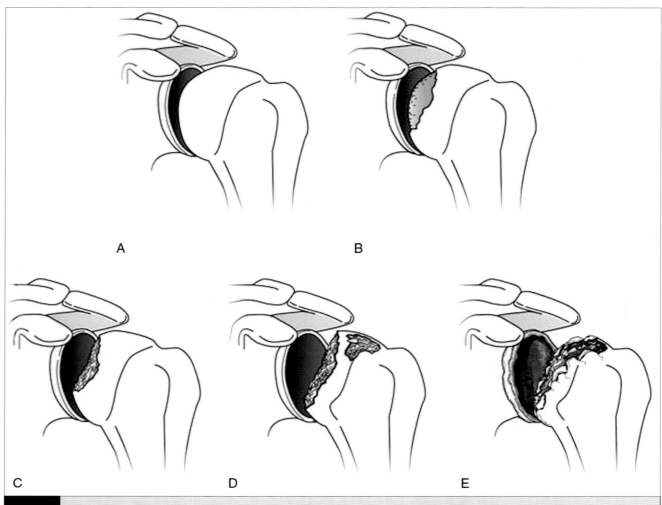

Figure 1 Schematic drawings showing the Cruess classification of proximal humeral osteonecrosis. **A,** Stage I: no radiographic evidence of shoulder osteonecrosis; the humeral head appears normal, with maintenance of curvature and no sclerosis. **B,** Stage II: signs of mottled sclerosis, but the curvature of the humeral head remains intact. **C,** Stage III: development of a crescent sign, which indicates a subchondral fracture with loss of sphericity of the humeral head. **D,** Stage IV: progression to collapse of the subchondral bone and humeral head. **E,** Stage V: progression to early degenerative changes of the glenoid. (Adapted from Harreld KL, Marker DR, Wiesler ER, Shafiz B, Mont MA: Osteonecrosis of the humeral head. *J Am Acad Orthop Surg* 2009;17:345-355.)

based on the severity of humeral head collapse (**Figure 1**). Stage I changes are not visible on plain radiographs and can be seen only as edema on MRI. Stage II changes are seen as a well-defined lesion on MRI and sclerosis on plain radiographs. A stage III lesion is a subchondral fracture with a loss of head sphericity. A stage IV or V lesion is characterized by humeral head collapse or glenoid involvement, respectively.

The recently described Sakai classification system was based on lesion size as well as extent of collapse.[14] The size of an osteonecrotic lesion was evaluated by defining the so-called necrotic angle on midoblique-coronal and midoblique-sagittal MRI. Of 46 shoulders with a Cruess stage I or II lesion, 12 shoulders had a necrotic angle of more than 90°. The humeral head later collapsed in 11 of these shoulders (92%); 4 shoulders progressed to Cruess stage III, and 7 progressed to

Cruess stage IV. None of the 34 shoulders with a necrotic angle of less than 90° progressed to a Cruess stage III, IV, or V lesion.[14]

Treatment Options

The treatment of posttraumatic osteonecrosis depends on three factors: the presence of symptoms, the stage of the lesion, and the extent of malunion. If the lesion is asymptomatic, observation is recommended, with follow-up radiographs to monitor the lesion. If the lesion is symptomatic, it is reasonable to institute treatment. The treatment options include nonsurgical measures, such as physical therapy and anti-inflammatory drugs, as well as surgery. The nonarthroplasty surgical options include core decompression, arthroscopy with or without core decompression, and vascularized bone graft. In general, these options are reserved for symptomatic stage I, II, and III lesions with minimal evidence of malunion, after unsuccessful nonsurgical treatment. Arthroplasty is reserved for symptomatic stage IV and V lesions as well as stage III lesions with significant malunion.

Natural History and Nonsurgical Treatment

The natural history of osteonecrotic lesions of the proximal humerus is poorly defined. The only available studies are of small, heterogeneous groups of patients with multiple etiologies and relatively poor radiographic categorization. The initial study reported that 78% of the patients with steroid-induced osteonecrosis had a satisfactory long-term outcome. Only 22% required surgical treatment (in the form of shoulder arthroplasty); all of these patients initially had a Cruess stage IV or V lesion.[13] Higher lesion stage and larger lesion size were found to have a significant negative effect on lesion progression and the need for surgery in a study of 151 patients (200 shoulders).[15] The patients were treated nonsurgically and initially did not require future surgery; 77% had no or mild pain at an average 8.6-year follow-up. Three years after initial treatment, 78% of the patients with traumatic osteonecrosis needed arthroplasty, compared with 47% with an atraumatic lesion. A study of 65 patients with osteonecrosis found worse long-term outcomes after nonsurgical treatment.[16] At a minimum 2-year follow-up, 20% of the patients had undergone immediate surgery, 34% had surgery during the evaluation period, 23% had a poor result after nonsurgical treatment, and only 23% had a satisfactory outcome after nonsurgical treatment. All of the patients who underwent surgery or had a poor outcome after continued nonsurgical treatment had a stage III, IV, or V lesion. Those with a stage I or II lesion did well long term, with limited progression or need for surgery.[16] Another study reported no progression of stage I and II lesions with necrotic angles of less than 90° on midoblique-coronal and midoblique-sagittal MRI.[14]

The primary goals of nonsurgical treatment include pain relief and maintenance of motion. Physical therapy is recommended to prevent adhesive capsulitis. Activity modification is necessary to limit heavy overhead lifting. In general, nonsurgical treatment can initially be considered for most patients. Initial nonsurgical treatment is most effective and therefore most appropriate for patients with stage I or II disease, especially if the lesion is small, and offers a good chance for a satisfactory result. A relatively small stage III lesion also may respond to nonsurgical treatment, although most stage III, IV, or V lesions require some form of surgical intervention.

Nonarthroplasty Surgical Treatment

A limited number of nonarthroplasty surgical options exist for osteonecrotic lesions of the humeral head, including core decompression, arthroscopic débridement alone, and arthroscopic débridement with core decompression. The indications include a stage I or II lesion that is resistant to nonsurgical treatment and a stage III lesion with limited collapse. A severe stage III lesion or a stage IV or V lesion should be treated with partial or complete shoulder replacement.

Data are limited regarding the use of arthroscopic débridement for osteonecrotic lesions. The primary goals are to improve the lesion stage and débride loose cartilage flaps or loose bodies. Short-term functional improvement and pain relief reasonably can be expected. In general, arthroscopic débridement is most useful for reducing pain from synovitis and relieving mechanical symptoms from chondral flaps or loose bodies, if it is performed in isolation without core decompression, even in a stage III or IV lesion.

Core decompression for osteonecrosis has been extensively studied in patients with femoral head osteonecrosis. The treatment effect is a result of a reduction in bone marrow pressure that can reduce pain and possibly incite revascularization and deposition of new bone in the necrotic region. The rates of success have varied. Although the procedure is somewhat controversial, it appears to be effective in patients with a stage I or II lesion in the hip.[12] Several limited evaluations have been performed in patients with proximal humeral osteonecrosis.[12,17,18] The surgical techniques described for core decompression in the proximal humerus are both open and arthroscopic.[9,10,12]

In general, stage I and II lesions resistant to nonsurgical treatment had excellent long-term functional results and limited radiographic progression after core decompression, and none required arthroplasty.[12,18] It is unclear whether a reduction in radiographic progression results from the decompression or the normal natural history of a stage I or II lesion. Some success has been reported after core decompression of stage III lesions; 70% of patients had a good or excellent result at an average 5.6-year follow-up, with the remaining 30% requiring arthroplasty.[12]

Several techniques have been described for proximal humeral core decompression. In an open decompression technique, a small incision is made in the inferior deltopectoral interval just above the pectoralis major with blunt dissection carried just lateral to the bicipital groove.[12] A small, lateral deltoid-splitting approach can also be used, in which biplane radiographs are used to locate the lesion and a 5-mm coring device is used to perform the decompression; a large biopsy cannula (6 to 10 mm) also can be used, depending on the size of the lesion.[18] A recently reported percutaneous decompression technique uses a 3.2-mm Steinmann pin with two or three passes in the lesion from a common entry site.[17] At a mean 32-month follow-up, 25 of 26 shoulders (96%) with stage I or II disease were successfully treated with the percutaneous technique, as measured on the University of California, Los Angeles (UCLA) scoring system. Only one patient had radiographic progression.[17] Reports of several arthroscopic techniques have emphasized the benefits of intra-articular

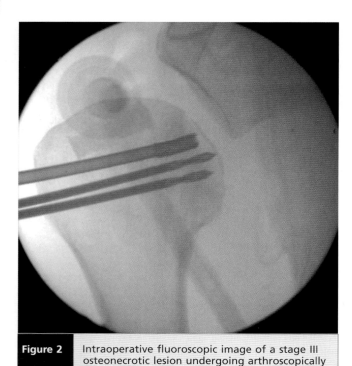

Figure 2 Intraoperative fluoroscopic image of a stage III osteonecrotic lesion undergoing arthroscopically assisted core decompression. (Courtesy of Pat Greis, MD, Salt Lake City, UT.)

visualization of the lesion to aid in staging, concomitant synovectomy, or débridement for pain relief; improve localization for decompression; and avoid joint penetration by the coring device (**Figure 2**). An anterior cruciate ligament (ACL) guide was used through the anterior portal, followed by a guidewire from the lateral portal, which was overreamed with a 7-mm cannulated reamer.[9] A similar technique used an ACL guide, with the placement of several 3.2-mm Steinmann pins followed by overdrilling with a 4-mm coring device.[10] All four patients in the two combined studies had uneventful recovery and immediate pain relief. In general, both arthroscopic and open techniques are safe and effective for treating symptomatic stage I and II and possibly stage III lesions.

Proximal Humeral Malunions

Malunion of the proximal aspect of the humerus after fracture can be the result of inadequate reduction during surgical fixation, loss of reduction after surgical fixation, or nonsurgical treatment if the fracture is displaced or becomes displaced during treatment. A recent systematic review found a 7% incidence of varus malunion in 650 nonsurgically treated proximal humerus fractures.[1] Patients with a malunited fracture often have pain, limited range of motion, and impaired strength, depending on the fracture pattern and the presence of concomitant humeral head collapse or arthritis. The final deformity of the malunited fracture is dictated by muscle pull on the fracture fragments. A

greater tuberosity malunion has superior and/or posterior displacement from the pull of the posterosuperior rotator cuff, which leads to subacromial impingement and weakness of the rotator cuff. The nonanatomic mechanics lead to pain and limited motion. Isolated surgical neck malunion typically results in varus and flexion deformity caused by the pull of the pectoralis major on the shaft fragment and the pull of the rotator cuff on the head fragment, leading to loss of flexion and abduction.

The clinical evaluation of a proximal humeral malunion should include the mechanism of injury and treatment history. Several conditions may predispose a patient to malunion, including osteoporotic bone, aggressive rehabilitation, or inadequate fixation. The radiographic evaluation should include plain radiographs (AP, AP in the plane of the scapula, axillary, and transscapular lateral views) as well as CT with three-dimensional reconstruction to allow accurate evaluation of the position and extent of any tuberosity displacement. MRI should be added if there is concern about early osteonecrosis or a lack of rotator cuff integrity, which may necessitate altering the surgical treatment plan.

Several classification systems have characterized proximal humeral malunions, although none are universally accepted. A modification of the Neer fracture classification using parts categorization probably is the most commonly used because of its simplicity. The Beredjiklian system evaluates both bony and soft-tissue abnormalities.[19] A bony deformity is classified as a malposition of the lesser or greater tuberosity of more than 1 cm (type I), a step-off of the articular surface of more than 5 mm (type II), or a malalignment of the proximal humeral articular segment of more than 45° (type III). Soft-tissue abnormalities include stiffness, rotator cuff tearing, or impingement. The Boileau system specifies the indications for treatment and the outcomes of unconstrained arthroplasty.[20] Type I sequelae include impacted proximal humeral fractures progressing to head collapse or necrosis; type II, chronic dislocations or fracture-dislocations; type III, surgical neck nonunions; and type IV, severe tuberosity malunions requiring greater tuberosity osteotomy. Type I and II sequelae were found to have a satisfactory result after unconstrained arthroplasty because no greater tuberosity osteotomy was performed. Type III and IV sequelae had a poor result after unconstrained arthroplasty because a greater tuberosity osteotomy was required.

Although malunion can occur after any proximal humeral fracture, very few are amenable to isolated correction. Typically, an isolated greater tuberosity malunion or surgical neck malunion with an intact rotator cuff and no concomitant arthritic changes is optimal for surgical treatment. The nonarthroplasty surgical options for these injuries include isolated arthroscopic débridement, débridement with tuberoplasty, and rotator cuff retensioning with osteotomy.[19,21-27] Malunion in a complex three- or four-part fracture or malunion with associated arthritic changes, humeral head collapse, insufficient bone stock, or rotator cuff deficiency is better treated with anatomic shoulder arthroplasty or reverse total shoulder arthroplasty.

Greater Tuberosity Malunion

Isolated greater tuberosity malunion probably is the most common proximal humeral malunion. The surgical indications for fixation of greater tuberosity fractures include displacement of more than 1 cm; however, some surgeons suggest surgical fixation of fractures with more than 5 mm of displacement.[28,29] Symptomatic malunion can occur with a neglected fracture having more than 1 cm of displacement, failure of fixation of an internally fixed tuberosity, or unsuccessful nonsurgical treatment of a fracture having less than 1 cm of displacement. Posterior displacement often causes a rigid block to external rotation, and superior displacement can cause loss of abduction, impingement, and rotator cuff weakness. Indications for surgical treatment of the malunion include more than 5 mm of superior displacement or 1 cm of posterior displacement with pain, loss of motion, and impingement.

The surgical options for a malunited greater tuberosity fracture include open osteotomy, arthroscopic débridement, or arthroscopic tuberoplasty with rotator cuff repair. In a study of 11 patients with an isolated greater tuberosity malunion, 2 patients with superior displacement of 1 to 1.5 cm had a satisfactory result after treatment with arthroscopic acromioplasty alone.[19] The remaining nine patients had more than 1.5 cm of displacement and were treated with isolated osteotomy, rotator cuff repair, and capsular release to within 5 mm of anatomic restoration. The surgical repairs primarily used suture fixation.

Several recent reports have described the arthroscopic treatment of isolated superiorly displaced greater tuberosity fractures using rotator cuff takedown, tuberoplasty, and repair. Four patients with isolated greater tuberosity malunion were treated with capsular release, lysis of subacromial adhesions, and subacromial decompression and rotator cuff takedown with tuberoplasty and rotator cuff repair.[23] The result was an average 52-point improvement in mean score on the American Shoulder and Elbow Surgeons Disability Index and a 4.5 point reduction in the visual analog scale pain score. Eight patients were treated in a similar fashion for 5- to 10-mm posterosuperior displacement of the greater tuberosity; seven of the patients had a good or excellent result and returned to their previous occupation without restrictions.[24] Arthroscopic tuberoplasty and rotator cuff repair were recommended for symptomatic malunited greater tuberosity fractures with more than 5 mm of displacement.[30] A delay of at least 6 months after fracture was recommended to allow complete maturation of the malunion before tuberoplasty and rotator cuff repair.

Greater tuberosity malunion with substantial (more than 1 cm) posterior displacement often requires open osteotomy, capsular and rotator cuff interval release, and fixation with suture or screws if the fragments are large enough. Preoperative CT with three-dimensional reconstruction is useful for planning the osteotomy. A deltopectoral approach is routinely used, but a second posterior approach may be required for mobilizing and detaching the fragment. A symptomatic malunion with 5 to 10 mm of superior displacement should be considered for arthroscopic acromioplasty, with or without tuberoplasty and rotator cuff reattachment.

Surgical Neck Malunion

Isolated surgical neck malunion is relatively uncommon, and limited data are available on both treatment indications and surgical options. Deformity typically results from acceptance of an imperfect open or closed reduction or a loss of reduction during nonsurgical treatment. A neck-shaft angle of less than 120° is sufficient to reduce active shoulder range of motion and increase pain.[31] Neer considered angulation of more than 45° to be an indication for surgical repair, which would result in a neck-shaft angle of approximately 90° to 100°.[28] All reported neck-shaft angles were less than 110°, and most were 90° to 105°; these reports can be used as a guide for the amount of proximal humeral varus necessary before corrective osteotomy is considered.[21,25,27]

Most surgeons recommend a simple lateral closing-wedge valgus osteotomy to restore a normal neck-shaft angle of 130° to 140°.[21,25,27] Although flexion and rotational deformity are common, restoration of valgus is of primary importance. The instrumentation options include a blade plate, a T-plate, or a locking proximal humeral plate, but the locking plate appears to be the current instrument of choice (**Figure 3**). Preoperative templating using both radiography and CT is critical for exactly measuring the appropriate wedge size. Capsular release should be considered to restore passive motion before osteotomy. The osteotomized closing wedge can be used as bone graft. The osteotomy should be performed in the metaphyseal region at the location of greatest deformity.[21,25] Improvement of the neck-shaft angle by 20° has resulted after osteotomy, with a corresponding increase of 90° of forward flexion.[21] A more modest average improvement in elevation of 56° also has been reported.[27] Consequently, a valgus closing-wedge osteotomy is a reasonable treatment option for improving pain, range of motion, and function in patients with an isolated surgical neck malunion of the proximal humerus and a neck-shaft angle of less than approximately 110°.

Surgical Neck Nonunion

Surgical neck nonunions after a proximal humeral fracture are relatively uncommon but can cause significant disability and can be extremely challenging to treat. Surgical neck nonunion was found to occur in 1.1% of

6: Trauma and Fractures

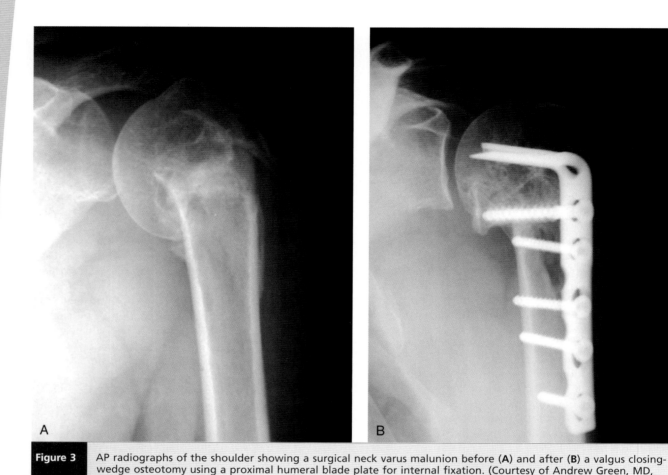

Figure 3   AP radiographs of the shoulder showing a surgical neck varus malunion before (**A**) and after (**B**) a valgus closing-wedge osteotomy using a proximal humeral blade plate for internal fixation. (Courtesy of Andrew Green, MD, Providence, RI.)

all proximal humeral fractures.[32] Successful surgical treatment dramatically improves function from that of a flail shoulder to that of a competent upper extremity.[33] The treatment options for surgical neck nonunions can be broadly categorized as open reduction and fixation (typically with associated bone grafting) or arthroplasty (anatomic and reverse).

Surgical neck nonunion can be classified as hypertrophic, in which the bone ends are viable with abundant callus formation, or atrophic, in which the bone ends have limited biologic viability. The predisposing factors include displacement, comminution, soft-tissue interposition of the biceps, systemic disease, osteopenia, or aggressive early rehabilitation.[32-34] Metaphyseal comminution or translation of more than one third of the surgical neck increases the prevalence to 8% or 10%, respectively.[32] In the Boileau classification, proximal humeral nonunion is a type III sequela.[20] Based on this classification, unconstrained arthroplasty for surgical neck nonunion is likely to have a poor result because the greater tuberosity often needs to be osteotomized. Open reduction and internal fixation is recommended if the head remains viable, and reverse arthroplasty is recommended if the head is compromised in a patient older than 70 years with low physi-

cal demands. Surgical neck nonunion with a nonviable humeral head is difficult to manage in relatively young patients; unconstrained arthroplasty with a greater tuberosity osteotomy typically is the only available option, with an expectation of poor function.[20] Better results, specifically in forward elevation, have been shown when surgical neck nonunion was treated with unconstrained arthroplasty using calcar grafting and avoiding a greater tuberosity osteotomy.[35]

The management of a surgical neck nonunion depends on various factors, including patient age, bone quality, humeral head bone viability, glenohumeral arthritis, and status of the rotator cuff. In general, the three primary treatment options for a surgical neck nonunion are open reduction and internal fixation with bone grafting, anatomic shoulder arthroplasty (total shoulder arthroplasty or humeral head replacement), or reverse total shoulder arthroplasty.

Open reduction and internal fixation with a plate is a reliable option in treating patients with a surgical neck nonunion who have sufficient humeral head bone stock and do not have arthritis. Twelve of 13 patients healed after open reduction and internal fixation using a T-plate and rotator cuff tension banding with autogenous bone grafting.[34] Nine of the patients reported a good result, with no pain and a return to prefracture function, and four patients reported a fair result, with mild to moderate pain and without a return to prefracture work or function. In 25 patients who underwent blade plate fixation and autogenous bone grafting for a proximal humeral nonunion, the nonunion healed in 23 (92%), and 20 (80%) had a good or excellent outcome.[36] Most recently, 18 patients with a symptomatic proximal humeral nonunion were treated with open reduction and internal fixation using a proximal humeral locking plate augmented with an intramedullary cortical allograft.[37] Union was achieved in 17 patients (94%) at an average 5.4-month follow-up, and active forward elevation averaged 115°. Demineralized bone matrix and morcellized allograft cancellous bone were used as an adjunct in four patients. Suture fixation of the tuberosities with attachment to the plate was used to augment fixation.

Several options exist to enhance bone healing in a repair of surgical neck nonunion, including bone grafting (autograft or structural allograft), extracorporeal shock wave therapy, pulsed electromagnetic field therapy, low-intensity pulsed ultrasound, and bone morphogenetic proteins (BMPs). Autograft is the gold standard for grafting because it has osteoconductive, osteoinductive, and osteogenic properties. Autograft should be considered in the treatment of all surgical neck nonunions. Structural intramedullary cortical allograft is efficacious for augmenting the repair construct, and its use also should be considered.[37] Some evidence suggests a positive role for low-intensity pulsed ultrasound, pulsed electromagnetic field therapy, and extracorporeal shock wave therapy in treating long-bone nonunions, but there are no data specifically on the use of these therapies after the treatment of proximal humeral nonunions. The data in favor of low-intensity pulsed ultrasound and extracorporeal shock wave therapy are stronger than the data for pulsed electromagnetic field therapy.[38-40] These therapies should be considered as reasonable adjuncts to treatment because of their low risk profile and potential for stimulating healing.

BMP-7 was found safe and effective for the treatment of tibial nonunion in a type I collagen carrier.[41] The clinical and radiographic results of BMP-7 treatment were comparable to those of autograft, without graft site morbidity. BMP-2 has been shown to lower the risk of nonunion and infection in the treatment of fresh open tibial shaft fractures.[42] BMP-2 is approved by the FDA for use only in acute open tibial fracture and anterior lumbar interbody fusion; BMP-7 is approved for the treatment of recalcitrant long-bone nonunion. BMP-7 has been taken off the market for clinical use, however, and off-label use of BMP-2 is the only available option for augmenting the treatment of surgical neck nonunions.

The recommended current approach to internal fixation of a surgical neck nonunion with a viable rotator cuff, humeral head, and glenohumeral cartilage is the use of a locking proximal humeral plate with autograft

or allograft. A preoperative infection workup, including the erythrocyte sedimentation rate and C-reactive protein level, should be done if the nonunion resulted from earlier unsuccessful internal fixation. A deltopectoral approach is typical and can be extended distally into an anterolateral approach for greater exposure of the humeral shaft. A complete nonunion takedown with intramedullary reaming distally and proximally into the humeral head should be performed until bleeding bone is achieved. Tissue cultures and pathology specimens should be obtained to detect signs of acute inflammation if the nonunion resulted from earlier unsuccessful internal fixation, and all hardware and other foreign material should be removed. Intramedullary cortical fibula allograft frequently is shaped to fit the intramedullary canal[37] (**Figure 4**). A proximal humeral locking plate often is used with an articulated tensioning device to aid in compression across the nonunion site. Suture augmentation through the rotator cuff and the locking plate routinely is used. Autogenous bone graft is packed around the nonunion site, often with the addition of BMP-2 (used in an off-label manner). Low-intensity pulsed ultrasound is used after surgery with a protective physical therapy regimen.

The initial choice of surgical treatment for a surgical neck nonunion should be based on the patient's age as well as shoulder-related factors. Open reduction and internal fixation with bone grafting should be considered if the patient is younger than 70 years and has an intact rotator cuff, a viable humeral head, and no arthritis. Reverse total shoulder arthroplasty should be considered if the patient is older than 70 years. If the patient is older than 70 years and has a surgical neck nonunion and either a deficient rotator cuff or a nonviable humeral head, reverse total shoulder arthroplasty should be the surgical treatment of choice. Reverse total shoulder arthroplasty also can be considered if the patient is age 60 to 70 years and has relatively low physical demands as well as a deficient rotator cuff or a nonviable or arthritic humeral head. Hemiarthroplasty, with avoidance of a greater tuberosity osteotomy and calcar grafting, can be considered for a patient age 60 to 70 years who has higher demands. An unconstrained arthroplasty can be performed, with calcar grafting and avoidance of a tuberosity osteotomy. However, a patient who is younger than 60 years and has a deficient rotator cuff, a nonviable humeral head, or an arthritic glenohumeral joint is likely to have less active and passive motion and decreased function after this procedure than after a standard hemiarthroplasty.

Glenohumeral Arthritis

Posttraumatic glenohumeral arthritis can be difficult to treat, especially in relatively young patients for whom arthroplasty is not desirable. The nonarthroplasty surgical options include arthroscopic débridement with or without capsular release as well as arthroscopic bio-

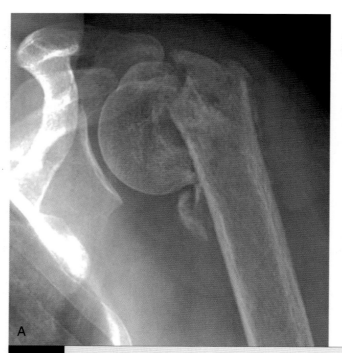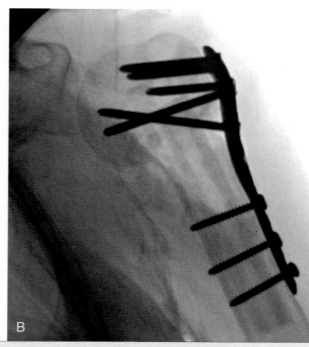

Figure 4 True AP radiographs of the shoulder showing a surgical neck nonunion with a viable humeral head and no arthritic changes before (**A**) and after (**B**) internal fixation using a locking proximal humeral plate augmented with intramedullary fibula and iliac crest allograft.

logic glenoid resurfacing. Several factors are used in making a decision, including patient age, work demands, the presence of limited motion or neurologic defects, the amount of joint space loss, the concentricity of wear, the presence of bipolar (humeral head and glenoid) disease, and the size and grade of osteochondral lesions. Each of these factors can affect the outcome of an arthroscopic procedure and should be considered in choosing prosthetic or nonprosthetic surgical treatment of posttraumatic glenohumeral arthritis.

The history of a patient with posttraumatic arthritis should include information regarding earlier surgical treatment, patient age and activity level, hand dominance, severity of symptoms, mechanical symptoms, and future demands on the shoulder (such as physical labor or sports). The physical examination should specifically include an evaluation of range-of-motion loss, which is likely to influence the choice of surgical treatment and its outcome. A comprehensive neurologic examination should be performed, including the axillary nerve and the rotator cuff. The radiographic evaluation should include AP, true AP, scapular lateral, and axillary lateral plain radiographs. True AP radiographs should be used to evaluate joint space narrowing as well as the extent of any malunited fragments. The axillary radiograph should be used to evaluate the glenoid morphology and detect an asymmetric wear pattern, such as posterior subluxation or a posteriorly eroded glenoid. MRI can be useful for determining the status of the rotator cuff as long as no metallic fixation devices have been implanted. Otherwise, ultrasonography

or CT arthrography can be used. Both MRI and CT can be useful for further classifying glenoid morphology.

The early stages of posttraumatic osteoarthritis often can be treated nonsurgically with activity modification, NSAIDs, physical therapy, and corticosteroid injections. The American Academy of Orthopaedic Surgeons (AAOS) evaluated these treatment methods and concluded that current literature neither supports nor refutes their usefulness.[43] Consequently, it is reasonable to use these methods. Because evidence is lacking to support the efficacy of corticosteroid injections, it is recommended that injections into a single joint be limited to three unless there are special circumstances.[44] The AAOS also determined that viscosupplementation can be considered for patients with glenohumeral osteoarthritis.[43] Patients with glenohumeral osteoarthritis who were treated with hylan G-F 20 (Synvisc; Genzyme) reported improvements in pain relief, range of motion, and quality of life lasting up to 6 months after three weekly injections.[45] Patients with glenohumeral osteoarthritis who were treated with three to five nonguided intra-articular sodium hyaluronate injections had a statistically significant improvement in pain relief compared with those treated with a placebo. Despite the statistical significance of the improvement (7.8 mm on a 100-mm visual analog scale), its clinical importance is questionable.[46]

If nonsurgical treatment is unsuccessful, a patient with glenohumeral arthritis can be treated with arthroscopic débridement with or without capsular release,

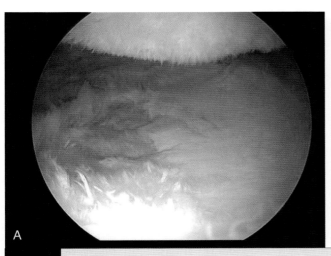 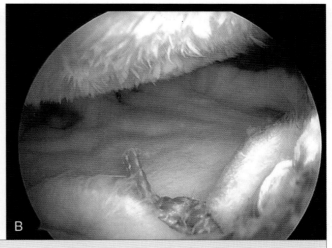

Figure 5   Arthroscopic images showing bipolar grade III humeral and grade IV glenoid osteochondral lesions before (**A**) and after (**B**) humeral débridement with arthroscopic biologic glenoid resurfacing. (Courtesy of Robert T. Burks, MD, Salt Lake City, UT.)

arthroscopic biologic glenoid resurfacing, or arthroplasty. The AAOS did not make a recommendation for or against arthroscopic treatment or biologic interposition in patients with glenohumeral osteoarthritis because of a lack of high-level evidence.[43]

Twenty-five patients with early glenohumeral arthritis underwent arthroscopic chondral and labral débridement with loose body removal, synovectomy, lavage, and subacromial bursectomy.[47] At 3-year follow-up, 80% had a good or excellent result. The researchers recommended arthroscopy only if some joint space was visible and the arthritis was concentric. Another study reported that 88% of the patients had pain relief at a minimum 2-year follow-up after arthroscopic débridement of grade IV osteochondral lesions.[48] If shoulder motion was within 15° of that of the opposite side, a capsular release was not performed. If decreased range of motion was found on examination (more than 15° of motion loss in elevation or external rotation compared with the opposite side), a capsular release was performed with the débridement. The average improvements in forward elevation and external rotation were 23° and 38°, respectively, in patients who received capsular release. The researchers recommended avoiding the procedure if the lesion was larger than 2 cm² because large size appeared to be associated with a return of pain and treatment failure. Another study reported similar increases in forward elevation and external rotation (of 21° and 17°, respectively) after capsular release.[49] The reduction in joint contact pressures after the release was believed to be the primary mechanism of pain relief. Reasonable results also were reported in a study of 36 patients, with significantly better results if the patient's Outerbridge changes were lower than grade IV.[50] Conversely, an evaluation of the extent of cartilage lesions found that monopolar Outerbridge grade IV lesions did just as well as lower

grade lesions.[51] Bipolar lesions had significantly worse outcomes than monopolar lesions. Similarly, the risk of failure after arthroscopic débridement was significant if the patient had bipolar grade IV lesions; 87% of the patients with bipolar grade IV disease later required arthroplasty.[52] Other risk factors for failure included a joint space of less than 2 mm and large osteophytes (Samilson-Prieto grade 2; 3 to 7 mm on the humerus or the glenoid).

Based on published studies, it is reasonable to consider arthroscopic débridement for a patient with concentric glenohumeral arthritis, at least 2 mm of preserved joint space, and relatively small unipolar lesions, up to and including grade IV lesions with small humeral osteophytes. Capsular release may be added to reliably improve elevation and external rotation in a patient with stiffness and arthritis. Débridement is likely to have an inferior result, and later arthroplasty is more likely to be required if the patient has nonconcentric wear, less than 2 mm of preserved joint space, large (3- to 7-mm) osteophytes on the humerus or the glenoid, and bipolar grade IV lesions. Arthroscopic débridement alone should be avoided for such a patient.

Arthroscopic glenoid resurfacing recently was described as an option for patients who have severe disease and for whom arthroscopic débridement alone is unsuitable. During the procedure, arthroscopic débridement is followed by suturing of an interposition graft to the face of the glenoid (**Figure 5**). Thirty-two patients who underwent arthroscopic débridement and biologic glenoid resurfacing with an acellular dermal matrix had significant improvement in pain and functional outcomes, with a 72% success rate an average 3-year follow-up.[53] Ninety-four percent of these patients had a concentric wear pattern; 59% had moderate osteophytes and joint space narrowing; and 41% had large osteophytes, marked joint space narrowing, and severe sclerosis. Hand dominance in the affected extremity and systemic disease such as diabetes, rheumatoid arthritis, or osteoarthritis were correlated with a poorer outcome, but radiographic grading was not. A study of 20 patients after arthroscopic glenoid resurfacing with a porcine small intestine submucosa patch found a 75% success rate at 3- to 6-year follow-up.[54] All patients had grade IV bipolar lesions, and 25% had posterior subluxation on initial radiographs. Twenty-five percent required arthroplasty 1 to 5 years after the resurfacing. The data from these studies suggest that arthroscopic débridement with glenoid biologic resurfacing may be an alternative for a young patient who has bipolar grade IV osteochondral changes with severe narrowing of a concentrically worn glenohumeral joint. It must be understood, however, that approximately 25% are likely to require arthroplasty within 3 to 5 years of the procedure.

Posttraumatic Stiffness Without Arthritis

Range-of-motion loss is common after treatment of proximal humeral fractures and occurs in approximately 3% of surgically treated proximal humeral fractures.[55] The range-of-motion deficit typically is mild. At an average 3.5-year follow-up after a minimally displaced proximal humeral fracture, forward elevation and external rotation averaged 89% and 87%, respectively, compared with the opposite shoulder.[56] This finding suggests mild permanent motion limitations. Such limitations are common after internal fixation of proximal humeral fractures. An average elevation of 156° and external rotation of 46° were reported after open reduction and internal fixation of proximal humeral fractures with a locking proximal humeral plate.[57]

Despite the acceptable results of both nonsurgical and surgical treatment, a small percentage of patients later have pathologic stiffness or adhesive capsulitis. Adhesive capsulitis can result from an extra-articular or an intra-articular etiology. The intra-articular etiologies of stiffness include capsular contracture, arthritis, osteonecrosis, and articular malunion. The extra-articular etiologies include subacromial adhesions, hardware impingement, and tuberosity or surgical neck malunion. The appropriate management of posttraumatic adhesive capsulitis requires an understanding of the sources of stiffness.

A careful history for a patient with a nonsurgically treated fracture should include the duration of immobilization. Although the topic is controversial, some evidence suggests that immediate mobilization for a minimally displaced proximal humeral fracture treated nonsurgically leads to faster functional recovery, better short-term pain relief and range of motion, and better long-term final function and range of motion compared with an initial 2- to 3-week period of sling immobilization.[56,58,59] A patient with stiffness should receive a thorough physical examination to evaluate earlier open

surgical incisions and a neurologic examination to specifically evaluate the axillary and suprascapular nerves. The status of the rotator cuff and the passive and active range of motion should be documented. Patients typically report restricted motion and pain at the end range of motion. Concomitant impingement-related symptoms are common with postfracture stiffness, especially in patients treated with open reduction and internal fixation using a locking proximal humeral plate.

The shoulder radiographs should include AP, scapula plane AP, axillary, and scapular lateral views. The radiographs should be used to evaluate the presence and location of hardware from earlier surgical fixation, malunion of the tuberosities or surgical neck, or any articular cartilage injury resulting from arthritis or osteonecrosis. MRI can be obtained if there is concern about a concomitant rotator cuff injury or early osteonecrosis, especially if the patient has mechanical symptoms or pain with resisted rotator cuff testing. CT is helpful only if there is concern that malunion may be a source of pain or limited motion. CT arthrography may be beneficial for evaluating rotator cuff integrity if hardware is present from earlier internal fixation.

A treatment plan for a stiff postfracture shoulder should take into account all intra-articular or extra-articular etiologies. Nonsurgical treatment usually should be considered before surgical intervention. Physical therapy should focus on global passive and active-assisted stretching. NSAIDs can reduce intra-articular inflammation, thereby limiting pain and improving motion. Intra-articular steroid injections can be used to limit inflammation and provide early pain relief. Intra-articular sodium hyaluronate injection is not recommended for treating isolated adhesive capsulitis because it has no apparent benefit compared with placebo.[46]

Nonsurgical treatment should extend over a minimum of 2 to 3 months. At least 4 to 6 months should elapse after the fracture before surgical treatment is considered. Arthroplasty should be considered if substantial osteonecrosis or arthritis is present. Corrective osteotomy should be considered, in conjunction with capsular release, if there is a tuberosity or surgical neck malunion without articular injury. Surgical release of the capsular contracture can be considered if the fracture has healed with reasonable alignment and there is no substantial articular cartilage injury.

Arthroscopic surgical release of a stiff posttraumatic shoulder has proved to be a reliable surgical solution leading to improvement in pain, function, and range of motion.[60-62] The first step in an arthroscopic release is diagnostic glenohumeral arthroscopy. The arthroscope initially is in a standard posterior portal; an anterior rotator cuff interval portal initially is developed as the working portal. The release is initiated by defining the anterior border of the supraspinatus and the superior margin of the subscapularis. An arthroscopic tissue ablator is used to remove all scarred rotator cuff interval tissue in the window until the underlying coracoacromial ligament can be identified to mark the superficial

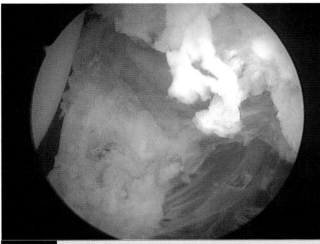

Figure 6 Arthroscopic image showing release of the posteroinferior glenohumeral ligament and capsule. The humeral head is on the left, and the glenoid on the right (in approximately the 6:30 position).

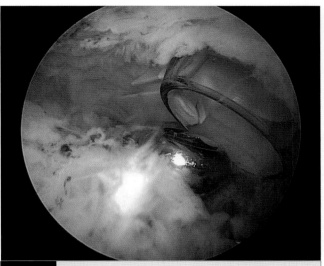

Figure 7 Arthroscopic image showing subacromial bursectomy and hardware removal after glenohumeral arthroscopic capsular release.

extent of the release. Care should be taken to avoid involving the bicipital sling and laterally destabilizing the biceps. Next, the interval between the subscapularis and the middle glenohumeral ligament is bluntly developed using a blunt instrument. The middle and inferior glenohumeral ligaments and capsule are released just adjacent to the labrum. Caution should be used inferiorly because the dissection approaches the axillary nerve; proximity can be gauged by using electrocautery if the patient is not paralyzed. Visualization of the underlying subscapularis muscle indicates a complete release. The release should be continued inferior to the 6-o'clock position. The arthroscope should be placed anteriorly, and release of the posteroinferior capsule is continued with the cautery in the posterior portal (**Figure 6**). Subacromial débridement should be performed by removing subacromial adhesions. Any screws used for internal fixation can be removed arthroscopically (**Figure 7**). If plate fixation was used at least 12 months earlier and the fracture has healed, a deltopectoral incision can be made to remove the plate after completing the arthroscopic release and débridement. Manipulation under anesthesia may have a role in the treatment of idiopathic adhesive capsulitis, but it is not recommended for the treatment of posttraumatic adhesive capsulitis because most patients have both intra-articular and extra-articular mechanisms of stiffness.

Physical therapy is initiated immediately after surgery, with a focus on passive and active-assisted stretching. Interscalene blocks using catheters typically provide pain relief for 24 to 48 hours and allow immediate physical therapy. In 200 consecutive patients, the use of an indwelling catheter placed under ultrasound guidance had a reported 99% success rate and a 1% rate of transient neurologic deficit, with no permanent deficits.[63] Alternatively, NSAIDs, narcotics, and pregabalin

can be prescribed for pain modulation. Continuous passive motion can be used as an adjunct to postoperative physical therapy, especially if the patient has limited social support for assistance with therapy.

Several studies have examined the results of arthroscopic capsular release for posttraumatic stiffness. A review of 21 patients with posttraumatic stiffness included 14 patients with stiffness after proximal humeral fracture.[61] The patients were treated with arthroscopic circumferential capsular and subacromial release of adhesions under interscalene block, with immediate physical therapy. At a mean 33-month follow-up (minimum follow-up, 12 months), 95% of the patients were satisfied with the final result. The patients had lost 48% of their gained motion 6 months after surgery, although at final follow-up they were able to recover 110% of immediate postoperative motion. Fifty patients underwent arthroscopic capsular release for adhesive capsulitis classified as postoperative (33 patients), postfracture (2 patients with glenoid fracture, 2 with proximal humeral fracture, and 2 with proximal humeral fracture-dislocation), or idiopathic (11 patients).[60] At an average 20-month follow-up after surgery, all patients had a similar gain in range of motion; the patients with postfracture stiffness gained 39° of elevation and 38° of external rotation. Patients with postoperative stiffness had worse pain, satisfaction, and functional activity scores than those with postfracture or idiopathic stiffness. Stiffness in 68 shoulders was categorized as idiopathic, posttraumatic, postoperative, diabetic, or impingement. After arthroscopic release, the differences in pain, motion, and function were limited, except that patients with diabetes had significantly worse outcomes than patients in the other groups.[62] In general, arthroscopic release of a posttraumatic frozen shoulder provides predictable pain relief and motion

6: Trauma and Fractures

improvement (approximately 40° of elevation and 40° of external rotation), which is comparable to that for an idiopathic frozen shoulder. After surgery, the final improvements take more than 1 year to achieve.

Summary

A variety of complications can result from the surgical or nonsurgical treatment of proximal humeral fractures. Osteonecrosis typically can be treated nonsurgically, with good results in stage I or II lesions and a limited risk of progression, but stage III or IV lesions typically requires surgical treatment. Arthroscopic débridement and core decompression are reasonable alternatives for persistently symptomatic stage I, II, or III lesions, with the most promising results in stage I or II lesions. Proximal humeral malunion is uncommon. Persistently symptomatic surgical neck malunion with a neck-shaft angle of less than 110° can be treated with a surgical neck osteotomy. Greater tuberosity malunion can be treated with osteotomy (usually for posterior displacement) or tuberoplasty with rotator cuff repair (for superior displacement). In a patient younger than 70 years, surgical neck nonunion with a viable humeral head and no arthritis can be treated with open reduction and internal fixation with intramedullary strut graft and a locking proximal humeral plate. Mild to moderate posttraumatic glenohumeral arthritis in a shoulder with concentric wear, some preserved joint space, and minimal, primarily unipolar osteophytes can be effectively treated with arthroscopic débridement and capsular release. Arthroscopic release is an excellent option for restoring motion and function in a patient who has posttraumatic adhesive capsulitis with minimal residual bony deformity or arthritic changes. The restoration of function is similar to that of patients with idiopathic adhesive capsulitis.

Annotated References

1. Iyengar JJ, Devcic Z, Sproul RC, Feeley BT: Nonoperative treatment of proximal humerus fractures: A systematic review. *J Orthop Trauma* 2011;25(10):612-617.

   A systematic review of 12 studies with 650 patients examined the results of nonsurgical treatment of proximal humeral fractures. The healing rate was 98%, and the complication rate was 13%, with varus malunion most common and osteonecrosis relatively rare (2%).

2. Harreld KL, Marker DR, Wiesler ER, Shafiq B, Mont MA: Osteonecrosis of the humeral head. *J Am Acad Orthop Surg* 2009;17(6):345-355.

   The etiology, diagnosis, evaluation, staging, natural history, and treatment of humeral head osteonecrosis were reviewed.

3. Gerber C, Werner CM, Vienne P: Internal fixation of complex fractures of the proximal humerus. *J Bone Joint Surg Br* 2004;86(6):848-855.

4. Thanasas C, Kontakis G, Angoules A, Limb D, Giannoudis P: Treatment of proximal humerus fractures with locking plates: A systematic review. *J Shoulder Elbow Surg* 2009;18(6):837-844.

   A systematic review of 12 studies with 791 patients evaluated the efficacy and early results of using locking plates for proximal humeral fractures. Osteonecrosis occurred in 7.9% of the patients, and screw cutout occurred in 11.6%. Further surgery was needed in 13.7% of the patients.

5. Yüksel HY, Yimaz S, Akşahin E, Celebi L, Muratli HH, Biçimoğlu A: The results of nonoperative treatment for three- and four-part fractures of the proximal humerus in low-demand patients. *J Orthop Trauma* 2011;25(10):588-595.

   A retrospective review of 18 patients with a nonsurgically treated three- or four-part proximal humeral fracture found osteonecrosis in 28%. The results were satisfactory in patients older than 65 years, but the best results were found in younger patients who had a three-part fracture. Level of evidence: IV.

6. Gerber C, Hersche O, Berberat C: The clinical relevance of posttraumatic avascular necrosis of the humeral head. *J Shoulder Elbow Surg* 1998;7(6):586-590.

7. Lee CK, Hansen HR: Post-traumatic avascular necrosis of the humeral head in displaced proximal humeral fractures. *J Trauma* 1981;21(9):788-791.

8. Boileau P, Chuinard C, Le Huec JC, Walch G, Trojani C: Proximal humerus fracture sequelae: Impact of a new radiographic classification on arthroplasty. *Clin Orthop Relat Res* 2006;442:121-130.

9. Chapman C, Mattern C, Levine WN: Arthroscopically assisted core decompression of the proximal humerus for avascular necrosis. *Arthroscopy* 2004;20(9):1003-1006.

10. Dines JS, Strauss EJ, Fealy S, Craig EV: Arthroscopic-assisted core decompression of the humeral head. *Arthroscopy* 2007;23(1):e1-e4.

    An arthroscopic technique used an ACL drill guide to locate and drill humeral head osteonecrosis.

11. Hardy P, Decrette E, Jeanrot C, Colom A, Lortat-Jacob A, Benoit J: Arthroscopic treatment of bilateral humeral head osteonecrosis. *Arthroscopy* 2000;16(3):332-335.

12. Mont MA, Maar DC, Urquhart MW, Lennox D, Hungerford DS: Avascular necrosis of the humeral head treated by core decompression: A retrospective review. *J Bone Joint Surg Br* 1993;75(5):785-788.

13. Cruess RL: Experience with steroid-induced avascular necrosis of the shoulder and etiologic considerations regarding osteonecrosis of the hip. *Clin Orthop Relat Res* 1978;130(130):86-93.

14. Sakai T, Sugano N, Nishii T, Hananouchi T, Yoshikawa H: Extent of osteonecrosis on MRI predicts humeral head collapse. *Clin Orthop Relat Res* 2008; 466(5):1074-1080.

    MRI was used to evaluate the necrotic angle (the extent of the necrotic lesion on midoblique-coronal and midoblique-sagittal studies) in 46 patients with humeral head osteonecrosis. No lesions collapsed if the necrotic angle was less than 90°, but 92% of the lesions collapsed if the angle was greater than 90°.

15. Hattrup SJ, Cofield RH: Osteonecrosis of the humeral head: Relationship of disease stage, extent, and cause to natural history. *J Shoulder Elbow Surg* 1999;8(6): 559-564.

16. L'Insalata JC, Pagnani MJ, Warren RF, Dines DM: Humeral head osteonecrosis: Clinical course and radiographic predictors of outcome. *J Shoulder Elbow Surg* 1996;5(5):355-361.

17. Harreld KL, Marulanda GA, Ulrich SD, Marker DR, Seyler TM, Mont MA: Small-diameter percutaneous decompression for osteonecrosis of the shoulder. *Am J Orthop (Belle Mead NJ)* 2009;38(7):348-354.

    Twenty-six shoulders underwent decompression with a surgical technique that used small-diameter (3-mm) percutaneous perforations. The radiographic progression rate was 4% compared with a 48% rate in nonsurgically treated shoulders.

18. LaPorte DM, Mont MA, Mohan V, Pierre-Jacques H, Jones LC, Hungerford DS: Osteonecrosis of the humeral head treated by core decompression. *Clin Orthop Relat Res* 1998;355:254-260.

19. Beredjiklian PK, Iannotti JP, Norris TR, Williams GR: Operative treatment of malunion of a fracture of the proximal aspect of the humerus. *J Bone Joint Surg Am* 1998;80(10):1484-1497.

20. Boileau P, Trojani C, Walch G, Krishnan SG, Romeo A, Sinnerton R: Shoulder arthroplasty for the treatment of the sequelae of fractures of the proximal humerus. *J Shoulder Elbow Surg* 2001;10(4):299-308.

21. Benegas E, Zoppi Filho A, Ferreira Filho AA, et al: Surgical treatment of varus malunion of the proximal humerus with valgus osteotomy. *J Shoulder Elbow Surg* 2007;16(1):55-59.

    Five patients with a proximal humeral surgical neck varus malunion underwent a valgus wedge osteotomy of the proximal humerus with plate and screws. All patients had union at 6 weeks and were satisfied.

22. Calvo E, Merino-Gutierrez I, Lagunes I: Arthroscopic tuberoplasty for subacromial impingement secondary

to proximal humeral malunion. *Knee Surg Sports Traumatol Arthrosc* 2010;18(7):988-991.

    An arthroscopic tuberoplasty technique for isolated greater tuberosity malunion with severe upward displacement included intra-articular and extra-articular transtendinous abrasion of the greater tuberosity with rotator cuff insertion preservation.

23. Lädermann A, Denard PJ, Burkhart SS: Arthroscopic management of proximal humerus malunion with tuberoplasty and rotator cuff retensioning. *Arthroscopy* 2012;28(9):1220-1229.

    Nine patients underwent arthroscopic tuberoplasty and rotator cuff advancement for malunion of a proximal humeral fracture. At 50-month follow-up, there was significant improvement in pain, range of motion, and outcome, with 89% able to return to their previous sport and 100% satisfied.

24. Martinez AA, Calvo A, Domingo J, Cuenca J, Herrera A: Arthroscopic treatment for malunions of the proximal humeral greater tuberosity. *Int Orthop* 2010; 34(8):1207-1211.

    Eight patients underwent arthroscopic rotator cuff detachment, tuberoplasty, rotator cuff repair, and acromioplasty. All patients had improved pain, and seven returned to their previous occupations without restrictions.

25. Gill TJ, Waters P: Valgus osteotomy of the humeral neck: A technique for the treatment of humerus varus. *J Shoulder Elbow Surg* 1997;6(3):306-310.

26. Porcellini G, Campi F, Paladini P: Articular impingement in malunited fracture of the humeral head. *Arthroscopy* 2002;18(8):E39.

27. Solonen KA, Vastamäki M: Osteotomy of the neck of the humerus for traumatic varus deformity. *Acta Orthop Scand* 1985;56(1):79-80.

28. Neer CS II: Displaced proximal humeral fractures: I. Classification and evaluation. *J Bone Joint Surg Am* 1970;52(6):1077-1089.

29. Park TS, Choi IY, Kim YH, Park MR, Shon JH, Kim SI: A new suggestion for the treatment of minimally displaced fractures of the greater tuberosity of the proximal humerus. *Bull Hosp Jt Dis* 1997;56(3): 171-176.

30. Kim KC, Rhee KJ, Shin HD: Arthroscopic treatment of symptomatic malunion of the greater tuberosity of the humerus using the suture-bridge technique. *Orthopedics* 2010;33(4):242-245.

    An arthroscopic technique for rotator cuff takedown, tuberoplasty, and double-row suture-bridge repair of symptomatic greater tuberosity malunion was described.

31. Paavolainen P, Björkenheim JM, Slätis P, Paukku P: Operative treatment of severe proximal humeral fractures. *Acta Orthop Scand* 1983;54(3):374-379.

6: Trauma and Fractures

32. Court-Brown CM, McQueen MM: Nonunions of the proximal humerus: Their prevalence and functional outcome. *J Trauma* 2008;64(6):1517-1521.

A prospective study of 1,027 consecutive proximal humeral fractures found a 1.1% nonunion rate. Risk factors included metaphyseal comminution and 33% to 100% surgical neck translation.

33. Galatz LM, Iannotti JP: Management of surgical neck nonunions. *Orthop Clin North Am* 2000;31(1):51-61.

34. Healy WL, Jupiter JB, Kristiansen TK, White RR: Nonunion of the proximal humerus: A review of 25 cases. *J Orthop Trauma* 1990;4(4):424-431.

35. Lin JS, Klepps S, Miller S, Cleeman E, Flatow EL: Effectiveness of replacement arthroplasty with calcar grafting and avoidance of greater tuberosity osteotomy for the treatment of humeral surgical neck nonunions. *J Shoulder Elbow Surg* 2006;15(1):12-18.

36. Ring D, McKee MD, Perey BH, Jupiter JB: The use of a blade plate and autogenous cancellous bone graft in the treatment of ununited fractures of the proximal humerus. *J Shoulder Elbow Surg* 2001;10(6):501-507.

37. Badman BL, Mighell M, Kalandiak SP, Prasarn M: Proximal humeral nonunions treated with fixed-angle locked plating and an intramedullary strut allograft. *J Orthop Trauma* 2009;23(3):173-179.

Eighteen patients with a surgical neck proximal humeral nonunion were treated using internal fixation with a locked plate augmented with an intramedullary cortical allograft. At an average 26.5-month follow-up, 94% of the nonunions had healed.

38. Goldstein C, Sprague S, Petrisor BA: Electrical stimulation for fracture healing: Current evidence. *J Orthop Trauma* 2010;24(suppl 1):S62-S65.

39. Watanabe Y, Matsushita T, Bhandari M, Zdero R, Schemitsch EH: Ultrasound for fracture healing: Current evidence. *J Orthop Trauma* 2010;24(suppl 1):S56-S61.

40. Zelle BA, Gollwitzer H, Zlowodzki M, Bühren V: Extracorporeal shock wave therapy: Current evidence. *J Orthop Trauma* 2010;24(suppl 1):S66-S70.

41. Friedlaender GE, Perry CR, Cole JD, et al: Osteogenic protein-1 (bone morphogenetic protein-7) in the treatment of tibial nonunions. *J Bone Joint Surg Am* 2001; 83(suppl 1 pt 2):S151-S158.

42. Govender S, Csimma C, Genant HK, et al; BMP-2 Evaluation in Surgery for Tibial Trauma (BESTT) Study Group: Recombinant human bone morphogenetic protein-2 for treatment of open tibial fractures: A prospective, controlled, randomized study of four hundred and fifty patients. *J Bone Joint Surg Am* 2002; 84-A(12):2123-2134.

43. Izquierdo R, Voloshin I, Edwards S, et al; American Academy of Orthopedic Surgeons: Treatment of glenohumeral osteoarthritis. *J Am Acad Orthop Surg* 2010; 18(6):375-382.

The AAOS guidelines on the treatment of glenohumeral osteoarthritis were reviewed.

44. Denard PJ, Wirth MA, Orfaly RM: Management of glenohumeral arthritis in the young adult. *J Bone Joint Surg Am* 2011;93(9):885-892.

Current management strategies for young, active patients with glenohumeral osteoarthritis include nonsurgical treatment, arthroscopic débridement, and arthroplasty.

45. Silverstein E, Leger R, Shea KP: The use of intra-articular hylan G-F 20 in the treatment of symptomatic osteoarthritis of the shoulder: A preliminary study. *Am J Sports Med* 2007;35(6):979-985.

Thirty patients with glenohumeral osteoarthritis were treated with three weekly intra-articular hylan injections. At 6-month follow-up, there was significant improvement in UCLA and visual analog pain scores as well as sleeping ability.

46. Blaine T, Moskowitz R, Udell J, et al: Treatment of persistent shoulder pain with sodium hyaluronate: A randomized, controlled trial. A multicenter study. *J Bone Joint Surg Am* 2008;90(5):970-979.

In a prospective randomized study, 456 patients with persistent shoulder pain of different etiologies were treated using sodium hyaluronate or saline. At 26-week follow-up, pain relief was significantly greater in the patients with glenohumeral osteoarthritis than in other patients.

47. Weinstein DM, Bucchieri JS, Pollock RG, Flatow EL, Bigliani LU: Arthroscopic debridement of the shoulder for osteoarthritis. *Arthroscopy* 2000;16(5):471-476.

48. Cameron BD, Galatz LM, Ramsey ML, Williams GR, Iannotti JP: Non-prosthetic management of grade IV osteochondral lesions of the glenohumeral joint. *J Shoulder Elbow Surg* 2002;11(1):25-32.

49. Richards DP, Burkhart SS: Arthroscopic debridement and capsular release for glenohumeral osteoarthritis. *Arthroscopy* 2007;23(9):1019-1022.

After arthroscopic débridement and capsular release in eight patients, motion significantly improved in forward elevation (21°), external rotation (17°), and internal rotation (31°).

50. Guyette TM, Bae H, Warren RF, Craig E, Wickiewicz TL: Results of arthroscopic subacromial decompression in patients with subacromial impingement and glenohumeral degenerative joint disease. *J Shoulder Elbow Surg* 2002;11(4):299-304.

51. Kerr BJ, McCarty EC: Outcome of arthroscopic débridement is worse for patients with glenohumeral arthritis of both sides of the joint. *Clin Orthop Relat Res* 2008;466(3):634-638.

6: Trauma and Fractures

In 19 patients retrospectively reviewed at an average 20 months after arthroscopic débridement for glenohumeral osteoarthritis, the grade of the lesion was found not to influence outcome scores. Patients with unipolar lesions did better than those with bipolar lesions.

52. Van Thiel GS, Sheehan S, Frank RM, et al: Retrospective analysis of arthroscopic management of glenohumeral degenerative disease. *Arthroscopy* 2010; 26(11): 1451-1455.

    In 81 patients retrospectively evaluated after arthroscopic débridement for glenohumeral osteoarthritis, the procedure was found to allow patients with residual joint space and no large osteophytes to avoid arthroplasty. The risks for failure included bipolar grade IV disease and a joint space of less than 2 mm.

53. de Beer JF, Bhatia DN, van Rooyen KS, Du Toit DF: Arthroscopic debridement and biological resurfacing of the glenoid in glenohumeral arthritis. *Knee Surg Sports Traumatol Arthrosc* 2010;18(12):1767-1773.

    Thirty-two patients underwent arthroscopic débridement and glenoid resurfacing with an acellular human dermal scaffold. At a minimum 2-year follow-up, the procedure was successful in 72% of patients. Five patients underwent conversion to arthroplasty.

54. Savoie FH III, Brislin KJ, Argo D: Arthroscopic glenoid resurfacing as a surgical treatment for glenohumeral arthritis in the young patient: Midterm results. *Arthroscopy* 2009;25(8):864-871.

    Twenty patients underwent arthroscopic glenoid resurfacing with a biologic patch for glenohumeral arthritis. At a minimum 3-year follow-up, 75% of patients were satisfied, with the other patients proceeding to shoulder replacement. Level of evidence: IV.

55. Faraj D, Kooistra BW, Vd Stappen WA, Werre AJ: Results of 131 consecutive operated patients with a displaced proximal humerus fracture: An analysis with more than two years follow-up. *Eur J Orthop Surg Traumatol* 2011;21(1):7-12.

    Ninety-two patients were treated with open reduction and internal fixation of a proximal humeral fracture with a locking proximal humeral plate or a PHILOS plate. At a median of 2.4 years after surgery, 39.1% of patients had a complication including loss of reduction or screw cutout (6.5%), impingement (11.9%), plate breakage (6.5%), and frozen shoulder (3.3%). Reoperations were required in 29% of patients due to a complication.

56. Koval KJ, Gallagher MA, Marsicano JG, Cuomo F, McShinawy A, Zuckerman JD: Functional outcome after minimally displaced fractures of the proximal part of the humerus. *J Bone Joint Surg Am* 1997;79(2): 203-207.

57. Duralde XA, Leddy LR: The results of ORIF of displaced unstable proximal humeral fractures using a locking plate. *J Shoulder Elbow Surg* 2010;19(4): 480-488.

    Twenty-two patients underwent open reduction and internal fixation with a locking proximal humeral plate. At a minimum 2-year follow-up, all fractures had healed. Anatomic alignment was maintained in 72%, and osteonecrosis had developed in 9%. Level of evidence: IV.

58. Hodgson SA, Mawson SJ, Saxton JM, Stanley D: Rehabilitation of two-part fractures of the neck of the humerus (two-year follow-up). *J Shoulder Elbow Surg* 2007;16(2):143-145.

    In a prospective randomized study, patients treated with immediate therapy after a two-part humeral neck fracture had better function at 1-year follow-up than those treated with 3 weeks of immobilization, but there was no difference at 2-year follow-up.

59. Lefevre-Colau MM, Babinet A, Fayad F, et al: Immediate mobilization compared with conventional immobilization for the impacted nonoperatively treated proximal humeral fracture: A randomized controlled trial. *J Bone Joint Surg Am* 2007;89(12):2582-2590.

    Seventy-four patients with an impacted proximal humeral fracture were randomly assigned to early passive motion or 3 weeks of immobilization. Early mobilization led to better Constant scores, better active mobility, and less pain at 3-month follow-up, with no displacement or nonunion.

60. Holloway GB, Schenk T, Williams GR, Ramsey ML, Iannotti JP: Arthroscopic capsular release for the treatment of refractory postoperative or post-fracture shoulder stiffness. *J Bone Joint Surg Am* 2001;83-A(11):1682-1687.

61. Levy O, Webb M, Even T, Venkateswaran B, Funk L, Copeland SA: Arthroscopic capsular release for posttraumatic shoulder stiffness. *J Shoulder Elbow Surg* 2008;17(3):410-414.

    Twenty-one patients underwent arthroscopic capsular release for a posttraumatic stiff shoulder. At 33-month follow-up, the patients achieved a final mean net gain of 110% of motion compared with immediate postsurgical motion, and 95% were satisfied.

62. Nicholson GP: Arthroscopic capsular release for stiff shoulders: Effect of etiology on outcomes. *Arthroscopy* 2003;19(1):40-49.

63. Davis JJ, Swenson JD, Greis PE, Burks RT, Tashjian RZ: Interscalene block for postoperative analgesia using only ultrasound guidance: The outcome in 200 patients. *J Clin Anesth* 2009;21(4):272-277.

    Two hundred patients undergoing shoulder or elbow surgery had ultrasonographically guided interscalene blocks. The success rate was 99%; 6% had needle paresthesia, and 1% had a transient neurologic deficit. There were no permanent deficits.

6: Trauma and Fractures

Chapter 36

Clavicle Fractures

James M. Dunwoody, MD, FRCSC   Michael D. McKee, MD, FRCSC

Epidemiology

Clavicle fractures have a reported annual incidence of 29.14 per 100,000 population.[1] Men and boys younger than 20 years are most commonly affected. Middle third fractures, usually displaced, account for 80%, lateral fractures account for 15%, and medial third fractures are only 5%.

Anatomy

The clavicle is in close proximity to the apical pleura, the brachial plexus, the subclavian artery, and the subclavian vein. These structures can be injured by a fracture fragment or screw placement. The subclavian vein is most at risk during internal fixation.[2,3] In the medial third of the clavicle, the subclavian vein may be in intimate contact with the posterior aspect of the bone, and this proximity makes anterior-to-posterior screw placement perilous.[2] In the middle third of the bone, the vessels assume a posteroinferior position. Abduction of the arm to 90° can increase the margin of safety during screw placement.[3] Instrumentation can be most safely used in the lateral third of the clavicle.

The cutaneous branches of the medial, intermediate, and lateral supraclavicular nerves fan out to cover the subcutaneous surface of the entire clavicle. These nerves are at risk from a transverse incision or intraoperative traction. Chest wall numbness inferior to the incision is common after surgery.[4,5]

Dr. Dunwoody or an immediate family member has stock or stock options held in Pfizer and Procter & Gamble. Dr. McKee or an immediate family member serves as a board member, owner, officer, or committee member of the American Shoulder and Elbow Surgeons, the Orthopaedic Trauma Society, and the Canadian Orthopedic Association; has received royalties from Stryker; is a member of a speakers' bureau or has made paid presentations on behalf of Synthes and Zimmer; serves as a paid consultant to or is an employee of Synthes and Zimmer; and has received research or institutional support from Wright Medical Technology and Zimmer.

Classification

The most common comprehensive classification of clavicle fractures is the Edinburgh system. In this reliable and reproducible system, the fracture is classified based on its location, displacement, comminution, and intra-articular extension.[1] In the less commonly used AO/Orthopaedic Trauma Association system, fractures are divided into types based on location and further subdivided into groups and subgroups based on the specific fracture pattern (**Figure 1**).[6]

Clinical Examination

Open fractures and true skin tenting are rare but can occur in patients older than 65 years or after high-energy trauma[7] (**Figure 2**). Clavicular shortening can be clinically assessed by measuring from the suprasternal notch to the acromioclavicular joint and comparing the measurement to that of the contralateral side. Scapular winging and dyskinesia may be present with a malunion with shortening.[8]

A careful neurologic and vascular examination always should be performed. Injuries to the subclavian vessels and the brachial plexus can occur, and associated shoulder girdle, chest wall, and upper extremity injuries should be sought.[5]

Imaging

AP and 20° cephalad upshot views of the shoulder should be routinely obtained.[9] CT may be useful in medial fractures but is not routinely used for other fractures. Angiography may be obtained if vascular trauma is suspected.

Nonsurgical Treatment

Nonsurgical treatment leads to uneventful healing in most patients with an nondisplaced clavicle fracture.[10] The figure-of-8 bandage has been used in the past but has no advantage over simple treatment using a sling for comfort.[11] Most patients will be able to remove the sling and begin range-of-motion exercises at 2 to 3 weeks.

6: Trauma and Fractures

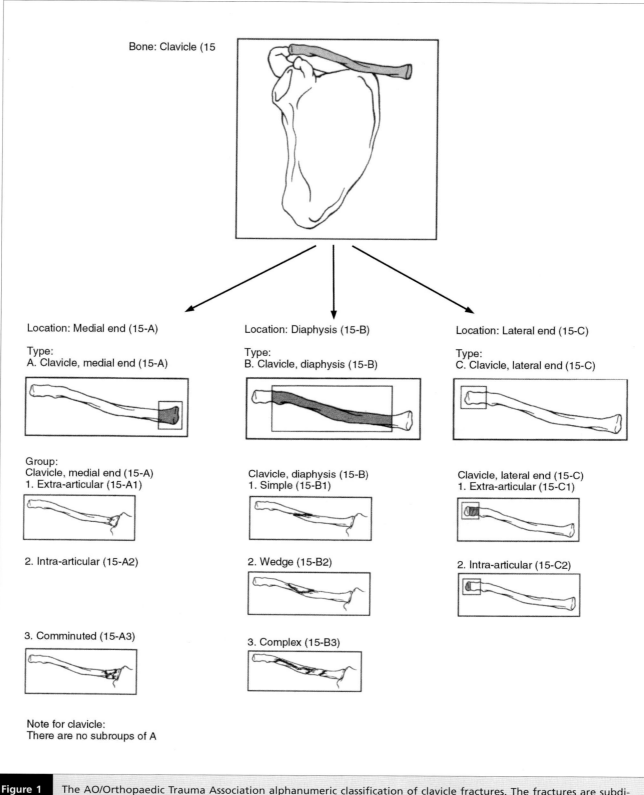

Bone: Clavicle (15

Location: Medial end (15-A)

Type:
A. Clavicle, medial end (15-A)

Group:
Clavicle, medial end (15-A)
1. Extra-articular (15-A1)

2. Intra-articular (15-A2)

3. Comminuted (15-A3)

Note for clavicle:
There are no subroups of A

Location: Diaphysis (15-B)

Type:
B. Clavicle, diaphysis (15-B)

Clavicle, diaphysis (15-B)
1. Simple (15-B1)

2. Wedge (15-B2)

3. Complex (15-B3)

Location: Lateral end (15-C)

Type:
C. Clavicle, lateral end (15-C)

Clavicle, lateral end (15-C)
1. Extra-articular (15-C1)

2. Intra-articular (15-C2)

Figure 1 The AO/Orthopaedic Trauma Association alphanumeric classification of clavicle fractures. The fractures are subdivided into type, group, and subgroup based on location and pattern. Subgroupings are not shown. Reproduced with permission from Marsh JL, Slongo TF, Asel J, et al: Fracture and dislocation classification compendium - 2017: Orthopaedic Trauma Association classification, database and outtcomes committee. *J Orthop Trauma* 2007; 21(suppl 10): S1-S133.

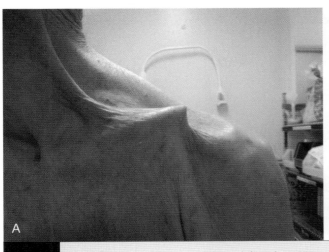
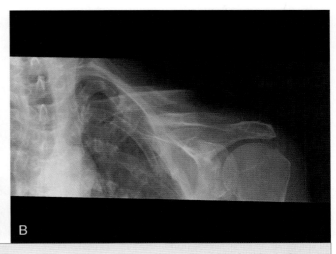

Figure 2   Photograph showing skin tenting (**A**) and AP 20° cephalad radiograph showing a displaced midshaft clavicle fracture (**B**) in a 79-year-old man 5 months after a fall down stairs. The patient also had fracture of ipsilateral ribs 2 through 10 and a hemothorax requiring tube thoracostomy drainage. Only the most superficial layer of skin was present over the medial spike of bone. True skin tenting with potential skin compromise, as seen in **A**, is rare.

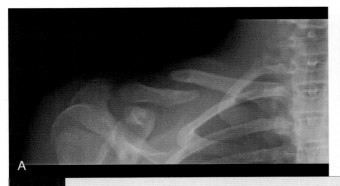
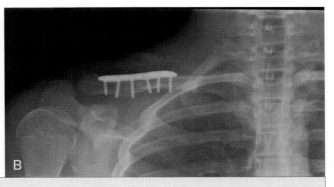

Figure 3   AP 20° cephalad radiograph showing a displaced midshaft clavicle fracture with significant shortening in a 16 year old before (**A**) and after (**B**) open reduction and internal fixation using a superiorly positioned, precontoured plate.

Not all displaced fractures require surgical intervention. Children have greater healing potential than adults, and patients older than 65 years may achieve satisfactory function in the setting of a nonunion.[12] Higher rates of functional deficit and complications have been reported after nonsurgical treatment of a displaced midshaft clavicle fracture than after surgical treatment.[10,13,14]

Surgical Treatment

The benefit of treating displaced midshaft clavicle fractures with open reduction and internal fixation has been shown in multiple studies. Patients age 16 to 60 years had better outcomes with lower rates of nonunion or malunion if treated surgically with open reduction and internal fixation rather than nonsurgically. The rate of complications was 37% in the surgically treated patients and 63% in the nonsurgically treated patients.[13]

If plating is chosen, the plate can be placed superiorly or anteroinferiorly (**Figure 3**). The advantages of the anteroinferior position include the ability to use longer screws, a potentially safer screw trajectory, less hardware prominence, and possible biomechanical superiority.[15-17] The 3.5-mm reconstruction plate should be avoided, especially in a relatively large and active patient, because it has less resistance to bending and torque than a precontoured or compression plate.[18]

Locking plates have become popular, but their use in clavicle fixation remains controversial.[17,19,20] The shallow threads used in locking plates may be more susceptible to failure when loads are applied in an axial direction.[19] No prospective randomized clinical studies have compared locking to conventional plates, and their use remains unclear.

Intramedullary devices have the theoretic advantage of causing less soft-tissue disruption, smaller scars, and less chest wall numbness compared with formal open reduction and plating techniques (**Figure 4**). Three

6: Trauma and Fractures

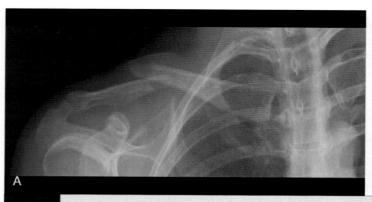
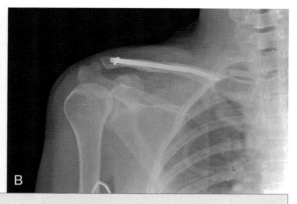

Figure 4 AP 20° cephalad radiograph showing a simple displaced midshaft clavicle fracture in a 28-year-old woman before (**A**) and after (**B**) treatment using a flexible, locked intramedullary nail. The advantages of this technique compared with formal open reduction and plate fixation include a smaller incision, less chest wall numbness, and minimal hardware prominence.

classes of intramedullary implants are in current use. Titanium elastic intramedullary nails are typically inserted antegrade. Straight, larger diameter pins are inserted using a retrograde technique. A retrograde flexible locked nail has been introduced, although clinical data are lacking. Unlocked intramedullary devices are biomechanically inferior to plates, especially in rotation. In most clinical studies, the use of straight, larger diameter pins leads to a higher complication rate (5% to 40%) than plating.[18,21,22] Few studies have compared plate to intramedullary fixation.[23,24] At this time, intramedullary fixation may be best reserved for patients with a simple fracture pattern and minimal comminution.[25]

Anatomically precontoured plates in a superior configuration often are preferred. Branches of the supraclavicular nerves are spared whenever possible, and attempts are made to achieve lag screw fixation followed by fracture stabilization, with a minimum of six cortices of fixation per fragment. A careful two-layer closure is performed, and the arm is kept in a sling for comfort. Contact sports are avoided for 3 months.[9] Plate removal is required in a few patients but is deferred at least 1 to 2 years to avoid refracture.[5]

Malunion

Symptomatic malunion of a displaced midshaft clavicle fracture is uncommon.[8,26] The typical deformity includes shortening, inferior translation, and anterior rotation of the distal fragment. Shortening has the most clinical significance; the symptoms are related to alterations in the musculotendinous relationships of the shoulder and narrowing of the costoclavicular space. Patients typically experience pain, easy fatigue of the shoulder musculature, and neurologic dysfunction. Unacceptable cosmesis may result from the ptotic, driven-in appearance of the clavicle.

During surgical planning, the clinical measurement of clavicular shortening is compared with the amount of radiographic overlap. If the clinical shortening is greater than the amount of radiographic overlap, an interpositional iliac crest bone graft may be required to restore adequate length.[8] In most patients, surgery is successful for restoring function and relieving pain. The clavicle is osteotomized in the plane of the healed fracture, the fracture is re-created, and the deformity is corrected. Local bone graft can be used in almost all patients, and iliac crest bone graft is not necessary unless the clinical shortening exceeds that seen radiographically (for example, osteotomy and reorientation of the clavicle to its preinjury position will leave a significant bone defect at the osteotomy site). The preferred osteotomy stabilization is with a precontoured clavicle plate in a superior position and at least six cortices on each side of the osteotomy, if possible. Compression through the plate is applied whenever possible. Strengthening and resistance activities are allowed at 6 to 8 weeks. In one study, the average shortening was 2.9 cm before surgery and 0.4 cm after surgery.[8] Fourteen of the 15 patients healed at the osteotomy site, and 1 patient had a nonunion. No iliac crest bone graft was needed. All patients with a healed osteotomy were satisfied with their surgery and functional outcome.

Nonunion

Nonunion has been defined as a condition in which bony union will not occur without surgical intervention. The exact timing of surgical intervention to correct a nonunion is a matter of debate and has been defined as both 24 weeks and 1 year.[13,27] Nonsurgically treated displaced midshaft clavicle fractures have a reported nonunion rate of approximately 15%; in comparison, the nonunion rate after plating is 1% to 2%.[10,13] Factors associated with the development of midshaft nonunion include female sex, advanced age, fracture displacement, and comminution.[27] Although smoking is believed to be a risk factor for nonunion af-

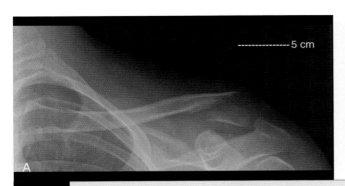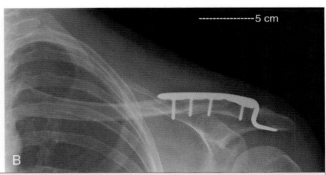

Figure 5	AP 20° cephalad radiograph showing a displaced type II lateral clavicle fracture in a 26-year-old man treated with open reduction and internal fixation using a 3.5-mm LCP clavicle hook plate (Synthes, West Chester, PA). A hook plate was needed because of inadequate screw purchase in the distal fragment.

ter fracture, little specific information is available on the effect of smoking on the clavicle.

In patients with a painful nonunion, surgery can be expected to have a high rate of success. Bone graft is required in a few patients.[28,29] Careful comparison of clinically assessed shortening with radiologic overlap may be helpful in predicting whether the patient requires an intercalary segment of iliac crest autograft. The bony ends are prepared by re-creating the medullary canals and feathering the edges. Local bone is saved and packed within the nonunion site. The use of superior anatomic plates with a minimum of six cortices per side is the treatment of choice. Interfragmentary compression with lag screws is performed if possible.

In the rare patient with failure of internal fixation, the possibility of infection must be considered. A two-stage approach may be necessary, in which eradication of the infection is followed by definitive reconstruction. These challenging procedures almost always require autogenous bone graft, occasionally augmented by osteoinductive osteobiologic material (bone morphogenetic protein).

Lateral Clavicle Fractures

Fractures of the lateral clavicle are less common than those of the midshaft clavicle, and they tend to occur in adults older than 65 years. The prevalence of nonunion in displaced lateral fractures is 28% to 44%,[1,12,30] but the number of symptomatic nonunions is lower than after a midshaft fracture. A patient who is older than 65 years and has low physical demands may have satisfactory function after nonsurgical treatment.

The most commonly used classification for lateral clavicle fractures is the modified Neer system.[30] The treatment of Neer types IIA, IIB, and V is the most controversial. Other comprehensive classifications are the AO/Orthopaedic Trauma Association and Edinburgh systems.[1,6]

The treatment of a nondisplaced lateral clavicle fracture is nonsurgical, and good results can be expected.

Displaced fractures may be amenable to surgical treatment. Although some authors prefer initial nonsurgical treatment for all fractures, there is evidence that more complications can be expected if fixation is delayed.[30] A myriad of fixation options has been described; the most popular and widely studied modern techniques involve the use of superior precontoured locking plates and hook plates.[30-34]

Hook plates have been in use since the 1980s for fractures in which there is inadequate purchase in the distal fragment. Care must be taken to appropriately size the hook to the morphology of the clavicle. In some instances, bending the hook down a few degrees may allow a better fit. The hook is placed under the acromion, posterior to the acromioclavicular joint. As the plate is reduced to the shaft of the clavicle, the fracture is reduced. The plate should be removed within 6 months. The use of a hook plate may be associated with shoulder pain, acromion osteolysis, and even fracture of the shaft of the clavicle medial to the plate. Symptoms are usually relieved by plate removal, and a high rate of union can be expected.[31,33-35] Although the hook plate is useful for treating very distal fractures, the complication rate is high, and usually the plate must be removed to reestablish a full range of shoulder motion.

Locking anatomic distal clavicle plates are the other common method of fixation. If the distal fragment is small or bone quality is poor, fixation into the coracoid can be beneficial, although this is uncommon. This can be achieved with a screw through the plate or sutures around the coracoid.[32,34] A hook plate can be used in these situations of questionable bone stock for plate fixation (**Figure 5**). It is preferable to fix most displaced lateral clavicle fractures in active, healthy patients. A rate of union higher than 90% and satisfactory functioned outcomes can be expected with this approach. Patients are informed not to expect normal shoulder motion until the plate is removed after fracture union.

Subcoracoid fixation is an alternative method of fixation for lateral clavicular fractures with inadequate or tenuous fixation of the distal fragment. In this tech-

6: Trauma and Fractures

nique, a sling of heavy suture (such as size 5 Mersilene [Ethicon, Somerville, NJ]) or tendon (hamstring is preferred) is used around the coracoid to secure the shaft fragment to the coracoid, thus indirectly reducing it to the distal fragment. Alternatively, suture anchors can be embedded into the coracoid, with the suture passed around the clavicle. This technique, alone or in combination with standard methods, resulted in a high rate of union with excellent shoulder function and minimal hardware-related complications.[36]

Medial Clavicle Fractures

Medial fracture is the least common clavicle fracture pattern. These fractures occur in fewer than 5% of patients with clavicle fracture and may be associated with high-energy trauma.[1,37] Reports in the literature are sparse and largely consist of small retrospective reviews. A medial fracture often is a fracture-dislocation of the sternoclavicular joint. Radiographs often are unclear, and CT is beneficial for defining a medial clavicle fracture. Surgery may be considered for a displaced fracture, particularly if nearby vital structures are compressed. Screws placed from anterior to posterior are at particular risk of causing injury to the subclavian vein.[2] These injuries must be approached on an individual basis.

Summary

Most fractures of the clavicle can be treated nonsurgically. However, randomized clinical studies have found that primary surgical repair of a completely displaced midshaft fracture of the clavicle in a healthy, active individual younger than 60 years was superior to nonsurgical treatment in functional outcomes and nonunion rates. As for other fractures, careful patient selection and meticulous attention to surgical technique are mandatory for success. Open reduction and plate fixation with an anatomic plate is the most popular method of treatment, although intramedullary fixation has theoretic advantages and has had good results in some studies. Displaced lateral clavicle fractures have a high rate of nonunion, often with minimal symptoms in patients older than 65 years. A variety of surgical options, including precontoured distal plate fixation, hook plate fixation, and subcoracoid or coracoid repair, have had high rates of success in studies of relatively young, active patients.

Annotated References

1. Robinson CM: Fractures of the clavicle in the adult: Epidemiology and classification. *J Bone Joint Surg Br* 1998;80(3):476-484.

2. Sinha A, Edwin J, Sreeharsha B, Bhalaik V, Brownson P: A radiological study to define safe zones for drilling during plating of clavicle fractures. *J Bone Joint Surg Br* 2011;93(9):1247-1252.

   Three-dimensional CT angiography was used to determine the relationship of vascular structures to the clavicle. The subclavian vein was most at risk, particularly with anterior-to-posterior screw placement in the medial third. Anteroinferior plating was considered safer than superior plating in the middle and lateral thirds.

3. Werner SD, Reed J, Hanson T, Jaeblon T: Anatomic relationships after instrumentation of the midshaft clavicle with 3.5-mm reconstruction plating: An anatomic study. *J Orthop Trauma* 2011;25(11):657-660.

   A cadaver study found increased distance of the subclavian vein, the subclavian artery, and the brachial plexus from the clavicle when the arm was abducted to 90°.

4. Wang K, Dowrick A, Choi J, Rahim R, Edwards E: Post-operative numbness and patient satisfaction following plate fixation of clavicular fractures. *Injury* 2010;41(10):1002-1005.

   In a retrospective review of patients treated with plate fixation of a clavicle fracture using a horizontal or a vertical incision, less chest wall numbness occurred in those with a vertical incision. Level of evidence: IV.

5. Hsu SH, Ahmad CS, Henry PD, McKee MD, Levine WN: How to minimize complications in acromioclavicular joint and clavicle surgery. *Instr Course Lect* 2012;61:169-183.

   Complications related to clavicle fracture treatment and their avoidance are summarized.

6. Marsh JL, Slongo TF, Agel J, et al: Fracture and dislocation classification compendium—2007: Orthopaedic Trauma Association classification, database and outcomes committee. *J Orthop Trauma* 2007;21(10, suppl):S1-S133.

   The Orthopaedic Trauma Association classification of clavicle fractures is provided.

7. Gottschalk HP, Dumont G, Khanani S, Browne RH, Starr AJ: Open clavicle fractures: Patterns of trauma and associated injuries. *J Orthop Trauma* 2012;26(2):107-109.

   The largest study of open clavicle fractures found that these rare injuries may be associated with severe head injury and great vessel trauma. Level of evidence: IV.

8. McKee MD, Wild LM, Schemitsch EH: Midshaft malunions of the clavicle. *J Bone Joint Surg Am* 2003;85-A(5):790-797.

9. McKee MD, Hall JA: Open reduction and internal fixation of displaced clavicle fractures, in Schemitsch EH, McKee MD, eds: *Operative Techniques: Orthopaedic Trauma Surgery*. Philadelphia, PA, WB Saunders, 2010, pp 3-10.

   The technical details of open reduction and internal

fixation of midshaft clavicle fractures with a superior plate are described.

10. McKee RC, Whelan DB, Schemitsch EH, McKee MD: Operative versus nonoperative care of displaced midshaft clavicular fractures: A meta-analysis of randomized clinical trials. *J Bone Joint Surg Am* 2012;94(8): 675-684.

    A meta-analysis of six randomized clinical studies found a higher rate of symptomatic malunion and nonunion in nonsurgically treated patients. Functional outcomes at 1 year were only marginally better after surgery. Displaced midshaft clavicle fractures will heal with few consequences in approximately 75% of patients. Level of evidence: I.

11. Andersen K, Jensen PO, Lauritzen J: Treatment of clavicular fractures: Figure-of-eight bandage versus a simple sling. *Acta Orthop Scand* 1987;58(1):71-74.

12. Robinson CM, Cairns DA: Primary nonoperative treatment of displaced lateral fractures of the clavicle. *J Bone Joint Surg Am* 2004;86-A(4):778-782.

13. Canadian Orthopaedic Trauma Society: Nonoperative treatment compared with plate fixation of displaced midshaft clavicular fractures: A multicenter, randomized clinical trial. *J Bone Joint Surg Am* 2007;89(1): 1-10.

    A prospective, randomized clinical study compared plate fixation with nonsurgical treatment of displaced midshaft clavicle fractures. Open reduction and internal fixation led to better outcomes and a lower rate of complications at 1-year follow-up. Level of evidence: I.

14. McKee MD, Pedersen EM, Jones C, et al: Deficits following nonoperative treatment of displaced midshaft clavicular fractures. *J Bone Joint Surg Am* 2006;88(1): 35-40.

15. Collinge C, Devinney S, Herscovici D, DiPasquale T, Sanders R: Anterior-inferior plate fixation of middle-third fractures and nonunions of the clavicle. *J Orthop Trauma* 2006;20(10):680-686.

16. Favre P, Kloen P, Helfet DL, Werner CM: Superior versus anteroinferior plating of the clavicle: A finite element study. *J Orthop Trauma* 2011;25(11):661-665.

    A finite element study found that anteroinferior plating had better resistance to cantilever bending than superior plating.

17. Celestre P, Roberston C, Mahar A, Oka R, Meunier M, Schwartz A: Biomechanical evaluation of clavicle fracture plating techniques: Does a locking plate provide improved stability? *J Orthop Trauma* 2008; 22(4):241-247.

    A biomechanical comparison of plate position and locking used synthetic clavicle bones. Superior locking plates were found to have better properties than conventional or anteroinferiorly placed plates.

18. Drosdowech DS, Manwell SE, Ferreira LM, Goel DP, Faber KJ, Johnson JA: Biomechanical analysis of fixation of middle third fractures of the clavicle. *J Orthop Trauma* 2011;25(1):39-43.

    A cadaver study compared the resistance to bending and torque of a clavicular pin and three superior plates. The 3.5-mm locking plate and dynamic compression plate were superior to the pin and 3.5-mm reconstruction plate, especially with simulated comminution.

19. Brouwer KM, Wright TC, Ring DC: Failure of superior locking clavicle plate by axial pull-out of the lateral screws: A report of four cases. *J Shoulder Elbow Surg* 2009;18(1):e22-e25.

    In a case study of four unsuccessful procedures using superiorly placed locking plates, failure was attributed to axial loading of screws and a shallow thread profile. The recommendations included using an anteroinferior plate position or conventional plating. Level of evidence: IV.

20. Pai HT, Lee YS, Cheng CY: Surgical treatment of midclavicular fractures in the elderly: A comparison of locking and nonlocking plates. *Orthopedics* 2009; 32(4).

    In a prospective study, patients older than 60 years with a midshaft clavicle fracture were treated with locked or conventional plating. Patients in the locked plating group had a lower complication rate. Level of evidence: II.

21. Millett PJ, Hurst JM, Horan MP, Hawkins RJ: Complications of clavicle fractures treated with intramedullary fixation. *J Shoulder Elbow Surg* 2011;20(1): 86-91.

    In a retrospective review of diaphyseal clavicle fractures treated with the Rockwood clavicle pin, all pins were removed at an average of 67 days. The rate of nonunion was 8.6%. Level of evidence: IV.

22. Mudd CD, Quigley KJ, Gross LB: Excessive complications of open intramedullary nailing of midshaft clavicle fractures with the Rockwood Clavicle Pin. *Clin Orthop Relat Res* 2011;469(12):3364-3370.

    In a retrospective review of clavicle fractures treated with the Rockwood clavicle pin, high rates of nonunion, repeat surgery, and soft-tissue complications were observed. Level of evidence: IV.

23. Ferran NA, Hodgson P, Vannet N, Williams R, Evans RO: Locked intramedullary fixation vs plating for displaced and shortened mid-shaft clavicle fractures: A randomized clinical trial. *J Shoulder Elbow Surg* 2010; 19(6):783-789.

    A small, single-center, randomized controlled study compared intramedullary fixation with a Rockwood pin to open reduction and internal fixation with plates. The results were equivalent. All pins required removal, and 53% of the plates were removed. Level of evidence: I.

24. Kleweno CP, Jawa A, Wells JH, et al: Midshaft clavicular fractures: Comparison of intramedullary pin and

plate fixation. *J Shoulder Elbow Surg* 2011;20(7): 1114-1117.

In a retrospective review of patients with an uncommunuted fracture who were treated with plating or intramedullary fixation using a Rockwood pin, comparable rates of complications were found. Level of evidence: III.

25. Smekal V, Irenberger A, Attal RE, Oberladstaetter J, Krappinger D, Kralinger F: Elastic stable intramedullary nailing is best for mid-shaft clavicular fractures without comminution: Results in 60 patients. *Injury* 2011;42(4):324-329.

A prospective, randomized, single-center study recommended elastic stable intramedullary nailing over nonsurgical treatment of simple displaced midshaft clavicle fractures. Level of evidence: I.

26. Hill JM, McGuire MH, Crosby LA: Closed treatment of displaced middle-third fractures of the clavicle gives poor results. *J Bone Joint Surg Br* 1997;79(4): 537-539.

27. Robinson CM, Court-Brown CM, McQueen MM, Wakefield AE: Estimating the risk of nonunion following nonoperative treatment of a clavicular fracture. *J Bone Joint Surg Am* 2004;86-A(7):1359-1365.

28. Endrizzi DP, White RR, Babikian GM, Old AB: Nonunion of the clavicle treated with plate fixation: A review of forty-seven consecutive cases. *J Shoulder Elbow Surg* 2008;17(6):951-953.

In a large study of surgically treated clavicular nonunions, all patients were treated with a superiorly placed plate. Iliac crest autograft was rarely required. Level of evidence: IV.

29. Rosenberg N, Neumann L, Wallace AW: Functional outcome of surgical treatment of symptomatic nonunion and malunion of midshaft clavicle fractures. *J Shoulder Elbow Surg* 2007;16(5):510-513.

A retrospective review of 11 patients with surgically treated symptomatic nonunion of midshaft clavicle fracture found that residual symptoms were common. Bone graft was used in all patients. Level of evidence: IV.

30. Banerjee R, Waterman B, Padalecki J, Robertson W: Management of distal clavicle fractures. *J Am Acad Orthop Surg* 2011;19(7):392-401.

Distal clavicle fractures were comprehensively reviewed.

31. Tiren D, van Bemmel AJ, Swank DJ, van der Linden FM: Hook plate fixation of acute displaced lateral clavicle fractures: Mid-term results and a brief literature overview. *J Orthop Surg Res* 2012;7(1):2.

Complications of osteolysis around the tip of the hook and subacromial impingement were common but resolved with removal of the implant, typically at 6 months. A high rate of union was observed. Level of evidence: IV.

32. Andersen JR, Willis MP, Nelson R, Mighell MA: Precontoured superior locked plating of distal clavicle fractures: A new strategy. *Clin Orthop Relat Res* 2011; 469(12):3344-3350.

In a retrospective review of 20 patients treated with precontoured locked plating for distal clavicle fractures, approximately half of the patients required additional fixation to the coracoid. A high rate of union was observed. Level of evidence: IV.

33. Good DW, Lui DF, Leonard M, Morris S, McElwain JP: Clavicle hook plate fixation for displaced lateral-third clavicle fractures (Neer type II): A functional outcome study. *J Shoulder Elbow Surg* 2012;21(8):1045-1048.

A review of hook plate fixation for displaced lateral clavicle fractures found predictable union and good functional outcomes. Plate removal before 6 months was recommended. Level of evidence: IV.

34. Klein SM, Badman BL, Keating CJ, Devinney DS, Frankle MA, Mighell MA: Results of surgical treatment for unstable distal clavicular fractures. *J Shoulder Elbow Surg* 2010;19(7):1049-1055.

There was a higher complication rate after delayed treatment than after early treatment of distal clavicle fractures using a hook plate or a superior locking plate with suture augmentation. Level of evidence: IV.

35. ElMaraghy AW, Devereaux MW, Ravichandiran K, Agur AM: Subacromial morphometric assessment of the clavicle hook plate. *Injury* 2010;41(6):613-619.

A cadaver study found that tip contact with the under-surface of the acromion, base-of-hook contact with the supraspinatus muscle, and penetration of the subacromial bursa were common after hook plate insertion.

36. Shin SJ, Roh KJ, Kim JO, Sohn HS: Treatment of unstable distal clavicle fractures using two suture anchors and suture tension bands. *Injury* 2009;40(12):1308-1312.

A retrospective review of 19 patients treated with suture anchor fixation into the coracoid found that 18 had union, with a mean Constant Shoulder Score of 94. Level of evidence: IV.

37. Throckmorton T, Kuhn JE: Fractures of the medial end of the clavicle. *J Shoulder Elbow Surg* 2007;16(1): 49-54.

A retrospective review of medial clavicle fractures found that treatment usually was nonsurgical, and most patients had multisystem trauma. Level of evidence: IV.

Chapter 37

Fractures of the Shaft of the Humerus

Robert M. Beer, MD   Robert V. O'Toole, MD

Introduction

The first recorded treatment of a humerus fracture dates to 1600 BC, when reduction and application of linen bandages were described for three patients.[1] This treatment has not greatly changed, although the recommended daily application of honey and alum has fallen out of favor. Most humeral shaft fractures still are treated nonsurgically with the use of a functional brace. The result appears to be a relatively high rate of fracture union, with few complications. However, there are many relative indications for surgical management of these fractures. Advocates of surgical fixation argue that nonsurgical treatment produces worse functional outcomes and higher nonunion rates than has been believed, particularly with certain fracture types.[2-8] As yet no published randomized studies are available to guide the decision as to surgical or nonsurgical treatment of humeral shaft fractures. The ideal treatment remains controversial.[9]

Epidemiology

Humeral shaft fractures are relatively uncommon and are reported to constitute only 1% to 3% of all fractures, depending on the study and population.[10] As is typical of many fractures, the population distribution is bimodal, with one peak occurring during the third decade of life in men who sustain high-energy trauma and another peak occurring during the eighth decade of life in individuals who sustain a low-energy fall. Proximal or middle shaft fractures each account for slightly more than 40% of such fractures, and distal shaft fractures account for 16%.[10]

Neither Dr. Beer nor any immediate family member has received anything of value from or owns stock in a commercial company or institution related directly or indirectly to the subject of this chapter. Dr. O'Toole or an immediate family member serves as a paid consultant to Synthes; has received research or institutional support from Synthes and Stryker; and serves as a board member, owner, officer, or committee member of the Orthopaedic Trauma Association.

Classification

The classification of humeral shaft fractures may have some clinical importance. Fractures of certain types are believed to have a higher rate of nonunion with nonsurgical treatment and to be more likely to incur radial nerve injury.[4,11] The AO-Orthopaedic Trauma Association (AO-OTA) classification system defines three fracture types. An AO-OTA type A fracture is a simple spiral, oblique, or transverse pattern; a type B fracture has a wedge fragment; and a type C fracture has comminution with no contact between proximal and distal fragments. The fractures often are described in terms of location (most commonly, as proximal, medial, and distal). The Holstein-Lewis fracture, a diaphyseal fracture in the distal third of the humerus with the distal segment laterally displaced, is frequently discussed because it is believed to have an association with radial nerve palsy.[12]

Nonsurgical Treatment

Multiple studies have found that nonsurgical treatment of a humeral shaft fracture with the use of a fracture brace produces consistently high fracture union rates[2,3,5,7] (**Figure 1**). A recent systematic review of all studies published in English found that the average nonunion rate with functional bracing was 5.5% (79 of 1,438 fractures) at an average of 11 weeks after fracture.[2] Interpreting this review requires caution because 97% of the patients were identified in retrospective case studies. In addition, the largest study in this review, a single retrospective case study with 620 patients, reported a very low nonunion rate (2.6%) based on a follow-up rate of only 67%.[2,13] Excluding the results of this study has the effect of increasing the overall nonunion rate to 10.7%, which still could be considered acceptable. Several authors believe that fractures of some types have a higher risk of nonunion when treated nonsurgically. Some believe that simple spiral, oblique, and transverse fractures (AO-OTA type A) have a higher rate of nonunion than comminuted fractures (AO-OTA types B and C), but not all studies have found the differences to reach statistical

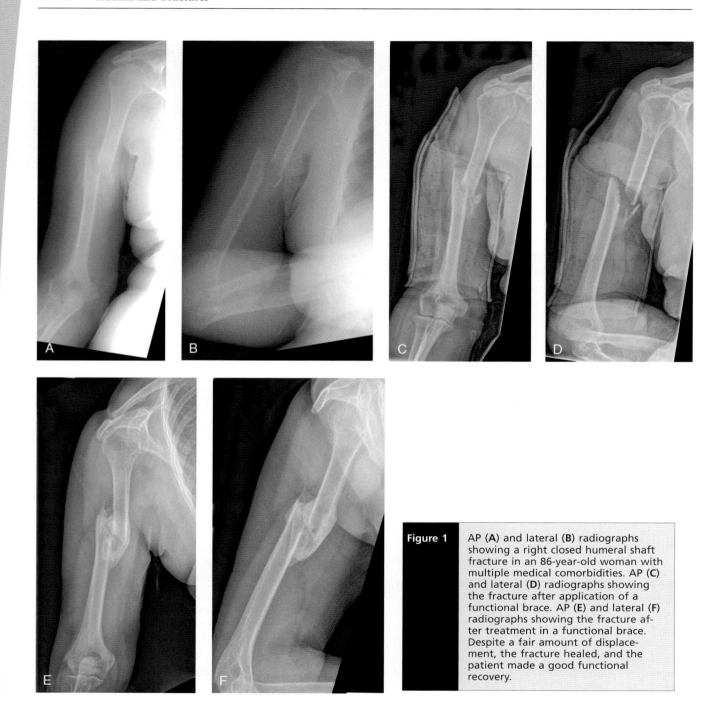

Figure 1 AP (**A**) and lateral (**B**) radiographs showing a right closed humeral shaft fracture in an 86-year-old woman with multiple medical comorbidities. AP (**C**) and lateral (**D**) radiographs showing the fracture after application of a functional brace. AP (**E**) and lateral (**F**) radiographs showing the fracture after treatment in a functional brace. Despite a fair amount of displacement, the fracture healed, and the patient made a good functional recovery.

significance.[2,5-7] Although some studies also have found that proximal third fractures are at a relatively high risk of nonunion, with nonunion rates approaching 32%, such findings have not been consistent.[2,3,5-7] A rare prospective study found that in 110 fractures, the only significant independent factors predicting nonunion after nonsurgical treatment were a proximal diaphyseal fracture and a poor Neer score at 8 and 12 weeks.[4]

A recent retrospective case control study comparing nonsurgical and surgical treatment of distal third fractures found excellent outcomes after treatment with functional bracing, despite previous reservations that these fractures were more prone to malunion or poor elbow function if treated nonsurgically. The data indicate that surgically treated distal third fractures have a higher rate of complications, including radial nerve palsy and infection, and that outcomes, including final shoulder or elbow range of motion, were the same as for fractures managed nonsurgically.[14]

Although functional bracing is by far the most common treatment of humeral shaft fractures, it should be noted that this treatment requires a high level of patient compliance and involvement. The treatment of patients who have dementia or are otherwise unable to cooperate can be difficult. The patient is asked to wear the sleeve at all times except when bathing, to adjust it frequently, initially to sleep in an upright position, and in many protocols to avoid active shoulder abduction and forward flexion. Normally a 1- to 2-week period of immobilization in a coaptation splint is followed by application of a functional brace (consisting of a prefabricated adjustable plastic sleeve) or a custom thermoplastic brace. The patient is instructed to tighten the straps as the swelling subsides. Range-of-motion exercises for the elbow, wrist, and digits are begun immediately, and a progressive program of active shoulder motion is prescribed.

Functional bracing appears to have a very low rate of complications. Patients who are unable to comply with the bracing instructions, particularly patients with dementia, may be at particular risk for skin breakdown and must be closely monitored. However, the most commonly reported skin complication is minor skin irritation; rates range from 1% to 5%.[2,13,15]

Varus and extension deformities are most commonly encountered after humeral shaft fracture. Nonsurgical treatment leads to varus or sagittal plane deformity of 10° or less in approximately 85% of patients.[2] The acceptable limits of residual angulation usually are considered to be 30° or less of varus or valgus, 20° or less of anterior or posterior angulation, and 2 to 3 cm of shortening.[16] These limits are derived from older studies, and few data exist on how deformity is related to functional impairment. The shoulder's extensive range of motion appears to enable it to compensate for a large deformity in the humeral shaft without obvious limits in function.

Shoulder range of motion reportedly is restored in 80% of patients.[2] Some shoulder motion impairment is expected, but usually the deficit is less than 10° in flexion-extension and external or internal rotation. The importance of this deficit has been debated. One prospective nonrandomized study found that function was not affected by the extent of malunion, but another study reported significantly lower Constant scores in the injured shoulder than in the uninjured shoulder after functional brace treatment of humeral shaft fractures.[4,8]

Further research is needed to ascertain whether certain types of fractures are more susceptible than others to nonunion or delayed union and whether early surgery in patients with these fractures results in an earlier return to full function or a better functional outcome. Most published assessments of nonsurgical treatment outcomes focus on union, deformity, and loss of shoulder and elbow motion. Less frequently, shoulder function is assessed using standardized outcome scores. A recent Cochrane review found no published randomized studies and only one prospective nonrandomized study comparing surgical and nonsurgical treatment.[9] The evidence is not strong for clinicians' widespread support for nonsurgical rather than surgical treatment of most humeral shaft fractures.

Surgical Treatment

Many indications for surgically treating humeral shaft fractures have been proposed, including unsuccessful nonsurgical management, open fracture, vascular injury, pathologic fracture, severe soft-tissue injury, ipsilateral forearm or hand fracture, lower extremity fracture requiring crutch weight bearing, and polytrauma (such as brain or lung injury) that would make nonsurgical treatment difficult. Radial nerve palsy resulting from closed fracture manipulation formerly was considered to be a surgical indication, but this belief has fallen out of favor. All of these indications should be considered relative, except that surgical treatment may be required to protect a vascular repair.[3] Even an open fracture can be successfully treated with functional bracing after appropriate surgical wound care, although this treatment is rarely used except with a civilian ballistic injury. In all instances, the overall care and function of the patient must be considered, and specifically the ways in which nonsurgical treatment will affect the patient.

No level I studies are available to guide the decision as to whether a patient should receive surgical or nonsurgical treatment.[9] The methods of surgical stabilization of the humeral diaphysis include external fixation, intramedullary nailing, and plate osteosynthesis. Whether plate or nail fixation provides a better outcome is the subject of much debate.

External Fixation

External fixation is rarely used for humeral shaft fractures and typically is reserved for patients whose fracture is accompanied by severe soft-tissue loss or damage, a vascular injury necessitating repair, or another condition requiring temporary fracture stabilization before definitive fixation[17] (**Figure 2**). In a recent study of 84 patients, external fixation was definitively used for patients who might have been treated nonsurgically at other centers. The resulting 0% nonunion rate and good shoulder and elbow outcomes suggest that the technique may have broader applicability.[18]

Intramedullary Nailing

Intramedullary nailing is commonly used to surgically treat humeral shaft fractures. The reported union rates are higher than 90%.[19,20] This technique involves percutaneous incision and a stable mechanical construct. In general, intramedullary nailing is advantageous to stabilize a large portion of the bone in a pathologic fracture. Nailing may be preferred to plate fixation if the surgical approach for plating is compromised by poor tissue quality or if the more extensive dissection for plating poses an inordinate risk (**Figure 3**).

Antegrade techniques are more commonly used than retrograde techniques because of the ability to provide mechanical stability with interlocking nails, in comparison with flexible retrograde wires, as well as the belief that antegrade techniques are technically easier. Ante-

6: Trauma and Fractures

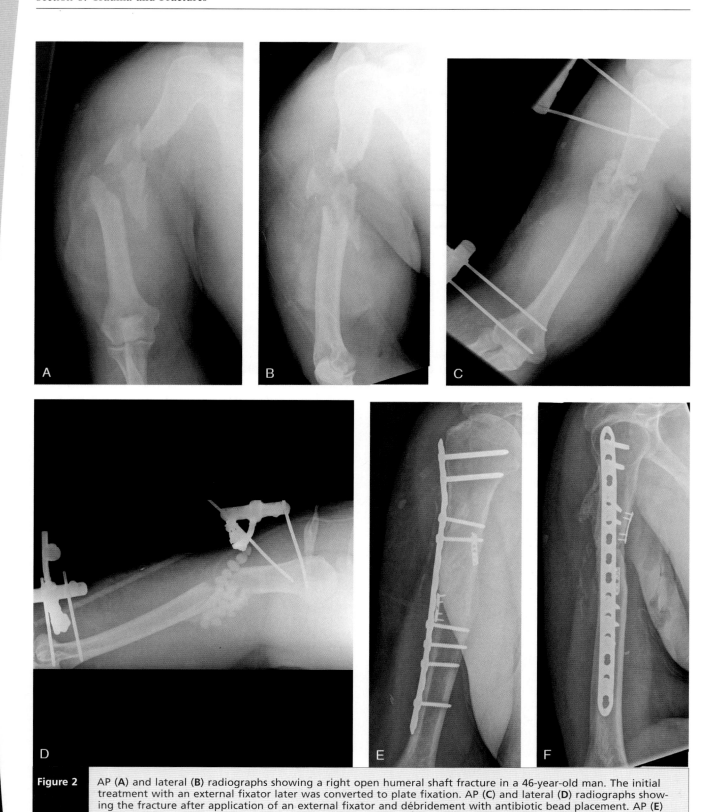

Figure 2 AP (**A**) and lateral (**B**) radiographs showing a right open humeral shaft fracture in a 46-year-old man. The initial treatment with an external fixator later was converted to plate fixation. AP (**C**) and lateral (**D**) radiographs showing the fracture after application of an external fixator and débridement with antibiotic bead placement. AP (**E**) and lateral (**F**) radiographs showing the fracture after conversion to plate osteosynthesis.

grade nails are believed to cause more shoulder pain, and retrograde nails are believed to cause more elbow pain.[19] A recent prospective randomized controlled study compared locked antegrade and locked retrograde nailing in 92 patients, finding no difference in time to union or perioperative complications.[19] The an-

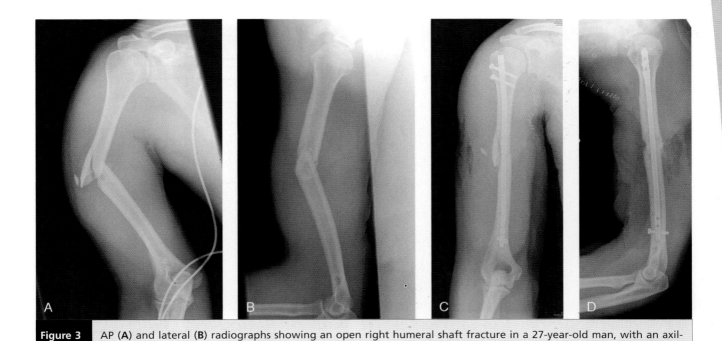

Figure 3 AP (**A**) and lateral (**B**) radiographs showing an open right humeral shaft fracture in a 27-year-old man, with an axillary artery injury requiring revascularization. The initial treatment with an external fixator later was converted to intramedullary nailing. AP (**C**) and lateral (**D**) radiographs showing the fracture after antegrade intramedullary nailing. (Courtesy of Andrew Egleseder, MD, Baltimore, MD.)

tegrade method required approximately 13 minutes less surgical time, but this finding probably has limited clinical importance. Patients in the antegrade group had more postoperative shoulder symptoms that were more pronounced in patients older than 75 years. The study authors concluded that the two techniques offer roughly similar clinical results.

Shoulder pain is the most prevalent complication of antegrade nailing and is the main disadvantage cited when its outcomes are compared to those of open reduction and internal fixation.[21] A recent study reviewed bilateral MRI taken within 11 days of humeral shaft fracture in 33 patients.[22] An abnormal condition was seen in 21 of the shoulders on the fracture side (64%) and none on the contralateral side. Although the study authors argued that the reasons for shoulder pain after humeral shaft fracture may be unrelated to intramedullary nail placement, antegrade nailing has consistently been found to lead to higher rates of shoulder pain than open reduction and internal fixation.[23]

Plate Osteosynthesis

Plate fixation of humeral shaft fractures typically leads to union rates higher than 90%.[20,21,24] The most important risks of open reduction and internal fixation are infection, iatrogenic injury to the radial nerve, and hardware failure. The typically reported complication rates are 2% to 4% for infection and 2% to 5% for radial nerve injury.[21]

The choice of an anterolateral or posterior surgical approach is based on the location of the fracture, the condition of the soft tissue, and the surgeon's desire to explore the radial nerve. The anterolateral approach is an extension of the deltopectoral interval that provides access to the proximal two thirds of the humerus. The anterolateral approach therefore is advantageous for a relatively proximal fracture. The patient's supine position allows another procedure to be simultaneously performed on another limb. The disadvantages include a lack of access to the radial nerve and the large anterior incision, which can be undesirable from a cosmetic standpoint. The posterior approach uses a triceps-sparing or triceps-splitting technique and can provide access to almost the entire diaphysis when the triceps is elevated from lateral to medial after the radial nerve is mobilized.[25] The posterior approach generally is preferred if the fracture is relatively distal, if it is advantageous to visualize the nerve, or if it is desirable to hide the scar posteriorly on the arm. The main disadvantages of this approach are the need to dissect out the radial nerve and the difficulty of performing simultaneous procedures if a patient with polytrauma is in the lateral position.

In an effort to minimize the morbidity associated with the surgical approach, minimally invasive percutaneous plate osteosynthesis (MIPPO) techniques for stabilizing the humerus continue to be examined. MIPPO involves inserting a plate anteriorly along the humeral shaft using small incisions proximally and distally. Anatomic studies found that the radial nerve with the arm in full supination is at least 2.5 cm from plates placed on the usually broad surface of the anterior humerus and is protected by the lateral half of the brachialis.[26] Three retrospective studies examined the results of us-

6: Trauma and Fractures

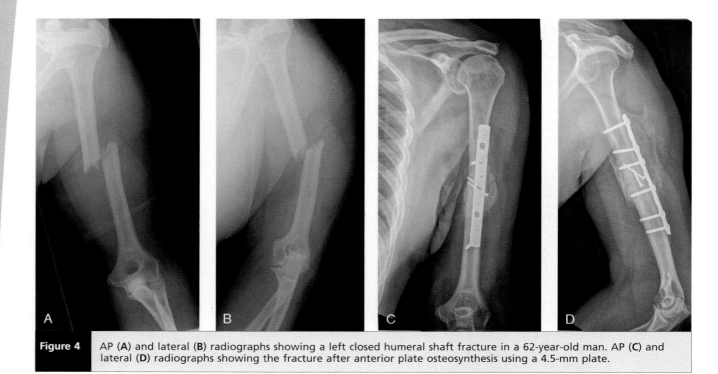

Figure 4 AP (**A**) and lateral (**B**) radiographs showing a left closed humeral shaft fracture in a 62-year-old man. AP (**C**) and lateral (**D**) radiographs showing the fracture after anterior plate osteosynthesis using a 4.5-mm plate.

ing MIPPO and found generally encouraging results.[26-28] This technique has not yet gained popularity in North America, however.

Biomechanics of Plate Fixation

The most effective plate-and-screw configuration is the subject of much recent biomechanical research. Large fragment plates have an established track record in treating humeral diaphyseal fractures. Broad and narrow 4.5-mm plates are used, if the patient's morphology is able to accommodate a large plate (**Figure 4**), although 3.5-mm plates also are used routinely at large trauma centers, with apparent success.

One rationale for plate fixation of a humeral shaft fracture in patients who also have a lower extremity fracture is the need for early mobilization using the plated arm for weight bearing with crutches (**Figure 5**). Recent studies examined the mechanical basis for this practice. A comparison of 4.5-mm and 3.5-mm plates found that in patients heavier than 50 kg, both nonlocking constructs deformed at the expected loads during crutch walking.[29] The large-fragment construct did not catastrophically fail under crutch-walking forces generated by patients weighing less than 90 kg, and small-fragment plate failure did not occur in patients weighing less than 70 kg. A second study used both synthetic and cadaver bone models to compare the effect of locking and nonlocking screws on the biomechanical properties of a 3.5-mm plate construct.[30] The locking screws offered no biomechanical advantage in either model. Both plate constructs failed at loads well above the anticipated physiologic loads for crutch weight bearing. This study contradicted the findings of

the earlier study, perhaps because of a difference in the definition of failure. Both study models assumed a worst-case fracture with no cortical contact between fragments. Plates may experience less extreme loading in a typical application (**Figure 6**). This fact may explain the low reported failure rates with the use of 4.5- and even 3.5-mm plates.[31]

It has become increasingly important to determine the optimal plate-and-screw configuration in osteoporotic bone. Two recent biomechanical studies found mechanical advantages to locking plates in an osteoporotic cadaver and synthetic bone model.[32,33] Another biomechanical study found that a third locking screw on each side of the fracture did not increase axial stability or load to bending in osteoporotic cadaver specimens.[34] Based on these and other biomechanical studies, the general recommendation is that the plate should be as long as practical to increase working length, and it should be fixed to the bone with at least three bicortical screws in each segment. Osteoporotic bone may benefit from locking screw fixation.

Nail Versus Plate Fixation

Both nail and plate fixation are reasonable options for treating most diaphyseal humerus fractures, but debate continues as to the ideal treatment. The ostensible advantages of plate fixation over intramedullary nailing include anatomic fracture reduction, the potential for direct radial nerve visualization, and less injury to the shoulder or elbow. Advocates of nail fixation cite the mechanical advantage of the intramedullary implant and the ability to avoid disrupting the periosteal blood supply and soft tissue.

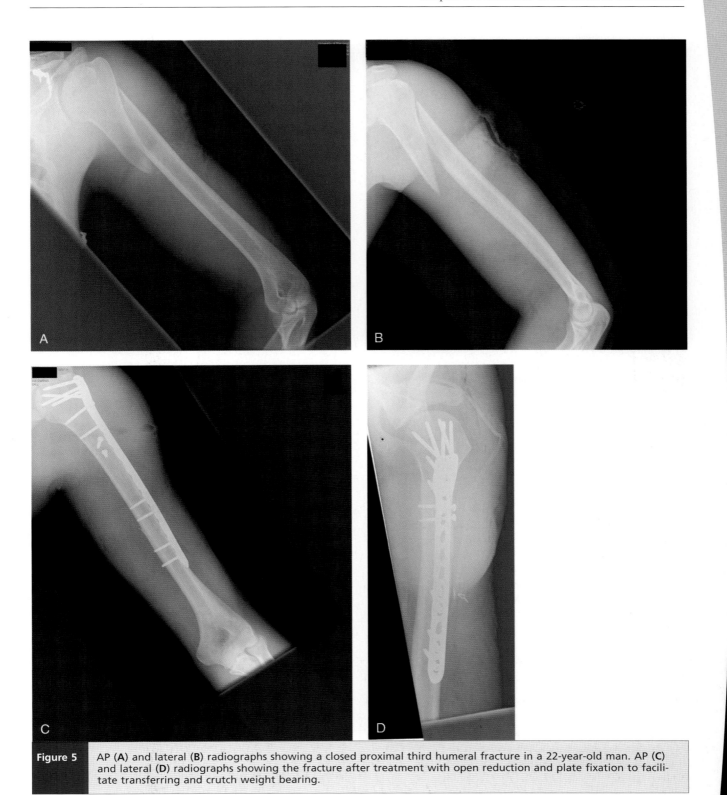

Figure 5 AP (**A**) and lateral (**B**) radiographs showing a closed proximal third humeral fracture in a 22-year-old man. AP (**C**) and lateral (**D**) radiographs showing the fracture after treatment with open reduction and plate fixation to facilitate transferring and crutch weight bearing.

Meta-analysis conclusions have changed over time regarding the outcomes of plates versus nails for humeral shaft fractures. Data from early randomized controlled studies suggested an advantage for plate fixation. A meta-analysis in 2006 found higher rates of reoperation, radial nerve injury, iatrogenic fracture, and shoulder pain when intramedullary nailing was used.[35] In 2010 an updated meta-analysis concluded that no statistically significant difference existed in the relative risk of a complication after intramedullary nail-

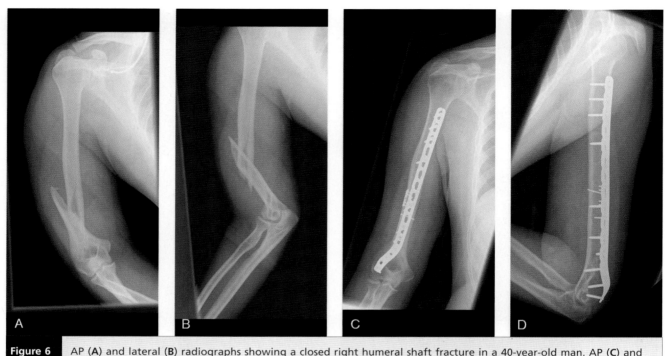

Figure 6 AP (**A**) and lateral (**B**) radiographs showing a closed right humeral shaft fracture in a 40-year-old man. AP (**C**) and lateral (**D**) radiographs showing the fracture after plate osteosynthesis.

ing or plate fixation. This analysis reflected the addition of recent data to expand the review to four studies and 203 patients.[36,37] The 2010 meta-analysis included a randomized controlled study of 34 patients that found a higher complication rate with intramedullary nailing.[20,37] The limitations of the relevant current literature are suggested by the fact that a single study of 34 patients could tip the balance related to complication rates from "no difference" to a risk ratio of 0.52 in favor of plate fixation. Further complicating the issue is a recent Cochrane review of five randomized controlled studies with 260 patients, which found no statistically significant difference in rates of nonunion or surgical complications.[23] This review did not include the most recent studies, however.

The 2010 meta-analysis noted that the individual studies were underpowered and that the heterogeneity of the study population was high.[37] The authors calculated that 470 patients per comparison group would be required for an adequate randomized controlled study. The literature supports the conclusion that both methods lead to high union rates and low complication rates. The debate on efficacy is not yet settled.

Radial Nerve Palsy

Palsy of the radial nerve is the most common nerve injury associated with fractures of the humeral shaft. Primary radial nerve palsy occurs in approximately 12% of all humeral shaft fractures (532 palsies in 4,517 fractures, in 21 studies). Middle and distal third fracture locations as well as transverse and spiral patterns have a significantly increased correspondence with radial nerve palsy. The Holstein-Lewis injury pattern (a spiral fracture of the distal third of the humerus) also has an increased association with radial nerve palsy. A consensus is beginning to emerge regarding management of these nerve palsies.[11,12]

A systematic review found a 70.7% rate of spontaneous recovery of radial nerve palsies treated with an initial observation strategy. Late exploration of radial nerve palsies that did not spontaneously recover led to a 69.2% recovery rate in these patients. The resulting overall recovery rate of initial observation and late exploration was 89%. This rate did not differ significantly from the recovery rate of 84.7% in nerves that were explored early.[11,38]

When data from a systematic review were analyzed in conjunction with a decision-making model, initial observation was found to be the best course of action for closed fractures with palsy.[39] In this model, initial exploration would not be favored unless the rate of spontaneous recovery fell to 40%, which is well below the current rate of 71%. The authors stressed that some patients might benefit from early surgery if the likelihood of nerve recovery is low; this would be true, for example, in an open fracture with a high risk of nerve laceration.[39]

The time required for the nerve to recover can vary, and clinical signs may be absent as long as 6 months. Electromyography and nerve conduction velocity studies may show evidence of nerve recovery as early as 1 month before clinical signs appear. The brachioradialis and the extensor carpi radialis longus are the first muscles to be reinnervated. Full return of function can take as long as 1 year. In the absence of clinical signs of recovery, it is generally recommended that the nerve be explored after 4 to 6 months.[40,41]

Summary

Most humeral shaft fractures can be safely managed nonsurgically using a functional brace. This method has led to high rates of union, low complication rates, and restoration of reasonable function, although recent studies have not been able to reproduce the very high union rates of earlier studies. Proximal third and simple humeral shaft fractures may be relatively likely to lead to nonunion with nonsurgical treatment, and fractures of these types may be less effectively treated in a fracture brace than with surgery. There are many relative indications for surgical fixation of humeral shaft fractures, but few absolute indications. The literature supports the use of nail or plate fixation, with good outcomes. Some data show higher rates of shoulder symptoms with nail fixation. Larger randomized studies are necessary to adequately compare the two forms of fixation. The treatment of radial nerve palsy with initial observation in most patients has gained an increasingly secure footing in the literature and is appropriate for most patients, with the exception of those at particularly high risk of nerve laceration. Research is ongoing to determine whether some patients would benefit from surgical fixation and which surgical treatment is most efficacious.

Annotated References

1. Brorson S: Management of fractures of the humerus in Ancient Egypt, Greece, and Rome: An historical review. *Clin Orthop Relat Res* 2009;467(7):1907-1914.

   Early writings on the treatment of humeral shaft fractures are described.

2. Papasoulis E, Drosos GI, Ververidis AN, Verettas DA: Functional bracing of humeral shaft fractures: A review of clinical studies. *Injury* 2010;41(7):e21-e27.

   A review of all published clinical studies of nonsurgical treatment of humeral shaft fractures found that the aggregate union rate is 94.5%. The nonunion rate rises to 10.7% if the largest study is excluded. Level of evidence: III.

3. Toivanen JA, Nieminen J, Laine HJ, Honkonen SE, Järvinen MJ: Functional treatment of closed humeral shaft fractures. *Int Orthop* 2005;29(1):10-13.

4. Broadbent MR, Will E, McQueen MM: Prediction of outcome after humeral diaphyseal fracture. *Injury* 2010;41(6):572-577.

   In a prospective study of 110 patients with a fracture of the humeral shaft, a proximal third fracture and a poor Neer score at 8 and 12 weeks were significant predictors of nonunion. Level of evidence: II.

5. Rutgers M, Ring D: Treatment of diaphyseal fractures of the humerus using a functional brace. *J Orthop Trauma* 2006;20(9):597-601.

6. Ring D, Chin K, Taghinia AH, Jupiter JB: Nonunion after functional brace treatment of diaphyseal humerus fractures. *J Trauma* 2007;62(5):1157-1158.

   A retrospective study found that short oblique fractures may have a higher rate of nonunion. A historical control group was used. Level of evidence: III.

7. Ekholm R, Tidermark J, Törnkvist H, Adami J, Ponzer S: Outcome after closed functional treatment of humeral shaft fractures. *J Orthop Trauma* 2006;20(9):591-596.

8. Rosenberg N, Soudry M: Shoulder impairment following treatment of diaphysial fractures of humerus by functional brace. *Arch Orthop Trauma Surg* 2006;126(7):437-440.

9. Gosler MW, Testroote M, Moorenhof JW, Janzing HM: Surgical versus non-surgical interventions for treating humeral shaft fractures in adults. *Cochrane Database Syst Rev* 2012;1:D008832.

   This review found insufficient evidence from randomized controlled studies to make recommendations regarding surgical or nonsurgical treatment of humeral shaft fractures. Level of evidence: III.

10. Ekholm R, Adami J, Tidermark J, Hansson K, Törnkvist H, Ponzer S: Fractures of the shaft of the humerus: An epidemiological study of 401 fractures. *J Bone Joint Surg Br* 2006;88(11):1469-1473.

11. Shao YC, Harwood P, Grotz MR, Limb D, Giannoudis PV: Radial nerve palsy associated with fractures of the shaft of the humerus: A systematic review. *J Bone Joint Surg Br* 2005;87(12):1647-1652.

12. Ekholm R, Ponzer S, Törnkvist H, Adami J, Tidermark J: The Holstein-Lewis humeral shaft fracture: Aspects of radial nerve injury, primary treatment, and outcome. *J Orthop Trauma* 2008;22(10):693-697.

   A retrospective analysis of 27 patients with the Holstein-Lewis fracture pattern found a higher rate of acute radial nerve palsy with these distal third humeral shaft fractures (22% versus 8%). Level of evidence: III.

13. Sarmiento A, Zagorski JB, Zych GA, Latta LL, Capps CA: Functional bracing for the treatment of fractures of the humeral diaphysis. *J Bone Joint Surg Am* 2000;82(4):478-486.

14. Jawa A, McCarty P, Doornberg J, Harris M, Ring D: Extra-articular distal-third diaphyseal fractures of the humerus: A comparison of functional bracing and plate fixation. *J Bone Joint Surg Am* 2006;88(11):2343-2347.

6: Trauma and Fractures

15. Woon CY: Cutaneous complications of functional bracing of the humerus: A case report and literature review. *J Bone Joint Surg Am* 2010;92(8):1786-1789.

    This is a case report of skin ulceration with bone protrusion during functional brace treatment of a closed humeral shaft fracture. A review of complications of functional bracing found low complication rates in earlier studies. Level of evidence: IV.

16. Klenerman L: Fractures of the shaft of the humerus. *J Bone Joint Surg Br* 1966;48(1):105-111.

17. Suzuki T, Hak DJ, Stahel PF, Morgan SJ, Smith WR: Safety and efficacy of conversion from external fixation to plate fixation in humeral shaft fractures. *J Orthop Trauma* 2010;24(7):414-419.

    Conversion of external fixation to plate fixation in 17 patients led to few complications. Level of evidence: IV.

18. Catagni MA, Lovisetti L, Guerreschi F, et al: The external fixation in the treatment of humeral diaphyseal fractures: Outcomes of 84 cases. *Injury* 2010;41(11):1107-1111.

    Definitive external fixation led to few complications and no nonunions in humeral shaft fractures. Level of evidence: IV.

19. Cheng H-R, Lin J: Prospective randomized comparative study of antegrade and retrograde locked nailing for middle humeral shaft fracture. *J Trauma* 2008;65(1):94-102.

    Antegrade and retrograde nailing had similar outcomes, with antegrade nailing requiring an average 13 minutes less time to perform. Level of evidence: II.

20. Putti AB, Uppin RB, Putti BB: Locked intramedullary nailing versus dynamic compression plating for humeral shaft fractures. *J Orthop Surg (Hong Kong)* 2009;17(2):139-141.

    A randomized controlled study with 34 patients found a similar union rate but a higher complication rate in patients who received nailing compared with those who received plating. Level of evidence: II.

21. McCormack RG, Brien D, Buckley RE, McKee MD, Powell J, Schemitsch EH: Fixation of fractures of the shaft of the humerus by dynamic compression plate or intramedullary nail: A prospective, randomised trial. *J Bone Joint Surg Br* 2000;82(3):336-339.

22. O'Donnell TM, McKenna JV, Kenny P, Keogh P, O'Flanagan SJ: Concomitant injuries to the ipsilateral shoulder in patients with a fracture of the diaphysis of the humerus. *J Bone Joint Surg Br* 2008;90(1):61-65.

    An MRI study found that the rate of ipsilateral shoulder injury is higher than previously known. This finding may explain some of the shoulder pain ascribed to nail insertion. Level of evidence: IV.

23. Kurup H, Hossain M, Andrew JG: Dynamic compression plating versus locked intramedullary nailing for humeral shaft fractures in adults. [Review]. *Cochrane Database Syst Rev* 2011;6(6):CD005959.

    This meta-analysis found no difference in outcomes after plating or nailing of humeral shaft fractures. Level of evidence: II.

24. Denard A Jr, Richards JE, Obremskey WT, Tucker MC, Floyd M, Herzog GA: Outcome of nonoperative vs operative treatment of humeral shaft fractures: A retrospective study of 213 patients. *Orthopedics* 2010;33(8).

    A nonrandomized study of surgical and nonsurgical treatment found no between-group difference in time to union or final range of motion. Nonsurgical treatment had a significantly higher rate of nonunion and malunion (20.6% versus 8.7% and 12.7% versus 1.3%, respectively). Level of evidence: III.

25. Gerwin M, Hotchkiss RN, Weiland AJ: Alternative operative exposures of the posterior aspect of the humeral diaphysis with reference to the radial nerve. *J Bone Joint Surg Am* 1996;78(11):1690-1695.

26. López-Arévalo R, de Llano-Temboury AQ, Serrano-Montilla J, de Llano-Giménez EQ, Fernández-Medina JM: Treatment of diaphyseal humeral fractures with the minimally invasive percutaneous plate (MIPPO) technique: A cadaveric study and clinical results. *J Orthop Trauma* 2011;25(5):294-299.

    The results of the MIPPO technique were retrospectively reviewed in 86 patients, and the position of the radial nerve was examined in 10 arms in five cadavers. Three nonunions and three transitory radial nerve palsies were reported. The cadaver study found that with the extended arm in full supination, the radial nerve is located 2.5 cm from the center of the humerus on average. Level of evidence: IV.

27. Zhiquan A, Bingfang Z, Yeming W, Chi Z, Peiyan H: Minimally invasive plating osteosynthesis (MIPO) of middle and distal third humeral shaft fractures. *J Orthop Trauma* 2007;21(9):628-633.

    In a prospective study of 13 patients treated with minimally invasive plating osteosynthesis using a 4.5-mm plate, the time to union averaged 16 weeks, and no nonunions, radial palsies, or implant failures occurred. Level of evidence: IV.

28. Kobayashi M, Watanabe Y, Matsushita T: Early full range of shoulder and elbow motion is possible after minimally invasive plate osteosynthesis for humeral shaft fractures. *J Orthop Trauma* 2010;24(4):212-216.

    A study of minimally invasive plating osteosynthesis in 14 patients found that elbow motion took longer to return than shoulder motion. Level of evidence: IV.

29. Patel R, Neu CP, Curtiss S, Fyhrie DP, Yoo B: Crutch weightbearing on comminuted humeral shaft fractures: A biomechanical comparison of large versus small fragment fixation for humeral shaft fractures. *J Orthop Trauma* 2011;25(5):300-305.

    A synthetic bone model study found that the performance of 4.5-mm plates was superior to that of

3.5-mm plates but questioned whether either is mechanically able to withstand crutch weight bearing after a comminuted fracture.

30. O'Toole RV, Andersen RC, Vesnovsky O, et al: Are locking screws advantageous with plate fixation of humeral shaft fractures? A biomechanical analysis of synthetic and cadaveric bone. *J Orthop Trauma* 2008; 22(10):709-715.

    Locking screws offered no mechanical advantage over nonlocking screws in the plating of humeral shaft fractures in synthetic and cadaver fracture models.

31. Sheerin DV, Sciadini MF, Halpern JL, Nascone JN, Eglseder WA: The use of locking small-fragment plates for treatment of humeral shaft fractures. *Final Program: 2004 Annual Meeting*. Rosemont, IL, Orthopaedic Trauma Association, 2004, poster 36. http://www.ota.org/education/archives.html. Accessed October 22, 2012.

32. Davis C, Stall A, Knutsen E, et al: Locking plates in osteoporosis: A biomechanical cadaveric study of diaphyseal humerus fractures. *J Orthop Trauma* 2012; 26(4):216-221.

    A study of osteoporotic cadaver bone found that locking plates confer a mechanical advantage over nonlocking plates.

33. Gardner MJ, Griffith MH, Demetrakopoulos D, et al: Hybrid locked plating of osteoporotic fractures of the humerus. *J Bone Joint Surg Am* 2006;88(9):1962-1967.

34. Hak DJ, Althausen P, Hazelwood SJ: Locked plate fixation of osteoporotic humeral shaft fractures: Are two locking screws per segment enough? *J Orthop Trauma* 2010;24(4):207-211.

    A biomechanical study found that the addition of a third locking screw on each side of a humeral shaft fracture may offer no mechanical advantage.

35. Bhandari M, Devereaux PJ, McKee MD, Schemitsch EH: Compression plating versus intramedullary nailing of humeral shaft fractures: A meta-analysis. *Acta Orthop* 2006;77(2):279-284.

36. Changulani M, Jain UK, Keswani T: Comparison of the use of the humerus intramedullary nail and dynamic compression plate for the management of diaphyseal fractures of the humerus: A randomised controlled study. *Int Orthop* 2007;31(3):391-395.

    No difference was found in scores on the American Shoulder and Elbow Surgeons Shoulder Index after nail or plate fixation, but the average time to union was significantly lower after nailing. The infection rate was higher after plating. Shortening and shoulder pain were more likely after nailing.Level of evidence: II.

37. Heineman DJ, Poolman RW, Nork SE, Ponsen K-J, Bhandari M: Plate fixation or intramedullary fixation of humeral shaft fractures. *Acta Orthop* 2010;81(2): 216-223.

    An addition of one study to a 2006 meta-analysis changed the conclusion so that similar outcomes were found after plate or nail fixation of humeral shaft fractures. Level of evidence: II.

38. Ring D, Chin K, Jupiter JB: Radial nerve palsy associated with high-energy humeral shaft fractures. *J Hand Surg Am* 2004;29(1):144-147.

39. Bishop J, Ring D: Management of radial nerve palsy associated with humeral shaft fracture: A decision analysis model. *J Hand Surg Am* 2009;34(6):991-996, e1.

    Expected-value decision analysis was used to examine strategies for managing humeral shaft fractures. Initial observation was found to be the preferred option for radial nerve palsy with a closed humeral shaft fracture. Early surgical exploration may be appropriate in some situations, such as an open fracture with a high risk of laceration.

40. Shah A, Jebson PJ: Current treatment of radial nerve palsy following fracture of the humeral shaft. *J Hand Surg Am* 2008;33(8):1433-1434.

    A literature review recommends initial nonsurgical management after closed primary or secondary radial nerve palsies. Initial exploration is recommended only for an open humerus fracture. Exploration at 6 months is recommended if clinical signs of function do not return.

41. Venouziou AI, Dailiana ZH, Varitimidis SE, Hantes ME, Gougoulias NE, Malizos KN: Radial nerve palsy associated with humeral shaft fracture: Is the energy of trauma a prognostic factor? *Injury* 2011;42(11):1289-1293.

    Eighteen patients with a humeral shaft fracture and associated radial nerve palsy underwent open reduction and internal fixation. Retrospective review found that a high-energy fracture mechanism is most likely to lead to laceration.

6: Trauma and Fractures

Chapter 38

Classification and Treatment of Acromioclavicular Separations

Steven Klepps, MD

Mechanism of Injury and Classification

The acromioclavicular (AC) joint frequently is injured in physically active individuals, including athletes who participate in contact sports. The most common mechanism of injury is a direct blow onto the superior aspect of the shoulder. The most commonly used classification, the Rockwood system, is based on the anatomic structures injured. Rockwood type I and II injuries involve the AC joint capsule; types III, IV, and V injuries involve the coracoclavicular (CC) ligaments as well as the capsule. A type III injury is displaced superiorly, and a type IV injury is displaced posteriorly. In addition to the CC ligament and capsular injuries, a type V injury involves deltotrapezial disruption leading to increased separation and often to incarceration of the clavicle into the deltotrapezial fascia. Type III and V separations that result in superior displacement of the clavicle are believed to be caused by drooping (ptosis) of the arm rather than by the clavicle's rising superiorly. Therefore, a sling that bears part of the weight of the arm often reduces the separation. A type VI injury is rare and involves clavicular displacement inferiorly in a subcoracoid position.[1,2]

Clinical Evaluation

History and Physical Examination

The patient often describes a direct injury to the superior aspect of the shoulder, as in forceful contact with the ground or a fall from a height. There is pain and swelling in the superior aspect of the shoulder. The pain usually precludes the patient from raising the arm or continuing to be involved in sports. There may be associated neck pain or numbness and tingling.

The components of the examination depend on the level of separation. With a type I or II injury, the pa-

Neither Dr. Klepps nor any immediate family member has received anything of value from or has stock or stock options held in a commercial company or institution related directly or indirectly to the subject of this chapter.

tient has pain with palpation of the AC joint. Cross-body adduction testing also is painful. The only deformity is slight swelling. With a type III or V injury, the patient has a painful deformity of the AC joint in which the clavicle sits superior to the acromion because of the downward force of the arm. A type III injury often can be reduced when the arm is simply pushed upward while the distal clavicle is held down or when the patient shrugs his or her shoulders. A type V injury usually cannot be reduced with this maneuver because the clavicle is trapped within the trapezius.[1,2] This distinction is helpful in initial surgical decision making: a type V injury is best treated surgically, and a type III injury still is considered to be best treated nonsurgically.[3,4] However, the preferred treatment of type III injuries is controversial. A type IV injury is notable for the posterior protrusion of the clavicle. Often the protrusion is subtle and best seen radiographically, but in some patients it can be seen on physical examination if the patient is closely evaluated for horizontal instability.

Imaging

Injury to the AC joint generally can be definitively diagnosed through radiographs. The AC joint view (also called the Zanca view) typically shows the separation well (**Figure 1, A**). This view is obtained with reduced radiation, and the x-ray beam is directed 15° cephalad to avoid overlap between the spine of the scapula and the AC joint. An axillary view is essential to detect posterior displacement in a type IV injury (**Figure 1, B**). Radiographs also are important in ruling out the main differential diagnosis, which is a distal clavicle fracture that can mimic an AC joint separation. In a young adolescent patient, a periosteal sleeve fracture can be identified if only a thin line of calcification from the periosteum is noted around a displaced distal clavicle. Imaging of the entire clavicle and scapula may be indicated to ensure the patient does not have an associated sternoclavicular injury (a bipolar clavicle) or a fracture within the clavicle or the scapula (a floating shoulder), especially if tenderness or swelling is noted within these areas.

In a type I injury, there is no evidence of separation on plain radiographs. In a type II injury, often there is slight widening or superior elevation that can be appre-

6: Trauma and Fractures

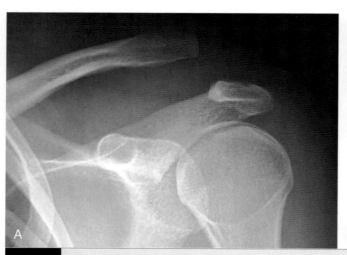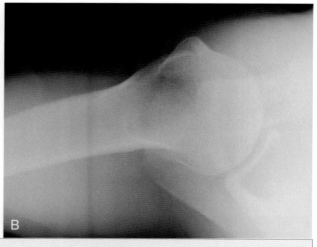

Figure 1 **A,** AP (Zanca) radiograph of the AC joint showing a type III separation with 100% displacement of the clavicle superior to the acromion. **B,** Axillary radiograph of the shoulder showing the clavicle posteriorly displaced relative to the anterior edge of the acromion.

ciated only by radiographically comparing the injured and contralateral AC joints. For a thin patient, one radiograph often is sufficient for obtaining an image of both joints. For a larger patient, bilateral views can be helpful if a type II separation is suspected. Although bilateral views showing type II separation do not significantly affect management, they can be useful for confirming the diagnosis for the patient. Weighted radiographs generally are not helpful and have fallen out of favor. The increase in CC distance (best seen on contralateral radiographs) is 25% to 100% in a type III injury and 100% to 300% in a type V injury.[1] Type IV injuries are best seen on axillary views with the clavicle sitting posterior to the anterior edge of the acromion.

Surgical Versus Nonsurgical Treatment

Type I and II separations are treated nonsurgically to achieve symptom relief and a gradual return to activity. Generally, these injuries heal well with a short course of rehabilitation. However, type II separations have been associated with persistent pain, and degenerative changes have been reported to develop 5 to 10 years after injury.[5] The patient should be made aware of these possible outcomes, but generally they do not affect the initial treatment. Distal clavicle resection can be considered for a patient with a type II separation who remains symptomatic. If instability is noted at the time of surgery, AC joint reconstruction also may be necessary; distal clavicle resection alone has been associated with persistent pain believed to result from the underlying instability.[5] For this reason, open resection should be considered for distal clavicle resection following type II separations because it allows manual evaluation for subtle instability.

Although type III separations are controversial, in the United States they are usually treated nonsurgically,

with some exceptions.[4] For instance, patients who are overhead athletes or do heavy manual labor have been considered for early repair, but studies have reported good results with nonsurgical treatment even in these patients.[4,6-8] In some countries including Germany and Spain, type III separations generally receive initial surgical treatment.[6,7] There is still no definitive study to show better results after surgical or nonsurgical treatment. A recent meta-analysis did find that surgical treatment led to better cosmesis but not to better results related to throwing, pain, or function.[9] Another attempted meta-analysis did not find sufficient randomized controlled studies to form an outcome-based conclusion.[10] One of the six studies examined within this study found that nonsurgical treatment led to an earlier return to sport or work and lower rates of complications, such as infection or hardware failure, but surgical treatment led to higher Constant scores. Unfortunately, the studies in this meta-analysis involved treatment using Kirschner wires (five studies) and hook plates (one study), neither of which is currently considered the best reconstructive option. The question remains as to whether a more modern reconstruction method would outperform nonsurgical treatment for type III injuries.

Nonsurgically treated patients with a type III injury generally require a longer time for complete recovery than those with a type I or II injury; as long as 3 months may be needed for return to full function and return to sport or work. For this reason, there is some question about the advisability of acute repair in athletes injured near the end of the season because a full course of nonsurgical treatment followed by surgery might not provide adequate time for recovery before the next season begins. Arthroscopic surgery and repair options, such as the use of cerclage sutures or hook plates, are less invasive than the typical reconstruction and have led to more early repairs being performed.

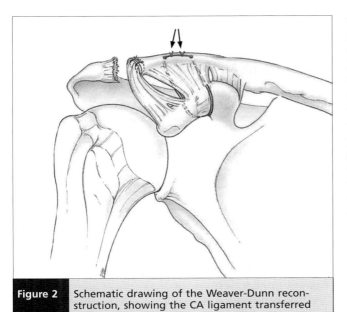

Figure 2 Schematic drawing of the Weaver-Dunn reconstruction, showing the CA ligament transferred to the distal end of the clavicle, with suture augmentation beneath the coracoid and through drill holes in the clavicle *(arrows)*.

These methods have replaced fixation with Kirschner wires or Bosworth screws, although they work on the same principle. In general, type IV and V separations are initially treated surgically in a healthy patient because these injuries tend to remain symptomatic if treated nonsurgically.

Surgical Treatment

Hundreds of surgical techniques have been described, and it can be difficult to determine which surgical option is best. Surgeons should be aware of the various techniques so as to make an informed decision on the best option for an individual patient. Regardless of the surgical technique, the surgeon must decide whether the distal clavicle needs to be resected as part of the reconstruction. In general, the distal clavicle can be left in place during an acute repair because it has not developed significant hypertrophy or irregularity. Some authors describe removing the intra-articular disk, especially if it is torn.[11] There is some risk of long-term pain or osteoarthritis at the AC joint if the distal clavicle is not resected, but in the short term, patients appear to do well regardless of whether distal clavicle resection is done with the reconstruction. Removing the distal clavicle is believed to add to horizontal instability after repair.[6,11] For chronic separations, the distal clavicle typically is resected, especially if significant irregularity or hypertrophic changes are present.

Several important technical points apply to all AC joint reconstruction techniques; these were developed in part from recent biomechanic and clinical studies. To avoid slippage, it is important to place the sutures or

the grafts that wrap around the coracoid at the base of the coracoid rather than at the tip. Placing suture anchors into the coracoid or a hole through the coracoid has been proposed as a means of avoiding slippage, but this technique is associated with an added cost for anchor placement and a risk of coracoid fracture because the hole weakens the coracoid.[12,13] When placing sutures or graft around the coracoid, it is important to pass them from medial to lateral to reduce the risk of neurologic injury.[14] Augmentation with tape (rather than suture fixation) has become common but can lead to coracoid or clavicle fracture because tape is stronger than suture and can cut through bone. The risk of suture failure has led to the use of multiple sutures; a 91% success rate was reported in suture-only acute repairs in which the suture was placed both in a cerclage fashion beneath the coracoid and either over or through the distal clavicle.[11] The clavicle holes for suture augmentation should not be placed too distally within the clavicle because doing so can lead to widening of the AC joint space as it pulls the clavicle medially. Essentially, the same clavicle drill hole location should be used for a Weaver-Dunn and an anatomic reconstruction. Overreduction of the clavicle is useful in compensating for stretching of the reconstruction.[2] Wide stripping of the clavicle periosteum with débridement of any scar tissue below the clavicle is essential to allow mobilization and anatomic reduction before the repair.[2] Oversewing the deltotrapezial fascia at the end of the procedure is important for stability, and, therefore, large, thick flaps of tissue should be mobilized during the exposure.

The Modified Weaver-Dunn Reconstruction

The modified Weaver-Dunn reconstruction has become the standard surgical option, although many variations of AC reconstruction have been proposed over the years. This method involves transferring the coracoacromial (CA) ligament from the acromion to the distal clavicle, with supplementation placed between the coracoid and the clavicle using heavy sutures or suture tapes (**Figure 2**). The modified Weaver-Dunn reconstruction has performed well, but its association with postoperative loosening has led to the development of multiple modifications, such as the Chuinard reconstruction (transfer of the acromion bone fragment with the CA ligament), conjoined tendon transfer, and anatomic reconstruction (free graft transfer).[15]

There are many potential advantages to performing reconstructions using local tissue. For instance, the use of local tissue with its vascular supply for the graft may maximize the healing potential. The sacrifice is minimal; the CA ligament often is taken down to treat impingement without significant effect. The conjoined tendon is transferred in shoulder stabilization procedures such as the Latarjet, with minimal effect. The use of local tissue also avoids the risk of reaction and the cost of using foreign material.

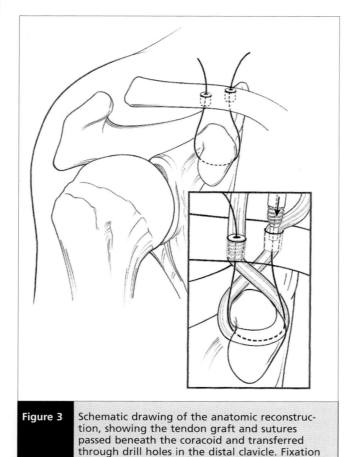

Figure 3 Schematic drawing of the anatomic reconstruction, showing the tendon graft and sutures passed beneath the coracoid and transferred through drill holes in the distal clavicle. Fixation is accomplished with interference screws *(inset)*.

The Anatomic Reconstruction

The anatomic reconstruction has become popular during the past 5 to 10 years, primarily as a reaction to the risk of loosening after the Weaver-Dunn reconstruction. Anatomic reconstruction involves transferring a tendinous graft, such as the semitendinosus or gracilis, around or through the coracoid and through drill holes in the clavicle (**Figure 3**). The main advantages of graft placement below the coracoid is that it provides a stronger construct than a CA ligament transfer and is technically easier than the Weaver-Dunn reconstruction because mobilizing the CA ligament often leaves inadequate tissue for the reconstruction. Autograft or allograft can be used. The graft can be fixed with either sutures or interference screws in the clavicle. Often, the graft is woven onto itself to avoid screw placement. Screws have been shown to provide the biomechanically strongest fixation, but the use of absorbable screws can lead to a reaction (osteolysis) and subsequent fracture. This factor has led some surgeons to use only sutures for fixation.[12,16]

Often, the tendon is extended over the AC joint and attached to the acromion to further strengthen the construct, especially in the anterior-posterior plane. The reconstruction of coracoclavicular ligaments has been shown to provide good superior-inferior stability but leaves anterior-posterior instability, which has been considered a limitation of standard reconstructions. In one new concept, intramedullary graft placed between the acromion and the clavicle is combined with the anatomic reconstruction; this technique has been shown to provide better anterior-posterior stabilization than the anatomic and Weaver-Dunn reconstructions.[16] In cadaver studies, the AC joint capsule has been shown to provide most of the anterior-posterior stability, and superior or intramedullary placement of the AC joint graft is designed to make up for this capsular insufficiency.

As with the Weaver-Dunn reconstruction, it is important to avoid too-distal placement of the clavicle screw holes, which can lead to a widened AC joint. Based on anatomic study, the entire clavicle length is measured as a straight line to determine drill hole placement. The holes are placed at 20% and 30% of the clavicle length from the distal end of the clavicle.[17] Keeping the tunnels at least 15 mm apart also is believed to be useful for decreasing the risk of fracture.[12] Some authors promote a single-tunnel or no-tunnel reconstruction as a means of further decreasing the risk of fracture, but this technique could lead to sawing through or loosening of the tendon.[2,18] Decreasing the size of the clavicle holes, with suture fixation only, also has been recommended.[12] Although several biomechanical cadaver studies have compared the anatomic reconstruction with the Weaver-Dunn reconstruction,[1,2,16,19] these have been time-zero studies using a variety of techniques, and they have not resolved the question of whether the anatomic reconstruction is clinically better than the Weaver-Dunn reconstruction.

One prospective clinical study directly compared the Weaver-Dunn and anatomic reconstructions in 24 patients.[20] The 12 anatomically treated patients had better American Shoulder and Elbow Surgeons Shoulder Index and Constant scores as well as a reduced CC interval. However, patients in both treatment groups had excellent results. Despite these positive results, the question remains as to whether the clinical benefit of anatomic reconstruction justifies the cost of graft and screws, donor site morbidity, and a possible foreign tissue reaction. Further studies are warranted before the anatomic reconstruction can be strongly recommended over the classic Weaver-Dunn reconstruction.

Arthroscopic Reconstruction

Arthroscopic techniques have been developed for AC joint repair and reconstruction. Acute repair fixation is performed using heavy sutures and locking metal clips, such as the Tightrope device (Arthrex, Naples, FL), placed between the clavicle and the coracoid. This fixation device allows motion through the sutures; unlike screw fixation, it is not rigid, and device removal therefore is not required. The principle is to place the clavicle in its native position in the hope that the CC ligaments will reconstitute themselves. This concept is similar to that of Bosworth screw or Kirschner wire fixation, which is left in place for 6 weeks before removal, but with the advantage of not requiring a second surgery. The Bosworth screw and Kirschner wire fixation methods also carried a risk of screw failure, pin migration, infection, or pullout. Unfortunately, disruption of Tightrope-like devices has occurred.[14] As a result, these fixation devices have been modified by changing the shape or size of the button (for example, to a dog bone shape) or increasing the amount of fixation (as with the double-tunnel technique).[21] Some manufacturers have added tendon to a flip-button device, which can still be placed arthroscopically.[22]

Arthroscopic methods for reconstructing chronic separations also have been developed. These techniques include the GraftRope system and tendon or CA ligament transfer technique (with or without a fleck of acromion).[22,23] A study of 10 patients treated with an arthroscopic Weaver-Dunn procedure for chronic instability reported a 90% success rate.[23] However, no studies have shown a significant advantage to any of the various arthroscopic techniques. There is concern that arthroscopic surgery is inferior to open surgery in the ability to mobilize the distal clavicle or oversew the deltotrapezial fascia; these are believed to be key surgical components, especially for chronic instability. The technical challenges of the arthroscopic techniques have probably prevented them from being more widely used.

One advantage of the arthroscopic technique is that it allows the shoulder to be evaluated for intra-articular pathology at the time of the AC joint repair and reconstruction. One study found a 15% rate of pathology, such as rotator cuff and labral tearing, that can be corrected at the time of AC joint surgery.[24]

Hook Plates

Hook plates have been used for the treatment of AC separations, although in general they are more commonly used for distal clavicle fractures. As with Bosworth screw fixation, short-term placement allows the CC ligaments and other structures to stabilize.[25] However, hook plates did not improve outcomes when compared with suture augmentation, and they required removal. The role of hook plate placement in primary AC joint separations was further called into question by a report of hook plate–specific complications in a study of 313 patients. These complications included hook plate erosion into the acromion with possible acromial fracture (1 patient), hook plate fracture (4 patients), infection (6 patients), and redislocation after hook plate removal (7 patients).[25,26] Hook plates were found to perform best when used with a soft-tissue graft, but this method appears to defeat the purpose of minimally invasive plate placement. A comparison study found better results after Weaver-Dunn reconstruction than after hook plate treatment, including less pain at rest and better Constant scores.[27]

Although hook plates do not appear to have a major role in acute, isolated AC joint injuries, they may have a role in specific patients. For instance, hook plates may be useful for AC separations associated with coracoid or scapula fracture, in which fixation cannot be placed between the coracoid and the clavicle (**Figure 4**). The hook plate is placed along the distal clavicle and under the spine of the acromion, with the acromion rather than coracoid relied on for stability. Hook plates also have been used for revision AC reconstruction, especially if excess distal clavicle was resected and poor soft-tissue quality remains.

Rehabilitation

In patients who are nonsurgically treated, the higher grade type III, IV, and V injuries typically require more time for recovery than the lower grade type I and II injuries. A type I or II injury typically requires 2 to 3 weeks of nonsurgical treatment followed by a gradual return to sport, and a type III injury typically requires 4 to 6 weeks. Return to sport requires full range of motion and full strength as well as a nontender AC joint. Nonsurgical treatment is considered unsuccessful if the patient is unable to return to sport or work at 3 months; then surgery should be considered.[28]

A recently developed program of progressive rehabilitation is organized into four phases.[29,30] In phase I, ice, NSAIDs, and minimal immobilization are used in an effort to reduce pain and swelling. Scapula stabilization treatment and lower extremity strengthening are begun. A sling is used for comfort only; patients having a type III injury typically require a longer period of sling use than those with a lower grade injury. Patients advance to phase II when they are at 75% of normal range of motion. Phase II treatment consists of restoring full range of motion, and early strengthening exercises are allowed. Patients proceed to phase III when 75% of strength returns. The goal of phase III is to regain full strength; power and endurance are emphasized. Patients advance to phase IV when the strength of the injured arm equals that of the contralateral arm. Phase IV involves sport-specific training. Patients who do not fully recover after 6 weeks of nonsurgical treatment are more likely to require surgery than patients who do recover.

Many different postoperative rehabilitation protocols have been proposed. Typically, the shoulder is immobilized for the first 6 weeks. During the next 6 weeks, full active and passive range of motion is pursued, with limited lifting. Strengthening is initiated at 3 months, with moderate lifting. Full activity and throwing begins at 4 months, with return to contact sports at 6 months.

Summary

AC joint injuries are common among physically active individuals. Most patients recover well with nonsurgical management and regain full function. A stepwise

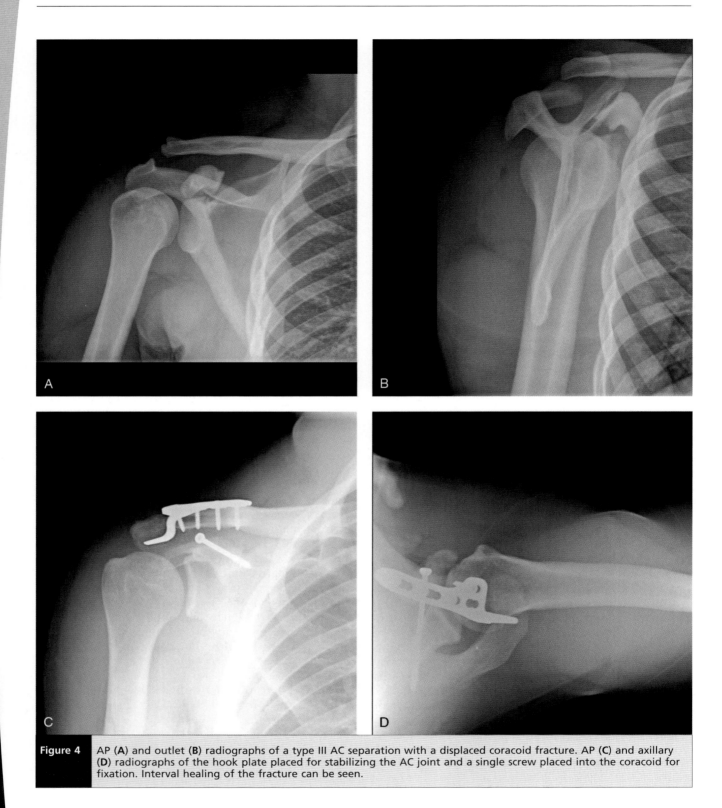

Figure 4   AP (**A**) and outlet (**B**) radiographs of a type III AC separation with a displaced coracoid fracture. AP (**C**) and axillary (**D**) radiographs of the hook plate placed for stabilizing the AC joint and a single screw placed into the coracoid for fixation. Interval healing of the fracture can be seen.

approach to rehabilitation appears to best restore patient function. However, certain injury patterns, such as types IV, V, and VI, are best treated surgically. In addition, patients who do not recover after 3 months of nonsurgical treatment also are best treated surgically. Controversy still exists as to the best surgical option,

but good outcomes can be expected as long as principles including adequate mobilization, augmented fixation with appropriately placed screw holes and suturing or taping, and appropriate rehabilitation are adhered to. Anatomic reconstruction provides a biomechanically strong reconstruction. Some surgeons have reported the use of less invasive techniques, which may become more popular as better fixation devices are developed or midterm results are reported. Hook plates have become more popular as a method of fixation, but their role in the treatment of AC joint injuries still is being developed.

Annotated References

1. Johansen JA, Grutter PW, McFarland EG, Petersen SA: Acromioclavicular joint injuries: Indications for treatment and treatment options. *J Shoulder Elbow Surg* 2011;20(2, suppl):S70-S82.

   The management of AC joint injuries is summarized, with a focus on diagnosis and treatment. The role of surgical management is discussed, with indications for surgery based on current literature.

2. Hsu SH, Ahmad CS, Henry PD, McKee MD, Levine WN: How to minimize complications in acromioclavicular joint and clavicle surgery. *Instr Course Lect* 2012;61:169-183.

   The treatment of AC joint injuries is summarized, with a focus on avoiding complications of surgical treatment. Methods for managing and evaluating patients postoperatively are discussed in terms of complications and patient outcome.

3. Nissen CW, Chatterjee A: Type III acromioclavicular separation: Results of a recent survey on its management. *Am J Orthop (Belle Mead NJ)* 2007;36(2):89-93.

   Members of the American Orthopaedic Society for Sports Medicine and orthopedic residency directors were surveyed concerning treatment of type III AC joint separations. More than 80% of the respondents recommended nonsurgical treatment.

4. Schlegel TF, Burks RT, Marcus RL, Dunn HK: A prospective evaluation of untreated acute grade III acromioclavicular separations. *Am J Sports Med* 2001;29(6):699-703.

5. Mouhsine E, Garofalo R, Crevoisier X, Farron A: Grade I and II acromioclavicular dislocations: Results of conservative treatment. *J Shoulder Elbow Surg* 2003;12(6):599-602.

6. Lizaur A, Sanz-Reig J, Gonzalez-Parreño S: Long-term results of the surgical treatment of type III acromioclavicular dislocations: An update of a previous report. *J Bone Joint Surg Br* 2011;93(8):1088-1092.

   At an average 24-year follow-up of 38 patients treated with Kirschner wire fixation for acute AC joint separation, 35 patients were satisfied. Two patients had redisplacement, and 1 had osteoarthritis of the AC joint.

7. Bäthis H, Tingart M, Bouillon B, Tiling T: The status of therapy of acromioclavicular joint injury: Results of a survey of trauma surgery clinics in Germany. *Unfallchirurg* 2001;104(10):955-960.

8. Bannister GC, Wallace WA, Stableforth PG, Hutson MA: The management of acute acromioclavicular dislocation: A randomised prospective controlled trial. *J Bone Joint Surg Br* 1989;71(5):848-850.

9. Smith TO, Chester R, Pearse EO, Hing CB: Operative versus non-operative management following Rockwood grade III acromioclavicular separation: A meta-analysis of the current evidence base. *J Orthop Traumatol* 2011;12(1):19-27.

   A meta-analysis of six studies attempted to determine whether surgical or nonsurgical treatment of type III AC separation was preferable. Only one study found better results with surgery. The older Kirschner wire technique was used in five studies. Surgical treatment had a better cosmetic result, but nonsurgical treatment was associated with less time to recovery. No difference was found related to strength, pain, or throwing.

10. Ceccarelli E, Bondì R, Alviti F, Garofalo R, Miulli F, Padua R: Treatment of acute grade III acromioclavicular dislocation: A lack of evidence. *J Orthop Traumatol* 2008;9(2):105-108.

    A literature review of the outcomes of surgical and nonsurgical treatment found only five randomized controlled studies. Patients had a similar result regardless of whether they were treated with or without surgery, but those treated surgically had a higher complication rate. Therefore, nonsurgical treatment was found to be valid for these patients.

11. Lädermann A, Grosclaude M, Lübbeke A, et al: Acromioclavicular and coracoclavicular cerclage reconstruction for acute acromioclavicular joint dislocations. *J Shoulder Elbow Surg* 2011;20(3):401-408.

    An excellent result was reported for 34 of 37 patients who underwent AC and CC suture fixation using nonabsorbable sutures for acute AC separation, with no soft-tissue transfer. Isokinetic study found normal function. There was no need for hardware removal.

12. Turman KA, Miller CD, Miller MD: Clavicular fractures following coracoclavicular ligament reconstruction with tendon graft: A report of three cases. *J Bone Joint Surg Am* 2010;92(6):1526-1532.

    Three patients had clavicle fracture after CC ligament reconstruction with tendon graft. This complication may be avoidable with preoperative counseling to avoid postoperative overactivity, the use of small-diameter tunnels, maintenance of an adequate bone bridge, and avoidance of posterior cortical breach.

13. Gerhardt DC, VanDerWerf JD, Rylander LS, McCarty EC: Postoperative coracoid fracture after transcoracoid acromioclavicular joint reconstruction. *J Shoulder Elbow Surg* 2011;20(5):e6-e10.

    The risk of coracoid fracture after AC joint reconstruction using transcoracoid fixation should be considered in choosing the best reconstructive method.

14. Motta P, Maderni A, Bruno L, Mariotti U: Suture rupture in acromioclavicular joint dislocations treated with flip buttons. *Arthroscopy* 2011;27(2):294-298.

6: Trauma and Fractures

Four of 20 patients undergoing acute AC joint repair using flip buttons had postoperative suture rupture. All patients had hyperlaxity. Horizontal instability of repair may lead to shearing of the suture and subsequent failure of repair.

15. Jiang C, Wang M, Rong G: Proximally based conjoined tendon transfer for coracoclavicular reconstruction in the treatment of acromioclavicular dislocation: Surgical technique. *J Bone Joint Surg Am* 2008; 90(suppl 2, pt 2):299-308.

The lateral half of the conjoined tendon was used, rather than the CA ligament, for AC joint reconstruction in 38 patients. The results were good or excellent in 89% of the patients. The main advantage is adequate soft tissue, with no sacrifice of the CA arch or the need for soft-tissue transfer.

16. Gonzalez-Lomas G, Javidan P, Lin T, Adamson GJ, Limpisvasti O, Lee TQ: Intramedullary acromioclavicular ligament reconstruction strengthens isolated coracoclavicular ligament reconstruction in acromioclavicular dislocations. *Am J Sports Med* 2010;38(10):2113-2122.

A cadaver study compared CC anatomic reconstruction alone and with intramedullary graft placement in the AC joint. The intramedullary graft improved horizontal stability.

17. Rios CG, Mazzocca AD: Acromioclavicular joint problems in athletes and new methods of management. *Clin Sports Med* 2008;27(4):763-788.

The relevant anatomy, classification, evaluation, and treatment of AC joint pathology is systematically reviewed.

18. Grutter PW, Petersen SA: Anatomical acromioclavicular ligament reconstruction: A biomechanical comparison of reconstructive techniques of the acromioclavicular joint. *Am J Sports Med* 2005;33(11):1723-1728.

19. Thomas K, Litsky A, Jones G, Bishop JY: Biomechanical comparison of coracoclavicular reconstructive techniques. *Am J Sports Med* 2011;39(4):804-810.

A cadaver study compared Weaver-Dunn, nonanatomic allograft, anatomic allograft, anatomic suture, and GraftRope reconstructions. In comparison with native control shoulders, the anatomic allograft had the highest load to failure, which was significantly higher than those of the other subgroups. The nonanatomic allograft technique did not bring the tendon through the clavicle and did not weave the tendon on itself. No significant difference was found among other subgroups.

20. Tauber M, Gordon K, Koller H, Fox M, Resch H: Semitendinosus tendon graft versus a modified Weaver-Dunn procedure for acromioclavicular joint reconstruction in chronic cases: A prospective comparative study. *Am J Sports Med* 2009;37(1):181-190.

A retrospective study of 24 patients compared the Weaver-Dunn and anatomic reconstructions. The 12 patients who received the anatomic reconstruction had superior clinical and radiographic outcomes.

21. Scheibel M, Dröschel S, Gerhardt C, Kraus N: Arthroscopically assisted stabilization of acute high-grade acromioclavicular joint separations. *Am J Sports Med* 2011;39(7):1507-1516.

Arthroscopically assisted stabilization of acute AC separation using a double TightRope technique had excellent clinical results in 28 patients, despite greater CC distance compared with the contralateral side. Patients' fairly high rate of horizontal instability did not appear to affect the clinical results.

22. DeBerardino TM, Pensak MJ, Ferreira J, Mazzocca AD: Arthroscopic stabilization of acromioclavicular joint dislocation using the AC graftrope system. *J Shoulder Elbow Surg* 2010;19(2, suppl):47-52.

Early results are reported for the AC flip button device with incorporated allograft as used for arthroscopic repair of acute AC joint separations. No complications were reported, and patients had an early return to function.

23. Boileau P, Old J, Gastaud O, Brassart N, Roussanne Y: All-arthroscopic Weaver-Dunn-Chuinard procedure with double-button fixation for chronic acromioclavicular joint dislocation. *Arthroscopy* 2010;26(2):149-160.

Ten patients with chronic AC joint instability underwent arthroscopic CA ligament transfer along with a fleck of acromion. All patients were satisfied, and 9 returned to sport. One patient had a superficial infection. The bone fragment healed in 8 patients. Level of evidence: IV.

24. Pauly S, Gerhardt C, Haas NP, Scheibel M: Prevalence of concomitant intraarticular lesions in patients treated operatively for high-grade acromioclavicular joint separations. *Knee Surg Sports Traumatol Arthrosc* 2009; 17(5):513-517.

Forty patients underwent diagnostic arthroscopy during surgery for high-grade AC separation. Six patients (15%) were found to have pathology, including 2 with subscapularis tears, 3 with superior labrum anterior and posterior tears, and 1 with a combined supraspinatus-subscapularis tendon tear.

25. Kienast B, Thietje R, Queitsch C, Gille J, Schulz AP, Meiners J: Mid-term results after operative treatment of Rockwood grade III-V acromioclavicular joint dislocations with an AC-hook-plate. *Eur J Med Res* 2011;16(2):52-56.

Midterm results were reported for an AC hook plate used to treat of 313 acute AC joint separations. The results were excellent in 89%, with an average Constant score of 92.4. The complication rate was 10.6%, with six infections, one acromial fracture, and seven redislocations.

26. Chiang CL, Yang SW, Tsai MY, Kuen-Huang Chen C: Acromion osteolysis and fracture after hook plate fixation for acromioclavicular joint dislocation: A case report. *J Shoulder Elbow Surg* 2010;19(4):e13-e15.

Acromial osteolysis followed by fracture developed after hook plate placement for AC separation. The patient did not have the plate removed 4 months after surgery, as recommended, and the complication developed at 8 months. Early plate removal is recommended.

27. Boström Windhamre HA, von Heideken JP, Une-Larsson VE, Ekelund AL: Surgical treatment of chronic acromioclavicular dislocations: A comparative study of Weaver-Dunn augmented with PDS-braid or hook plate. *J Shoulder Elbow Surg* 2010;19(7):1040-1048.

A retrospective study compared Weaver-Dunn reconstructions with polydioxanone braid or a hook plate for augmentation. The clinical results were similar, but the necessity of an additional surgical procedure for hook plate removal led to a recommendation for suture augmentation.

28. Trainer G, Arciero RA, Mazzocca AD: Practical management of grade III acromioclavicular separations. *Clin J Sport Med* 2008;18(2):162-166.

A protocol is presented for the initial treatment of grade III AC joint separations depending on the timing of injury (in-season or off-season) and the response to initial nonsurgical treatment. Surgery was recommended after 3 months of unsuccessful nonsurgical treatment.

29. Cote MP, Wojcik KE, Gomlinski G, Mazzocca AD: Rehabilitation of acromioclavicular joint separations: Operative and nonoperative considerations. *Clin Sports Med* 2010;29(2):213-228, vii.

The anatomy and biomechanics of the AC joint are considered in determining a rehabilitation protocol for patients treated nonsurgically or surgically.

30. Lervick GN, Klepps SK: Shoulder dislocations, clavicle fractures, and acromioclavicular separations. *Orthopaedic Knowledge Online Journal*. March 1, 2011. http://orthoportal.aaos.org/oko/article.aspx?article=OKO_SHO042#abstract. Accessed September 6, 2012.

A practical method is provided for enabling athletes to return to play after AC joint and clavicle injuries based on rehabilitation protocols and biomechanical studies.

6: Trauma and Fractures

Elbow Trauma, Fracture, and Reconstruction

SECTION EDITOR:
MARK S. COHEN, MD

Tendon Injuries and Conditions of the Elbow: Biceps, Triceps, and Lateral and Medial Epicondylitis

Brandon Cincere, MD   Robert P. Nirschl, MD, MS

Elbow Trauma, Fracture, and Reconstruction

Introduction

Elbow tendon injuries typically are categorized as resulting from single-event macrotrauma (acute injury), single-event trauma superimposed on tissue made vulnerable by overuse (acute-on-chronic injury), or multiple repetition overuse (chronic injury). Numerous pathologic conditions, ranging from acute to chronic injury, can occur around the circumference of the elbow. Ligament dysfunction, nerve dysfunction, and osteochondral injury may be associated with the condition. Elbow tendon overuse injury often is not an isolated event, and the entire extremity, from the cervical and thoracic spine to the shoulder and hand, should be evaluated.

Biceps Injuries

Evaluation

The distal biceps has two insertions on the radial tuberosity. The short head attaches distally on the tuberosity, allowing it to be a powerful elbow flexor. The long head attaches more proximally and ulnarly, farther from the axis of rotation of the forearm. This attachment enhances supination by increasing leverage. The biceps tendon spirals like a ribbon; its direction is clockwise in the left arm and counterclockwise in the right arm.[1]

Most distal bicep injuries occur as an acute avulsion from the radial tuberosity after sudden eccentric extension force while the elbow is in midflexion. The symptoms may include a tearing sensation and acute pain.

Most such injuries occur in the dominant extremity in men aged 40 to 60 years. The risk of rupture is 7.5 times greater in people who use tobacco.[2] Pain and ecchymosis in the antecubital fossa are common findings, and tenderness and weakness with resisted supination and elbow flexion also may be found. Palpation of a defect, a positive O'Driscoll hook test, or a positive squeeze test can reveal the injury unless there is a partial tear, an intact bicipital aponeurosis (a lacertus fibrosus), or bicipital tendinosis.[3,4] The O'Driscoll hook test was found to have 100% sensitivity and specificity.[3] A complete tear is diagnosed as acute if it occurred within the past 4 weeks or chronic if it occurred earlier. Radiographic evaluation typically does not reveal an osseous injury but occasionally may show an irregularity, enlargement of the radial tuberosity, or avulsion.[5] Bicipital tendinosis without rupture can occur in isolation or in association with a cubital bursitis or a partial rupture. A partial tear is less common and can occur within the tendon or at its insertion (**Figure 1**). A clicking sensation near the tendon insertion during forearm rotation may be caused by inflammation of the bursa between the tendon and the tuberosity. MRI can be

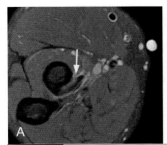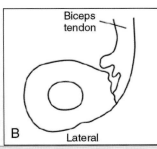

Figure 1   T2-weighted MRI (**A**) and line drawing (**B**) showing a partial-thickness tear at the radial side attachment of the distal biceps tendon (arrow). (Reproduced from Sutton KM, Dodds SD, Ahmad CS, Sethi PM: Surgical treatment of distal biceps rupture. J Am Acad Orthop Surg 2010;18[3]:139-148.)

Dr. Nirschl or an immediate family member has received royalties from Medical Sports; is a member of a speakers' bureau or has made paid presentations on behalf of Norvartis; and has stock or stock options held in Tenex and Medical Sports. Neither Dr. Cincere nor any immediate family member has received anything of value from or in a commercial company or institution related directly or indirectly to the subject of this chapter.

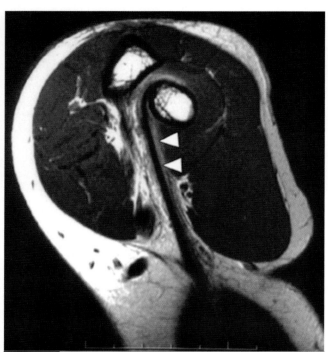

Figure 2 Proton density–weighted MRI taken from the FABS position showing a partial tear of the right distal biceps (*arrowheads*, indicating a linear abnormal signal). The full tendon length can be seen from the FABS position. (Reproduced with permission from Giuffrè BM, Moss MJ: Optimal positioning for MRI of the distal biceps brachii tendon: Flexed abducted supinated view. *AJR Am J Roentgenol* 2004;182 [4]:944-946.)

helpful in identifying integrity and intrasubstance changes, but these are not always apparent.[5] MRI in the prone flexion, abduction, supinated (FABS) position shows the full length of the biceps from the tuberosity to the musculocutaneous junction[6] (**Figure 2**). Diagnostic ultrasound also can be considered.

Treatment

Most acute and complete distal biceps ruptures can be treated by reattachment. A variety of techniques have predictably good results superior to those of nonsurgical management.[5] The treatment of a chronic rupture can be challenging and is based on whether the bicipital aponeurosis is disrupted or intact. An intact tendon may be prevented from retracting more proximally. As time passes, retraction and scarring of the brachialis may limit the ability to achieve enough surgical length for a satisfactory primary repair. Semitendinosus graft reconstruction has been used to treat a chronic injury with inadequate length.[7] Repair and reconstruction to the radial tuberosity are less predictable in chronic injury and carry greater neurovascular risk. In such circumstances, a compromise method of soft-tissue attachment to the brachialis may be considered.

Partial tears can occur in association with tendinosis and bursitis. MRI can be useful in the diagnosis by showing partial tearing at the radial insertion of the radial tuberosity.[5] Endoscopy has been used to evaluate the potential for repairing a partial tear.[8] Injuries are considered for surgical intervention after unsuccessful nonsurgical management. Most partial ruptures can be successfully treated with release, débridement, and reattachment of the tendon, especially if the tear exceeds 50%. Débridement alone is less likely to have a successful outcome. Repair of a complete rupture is most likely to restore supination and flexion strength if it is done within 2 weeks of injury.[5]

Better functional and objective outcomes were found in patients treated surgically rather than nonsurgically.[2] Supination strength but not flexion strength was significantly improved in patients who underwent repair.[2] Patients treated nonsurgically had a higher incidence of activity pain and had decreased strength and endurance that was more severe in supination than in flexion. In general, nonsurgical treatment should be considered for a patient who has a chronic complex rupture, has a serious medical comorbidity, and is sedentary.[2]

Single- and two-incision techniques have been described. The Boyd-Anderson two-incision technique was developed to avoid the neurologic complications associated with a single incision. However, the use of this technique has led to various complications, including radioulnar synostosis and heterotopic ossification. Modification of the Boyd-Anderson technique into a muscle-splitting approach that does not violate the periosteum of the ulna has reduced the incidence of complications.[5] With this technique, "virtually 100%" improvement was reported in restoring flexion and supination strength, without loss of motion or rerupture.[9] Several other studies also reported that the technique led to successful results.[10-12] A systematic review documented an overall 16% complication rate with the two-incision technique and an 18% rate with the single-incision technique.[13] Patients who underwent a two-incision procedure were more likely to have a poor result compared with those who underwent a single-incision procedure (31% and 6%, repectively[13] (**Table 1**).

The single-incision method has evolved with improvements in technique, devices, and repairs. Complications related to single-incision techniques include injuries to the posterior interosseous and lateral antebrachial cutaneous nerves.[2] The risk of nerve injury has been reduced by identifying the cutaneous nerve, maintaining the arm in supination, and using less invasive incisions. Multiple studies found a minimal risk of complications and good outcomes when cortical button fixation was used with single-incision techniques.[14-16] A meta-analysis found a 69% rate of satisfactory outcomes with the two-incision technique and a 94% rate with the single-incision technique.[13] The lower rate of satisfactory outcomes with the two-incision technique was attributable to loss of forearm rotation or rotational

Table 1

Complications After Two-Incision and Single-Incision Elbow Repairs

| | Technique | | |
	Two-Incision (N = 142)	Single-Incision (N = 165)	P
Complication			
Heterotopic ossification[a]	8 (6%)	5 (3%)	0.45
Nerve palsy[b]	10 (7%)	20 (12%)	0.12
Loss of forearm rotation	13 (9%)	3 (2%)	0.01
Infection	0	3 (2%)	0.25
Flexion contracture	2 (1%)	1 (1%)	0.61
Total elbows with a complication	23 (16%)	29 (18%)	0.88

[a] Resulting in motion loss
[b] Transient or permanent
(Adapted with permission from Chavan PR, Duquin TR, Bisson LJ: Repair of the ruptured distal biceps tendon: A systematic review. *Am J Sports Med* 2008;36:1618-1624.)

Table 2

Biomechanical Studies of Distal Biceps Fixation

| | Single Load to Failure Testing | | Cyclic Testing | |
Fixation Method	Ultimate Tensile Load (N)	Stiffness (N/mm)	Ultimate Tensile Load (N)	Displacement (mm)
Transosseous tunnel	125 to 210	15.9	195 to 310	3.55
Interference screw	131 to 192	30.4	232	2.15
EndoButton	159	—	249 to 440	2.58 to 3.42
Suture anchor	105 to 263	—	209 to 381	2.06 to 2.38

(Adapted with permission from Chavan PR, Duquin TR, Bisson LJ: Repair of the ruptured distal biceps tendon: A systematic review. *Am J Sports Med* 2008;36:1618-1624.)

strength. The surgeon's level of training and experience should guide the decision as to the preferred technique.

A delay in diagnosis and treatment may complicate an anatomic repair. An intact bicipital aponeurosis can mask an acute rupture but also can limit proximal retraction and possibly allow a direct repair. Inadequate length should be anticipated in a chronic injury, and graft material should be available for reconstruction. The semitendinosus is anatomically similar to the distal biceps tendon.[7] A more extensive dissection is warranted, and nearby neurovascular structures should be identified and protected. Tenodesis to the brachialis also should be considered as a reasonable backup technique for treating a patient with a chronic injury and activity-related pain, with the expectation that supination strength may not improve.[5] This technique usually allows accelerated rehabilitation. At the time of repair or reconstruction, tension should be tested in elbow extension to assess the security of the repair as well as any limitations pertaining to the progression of the postoperative rehabilitation program.

Multiple studies have evaluated methods of radial tuberosity fixation. In a comparison of fixation strength

in cyclic loading when transosseous tunnels and suture anchors were used, there was no specimen failure at 50 N over 3,600 cycles; the mean load to failure was significantly higher for osseous tunnels.[17] These results were confirmed in a second study.[18] A comparison of intact tendons and injured tendons repaired with interference screws found no significant difference, and interference screws had significantly higher mean failure strength and stiffness in comparison with interosseous tunnels.[19] An evaluation of several fixation techniques found that the use of cortical buttons achieved the highest load, stiffness, and cyclical load to failure, possibly allowing an earlier and more aggressive rehabilitation.[20,21] A systematic review of biomechanical studies found that the EndoButton (Smith and Nephew) was the best performing fixation device[13] (**Table 2**). When a cortical button and an interference screw were used for dual fixation to allow an aggressive rehabilitation protocol, most patients returned to normal daily activity within 4 weeks of surgery.[22]

After surgery, the elbow is immobilized for 7 to 10 days in 90° of flexion and supination. A hinged elbow brace may be used to protect the repair and block full

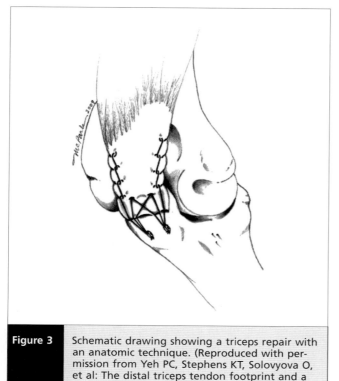

Figure 3 Schematic drawing showing a triceps repair with an anatomic technique. (Reproduced with permission from Yeh PC, Stephens KT, Solovyova O, et al: The distal triceps tendon footprint and a biomechanical analysis of 3 repair techniques. *Am J Sports Med* 2010;38[5]:1025-1033.)

extension for 6 to 8 weeks, based on the identified postrepair intraoperative tension. At this point, periods of unrestricted motion gradually are increased with the use of strengthening exercises. The patient usually is able to resume unrestricted activities 5 to 6 months after surgery, depending on the symptoms, strength, and endurance. Patients follow a similar course after repairs or reconstruction of a chronic injury. A patient who has undergone soft-tissue tenodesis to the brachialis often is able to resume unrestricted activities at 3 to 4 months.

Triceps Injuries

Evaluation

Approximately 0.8% of all tendon ruptures involve the distal triceps.[23] Most distal triceps ruptures occur in men and are associated with anabolic steroid use or weightlifting. The condition also is associated with metabolic bone disease, renal osteodystrophy, olecranon bursitis, Marfan syndrome, osteogenesis imperfecta, rheumatoid arthritis, and diabetes. The three heads of the triceps converge to insert over a wide footprint (average, 466 mm²) on the olecranon, and most injuries occur at this osseous insertion.[23] The most common mechanism of injury is a sudden eccentric load to a contracted triceps. The patient has pain, swelling, and ecchymosis, with a palpable defect. Not all complete tears prevent active extension, but an ab-

sence of active extension signifies a complete tear. An intact lateral expansion or compensatory anconeus may allow active extension. A modified Thompson squeeze test may be positive if the patient is in the prone position with the arm hanging over the edge of the table. AP and lateral radiographs may reveal flecks of bone. MRI can be helpful in determining whether the rupture is complete or partial.[23] Eight of 10 partial ruptures were found to involve the medial insertion.[24] In 801 consecutive elbow MRI examinations, a triceps tear was found in 28 patients, including 5 women and 23 men. Partial tears were more common than complete tears.[25] The most common symptom was pain, typically after an athletic injury.

Treatment

The management of a triceps tear is dictated by patient-specific factors as well as the tear location and completeness and the patient's functional extension strength. A partial tear in a patient who is debilitated and has low physical demands can be managed nonsurgically. In general, tears smaller than 50% have been managed nonsurgically with satisfactory results.[24,26] A nonsurgically treated weightlifter with bilateral partial ruptures had normal function at 41 weeks and fatigue with lifting at 55 weeks.[27] Complete tears or tears of more than 50% are best treated surgically in an active patient. Chronic ruptures (of more than 6 weeks' duration) are more challenging, and multiple repair and reconstruction techniques have been described.[23]

Early primary repair (within 2 weeks of injury) is recommended for a complete tear with substantial loss of strength. Most commonly, transosseous holes are drilled, and whipstitch sutures are tied over a bone bridge. As an alternative, a bone anchor technique may be considered. An anatomic footprint repair technique has been described that resembles the suture-bridge technique for the rotator cuff[28] (**Figure 3**). When cylindrically loaded, this repair configuration had less repair site motion than a cruciate or a suture anchor repair, possibly allowing earlier rehabilitation.

The elbow is immobilized in 30° to 45° of flexion for 2 weeks after surgery. Passive extension and active guided flexion are begun at 2 weeks, with full active range of motion attained by 4 weeks. Aggressive weightlifting should be avoided for 4 to 6 months. Complications such as bursitis, flexion contractures, and rerupture can occur.

Posterior Elbow (Triceps) Tendinosis

Triceps tendinosis or posterior tennis elbow also is called boxer's elbow. This relatively uncommon overuse condition involves the insertion of the triceps into the posterior elbow with synovitis of the olecranon fossa. Repetitive rapid extensions of the elbow, such as in throwing, punching, blocking (in football linemen), tennis serving, and weightlifting are implicated in the

7: Elbow Trauma, Fracture, and Reconstruction

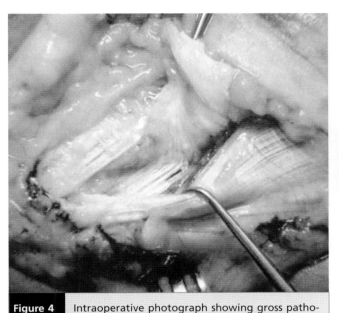

Figure 4 | Intraoperative photograph showing gross pathologic angiofibroblastic hyperplastic tendinosis tissue. (Courtesy of Nirschl RP, Photo file.)

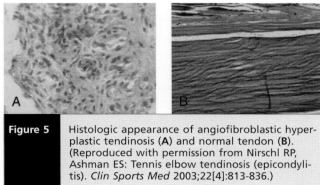

Figure 5 | Histologic appearance of angiofibroblastic hyperplastic tendinosis (**A**) and normal tendon (**B**). (Reproduced with permission from Nirschl RP, Ashman ES: Tennis elbow tendinosis (epicondylitis). *Clin Sports Med* 2003;22[4]:813-836.)

pathology. Osteophyte and loose body formation with synovitis in the olecranon fossa frequently coexist as a result of the rapid and violent extension characteristic of boxing and overhead sports motions. Bursitis, posterior medial impingement, olecranon stress fracture, or olecranon apophysitis (in an adolescent) should be included in the differential diagnosis. The histopathology of triceps tendinosis is identical to that of medial and lateral tendinosis, with the potential for associated olecranon fossa synovitis and loose bodies. Extension blockade and flexion contractures may be encountered. The nonsurgical physical therapy methods are similar to those used for tennis elbow, but with extension blockade, the treatment plan should include posterior, medial, and lateral gliding of the ulna on the humerus.[29-31]

The recommended surgical approach for posterior tennis elbow is a small longitudinal posterior incision centered over the palpably sensitive area. An elliptical excision of the tissue with angiofibroblastic tendinosis changes is undertaken. A spur at the tip of the olecranon, if any, should be removed. In the throwing athlete, triceps tendinosis most commonly is associated with olecranon fossa synovitis, chondromalacia, osteophytes, and/or loose bodies, and it should be surgically treated.[32] The postoperative management is similar to that of lateral and medial elbow conditions.

Lateral Elbow Tendinosis

Lateral elbow tendinosis or tennis elbow most commonly is caused by tendon overuse and failure of tendon healing. This condition typically occurs during the fourth or fifth decade of life, affects the dominant extremity, and is equally common in men and women. The pathoanatomy is a noninflammatory, degenerative angiofibroblastic hyperplasia, possibly attributable to an inadequate healing response to microtearing. The tissue typically is dull, gray, and friable, and on gross examination, it often is edematous (**Figures 4** and **5**). The specific areas of the lateral elbow involve the extensor carpi radialis brevis (ECRB)–extensor digitorum communis (EDC) complex. The ECRB is involved in 100% of incidences, and the anterior edge of the EDC is involved in 35%. The primary goal of nonsurgical treatment is to revitalize the pain-producing unhealthy tissue so that it becomes healthy and does not produce pain. The patient risk factors for tendon overuse include age older than 35 years, a high activity level, a demanding activity technique, and an inadequate fitness level. Activities that can lead to lateral elbow tendinosis are listed in **Table 3**. The associated conditions include medial epicondylitis, cubital tunnel syndrome, carpal tunnel syndrome, and rotator cuff tendinosis. A patient with all of these conditions is said to have mesenchymal syndrome. In approximately 5% of patients, anterolateral joint chondromalacia and synovitis are associated with lateral tennis elbow.[30,33-35]

Evaluation

An insidious onset of activity-related pain is followed by pain at rest and dysfunction as the pathologic change becomes extensive. The maximal tenderness on palpation is slightly (5 mm) distal and anterior to the lateral epicondyle. The patient has pain with provocative manual stress testing, such as resisted wrist and finger extension with the elbow in extended and flexed positions. Pain with the elbow flexed suggests substantial tendinosis damage. Functional strength loss can be measured using a dynamometer. Range of motion typically is within normal limits. The medial and posterior tendons should be assessed, with evaluation of the cubital tunnel, any posterior interosseous nerve (PIN) entrapment (3 to 4 cm distal), the cervical spine, and the carpel tunnel (a 10% association), each of which may represent an associated finding.[30] The strength of the rotator cuff should be assessed because weakness on the ipsilateral side is common and should be treated during rehabilitation. Elbow stability also should be

Table 3

Common Activities Leading to Epicondylitis

Activity	Lateral Epicondylitis	Medial Epicondylitis
Sports	Tennis (groundstrokes) Racquetball Squash Fencing	Golf Rowing Baseball (pitching) Javelin throwing Tennis (serving)
Occupational or other	Meat cutting Plumbing Painting Raking Weaving	Bricklaying Hammering Typing Textile production

(Adapted from Jobe FW, Ciccotti MG: Lateral and medial epicondylitis of the elbow. *J Am Acad Orthop Surg* 1994;2[1]:1-8.)

evaluated and treated. The cervical and thoracic spine, the upper extremity, and sports mechanics should be assessed. Radiographic evaluation is recommended because 20% of patients have tendon calcification or lateral epicondyle reactive exostosis.[30] MRI is rarely needed for diagnosis, but it reveals edema and thickening at the extensor origin in 90% of patients with symptoms. Ultrasound has moderate sensitivity and variable specificity, depending on the study and the examiner.[34]

The Posterior Interosseous Nerve

A 1972 report described surgical treatment of presumed tennis elbow by decompressing the PIN at the canal of Froshe, and lateral tennis elbow has been linked to PIN entrapment.[36] Nonetheless, there is no compelling evidence that PIN entrapment is a cause of lateral elbow tendinosis. Although the PIN is anatomically adjacent to the location of lateral elbow tendinosis, the possibility of an independent PIN condition should be considered. PIN entrapment is difficult to diagnose. The symptoms include a vague aching sensation over the extensor muscle mass and pain with resisted supination. Electromyography and a xylocaine block may aid in the diagnosis. Surgical nerve decompression often is unsuccessful, in part perhaps because of misdiagnosis.

Nonsurgical Treatment

The treatment of lateral elbow tendinosis should complement the natural biologic healing response in an ordered progression to enhance the sequence of neovascularization and collagen production. Treatment should begin by controlling inflammatory exudation and hemorrhage to relieve pain and then promoting specific tissue healing, general fitness, and control of force loads or violence. Some patients may require surgical removal of pathologic tissue, but the initial treatment should consist of protection, rest, ice, compression, ele-

vation, medications (specifically, NSAIDs), and activity modification. Lateral elbow tendinosis histologically is not an inflammatory condition, but anti-inflammatory medications can control pain caused by chemical mediators and relieve associated synovitis or inflammation in the surrounding adipose and connective tissue.[30,32] When diclofenac was compared with placebo, patients receiving diclofenac reported lower levels of pain.[37] There was no significant difference when naproxen was compared with placebo.[38] Healing is promoted through concentric and eccentric rehabilitative exercise, high-voltage transcutaneous electrical nerve stimulation, aerobic and general conditioning exercise, absence from abuse, and possibly ultrasound. General body conditioning can maintain or improve body fitness and stimulate healing of the injured tissue. Force load control is used to minimize potential injury-producing activities by counterforce bracing, improvement in sports technique, control of the intensity and the duration of activity, and equipment evaluation.[30]

Steroid injections have been used for pain control but cannot be considered capable of tissue healing. Although steroid injections led to early good results, at 1-year follow-up, the results were no better or even worse than those of treatment with NSAIDs or physical therapy.[39] The excessive use of steroid injections (more than three focused injections) could cause harm to the underlying tissue, leading to further weakness and possibly tendon rupture. The injection technique is important; the needle should be placed under the ECRB, not at the epicondyle. The use of botulinum toxin A for pain control had conflicting results at 3 months, with no significant improvement in patients' grip strength.[40] It is possible that the use of botulinum toxin–A could lead to muscle atrophy because of loss of use and worsening symptoms. A recent level I study found significant improvement in scores on the visual analog and Disabilities of the Arm, Shoulder and Hand scales when platelet-rich plasma (PRP) was used compared with steroid injection.[41] Patients treated with steroid injection had improved early results that were not sustained; patients treated with PRP had progressively improving results, with continued significant improvement at 1-year follow-up and no complications. A similar level I study reported similar results at 2-year follow-up.[42] PRP also was found to offer greater improvement than autologous whole blood.[43] A long-term biologic cure has yet to be found.

Extracorporeal shock wave therapy has been used for a variety of tendinopathies, but meta-analysis of nine placebo-controlled studies found conflicting results and no significant benefit over placebo.[44] Ultrasound-guided percutaneous radiofrequency lesioning led to a 78% reduction in symptoms.[45] Nitric oxide delivered with glyceryl trinitrate patches was found to offer no benefit over placebo in a 5-year prospective study.[46] General studies of nonsurgical treatment reported that 83% of patients had improvement at 1-year follow-up, but 40% continued to have minor discomfort at 5-year follow-up.[47,48] The negative prognostic indicators included manual work and a high level of baseline pain.

Surgical Treatment and Indications

Pain is the major indication for surgery. The answers to three questions should be considered: Is the pain of significant intensity to limit function? Does the pain interfere with the patient's daily activity or occupation? Is the pain and tenderness precisely located at the origin of the ECRB adjacent to the lateral epicondyle? Surgery may be considered after a period of high-quality nonsurgical management, usually of approximately 6 months' duration. Surgery may be contraindicated, and a careful reevaluation is necessary if the nonsurgical program was inadequate, the patient has been noncompliant, or the patient has a workers' compensation claim with a secondary gain component.[35]

The Nirschl miniopen techniques have gradually been refined since being originally described in 1979[35,49] (Figure 6). A 2.5-cm straight lateral incision is made, passing just anteromedial to the lateral epicondyle. A too-distal or too-medial incision is common and should be avoided. The interface between the extensor carpi radialis longus (ECRL) and the aponeurosis of the EDC should be identified after dissection of bursal and adipose tissue; the ECRL typically is less firm than the extensor aponeurosis, and the fibers of the ECRL run more obliquely. The ECRL-EDC interval is vertically incised to a depth of 1 to 2 mm, just anteromedial to the epicondyle and in line with the EDC fibers. Sharp dissection proceeds in a more horizontal plane to allow the pathologic tissue to be identified. Dissection of the ECRL-EDC interval vertically beyond the 1- to 2-mm depth is a common error that distorts a clean exposure and identification of the ECRB. With anteromedial retraction of the ECRL, the diagonally oriented fibers of the ECRB come into view as they attach to the EDC and the anteromedial edge of the lateral epicondyle. The pathologic tissue can be identified in the ECRB as dull, gray, friable, and often edematous. This tissue is incised en block in an elliptical fashion, leaving the distal attachments of the ECRB. The ECRB has remaining distal attachments to the capsule, the orbicular ligament, the distal anterior extensor aponeurosis, and the underside of the ECRL and, as a result, does not retract more than 1 to 2 mm. An essentially normal mechanical ECRB working length thus is maintained. Any questionable tissue can be evaluated using the Nirschl scratch maneuver; normal tissue appears shiny and firm, with a yellowish white hue. Thirty-five percent of patients have changes to the anteromedial underside edge of the EDC, which constitutes approximately 15% of the EDC volume. Under no circumstances should the origin of the EDC be released from the epicondyle. Epicondyle bony exostosis is present in approximately 20% of patients and almost always is anteromedial; therefore, it is unnecessary to remove most of the epicondyle. When all pathologic tissue has been resected, one small hole can be drilled in the exposed cortical bone distal to the epicondyle but not in the epicondyle itself to enhance the vascular supply. If intra-articular pathology is suspected, the incision can be extended 0.5 cm distally, and a small longitudinal joint opening can be made in the capsule anterior to the radial collateral ligament.

Associated intra-articular pathology (most commonly synovitis or a plica) is found in only approximately 5% of patients with lateral tendinosis. Occasionally, a full-thickness tear of the ECRB extends into the joint. If this is present, the intra-articular pathology can be evaluated. The capsule should be repaired to prevent postoperative leakage of synovial fluid. The ECRB still has firm distal attachments to bone, and therefore repair is unnecessary. A side-to side suture repair of the ECRL to the EDC is performed, burying the knots or using the Quill knotless closure device (Angiotech). In the uncommon situation in which the joint is opened, the capsule is closed with absorbable suture. A subcuticular closure is performed, and a sterile dressing is applied.[35] The postoperative management is similar to that of lateral, medial, or posterior tendinosis.

The Role of Arthroscopy

In comparison with an open or a miniopen procedure, arthroscopic débridement and release are reported to require less postoperative physical therapy, allow an earlier return to work, and provide the ability to treat associated intra-articular pathology.[50-54] The arthroscopic appearance of the lateral capsule was classified by Baker et al.[55] The degenerative capsule and the undersurface of the ECRB are released from the lateral epicondyle by a mechanical shaver. The major concerns are iatrogenic cartilage injury, neurovascular injury, and inadequate débridement of the pathologic tissue. Open inspection after arthroscopic débridement revealed that 10 of 18 patients had residual gross pathologic tissue during the first year of the investigation, and an additional 4 patients had residual microscopic pathology.[56] In response, the technique was altered to use a curved radiofrequency probe rather than a shaver.[57] Other negative aspects of the arthroscopic technique compared with an open or a miniopen technique include increases in instrument costs, setup time, surgical time, and the learning curve. In comparison with the miniopen technique, the arthroscopic technique has no demonstrated advantages related to results or rehabilitation times.

Surgical Results

The ECRB open resection technique was found to lead to complete pain relief and return of full forearm strength in 85% of patients, and an additional 12% had significant pain relief.[49] The remaining 3% reported no pain relief or strength improvement; these patients included those with a workers' compensation claim. Complications were reported in 1% of patients. At 10- to 14-year follow-up after ECRB resection, the success rate was 97%.[58] A study of 19 patients who un-

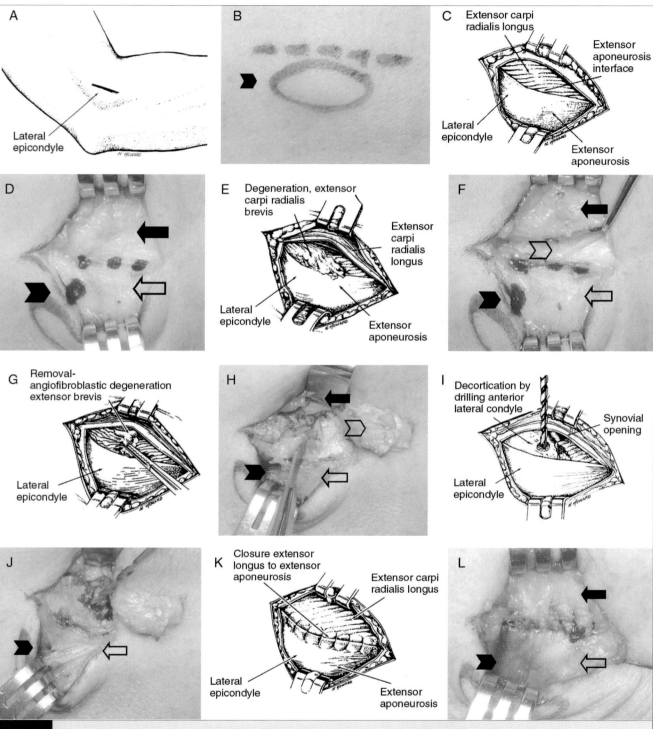

Figure 6 Matched schematic drawings and photographs showing the miniopen Nirschl technique for treating lateral tennis elbow. **A** and **B,** The 2.5-cm incision passes just anteromedial to the lateral epicondyle. **C** and **D,** The interface between the ECRL and the extensor aponeurosis is identified. **E** and **F,** The incision is deepened to 2 to 3 mm, and the ECRL is retracted as the ECRB is seen. Grayish edematous pathologic tissue should be visible. **G** and **H,** Degenerated ECRB is removed. **I** and **J,** A hole is drilled through the cortical bone of the anterior lateral condyle to the cancellous bone level to enhance the vascular supply. **K** and **L,** The ECRL is firmly repaired to the anterior margin of the EDC. Because the ECRB is still attached to adjacent tissues, it is not necessary to suture the distal brevis. Black arrowheads = lateral epicondyle, black arrows = ECRL, clear arrowheads = tendinosis tissue, clear arrows = extensor aponeurosis. (Reproduced with permission from Nirschl RP, Ashman ES: Tennis elbow tendinosis (epicondylitis). *Clin Sports Med* 2003:22[4]:813-836.)

derwent open EDC release, excision, and reattachment found improvement in 18 patients, but 60% of those who played a high-demand sport and 15% of those with a high-demand job had changed their sport or job after the surgery.[59] A long-term prospective study of lateral EDC release found that 40% had persistent pain 6 weeks after surgery, 24% had persistent pain at 1 year, and 9% had persistent pain at 5 years.[60] A comparison of the open Nirschl technique with a percutaneous EDC release technique found greater improvement in Disabilities of the Arm, Shoulder and Hand scores and patient satisfaction as well as a more rapid return to work in patients treated with the percutaneous technique.[61] Three studies of arthroscopic techniques found that 93% to 100% of patients had improvement at 2-year follow-up, but only 62% to 80% achieved complete pain relief.[51,52,54] At a minimum 2-year follow-up, a comparison of 44 patients treated with an arthroscopic procedure, 41 treated with an open procedure, and 24 treated with a percutaneous release identified no statistically significant differences; the 5.8% of patients who experienced a recurrence included three patients in the percutaneous group, one in the arthroscopic group, and two in the open group.[62] A comparison of open release and arthroscopic procedures found no statistically significant difference at 6-month follow-up; 70% of patients had a good or excellent result.[53] Patients who underwent an arthroscopic procedure returned to work earlier and required less postoperative physical therapy.

The most common reason surgery is unsuccessful and the patient continues to have pain is the surgeon's failure to adequately remove the pathologic tendinosis tissue. This situation is common in an extensor release procedure, which is intended to weaken the force generator rather than resect pathologic tissue. Revision surgery, in which residual ECRB tendinosis tissue was resected, had an 83% success rate in 35 patients.[63] Other complications reflecting inadequate technique include excessive débridement with harm to the collateral ligament, which compromised stability; neuroma of a cutaneous radial branch as it crosses 1.5 cm anterior to the lateral epicondyle; reactive bone formation; and lateral epicondylar pain associated with epicondyle excision.[33]

Medial Elbow Tendinosis

Medial tendinosis (golfer's elbow) is caused by overuse-induced trauma to the wrist flexor-pronator muscle group. Pain and tenderness are centered about the common flexor origin at the medial epicondyle, which serves as the attachment point for the wrist flexor-pronator muscle groups and the ulnar collateral ligament. The primary tendons involved in the pathology are the flexor carpi radialis, the pronator teres, and, to a lesser extent, the flexor carpi ulnaris (in 5% of patients).[33,35] These three tendons have a confluent attachment site. The histologic changes are the same as in lateral tendinosis. The incidence of medial elbow tendinosis is approximately one fifth that of lateral tendinosis. Young and middle-aged athletes are affected, and the condition has a peak incidence during the fourth and fifth decades of life.

Evaluation

Pain in medial elbow tendinosis can be reproduced with resisted wrist flexion and pronation, in which the elbow is extended while the wrist is extended and supinated. Palpable tenderness is present at and slightly distal to the epicondyle. Full range of motion is typical, but a slight loss of extension can occur. As with lateral elbow tendinosis, the medial elbow injury occurs as a result of failure of the tendon to adapt to overuse activity. Associated conditions include ulnar collateral ligament injury with valgus instability, which should be suspected in an overhead throwing athlete, and cubital tunnel syndrome. Ulnar nerve involvement, most notably in zone 3 of the medial epicondylar groove, is found in as many as 40% of patients and should be carefully evaluated.[33,35] The mechanics of overuse include repetitive wrist flexion and forearm pronation, as are common in racquet and throwing sports and in golf, in which the trailing arm is affected. Pronator syndrome and anterior interosseous nerve compression syndrome are uncommon but are included in the differential diagnosis. An adolescent athlete with medial elbow pain should be evaluated for Little Leaguer's elbow (medial apophysitis and lateral radial capitellar compression). The radiographs typically are normal but may reveal intra-articular issues, such as osteophytic spurs, in a high-demand athlete. MRI usually is unnecessary but may be helpful if an ulnar collateral ligament abnormality is suspected.[30,33,35]

Nonsurgical Treatment

The management of medial elbow tendinosis begins with nonsurgical treatment similar to that of lateral tendinosis, which has reported success rates of 88% to 96%.[64] In a level I comparison study, pain control was significantly improved at 6-week follow-up in patients treated with steroid injection rather than saline, but there was no difference at 3 months or 1 year.[65] Ultrasound-guided autologous blood injection led to improvement in scores on the visual analog and modified Nirschl scales at 4-week and 10-month follow-up.[66]

Surgical Treatment

A patient whose condition does not respond to high-quality nonsurgical management within 6 months can be considered for surgery. Surgical intervention through a miniopen approach is used to excise the degenerative tissue and reapproximate the normal healthy tissue (**Figure 7**). The skin incision is 4 cm long and parallels the medial epicondylar groove just posterior to the medial epicondyle, extending from 1 cm proximal to 3 cm

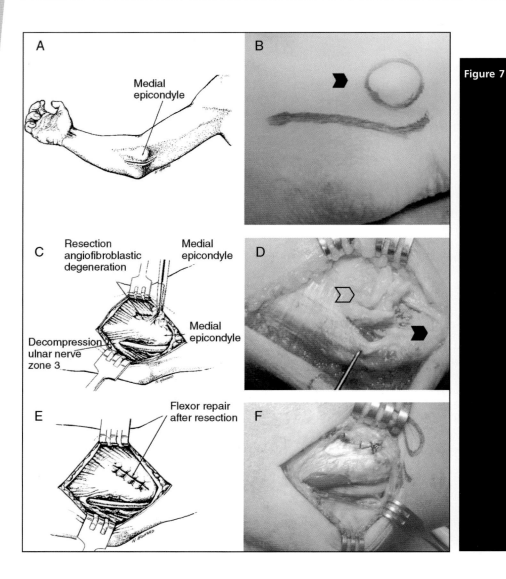

Figure 7 Matched schematic drawings and photographs showing the miniopen Nirschl technique for treating medial tennis elbow. **A** and **B,** The incision is made from the tip of the medial epicondyle distally for 3 to 4 cm, with care to avoid harming the sensory cutaneous nerve (medial antebrachial nerve) just anterior to the medial epicondyle. **C** and **D,** Resection of the angiofibroblastic tendinosis. The angiofibroblastic changes usually are located in the origin of the pronator teres and the flexor carpi radialis. The pathologic tissue is removed in a longitudinal and elliptical fashion, leaving normal tissue attachments intact. Ulnar nerve dysfunction is clinically detected in 60% of patients, and the ulnar nerve in zone 3 is decompressed. **E** and **F,** Repair of the common flexor origin. The medial epicondylar attachments of normal tissue are not disturbed. Black arrowheads = medial epicondyle, clear arrowheads = tendinosis tissue. (Reproduced with permission from Nirschl RP, Ashman ES: Tennis elbow tendinosis (epicondylitis). *Clin Sports Med* 2003;22[4]:813–836.)

distal. This incision avoids branches of the medial antebrachial cutaneous nerve. The dissection is carried through the subcutaneous tissue to the deep fascia covering the ulnar head of the flexor carpi ulnaris, and then progresses anterolaterally, with retraction of subcutaneous tissue and skin over the medial epicondyle to expose the common flexor origin. Pathologic changes often are intratendinous, and most of the tendinosis may not be visible at this time. However, some tendinosis and softening almost always is detectable at the superficial layer. The most common pathologic areas are at the interface of the pronator teres and the flexor carpi radialis extending 2 to 3 cm distally from the tip of the epicondyle. It is important to understand the patient's primary area of palpable tenderness before anesthesia is administered because this information is useful for identifying the probable location of the tendinosis. A longitudinal split is made in the tendon at its origin and extending 2 to 3 cm distally, in line with the fibers. The tendon is separated, and the hidden pathologic tissue can be observed. This tissue is elliptically excised, and the scratch test is performed to evaluate the surrounding tissue. All normal tissue is left intact. The common flexor origin is a key medial elbow stabilizer, and total release of a normal common flexor tendon is to be avoided. To enhance the potential for neovascularization, a drill bit no larger than 5/64 inch is use to drill one hole though the cortical bone distal to the epicondyle. Drilling into the epicondyle itself may lead to increased postoperative pain and is to be avoided.[30]

Forty percent of patients have concomitant cubital tunnel syndrome, for which decompression of zone 3 of the medial epicondylar groove is undertaken. Zone 3 is distal to the epicondyle, and compression neurapraxia is most common in this zone (**Figure 8**). Nerve compression rarely occurs in zone 1 (proximal to the epicondyle) or zone 2 (at the epicondyle). Release of the cubital tunnel retinaculum and the flexor carpi ulnaris arcade is essential for adequately decompressing zone 3. After decompression, elbow flexion and exten-

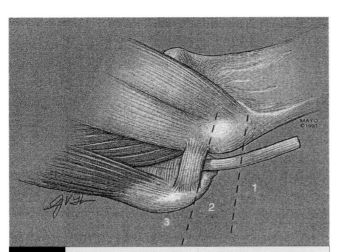

Figure 8 Schematic drawing showing the cubital tunnel zones of the ulnar nerve. Zone 1 is proximal to the epicondyle, zone 2 is at the medial epicondyle, and zone 3 is distal to the medial epicondyle (cubital tunnel retinaculum). Most ulnar nerve compression associated with medial elbow tendinosis occurs as compression of the cubital tunnel retinaculum in zone 3. (Reproduced with permission from Nirschl RP: Lateral and medial epicondylitis, in Morrey BF, ed: *Master Techniques in Orthopaedic Surgery: The Elbow.* New York, NY, Raven, 1994, pp 129-148.)

sion are performed to ensure the nerve does not dislocate from the groove and is not under tension. If this uncommon instability is present or if nerve dysfunction is secondary to tension, full anterior ulnar nerve transfer can be considered.[33] The elliptical resection tendon defect is closed with a side-to-side suture repair while the knots are buried. This closure tends to enhance the decompression of the ulnar nerve at zone 3. A subcutaneous closure is performed, and a sterile dressing is applied.

A medial epicondylectomy and a complete common flexor origin release are alternatives that may be considered but are not recommended for treating most patients.

Reports on the outcomes of medial elbow tendinosis surgery are limited. One study found involvement of the ulnar nerve in 23% of the patients and concomitant lateral epicondylitis in 20%. Objective function scores improved from 38% to 98% after surgery. In 86% of the patients, use of the elbow was not limited during daily activities or sports activities.[67] A 90% improvement also has been reported.[33] At 7-year follow-up, 87% of the patients had a good or excellent result after débridement of the common flexor origin and decompression of the ulnar nerve (53% involvement); before surgery, 62% of these patients had a predisposition to overuse syndromes, as indicated by a concomitant musculotendinous dysfunction or a history of such dysfunc-

tion.[64] These findings emphasize the importance of evaluating and treating the entire patient and, specifically, the entire upper extremity.

Postoperative Management

Lateral, medial, and posterior elbow tendinosis require similar postoperative management. The arm is immobilized in 90° of flexion and neutral rotation for 48 hours, and active motion exercises are started after this time. The elbow immobilizer is used as needed during the next 3 to 5 days, with activities of daily living initiated at 3 to 4 days. Active range of motion without resistance is begun within 3 to 4 days, as are neck and shoulder exercises. At 3 weeks, resistance exercise is started with 1-lb weights. A counterforce brace is used during the next 2 months and later at the patient's discretion. A gradual return to high-demand activities begins 6 to 8 weeks after surgery. A full return to unrestricted activities usually is possible by 4 to 6 months. **Table 4** presents the three phases of rehabilitation after elbow tendinosis surgery.

Combined Medial and Lateral Elbow Tendinosis

The signs and symptoms of elbow tendinosis often simultaneously include those of both medial and lateral tendinosis. This condition is most commonly diagnosed in recreational golfers and tennis players and is known as country club elbow. After unsuccessful nonsurgical treatment of this condition, 53 elbows were surgically treated and followed for an average of 11.7 years (minimum, 5 years).[68] The average score on the Nirschl Tennis Elbow Scale, the Numeric Pain Intensity Scale, and the American Shoulder and Elbow Surgeons scale improved significantly, and 96% of the patients had returned to sports. No patients required revision surgery, and one postoperative infection had resolved at 1 month.

Summary

As the understanding of acute and chronic elbow tendon injuries becomes more complete, treatments are evolving to provide definitively satisfactory results with little morbidity. The development of miniopen surgical techniques is an example of this progress. The successful nonsurgical treatment of tendinosis begins with a correct diagnosis, an understanding of the injury, and a revitalization of the tissue through appropriate rehabilitation. Successful surgical intervention focuses on identification of the pathologic tissue and appropriate resection. Further studies on PRP and sclerosing polidocanol as well as basic science research may lead to treatment at a cellular level and provide improved outcomes for patients with tendinopathy.

Table 4

Physical Therapy Program for Medial and Lateral Elbow Tendinosis

Stage 1

Elbow position: Flexed to 90° and supported on the patient's lower extremities

Frequency: Once daily

Exercises: Isotonic wrist flexion, extension, and pronation-supination

Progression: Repetitions and resistance are increased as tolerated without an increase in symptoms until 30 repetitions with a 3-lb weight can be performed on two consecutive days without an increase in symptoms.

Stage 2

Elbow position: More extended position with less support from the lower extremities

Frequency: Once daily

Exercises: Isotonic wrist flexion, extension, and pronation-supination. Resistance is decreased from 3 lb to 2 lb or 1 lb, depending on patient tolerance.

Progression: Repetitions and resistance are increased as tolerated without an increase in symptoms until 30 repetitions with a 3-lb weight can be performed on two consecutive days without an increase in symptoms.

Stage 3

Elbow position: Fully extended and unsupported

Frequency: Once daily

Exercises: Wrist flexion, extension, and pronation-supination. Resistance is decreased from 3 lb to 2 lb or 1 lb, depending on patient tolerance.

Progression: Repetitions and resistance are increased as tolerated without an increase in symptoms until 30 repetitions with a 3-lb weight can be performed on two consecutive days without an increase in symptoms. At this point, the frequency can be decreased to three or four times per week.

Additional Exercise

Finger abduction (splaying) against the resistance of a rubber band and squeezing of an egg, putty, or a stress ball frequently throughout the day to tolerance. Submaximal squeezes are recommended at first, with progressive intensity as the patient advances.

Modification

If the patient has pain during or after exercise persisting longer than 24 hours, the weight, the number of repetitions, or the range of motion is decreased.

(Adapted with permission from Johnson B, Nirschl RP: Overuse injuries of the elbow. *Orthop Phys Ther Clin N Am* 2001;10[4]:617-634.)

Annotated References

1. Kulshreshtha R, Singh R, Sinha J, Hall S: Anatomy of the distal biceps brachii tendon and its clinical relevance. *Clin Orthop Relat Res* 2007;456:117-120.

   An anatomic cadaver study analyzed the complex fiber arrangement of the distal biceps.

2. Miyamoto RG, Elser F, Millett PJ: Distal biceps tendon injuries. *J Bone Joint Surg Am* 2010;92(11):2128-2138.

   This is a current concepts review of distal biceps tendon injuries.

3. O'Driscoll SW, Goncalves LB, Dietz P: The hook test for distal biceps tendon avulsion. *Am J Sports Med* 2007;35(11):1865-1869.

   A cohort study evaluated the hook test for complete distal biceps injuries, finding that it is more sensitive and specific than MRI. Level of evidence: II.

4. Ruland RT, Dunbar RP, Bowen JD: The biceps squeeze test for diagnosis of distal biceps tendon ruptures. *Clin Orthop Relat Res* 2005;437:128-131.

5. Ramsey ML: Distal biceps tendon injuries: Diagnosis and management. *J Am Acad Orthop Surg* 1999;7(3):199-207.

6. Giuffrè BM, Moss MJ: Optimal positioning for MRI of the distal biceps brachii tendon: Flexed abducted supinated view. *AJR Am J Roentgenol* 2004;182(4):944-946.

7. Hang DW, Bach BR Jr, Bojchuk J: Repair of chronic distal biceps brachii tendon rupture using free autogenous semitendinosus tendon. *Clin Orthop Relat Res* 1996;323:188-191.

8. Bain GI, Johnson LJ, Turner PC: Treatment of partial distal biceps tendon tears. *Sports Med Arthrosc* 2008;16(3):154-161.

7: Elbow Trauma, Fracture, and Reconstruction

Partial tears of the biceps were described and defined, with treatment options.

9. Morrey BF, ed: *Master Techniques in Orthopaedic Surgery: The Elbow.* New York, NY, Raven, 1994, pp 115-128.

10. D'Alessandro DF, Shields CL Jr, Tibone JE, Chandler RW: Repair of distal biceps tendon ruptures in athletes. *Am J Sports Med* 1993;21(1):114-119.

11. Baker BE, Bierwagen D: Rupture of the distal tendon of the biceps brachii: Operative versus non-operative treatment. *J Bone Joint Surg Am* 1985;67(3):414-417.

12. Davison BL, Engber WD, Tigert LJ: Long term evaluation of repaired distal biceps brachii tendon ruptures. *Clin Orthop Relat Res* 1996;333:186-191.

13. Chavan PR, Duquin TR, Bisson LJ: Repair of the ruptured distal biceps tendon: A systematic review. *Am J Sports Med* 2008;36(8):1618-1624.

   A systematic review evaluated the outcomes of single- and two-incision distal biceps injury treatment. EndoButton fixation performed best in biomechanical studies. The eight studies reported comparable complication rates. Each technique had specific complications. Level of evidence: IV.

14. Bain GI, Prem H, Heptinstall RJ, Verhellen R, Paix D: Repair of distal biceps tendon rupture: A new technique using the Endobutton. *J Shoulder Elbow Surg* 2000;9(2):120-126.

15. Greenberg JA, Fernandez JJ, Wang T, Turner C: EndoButton-assisted repair of distal biceps tendon ruptures. *J Shoulder Elbow Surg* 2003;12(5):484-490.

16. Peeters T, Ching-Soon NG, Jansen N, Sneyers C, Declercq G, Verstreken F: Functional outcome after repair of distal biceps tendon ruptures using the endobutton technique. *J Shoulder Elbow Surg* 2009;18(2):283-287.

   A retrospective clinical study found that EndoButton fixation of distal biceps repairs is safe and efficacious, with 80% flexion and 91% supination strength regained. Level of evidence: IV.

17. Berlet GC, Johnson JA, Milne AD, Patterson SD, King GJ: Distal biceps brachii tendon repair: An in vitro biomechanical study of tendon reattachment. *Am J Sports Med* 1998;26(3):428-432.

18. Pereira DS, Kvitne RS, Liang M, Giacobetti FB, Ebramzadeh E: Surgical repair of distal biceps tendon ruptures: A biomechanical comparison of two techniques. *Am J Sports Med* 2002;30(3):432-436.

19. Idler CS, Montgomery WH III, Lindsey DP, Badua PA, Wynne GF, Yerby SA: Distal biceps tendon repair: A biomechanical comparison of intact tendon and 2 repair techniques. *Am J Sports Med* 2006;34(6):968-974.

20. Kettler M, Lunger J, Kuhn V, Mutschler W, Tingart MJ: Failure strengths in distal biceps tendon repair. *Am J Sports Med* 2007;35(9):1544-1548.

   A controlled laboratory study compared 13 fixation options for the distal biceps and found that the EndoButton had a substantially higher load to failure.

21. Mazzocca AD, Burton KJ, Romeo AA, Santangelo S, Adams DA, Arciero RA: Biomechanical evaluation of 4 techniques of distal biceps brachii tendon repair. *Am J Sports Med* 2007;35(2):252-258.

   A controlled cadaver laboratory study compared the dual-incision bone tunnel, suture anchor repair, interference screw, and EndoButton techniques for distal biceps repair. The load to failure was substantially greater with the EndoButton technique than with the other options.

22. Heinzelmann AD, Savoie FH III, Ramsey JR, Field LD, Mazzocca AD: A combined technique for distal biceps repair using a soft tissue button and biotenodesis interference screw. *Am J Sports Med* 2009;37(5):989-994.

   A clinical study found that dual fixation of the distal biceps tendon with a soft-tissue button and biotenodesis screw may allow earlier return to function, with minimal complications. Level of evidence: IV.

23. Yeh PC, Dodds SD, Smart LR, Mazzocca AD, Sethi PM: Distal triceps rupture. *J Am Acad Orthop Surg* 2010;18(1):31-40.

   Distal triceps injuries were reviewed.

24. Mair SD, Isbell WM, Gill TJ, Schlegel TF, Hawkins RJ: Triceps tendon ruptures in professional football players. *Am J Sports Med* 2004;32(2):431-434.

25. Koplas MC, Schneider E, Sundaram M: Prevalence of triceps tendon tears on MRI of the elbow and clinical correlation. *Skeletal Radiol* 2011;40(5):587-594.

   An MRI-based retrospective study found a 3.8% prevalence of triceps tendon tearing. The most common was a partial tear from an athletic injury. Pain was the initial symptom.

26. Vidal AF, Drakos MC, Allen AA: Biceps tendon and triceps tendon injuries. *Clin Sports Med* 2004;23(4):707-722, xi.

27. Harris PC, Atkinson D, Moorehead JD: Bilateral partial rupture of triceps tendon: Case report and quantitative assessment of recovery. *Am J Sports Med* 2004;32(3):787-792.

28. Yeh PC, Stephens KT, Solovyova O, et al: The distal triceps tendon footprint and a biomechanical analysis of 3 repair techniques. *Am J Sports Med* 2010;38(5):1025-1033.

   A controlled cadaver laboratory study described the 466-mm^2 footprint anatomy of the triceps insertion on the olecranon. An anatomic footprint repair using the suture bridge technique, similar to the rotator cuff repair technique, was compared with two other techniques and found to better restore anatomy and allow less repair site motion when cyclically loaded.

29. Johnson B, Nirschl RP: Overuse injuries of the elbow. *Orthop Phys Ther Clin N Am* 2001;10(4):617-634.

30. Nirschl RP, Ashman ES: Tennis elbow tendinosis (epicondylitis). *Instr Course Lect* 2004;53:587-598.

31. Ellenbecker TS, Mattalino AJ: *The Elbow in Sport: Injury Treatment and Rehabilitation*. Champaign, IL, Human Kinetics, 1997.

32. Nirschl RP: Elbow tendinosis/tennis elbow. *Clin Sports Med* 1992;11(4):851-870.

33. Nirschl RP, Davis L: *Wrist and Elbow Reconstruction and Arthroscopy*. Rosemont, IL, American Society for Surgery of the Hand, 2006, pp 513-521.

34. Calfee RP, Patel A, DaSilva MF, Akelman E: Management of lateral epicondylitis: Current concepts. *J Am Acad Orthop Surg* 2008;16(1):19-29.

    This is a current concepts review of the management of lateral epicondylitis.

35. Nirschl RP: *Master Techniques in Orthopaedic Surgery: The Elbow*. New York, NY, Raven, 1994, pp 129-148.

36. Roles NC, Maudsley RH: Radial tunnel syndrome: Resistant tennis elbow as a nerve entrapment. *J Bone Joint Surg Br* 1972;54(3):499-508.

37. Labelle H, Guibert R; The University of Montreal Orthopaedic Research Group: Efficacy of diclofenac in lateral epicondylitis of the elbow also treated with immobilization. *Arch Fam Med* 1997;6(3):257-262.

38. Hay EM, Paterson SM, Lewis M, Hosie G, Croft P: Pragmatic randomised controlled trial of local corticosteroid injection and naproxen for treatment of lateral epicondylitis of elbow in primary care. *BMJ* 1999; 319(7215):964-968.

39. Smidt N, van der Windt DA, Assendelft WJ, Devillé WL, Korthals-de Bos IB, Bouter LM: Corticosteroid injections, physiotherapy, or a wait-and-see policy for lateral epicondylitis: A randomised controlled trial. *Lancet* 2002;359(9307):657-662.

40. Wong SM, Hui AC, Tong PY, Poon DW, Yu E, Wong LK: Treatment of lateral epicondylitis with botulinum toxin: A randomized, double-blind, placebo-controlled trial. *Ann Intern Med* 2005;143(11):793-797.

41. Peerbooms JC, Sluimer J, Bruijn DJ, Gosens T: Positive effect of an autologous platelet concentrate in lateral epicondylitis in a double-blind randomized controlled trial: Platelet-rich plasma versus corticosteroid injection with a 1-year follow-up. *Am J Sports Med* 2010; 38(2):255-262.

    Both corticosteroid injection and PRP use led to lateral epicondylitis improvement. Improvement was progressive in patients treated with PRP but declined over time in those treated with corticosteroid. Level of evidence: I.

42. Gosens T, Peerbooms JC, van Laar W, den Oudsten BL: Ongoing positive effect of platelet-rich plasma versus corticosteroid injection in lateral epicondylitis: A double-blind randomized controlled trial with 2-year follow-up. *Am J Sports Med* 2011;39(6):1200-1208.

    At 2-year follow-up, patients treated with PRP had greater improvement than those treated with corticosteroid. Level of evidence: I.

43. Thanasas C, Papadimitriou G, Charalambidis C, Paraskevopoulos I, Papanikolaou A: Platelet-rich plasma versus autologous whole blood for the treatment of chronic lateral elbow epicondylitis: A randomized controlled clinical trial. *Am J Sports Med* 2011; 39(10):2130-2134.

    A comparison of PRP and autologous whole blood treatments of chronic lateral epicondylitis found PRP to be effective and superior to whole blood at 6-week follow-up. Level of evidence: I.

44. Buchbinder R, Green SE, Youd JM, Assendelft WJ, Barnsley L, Smidt N: Shock wave therapy for lateral elbow pain. *Cochrane Database Syst Rev* 2005;4(4): CD003524.

45. Lin CL, Lee JS, Su WR, Kuo LC, Tai TW, Jou IM: Clinical and ultrasonographic results of ultrasonographically guided percutaneous radiofrequency lesioning in the treatment of recalcitrant lateral epicondylitis. *Am J Sports Med* 2011;39(11):2429-2435.

    An evaluation of a new, minimally invasive procedure for recalcitrant lateral epicondylitis found improvement of 78% at an average 14.3-month follow-up, with no major complications. Level of evidence: IV.

46. Bokhari AR, Murrell GA: The role of nitric oxide in tendon healing. *J Shoulder Elbow Surg* 2012;21(2): 238-244.

    The basic science of nitric oxide use is reviewed for various tendinopathies.

47. Haahr JP, Andersen JH: Prognostic factors in lateral epicondylitis: A randomized trial with one-year follow-up in 266 new cases treated with minimal occupational intervention or the usual approach in general practice. *Rheumatology (Oxford)* 2003;42(10):1216-1225.

48. Binder AI, Hazleman BL: Lateral humeral epicondylitis—a study of natural history and the effect of conservative therapy. *Br J Rheumatol* 1983;22(2):73-76.

49. Nirschl RP, Pettrone FA: Tennis elbow: The surgical treatment of lateral epicondylitis. *J Bone Joint Surg Am* 1979;61(6):832-839.

50. Kuklo TR, Taylor KF, Murphy KP, Islinger RB, Heekin RD, Baker CL Jr: Arthroscopic release for lateral epicondylitis: A cadaveric model. *Arthroscopy* 1999;15(3):259-264.

51. Owens BD, Murphy KP, Kuklo TR: Arthroscopic release for lateral epicondylitis. *Arthroscopy* 2001;17(6):582-587.

52. Mullett H, Sprague M, Brown G, Hausman M: Arthroscopic treatment of lateral epicondylitis: Clinical and cadaveric studies. *Clin Orthop Relat Res* 2005;439:123-128.

53. Peart RE, Strickler SS, Schweitzer KM Jr: Lateral epicondylitis: A comparative study of open and arthroscopic lateral release. *Am J Orthop (Belle Mead NJ)* 2004;33(11):565-567.

54. Baker CL Jr , Baker CL III: Long-term follow-up of arthroscopic treatment of lateral epicondylitis. *Am J Sports Med* 2008;36(2):254-260.

    After 42 elbow arthroscopies for lateral epicondylitis, 77% of patients had improvement, and the satisfaction rating was 87%. Level of evidence: IV.

55. Baker CL Jr, Murphy KP, Gottlob CA, Curd DT: Arthroscopic classification and treatment of lateral epicondylitis: Two-year clinical results. *J Shoulder Elbow Surg* 2000;9(6):475-482.

56. Cummins CA: Lateral epicondylitis: In vivo assessment of arthroscopic debridement and correlation with patient outcomes. *Am J Sports Med* 2006;34(9):1486-1491.

57. Baker CL Jr, Baker CL III: Arthroscopy remains a viable, reliable method for treating lateral epicondylitis. *Orthopedics Today* February 2012. http://www.helio.com/orthopedics/arthroscopy/news/print/orthopedics-today. Accessed October 1, 2012.

    Enhancements to the arthroscopic technique for lateral epicondylitis were described.

58. Dunn JH, Kim JJ, Davis L, Nirschl RP: Ten- to 14-year follow-up of the Nirschl surgical technique for lateral epicondylitis. *Am J Sports Med* 2008;36(2):261-266.

    A clinical study with long-term follow-up found an overall improvement rate of 97% and patient satisfaction of 8.9 out of 10 when the Nirschl technique for lateral epicondylitis was used; 93% of the patients returned to their sport. Level of evidence: IV.

59. Rosenberg N, Henderson I: Surgical treatment of resistant lateral epicondylitis: Follow-up study of 19 patients after excision, release and repair of proximal common extensor tendon origin. *Arch Orthop Trauma Surg* 2002;122(9-10):514-517.

60. Verhaar J, Walenkamp G, Kester A, van Mameren H, van der Linden T: Lateral extensor release for tennis elbow: A prospective long-term follow-up study. *J Bone Joint Surg Am* 1993;75(7):1034-1043.

61. Dunkow PD, Jatti M, Muddu BN: A comparison of open and percutaneous techniques in the surgical treatment of tennis elbow. *J Bone Joint Surg Br* 2004;86(5):701-704.

62. Szabo SJ, Savoie FH III, Field LD, Ramsey JR, Hosemann CD: Tendinosis of the extensor carpi radialis brevis: An evaluation of three methods of operative treatment. *J Shoulder Elbow Surg* 2006;15(6):721-727.

63. Organ SW, Nirschl RP, Kraushaar BS, Guidi EJ: Salvage surgery for lateral tennis elbow. *Am J Sports Med* 1997;25(6):746-750.

64. Gabel GT, Morrey BF: Operative treatment of medical epicondylitis: Influence of concomitant ulnar neuropathy at the elbow. *J Bone Joint Surg Am* 1995;77(7):1065-1069.

65. Stahl S, Kaufman T: The efficacy of an injection of steroids for medial epicondylitis: A prospective study of sixty elbows. *J Bone Joint Surg Am* 1997;79(11):1648-1652.

66. Suresh SP, Ali KE, Jones H, Connell DA: Medial epicondylitis: Is ultrasound guided autologous blood injection an effective treatment? *Br J Sports Med* 2006;40(11):935-939, discussion 939.

67. Vangsness CT Jr, Jobe FW: Surgical treatment of medial epicondylitis: Results in 35 elbows. *J Bone Joint Surg Br* 1991;73(3):409-411.

68. Schipper ON, Dunn JH, Ochiai DH, Donovan JS, Nirschl RP: Nirschl surgical technique for concomitant lateral and medial elbow tendinosis: A retrospective review of 53 elbows with a mean follow-up of 11.7 years. *Am J Sports Med* 2011;39(5):972-976.

    At long-term follow-up, a combined surgical procedure for concurrent lateral and medial epicondylitis was found to improve surgical outcome scores, with 85% good to excellent results and 96% of the patients returning to their sport. Level of evidence: IV.

7: Elbow Trauma, Fracture, and Reconstruction

Chapter 40

Elbow Injuries and the Throwing Athlete

James Hammond, DO, ATC   Brian J. Cole, MD, MBA

Introduction

Overhead throwing imparts substantial stress to the elbow and can cause unique injuries. Biomechanical and clinical studies have elucidated the causative factors in these injuries and have allowed prevention and treatment strategies to evolve. The diagnosis of an elbow condition is facilitated by specific examination maneuvers, and radiography is useful for confirming the diagnosis. Prevention strategies, such as the monitoring of pitch counts, have been developed to decrease the risk of injury in young athletes. Evolving surgical strategies have contributed to changes in techniques for treating certain conditions in the throwing athlete.

Throwing-Related Elbow Anatomy and Biomechanics

The medial or ulnar collateral ligament (UCL) is the most clinically relevant anatomic structure in the elbow of the throwing athlete. The UCL is a complex composed of the anterior oblique, posterior oblique, and transverse ligaments. The anterior oblique ligament is the strongest ligament of the complex and the most important stabilizer to valgus stress in the throwing athlete. The anterior oblique ligament originates in the medial epicondyle. A recent evaluation of the ulnar insertion of the anterior oblique ligament found that it extends distal to the sublime tubercle along a previously unnamed ridge and was present on all skeletal specimens.[1] Within the anterior oblique ligament, the anterior band and the posterior band alternately have primary responsibility for valgus stress throughout the ranges of flexion and extension; the anterior band is tight during extension, and the posterior band is tight during flexion.

The UCL receives dynamic support from the surrounding musculature. The flexor carpi ulnaris is the primary dynamic contributor to valgus stabilization of the elbow, and the flexor digitorum superficialis is a secondary stabilizer.[2] These two muscles help disseminate the substantial forces across the elbow during the throwing motion and thereby protect the UCL. Their relationship has implications for preventing and managing UCL injuries.

The throwing motion creates substantial energy and subsequent forces that are mediated by structures about the elbow. Angular velocities as high as 3,000° per second have been observed at the elbow during the acceleration phase of the throwing motion. This velocity translates into 64 N/m of valgus torque. Because the tensile strength of the UCL is only 34 N/m, the other stabilizers of the elbow also are important for avoiding or minimizing injury.[3] The valgus load creates stress about the other aspects of the elbow: tensile forces occur on the medial aspect, shear and compressive stresses occur in the olecranon fossa as the elbow reaches extension, and compression forces occur laterally, primarily at the radiocapitellar joint. A recent cadaver study found that lateral contact pressures increased 67% after the UCL was transected.[4] Understanding these forces increases the ability to understand the relationships among the conditions that occur about the elbow.

Clinical Evaluation

History

A specific, detailed patient history is vital to understanding elbow pathology in a throwing athlete. Arm dominance and the duration, intensity, and location of symptoms should be noted as well as the type of activity that elicits symptoms (for example, does the pain occur at rest, with activities of daily living, or only with throwing?). Information should be elicited as to

Dr. Cole or an immediate family member has received royalties from Arthrex and DJ Orthopaedics; is a member of a speakers' bureau or has made paid presentations on behalf of Genzyme; serves as a paid consultant to or is an employee of Zimmer, Arthrex, Carticept, Biomimmetic, Allosource, and DePuy; and has received research or institutional support from Regentis, Arthrex, Smith & Nephew, and DJ Orthopaedics. Neither Dr. Hammond nor any immediate family member has received anything of value from or has stock or stock options held in a commercial company or institution related directly or indirectly to the subject of this chapter.

associated mechanical symptoms, paresthesias, or pain in other joints, especially the shoulder. It is important to determine the point in the throwing motion during which symptoms occur (windup, early cocking, late cocking, acceleration, deceleration, or follow through). The types of pitches, the number of pitches thrown per outing, and the throwing schedule should be determined. The curveball generates the greatest valgus stress at the elbow, the fastball and slider generate the greatest force, and the changeup generates less stress on the elbow and is considered a relatively safe pitch for athletes of all ages. However, skilled players are more likely to throw the fastball or the curveball, play on more teams, and pitch more frequently than other players.[5]

Physical Examination

General observations are easy to overlook during an evaluation of the elbow, but they can provide insight into stresses about the elbow. The patient's carrying angle should be observed to identify any side-to-side difference. The exact location and the medial, lateral, or posterior character of the pain should be determined. The range of motion should be evaluated; a lack of full extension is common in throwers.

Typically, the focus of the examination in a throwing athlete is on the medial elbow. An acute avulsion injury of the UCL usually occurs proximally at the medial epicondyle, and tenderness there or along the length of the anterior oblique ligament should be determined. Resisted strength testing of the flexor-pronator mass is done. Valgus stress at 0° and 30° of flexion also is typically assessed, but the instability is often more subtle in a throwing athlete. This test lacks the sensitivity needed to reliably identify a chronic injury. The milking maneuver and the moving valgus stress test also are used to assess valgus instability and UCL injury. The milking maneuver is performed by pulling on the patient's thumb with the forearm supinated and the elbow flexed beyond 90°. The moving valgus stress test begins in the same position, and the patient's thumb is pulled until the limit of external rotation is reached at the shoulder. The elbow is taken through a range of motion while the torque created by pulling on the thumb remains constant. Pain typically is most intense when the elbow is between 70° and 120° (**Figure 1**). The sensitivity of the moving valgus stress test is reported to be 100%, with 75% specificity.[6]

A patient with suspected UCL injury should be assessed for ulnar nerve pathology. Evidence of nerve subluxation, a positive Tinel sign, or symptoms with elbow hyperflexion testing should be noted. Pain associated with a flexor-pronator injury, as indicated by pain with resistance testing, should be differentiated from pain associated with medial epicondylitis, as indicated by tenderness over only the epicondyle with normal moving valgus stress.

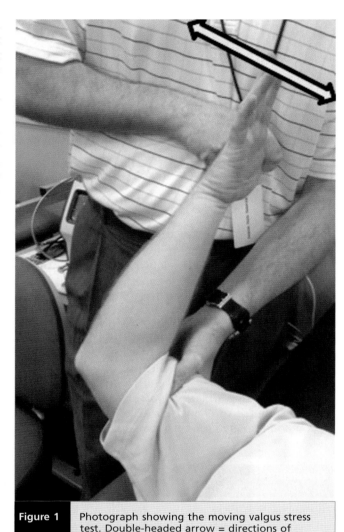

| Figure 1 | Photograph showing the moving valgus stress test. Double-headed arrow = directions of motion. |

Imaging

The initial imaging studies are plain radiographs in the AP, lateral, radiocapitellar, and axillary views. Valgus stress radiographs can be used to identify a medial joint line opening; an opening of more than 3 mm has been considered diagnostic.[7] The radiographs can be assessed for evidence of osteophytes, loss of joint space, loose bodies, or osteochondral defects. MRI can be used to confirm several diagnoses about the elbow, including osteochondritis dissecans, a UCL injury, avulsion of the flexor-pronator mass, and chronic thickening of the UCL. A recent study found that signal intensity on MRI can be used to predict rehabilitation outcomes; patients with a complete or high-grade UCL tear were most likely to require surgery[8] (**Figure 2**).

Ultrasonography and dynamic ultrasonographic examination have been described for defining UCL injury, but most available studies are small case studies or case reports. Several studies have found differences in UCL laxity among overhead throwing athletes as well as

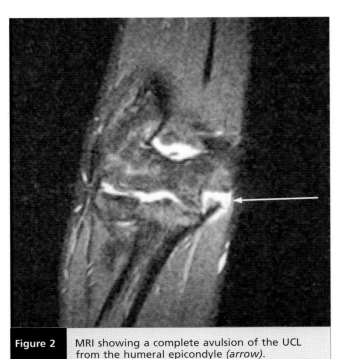

Figure 2 MRI showing a complete avulsion of the UCL from the humeral epicondyle (arrow).

side-to-side differences between the athletes' throwing and nonthrowing arms.[9,10]

Arthroscopy has been used as a diagnostic tool primarily for closely evaluating a joint line opening with stress; 1 to 2 mm of joint line opening indicate a partial-thickness tear, and 4 to 10 mm of opening indicate a full-thickness tear. The ulnohumeral joint is viewed from the anterolateral portal, and the joint is stressed at 65° to 70° of elbow flexion with the forearm pronated.[11]

Conditions Causing Medial Elbow Pain

Medial Epicondylitis

Medial epicondylitis is less common than lateral epicondylitis and usually occurs as a result of repetitive wrist flexion and forceful pronation during golf, a racquet sport, or overhead throwing. Pain typically is elicited over the medial elbow and exacerbated by resisted forearm flexion and pronation. The diagnosis is primarily clinical, but ultrasonography and MRI are reported to be useful.[12] On MRI, increased signal is seen in the flexor muscular origin about the medial epicondyle.[13] Nonsurgical treatments have high success rates. The components of a typical nonsurgical treatment program include NSAIDs, flexibility exercises, ice, and guided physical therapy. Steroid injections have also been used. The use of iontophoresis was found to improve pain relief in a comparative study.[14] Ultrasound-guided autologous blood injection led to improved scores on the visual analog and modified Nirschl Pain Phase scales.[15] Surgical intervention typically involves

resection of a portion of the diseased tendon by open, miniopen, or arthroscopic means. If the surgical goal has been accomplished, pain relief can be expected, but a strength deficit may remain.

UCL Injury

The initial management of a UCL injury in an overhead throwing athlete should be nonsurgical. The regimen includes a 6-week period of rest from throwing as well as strengthening of the flexor-pronator musculature.[2] The athlete should be asymptomatic and have a normal examination before throwing activities are resumed. At that time, the athlete should optimize throwing mechanics and offset stress from the medial elbow. Late trunk rotation, reduced shoulder external rotation, and increased elbow flexion have been shown to increase valgus stress at the elbow.[16] A 42% return-to-sport rate was reported for overhead throwing athletes at a mean 24.5-week follow-up.[17]

In the original Jobe technique for reconstructing the UCL, a figure-of-8 tendon graft was woven through bone tunnels and sutured back onto itself. This technique required takedown of the flexor-pronator mass and exposure of the posterior humeral cortex for one of the tunnels. An ulnar nerve transposition always was performed. The substantial morbidity of the exposure led to modification of this technique and development of new techniques. The modified Jobe technique consists of a muscle-splitting approach to decrease morbidity to the flexor-pronator musculature, a change in humeral tunnel direction, and ulnar nerve transposition only if the patient has preoperative symptoms. The humeral tunnel is directed somewhat anteriorly to avoid ulnar nerve injury with graft passage and decrease the dissection necessary for exposure. The outcomes and the biomechanical strength resulting from using the modified Jobe technique have become the standard for comparison with any other technique. A 93% return-to-sport rate was reported for overhead throwing athletes.[7] Another study reported an 83% return to the previous level of throwing at a minimum 2-year follow-up after a modified Jobe technique was used.[18]

The commonly described docking technique also uses a muscle-splitting approach and two converging tunnels in the ulna. Only one primary tunnel is drilled in the humerus, and two smaller holes are drilled in the humerus to facilitate suture passage. One limb of the tendon graft is passed into the tunnel in the humerus. The second limb of the tendon graft is assessed for length and tension, sectioned to the appropriate length, and docked in the humeral socket. The sutures from each limb of the tendon graft are tied over a bone bridge after final tensioning. The use of the docking technique led to a good or excellent outcome in 19 of 21 athletes (90%).[19] An excellent result was defined as a return to previous level of play for at least 1 year, and a good result was defined as a return to throwing at a lower level for at least 1 year or the ability to throw at daily batting practice. A 92% rate of return to the preinjury level of throwing was reported at an 11.5-month follow-up after a quadrupled palmaris graft was used with the docking technique.[20]

Several techniques can be categorized as hybrid. A relatively new technique uses a single drill hole at the sublime tubercle and a single drill hole in the medial epicondyle. An interference screw is used at the sublime tubercle, with a docking technique on the humeral attachment. At 3-year follow-up after this technique was used, 19 of 22 patients (86%) had an excellent result.[21] Another technique uses the same single drill holes on the sublime tubercle and the medial epicondyle, with interference screws on each end of the construct. In a biomechanical study, this technique led to stability similar to that of intact UCL specimens.[3]

Ulnar Neuritis

Approximately 40% of patients with UCL insufficiency have ulnar neuritis. A substantial valgus stress can create traction, friction, and compression on the nerve and induce neuritis. The presence of adhesions and/or osteophytes, nerve subluxation, a thickened medial triceps, or UCL injury also can increase stress on the nerve. Night pain and paresthesias into the ulnar nerve distribution can occur. Ulnar nerve symptoms can occur with throwing. On physical examination, a positive Tinel sign at the cubital tunnel, a positive elbow hyperflexion test, and/or evidence of ulnar nerve subluxation can be observed. Nonsurgical measures, including the use of night splinting, ice, NSAIDs, and activity modification, can be successful. Surgical treatment typically involves transposing the ulnar nerve into a subcutaneous position. This procedure has had great success with appropriate rehabilitation and a graduated return to throwing activities. The time to return to play with isolated ulnar nerve transposition is approximately 12 weeks.[22] If the patient has ulnar nerve symptoms associated with a UCL injury requiring reconstruction, ulnar nerve transposition should be done at the time of reconstruction.

Conditions Causing Posterior Elbow Pain

Posteromedial Impingement or Valgus Extension Overload

Valgus extension overload is a relatively common condition in overhead throwing athletes in which posterior and, commonly, medial osteophytes impinge within the olecranon fossa as the elbow reaches extension. A review of 72 professional baseball players who underwent elbow surgery found that 65% had posterior olecranon osteophytes.[23] Athletes typically report posterior pain at the elbow during ball release and as the elbow reaches extension; this is the point at which osteophytes from the olecranon impinge within the fossa. The patient also commonly has some loss of terminal extension on examination. When valgus stress on the elbow is applied at 20° to 30° of flexion and the elbow is quickly taken to extension, a positive test re-creates the pain in the posteromedial elbow. Care must be taken to determine whether there is a concomitant UCL injury because there is a significant relationship between these diagnoses. Plain radiographs can reveal the posterior osteophyte.

Nonsurgical treatment begins with rest and 10 to 14 days of throwing restrictions followed by an interval throwing program to allow a gradual return to throwing. Pitching mechanics must be corrected during the interval throwing program to minimize stress at the elbow. A longer period of rest is recommended if symptoms persist or the patient cannot return to throwing at the earlier level. Intra-articular injection is not particularly helpful in patients with posteromedial impingement and should not be repeated.

Surgical treatment should be carefully considered. The medial elbow endures substantial valgus forces in the throwing athlete, and engagement of the olecranon in its fossa provides secondary stabilization to the elbow, particularly during extension. Any subtle laxity in the UCL may transfer stress to the posteromedial olecranon and cause it to impinge on the fossa as the elbow reaches extension. This stress induces osteophyte formation, which then increases impingement by shear mass effect. Overresection of the posteromedial olecranon can unmask or exacerbate symptoms of UCL injury. Twenty-five percent of professional baseball players who underwent osteophyte excision later had valgus instability requiring UCL reconstruction.[23] Studies conflict as to the amount of olecranon that can be excised before increased strain is seen at the UCL, and there is debate as to whether any excision of normal olecranon should be done. The procedure can be done in an arthroscopic or open fashion. In an open procedure, an osteotome is used to resect a portion of the olecranon tip, and a portion of the medial olecranon is removed. The arthroscopic procedure can be accomplished using a posterolateral portal for viewing and a central posterior portal for working. Care must be taken to remove osteophytes and minimize resection of normal olecranon. In addition, care must be taken to avoid ulnar nerve injury when resecting the medial aspect of the osteophyte as the ulnar nerve enters the cubital tunnel. A recent study reported an excellent outcome in seven of nine patients who underwent arthroscopic treatment of valgus extension overload.[24]

Olecranon Stress Fracture

Stress fractures of the olecranon have been described in javelin throwers and other throwing athletes.[25,26] These fractures are primarily described as transverse or oblique, with a mechanism of injury similar to that of a valgus extension overload injury. The olecranon is subject to increased stress as the elbow undergoes a valgus load and approaches extension. The substantial triceps forces at extension also have been implicated in this condition.

On physical examination, the athlete may have tenderness over the physis (if it is open), the posterior olecranon, or the posteromedial olecranon. Symptoms may be elicited by forceful extension of the elbow or resisted triceps muscle testing. Typically, the patient has less extension than in the contralateral elbow. Plain radiographs may show a sclerotic line of remodeling fracture if the condition is chronic. If the physis is open, it may be beneficial to obtain radiographs of the contralateral side to detect any physeal widening. A bone scan will reveal increased uptake in the area. MRI will show edema within the bone and allow characterization of the fracture line. MRI also is beneficial if an associated UCL injury is suspected.

The treatment of an olecranon stress fracture is somewhat controversial. Nonsurgical measures require rest from throwing and possibly temporary splinting. The return to an interval throwing program is delayed until symptoms have subsided and there is radiographic evidence of fracture healing. As a result, throwing can be restricted for as long as 6 months. Stress fractures may respond to bone stimulators, but this treatment has not been well defined.

Some experts recommend early surgical treatment to reduce the time to resumption of throwing.[27] Surgical treatment also is recommended if nonsurgical management is unsuccessful. Tension-band wiring, tension-band wiring with a compression screw, and the use of a compression screw alone have been described. A 6.5- or 7.3-mm cannulated compression screw typically is used. A recent case report described a persistent fracture after fixation in a college pitcher, in which bone grafting ultimately was required for healing.[28]

Persistent Olecranon Physis

The persistent olecranon physis is similar to an olecranon stress fracture and may be responsible for an athlete's posterior elbow pain. The olecranon physis has two ossification centers: the posterior center is oriented transverse to the longitudinal axis of the ulna and contributes to longitudinal growth; a second center is more anterior at the olecranon tip, contributing to the joint surface but not to longitudinal growth. These two centers fuse and create a single physis that persists until approximately age 14 years in girls and age 16 years in boys. This physis can become sclerotic during the process of closing and can be as wide as 5 mm.

Posterior elbow pain typically develops during the years from adolescence through the late teens. The pain occurs at terminal extension in the follow-through phase of throwing, and it can be relieved with rest. The physical examination may be benign; motion is normal, the elbow is stable, and there is no tenderness to palpation. Plain radiographs reveal a persistent physis in the olecranon that may be wider on the involved side than on the contralateral side. There may be evidence of sclerosis about the physis that is unexpected for the patient's age. T2-weighted MRI may show edema about the physis, but this finding is not diagnostic.

Treatment starts with nonsurgical measures, including a period of relative rest and cessation of throwing activities. NSAIDs and ice may be used as needed. Nonsurgical measures appear to be successful in most patients but may require as long as 4 months. The options for surgical treatment include open reduction and internal fixation, bone grafting, and open reduction and internal fixation with bone grafting. The fixation techniques include tension-band wiring, compression screws, and a combination of screws and tension-band wiring. The available studies are largely limited to case reports and small case studies.[29,30] It appears that the highest rates of successful union were in patients who underwent bone grafting with or without fixation. Those undergoing fixation alone had an approximately 66% failure rate. A recent study found that those with a persistent olecranon physis and evidence of sclerosis had a 100% failure rate with nonsurgical measures.[31]

Conditions Causing Lateral Elbow Pain

Capitellar Osteochondritis Dissecans

Osteochondritis dissecans (OCD) is a local disorder of the subchondral bone that results in separation and fragmentation of articular cartilage and its underlying bone. It is important to differentiate this condition from Panner disease, which occurs in younger patients, is idiopathic, usually is self-limiting, and improves without surgical intervention. OCD typically occurs at the elbow in adolescents who are high-demand, repetitive overhead throwing athletes. The pathogenesis is not completely understood. Genetic factors, blood supply, repetitive trauma, and a vulnerable epiphysis have been implicated. The underlying bone undergoes degradation and can destabilize the overlying cartilage. Probably a combination of factors contributes to the process by which the lesion is created.

Typically, the athlete has elbow pain during activity. The pain is insidious in onset, is relieved by rest, and progresses if the activity is continued. The pain is difficult to localize and often is accompanied by loss of motion. Occasionally, the symptoms are mechanical, with catching or locking of the elbow joint. The most common finding on examination is tenderness over the radiocapitellar joint. Crepitus can be elicited in the lateral joint with pronation and supination, and there is loss of motion of 15° to 30°. In the active radiocapitellar compression test, the elbow is fully extended while the patient actively pronates and supinates the forearm and contracts the muscles about the elbow. A positive test reproduces the athlete's symptoms.

The initial imaging is with plain radiographs. The standard AP view in full extension and lateral views in 90° of flexion show typical capitellar radiolucency and flattening of the joint surface (**Figure 3**). The lesion commonly occurs in the anterolateral aspect of the capitellum. In the Minami classification system, a grade I lesion is a translucent cystic shadow in the mid-

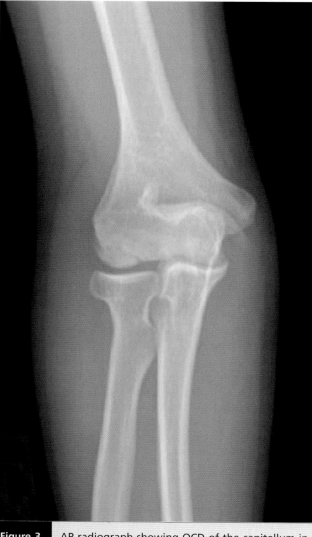

Figure 3 AP radiograph showing OCD of the capitellum in which there is a complete fragment with subtle displacement. Such a lesion often has a relatively normal arthroscopic appearance because the articular cartilage is intact.

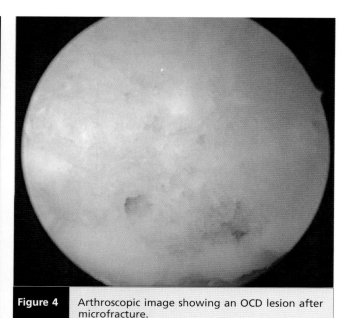

Figure 4 Arthroscopic image showing an OCD lesion after microfracture.

dle or lateral capitellum, a grade II lesion has a split line or clear zone between the lesion and its subchondral bone, and loose bodies are present in a grade III lesion.[32]

MRI has become the modality of choice for evaluating these lesions. Early changes not found on plain radiographs can be detected on MRI, and the size, location, and stability of the lesion can be assessed. The key to making a treatment decision is to determine whether the articular surface is intact and the lesion is stable as seen on MRI. A peripheral ring of fluid or fluid under the articular surface suggests an unstable lesion; these findings are similar to those of an OCD lesion in another area of the body. The diagnosis sometimes is facilitated by the addition of arthrographically or intravenously administered gadolinium.

OCD lesions are amenable to healing, and nonsurgical regimens are an option. The treatment begins with 6 months of elbow rest without throwing activity. Anti-inflammatory medications are used, and physical therapy is implemented to optimize motion and strength. Radiographs are assessed at 6-week intervals to ensure that the lesion is healing or is not progressing. MRI is repeated as needed at an approximately 3-month interval and compared with the initial studies. An interval throwing program is initiated at 6 months if the athlete has good motion, is asymptomatic, and has evidence of healing. Pitch counts initially should be monitored.[33] Patients with capitellar lucency or flattening have healing rates of 88% to 91%.[34,35] Those with open capitellar physes have a higher rate of healing. Advanced lesions have less capacity for nonsurgical healing. A stable lesion is characterized by an open capitellar growth plate, localized flattening or radiolucency of the subchondral bone, and good elbow motion. In an unstable lesion, the physis is closed, with radiographic fragmentation and loss of elbow motion of more than 20°.[36]

Surgical management is indicated if the patient has an unstable lesion or loose bodies or if nonsurgical treatment has been unsuccessful. Several surgical procedures have been described. Simple débridement can be effective for a contained lesion involving less than 50% of the capitellar surface. Microfracture or trephination of the subchondral base with a Kirschner wire also can be used after fragment excision and bed preparation (**Figure 4**). Fixation of a relatively large, unfragmented lesion can be achieved through different methods. Pull-out wires, bone grafting, and Herbert screws have been successfully used. Several options exist for cartilage replacement, mirroring the options used in the knee and other joints. Mosaicplasty, osteochondral allograft, and autograft transplantation have been used to treat a relatively large OCD lesion or an uncontained lesion (in which there is loss of lateral column support).

Radiocapitellar Plica

Radiocapitellar plica, first described as a cause of a snapping elbow, essentially is a hypertrophic synovial plica that snaps over the edge of the radial head as the elbow moves from flexion to extension. The differential diagnosis includes intra-articular loose bodies, instability, lateral epicondylitis, and subluxation of the medial triceps over the medial epicondyle. Some of these conditions can be ruled out on the basis of location. The elbow examination typically is otherwise benign, with stability, full motion, and normal strength. The patient may have tenderness posterior to the lateral epicondyle and centered over the joint. Plain radiographs usually are not informative, and the plica frequently is missed on MRI.

Nonsurgical measures should be initially considered, including relative rest, NSAIDs, and gentle motion. Intra-articular steroid injections have been used in an attempt to relieve inflammation and decrease pain. Surgical treatment with an arthroscopic procedure has yielded good results. The snapping of the plica typically can be replicated on arthroscopic examination and allows the surgeon to locate the area to be released. The goal is to adequately release the synovial plica so that it no longer snaps over the radial head. The examination is repeated to ensure the release is complete. Postoperative management allows early range of motion and advancement of strength. An interval throwing program typically is started at 8 weeks and can advance as long as the patient remains asymptomatic.

Summary

The elbow of a throwing athlete endures substantial stress during the phases of the throwing motion. The key to the correct diagnosis is to analyze the condition by elbow region, obtain a detailed history, apply specific examination maneuvers, and obtain appropriate imaging studies. Nonsurgical measures can be successful during specific phases of the disease process, and advances in surgical techniques have improved patient outcomes. Arthroscopic procedures have an increasing role in treating many conditions, with acceptable outcomes and return-to-play rates. Postoperative management is stepwise and specific to restore optimal mechanics, flexibility, and strength to the affected muscle groups.

Annotated References

1. Farrow LD, Mahoney AJ, Stefancin JJ, Taljanovic MS, Sheppard JE, Schickendantz MS: Quantitative analysis of the medial ulnar collateral ligament ulnar footprint and its relationship to the ulnar sublime tubercle. *Am J Sports Med* 2011;39(9):1936-1941.

   The anterior band of the UCL was evaluated in 10 fresh-frozen cadaver specimens. The mean length was 53.0 mm, and the mean length of the footprint on the ulna was 29.2 mm. The ridge was present in all specimens and had a mean measurement of 24.5 mm.

2. Park MC, Ahmad CS: Dynamic contributions of the flexor-pronator mass to elbow valgus stability. *J Bone Joint Surg Am* 2004;86-A(10):2268-2274.

3. Ahmad CS, Lee TQ, ElAttrache NS: Biomechanical evaluation of a new ulnar collateral ligament reconstruction technique with interference screw fixation. *Am J Sports Med* 2003;31(3):332-337.

4. Duggan JP Jr, Osadebe UC, Alexander JW, Noble PC, Lintner DM: The impact of ulnar collateral ligament tear and reconstruction on contact pressures in the lateral compartment of the elbow. *J Shoulder Elbow Surg* 2011;20(2):226-233.

   Six cadaver specimens were tested under a valgus load of 1.75 N/m and 5.25 N/m torque to simulate late cocking and the release phase. The average valgus laxity was doubled after UCL transection and restored after reconstruction.

5. Fleisig GS, Kingsley DS, Loftice JW, et al: Kinetic comparison among the fastball, curveball, change-up, and slider in collegiate baseball pitchers. *Am J Sports Med* 2006;34(3):423-430.

6. O'Driscoll SW, Lawton RL, Smith AM: The "moving valgus stress test" for medial collateral ligament tears of the elbow. *Am J Sports Med* 2005;33(2):231-239.

7. Thompson WH, Jobe FW, Yocum LA, Pink MM: Ulnar collateral ligament reconstruction in athletes: Muscle-splitting approach without transposition of the ulnar nerve. *J Shoulder Elbow Surg* 2001;10(2):152-157.

8. Kim NR, Moon SG, Ko SM, Moon WJ, Choi JW, Park JY: MR imaging of ulnar collateral ligament injury in baseball players: Value for predicting rehabilitation outcome. *Eur J Radiol* 2011;80(3):e422-e426.

   Thirty-nine baseball players with clinical evidence of UCL injury were evaluated with MRI. After nonsurgical treatment, 27 required surgery. The patients who responded to nonsurgical treatment had a less severe injury on MRI, and those with a higher-grade injury required surgery.

9. Nazarian LN, McShane JM, Ciccotti MG, O'Kane PL, Harwood MI: Dynamic US of the anterior band of the ulnar collateral ligament of the elbow in asymptomatic major league baseball pitchers. *Radiology* 2003;227(1):149-154.

10. Sasaki J, Takahara M, Ogino T, Kashiwa H, Ishigaki D, Kanauchi Y: Ultrasonographic assessment of the ulnar collateral ligament and medial elbow laxity in college baseball players. *J Bone Joint Surg Am* 2002;

84-A(4):525-531.

11. Field LD, Altchek DW: Evaluation of the arthroscopic valgus instability test of the elbow. *Am J Sports Med* 1996;24(2):177-181.

12. Park GY, Lee SM, Lee MY: Diagnostic value of ultrasonography for clinical medial epicondylitis. *Arch Phys Med Rehabil* 2008;89(4):738-742.

     An ultrasonographic assessment of 21 elbows with a clinical diagnosis of medial epicondylitis had sensitivity, specificity, accuracy, positive predictive value, and negative predictive value > 90%. This study reinforced the value of the physical examination and moved toward validating ultrasonography for diagnosing medial epicondylitis.

13. Kijowski R, De Smet AA: Magnetic resonance imaging findings in patients with medial epicondylitis. *Skeletal Radiol* 2005;34(4):196-202.

14. Nirschl RP, Rodin DM, Ochiai DH, Maartmann-Moe C; DEX-AHE-01-99 Study Group: Iontophoretic administration of dexamethasone sodium phosphate for acute epicondylitis: A randomized, double-blinded, placebo-controlled study. *Am J Sports Med* 2003; 31(2):189-195.

15. Suresh SP, Ali KE, Jones H, Connell DA: Medial epicondylitis: Is ultrasound guided autologous blood injection an effective treatment? *Br J Sports Med* 2006; 40(11):935-939, discussion 939.

16. Aguinaldo AL, Chambers H: Correlation of throwing mechanics with elbow valgus load in adult baseball pitchers. *Am J Sports Med* 2009;37(10):2043-2048.

     Three-dimensional motion analysis was used to evaluate 69 adult baseball pitchers at an indoor mound. The variables most associated with elbow valgus included late trunk rotation, reduced shoulder external rotation, and increased elbow flexion. Sidearm pitchers were less susceptible to elbow valgus than those with a higher arm slot.

17. Rettig AC, Sherrill C, Snead DS, Mendler JC, Mieling P: Nonoperative treatment of ulnar collateral ligament injuries in throwing athletes. *Am J Sports Med* 2001; 29(1):15-17.

18. Cain EL Jr, Andrews JR, Dugas JR, et al: Outcome of ulnar collateral ligament reconstruction of the elbow in 1281 athletes: Results in 743 athletes with minimum 2-year follow-up. *Am J Sports Med* 2010;38(12): 2426-2434.

     Prospective data were collected for a 2-year minimum on 942 patients, most of whom underwent UCL reconstruction with a palmaris longus or gracilis graft using the modified Jobe technique. All patients underwent subcutaneous nerve transposition. The rate of return to previous level of function was 83%. The average time to return to throwing was 4.4 months, and the average return to competition was 11.6 months.

19. Bowers AL, Dines JS, Dines DM, Altchek DW: Elbow medial ulnar collateral ligament reconstruction: Clinical relevance and the docking technique. *J Shoulder Elbow Surg* 2010;19(2, suppl):110-117.

     Of 21 overhead athletes who underwent UCL reconstruction with a modified docking technique using a three-strand graft, 90% had a good or excellent result. This technique is acceptable for UCL reconstruction.

20. Paletta GA Jr, Wright RW: The modified docking procedure for elbow ulnar collateral ligament reconstruction: 2-year follow-up in elite throwers. *Am J Sports Med* 2006;34(10):1594-1598.

21. Dines JS, ElAttrache NS, Conway JE, Smith W, Ahmad CS: Clinical outcomes of the DANE TJ technique to treat ulnar collateral ligament insufficiency of the elbow. *Am J Sports Med* 2007;35(12):2039-2044.

     Twenty-two athletes underwent UCL reconstruction with a hybrid variation of the docking technique in which an interference screw is used in a single tunnel on the ulna to avoid the fracture risk of the two-tunnel technique. Nineteen patients had an excellent result, as did patients requiring revision for sublime tubercle avulsions.

22. Rettig AC, Ebben JR: Anterior subcutaneous transfer of the ulnar nerve in the athlete. *Am J Sports Med* 1993;21(6):836-839, discussion 839-840.

23. Andrews JR, Timmerman LA: Outcome of elbow surgery in professional baseball players. *Am J Sports Med* 1995;23(4):407-413.

24. Cohen SB, Valko C, Zoga A, Dodson CC, Ciccotti MG: Posteromedial elbow impingement: Magnetic resonance imaging findings in overhead throwing athletes and results of arthroscopic treatment. *Arthroscopy* 2011;27(10):1364-1370.

     After unsuccessful nonsurgical treatment, nine patients with posteromedial impingement underwent arthroscopy followed by rehabilitation and an interval throwing program. The results were excellent at a mean 68-month follow-up.

25. Hulkko A, Orava S, Nikula P: Stress fractures of the olecranon in javelin throwers. *Int J Sports Med* 1986; 7(4):210-213.

26. Nuber GW, Diment MT: Olecranon stress fractures in throwers: A report of two cases and a review of the literature. *Clin Orthop Relat Res* 1992;278:58-61.

27. Suzuki K, Minami A, Suenaga N, Kondoh M: Oblique stress fracture of the olecranon in baseball pitchers. *J Shoulder Elbow Surg* 1997;6(5):491-494.

28. Stephenson DR, Love S, Garcia GG, Mair SD: Recurrence of an olecranon stress fracture in an elite pitcher after percutaneous internal fixation: A case report. *Am J Sports Med* 2012;40(1):218-221.

     A collegiate pitcher with an olecranon stress fracture was successfully treated nonsurgically but had a recurrence on return to full activity. Seven months after surgical treatment with a single cannulated screw, he had posterior elbow pain with bullpen throwing. Revision fixation was with repeat screw fixation and a second smaller screw. After an interval throwing program, the patient returned to pitching without symptoms at 17-month follow-up.

29. Charlton WP, Chandler RW: Persistence of the olecranon physis in baseball players: Results following operative management. *J Shoulder Elbow Surg* 2003;12(1): 59-62.

30. Skak SV: Fracture of the olecranon through a persistent physis in an adult: A case report. *J Bone Joint Surg Am* 1993;75(2):272-275.

31. Matsuura T, Kashiwaguchi S, Iwase T, Enishi T, Yasui N: The value of using radiographic criteria for the treatment of persistent symptomatic olecranon physis in adolescent throwing athletes. *Am J Sports Med* 2010;38(1):141-145.

    In a retrospective analysis of persistent olecranon physis in 16 male baseball players, the lesions were classified as stage I (a widened physis compared with the contralateral elbow) or stage II (radiographic lesion). Nonsurgical treatment was successful in 92% of those with a stage I lesion but none with a stage II lesion.

32. Minami M, Nakashita K, Ishii S, et al: Twenty-five cases of osteochondritis dissecans of the elbow. *Rinsho Seikei Geka* 1979;14(8):805-810.

33. Baker CL III, Romeo AA, Baker CL Jr: Osteochondritis dissecans of the capitellum. *Am J Sports Med* 2010; 38(9):1917-1928.

    OCD of the capitellum was reviewed, including pathoanatomy, clinical presentation, diagnostic studies, nonsurgical and surgical treatments, and a rehabilitation program.

34. Mihara K, Tsutsui H, Nishinaka N, Yamaguchi K: Nonoperative treatment for osteochondritis dissecans of the capitellum. *Am J Sports Med* 2009;37(2): 298-304.

    Retrospective review of 39 patients with OCD of the capitellum who were treated nonsurgically led to the recommendation that patients with an advanced lesion undergo surgical intervention because of poor healing rates and evidence of progression with nonsurgical management.

35. Matsuura T, Kashiwaguchi S, Iwase T, Takeda Y, Yasui N: Conservative treatment for osteochondrosis of the humeral capitellum. *Am J Sports Med* 2008;36(5): 868-872.

    Retrospective review of 176 patients with OCD of the humeral capitellum found that 90.5% of stage I and 53% of stage II lesions healed with nonsurgical measures. Mean time to healing was 14.9 months and 12.3 months for stage I and II lesions, respectively, and return-to-throwing rates were 78.6% and 52.9%, respectively.

36. Takahara M, Mura N, Sasaki J, Harada M, Ogino T: Classification, treatment, and outcome of osteochondritis dissecans of the humeral capitellum. *J Bone Joint Surg Am* 2007;89(6):1205-1214.

    In a retrospective review of 106 patients with OCD of the humeral capitellum, treatment was nonsurgical or surgical fragment removal, fragment fixation with bone grafting, or mosaicplasty with plugs from the lateral femoral condyle. Lesions were classified as stable or unstable at 7.2-year follow-up. Stable lesions responded well to nonsurgical measures, and unstable lesions responded to surgical intervention.

Chapter 41

Medial and Lateral Recurrent Elbow Instability

April D. Armstrong, BSc(PT), MSc, MD, FRCSC

Introduction

Recurrence of medial or lateral elbow instability is uncommon. The patient often describes pain in the elbow but not instability, and therefore the diagnosis is difficult. The patient history, the physical examination findings, and a high index of suspicion are more critical in making an accurate diagnosis than are static imaging studies, which may appear normal. Lateral collateral ligament insufficiency is poorly tolerated because most normal activities of daily living require varus loading of the elbow. In contrast, medial collateral ligament (MCL) insufficiency is well tolerated by most patients because valgus loading is uncommon during daily routines. Overhead throwing athletes, particularly baseball pitchers, cannot tolerate MCL insufficiency and often require reconstructive surgery.

Valgus Elbow Instability

In the past 5 to 10 years, the understanding of medial elbow instability has dramatically improved. MCL injury most often is the result of repetitive overloading during overhead throwing, and most such injuries occur in baseball players. During the late cocking and early acceleration phase of throwing, the valgus load applied to the elbow exceeds the tensile strength of the anterior bundle of the MCL.[1,2] Professional athletes with a high pitch velocity are at relatively high risk for MCL injury.[3] A tall, heavy high school baseball player may be susceptible to MCL injury because of the ability to generate great valgus forces.[4] Compared with baseball pitchers, javelin throwers have a distinctly different throwing motion, and their postoperative rehabilitation needs are different.[5] Because of the weight of the javelin, 10 javelin throwers required a longer delay than

Dr. Armstrong or an immediate family member has received nonincome support (such as equipment or services), commercially derived honoraria, or other non–research-related funding (such as paid travel) from Zimmer and serves as a board member, owner, officer, or committee member of the American Shoulder and Elbow Surgeons.

baseball pitchers before starting an interval throwing program after MCL reconstruction, with a return-to-sport time of 15 months (a 1-year period is traditionally reported for baseball pitchers). Javelin throwers should be counseled to expect a lengthy recovery.[5] MCL injury has been reported in football quarterbacks, but a recent review of the National Football League Injury Surveillance System revealed only 10 reported incidences from 1994 to 2008.[6] These athletes were successfully treated nonsurgically; in contrast, baseball players often require surgical reconstruction. MCL injury also can develop after trauma, such as an elbow dislocation. Such an injury typically can be treated nonsurgically because in most patients little valgus load is applied to the elbow during activities of daily living.

Biomechanical studies have established that the anterior bundle of the MCL is the primary stabilizer for valgus load of the elbow.[7-9] A recent biomechanical cadaver study looked at the contact pressure of the radiocapitellar joint during simulation of two critical phases of the throwing motion during pitching.[10] MCL reconstruction restored the average articular pressures of the radiocapitellar joint to within 20% of intact elbow values. This study supported the primary role of the anterior bundle and MCL reconstruction as providing valgus stability.

Overhead athletes with valgus elbow instability describe pain with throwing localized to the medial aspect of the elbow. They may describe a distinct popping sensation during throwing or an insidious onset of increasing pain and decreasing velocity and accuracy during throwing. Occasionally, a patient also describes transient ulnar nerve symptoms. Some athletes describe pain in the posterior aspect of the elbow related to posteromedial osteophytosis or valgus extension overload (**Figure 1**). The athlete may describe increased pain during deceleration and release of the ball. Some surgeons think that posteromedial impingement occurs at lower flexion angles, with resultant increased contact forces at the posteromedial compartment of the elbow secondary to valgus instability.[11,12] A more recent biomechanical study proposed that this impingement occurs throughout the entire arc of motion, not solely at the lower flexion angles, and that it coincides with an ulnohumeral chondral injury.[13]

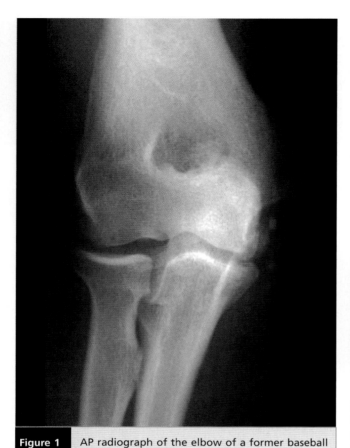

Figure 1 AP radiograph of the elbow of a former baseball pitcher showing posteromedial osteophytosis related to chronic valgus extension overload.

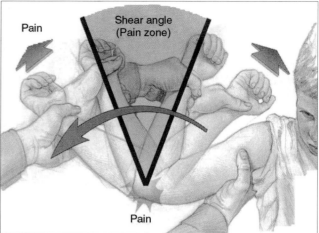

Figure 2 Schematic drawing showing the moving valgus stress test, in which a valgus load is applied to the elbow throughout an arc of motion. A patient with an MCL tear will describe pain through the middle of the arc of motion, typically between 70° and 120° of flexion (the shear angle). (Reproduced with permission from The Mayo Foundation for Medical Education and Research, Rochester, MN.)

The diagnosis of valgus elbow instability can be challenging, and the physical examination findings can be subtle. The patient often has point tenderness over the medial epicondyle and the flexor pronator mass. If the patient has valgus extension overload with posterior osteophytosis, palpation along the posteromedial olecranon may elicit pain. The patient also may report pain with forced extension of the elbow. Sometimes a throwing athlete has a slight flexion contracture and is asymptomatic despite posterior osteophytosis. Physical examination findings and ulnar nerve symptoms, particularly nerve subluxation, should be documented. Provocative physical examination testing should include the valgus stress test, the milking maneuver, and the moving valgus stress test.[14] The valgus stress test is performed with the elbow flexed at 30° to unlock the olecranon from the olecranon fossa. Shoulder rotation must be controlled, and gapping should be compared with the opposite limb. Palpation at the medial joint line during the valgus stress test can elicit pain and may allow a better appreciation of the gapping at the joint. The milking maneuver statically loads the MCL. While shoulder rotation is being controlled, the patient's elbow is flexed to 90°, and the forearm is fully supinated. The examiner or the patient then pulls on the thumb to apply valgus stress. Pain at the MCL is considered a

positive test result. The moving valgus stress test is a dynamic test that applies a constant valgus load to the elbow during an arc of motion of the elbow.[14] Patients with MCL injury describe pain at the medial elbow, typically at 70° to 120° of flexion (**Figure 2**).

Examination for valgus elbow instability should not be restricted to the elbow. The ipsilateral shoulder should be examined for associated rotator cuff disease or a glenohumeral internal rotation deficit with a tight posterior capsule. Injured throwing athletes with MCL insufficiency had a higher incidence of glenohumeral rotation deficit than matched uninjured athletes.[15] It is also important to assess the athlete's core musculature strength. The throwing mechanism includes a transfer of force from the legs to the trunk to the upper extremity, and core weakness can increase the load on the upper extremity. A one-leg stance can be quickly and easily used to test core weakness. When the patient stands on one leg and is asked to do a deep knee bend, a patient with core weakness becomes unbalanced or must lean toward the supporting leg to maintain balance.[16] A formal assessment of the athlete's pitching mechanics also can be informative. Younger pitchers in particular tend to open up the trunk too early in the pitch, leaving the elbow behind. This so-called dropped elbow pitch increases the valgus load on the elbow.

The diagnosis of valgus elbow instability relies mostly on the patient's history and physical examination findings, but imaging studies can be helpful. Static elbow radiographs often appear normal, but stress radiographs may show asymmetric gapping of more than 2 to 3 mm at the ulnohumeral joint. MRI with or without arthrography and CT arthrography are advantageous in that they allow identification of associated pathologies such as an osteochondral lesion. A study found that thickening of the MCL and posteromedial subchondral sclerosis of the trochlea are common in asymptomatic high school pitchers, which suggests that these conditions may be normal adaptations resulting from throwing.[17] Higher peak internal elbow adduction moments were found to be associated with MCL thickening and adaptations on MRI.[18] Dynamic ultrasonographic assessment is becoming increasingly popular.[19]

The initial treatment of an athlete with MCL insufficiency is a dedicated 3- to 6-month period of rest and rehabilitation. After nonsurgical treatment of MCL injury, 42% of patients returned to sport.[20] The focus should be on improving the strength and endurance of the flexor pronator muscles, reducing the tightness of the posterior capsule of the shoulder, and increasing core strength and stability.

Ligament reconstruction is the classic surgical treatment of MCL insufficiency in a throwing athlete. It has been proposed that MCL repair may be a reasonable alternative for relatively young athletes, who have better tissue quality and less likelihood of chronic attritional change to the ligament.[21] Repairs limited to a proximal or distal injury led to a 91% rate of return to sport; 97% returned to full athletic activity within 6 months compared with 1 year for a reconstruction procedure. MCL repair is an important technique to consider in younger athletes.

Ligament reconstruction is still the preferred treatment for a throwing athlete after unsuccessful nonsurgical management. MCL procedures have focused on reconstruction of the anterior bundle of the MCL. Almost-isometric fibers have been identified in the anterior bundle, originating on the humeral side close to the anatomic axis of rotation.[22] A recent study identified four unique isometric ligaments in the anterior bundle of the MCL and described their origins as broadly aligned along the axis of rotation in the coronal plane.[23] The isometric fibers extend more medially in the coronal plane and are more predominant than previously believed, constituting almost one half of the fibers of the anterior bundle of the MCL. As in past studies, isometricity was observed on the humeral rather than the ulnar side of the anterior bundle of the MCL.[22]

Numerous MCL ligament reconstruction techniques have been described, based on either a double- or a single-strand construct.[24-34] Good results have been reported for both constructs. The average reported return-to-sport rate is 83% (range, 68% to 95%).[35] Single-strand reconstruction may be more feasible for revision surgery after unsuccessful MCL reconstruction.[36,37] The largest outcome study of MCL reconstruction described the use of a modified Jobe (figure-of-8) technique, with subcutaneous ulnar nerve transposition and exposure through elevation of the flexor pronator muscle mass without detachment.[38] At 2-year follow-up for 743 patients, the return-to-sport rate was 83%, the

average time to full competition was 11.6 months, and 20% experienced a complication (16% minor, 4% major). Ulnar nerve symptoms, including transient neurapraxia, were the most common minor complications. The results were improved by modifying the subcutaneous ulnar nerve transposition from a two-sling to a one-sling technique, using a sleeve of the intermuscular septum rather than the flexor muscle fascia. Clear indications for ulnar nerve transposition are still undetermined. Also reported was the treatment of five medial epicondyle fractures, in which the humeral tunnel placement was modified so that it was deeper (more lateral) on the epicondyle. Open excision of posteromedial olecranon osteophytes was required in 34% of the patients.

More recent advances in MCL reconstruction include a flexor-pronator muscle-splitting technique without transposition of the ulnar nerve, which is reported to lead to decreased incidence of ulnar neuropathy.[39] The docking technique for MCL reconstruction has relatively high rates of return to sport[28-30,34] (**Figures 3 and 4**). Patients older than 30 years are at higher risk for the development of a combined MCL and flexor-pronator muscle injury, which is associated with a poor rate of return to sport (12.5%).[40]

There is growing concern about the increasing incidence of MCL injury, particularly in collegiate and high school athletes. Prevention is key, particularly for younger athletes. Appropriate rehabilitation is essential, as are diligence in restricting the number of pitches and enforcing strict rest periods for pitchers. The guidelines for limiting pitch counts and cumulative counts published by the USA Baseball Medical and Safety Advisory Committee stress that these factors are linearly associated with the risk of injury.[41] The number of pitches was found to be a stronger risk factor for injury than the type of pitch thrown.[42] The guidelines also provided recommendations for proper pitching mechanics and a minimum of 3 months of rest, with no throwing, after the baseball season. Fatigue was the factor most strongly correlated with arm injury.[41]

Posterolateral Rotatory Instability

Unlike valgus elbow instability, posterolateral rotatory instability (PLRI) does not occur exclusively in athletes. PLRI can be debilitating for patients whose demands include only normal activities of daily living because it places the lateral collateral ligament complex (LCLC) under continual stress. PLRI typically develops after an elbow dislocation or a traumatic fall onto an outstretched hand, followed by inadequate healing of the LCLC. Although other mechanisms have been described, the classic mechanism for elbow dislocation is an axial compressive, external rotatory, and valgus load to the elbow.[43,44] An MRI investigation of simple elbow dislocations proposed that healing of the LCLC is more likely after posterolateral dislocation because the

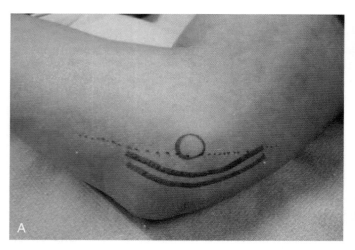
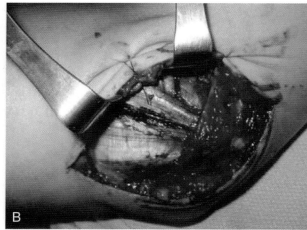
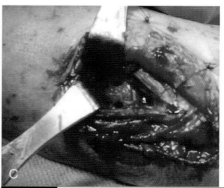
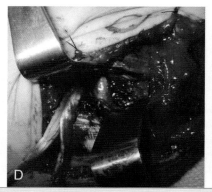
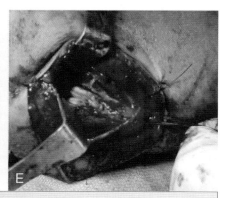

Figure 3   Photographs showing the docking technique for MCL reconstruction. **A,** The medial-based incision *(dotted line)*, the medial epicondyle *(circle)*, and the ulnar nerve path *(solid lines)* are marked. **B,** The muscle-splitting approach requires care to protect the medial antebrachial cutaneous nerve. **C,** Two holes are drilled in the ulna, bridging the sublime tubercle. **D,** The medial epicondyle is exposed to drill one hole at the point of isometry, and the tendon graft is passed through ulna drill holes. **E,** In the completed reconstruction, both tendon ends are docked into the humerus with sutures passed through smaller drill holes placed more proximal than the isometric drill hole.

lateral-side injury tends to be a stripping injury. After reduction of the elbow, the injured LCLC was found to return to its position next to the bone and was postulated to have an improved chance of healing and, therefore, less likelihood for PLRI. Posteromedial dislocation resulted in a distraction injury with medial bony contusions, resulting in more severe lateral soft-tissue injury. The authors of a 2012 study postulated that posteromedial dislocation may be associated with a higher risk for PLRI and recurrent instability because of the distraction inherent in the lateral injury.[45] PLRI also can develop from an iatrogenic cause, such as an aggressive lateral epicondylar release or multiple steroid injections for recalcitrant lateral epicondylitis.[46] Other reported causes are chronic cubitus varus deformity, such as malunion after a childhood supracondylar fracture, and radial head resection because tension on the LCLC from the radial head is removed.[47-49]

The LCLC is composed of the lateral ulnar collateral ligament (LUCL), the radial collateral ligament (RCL), the annular ligament, and the accessory collateral ligament. The LUCL is classically described as the primary restraint to PLRI, but biomechanical studies have suggested a significant role for the RCL in providing stability against PLRI.[43,50,51] One study suggested that the RCL, but not the LUCL, is an isometric bundle.[52] However, another study found that no truly isometric point exists for the LCLC; in addition, significant variability was seen among individual elbows in the maximal isometric graft insertion point for LCLC reconstruction.[53] Stability against PLRI most likely is provided by a combined effort of the LUCL and the RCL. A dual reconstruction of the RCL and the LUCL has recently been reported for the management of PLRI.[54]

The diagnosis of PLRI can be difficult. Patients often describe only pain or a nonspecific sensation of "something not right" in the elbow. Some patients describe a painful locking or clicking and may notice elbow subluxation is occurring when the elbow is extended or weight is borne through the arm. The classic examination test for PLRI is the lateral pivot-shift test. This test typically is performed under anesthesia because the patient is otherwise unable to tolerate the testing position[55] (**Figure 5**). The patient is supine, the arm is bent

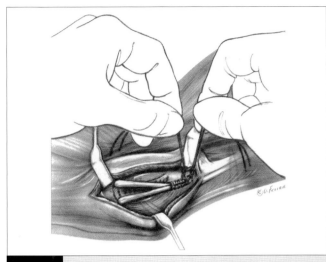

Figure 4 Drawing showing the docking technique for MCL reconstruction, as it was first described. The tendon graft is passed through two drill holes in the ulna and one docking drill hole at the isometric point on the humerus. Sutures are passed through two smaller holes drilled more proximally. (© Hospital for Special Surgery, New York, NY.)

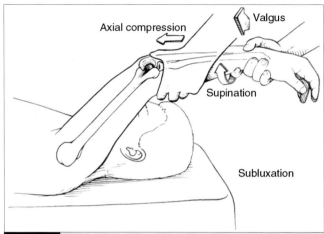

Figure 5 Drawing showing the lateral pivot-shift test, which is the classic instability test for LCLC insufficiency. An axial load is applied to the elbow at the same time as a forced supinated and valgus load. The elbow is subluxated when it is in extension, and often it is possible to visually and audibly observe elbow flexion to reduce the joint. (Reproduced with permission from O'Driscoll SW, Bell DF, Morrey BF: Posterolateral rotatory instability of the elbow. *J Bone Joint Surg Am* 1991;73[3]:440-446.)

overhead, and the elbow is extended with an axial and valgus load while the forearm is maximally supinated. The elbow is subluxated at this point. Fluoroscopic analysis shows the radial head posterior to the capitellum, and the ulnohumeral joint is widened. The elbow is moved into flexion to elicit an appreciable clunk and reduction of the joint. The lateral pivot-shift test is highly reproducible and not dependent on the examiner's level of training or experience.[56]

The posterolateral drawer test, the chair push-up test, the floor push-up test, and the tabletop relocation test are more easily tolerated by the patient.[57,58] Each of these tests mimics the lateral pivot-shift test by producing an extended, supinated, axially, and valgus-loaded elbow joint, with subsequent subluxation. With a positive test result, the patient identifies a reproduction of the symptoms or shows apprehension.

PLRI is a clinical diagnosis. Static radiographs often appear normal, but advanced imaging studies may be helpful, particularly for PLRI with an iatrogenic cause. If the original reason for LCLC insufficiency was not instability, detection of the classic instability pattern may be difficult. MRI (with or without arthrography) and ultrasonography have been described.[59,60] A posterior capitellar impression fracture may be associated with elbow dislocation and is similar to a Hill-Sachs deformity of the shoulder.[61] MRI may show a so-called pseudodefect of the capitellum, which should not be confused with a posterior capitellar impression fracture, or a so-called Osborne-Cotterill lesion, which is an osteochondral fracture of the posterolateral capitellum similar to a Bankart lesion of the glenoid and believed to indicate PLRI.[62-64]

Symptomatic PLRI most often is treated with surgical reconstruction of the LCLC using a tendon graft. Yet, surgical repair provides inferior results, probably because the ligament often is attenuated.[65,66] The classic LCLC reconstruction involved creating a figure-of-8 construct from the humerus to the ulna, with two holes drilled in the ulna at the crista supinatoris, three holes drilled in the humerus, and one critical hole drilled at the isometric insertion of the LCLC.[55] The tendon graft is passed in a figure-of-8 fashion and sutured to itself. At a mean follow-up of 6 years after 12 direct repairs and 33 reconstructions using the figure-of-8 technique, 86% of the patients were subjectively satisfied with the outcome of the operation.[66] Seven patients had instability. Reconstruction yielded better results than ligament repair. Patients with a posttraumatic etiology and subjective symptoms of instability also had better results. Smaller studies reported on other reconstruction options, such as using the triceps tendon, arthroscopic techniques,[67] and an interference single-strand construct.[67-71]

The use of a docking technique similar to the technique used for MCL reconstruction is increasing for LCLC reconstruction[72] (**Figure 6**). The elbow is approached through a Kocher interval. Two holes are drilled into the ulna to bridge the supinator crest with an approximately 2-cm osseous bridge; one hole is on the supinator crest, and the second is more proximal, near the base of the annular ligament. The tendon graft is passed through the drill holes, and both ends of the graft are docked into the isometric point on the humerus. Two smaller exit holes are drilled proximal to

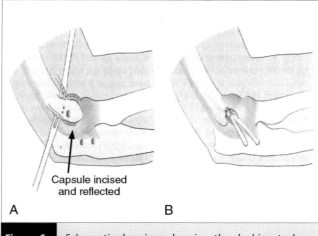

A   **B**

Capsule incised
and reflected

Figure 6   Schematic drawings showing the docking technique for reconstruction of the lateral collateral ligament complex. **A,** Two drill holes are created in the ulna, and one drill hole is created at the isometric point on the humerus, with two smaller exit drill holes proximal in the humerus for suture passage. **B,** In the completed reconstruction, the underlying capsuloligamentous complex is repaired, and tendon graft is passed through two ulnar drill holes and docked into a humeral drill hole. (Reproduced with permission from Jones KJ, Dodson CC, Osbahr DC, et al: The docking technique for lateral ulnar collateral ligament reconstruction: Surgical technique and clinical outcomes. *J Shoulder Elbow Surg* 2012;21[3]:389-395.)

the humeral isometric point to allow the sutures to be passed from the isometric tunnel to tie over a 1-cm osseous bridge. Stitches placed through the attenuated capsuloligamentous complex are passed with the tendon graft stitches to reinforce the repair. One of the critical aspects of the ligament reconstruction is placement of the isometric tunnel on the humerus. The isometric tunnel should be placed at the center of the capitellum, which is the center of the axis of rotation. Because the elbow becomes unstable in a supinated and extended position, maximal tension is important with the ligament reconstruction in this position. Eccentric drilling of the humeral isometric point is required for this purpose. A biomechanical study found that a truly isometric point could not be identified for tunnel placement in LCLC reconstruction, and there was significant variation among cadaver specimens.[53] However, a location between the 3-o'clock and 4:30 positions was considered ideal for humeral tunnel placement. The hole on the humeral side should be drilled slightly more anterior and proximal than the isometric point so that the distal posterior wall of the humeral tunnel maintains its isometry, particularly in elbow extension. At a mean follow-up of 7 years of the docking technique in eight patients, 75% (six patients) had no recurrent instability and 25% (two patients) reported occasional instability during activities of daily living.[72] All patients were satisfied with the outcome.

Summary

Medial or lateral recurrent elbow instability is uncommon but can be disabling. Nonsurgical treatment is unlikely to be effective. The diagnosis relies on a high level of clinical suspicion and a focused clinical examination. Ligament reconstruction is the preferred treatment and has had high rates of success.

Annotated References

1. Fleisig GS, Andrews JR, Dillman CJ, Escamilla RF: Kinetics of baseball pitching with implications about injury mechanisms. *Am J Sports Med* 1995;23(2): 233-239.

2. Dillman CJ, Fleisig GS, Andrews JR: Biomechanics of pitching with emphasis upon shoulder kinematics. *J Orthop Sports Phys Ther* 1993;18(2):402-408.

3. Bushnell BD, Anz AW, Noonan TJ, Torry MR, Hawkins RJ: Association of maximum pitch velocity and elbow injury in professional baseball pitchers. *Am J Sports Med* 2010;38(4):728-732.

   A significant association was found between maximum pitch velocity and elbow injury in 23 professional baseball pitchers. Level of evidence: III.

4. Han KJ, Kim YK, Lim SK, Park JY, Oh KS: The effect of physical characteristics and field position on the shoulder and elbow injuries of 490 baseball players: Confirmation of diagnosis by magnetic resonance imaging. *Clin J Sport Med* 2009;19(4):271-276.

   An analysis of baseball-related injuries in 490 baseball players referred to a shoulder and elbow institute for rehabilitation revealed that high school and collegiate players were more likely to have an MCL injury or superior labrum anterior to posterior injury than junior high school players. Pitchers and outfielders were more likely to have MCL injury than infielders. Players who were relatively tall and heavy had a higher incidence of MCL injury.

5. Dines JS, Jones KJ, Kahlenberg C, Rosenbaum A, Osbahr DC, Altchek DW: Elbow ulnar collateral ligament reconstruction in javelin throwers at a minimum 2-year follow-up. *Am J Sports Med* 2012;40(1): 148-151.

   MCL reconstruction in 10 javelin throwers highlighted that the rehabilitation needs of javelin throwers are different from those of baseball players. Level of evidence: IV.

6. Dodson CC, Slenker N, Cohen SB, Ciccotti MG, DeLuca P: Ulnar collateral ligament injuries of the elbow in professional football quarterbacks. *J Shoulder Elbow Surg* 2010;19(8):1276-1280.

   A review of the National Football League Injury Surveillance System found that MCL injuries are uncommon in quarterbacks, and most are treated nonsurgically. Level of evidence: IV.

7. Hotchkiss RN, Weiland AJ: Valgus stability of the elbow. *J Orthop Res* 1987;5(3):372-377.

8. Søjbjerg JO, Ovesen J, Nielsen S: Experimental elbow instability after transection of the medial collateral ligament. *Clin Orthop Relat Res* 1987;218:186-190.

9. Morrey BF, An KN: Articular and ligamentous contributions to the stability of the elbow joint. *Am J Sports Med* 1983;11(5):315-319.

10. Duggan JP Jr, Osadebe UC, Alexander JW, Noble PC, Lintner DM: The impact of ulnar collateral ligament tear and reconstruction on contact pressures in the lateral compartment of the elbow. *J Shoulder Elbow Surg* 2011;20(2):226-233.

    A biomechanical cadaver study found that MCL reconstruction restored valgus stability and decreased radiocapitellar contact pressures almost to normal levels.

11. Ahmad CS, Park MC, ElAttrache NS: Elbow medial ulnar collateral ligament insufficiency alters posteromedial olecranon contact. *Am J Sports Med* 2004; 32(7):1607-1612.

12. Kamineni S, ElAttrache NS, O'Driscoll SW, et al: Medial collateral ligament strain with partial posteromedial olecranon resection: A biomechanical study. *J Bone Joint Surg Am* 2004;86-A(11):2424-2430.

13. Osbahr DC, Dines JS, Breazeale NM, Deng XH, Altchek DW: Ulnohumeral chondral and ligamentous overload: Biomechanical correlation for posteromedial chondromalacia of the elbow in throwing athletes. *Am J Sports Med* 2010;38(12):2535-2541.

    The authors examine, using a biomechanical model, the contact area and pressure across the posteromedial elbow before and after sectioning the anterior bundle of the medial collateral ligament. They reported that valgus laxity increased contact pressures, with the elbow held at 90 degrees, across the posteromedial elbow. They suggested that posteromedial impingement and the potential for chondral damage is possible throughout the entire arc of flexion and not just in extension.

14. O'Driscoll SW, Lawton RL, Smith AM: The "moving valgus stress test" for medial collateral ligament tears of the elbow. *Am J Sports Med* 2005;33(2):231-239.

15. Dines JS, Frank JB, Akerman M, Yocum LA: Glenohumeral internal rotation deficits in baseball players with ulnar collateral ligament insufficiency. *Am J Sports Med* 2009;37(3):566-570.

    In a comparison of 29 baseball players with MCL insufficiency with a matched control group of 29 baseball players with no insufficiency, the injured players were found to have significantly less glenohumeral internal rotation motion. Level of evidence: III.

16. Ben Kibler W, Sciascia A: Kinetic chain contributions to elbow function and dysfunction in sports. *Clin Sports Med* 2004;23(4):545-552, viii.

17. Hurd WJ, Kaufman KR, Murthy NS: Relationship between the medial elbow adduction moment during pitching and ulnar collateral ligament appearance during magnetic resonance imaging evaluation. *Am J Sports Med* 2011;39(6):1233-1237.

    A comparison of elbow MRI with three-dimensional motion analysis testing in 20 uninjured, asymptomatic high school baseball pitchers found that MCL thickening was associated with higher peak internal elbow adduction moments. Level of evidence: II.

18. Hurd WJ, Eby S, Kaufman KR, Murthy NS: Magnetic resonance imaging of the throwing elbow in the uninjured, high school-aged baseball pitcher. *Am J Sports Med* 2011;39(4):722-728.

    Thickening of the anterior band of the MCL and posteromedial subchondral sclerosis was found in 23 uninjured, asymptomatic high school baseball pitchers. These findings may be considered normal or warn of risk for injury. Level of evidence: III.

19. Smith W, Hackel JG, Goitz HT, Bouffard JA, Nelson AM: Utilization of sonography and a stress device in the assessment of partial tears of the ulnar collateral ligament in throwers. *Int J Sports Phys Ther* 2011; 6(1):45-50.

    An ultrasonographic technique for assessing valgus elbow instability is described.

20. Rettig AC, Sherrill C, Snead DS, Mendler JC, Mieling P: Nonoperative treatment of ulnar collateral ligament injuries in throwing athletes. *Am J Sports Med* 2001;29(1):15-17.

21. Savoie FH III, Trenhaile SW, Roberts J, Field LD, Ramsey JR: Primary repair of ulnar collateral ligament injuries of the elbow in young athletes: A case series of injuries to the proximal and distal ends of the ligament. *Am J Sports Med* 2008;36(6):1066-1072.

    Acute repair of the MCL is proposed as a viable alternative to reconstruction in young nonprofessional athletes. Level of evidence: IV.

22. Armstrong AD, Ferreira LM, Dunning CE, Johnson JA, King GJ: The medial collateral ligament of the elbow is not isometric: An in vitro biomechanical study. *Am J Sports Med* 2004;32(1):85-90.

23. Miyake J, Moritomo H, Masatomi T, et al: In vivo and 3-dimensional functional anatomy of the anterior bundle of the medial collateral ligament of the elbow. *J Shoulder Elbow Surg* 2012;21(8):1006-1012.

    Four unique isometric bands of the anterior bundle of the MCL were found to broadly align along the axis of rotation in the coronal plane.

24. Jobe FW, Stark H, Lombardo SJ: Reconstruction of the ulnar collateral ligament in athletes. *J Bone Joint Surg Am* 1986;68(8):1158-1163.

25. Conway JE, Jobe FW, Glousman RE, Pink M: Medial instability of the elbow in throwing athletes: Treatment by repair or reconstruction of the ulnar col-

7: Elbow Trauma, Fracture, and Reconstruction

lateral ligament. *J Bone Joint Surg Am* 1992;74(1): 67-83.

26. Azar FM, Andrews JR, Wilk KE, Groh D: Operative treatment of ulnar collateral ligament injuries of the elbow in athletes. *Am J Sports Med* 2000;28(1):16-23.

27. Thompson WH, Jobe FW, Yocum LA, Pink MM: Ulnar collateral ligament reconstruction in athletes: Muscle-splitting approach without transposition of the ulnar nerve. *J Shoulder Elbow Surg* 2001;10(2): 152-157.

28. Rohrbough JT, Altchek DW, Hyman J, Williams RJ III, Botts JD: Medial collateral ligament reconstruction of the elbow using the docking technique. *Am J Sports Med* 2002;30(4):541-548.

29. Paletta GA Jr, Wright RW: The modified docking procedure for elbow ulnar collateral ligament reconstruction: 2-year follow-up in elite throwers. *Am J Sports Med* 2006;34(10):1594-1598.

30. Koh JL, Schafer MF, Keuter G, Hsu JE: Ulnar collateral ligament reconstruction in elite throwing athletes. *Arthroscopy* 2006;22(11):1187-1191.

31. Dines JS, ElAttrache NS, Conway JE, Smith W, Ahmad CS: Clinical outcomes of the DANE TJ technique to treat ulnar collateral ligament insufficiency of the elbow. *Am J Sports Med* 2007;35(12):2039-2044.

    Patients who underwent a single-strand MCL ligament reconstruction technique had an 86% rate of return to sport. Level of evidence: IV.

32. Bowers AL, Dines JS, Dines DM, Altchek DW: Elbow medial ulnar collateral ligament reconstruction: Clinical relevance and the docking technique. *J Shoulder Elbow Surg* 2010;19(suppl 2):110-117.

    A modified docking technique for MCL reconstruction had an excellent result in 90% of patients. Level of evidence: IV.

33. Hechtman KS, Zvijac JE, Wells ME, Botto-van Bemden A: Long-term results of ulnar collateral ligament reconstruction in throwing athletes based on a hybrid technique. *Am J Sports Med* 2011;39(2):342-347.

    At an average follow-up of 6.9 years, patients treated with a hybrid technique for MCL reconstruction had an 85% recovery to preinjury level of performance. Level of evidence: IV.

34. Dodson CC, Thomas A, Dines JS, Nho SJ, Williams RJ III, Altchek DW: Medial ulnar collateral ligament reconstruction of the elbow in throwing athletes. *Am J Sports Med* 2006;34(12):1926-1932.

35. Vitale MA, Ahmad CS: The outcome of elbow ulnar collateral ligament reconstruction in overhead athletes: A systematic review. *Am J Sports Med* 2008;36(6): 1193-1205.

Articles published from 1950 to 2007 on ulnar collateral ligament reconstruction were systematically reviewed.

36. Dines JS, Yocum LA, Frank JB, ElAttrache NS, Gambardella RA, Jobe FW: Revision surgery for failed elbow medial collateral ligament reconstruction. *Am J Sports Med* 2008;36(6):1061-1065.

    A retrospective review of 15 patients who required a revision MCL reconstruction procedure found that the rate of return to sport was lower and the complication rate was higher than after the initial procedure. Level of evidence: IV.

37. Lee GH, Limpisvasti O, Park MC, McGarry MH, Yocum LA, Lee TQ: Revision ulnar collateral ligament reconstruction using a suspension button fixation technique. *Am J Sports Med* 2010;38(3):575-580.

    A cadaver biomechanical study found successful restoration of elbow kinematics using a suspension button fixation technique.

38. Cain EL Jr, Andrews JR, Dugas JR, et al: Outcome of ulnar collateral ligament reconstruction of the elbow in 1281 athletes: Results in 743 athletes with minimum 2-year follow-up. *Am J Sports Med* 2010;38(12): 2426-2434.

    At a minimum follow-up of 2 years of 743 patients who underwent MCL reconstruction using a modified Jobe technique with subcutaneous ulnar nerve transposition, the rate of return to sport was 83%, the average time to competition was 11.6 months, and the rates of complications were 16% minor (mostly related to ulnar neuropathy) and 4% major. Level of evidence: IV.

39. Smith GR, Altchek DW, Pagnani MJ, Keeley JR: A muscle-splitting approach to the ulnar collateral ligament of the elbow: Neuroanatomy and operative technique. *Am J Sports Med* 1996;24(5):575-580.

40. Osbahr DC, Swaminathan SS, Allen AA, Dines JS, Coleman SH, Altchek DW: Combined flexor-pronator mass and ulnar collateral ligament injuries in the elbows of older baseball players. *Am J Sports Med* 2010;38(4):733-739.

    A study of 187 baseball players age 14 to 42 years who had undergone MCL reconstruction found that 4% were treated for a combined flexor-pronator and MCL injury. These patients were older and had a poorer prognosis than other patients; their rate of return to sport was only 12.5%. Level of evidence: IV.

41. Kerut EK, Kerut DG, Fleisig GS, Andrews JR: Prevention of arm injury in youth baseball pitchers. *J La State Med Soc* 2008;160(2):95-98.

    Concern exists about the increasing number of injuries in youth baseball pitchers. The injury prevention recommendations of the USA Baseball Medical and Safety Advisory Committee are described.

42. Dun S, Loftice J, Fleisig GS, Kingsley D, Andrews JR: A biomechanical comparison of youth baseball pitch-

es: Is the curveball potentially harmful? *Am J Sports Med* 2008;36(4):686-692.

A three-dimensional motion analysis system was used during different types of pitches thrown by 29 youth baseball pitchers. The shoulder and elbow loads were greatest during the fastball pitch and least during the change-up. The type of pitch was found to affect the risk of injury less than the number of pitches.

43. O'Driscoll SW, Morrey BF, Korinek S, An KN: Elbow subluxation and dislocation: A spectrum of instability. *Clin Orthop Relat Res* 1992;(280):186-197.

44. Deutch SR, Jensen SL, Olsen BS, Sneppen O: Elbow joint stability in relation to forced external rotation: An experimental study of the osseous constraint. *J Shoulder Elbow Surg* 2003;12(3):287-292.

45. Rhyou IH, Kim YS: New mechanism of the posterior elbow dislocation. *Knee Surg Sports Traumatol Arthrosc* 2012;20(12):2535-2541.

   Soft-tissue injury after simple elbow dislocation is described, with the mechanisms of injury. Level of evidence: IV.

46. Kalainov DM, Cohen MS: Posterolateral rotatory instability of the elbow in association with lateral epicondylitis: A report of three cases. *J Bone Joint Surg Am* 2005;87(5):1120-1125.

47. O'Driscoll SW, Spinner RJ, McKee MD, et al: Tardy posterolateral rotatory instability of the elbow due to cubitus varus. *J Bone Joint Surg Am* 2001;83-A(9):1358-1369.

48. Beuerlein MJ, Reid JT, Schemitsch EH, McKee MD: Effect of distal humeral varus deformity on strain in the lateral ulnar collateral ligament and ulnohumeral joint stability. *J Bone Joint Surg Am* 2004;86-A(10):2235-2242.

49. Hall JA, McKee MD: Posterolateral rotatory instability of the elbow following radial head resection. *J Bone Joint Surg Am* 2005;87(7):1571-1579.

50. Dunning CE, Zarzour ZD, Patterson SD, Johnson JA, King GJ: Ligamentous stabilizers against posterolateral rotatory instability of the elbow. *J Bone Joint Surg Am* 2001;83-A(12):1823-1828.

51. McAdams TR, Masters GW, Srivastava S: The effect of arthroscopic sectioning of the lateral ligament complex of the elbow on posterolateral rotatory stability. *J Shoulder Elbow Surg* 2005;14(3):298-301.

52. Moritomo H, Murase T, Arimitsu S, Oka K, Yoshikawa H, Sugamoto K: The in vivo isometric point of the lateral ligament of the elbow. *J Bone Joint Surg Am* 2007;89(9):2011-2017.

   The three-dimensional kinematics of the normal elbow were studied. The radial collateral ligament was found to be isometric, and the lateral collateral ligament was

not. The isometric point for a graft origin was 2 mm proximal to the center of the capitellum.

53. Goren D, Budoff JE, Hipp JA: Isometric placement of lateral ulnar collateral ligament reconstructions: A biomechanical study. *Am J Sports Med* 2010;38(1):153-159.

   A cadaver study found that the isometric position for LUCL reconstruction on the humerus is between the 3-o'clock and 4:30 positions on the lateral epicondyle for the posterior distal wall of the tunnel.

54. Rhyou IH, Park MJ: Dual reconstruction of the radial collateral ligament and lateral ulnar collateral ligament in posterolateral rotator instability of the elbow. *Knee Surg Sports Traumatol Arthrosc* 2011;19(6):1009-1012.

   A dual reconstruction technique is described for LCLC reconstruction. Level of evidence: IV.

55. O'Driscoll SW, Bell DF, Morrey BF: Posterolateral rotatory instability of the elbow. *J Bone Joint Surg Am* 1991;73(3):440-446.

56. Lattanza LL, Chu T, Ty JM, et al: Interclinician and intraclinician variability in the mechanics of the pivot shift test for posterolateral rotatory instability (PLRI) of the elbow. *J Shoulder Elbow Surg* 2010;19(8):1150-1156.

   Pivot-shift testing performed by three clinicians on five cadaver elbows was consistent and reproducible.

57. Regan W, Lapner PC: Prospective evaluation of two diagnostic apprehension signs for posterolateral instability of the elbow. *J Shoulder Elbow Surg* 2006;15(3):344-346.

58. Arvind CH, Hargreaves DG: Tabletop relocation test: A new clinical test for posterolateral rotatory instability of the elbow. *J Shoulder Elbow Surg* 2006;15(6):707-708.

59. Teixeira AA, Buffani A, Tavares A, et al: Effects of fluvastatin on insulin resistance and cardiac morphology in hypertensive patients. *J Hum Hypertens* 2011;25(8):492-499.

   The authors reported their technique and findings when imaging the LCLC in 10 cadaver elbows.

60. Stewart B, Harish S, Oomen G, Wainman B, Popowich T, Moro JK: Sonography of the lateral ulnar collateral ligament of the elbow: Study of cadavers and healthy volunteers. *AJR Am J Roentgenol* 2009;193(6):1615-1619.

   This effectiveness of ultrasonography was investigated for detecting LCLC in four cadaver elbows and subsequently in 35 healthy individuals. Level of evidence: IV.

61. Faber KJ, King GJ: Posterior capitellum impression fracture: A case report associated with posterolateral rotatory instability of the elbow. *J Shoulder Elbow Surg* 1998;7(2):157-159.

7: Elbow Trauma, Fracture, and Reconstruction

62. Rosenberg ZS, Blutreich SI, Schweitzer ME, Zember JS, Fillmore K: MRI features of a posterior capitellar impaction injuries. *AJR Am J Roentgenol* 2008; 190(2):435-441.

   The distinguishing features of posterior capitellar impression fracture and a pseudodefect of the capitellum are described. Level of evidence: IV.

63. Jeon IH, Micic ID, Yamamoto N, Morrey BF: Osborne-Cotterill lesion: An osseous defect of the capitellum associated with instability of the elbow. *AJR Am J Roentgenol* 2008;191(3):727-729.

   An association was proposed between the Osborne-Cotterill lesion and PLRI. Level of evidence: IV.

64. Jeon IH, Min WK, Micic ID, Cho HS, Kim PT: Surgical treatment and clinical implication for posterolateral rotatory instability of the elbow: Osborne-Cotterill lesion of the elbow. *J Trauma* 2011;71(3): E45-E49.

   A study of five patients with an Osborne-Cotterill lesion found that LCLC reconstruction may not be successful for such patients. Level of evidence: IV.

65. Lee BP, Teo LH: Surgical reconstruction for posterolateral rotatory instability of the elbow. *J Shoulder Elbow Surg* 2003;12(5):476-479.

66. Sanchez-Sotelo J, Morrey BF, O'Driscoll SW: Ligamentous repair and reconstruction for posterolateral rotatory instability of the elbow. *J Bone Joint Surg Br* 2005;87(1):54-61.

67. Savoie FH III, O'Brien MJ, Field LD, Gurley DJ: Arthroscopic and open radial ulnohumeral ligament reconstruction for posterolateral rotatory instability of the elbow. *Clin Sports Med* 2010;29(4):611-618.

   The authors' experience with open and arthroscopic LCLC reconstruction was described. Level of evidence: V.

68. Gong HS, Kim JK, Oh JH, Lee YH, Chung MS, Baek GH: A new technique for lateral ulnar collateral ligament reconstruction using the triceps tendon. *Tech Hand Up Extrem Surg* 2009;13(1):34-36.

   A technique for LCLC reconstruction uses a portion of the triceps tendon. Level of evidence: V.

69. Eygendaal D: Ligamentous reconstruction around the elbow using triceps tendon. *Acta Orthop Scand* 2004; 75(5):516-523.

70. Lehman RC: Lateral elbow reconstruction using a new fixation technique. *Arthroscopy* 2005;21(4):503-505.

71. King GJ, Dunning CE, Zarzour ZD, Patterson SD, Johnson JA: Single-strand reconstruction of the lateral ulnar collateral ligament restores varus and posterolateral rotatory stability of the elbow. *J Shoulder Elbow Surg* 2002;11(1):60-64.

72. Jones KJ, Dodson CC, Osbahr DC, et al: The docking technique for lateral ulnar collateral ligament reconstruction: Surgical technique and clinical outcomes. *J Shoulder Elbow Surg* 2012;21(3):389-395.

   The docking technique for LCLC reconstruction led to complete resolution in 75% of patients; 25% had occasional instability. Level of evidence: IV.

Chapter 42

Elbow Stiffness: Pathogenesis, Evaluation, and Open Treatment

Rudy Kovachevich, MD   Hill Hastings II, MD

Introduction

The function of the upper extremity largely depends on the ability of the elbow to position the hand in space. Loss of elbow motion, therefore, can seriously interfere with daily activities and the ability to take care of oneself. Contracture and stiffness of the elbow can result from trauma, heterotopic ossification, burn injury, neurologic spasticity, prolonged immobilization, or postoperative scarring. The propensity of the elbow to become stiff has been attributed to numerous factors, including the congruous nature of the joint, the presence of three articulations within a single synovial cavity, and the proximity of the articular surface and capsule to the intracapsular ligaments and extracapsular muscles.[1] The etiology of elbow stiffness has been classified as extrinsic (extra-articular), intrinsic (intra-articular), or mixed[2] (**Table 1**).

Etiology

The anatomic structures and pathophysiologic mechanisms involved in a patient's elbow stiffness dictate the treatment and affect the prognosis. Soft-tissue contractures around the elbow, particularly the capsule and collateral ligaments, play a critical role in the development of arthrofibrosis, in which structural and biochemical alterations lead to thickening, loss of motion, and decreased tissue compliance.[3] Basic science animal studies have found increased expression of transforming growth factor–β in rabbit elbow capsular tissue.[4] Transforming growth factor–β may have a role in the development of fibrotic scarring around the elbow secondary to cellular changes, such as elevated myofibroblast levels, increased extracellular matrix proliferation, and increased formation of collagen cross-links.[5-7]

Dr. Hastings or an immediate family member has received royalties from Biomet and serves as a paid consultant to or is an employee of Biomet. Neither Dr. Kovachevich nor any immediate family member has received anything of value from or has stock or stock options held in a commercial company or institution related directly or indirectly to the subject of this chapter.

Heterotopic ossification, defined as the inappropriate formation of mature lamellar bone in a nonosseous location, can contribute to the development of elbow stiffness, especially after traumatic injury. Heterotopic ossification must be distinguished from periarticular calcifications, which are amorphous calcium depositions in soft tissues that commonly occur after injury but do not necessarily affect motion.[8,9] The cause is not completely understood, but it involves an osteoblastic differentiation of pluripotent mesenchymal stem cells believed to occur after injury or surgery or in an inflammatory state. The bone formed in heterotopic ossification is histologically identical to native bone although more metabolically active and without a true periosteal layer.

Evaluation

Elbow contractures are challenging to treat. Therefore, prevention is of paramount importance. The treatment of a patient with an elbow contracture is nonsurgical, followed by surgical treatment if necessary. A thorough history and physical examination complemented by plain radiographs are prerequisites to a full assessment of the causes of a loss of elbow motion. The character of end point resistance to motion should be noted; a hard, sudden end point suggests a bony block, and a softer end point suggests a soft-tissue constraint to motion.

It is helpful to supplement standard AP and lateral radiographs with coronoid and radiocapitellar views to better evaluate the coronoid and radiocapitellar joints. Evaluation of joint surfaces in the contracted elbow require the AP view to be taken as two separate radiographs, one of which is perpendicular to the humerus and the other perpendicular to the radius and ulna. A lateral radiograph in full flexion can be useful for detecting bony impingement. Fluoroscopy can be used as an adjunct to distinguish between an osseous block to motion and a purely soft-tissue contracture. Advanced imaging studies, such as CT with two- or three-dimensional reconstruction, can identify the intra-articular blocks to range of motion for the purpose of surgical planning. MRI usually is not helpful.

Table 1

The Etiology of Elbow Stiffness

Classification	Types
Extrinsic (Extra-articular)	Skin contracture
	Subcutaneous tissue contracture
	Capsule contracture
	Medial or lateral collateral ligament contracture
	Myostatic contracture
	Extra-articular malunion
	Heterotopic ossification
Intrinsic (Intra-articular)	Articular malalignment
	Joint incongruity
	Arthritis
	Intra-articular adhesions
	Loose bodies
	Osteophyte impingement
	Coronoid
	Olecranon
	Fossa fibrosis
	Coronoid fossa
	Olecranon fossa
Mixed	Extrinsic contractures secondary to intrinsic pathology

Treatment Modalities

The goal of treatment for a patient with elbow stiffness and contracture is to provide and maintain a pain-free, functional, and stable joint. Nonsurgical measures can be helpful within the first 3 to 6 months after the contracture develops. These measures can include supervised physical therapy, static-progressive splinting, dynamic splinting, serial casting, and joint manipulation under anesthesia.

Surgical treatment is considered if the initial nonsurgical management is unsuccessful or if the patient has a significant osseous block to motion, as identified on examination and imaging studies. The typical indications for surgery include flexion contractures of more than 30° or the inability to flex the elbow to 130°. Patients who need greater motion for a vocational or sports activity may require surgical intervention for a smaller deficit.

The prerequisites for contracture release include a congruous joint with adequate ulnohumeral joint space, adequate soft-tissue coverage of the surgical site, resolution of soft-tissue posttraumatic inflammation,

maturation of any heterotopic ossification, and the ability to comply with an aggressive postoperative rehabilitation regimen. The development of an incongruous or an arthritic ulnohumeral joint is a contraindication to simple surgical release because the release could worsen pain but only minimally improve motion. Severe posttraumatic arthritic changes are an indication for a salvage procedure, such as soft-tissue interposition arthroplasty, hemiarthroplasty, or total elbow arthroplasty.

Open Treatment

Surgical release of the elbow has proved to be an effective measure to restore range of motion and can be achieved with an open or an arthroscopic procedure. Arthroscopic release is discussed in chapters 46 and 47. An open release typically is performed using an ultrasound-guided regional anesthetic block, with or without an indwelling catheter, and long-acting medications that provide postoperative pain control and muscular relaxation.

Open elbow contracture release should be tailored to the needs of the individual patient after determining whether the loss of elbow motion is in flexion, extension, or both. To improve elbow flexion, the posterior soft tissues that tether the joint, including the posterior joint capsule and triceps extensor mechanism, are released. Anterior bony restraints to flexion are removed, including loose bodies, osteophytes or overgrowth of the coronoid process, and scar or bone that may have filled the coronoid and radial fossae (Figure 1). There may be thickening and contracture of the posteromedial capsule (the posterior band of the ulnar collateral ligament), which requires release to restore full flexion. The steps for improving elbow extension are similar. Anteriorly, tethering soft tissues, such as joint capsule and brachialis adhesions, are released. Posterior impingement between the olecranon and olecranon fossa is corrected by partial olecranon excision and fossa débridement.

The ulnar nerve requires special consideration during contracture release. The normal tension and compression of the ulnar nerve during elbow flexion is more pronounced in a contracted elbow. If the patient has preoperative symptoms or ulnar nerve irritability, as shown by the Tinel sign, the elbow flexion test, or the ulnar nerve compression test, the nerve should be decompressed with or without transposition.

Numerous surgical approaches can be used for a contracture release. The skin incision to gain deep access to the joint can vary from a limited medial and/or lateral to a single extensile posterior approach that will provide access to both sides of the elbow. The approach typically is chosen based on the surgeon's preference, the presence of previous surgical incisions, the need for nerve decompression, and the location and extent of heterotopic ossification. A posterior incision is advisable if there is a possibility that elbow replacement eventu-

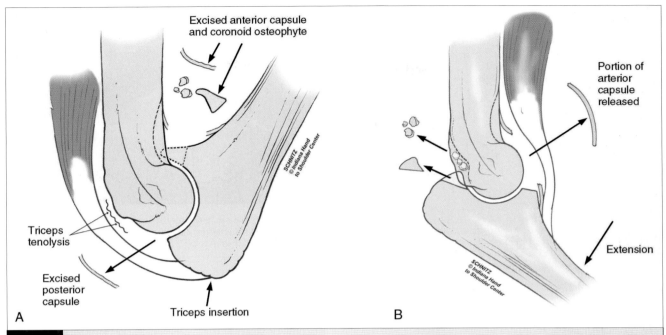

Figure 1 Schematic drawings showing anterior (**A**) and posterior (**B**) capsulectomy and débridement (© G. Schnitz, Indiana Hand to Shoulder Center, Indianapolis, IN.)

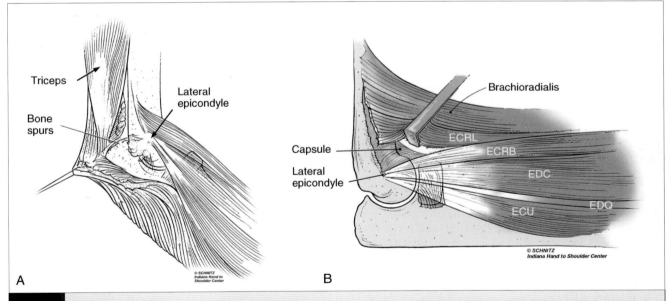

Figure 2 Schematic drawings showing the deep lateral (lateral collateral ligament–preserving) approach. **A,** Posterior exposure. **B,** Anterior exposure. ECRB = extensor carpi radialis brevis, ECRL = extensor carpi radialis longus, ECU = extensor carpi ulnaris, EDC = extensor digitorum communis, EDQ = extensor digiti quinti. (© G. Schnitz, Indiana Hand to Shoulder Center, Indianapolis, IN.)

ally will be needed. Elevation of flaps to obtain medial and lateral deep exposure usually carries a greater chance of seroma formation than separate medial and lateral incisions. Regardless of the approach, it is important to protect and avoid injury to the medial brachiocutaneous, ulnar, median, radial, posterior interosseous, and median nerves during all dissections and releases.

The deep lateral approach, described initially as the lateral collateral ligament–preserving approach and subsequently as the column procedure, consists of open arthrolysis through a limited (6-cm) skin incision through the proximal aspect of a standard Kocher interval[10-12] (**Figure 2**). Dissection is carried down to the lateral column of the humerus. The triceps and the

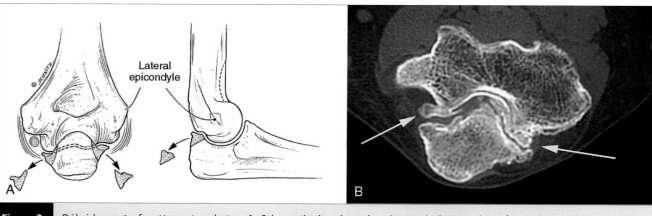

Figure 3 Débridement of gutter osteophytes. **A,** Schematic drawings showing typical osteophyte formations on the medial, lateral, and posterior aspects of the olecranon and proximal ulna. **B,** CT showing large medial and lateral gutter osteophytes *(arrows)*. (© G. Schnitz, Indiana Hand to Shoulder Center, Indianapolis, IN.)

most proximal portion of the anconeus are reflected posteriorly to expose the olecranon, the olecranon fossa, and the lateral gutter (lateral ulnohumeral joint). The posterior capsule and scar are excised. The fossa is cleared of loose bodies, bone, and scar, and areas of bony overgrowth on the humerus and the olecranon are excised. The capsule can be excised from the soft area proximal and posterior to the radiocapitellar joint to inspect the radial head and excise proliferative synovitis. Any osteophytes on the posterior capitellum or the lateral olecranon that may be blocking extension are removed (**Figure 3**).

Anteriorly, exposure is obtained by reflecting the distalmost brachioradialis and extensor carpi radialis longus muscle origins from the supracondylar ridge of the humerus and distally splitting for 2 to 3 cm between the extensor carpi radialis longus and the extensor carpi radialis brevis distal to the lateral epicondyle. This distal extension facilitates exposure and can be used as needed to release the proximal supinator for decompression of the posterior interosseous nerve. At this point, the coronoid, olecranon, and radial fossae are débrided, osteophytes are resected, and loose bodies are removed. It is essential to restore a capacious coronoid fossa and capitellar recess with respect to depth and width. The elbow is manipulated first by extending and then flexing the elbow under direct visualization, using firm pressure on the proximal forearm. In long-standing contractures, the brachialis and triceps muscles typically have undergone myostatic contraction and can limit full terminal elbow extension and flexion, which can be stretched at the time of surgical release.

The advantages of the lateral approach include its simplicity, the use of a muscular plane that allows superficial sensory nerves to be avoided, and access to all three joint articulations. The lateral approach is limited, however, because it does not allow the posteromedial capsule and the ulnar nerve to be treated. A separate limited medial approach may be necessary for complete release in some patients and for simple de-

compression of the ulnar nerve. This approach usually involves a 3- to 5-cm posteromedial incision for in situ cubital tunnel release. If the ulnar nerve is not transposed, posteromedial olecranon residual osteophytes are exposed and débrided through a longitudinal incision in the medial triceps 1.5 cm posterior to the ulnar nerve.

A conceptually similar medial approach (Hotchkiss) is chosen if there is substantial ulnar nerve pathology that requires anterior transposition.[12] A medial or posterior incision is made to expose the flexor-pronator origin (**Figure 4**). The medial antebrachial cutaneous nerve is protected, and the ulnar nerve is released, mobilized, and transposed anteriorly. The triceps is elevated posteriorly from the intermuscular septum and the humerus to expose the posteromedial joint. The posterior capsule, including the posterior band of the medial collateral ligament, is released with care to preserve and protect the important and more distal anterior band of the medial collateral ligament. The posterior joint and olecranon fossa then can be further débrided. The flexor pronator origin is longitudinally incised, and the anterior two thirds are reflected from the medial epicondyle. The brachialis and the anterior portion of the flexor pronator mass are reflected from the medial humerus to expose the anterior capsule. The capsule is excised, and the coronoid and radial fossa are débrided. Enlarged or overgrown portions of the coronoid are excised. At this point, the elbow can be manipulated.

The advantages of the medial approach include the less visible postoperative scar, the ability to expose and decompress the ulnar nerve, and access for a direct release of the posterior band of the ulnar collateral ligament. The medial approach is limited because it does not facilitate exposure of common lateral pathology. The limitations of both the medial and lateral approaches, especially in patients with considerable heterotopic ossification, have led to the use of a combined medial and lateral approach. The outcomes of elbow

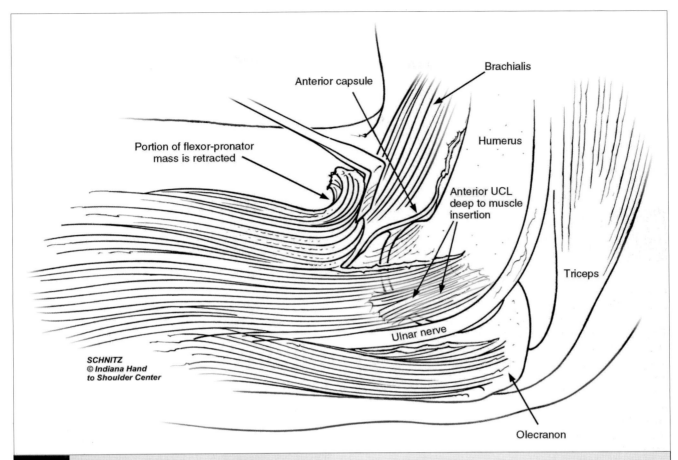

Figure 4	Schematic drawing showing the medial Hotchkiss approach. An anterior exposure through the flexor-pronator mass is used to gain access to the contracted anterior capsule. Care must be taken to preserve the anterior band of the ulnar collateral ligament (UCL). (© G. Schnitz, Indiana Hand to Shoulder Center, Indianapolis, IN.)

contracture release are better if there is a discrete mechanical (osseous) block to motion rather than soft-tissue contracture alone.[13,14]

Heterotopic Ossification

Heterotopic ossification of the elbow most often occurs after direct joint trauma, surgery, burns, or traumatic brain injury. Its development appears to be partially related to the severity of the injury and the time between injury and surgery. It has been reported to occur in approximately 3% of simple elbow dislocations and as many as 20% of periarticular fracture-dislocations.[15] After a closed head injury associated with elbow trauma, heterotopic ossification was documented to occur in 75% to 89% of patients.[11] Although heterotopic ossification around the elbow begins with the inciting insult, it is clinically manifested 2 to 12 weeks later. The initial findings include local soft-tissue swelling, tenderness, and warmth followed by progressive loss of elbow motion. Heterotopic ossification may be mistaken for infection during the perisurgical period. Its lo-

calized or diffuse pattern of formation may not follow anatomic tissue planes. The end points of elbow motion become rigid rather than compliant, as in soft-tissue contracture. Pain typically occurs with terminal flexion and/or extension rather than at the mid-arc of motion, as is indicative of joint incongruity or arthrosis. The classification system of Hastings and Graham is useful for defining surgical planning and treatment[16] (**Table 2**).

The maturity of the bone and the time since bone production onset are important factors in evaluating heterotopic ossification and considering surgical intervention. In the past, laboratory studies (serum calcium, inorganic phosphate, and alkaline phosphatase) and technetium bone scans were used to follow the progression of heterotopic ossification. The prognostic value of these tests has not been proven, and they are no longer used for evaluation.[17,18] Plain radiography is the most effective means of evaluating for heterotopic ossification and following its progression. In patients with extensive ectopic bone formation, CT, particularly CT with three-dimensional reconstruction, can be useful for defining the geometry of ectopic bone formation, assessing ulnohumeral joint congruity, and planning the

Table 2

The Classification of Heterotopic Ossification

Class	Characteristics
I	Clinically insignificant
	No functional elbow motion limitation
II	Functional limitation to elbow motion
IIA	Ulnohumeral motion plane deficit smaller than 100°
	Flexion arc from 30° to 130°
IIB	Forearm rotation motion plane deficit smaller than 100°
	Arc from 50° pronation to 50° supination
IIC	Motion deficits in both ulnohumeral and forearm rotation planes
III	Elbow joint ankylosis
IIIA	Ulnohumeral motion plane
IIIB	Forearm rotation plane
IIIC	Both ulnohumeral and forearm rotation planes

direction of surgical exposure. Within 4 to 6 weeks of the onset of heterotopic ossification, ill-defined fluffy periarticular densities can be identified radiographically. Over time, the margins become more distinct, and trabeculae appear. Smooth, well-demarcated cortical margins, the defining characteristic of radiographic maturity, typically do not appear for 3 to 6 months.[8] In most patients, surgical excision can be safely performed when the extent of heterotopic bone can be seen radiographically; it is not necessary to wait until full maturation. Early surgical intervention may be beneficial to limit capsular and ligamentous contracture, muscular atrophy, and cartilage degeneration, and it may be technically easier than later intervention.

Prevention of heterotopic ossification is key because there is no effective medical treatment. Bisphosphonate therapy was formerly used but was found to merely delay the mineralization of ectopic bone.[11] Prophylaxis consists of NSAIDs, such as indomethacin, ibuprofen, naproxen, or aspirin, and low-dosage external beam radiation. NSAIDs are effective if begun within 3 to 5 days of the inciting traumatic event. The treatment duration is controversial and ranges between 5 days and 6 weeks.[19] These agents work by inhibiting prostaglandin formation, and experimentally they have been found to inhibit stem cell differentiation and migration. Low-dosage external beam radiation therapy is administered using a limited-field technique, in a single dose of 600 to 700 cGy within 72 hours of surgery or trauma. The radiation therapy works by inhibiting the differentiation of stem cells.[16] Treatment with radia-

tion, NSAIDs, or both has been proven safe and effective for preventing heterotopic ossification after surgical contracture release.[16] Results have been mixed after acute elbow trauma, however. Multiple studies found the treatment to be safe and efficacious,[20,21] but a recent prospective randomized study was stopped because of increased rates of nonunion at fracture and olecranon osteotomy sites.[22]

Anteriorly located heterotopic ossification can be surgically resected using a medial, lateral, or combined approach. Anterior heterotopic ossification most commonly forms beneath the brachialis muscle and appears to be separated from the anterior articular surface by a radiolucent area. In contrast, posterior heterotopic ossification often forms in continuity with the articular surface beneath the triceps tendon. Care must be taken during resection to identify and protect the nearby radial, posterior interosseous, and median nerves. Burrs, curets, osteotomes, and rongeurs typically are used to excise the bone. Because of the continuity of posterior bone with the joint surface, partial or complete elevation of the triceps from the olecranon is required. The ulnar nerve can be intimately involved and must be located and protected. Extensive restriction from heterotopic ossification is not necessarily a negative prognostic factor; a recent study found comparable postoperative motion in completely ankylosed elbows and those with a partial motion restriction.[23]

Salvage Procedures

Elbow contracture release alone is contraindicated if the patient's elbow stiffness is associated with articular incongruity or arthrosis. In these patients, a salvage procedure typically is required for augmenting or replacing the damaged joint surface. Interposition arthroplasty is recommended to restore function and relieve pain in a patient who is physiologically young and has high physical demands. The goal of interposition arthroplasty is to improve and preserve functional stability and prevent reankylosis by placing a resurfacing material between the resected bone ends. Various interposition materials have been used to resurface the ulnohumeral joint, including fascia lata, cutis graft, Achilles tendon allograft, regenerative tissue matrix (AlloDerm [LifeCell]), bovine collagen, absorbable gelatin foam (Gelfoam [Pfizer]), and silicone. Patients with elbow instability have had poor results despite attempts at collateral ligament reconstruction.[24,25] A hinged external fixator can be used postoperatively to provide sufficient stability for soft-tissue healing without limiting early motion.[26] The use of external fixation to provide distraction on the interposed tissue had satisfactory results in 69% to 92% of patients by minimizing the load on the interposition material during early postoperative motion.[24,25,27] The complications can be significant and include bone resorption, nerve dysfunction, heterotopic ossification, triceps rupture, instability, and infection.

In patients who are older than approximately 60 years and have relatively low physical demands, hemiarthroplasty or total elbow arthroplasty should be considered for treating elbow contracture or arthrosis. Because such a patient may have poor bone stock, deformity, and capsuloligamentous instability, the use of a semiconstrained implant is recommended.[28] The surgical technique can be challenging because of anatomic distortion, and complications are likely, including mechanical failure, loosening, problematic wound healing, infection, triceps disruption, and fracture.[26] Despite these concerns, substantial functional improvement and pain relief can be expected.[27]

Postoperative Care

Numerous effective postoperative treatment programs have been described for patients who have undergone elbow contracture release surgery. The overall goals are to maintain a functional arc of motion, strengthen the muscles around the elbow, and reincorporate extremity use into functional activities.[1] Range-of-motion exercises are initiated postoperatively, with judicious use of regional anesthetic blockade, formal therapy, continuous passive motion, and/or static progressive splinting. Regional blockade is useful for immediate postoperative pain control and can facilitate the initiation of functional range-of-motion exercises. The use of continuous passive motion remains controversial; numerous authors have recommended this treatment despite the limited, low-level scientific evidence to support its use. A recent study examined the use of continuous passive motion in a matched split cohort of 32 patients after open elbow contracture release.[29] There was no demonstrable benefit to continuous passive motion in the postoperative management of contracture release at 6-month or final follow-up. The flexion-extension arc of motion improved a statistically nonsignificant average of 96° or 101° in the two groups.

The postoperative rehabilitation regimen should be continued until a plateau in motion has been reached, typically at 3 to 6 months. If the patient's functional range of motion continues to be limited, formal manipulation under anesthesia has been described; however, few studies have documented an improved range of motion without complications. A recently described examination under anesthesia, consisting of an evaluation of passive motion arc, gentle manipulation in extension and flexion; evaluation of joint stability; and an assessment of smoothness of motion arc for crepitus, catching or other surface irregularities, was performed in 51 patients at a mean 40 days after surgical release.[30] An average of 36° improved arc of motion was noted, with no permanent complications. The intent of this procedure is to overcome adhesions and contractures, thereby enhancing elbow motion, in patients undergoing external fixator removal or patients who have had limited progress in the first weeks after surgical release.

Summary

The elbow joint is of critical importance to overall upper extremity function. Its high degree of constraint and associated soft tissues predisposes it for the development of stiffness and contracture. Recent basic science and clinical research has shed light on the etiology and treatment options, although many questions remain unanswered. The prevention of elbow stiffness remains of paramount importance. Patient selection is essential when surgical intervention is being considered because the outcome partially depends on the patient's willingness and ability to participate in postoperative rehabilitation. In a properly selected patient, surgical release and débridement can restore a functional arc of elbow motion.

Annotated References

1. Modabber MR, Jupiter JB: Reconstruction for post-traumatic conditions of the elbow joint. *J Bone Joint Surg Am* 1995;77(9):1431-1446.

2. Morrey BF: Post-traumatic contracture of the elbow: Operative treatment, including distraction arthroplasty. *J Bone Joint Surg Am* 1990;72(4):601-618.

3. Cohen MS, Schimmel DR, Masuda K, Hastings H II, Muehleman C: Structural and biochemical evaluation of the elbow capsule after trauma. *J Shoulder Elbow Surg* 2007;16(4):484-490.

   Contractures around the elbow, particularly capsular and ligamentous, play a critical role in the development of arthrofibrosis secondary to structural and biochemical alterations. Traumatic injury was found to lead to capsular thickening, collagen fiber disorganization, and increased cytokine levels.

4. Hildebrand KA, Zhang M, Hart DA: Myofibroblast upregulators are elevated in joint capsules in posttraumatic contractures. *Clin Orthop Relat Res* 2007;456: 85-91.

   Growth factor mRNA levels in joint capsules of patients with posttraumatic elbow contracture were compared with those of organ donor control tissues. Increased myofibroblast upregulator levels (transforming growth factor–β1, connective tissue growth factor, and α-smooth muscle actin) were found.

5. Hildebrand KA, Zhang M, van Snellenberg W, King GJ, Hart DA: Myofibroblast numbers are elevated in human elbow capsules after trauma. *Clin Orthop Relat Res* 2004;419:189-197.

6. Unterhauser FN, Bosch U, Zeichen J, Weiler A: Alpha-smooth muscle actin containing contractile fibroblastic cells in human knee arthrofibrosis tissue: Winner of the AGA-DonJoy Award 2003. *Arch Orthop Trauma Surg* 2004;124(9):585-591.

7: Elbow Trauma, Fracture, and Reconstruction

7. Hildebrand KA, Zhang M, Hart DA: High rate of joint capsule matrix turnover in chronic human elbow contractures. *Clin Orthop Relat Res* 2005;439: 228-234.

8. Viola RW, Hastings H II: Treatment of ectopic ossification about the elbow. *Clin Orthop Relat Res* 2000; 370:65-86.

9. Summerfield SL, DiGiovanni C, Weiss AP: Heterotopic ossification of the elbow. *J Shoulder Elbow Surg* 1997; 6(3):321-332.

10. Cohen MS, Hastings H II: Post-traumatic contracture of the elbow: Operative release using a lateral collateral ligament sparing approach. *J Bone Joint Surg Br* 1998;80(5):805-812.

11. Cohen MS, Hastings H II: Operative release for elbow contracture: The lateral collateral ligament sparing technique. *Orthop Clin North Am* 1999;30(1): 133-139.

12. Mansat P, Morrey BF: The column procedure: A limited lateral approach for extrinsic contracture of the elbow. *J Bone Joint Surg Am* 1998;80(11):1603-1615.

13. Jupiter JB, O'Driscoll SW, Cohen MS: The assessment and management of the stiff elbow. *Instr Course Lect* 2003;52:93-111.

14. Kasparyan NG, Hotchkiss RN: Dynamic skeletal fixation in the upper extremity. *Hand Clin* 1997;13(4): 643-663.

15. Thompson HC III, Garcia A: Myositis ossificans: Aftermath of elbow injuries. *Clin Orthop Relat Res* 1967;50:129-134.

16. Hastings H II, Graham TJ: The classification and treatment of heterotopic ossification about the elbow and forearm. *Hand Clin* 1994;10(3):417-437.

17. Lindenhovius AL, Linzel DS, Doornberg JN, Ring DC, Jupiter JB: Comparison of elbow contracture release in elbows with and without heterotopic ossification restricting motion. *J Shoulder Elbow Surg* 2007;16(5): 621-625.

   Sixteen patients with elbow contracture and posttraumatic heterotopic ossification were compared with 21 patients with capsular contracture alone. The average flexion-extension arc for contractures with associated heterotopic bone was 116° compared with 98° for capsular contracture alone. Level of evidence: III.

18. Park MJ, Kim HG, Lee JY: Surgical treatment of posttraumatic stiffness of the elbow. *J Bone Joint Surg Br* 2004;86(8):1158-1162.

19. McAuliffe JA, Wolfson AH: Early excision of heterotopic ossification about the elbow followed by radiation therapy. *J Bone Joint Surg Am* 1997;79(5): 749-755.

20. Ellerin BE, Helfet D, Parikh S, et al: Current therapy in the management of heterotopic ossification of the elbow: A review with case studies. *Am J Phys Med Rehabil* 1999;78(3):259-271.

21. Strauss JB, Wysocki RW, Shah A, et al: Radiation therapy for heterotopic ossification prophylaxis afer high-risk elbow surgery. *Am J Orthop (Belle Mead NJ)* 2011;40(8):400-405.

   A retrospective study analyzed the outcomes of prophylactic single-fraction radiotherapy and NSAID use for preventing heterotopic ossification in high-risk elbow surgery. At a mean 136-day follow-up, radiographic heterotopic ossification that was small and not functionally significant had developed in 48% of the patients. No complications were noted. Level of evidence: IV.

22. Hamid N, Ashraf N, Bosse MJ, et al: Radiation therapy for heterotopic ossification prophylaxis acutely after elbow trauma: A prospective randomized study. *J Bone Joint Surg Am* 2010;92(11):2032-2038.

   A multicenter prospective randomized study compared prophylactic radiotherapy with no treatment after intra-articular distal humerus or elbow fracture-dislocation. The study was terminated early because of the high nonunion rate in the treated patients (38%) versus the control group patients (4%).

23. Brouwer KM, Lindenhovius AL, de Witte PB, Jupiter JB, Ring D: Resection of heterotopic ossification of the elbow: A comparison of ankylosis and partial restriction. *J Hand Surg Am* 2010;35(7):1115-1119.

   Eighteen patients with surgical release of complete elbow ankylosis were compared with 27 matched patients with partial restriction of motion by heterotopic bone. At an average 22-month follow-up, range of motion and outcomes scores were similar. Level of evidence: III.

24. Larson AN, Morrey BF: Interposition arthroplasty with an Achilles tendon allograft as a salvage procedure for the elbow. *J Bone Joint Surg Am* 2008;90(12): 2714-2723.

   Thirty-four elbows were evaluated at a mean 6-year follow-up after interposition arthroplasty for treatment of inflammatory or posttraumatic elbow arthritis. Patients with preoperative instability had a poor result. Thirteen patients had a good or excellent result, 14 had a fair result, and 11 had a poor result. Seven underwent revision. Level of evidence: IV.

25. Cheng SL, Morrey BF: Treatment of the mobile, painful arthritic elbow by distraction interposition arthroplasty. *J Bone Joint Surg Br* 2000;82(2):233-238.

26. Ring D, Jupiter JB: Operative release of complete ankylosis of the elbow due to heterotopic bone in patients without severe injury of the central nervous system. *J Bone Joint Surg Am* 2003;85(5):849-857.

27. Nolla J, Ring D, Lozano-Calderon S, Jupiter JB: Interposition arthroplasty of the elbow with hinged exter-

nal fixation for post-traumatic arthritis. *J Shoulder Elbow Surg* 2008;17(3):459-464.

In a review of 13 patients with posttraumatic elbow arthritis treated with interposition arthroplasty and hinged external fixation, 2 patients had early instability. The remaining 11 were followed for a mean of 4 years. Mean range of motion improved 48° to 110°, with five good or excellent, four fair, and four poor results. The poor results were secondary to severe postoperative instability. Level of evidence: IV.

28. Mansat P, Morrey BF: Semiconstrained total elbow arthroplasty for ankylosed and stiff elbows. *J Bone Joint Surg Am* 2000;82(9):1260-1268.

29. Lindenhovius AL, van de Luijtgaarden K, Ring D, Jupiter J: Open elbow contracture release: Postoperative management with and without continuous passive motion. *J Hand Surg Am* 2009;34(5):858-865.

A retrospective study compared 16 patients who received continuous passive motion after open elbow contracture release with 16 patients who did not use continuous passive motion. At an average 6-month follow-up, there was no difference in range of motion or other benefits. Level of evidence: III.

30. Araghi A, Celli A, Adams RA, Morrey BF: The outcome of examination (manipulation) under anesthesia on the stiff elbow after surgical contracture release. *J Shoulder Elbow Surg* 2010;19(2):202-208.

In 51 patients who underwent elbow examination under anesthesia a mean 40 days after open elbow contracture release, the range-of-motion arc improved an average of 38°, with 44 patients showing improvement, 3 with no change, and 1 with loss of motion. Level of evidence: IV.

7: Elbow Trauma, Fracture, and Reconstruction

Chapter 43

Elbow Arthritis

Julie Adams, MD   Scott P. Steinmann, MD

Introduction

Elbow arthritis continues to be a challenging condition to treat. Rheumatoid arthritis and other inflammatory arthritides formerly were the most common forms of arthritis requiring surgical management. These conditions are becoming less symptomatic because of the advent and widespread use of disease-modifying antirheumatic drugs, which have been successful in limiting symptomatic joint changes in many patients. However, osteoarthritis and posttraumatic arthritis continue to be problematic conditions. Patients with hemophilia also can be affected by elbow arthritis. Although the lives of these patients have been prolonged and improved by the widespread use of blood factor replacement, persistent subclinical or clinical instances of bleeding in the elbow may set off changes that can develop into arthrosis.

The changing epidemiology of the disease has led to a conundrum. Previously, most patients with symptomatic arthritis of the elbow who required surgical treatment were of advanced age and had low physical demands, often because of rheumatoid arthritis. Currently, many patients with symptomatic arthritis are relatively young and healthy, and they expect to live long and active lives. These patients may not be amenable to complying with the typical restrictions after total elbow arthroplasty (TEA). The implants used for the treatment of rheumatoid arthritis were designed for low activity levels and may not be optimal for a patient with higher demands. Recent strategies have focused on alternative procedures or implants for such patients.

Nonsurgical Treatment

The nonsurgical treatment for all types of arthrosis of the elbow includes rest, bracing, NSAIDs or oral analgesics, and injectable corticosteroids and hyaluronic acid. No benefit was seen 6 months after hyaluronic acid injection in the elbow joint.[1] A short-term benefit may be seen, as in other joints, but it may represent an anti-inflammatory effect.

Disease-modifying agents have altered the management of rheumatoid arthritis in the past few decades. Previously, a combination of NSAIDs and analgesics was used to reduce symptoms. The use of disease-modifying antirheumatic drugs has altered the course of disease treatment. These drugs are effective in reducing synovitis and systemic inflammation and in altering the course of joint destruction. Methotrexate, sulfasalazine, and leflunomide often are prescribed soon after diagnosis, and they may be used in combination. Corticosteroids often are used in the short term to alter joint inflammation or in the long term as an adjunctive treatment. The recent introduction of biologic agents to alter the inflammatory cascade in rheumatoid arthritis has revolutionized the treatment of this condition by targeting cytokines responsible for potentiating the disease process. The biologic drugs include tumor necrosis factor inhibitors such as adalimumab, etanercept, infliximab, certolizumab, and golimumab; interleukin-6 inhibitors such as tocilizumab; B-cell inhibitors such as rituximab; and T-cell costimulation inhibitors such as abatacept. These drugs can alter a patient's ability to mount an immune response to infection. Concern exists regarding the long-term effects of immunogenicity as well as the activation of latent viral infection and an increased risk of malignancy. To enhance surgical healing, most experts recommend discontinuing the use of these biologic agents for several half-lives before a planned procedure.[2]

The frequency and severity of intra-articular bleeding into the elbow in patients with hemophilic arthropathy may be decreased by the use of prophylactic and on-demand blood factor replacement. This treatment may limit synovitis and joint destruction in the long term and provide short-term symptomatic relief.[3]

Dr. Adams or an immediate family member has received royalties from DePuy; serves as a paid consultant to or is an employee of Arthrex, DePuy, and Articulinx; serves as an unpaid consultant to Synthes; and serves as a board member, owner, officer, or committee member of the American Association for Hand Surgery, the Minnesota Orthopaedic Society, the American Shoulder and Elbow Surgeons, the American Society for Surgery of the Hand, and the Arthroscopy Association of North America. Dr. Steinmann or an immediate family member has received royalties from DePuy; serves as a paid consultant to or is an employee of Arthrex, DePuy, and Articulinx; serves as an unpaid consultant to Synthes; and serves as a board member, owner, officer, or committee member of the American Association for Hand Surgery, the Minnesota Orthopaedic Society, the American Shoulder and Elbow Surgeons, the American Society for Surgery of the Hand, and the Arthroscopy Association of North America.

Primary degenerative osteoarthritis of the elbow typically involves the dominant arm in men who have a history of manual labor. The use of crutches or a wheelchair for ambulation also increases the risk of primary degenerative osteoarthritis of the elbow. Most patients are older than 40 to 50 years and have mechanical symptoms, including catching and locking of the joint, symptomatic loose bodies, and lack of motion, particularly in terminal extension. The patient often describes pain at the ends of the arc of motion, although in advanced disease the pain exists throughout the arc of motion, indicating severe articular changes that may not be treatable with simple débridement.

Evaluation

A patient with arthrosis of the elbow often has a concomitant cubital tunnel syndrome. It is important to specifically ask about symptoms and examine the patient with this condition in mind. The patient's symptoms sometimes are nerve related rather than explained by obvious radiographic findings. Plain radiographs in three views are helpful for the diagnosis. The osseous anatomy and subchondral cysts can be delineated on CT scans. CT with three-dimensional reconstruction is most helpful for understanding the three-dimensional anatomy, developing a surgical plan, and appropriately treating all areas of interest.

Surgical Options

Surgical intervention may be considered for a patient who has functional limitations after unsuccessful nonsurgical management. The factors in determining the appropriate surgical treatment include the patient's activity level and age, the patient's preferences, the surgeon's experience and preference, and the extent of pathologic changes.

Open and arthroscopic débridement and synovectomy are effective treatment options for rheumatoid arthritis, osteoarthritis, posttraumatic arthritis, and hemophilic arthropathy. These procedures are most effective during earlier disease stages, before the joint space and the cartilage are totally obliterated. Synovectomy may delay disease progression and reduce the incidence of painful synovitis in inflammatory arthritis or symptomatic bleeding episodes in hemophilia. Arthroscopic débridement may be considered desirable because it is perceived to be minimally invasive and requires a shorter, less painful recovery period than open débridement. However, the outcomes of arthroscopic débridement have not been shown to be superior to those of open débridement, and the risks of arthroscopy may be greater than those of traditional open surgery. Open débridement is preferred if the surgeon lacks arthroscopic experience, the patient has very restricted motion, or a concomitant open procedure will

be needed (although there is evidence that decompression of the ulnar nerve can be accomplished arthroscopically in selected patients).[4,5]

The approach for an open débridement can include a medial incision, a lateral incision, or both, depending on the pathology and the preference of the surgeon. A single posterior incision can be used, with the creation of full-thickness flaps to the medial and lateral sides. This approach necessitates a larger incision that can lead to seromas or wound complications.

TEA is a definitive means of improving pain and function in an arthritic elbow. However, TEA limits the use of the arm to light activity, and this restriction can be devastating for a young or an active patient. Therefore, TEA may be undesirable for such a patient.

Other options are being sought to alleviate pain while preserving extensive use of the arm. Interposition arthroplasty has been suggested as such an option. A variety of materials have been used for interposition arthroplasty, including allograft and autograft dermis, Achilles tendon, and fascia lata. Outcomes of interposition arthroplasty were reported at a mean 6-year follow-up.[6] Thirty-two of the 45 patients required revision surgery or had poor or fair results. Preoperative instability was associated with a relatively poor outcome. Several factors have been described as leading to a successful outcome after interposition arthroplasty, including preserved elbow stability, relatively well-preserved bony anatomy, intraoperative adequacy of joint release, stable resurfacing, and careful wound closure and management.[7] The patient should understand that improved motion and pain relief are the goals, but absolute improvement should not be expected.

Elbow Hemiarthroplasty and Arthroplasty

Humeral hemiarthroplasty of the elbow may be considered in selected patients (**Figure 1**). Most of the published reports are of single patients or small studies. However, the recent increased interest in this technique suggests that additional outcomes data are forthcoming. Hemiarthroplasty may be indicated for a patient with rheumatoid arthritis who wishes to remain active and has preserved humeral and ulnar bone stock, a patient with an unreconstructable distal humeral fracture with preserved ulnar articulation, or a patient with nonunion or unsuccessful fixation of a distal humeral fracture. Early results were promising after hemiarthroplasty with a Kudo humeral component (Biomet) for unreconstructable distal humeral fracture in four patients (mean age, 80 years).[8] At a mean 4-year follow-up after hemiarthroplasty, eight women (mean age, 79 years) had a good to excellent Mayo Elbow Performance Score.[9] One patient had a periprosthetic fracture at 3 years, and another patient had an unsatisfactory range of motion. Radiographs revealed ulnar arthritic changes, but these were not correlated with functional outcomes. One report described outcomes of hemiarthroplasty of the elbow for a comminuted distal humeral fracture in 10 women (mean age, 75 years).[10]

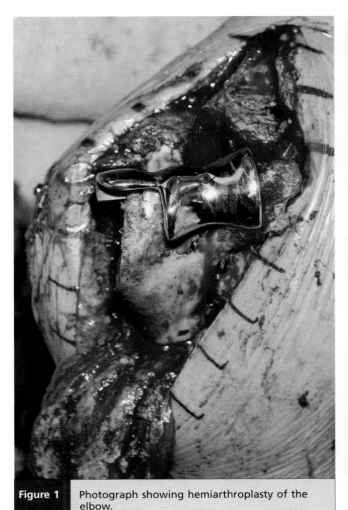

Figure 1 Photograph showing hemiarthroplasty of the elbow.

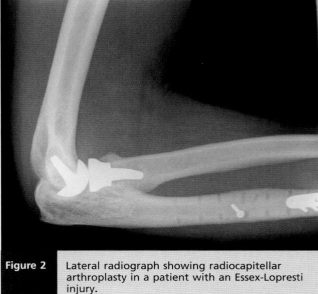

Figure 2 Lateral radiograph showing radiocapitellar arthroplasty in a patient with an Essex-Lopresti injury.

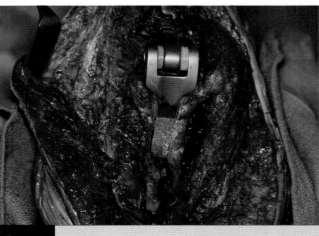

Figure 3 Photograph showing linked total elbow arthroplasty.

At 1-year follow-up, 9 patients had a good to excellent Mayo Elbow Performance Score. There were five complications, most of which were minor, including transient ulnar nerve irritation, heterotopic ossification, and arthrosis at the ulna. The use of a humeral component without an ulnar component, as in hemiarthroplasty, has not been approved by the FDA and is considered an off-label use.

Hemiarthroplasty of the lateral compartment of the elbow has been performed in selected patients (Figure 2). This procedure may be indicated for a patient with an Essex-Lopresti injury or a radial head fracture in association with articular impaction or a shear injury of the capitellum.[11] After an Essex-Lopresti injury, the native capitellar cartilage may not withstand surgical impaction of the radial neck, but a metallic articulation may be tolerated. Few reports have been published on the use of this procedure.[11,12]

Convertible prostheses recently have become available. One implant allows conversion from distal humeral hemiarthroplasty to unlinked or linked TEA without removal of the humeral component. Outcomes studies of these procedures are limited, but the outcomes of revision of unlinked TEA have been published.[12] Results were better after an unlinked prosthesis was revised to a linked prosthesis rather than to a second unlinked device, and overall survival was better when a primary procedure included a linked device rather than an unlinked device. However, the devices used in this study were older types, not the newer, currently available types of prostheses.[12,13]

Linked TEA is an acceptable option for a patient who is willing to comply with the severe restrictions placed on the activity of the arm (Figure 3). Patients who are relatively young must anticipate the need for revision of the prosthesis, and all patients must understand the high rate of complications associated with the procedure.[14,15]

Complications of TEA were studied in patients identified from a California discharge database.[16] High rates of short-term complications requiring inpatient treatment (10%) or reoperation within 90 days of the initial prosthesis placement (8%) were reported. At a mean 4-year follow-up, 120 of the 170 patients had undergone revision, amputation, or fusion; 48 of these patients required revision within 12 months. These study results should temper enthusiasm for prosthesis placement. Nonetheless, the increased use of TEA recently was reported in a study of data from New York state.[17] Between 1997 and 2006, the use of TEA increased for patients with traumatic injury and greatly decreased for those with inflammatory arthritis. Within 90 days of the procedure, 5.6% of the patients required hospital readmission for a prosthesis-rated complication. Revision rates were higher for patients who underwent a procedure for osteoarthritis (14.7%) rather than for trauma (4.8%) or inflammatory arthritis (8.3%). Revision may be required because of infection, bushing failure, fracture, or aseptic loosening. The failure of linked (semiconstrained) devices may be associated with the high demands the constraint places on the implant, which may be greatest in patients with posttraumatic arthritis or osteoarthritis.[18] A study of patients who underwent semiconstrained TEA for posttraumatic changes found a 70% survival rate at 15-year follow-up; 65% of the unsuccessful TEAs were in patients younger than 60 years. The use of unlinked implants may improve the durability of elbow arthroplasty, and further studies may provide additional information.[13,19]

Elbow Arthrodesis

Elbow arthrodesis is an option for the arthritic elbow if the patient is not a candidate for joint arthroplasty or if a salvage procedure is required after unsuccessful elbow arthroplasty. Most of the available studies are small. Elbow arthrodesis causes profound functional limitations, and some believe there is no good position for elbow fusion. Before planned, elective elbow arthrodesis, using casting to simulate the possible positions of fusion so that the patient can select the position allowing the best function, is often worthwhile. Typically, the patient must choose between functional positioning of the arm for general activity or for bringing the hand to the mouth. One experienced surgeon's study of elbow fusion in patients with acute trauma or posttraumatic arthritis found that 10 of 12 patients required an additional procedure, 42% of the elbows had nonunion or delayed union, and infection developed in 33% of the elbows. The report states, "For the most part, this is a procedure of last resort and should be performed when no other options . . . exist."[20]

Summary

Elbow arthritis can be challenging to treat. The surgical options continue to evolve, but many procedures still sacrifice durability or function in favor of pain relief.

Careful consideration of patient-specific and disease-specific factors is critical to successfully treating a patient with elbow arthritis.

Annotated References

1. van Brakel RW, Eygendaal D: Intra-articular injection of hyaluronic acid is not effective for the treatment of post-traumatic osteoarthritis of the elbow. *Arthroscopy* 2006;22(11):1199-1203.

2. Scott DL: Biologics-based therapy for the treatment of rheumatoid arthritis. *Clin Pharmacol Ther* 2012;91(1): 30-43.

   The medical treatment options for rheumatoid arthritis were reviewed, including an overview of current therapies and recent advances in treatment.

3. Adams JE, Reding MT: Hemophilic arthropathy of the elbow. *Hand Clin* 2011;27(2):151-163, v.

   Nonsurgical and surgical experience at a large center was described for treatment of the elbow in patients with hemophilia.

4. Kovachevich R, Steinmann SP: Arthroscopic ulnar nerve decompression in the setting of elbow osteoarthritis. *J Hand Surg Am* 2012;37(4):663-668.

   Outcomes were described for arthroscopic ulnar nerve decompression in patients with elbow arthritis. This technique, although technically challenging, was effective for treating symptomatic ulnar neuritis.

5. Adams JE, Wolff LH III, Merten SM, Steinmann SP: Osteoarthritis of the elbow: Results of arthroscopic osteophyte resection and capsulectomy. *J Shoulder Elbow Surg* 2008;17(1):126-131.

   Outcomes were described for elbow arthroscopy in patients with primary osteoarthritis of the elbow. Improvement in range of motion and pain was noted, with a low complication rate.

6. Larson AN, Morrey BF: Interposition arthroplasty with an Achilles tendon allograft as a salvage procedure for the elbow. *J Bone Joint Surg Am* 2008;90(12): 2714-2723.

   At a mean 6-year follow-up of interposition arthroplasty with Achilles tendon allograft in 45 elbows with posttraumatic or inflammatory arthritis, the average arc of motion had increased from 51° to 97° in surviving implants. Seven patients (15.5%) required revision surgery; 11 of the remaining patients (29%) had a poor result, and 14 (37%) had a fair result. Preoperative instability should be an exclusion criterion.

7. Chen DD, Forsh DA, Hausman MR: Elbow interposition arthroplasty. *Hand Clin* 2011;27(2):187-197, vi.

   Interposition arthroplasty of the elbow with a biologic material was described, with tips and techniques for the procedure as well as a discussion of patient selection factors.

8. Adolfsson L, Hammer R: Elbow hemiarthroplasty for acute reconstruction of intra-articular distal humerus fractures: A preliminary report involving 4 patients. *Acta Orthop* 2006;77(5):785-787.

9. Adolfsson L, Nestorson J: The Kudo humeral component as primary hemiarthroplasty in distal humeral fractures. *J Shoulder Elbow Surg* 2012;21(4):451-455.

   Eight women were treated with elbow hemiarthroplasty for distal humerus fracture. At a mean 4-year follow-up, all patients had a good or excellent outcome with an average range of motion of 31° to 126°. Radiographic changes occurred in the ulna but were not correlated with symptoms.

10. Burkhart KJ, Nijs S, Mattyasovszky SG, et al: Distal humerus hemiarthroplasty of the elbow for comminuted distal humeral fractures in the elderly patient. *J Trauma* 2011;71(3):635-642.

    Satisfactory short-term outcomes were described for hemiarthroplasty in 10 elderly women to treat osteoporotic or unreconstructable distal humerus fracture or failed fixation. Complications frequently occurred.

11. Heijink A, Morrey BF, Cooney WP III: Radiocapitellar hemiarthroplasty for radiocapitellar arthritis: A report of three cases. *J Shoulder Elbow Surg* 2008;17(2):e12-e15.

    Radiocapitellar replacement arthroplasty was performed in three patients, with an acceptable complication rate.

12. Steinmann SP: Hemiarthroplasty of the ulnohumeral and radiocapitellar joints. *Hand Clin* 2011;27(2):229-232, vi.

    The author's experience with hemiarthroplasty of the distal humerus and the radiocapitellar joint was described, with a literature review and discussion of the available evidence.

13. Levy JC, Loeb M, Chuinard C, Adams RA, Morrey BF: Effectiveness of revision following linked versus unlinked total elbow arthroplasty. *J Shoulder Elbow Surg* 2009;18(3):457-462.

    The outcomes of unlinked and linked arthroplasty were compared. Primary linked arthroplasty implants had longer survival than unlinked implants, but the unlinked implants were mostly of older designs.

14. Celli A, Morrey BF: Total elbow arthroplasty in patients forty years of age or less. *J Bone Joint Surg Am* 2009;91(6):1414-1418.

    At 7-year follow-up, a 22% revision rate was found in young patients undergoing TEA for posttraumatic or inflammatory arthritis. Those with posttraumatic arthritis had a poorer result than those with inflammatory arthritis.

15. Leclerc A, King GJ: Unlinked and convertible total elbow arthroplasty. *Hand Clin* 2011;27(2):215-227, vi.

    The indications and techniques for linked and unlinked arthroplasty were described.

16. Krenek L, Farng E, Zingmond D, SooHoo NF: Complication and revision rates following total elbow arthroplasty. *J Hand Surg Am* 2011;36(1):68-73.

    A comprehensive look at complication and revision rates after TEA was provided in this study of a statewide database.

17. Gay DM, Lyman S, Do H, Hotchkiss RN, Marx RG, Daluiski A: Indications and reoperation rates for total elbow arthroplasty: An analysis of trends in New York State. *J Bone Joint Surg Am* 2012;94(2):110-117.

    An analysis of TEA performed in New York state suggested increasing use for patients with trauma or osteoarthritis and decreasing use for those with inflammatory arthritis. Complication and revision rates were high.

18. Throckmorton T, Zarkadas P, Sanchez-Sotelo J, Morrey B: Failure patterns after linked semiconstrained total elbow arthroplasty for posttraumatic arthritis. *J Bone Joint Surg Am* 2010;92(6):1432-1441.

    TEA with a semiconstrained device was studied in patients with posttraumatic arthritis. The revision rate was high, and revisions were more common in patients younger than 60 years, probably because they placed relatively high demands on the arm. The 15-year survival rate was 70%.

19. Ring D, Kocher M, Koris M, Thornhill TS: Revision of unstable capitellocondylar (unlinked) total elbow replacement. *J Bone Joint Surg Am* 2005;87(5):1075-1079.

20. Reichel LM, Wiater BP, Friedrich J, Hanel DP: Arthrodesis of the elbow. *Hand Clin* 2011;27(2):179-186, vi.

    The results and complications of elbow arthrodesis were discussed.

Chapter 44

Radial Head and Neck Fractures

Albert Yoon, MBChB   Graham J.W. King, MD, MSc, FRCSC

Introduction

Radial head and neck fractures are the most common types of fracture around the elbow, with a combined incidence of 55.4 per 100,000 people per year. Radial head fractures are more common than radial neck fractures.[1] Although earlier studies found radial head fractures to be more common among men, more recent epidemiologic studies found either no sex-based difference in incidence or a 3:2 ratio of women to men.[1,2] The average age of patients with radial head fracture traditionally was reported as 30 to 40 years, but recent studies narrow the age range to an average 43 to 48 years.[1,2]

Nondisplaced fractures of the radial head and neck can be managed nonsurgically, but the treatment of displaced and comminuted fractures of the radial head and neck is controversial. Long-term outcome studies of the treatment options are emerging, and future randomized controlled studies may further guide patient management.

Anatomy and Biomechanics

The radial head has a variably elliptical shape at its concave proximal surface, where it articulates with the convex capitellum to form the radiocapitellar joint, and at its margin, where a slightly flatter portion articulates with the lesser sigmoid notch to form the proximal radioulnar joint. The noncircular anatomy of the radial head and the variable offset of the head from the neck mean that a small amount of translation occurs at both joints during rotation.[3-5] These anatomic features need to be considered in radial head fracture repair or arthroplasty. A safe zone for metalware placement on the rounder, nonarticular margin of the radial head has been described as a 110° arc centered on a point 10° anterior to the lateral aspect of the radial head with the forearm in neutral rotation.[6]

The radial head contributes to the valgus, varus, and posterolateral rotatory stability of the elbow, especially in the presence of associated elbow injury. The radial head also acts as an axial stabilizer of the forearm. Partial excision of radial head fracture fragments can reduce the stabilizing potential of the radial head, and total excision results in transfer of the normal radiocapitellar load transmission forces to the remaining ulnohumeral joint.[7,8]

The main extraosseous blood supply to the radial head is provided by a pericervical arterial ring formed around the radial neck by the radial recurrent artery (supplying the volar, lateral, and dorsal sides), and branches from the ulnar artery. Sequential plastination techniques have shown that this blood supply is more likely to be damaged by internal fixation with plates than by screws alone.[9]

Like other areas of the human skeleton, the microarchitecture of the radial head undergoes age- and sex-related changes.[10] Osteoporotic changes may be responsible for the high proportion of patients who are female and older than 50 years as well as the differences in mechanism of injury and severity between men and women. Women with a radial head fracture had a mean age of 52 years, and a simple fall was the mechanism in 73% of fractures.[1,2] These demographic considerations mean that the fractures met the criteria for fragility fracture, and considerations related to osteoporosis investigation and management therefore were relevant. In contrast, 60% of men with a radial head injury had a high-energy mechanism of injury, and the injury occurred at a younger age (mean, 40 years).[1,2]

Dr. King or an immediate family member serves as a board member, owner, officer, or committee member of the American Shoulder and Elbow Surgeons; has received royalties from Wright Medical Technology, Inc., Tornier, and Tenet Medical; is a member of a speakers' bureau or has made paid presentations on behalf of Wright Medical Technology, Inc.; and serves as a paid consultant to or is an employee of Wright Medical Technology, Inc. Neither Dr. Yoon nor any immediate family member has received anything of value from or has stock or stock options held in a commercial company or institution related directly or indirectly to the subject of this chapter.

Assessment

The patient history should include the mechanism of injury, the level of energy involved, and the likelihood of associated injuries. The patient should be asked about concomitant pain in the shoulder or wrist as well as the presence of an elbow dislocation or a feeling of subluxation at the time of injury. The possibility of a neurovascular injury should be investigated through the history and physical examination. Stability testing of the elbow is difficult in the acute setting because of pain. Palpation of the bony prominences of the elbow and the collateral ligament landmarks may provide clues as to the presence of associated injuries. The assessment of forearm range of motion is important and guides the treatment of a nondisplaced or displaced radial head fracture. If the elbow does not have full rotational movement, it is important to determine whether the pain is from joint hemarthrosis or a mechanical block. Reevaluation in 1 week or aspiration of the intra-articular hemarthrosis under an injected local anesthetic can allow examination for clicking, crepitus, or a mechanical block.

Plain radiographs should be used to evaluate a radial head or neck fracture. The presence of an anterior or posterior fat pad sign should lead to a high level of suspicion for a nondisplaced fracture. Shoulder, forearm, and wrist radiographs may be required depending on the patient history and physical examination findings. CT defines fracture characteristics and associated osseous injuries more accurately than plain radiographs, and MRI is useful for detecting associated ligament injuries.[11,12] The additional information from MRI has not been proved to change treatment, however, and MRI does not need to be routinely used.[13]

Classification

There is poor interobserver agreement regarding the classification of radial head fractures, despite the introduction of CT and three-dimensional reconstruction.[11] Three types of radial head fractures were described by Mason in 1954.[14] A type I fracture is a marginal sector or fissure fracture without displacement, a type II fracture is a marginal sector fracture with displacement, and a type III fracture is a comminuted fracture involving the entire radial head. A type IV fracture, as added by Johnston in 1962, is any fracture of the radial head associated with an elbow dislocation; type IV does not classify the injury sustained by the radial head itself.[15] Broberg and Morrey modified the original Mason classification to clarify the difference between types I and II by describing type II as displaced more than 2 mm and involving more than 30% of the articular surface.[16] Radial neck fractures also were included in this modification. In a further modification (the Mayo-Mason classification), a suffix is used to denote an associated bony, ligamentous, or dislocation injury.[17]

Associated Injuries

Associated injuries can be related to patient age, mechanism of injury, or fracture complexity.[1] A recent study found that 35 of 46 elbows with a radial head fracture (76%) had an associated injury on MRI.[12] All six Mason type III radial head fractures had associated injury (six lateral collateral ligament [LCL], one medial collat-

eral ligament [MCL], and two capitellar); 17 of 23 Mason type II and 12 of 17 Mason type I fractures had associated injury, of which LCL and capitellar injuries were most common. Although these associated injuries are important, usually they can be observed during surgery (if surgical intervention is required), and MRI appears not to alter treatment decision making.[13] Although the likelihood of capitellar cartilage injury increases with the amount of displacement in a radial head fracture, often it is less severe than capitellar injury associated with a less displaced fracture.[18] Capitellar cartilaginous fragments have been found interposed between radial head fragments in Mason type I and type II fractures, and they can contribute to preoperative restriction in forearm rotation.[18,19] In Mason type II fractures, a complete loss of cortical contact of any fracture fragment strongly predicts the presence of an associated elbow fracture or ligamentous injury.[20] An associated bony injury was identified in 12.4% of radial head fractures.[2] Elbow dislocation occurs in as many as 10% of radial head fractures and is called a terrible triad injury when accompanied by a coronoid fracture. These injuries are associated with a relatively poor outcome.[21]

Treatment

Nonsurgical Management
A nondisplaced or minimally displaced radial head or neck fracture can be managed nonsurgically, with a good long-term result in most patients.[22] Good long-term results also are reported for Mason type II radial head fractures that are moderately displaced (2 to 5 mm) without a block to rotation, although 12% of patients had a poor early outcome after nonsurgical management and subsequently were treated with radial head excision.[23] Elbow mobilization within 1 week of injury was found to lead to a significant decrease in pain, a better range of motion, and better elbow function, with none of the adverse effects related to longer immobilization.[24] Aspiration of the hematoma that accompanies a Mason type I radial head fracture was reported to decrease the mean level of pain from 5.5 to 2.5 on the visual analog scale.[25] A randomized study compared patients with nondisplaced radial head fracture who were treated with aspiration alone or with aspiration and bupivacaine injection. There was no functional benefit to local anesthetic use at any time from the first day through the first year after the procedure.[26]

Open Reduction and Internal Fixation
No studies have compared open reduction and internal fixation (ORIF) and nonsurgical management of displaced partial articular radial head fractures without mechanical block to rotation. If surgical intervention is elected because of the presence of a mechanical block or an associated elbow injury, ORIF of the fractured radial head has good results as long as stable fixation is

technically possible.[27,28] The results are better in a simple partial articular fracture than a complete articular fracture or a fracture with more than three displaced fragments, for which a primary radial head arthroplasty is recommended.[29,30] In a nonrandomized comparison, patients treated with radial head excision had poorer outcomes and a higher rate of osteoarthritis than those treated with ORIF.[28,31]

Low-profile fixation with countersunk screws, when feasible, is preferable to ORIF with plate and screw fixation, which is associated with more stiffness and high rates of hardware removal.[32,33] A posterior skin incision with elevation of a lateral full-thickness flap or a direct lateral skin incision can be used for any radial head surgery. If injury to the LCL is suspected on stress examination or visual examination of soft-tissue injury, using a Kocher approach simplifies the LCL repair as the surgery is completed. A common extensor origin–splitting approach is preferred in the setting of an intact LCL because it allows access to the commonly fractured anterolateral segment of the radial head. Keeping the forearm in pronation during the deep approach and avoiding the use of retractors on the anterior radial neck reduces the possibility of posterior interosseous nerve palsy. The fracture fragments are reduced while any soft-tissue attachments are maintained to preserve blood supply, and the fragments are provisionally held with Kirschner wires or pointed reduction forceps. Countersunk interfragmentary screws then can be used to maintain the reduction of a partial articular fracture (**Figure 1**). In a complete noncomminuted articular fracture or radial neck fracture, countersunk cannulated bouquet screws can be placed obliquely from the head to the neck in multiple planes to attain stability (**Figure 2**). The guidewire of the cannulated screw helps prevent the screw from glancing off the cortical bone of the radial neck during oblique placement. If there is significant radial neck comminution and a plate is required for stability, a low-profile plate should be placed on the nonarticular portion of the head, with minimal soft-tissue stripping. The radial head and neck anatomy is complex and variable, and no anatomically precontoured plate can provide a reproducible perfect fit. However, such plates can be adjusted to fit by additional contouring during the surgery.[34]

Radial Head Arthroplasty

Radial head arthroplasty is preferred to ORIF if stable fixation cannot be achieved in a comminuted fracture. Radial head replacement has had good early and medium-term results with the use of a variety of metal head designs.[35-39] Biomechanical testing revealed that monopolar radial head replacement stabilizes the radiocapitellar joint but that a bipolar prosthesis may facilitate subluxation.[40] Radiolucency is commonly seen around the stem of an uncemented smooth stem component but is not correlated with patient symptoms[41] (**Figure 3**). Radiolucency around a stem of a nonsmooth design is associated with pain and is a common

reason for reoperation.[42] Significant proximal radius osteolysis resulting from stress shielding was observed when a fully grit-blasted uncemented stem component was used.[43] Progressive osteolysis in cemented bipolar radial head replacement, presumably resulting from polyethylene wear, was reported to be common 8 years after surgery.[35] Uncemented smooth-stem bipolar radial head replacements had good results at 24- to 48-month follow-up, with no evidence of polyethylene wear and no reports of head-neck dissociation.[44] Additional reasons for the failure of metal radial head replacements include stiffness, instability, overlengthening, and infection.

Pyrocarbon, which has a similar modulus of elasticity to bone, is a new alternative to metal for the bearing surface in radial head replacement. Outcomes were good at a minimum 21-month follow-up, despite several early catastrophic failures at the head-neck junction.[45] Long-term follow-up is required for determining whether the theoretic advantages of pyrocarbon lead to satisfactory clinical outcomes.

Recent studies have improved the understanding of appropriate implant sizing in radial head arthroplasty. The diameter and thickness of the implant should be based on the size of the native radial head. To avoid lateral trochlear wear, the implant diameter should be similar to the minor diameter of the native radial head, which typically is 2 mm less than the maximum diameter of the radial head. The prosthesis should articulate so that its proximal aspect is level with the proximal aspect of the radial notch of the ulna, which is approximately 2 mm distal to the tip of the coronoid[46] (**Figure 4**). The gap between the capitellum and the radial head prosthesis should not be used to judge the optimal thickness of the radial head implant if the LCL was injured by the original fracture or the surgical approach. Intraoperative fluoroscopy and postoperative radiographs are useful for judging radial length. In uninjured elbows, the radiographically assessed lateral ulnohumeral joint space often is wider than the medial ulnohumeral joint space, and it may be nonparallel (becoming wider laterally). Therefore, the lateral ulnohumeral joint space is not a reliable measure of radial head arthroplasty overlengthening.[47] The medial ulnohumeral joint space usually is parallel in an uninjured elbow, but incongruity of the joint space may not be apparent on an AP radiograph until the radius is overlengthened at least 6 mm. In contrast, a dental mirror can be used during surgery to detect asymmetric widening of the lateral ulnohumeral joint space with as little as 2 mm of overlengthening of the radial head.[48] Contralateral radiographs are useful for quantifying radial head arthroplasty overlengthening because the measurements are consistent from side to side. A recently described radiographic measurement technique had sensitivity of 98% for measuring radial head implant overlengthening as small as 1 mm.[49]

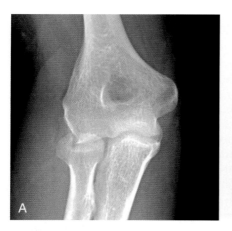
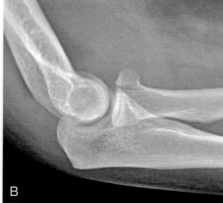
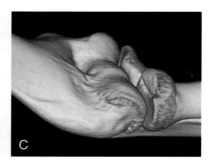
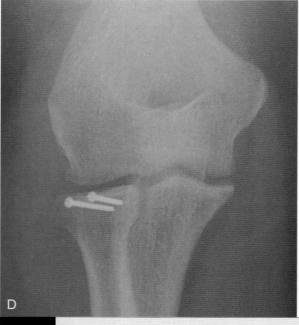
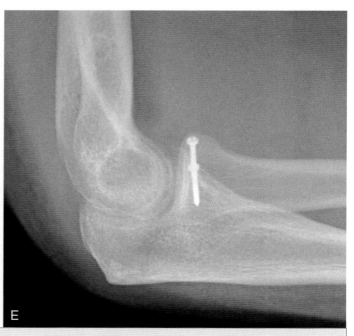

Figure 1   A partial articular radial head fracture in a 31-year-old man, as seen on an AP radiograph **(A)**, a lateral radiograph **(B)**, and three-dimensional CT **(C)**. The patient was treated with open reduction and internal fixation of the displaced fragment. A significant chondral injury to the capitellum was observed during surgery, as well as an avulsion of the lateral collateral ligament, which was repaired. AP **(D)** and **(E)** lateral radiographs 3 months after surgery showing anatomic fixation. The patient had occasional discomfort but had returned to work as a truck driver. The elbow range of motion was 0° to 135°, with 70° of pronation and 70° of supination.

Radial Head Excision

Primary excision of unreconstructable radial head fractures is not commonly performed because of the high incidence of associated ligamentous injuries with more complex radial head fractures and the understanding of the key roles of the radial head in stabilization of a ligament-deficient elbow and load transfer across the elbow. Despite the theoretic concerns, several recent long-term outcome studies found good functional outcomes after radial head excision for isolated fracture of the radial head or neck. Most of these elbows had degenerative changes on radiographs and a 7° to 11° increase in the carrying angle at the elbow.[50-52] Proximal radial migration is common after radial head excision

and may result in symptomatic ulnar impaction symptoms at the wrist.[53] Because delayed radial head excision can be performed with good results, it is reasonable to consider excision as a late treatment option after unsuccessful initial management.[54]

Rehabilitation

Active range-of-motion exercises should be initiated within 1 week of injury in a patient who is being treated nonsurgically.[24] Early active range-of-motion exercises also should be initiated after surgery to reduce the likelihood of stiffness. The range of motion may be restricted by the presence of associated bony or ligamentous elbow injury. If there is residual subluxation

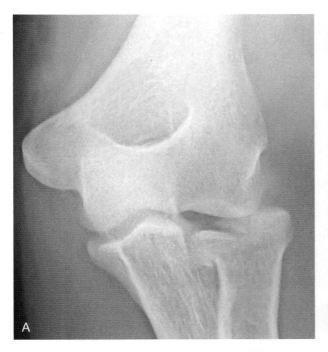

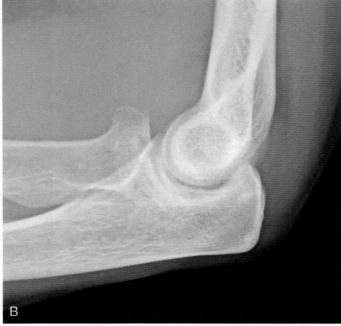

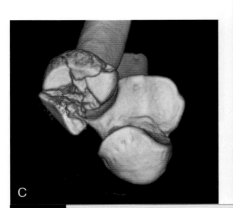

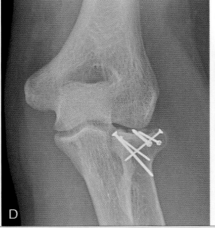

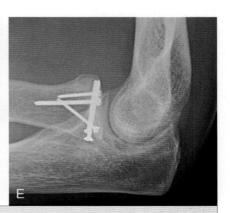

Figure 2 A full articular fracture of the radial head in a 31-year-old man who worked as heavy manual laborer, as seen on an AP radiograph **(A)**, a lateral radiograph **(B)**, and three-dimensional CT **(C)**. The patient was treated with ORIF with bouquet fixation of the radial head fragments to each other and to the shaft, as seen on AP **(D)** and lateral **(E)** radiographs 5 months after surgery. The patient had an elbow range of motion from 17° to 144°, with 70° of pronation and 85° of supination.

of the elbow with extension, rehabilitation is performed within the safe range, and a weekly increase of 10° to 15° of extension is allowed as muscle tone improves and ligaments heal.[55] Isometric muscle contractions are encouraged. If the LCL is deficient, supination is avoided and the elbow is splinted in pronation and 90° of flexion. The elbow should be extended only in pronation. Varus elbow stress, as is created by gravity in the common position of shoulder flexion and internal rotation with elbow flexion, should be avoided.[56] If the MCL is deficient, pronation is avoided and the elbow is splinted in supination and 90° of flexion. The elbow should be extended only in supination.[57] Valgus

elbow stress should be avoided. If both the medial and lateral sides of the elbow are deficient, the elbow is splinted at 90° of flexion in neutral rotation, and extension is done in neutral elbow rotation. With any ligament deficiency, permitted rotation initially should be performed with the elbow in flexion.

Radiographs should be used to monitor for fragment displacement and to determine when the bony union is sufficient to allow passive stretching and strengthening, typically at 6 weeks.[58] Patients who have residual instability or struggle with range of motion should receive formal physical therapy and splinting to reduce the risk of subluxation and stiffness.

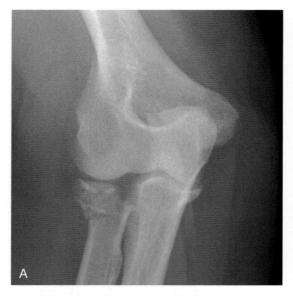
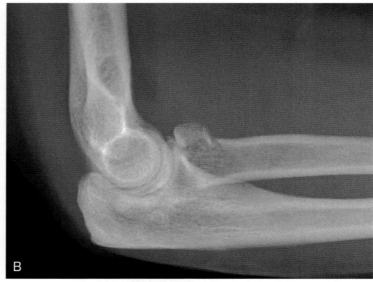
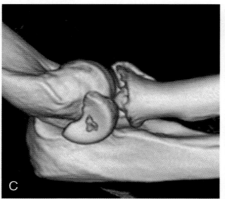
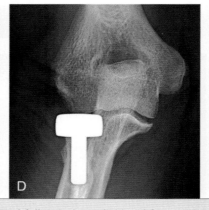
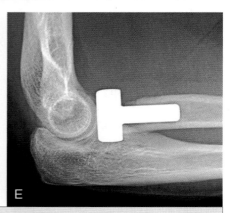

Figure 3   A highly comminuted and displaced full articular radial head fracture in the dominant arm of a 60-year-old woman, as seen on an AP radiograph (**A**), a lateral radiograph (**B**), and three-dimensional CT (**C**). At 3-month follow-up, AP (**D**) and lateral (**E**) radiographs show the radial head arthroplasty with a modular smooth-stemmed design. The implant length appears to be correct because the proximal aspect of the metal implant is articulating at the proximal aspect of the radial notch, the medial ulnohumeral joint is parallel, and there is no widening of the lateral ulnohumeral joint space. The typical mild radiolucency is seen around the implant stem. The patient had returned to all of her normal activities and had a full range of motion with no pain.

Complications

Stiffness after radial head fracture is most common with surgical intervention and can be caused by prominent hardware in ORIF, improper sizing or technique in radial head arthroplasty, or the patient's noncompliance with postoperative rehabilitation. Stiffness can develop because of capsular contracture or heterotopic ossification even if the fracture is appropriately managed and the patient complies with rehabilitation. Soft-tissue stiffness often can be managed with physical therapy and static or dynamic splinting, but a firm mechanical block to range of motion may require surgical management.[58]

Radiographic malunion or nonunion is common after nonsurgical management and less common after ORIF, but frequently it is asymptomatic. For significant pain or mechanical symptoms, radial head excision and arthroplasty are well-recognized treatment options. Good results can be expected.[53,59] Intra-articular osteotomy is reported to be safe and effective for treating a symptomatic malunion of partial articular radial head fracture in the absence of significant degenerative change.[60]

Long-term outcome studies found that radiographic osteoarthritic changes are common after radial head fracture but are not correlated with a poor functional outcome.[23] Clinically significant osteoarthritis can be managed with radial head excision if the ulnohumeral joint is uninvolved. Instability is uncommon if associated elbow injuries are appropriately managed and the radial head is not excised. Significant proximal migration of the radius after radial head excision can cause symptoms at both the wrist and elbow. This complication is complex and has no simple or reliable treatment.

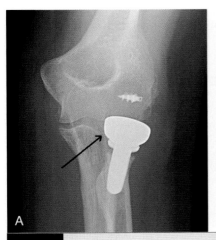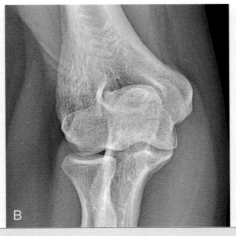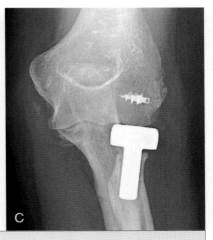

Figure 4 **A,** AP radiograph of a patient with significant pain and stiffness after radial head arthroplasty for fracture. Considerable overlengthening of the implant can be seen. The proximal aspect of the implant is proximal to both the proximal aspect of the radial notch *(arrow)* and the coronoid process. There is widening of the lateral ulnohumeral joint space but no widening of the medial ulnohumeral joint space. **B,** AP radiograph of the contralateral elbow shows the normal relationship of the radial head to the central ridge of the coronoid process in this patient. **C,** AP radiograph of the same patient 3 months after revision surgery with an appropriately sized implant. The ulnohumeral alignment and the relationship of the radial head implant to the radial notch and coronoid process have been restored.

Summary

Radial head and neck fractures are common and often are associated with other elbow injuries that may or may not require treatment. Nondisplaced fractures can be managed nonsurgically, with excellent results. Displaced fractures without significant comminution can be managed nonsurgically or with ORIF, with excellent expected results, but the optimal treatment remains unknown. Comminuted fractures can be managed with radial head arthroplasty, with good medium-term results, but long-term outcome studies are required. Radial head excision appears to be a good salvage option, although the patient should be warned that an increased carrying angle and degenerative radiographic changes are likely.

Recent long-term outcome studies have increased the understanding of some treatment options. There is a need for randomized controlled studies to guide the management of displaced and comminuted radial head and neck fractures.

Annotated References

1. Duckworth AD, Clement ND, Jenkins PJ, Aitken SA, Court-Brown CM, McQueen MM: The epidemiology of radial head and neck fractures. *J Hand Surg Am* 2012;37(1):112-119.

   A prospective trauma database containing 199 radial head fractures and 86 radial neck fractures revealed that male patients were younger on average than female patients, women commonly sustained their fracture from a low-energy fall, and 99% of radial neck fractures were nondisplaced or noncomminuted. Level of evidence: IV.

2. Kaas L, van Riet RP, Vroemen JP, Eygendaal D: The epidemiology of radial head fractures. *J Shoulder Elbow Surg* 2010;19(4):520-523.

   A retrospective database contained 328 radial head fractures. The incidence was calculated at 2.8 per 10,000 population per year. In patients older than 50 years, the number of women was significantly higher than the number of men. Level of evidence: IV.

3. King GJ, Zarzour ZD, Patterson SD, Johnson JA: An anthropometric study of the radial head: Implications in the design of a prosthesis. *J Arthroplasty* 2001; 16(1):112-116.

4. van Riet RP, Van Glabbeek F, Neale PG, Bortier H, An KN, O'Driscoll SW: The noncircular shape of the radial head. *J Hand Surg Am* 2003;28(6):972-978.

5. Galik K, Baratz ME, Butler AL, Dougherty J, Cohen MS, Miller MC: The effect of the annular ligament on kinematics of the radial head. *J Hand Surg Am* 2007; 32(8):1218-1224.

   In a cadaver study, the radial head was found to translate an average 2.1 mm in the anteroposterior plane and 1.6 mm in the mediolateral plane. Resection of the annular ligament increased the translation in both planes but did not change the location of the pronation-supination axis.

6. Smith GR, Hotchkiss RN: Radial head and neck fractures: Anatomic guidelines for proper placement of internal fixation. *J Shoulder Elbow Surg* 1996;5(2, pt 1): 113-117.

7. Beingessner DM, Dunning CE, Gordon KD, Johnson JA, King GJ: The effect of radial head fracture size on elbow kinematics and stability. *J Orthop Res* 2005; 23(1):210-217.

8. Beingessner DM, Dunning CE, Gordon KD, Johnson JA, King GJ: The effect of radial head excision and arthroplasty on elbow kinematics and stability. *J Bone Joint Surg Am* 2004;86(8):1730-1739.

9. Koslowsky TC, Schliwa S, Koebke J: Presentation of the microscopic vascular architecture of the radial head using a sequential plastination technique. *Clin Anat* 2011;24(6):721-732.

   Seventeen fresh human cadaver elbows were sequentially plastinated. The blood supply to the radial head was found to come from branches of the radial recurrent artery and a branch of the ulnar artery (ramus periostalis ulnaris), both of which form a pericervical arterial ring. A branch of the interosseus artery supports the neck, and the nutrient artery provides intraosseous blood supply.

10. Gebauer M, Barvencik F, Mumme M, et al: Microarchitecture of the radial head and its changes in aging. *Calcif Tissue Int* 2010;86(1):14-22.

    An equal number of left-side and right-side radial head cadaver specimens were examined from an equal number of males and females in three age categories. Age- and sex-related changes in bone structure were observed, with significantly worse trabecular parameters in older women compared with men.

11. Guitton TG, Ring D; Science of Variation Group: Interobserver reliability of radial head fracture classification: Two-dimensional compared with three-dimensional CT. *J Bone Joint Surg Am* 2011;93(21):2015-2021.

    Eighty-five orthopaedic surgeons evaluated and classified 12 radial head fractures with radiographs and two-dimensional or three-dimensional CT scans. Although three-dimensional CT led to a slightly more accurate classification, there is still considerable disagreement regarding classification of radial head fractures.

12. Kaas L, Turkenburg JL, van Riet RP, Vroemen JP, Eygendaal D: Magnetic resonance imaging findings in 46 elbows with a radial head fracture. *Acta Orthop* 2010;81(3):373-376.

    An associated elbow injury was found in 35 of 46 patients with a radial head fracture who underwent MRI within 16 days of injury, including 28 LCL and 1 MCL injuries, 18 capitellar injuries, and 1 coronoid fracture.

13. Kaas L, van Riet RP, Turkenburg JL, Vroemen JP, van Dijk CN, Eygendaal D: Magnetic resonance imaging in radial head fractures: Most associated injuries are not clinically relevant. *J Shoulder Elbow Surg* 2011;20(8):1282-1288.

    Retrospective review of 40 patients (42 radial head fractures) at a mean 13 months after injury found clinical MCL or LCL laxity in three elbows, which was not detected on initial MRI in two of the elbows. One patient had infrequent elbow locking.

14. Mason ML: Some observations on fractures of the

    head of the radius with a review of one hundred cases. *Br J Surg* 1954;42(172):123-132.

15. Johnston GW: A follow-up of one hundred cases of fracture of the head of the radius with a review of the literature. *Ulster Med J* 1962;31:51-56.

16. Broberg MA, Morrey BF: Results of treatment of fracture-dislocations of the elbow. *Clin Orthop Relat Res* 1987;216:109-119.

17. van Riet RP, Morrey BF: Documentation of associated injuries occurring with radial head fracture. *Clin Orthop Relat Res* 2008;466(1):130-134.

    Associated injury was seen in 88 of 333 radial head fractures at one institution. A expansion of the Mason classification was devised in which associated injuries were designated by a suffix (c for coronoid fracture, o for olecranon fracture, m for MCL injury, l for LCL injury, d for distal radioulnar disruption).

18. Nalbantoglu U, Gereli A, Kocaoglu B, Aktas S, Turkmen M: Capitellar cartilage injuries concomitant with radial head fractures. *J Hand Surg Am* 2008;33(9):1602-1607.

    Of 51 consecutive patients with Mason type II or type III fracture who were surgically treated, 10 had a capitellar cartilage injury. Although this injury was more common with higher grade radial head fracture, injury severity was worse in lower grade fractures because the more intact radial head was able to cause more damage to the capitellum. Level of evidence: IV.

19. Caputo AE, Burton KJ, Cohen MS, King GJ: Articular cartilage injuries of the capitellum interposed in radial head fractures: A report of ten cases. *J Shoulder Elbow Surg* 2006;15(6):716-720.

20. Rineer CA, Guitton TG, Ring D: Radial head fractures: Loss of cortical contact is associated with concomitant fracture or dislocation. *J Shoulder Elbow Surg* 2010;19(1):21-25.

    A retrospective review of 121 consecutive radial head fractures with displacement of more than 2 mm found that in 91 (75%), there was complete cortical loss of contact of a fracture fragment with the rest of the proximal radius. Only 6% of the fractures were isolated. In the fractures classified as having cortical contact, 88% had no other injuries or dislocation.

21. Regan W, Morrey B: Fractures of the coronoid process of the ulna. *J Bone Joint Surg Am* 1989;71(9):1348-1354.

22. Herbertsson P, Josefsson PO, Hasserius R, Karlsson C, Besjakov J, Karlsson MK: Displaced Mason type I fractures of the radial head and neck in adults: A fifteen- to thirty-three-year follow-up study. *J Shoulder Elbow Surg* 2005;14(1):73-77.

23. Akesson T, Herbertsson P, Josefsson PO, Hasserius R, Besjakov J, Karlsson MK: Primary nonoperative treatment of moderately displaced two-part fractures of the

radial head. *J Bone Joint Surg Am* 2006;88(9):1909-1914.

24. Liow RY, Cregan A, Nanda R, Montgomery RJ: Early mobilisation for minimally displaced radial head fractures is desirable: A prospective randomised study of two protocols. *Injury* 2002;33(9):801-806.

25. Ditsios KT, Stavridis SI, Christodoulou AG: The effect of haematoma aspiration on intra-articular pressure and pain relief following Mason I radial head fractures. *Injury* 2011;42(4):362-365.

    Intra-articular pressure monitoring was done before and after aspiration in 16 patients with a Mason type I radial head fracture. A mean 2.75 mL was aspirated, and intra-articular pressure was found to drop from between 49 and 120 mm Hg to between 9 and 25 mm Hg. Reported pain decreased from a mean 5.5 to 2.5 on the visual analog scale.

26. Chalidis BE, Papadopoulos PP, Sachinis NC, Dimitriou CG: Aspiration alone versus aspiration and bupivacaine injection in the treatment of undisplaced radial head fractures: A prospective randomized study. *J Shoulder Elbow Surg* 2009;18(5):676-679.

    A prospective randomized controlled study of 40 patients with Mason type I radial head fracture found no difference in range of motion, pain, and elbow function based on treatment with aspiration of hematoma alone or with aspiration and intra-articular local anesthetic injection. Level of evidence: I.

27. Lindenhovius AL, Felsch Q, Ring D, Kloen P: The long-term outcome of open reduction and internal fixation of stable displaced isolated partial articular fractures of the radial head. *J Trauma* 2009;67(1):143-146.

    Sixteen patients with a stable Mason type II radial head fracture received ORIF with screws (11 patients) or plate and screws (5 patients). At an average 22-year follow-up, 14 patients were found to have undergone routine removal of hardware an average 14 months after surgery. The average Disabilities of the Arm, Shoulder, and Hand (DASH) score was 12. Level of evidence: IV.

28. Lindenhovius AL, Felsch Q, Doornberg JN, Ring D, Kloen P: Open reduction and internal fixation compared with excision for unstable displaced fractures of the radial head. *J Hand Surg Am* 2007;32(5):630-636.

    Fifteen patients with an unstable displaced radial head fracture treated with excision were compared with 13 patients with a similar fracture treated with ORIF. There was no difference in range of motion at 1 year or 17 years after injury. At long-term follow, up the average DASH score was 5 in patients treated with ORIF and 15 in those treated with excision. Level of evidence: III.

29. Ring D, Quintero J, Jupiter JB: Open reduction and internal fixation of fractures of the radial head. *J Bone Joint Surg Am* 2002;84(10):1811-1815.

    At 2-year follow-up of 56 patients treated with ORIF

for a radial head fracture, patients with a comminuted fracture with more than three fragments had a relatively poor result. Level of evidence: III.

30. Chen X, Wang SC, Cao LH, Yang GQ, Li M, Su JC: Comparison between radial head replacement and open reduction and internal fixation in clinical treatment of unstable, multi-fragmented radial head fractures. *Int Orthop* 2011;35(7):1071-1076.

    A randomized controlled study of 45 patients with a Mason type III fracture compared ORIF and radial head replacement. Severely comminuted fractures were excluded. At 2-year follow-up, 91% of patients with arthroplasty had a good or excellent result, compared with 65% of those with ORIF. Level of evidence: II.

31. Ikeda M, Sugiyama K, Kang C, Takagaki T, Oka Y: Comminuted fractures of the radial head: Comparison of resection and internal fixation. *J Bone Joint Surg Am* 2005;87(1):76-84.

32. Smith AM, Morrey BF, Steinmann SP: Low profile fixation of radial head and neck fractures: Surgical technique and clinical experience. *J Orthop Trauma* 2007; 21(10):718-724.

    A retrospective review of 19 patients who underwent ORIF using a technique for low-profile fixation of radial head fracture found a trend toward reduced forearm rotation. Heterotopic ossification occurred in five patients who received ORIF with plate fixation and one with low-profile fixation. Level of evidence: III.

33. Neumann M, Nyffeler R, Beck M: Comminuted fractures of the radial head and neck: Is fixation to the shaft necessary? *J Bone Joint Surg Br* 2011;93(2):223-228.

    A retrospective review of 25 patients with Mason type III radial head fracture identified two groups at a mean 4-year follow-up, based on whether the radial head rotated as one with the neck and shaft after the head fracture was fixed with ORIF or required a plate to fix the head to the neck. Hardware was removed in 7 of 13 patients requiring plate fixation and 1 of 12 patients without plate fixation. Level of evidence: III.

34. Burkhart KJ, Nowak TE, Kim YJ, Rommens PM, Müller LP: Anatomic fit of six different radial head plates: Comparison of precontoured low-profile radial head plates. *J Hand Surg Am* 2011;36(4):617-624.

    Twenty-two human cadaver proximal radius specimens were used in assessing the fit and profile of six precontoured radial head plates. Although two plates appeared to have a better fit and lower profile than the others, none of the plates had a reproducibly perfect fit because of the complexity and variability of the proximal radius. The surgeon's ability to modify a plate may be important in achieving optimal fit.

35. Popovic N, Lemaire R, Georis P, Gillet P: Midterm results with a bipolar radial head prosthesis: Radiographic evidence of loosening at the bone-cement interface. *J Bone Joint Surg Am* 2007;89(11):2469-2476.

    At a mean 8.4-year follow-up of 51 patients with a cemented bipolar radial head replacement, the outcome on the Mayo Elbow Performance Index (MEPI) was excellent in 14, good in 25, fair in 9, and poor in 3. Osteolysis was seen on radiographs in 37 patients, and there were 10 complications. Level of evidence: IV.

36. Grewal R, MacDermid JC, Faber KJ, Drosdowech DS, King GJ: Comminuted radial head fractures treated with a modular metallic radial head arthroplasty: Study of outcomes. *J Bone Joint Surg Am* 2006; 88(10):2192-2200.

37. Dotzis A, Cochu G, Mabit C, Charissoux JL, Arnaud JP: Comminuted fractures of the radial head treated by the Judet floating radial head prosthesis. *J Bone Joint Surg Br* 2006;88(6):760-764.

38. Doornberg JN, Parisien R, van Duijn PJ, Ring D: Radial head arthroplasty with a modular metal spacer to treat acute traumatic elbow instability. *J Bone Joint Surg Am* 2007;89(5):1075-1080.

    At a mean 40-month follow-up of 27 patients with an uncemented smooth-stem modular radial head replacement, the average range of motion was from 20° of flexion to 131° of flexion, 73° of pronation, and 57° of supination. Seventeen patients had lucency around the neck of the prosthesis not associated with pain. Nine patients had radiographic changes around the capitellum. Level of evidence: IV.

39. Chapman CB, Su BW, Sinicropi SM, Bruno R, Strauch RJ, Rosenwasser MP: Vitallium radial head prosthesis for acute and chronic elbow fractures and fracture-dislocations involving the radial head. *J Shoulder Elbow Surg* 2006;15(4):463-473.

40. Moon JG, Berglund LJ, Zachary D, An KN, O'Driscoll SW: Radiocapitellar joint stability with bipolar versus monopolar radial head prostheses. *J Shoulder Elbow Surg* 2009;18(5):779-784.

    Bipolar and monopolar radial head prosthesis designs were tested using 12 human cadaver elbow specimens. The monopolar radial head replacement and the native radial head both resisted radiocapitellar subluxation. The bipolar radial head replacement facilitated subluxation.

41. Fehringer EV, Burns EM, Knierim A, Sun J, Apker KA, Berg RE: Radiolucencies surrounding a smooth-stemmed radial head component may not correlate with forearm pain or poor elbow function. *J Shoulder Elbow Surg* 2009;18(2):275-278.

    Radiolucency around the stem was detected in 16 of 17 patients assessed clinically and radiographically at a minimum 2 years after surgery. All elbows were stable, and radiolucency was not correlated with proximal forearm pain. Level of evidence: IV.

42. van Riet RP, Sanchez-Sotelo J, Morrey BF: Failure of metal radial head replacement. *J Bone Joint Surg Br* 2010;92(5):661-667.

    In 44 patients (47 elbows) who had removal of a metal radial head replacement, the most common indication for removal was painful loosening (31 elbows). The implant was revised for stiffness in 18 elbows and instability in 9 elbows. Overlengthening was seen before removal in 11 elbows. Degenerative changes were found in all but one elbow. Level of evidence: IV.

43. Chanlalit C, Fitzsimmons JS, Moon JG, Berglund LJ, An KN, O'Driscoll SW: Radial head prosthesis micromotion characteristics: Partial versus fully grit-blasted stems. *J Shoulder Elbow Surg* 2011;20(1):27-32.

    In a human cadaver biomechanical study, micromotion was comparable in partially and fully grit-blasted radial head replacement stems. Less stress shielding with a partially grit-blasted uncemented stem was believed to be advantageous.

44. Zunkiewicz MR, Clemente JS, Miller MC, Baratz ME, Wysocki RW, Cohen MS: Radial head replacement with a bipolar system: A minimum 2-year follow-up. *J Shoulder Elbow Surg* 2012;21(1):98-104.

    The results of using 30 smooth stem and telescoping radial neck bipolar radial head replacements were assessed a mean 34 months after surgery. The mean MEPI score was 92.1, and the DASH score was 13.8. Level of evidence: IV.

45. Sarris IK, Kyrkos MJ, Galanis NN, Papavasiliou KA, Sayegh FE, Kapetanos GA: Radial head replacement with the MoPyC pyrocarbon prosthesis. *J Shoulder Elbow Surg* 2012;21(9):1222-1228.

    At a mean 27-month follow-up of 32 patients with a pyrocarbon uncemented radial head replacement, the mean arc of flexion-extension was 130°, mean pronation was 74°, and mean supination was 72°. Broberg and Morrey scores were excellent in 33% of patients, good in 44%, and fair in 23%. Six patients had osteolysis, and 2 had early catastrophic failure at the stem-neck junction. Level of evidence: IV.

46. Doornberg JN, Linzel DS, Zurakowski D, Ring D: Reference points for radial head prosthesis size. *J Hand Surg Am* 2006;31(1):53-57.

47. Rowland AS, Athwal GS, MacDermid JC, King GJ: Lateral ulnohumeral joint space widening is not diagnostic of radial head arthroplasty overstuffing. *J Hand Surg Am* 2007;32(5):637-641.

    Evaluation of 50 AP radiographs of the elbow revealed that the lateral ulnohumeral joint space often is wider than the medial ulnohumeral joint space in a normal elbow. The medial joint space usually is parallel, but the lateral joint space can be nonparallel and wider laterally.

48. Frank SG, Grewal R, Johnson J, Faber KJ, King GJ, Athwal GS: Determination of correct implant size in radial head arthroplasty to avoid overlengthening. *J Bone Joint Surg Am* 2009;91(7):1738-1746.

    After implantation of a radial head replacement of a varying thickness in seven human cadaver specimens, a significant incongruity of the medial ulnohumeral joint appeared radiographically only after overlengthening of the radius by more than 6 mm. Overlengthening of

2 mm or more could be detected by intraoperative assessment of a lateral ulnohumeral joint space gap.

49. Athwal GS, Rouleau DM, MacDermid JC, King GJ: Contralateral elbow radiographs can reliably diagnose radial head implant overlengthening. *J Bone Joint Surg Am* 2011;93(14):1339-1346.

Examination of 100 radiographs of 50 elbow pairs revealed no difference in same-patient radiographic measurements. A measurement technique tested on a cadaver model was found to reliably predict overlengthening of as little as 1 mm (sensitivity, 98%).

50. Iftimie PP, Calmet Garcia J, de Loyola Garcia Forcada I, Gonzalez Pedrouzo JE, Giné Gomà J: Resection arthroplasty for radial head fractures: Long-term follow-up. *J Shoulder Elbow Surg* 2011;20(1):45-50.

Radial head excision was reviewed in 27 patients at an average 17-year follow-up. On the MEPI, the outcome was excellent in 81%, good in 15%, and fair in 4%. The mean DASH score was 4.9. Eighty-five percent of patients reported no pain. Their mean range of motion was 5° to 135°, mean pronation was 83°, and mean supination was 79°. Almost all patients had radiographic degenerative changes. Level of evidence: IV.

51. Antuña SA, Sánchez-Márquez JM, Barco R: Long-term results of radial head resection following isolated radial head fractures in patients younger than forty years old. *J Bone Joint Surg Am* 2010;92(3):558-566.

At a mean 25-year follow-up, radial head excision was retrospectively reviewed in 26 patients younger than 40 years at surgery. Eighty-one percent of patients reported no pain. Their mean arc of flexion was 9° to 139°. Mean pronation was 84°, and mean supination was 85°. The mean MEPI was 92, and 92% were classified as good or excellent. The mean DASH score was 6. The mean carrying angle of the elbow had increased by 11°. Level of evidence: IV.

52. Karlsson MK, Herbertsson P, Nordqvist A, Hasserius R, Besjakov J, Josefsson PO: Long-term outcome of displaced radial neck fractures in adulthood: 16-21 year follow-up of 5 patients treated with radial head excision. *Acta Orthop* 2009;80(3):368-370.

At a mean 18-year follow-up, retrospective review of three women and two men treated with radial head excision for a comminuted radial neck fracture found occasional weakness in two patients, a mean loss of 10° of terminal extension, and a mean loss of less than 5° of flexion, pronation, and supination. The mean difference in carrying angle was 2° between the injured and uninjured sides. Level of evidence: IV.

53. Schiffern A, Bettwieser SP, Porucznik CA, Crim JR, Tashjian RZ: Proximal radial drift following radial head resection. *J Shoulder Elbow Surg* 2011;20(3):426-433.

At a mean 72-month follow-up, 13 patients treated with radial head excision were retrospectively reviewed. The proximal radial stump had migrated medially and posteriorly, and resection of more than 2 cm resulted in increased posterior drift. Level of evidence: IV.

54. Broberg MA, Morrey BF: Results of delayed excision of the radial head after fracture. *J Bone Joint Surg Am* 1986;68(5):669-674.

55. Coonrad RW, Roush TF, Major NM, Basamania CJ: The drop sign, a radiographic warning sign of elbow instability. *J Shoulder Elbow Surg* 2005;14(3):312-317.

56. Dunning CE, Zarzour ZD, Patterson SD, Johnson JA, King GJ: Muscle forces and pronation stabilize the lateral ligament deficient elbow. *Clin Orthop Relat Res* 2001;388:118-124.

57. Armstrong AD, Dunning CE, Faber KJ, Duck TR, Johnson JA, King GJ: Rehabilitation of the medial collateral ligament-deficient elbow: An in vitro biomechanical study. *J Hand Surg Am* 2000;25(6):1051-1057.

58. Szekeres M, Chinchalkar SJ, King GJ: Optimizing elbow rehabilitation after instability. *Hand Clin* 2008;24(1):27-38.

59. Shore BJ, Mozzon JB, MacDermid JC, Faber KJ, King GJ: Chronic posttraumatic elbow disorders treated with metallic radial head arthroplasty. *J Bone Joint Surg Am* 2008;90(2):271-280.

At a mean 8-year follow-up, 32 patients treated with a metallic radial head arthroplasty on a delayed basis for a variety of indications had an average MEPI score of 83, with 53% of patients rated as excellent, 13% as good, 22% as fair, and 13% as poor. Posttraumatic arthritis was found in 74% on radiographs. None of the implants required revision. Level of evidence: IV.

60. Rosenblatt Y, Young C, MacDermid JC, King GJ: Osteotomy of the head of the radius for partial articular malunion. *J Bone Joint Surg Br* 2009;91(10):1341-1346.

Five patients were treated with intra-articular osteotomy for a malunited partial articular radial head fracture a mean 8 months after injury. At a mean 5.5-year follow-up, MEPI scores had improved from 74 to 88, and four patients had a good or excellent outcome. All osteotomies healed, and there were no complications. Level of evidence: IV.

Chapter 45

Fractures of the Distal Humerus

David Ring, MD, PhD

Introduction

Distal humeral fractures are complex injuries that are difficult to repair and prone to complications. However, long-term evaluations of patients with bicolumnar fractures and capitellum-trochlea fractures suggest that the results of surgical treatment are durable, and symptoms and disability are not correlated with arthrosis.

Between 2007 and 2011, published data confirmed the long-underappreciated complexity of many capitellum-trochlea fractures, discussed the use of distal humeral hemiarthroplasty, and compared total elbow arthroplasty with plate fixation of bicolumnar fractures for patients at least 65 years old. Several case studies of fixation techniques or surgical exposures found a higher rate of acknowledged ulnar neuropathy than previously noted. Three published studies specifically reported on ulnar neuropathy: one favored transposing the nerve, one favored not transposing, and one found no difference. This topic and many others continue to be debated.

Columnar Fractures

Single-column fractures of the distal humerus are uncommon. Few AO type B fractures were reported in some of the larger studies of plate fixation, and in the past 5 years, only a single study evaluated single-column fractures.[1] A review of medial column fractures treated over many years at one of two medical centers found complex articular fragmentation in 10 of 14 patients (71%) (**Figure 1**). An average flexion arc of 92° was achieved, and 10 patients had a good or excellent result on the Broberg-Morrey Functional Rating Index.[1]

Most fractures that involve the columns of the distal humerus (the bone on either side of the coronoid-olecranon fossae, between the base of the olecranon

Dr. Ring or an immediate family member has received royalties from Wright Medical Technology; serves as a paid consultant to or is an employee of Biomet, Skeletal Dynamics, and Wright Medical Technology; has stock or stock options held in Illuminos; and serves as a board member, owner, officer, or committee member of the American Shoulder and Elbow Surgeons and the American Society for Surgery of the Hand.

fossa and the humeral diaphysis) are fractures of both columns, which are called bicolumnar or supracondylar fractures. Current areas of interest with respect to bicolumnar fractures of the distal humerus include parallel versus perpendicular plate fixation, the role of angular stable fixation (with screws that lock to the plate), optimal exposure achieved while limiting the risk of adverse events, and the optimal handling of the ulnar nerve.

The Biomechanics of Plate-and-Screw Fixation

Fixation in two orthogonal planes is a basic engineering concept that has long been applied to the fixation of fractures of the distal humerus. However, placing the plates parallel to each other on the direct medial and lateral surfaces of the distal humerus allows for a higher number of screws and longer screws to engage the distal fracture fragments; each of these screws can go through a plate and contribute to stabilization across the columns, and can contribute to securing ar-

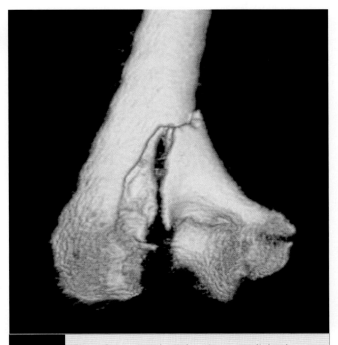

| **Figure 1** | Three-dimensional CT showing a medial column fracture of the distal humerus. The medial trochlea is a separate impacted fragment. |

ticular fragments. Particularly with the advent of plates with smaller distal screws, some surgeons think that parallel plates provide more options for securing articular fragments. Until approximately 2007, biomechanical testing did not show a clear advantage to orthogonal or parallel plate fixation. Within the past several years, orthogonal and parallel plating have been compared in several biomechanical studies, all of which found an advantage with using parallel plates.[2-6] Parallel plates allow the use of longer screws and more metal, which create a stronger fixation.

A study of an AO type C2.3 fracture model in 14 cadaver pairs used loading through an intact elbow joint.[2] Another study used artificial bone with an AO C2.3 fracture model to study one parallel plate configuration and two orthogonal plate configurations in flexion and extension loading models.[3] A third study used cadaver pairs with an AO type C2.3 fracture and compared interconnected parallel plates with orthogonal locking plates.[4] A fourth study used epoxy resin humera and tested failure with sagittal plane bending forces.[5] A fifth study simulated AO type C2 fractures in paired cadaver bones to compare orthogonal and parallel locking plates.[6]

Another biomechanical study used a cadaver supracondylar gap model with orthogonal plating and found greater stiffness when shifting a direct medial six-hole locking plate distally, so there were more screws in the distal fragment (three rather than one), even though the multiple distal screws were short.[7] Finally, conventional and locking reconstruction plates and distal humerus–specific locking plates were compared in an AO type C2.3 cadaver model; the only difference in the results was that screw loosening occurred with nonlocking plates in osteoporotic bones.[8]

Other Translational Research

In a study of sequential excision of the capitellum and the anterior trochlea in eight cadaver arms, kinematics were not notably affected until part of the trochlea was excised.[9] Loss of the lateral trochlea is tolerated if radiocapitellar contact is maintained. The elbow requires an intact medial ulnohumeral articulation and either an intact lateral trochlea or a radiocapitellar articulation, but not necessarily both.

A quantitative CT study of 14 cadaver distal humeri found the lowest bone volume and cortical thickness in the posterior part of the lateral condyle.[10] This finding, combined with the fact that screws directed from posterior to anterior on the distal part of the posterior lateral column must be short and unicortical, supports the clinical observation that the lateral condyle is a potential weak point for surgical fixation of the distal humerus with a posterolateral plate, especially if the bone is osteoporotic. The fact that the elbow encounters substantial varus stress during daily activity when an object is lifted away from the body (for example, when pouring milk) also should be taken into account when the use of a posterolateral plate is considered.

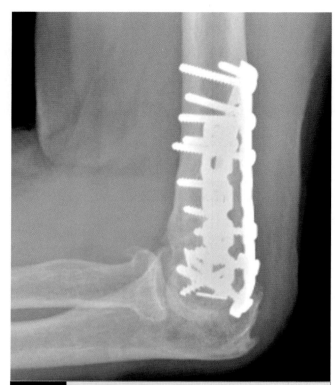

Figure 2   Lateral radiograph after open reduction and internal fixation of a distal humeral fracture, showing loss of the normal anterior translation of the distal humerus. The patient had only 90° of flexion.

A study of 141 patients more than 6 months after a fracture of the distal humerus identified a limited but significant correlation between flexion and anterior translation of the trochlea as a percentage of the humeral shaft diameter[11] (**Figure 2**). This study found that loss of the normal anterior translation of the trochlea can hinder elbow flexion by a mechanism that does not respond to exercise or capsular release. This loss of anterior translation results in earlier contact of the coronoid with the humeral shaft in flexion and a diminished space for the anterior arm musculature.

An injection study of nine fresh-frozen cadavers determined that the distal humeral diaphysis is supplied by a single nutrient artery, with the lateral column of the distal humeral metaphysis supplied predominantly by posterior segmental vessels.[12] This finding may partly explain the recently observed association between posterior column comminution and nonunion of capitellum-trochlea fractures.[13]

Bicolumnar Fractures: Case Studies

Many retrospective case studies of patients who were surgically treated for a columnar fracture of the distal humerus have been published in the past 5 years. In the long term, the healed fractures develop arthrosis but maintain function and do not require additional surgery. At an average of 19 years after plate-and-screw fixation of an AO type C fracture of the distal humerus in 30 patients, the average arc of flexion was 106°, and 26 patients had good or excellent results. The results were not correlated with the presence of arthrosis.[14]

Patient age and osteoporosis are not contraindications to open reduction and plate fixation using careful technique. It is generally agreed that the patient's health and functional demands are more important than chronologic age when considering treatment options. Among 14 patients older than 65 years who had a distal humeral fracture treated with plate-and-screw fixation, all 14 fractures united, the mean Mayo Elbow Performance Score was 83; the mean Disabilities of the Arm, Shoulder and Hand (DASH) score was 34.7; and the mean elbow flexion-extension arc was 20° to 120°.[15] All 32 patients at least 65 years of age healed and achieved an excellent result after plate fixation, with average motion from 22° to 125°.[16]

A persistent interest in Y-shaped plates is evident in published reports. Most nonunions occur in the supracondylar region, so this practice has potential risks. Of 34 patients whose fracture was fixed with a reverse Y-shaped plate (13 patients) or a double plate (21 patients), 71% had satisfactory results, but many complications and more difficulties were encountered in patients older than 65 years.[17] In another study, all 17 patients with an AO type C fracture healed after treatment with a Y-shaped plate; average flexion was 13° to 112°, and 14 patients had good or excellent results.[18]

Most studies examined variations of two-column conventional plate fixation. All 60 relatively young patients (mean age, 30 years) healed after fracture repair with a third tubular plate and a 3.5-mm reconstruction or dynamic compression plate; average flexion at 1-year follow-up was 20° to 110°.[19] A study of 184 patients found that 100% had union, the average flexion was from 20° to 110°, and 72% of the patients had excellent or good results.[20] Among 22 distal humeral fractures treated with perpendicular plate fixation, 86.4% had excellent or good results, the mean Quick-DASH score was 36.1, and the mean flexion ranged from 11° to 128°.[21] Of 56 patients whose fracture was fixed with two plates, 16% had a complication.[22] In 34 patients older than 60 years (mean, 77.6 years) who had surgical treatment of an AO type C fracture (plates were used in 24; 10 were treated with pins, screws, or external fixation), the mean Mayo elbow score was 73.3. Twenty-one patients had an excellent or good result, and the mean arc of flexion was 80°.[23]

Interest in attempting to work on either side of the triceps without elevating the triceps off the bone or cutting the olecranon is increasing. A retrospective review of 34 patients treated using a triceps-sparing approach and 33 treated with an olecranon osteotomy identified no significant differences in motion; however, a higher percentage of unsatisfactory results was reported among the patients older than 60 years who did not undergo osteotomy.[24] A paratricipital surgical exposure was used for plate fixation of fractures in 22 patients with an AO type C fracture. The results were good or excellent in 86% of the patients, and the average flexion arc was 120°. One deep infection and no nonunions occurred.[25] In another study, the paratricipital approach was used to treat seven type C fractures, all of which healed. The median arc of elbow motion was 90°, all patients had a good or excellent Mayo score, and the mean DASH score was 17.9.[26] When the paratricipital approach is used, there should be a low threshold for the addition of an olecranon osteotomy if unanticipated comminution is found or if visualization or reduction is difficult because of the size of the patient or metaphyseal bone loss. Distal humeral fractures are complex, and a second procedure to remove the olecranon osteotomy fixation devices may be a fair trade for an optimal fracture repair and avoidance of complications.

The emerging data on parallel plate fixation appear comparable to those for orthogonal plate fixation. Among 16 patients whose fracture was treated with precontoured parallel plating, 100% had union, the mean extension was 29°, the mean flexion was 132°, the mean Mayo score was 72.3, and the mean DASH score was 46.1.[27] In a study of 37 patients with an AO type C distal humeral fracture treated with parallel plates, all fractures healed, the mean arc of elbow flexion was 97°, the mean Mayo score was 82, and the mean DASH score was 24. Five patients (16%) had nerve dysfunction, and a total of 24 complications occurred in 17 patients (53%).[28] In 32 patients with an AO type C fracture repaired with parallel plates, 1 had nonunion, 5 underwent subsequent surgery for elbow stiffness, and 1 had a deep infection. The mean arc of flexion was 99°, the mean Mayo score was 85, and 27 patients had good or excellent results.[29] In a study from China, no significant differences were reported among 17 patients treated with perpendicular plating and 18 treated with parallel plating, although 2 of the patients treated with perpendicular plating had nonunion.[30]

The results of locked or angular stable plate fixation of the distal humerus also have been reported. In a review of 40 consecutive patients treated with locking distal humerus–specific plates, the results were good or excellent in 29 patients (72.5%). The median Mayo score was 84, and the mean flexion arc was 100°.[31] One patient experienced implant failure. Patients who were relatively young or had an injury without comminution of the articular surface tended to have better functional results. Five patients (12.5%) had ulnar neuropathy. All 14 patients (12 with an AO type C fracture and 2 with a type B fracture of the distal humerus) healed after treatment with distal humerus–specific locking plates. The average flexion arc was 121°, and all patients had a good or excellent Mayo score (mean, 91); the mean DASH score was 18.5.[32]

Open Bicolumnar Fractures

In a study of open fractures of the distal humerus, eight patients treated with initial external fixation followed

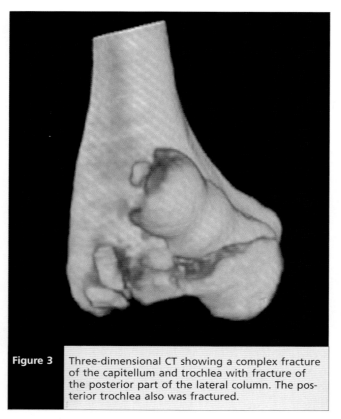

Figure 3 Three-dimensional CT showing a complex fracture of the capitellum and trochlea with fracture of the posterior part of the lateral column. The posterior trochlea also was fractured.

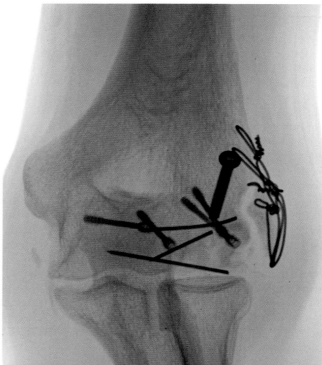

Figure 4 AP radiograph showing nonunion of the capitellum after open reduction and internal fixation of a complex Dubberley type 3B capitellum and trochlea fracture.

by later plate-and-screw fixation were compared with six patients treated with immediate plating.[33] The patients who received delayed treatment had less motion than those treated immediately (average arc of flexion, 74° and 94°, respectively), a lower Mayo score (mean, 56 and 84, respectively), and greater disability (mean Musculoskeletal Functional Assessment score, 33 and 12, respectively). In this small retrospective study, it is likely that the patients treated with external fixation had more severe injuries.

Capitellum-Trochlea Fractures

Capitellum fractures typically involve part of the lateral trochlea and often involve a greater part of the anterior trochlea, the posterior part of the lateral column, and even the posterior and medial parts of the trochlea. Considering these as so-called apparent capitellar fractures or capitellum-trochlea fractures to emphasize the potential complexity of the injuries can be useful, even if they appear relatively benign on radiographs (**Figure 3**). Recent studies confirmed the complexity of these injuries and documented that nonunion and osteonecrosis are much more problematic if both fragmentation of the capitellum-trochlea and fracture of the posterior aspect of the lateral column and the posterior trochlea are present.

A review of capitellum-trochlea fractures in the fracture database of the Royal Infirmary in Edinburgh,

Scotland, identified 79 patients and estimated an annual incidence of 1.5 per 100,000 population.[34] Twenty-four percent of the patients had a concomitant radial head fracture, and 59% had involvement of more than just the capitellum.

The 1-year results of 27 patients and the long-term results (median, 17 years) of 14 patients were reported after open reduction and internal fixation of a fracture of the capitellum and the trochlea.[35] Four patients had concomitant dislocation, 3 patients had a fracture of the proximal ulna, and 2 patients had a fracture of the radial head. Eight patients required a second procedure to treat an adverse event. In the 14 patients with long-term follow-up, the median arc of flexion improved from 106° at 1 year after fracture to 119°, and the median Broberg-Morrey scores were 93 and 95, respectively. The average final DASH score was 8. Nine patients had radiographic signs of arthrosis. Patients had a relatively poor result if they had a fracture of the posterior elements (a Dubberley type 3 fracture) or if the fracture involved fragmentation of the capitellum-trochlea.[36]

In 30 patients followed an average of 34 months after open reduction and internal fixation of a capitellum-trochlea fracture, 8 of the 18 patients with a Dubberley type 3B fracture (fragmentation of the capitellum and the trochlea and posterior fracture) had nonunion[13] (**Fig-**

ure 4). No patient with a simpler fracture had non-union. Eight of 26 patients (31%) had a fair result after open reduction and internal fixation of a capitellum-trochlea fracture related to posterior comminution.[37] Better results were reported after surgical treatment of 11 Dubberley type 1A injuries and 7 type 2A capitellum-trochlea fractures; 1 patient had an unsatisfactory result, and osteonecrosis developed in 3 patients.[38]

Arthroplasty

Hemiarthroplasty

Hemiarthroplasty often is discussed as an option for complex capitellum-trochlea fractures in older and less active patients. In these fractures, both columns are intact, the medial collateral ligament and the medial epicondyle usually are intact, and the lateral epicondyle fracture can be repaired, thus restoring the function of the lateral collateral ligament complex. Some surgeons also consider hemiarthroplasty for columnar fractures that can be repaired to restore collateral ligament function.

Eight women with an average age of 79 years were evaluated at a mean follow-up of 4 years after Kudo hemiarthroplasty for fracture of the distal humerus. Average flexion ranged from 31° to 126°, and all patients had a good or excellent outcome based on the Mayo score.[39] Of 10 women with a mean age of 75 years who were treated with hemiarthroplasty of the distal humerus for fracture (8 patients) or early failed internal fixation (2 patients), 9 had a good or excellent result on the Mayo score, mean flexion ranged from 18° to 125°, and the mean DASH score was 11.[40]

Total Elbow Arthroplasty

Arthroplasty for distal humeral fractures usually requires removing the entire distal humerus, including the condyles and the collateral ligament origins. This technique requires a linked arthroplasty. In the past 5 years, several studies, including a randomized study, examined using linked total elbow arthroplasty for distal humeral fractures.

The Canadian Orthopaedic Trauma Society completed a prospective randomized study comparing open reduction and internal fixation with primary semiconstrained total elbow arthroplasty in 42 patients age 65 years or older who had an AO type C fracture. Two patients died before sufficient evaluation, and 5 patients randomly assigned to open reduction and internal fixation underwent total elbow arthroplasty. An analysis of the 25 patients who underwent total elbow arthroplasty compared with the 15 who underwent open reduction and internal fixation found that total elbow arthroplasty was associated with a shorter surgical time as well as a better Mayo score but not with better motion or DASH scores. The between-group reoperation rates were similar.[41]

In a retrospective study, the results of 9 patients after linked total elbow arthroplasty were compared with those of 11 patients after plate-and-screw fixation at an average 15-month follow-up. All patients had an AO type B or C fracture of the distal humerus and were older than 60 years. The average flexion arcs were 92° and 98°, respectively; the Mayo score were 79 and 85, respectively; and the DASH scores were 30 and 32, respectively. Two patients in each group died, one plated fracture did not heal, and four patients with arthroplasty had radiographic loosening.[42]

At an average follow-up of 63 months after total elbow arthroplasty for distal humeral fracture in 26 patients (average age at surgery, 72 years), 3 patients had died, 1 had severe dementia, and 2 could not be contacted. The remaining 4 men and 16 women had an average age of 72 years at the time of surgery, had an average Mayo score of 92, and had an average flexion from 27° to 125°. Two patients had heterotopic ossification, and one had radiographic loosening.[43] In another study, 11 patients age 75 years or older had an average flexion arc of 107° and an average Mayo score of 90 at an average follow-up of 2.8 years after linked total elbow arthroplasty for distal humeral fracture. Eight patients had radiographic loosening.[44] At an average follow-up of 56 months after linked total elbow arthroplasty for fracture of the distal humerus in 32 patients (15 with early treatment and 17 with delayed treatment), no significant between-group differences were seen in Mayo scores, satisfaction, or implant survival. Two patients in the delayed-treatment group had a deep infection.[45]

A unique study reported on the use of unlinked total elbow arthroplasty for distal humeral fractures which is commonly used outside North America. The fractures in this study were primarily capitellum-trochlea fractures, for which hemiarthroplasty is an option. At an average follow-up of 3.5 years, the nine patients (average age, 73 years) had an average Mayo score of 95 (range, 65 to 100).[46]

Complications

A few uncommon complications that may be related to parallel plating have been reported in the past 5 years. One report described four incidences of osteonecrosis of the trochlea after parallel plate and screw fixation of a distal humeral fracture[47] (**Figure 5**). A second case report described distal humeral osteonecrosis reconstructed with a vascularized fibula graft.[48] A third case report described three patients with elbow dislocation after plate fixation of a bicolumnar fracture, possibly related to injury to the collateral ligament origins.[49]

A long-term follow-up study of elbow injuries found that posttraumatic arthrosis is more likely to develop in distal humeral fractures, both bicolumnar and capitellum-trochlea, than after other elbow injuries.[50] The arthrosis was not correlated with symptoms or dis-

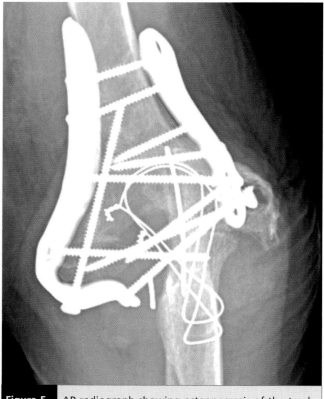

Figure 5 AP radiograph showing osteonecrosis of the trochlea after open reduction and internal fixation of the distal humerus.

humerus had preoperative ulnar nerve symptoms and were randomly assigned to subfascial transposition or in situ decompression of the ulnar nerve. No new ulnar neuropathies were reported in the 88 patients without preoperative symptoms, and transposition led to better ulnar nerve recovery than in situ decompression.[54]

A study of 59 patients found that the combination of an unstable elbow injury such as a displaced fracture of the distal humerus and a displaced fracture of the distal radius (9 patients), is associated with a risk of forearm compartment syndrome 50 times greater than that for a displaced fracture of the distal radius alone.[55]

Summary

Most data on distal humeral fractures are derived from numerous small retrospective case studies. Some advances have resulted from simple observations; for example, capitellum-trochlea fractures are often more complex than they appear. Areas of study that should be examined in future research include the results of parallel and perpendicular plate fixation, the role of locking screws, the risk factors for ulnar neuropathy, and the best method for handling the ulnar nerve. Because distal humeral fractures are uncommon, the participation of multiple centers in registries and randomized studies (as with the Canadian Orthopaedic Trauma Society study) is important to improving treatment.

ability and did not require additional surgery. A randomized study of radiation prophylaxis for heterotopic ossification was terminated before completion because of the relatively high rate of nonunion, primarily in patients with a distal humeral fracture.[51]

Three studies examined ulnar neuropathy, a relatively complex condition. Variability exists in the definition of ulnar neuropathy, its diagnosis, and the manner in which it is managed during surgery, particularly in retrospective studies. When 69 bicolumnar distal humeral fractures were treated with plate-and-screw fixation, the incidence of ulnar nerve dysfunction was 16%, but no demographic, injury, or treatment factors were associated with a risk of postoperative ulnar nerve dysfunction.[52] The second study of plate fixation of the distal humerus documented ulnar neuropathy in 16 of 48 patients treated with ulnar nerve transposition (33%), and 8 of 89 patients treated without transposition (9%).[53] In this retrospective study, it is possible that the patients treated with transposition underwent more extensive surgery on the medial side with more handling of the nerve and implants entering the cubital tunnel, necessitating transposition. The third study reported a high incidence of preoperative ulnar nerve dysfunction. Preoperative ulnar nerve dysfunction either is uncommon or is not commonly diagnosed. Twenty-nine of 117 patients with an AO type C fracture of the distal

Annotated References

1. Brouwer KM, Guitton TG, Doornberg JN, Kloen P, Jupiter JB, Ring D: Fractures of the medial column of the distal humerus in adults. *J Hand Surg Am* 2009; 34(3):439-445.

   Medial column fractures are uncommon in adults and often feature complex articular comminution.

2. Zalavras CG, Vercillo MT, Jun BJ, Otarodifard K, Itamura JM, Lee TQ: Biomechanical evaluation of parallel versus orthogonal plate fixation of intra-articular distal humerus fractures. *J Shoulder Elbow Surg* 2011; 20(1):12-20.

   Parallel plates were found to be stronger than perpendicular plates in a bicolumnar metaphyseal defect model.

3. Penzkofer R, Hungerer S, Wipf F, von Oldenburg G, Augat P: Anatomical plate configuration affects mechanical performance in distal humerus fractures. *Clin Biomech (Bristol, Avon)* 2010;25(10):972-978.

   Three different plate configurations offered adequate stability for active motion after open reduction and internal fixation of bicolumnar fractures.

4. Windolf M, Maza ER, Gueorguiev B, Braunstein V, Schwieger K: Treatment of distal humeral fractures using conventional implants: Biomechanical evaluation

of a new implant configuration. *BMC Musculoskelet Disord* 2010;11:172.

A cadaver study found that a new method of interlocking parallel plates was slightly stronger than conventional methods.

5. Arnander MW, Reeves A, MacLeod IA, Pinto TM, Khaleel A: A biomechanical comparison of plate configuration in distal humerus fractures. *J Orthop Trauma* 2008;22(5):332-336.

Parallel plates were found to be stronger than perpendicular plates in certain bending modes.

6. Stoffel K, Cunneen S, Morgan R, Nicholls R, Stachowiak G: Comparative stability of perpendicular versus parallel double-locking plating systems in osteoporotic comminuted distal humerus fractures. *J Orthop Res* 2008;26(6):778-784.

A biomechanical study found greater stability with parallel plating than with perpendicular plating.

7. Mehling I, Schmidt-Horlohé K, Müller LP, Sternstein W, Korner J, Rommens PM: Locking reconstruction double plating of distal humeral fractures: How many screws in the distal ulnar column segment in A3 fracture provide superior stability? A comparative biomechanical in vitro study. *J Orthop Trauma* 2009;23(8): 581-587.

Based on biomechanical analysis, the use of more than one locked screw was recommended in the distal humerus was recommended by the authors.

8. Schuster I, Korner J, Arzdorf M, Schwieger K, Diederichs G, Linke B: Mechanical comparison in cadaver specimens of three different 90-degree double-plate osteosyntheses for simulated C2-type distal humerus fractures with varying bone densities. *J Orthop Trauma* 2008;22(2):113-120.

Locking screws were found to make a difference only in distal humerus fractures in cadavers with poor quality bone.

9. Sabo MT, Fay K, McDonald CP, Ferreira LM, Johnson JA, King GJ: Effect of coronal shear fractures of the distal humerus on elbow kinematics and stability. *J Shoulder Elbow Surg* 2010;19(5):670-680.

Excision of the capitellum did not destabilize the elbow if the ligaments were intact, but any loss of the trochlea destabilized the elbow.

10. Park SH, Kim SJ, Park BC, et al: Three-dimensional osseous micro-architecture of the distal humerus: Implications for internal fixation of osteoporotic fracture. *J Shoulder Elbow Surg* 2010;19(2):244-250.

The lowest quality bone was found in the posterolateral distal humerus.

11. Brouwer KM, Lindenhovius AL, Ring D: Loss of anterior translation of the distal humeral articular surface is associated with decreased elbow flexion. *J Hand Surg Am* 2009;34(7):1256-1260.

Relative straightening of the distal humerus in the sag-

ittal plane hindered flexion after distal humeral fracture.

12. Kimball JP, Glowczewskie F, Wright TW: Intraosseous blood supply to the distal humerus. *J Hand Surg Am* 2007;32(5):642-646.

The blood supply to the distal humerus was found to be limited.

13. Brouwer KM, Jupiter JB, Ring D: Nonunion of operatively treated capitellum and trochlear fractures. *J Hand Surg Am* 2011;36(5):804-807.

Thirty patients underwent open reduction and internal fixation of a capitellum-trochlea fracture. At an average follow-up of 34 months, 8 of the 18 patients with a Dubberley type 3B fracture had nonunion. No patient with a simpler fracture had nonunion.

14. Doornberg JN, van Duijn PJ, Linzel D, et al: Surgical treatment of intra-articular fractures of the distal part of the humerus: Functional outcome after twelve to thirty years. *J Bone Joint Surg Am* 2007;89(7):1524-1532.

At an average follow-up of 19 years after plate-and-screw fixation of an AO type C fracture of the distal humerus in 30 patients, the average arc of flexion was 106°, the average DASH score was 7, and the average Mayo score was 91, with 26 good or excellent results. The results were not correlated with arthrosis.

15. Huang JI, Paczas M, Hoyen HA, Vallier HA: Functional outcome after open reduction internal fixation of intra-articular fractures of the distal humerus in the elderly. *J Orthop Trauma* 2011;25(5):259-265.

Distal humeral fracture was found to be an elbow-changing injury that causes pain and disability in the elderly.

16. Liu JJ, Ruan HJ, Wang JG, Fan CY, Zeng BF: Double-column fixation for type C fractures of the distal humerus in the elderly. *J Shoulder Elbow Surg* 2009; 18(4):646-651.

A retrospective study found acceptable results after open reduction and internal fixation of double-column fractures.

17. Frattini M, Soncini G, Corradi M, Panno B, Tocco S, Pogliacomi F: Mid-term results of complex distal humeral fractures. *Musculoskelet Surg* 2011;95(3): 205-213.

Another retrospective study found acceptable results after open reduction and internal fixation of double-column fractures.

18. Luegmair M, Timofiev E, Chirpaz-Cerbat JM: Surgical treatment of AO type C distal humeral fractures: Internal fixation with a Y-shaped reconstruction (Lambda) plate. *J Shoulder Elbow Surg* 2008;17(1):113-120.

The functional outcome of fixation of distal humeral fractures with a Y-shaped plate was analyzed.

19. Bhattacharyya A, Jha AK, Chatterjee D, Ghosh B, Roy SK, Banerjee D: Operative management of closed intra-articular fractures of distal end of humerus in adults. *J Indian Med Assoc* 2011;109(6):418-423, 423.

The fixation of type C distal humeral fractures using older methods had acceptable outcomes in India.

20. Babhulkar S, Babhulkar S: Controversies in the management of intra-articular fractures of distal humerus in adults. *Indian J Orthop* 2011;45(3):216-225.

The use of three different dual-plate configurations for distal humeral fractures had comparably good results.

21. Puchwein P, Wildburger R, Archan S, Guschl M, Tanzer K, Gumpert R: Outcome of type C (AO) distal humeral fractures: Follow-up of 22 patients with bicolumnar plating osteosynthesis. *J Shoulder Elbow Surg* 2011;20(4):631-636.

A retrospective study found acceptable outcomes after open reduction and internal fixation of bicolumnar fractures using dual plates.

22. Li SH, Li ZH, Cai ZD, et al: Bilateral plate fixation for type C distal humerus fractures: Experience at a single institution. *Int Orthop* 2011;35(3):433-438.

A retrospective study found acceptable outcomes after open reduction and internal fixation of bicolumnar fractures using a transolecranon approach.

23. Proust J, Oksman A, Charissoux JL, Mabit C, Arnaud JP: [Intra-articular fracture of the distal humerus: Outcome after osteosynthesis in patients over 60]. *Rev Chir Orthop Reparatrice Appar Mot* 2007;93(8):798-806.

Open reduction and internal fixation of bicolumnar fractures had a good or very good outcome in 59% of patients older than 60 years.

24. Chen G, Liao Q, Luo W, Li K, Zhao Y, Zhong D: Triceps-sparing versus olecranon osteotomy for ORIF: Analysis of 67 cases of intercondylar fractures of the distal humerus. *Injury* 2011;42(4):366-370.

Olecranon osteotomy was found to lead to better results than a triceps-sparing approach in patients older than 60 years.

25. Ali AM, Hassanin EY, El-Ganainy AE, Abd-Elmola T: Management of intercondylar fractures of the humerus using the extensor mechanism-sparing paratricipital posterior approach. *Acta Orthop Belg* 2008;74(6):747-752.

The use of the paratricipital approach in patients with an interarticular fracture of the distal humerus led to satisfactory results.

26. Ek ET, Goldwasser M, Bonomo AL: Functional outcome of complex intercondylar fractures of the distal humerus treated through a triceps-sparing approach. *J Shoulder Elbow Surg* 2008;17(3):441-446.

The use of the paratricipital approach in patients with an interarticular fracture of the distal humerus led to satisfactory results.

27. Theivendran K, Duggan PJ, Deshmukh SC: Surgical treatment of complex distal humeral fractures: Functional outcome after internal fixation using precontoured anatomic plates. *J Shoulder Elbow Surg* 2010;19(4):524-532.

The use of anatomic precontoured plates led to acceptable functional outcomes with complex distal humeral fractures.

28. Athwal GS, Hoxie SC, Rispoli DM, Steinmann SP: Precontoured parallel plate fixation of AO/OTA type C distal humerus fractures. *J Orthop Trauma* 2009;23(8):575-580.

The use of anatomic precontoured plates was effective, but more than one half of the patients experienced a complication.

29. Sanchez-Sotelo J, Torchia ME, O'Driscoll SW: Complex distal humeral fractures: Internal fixation with a principle-based parallel-plate technique. *J Bone Joint Surg Am* 2007;89(5):961-969.

After 32 AO type C fractures were repaired with parallel plates, 1 patient had nonunion, 5 underwent subsequent surgery for elbow stiffness, and 1 had a deep infection. The mean arc of flexion was 99°, and the mean Mayo score was 85, with 27 patients with good or excellent results.

30. Shin SJ, Sohn HS, Do NH: A clinical comparison of two different double plating methods for intraarticular distal humerus fractures. *J Shoulder Elbow Surg* 2010;19(1):2-9.

Perpendicular plating was less successful than parallel plating in achieving bony union for supracondylar fractures of the distal humerus.

31. Reising K, Hauschild O, Strohm PC, Suedkamp NP: Stabilisation of articular fractures of the distal humerus: Early experience with a novel perpendicular plate system. *Injury* 2009;40(6):611-617.

The use of locking precontoured plates led to stable fixation for articular fractures of the distal humerus.

32. Greiner S, Haas NP, Bail HJ: Outcome after open reduction and angular stable internal fixation for supra-intercondylar fractures of the distal humerus: Preliminary results with the LCP distal humerus system. *Arch Orthop Trauma Surg* 2008;128(7):723-729.

The use of locking precontoured plates led to stable fixation for supracondylar fractures of the distal humerus.

33. Min W, Ding BC, Tejwani NC: Staged versus acute definitive management of open distal humerus fractures. *J Trauma* 2011;71(4):944-947.

Patients with open distal humeral fractures who were treated with temporary external fixation and staged open reduction and internal fixation had worse results than those who underwent early definitive fixation, probably because these patients had more severe fractures.

34. Watts AC, Morris A, Robinson CM: Fractures of the distal humeral articular surface. *J Bone Joint Surg Br* 2007;89(4):510-515.

    This recent case study reported that fractures of the capitellum and the trochlea are more common than previously recognized.

35. Guitton TG, Doornberg JN, Raaymakers EL, Ring D, Kloen P: Fractures of the capitellum and trochlea. *J Bone Joint Surg Am* 2009;91(2):390-397.

    This case study provides data on long-term outcomes of fractures of the capitellum and the trochlea.

36. Dubberley JH, Faber KJ, Macdermid JC, Patterson SD, King GJ: Outcome after open reduction and internal fixation of capitellar and trochlear fractures. *J Bone Joint Surg Am* 2006;88(1):46-54.

37. Ashwood N, Verma M, Hamlet M, Garlapati A, Fogg Q: Transarticular shear fractures of the distal humerus. *J Shoulder Elbow Surg* 2010;19(1):46-52.

    The treatment of patients with a capitellum-trochlea fracture is described.

38. Mighell M, Virani NA, Shannon R, Echols EL Jr, Badman BL, Keating CJ: Large coronal shear fractures of the capitellum and trochlea treated with headless compression screws. *J Shoulder Elbow Surg* 2010;19(1):38-45.

    The treatment of patients with a capitellum-trochlea fracture is described.

39. Adolfsson L, Nestorson J: The Kudo humeral component as primary hemiarthroplasty in distal humeral fractures. *J Shoulder Elbow Surg* 2012;21(4):451-455.

    Eight women (average age, 79 years) who were evaluated at a mean 4-year follow-up after Kudo hemiarthroplasty for fracture of the distal humerus had an average flexion from 31° to 126°. All patients had good or excellent Mayo scores.

40. Burkhart KJ, Nijs S, Mattyasovszky SG, et al: Distal humerus hemiarthroplasty of the elbow for comminuted distal humeral fractures in the elderly patient. *J Trauma* 2011;71(3):635-642.

    Hemiarthroplasty for distal humeral fracture had good results in 10 patients (mean age, 75.2 years).

41. McKee MD, Veillette CJ, Hall JA, et al: A multicenter, prospective, randomized, controlled trial of open reduction—internal fixation versus total elbow arthroplasty for displaced intra-articular distal humeral fractures in elderly patients. *J Shoulder Elbow Surg* 2009;18(1):3-12.

    A Canadian Orthopaedic Trauma Society prospective randomized study compared open reduction and internal fixation with primary semiconstrained total elbow arthroplasty in 42 patients (minimum age, 65 years) with AO type C fracture. Total elbow arthroplasty was associated with shorter surgical times and better Mayo scores but not better motion or DASH scores.

42. Egol KA, Tsai P, Vazques O, Tejwani NC: Comparison of functional outcomes of total elbow arthroplasty vs plate fixation for distal humerus fractures in osteoporotic elbows. *Am J Orthop (Belle Mead NJ)* 2011;40(2):67-71.

    A retrospective study found that both open reduction and internal fixation and total elbow arthroplasty had good results in patients with an osteoporotic elbow.

43. Ali A, Shahane S, Stanley D: Total elbow arthroplasty for distal humeral fractures: Indications, surgical approach, technical tips, and outcome. *J Shoulder Elbow Surg* 2010;19(Suppl 2):53-58.

    Total elbow arthroplasty was described for patients with a bicolumnar fracture.

44. Chalidis B, Dimitriou C, Papadopoulos P, Petsatodis G, Giannoudis PV: Total elbow arthroplasty for the treatment of insufficient distal humeral fractures: A retrospective clinical study and review of the literature. *Injury* 2009;40(6):582-590.

    The treatment and outcomes of total elbow arthroscopy for distal humeral fracture were described.

45. Prasad N, Dent C: Outcome of total elbow replacement for distal humeral fractures in the elderly: A comparison of primary surgery and surgery after failed internal fixation or conservative treatment. *J Bone Joint Surg Br* 2008;90(3):343-348.

    A small comparative study found that delayed total elbow arthroscopy had less satisfactory outcomes than early arthroplasty, but the difference was not significant.

46. Kalogrianitis S, Sinopidis C, El Meligy M, Rawal A, Frostick SP: Unlinked elbow arthroplasty as primary treatment for fractures of the distal humerus. *J Shoulder Elbow Surg* 2008;17(2):287-292.

    The use of an unlinked total elbow prosthesis is described.

47. Wiggers JK, Ring D: Osteonecrosis after open reduction and internal fixation of a bicolumnar fracture of the distal humerus: A report of four cases. *J Hand Surg Am* 2011;36(1):89-93.

    Some patients experienced a complication related to osteonecrosis in the articular surface after open reduction and internal fixation.

48. Vigler M, Gargano F, Hausman MR: Trochlear reconstruction using vascularized lateral clavicle bone graft for posttraumatic osteonecrosis of the distal humerus. *J Shoulder Elbow Surg* 2008;17(5):e4-e8.

    The treatment of osteonecrosis of the distal humerus was reported.

49. Lu HT, Guitton TG, Capo JT, Ring D: Elbow instability associated with bicolumnar fracture of the distal humerus: Report of three cases. *J Hand Surg Am* 2010;35(7):1126-1129.

    Instability, presumably related to lateral collateral ligament injury during fixation, was found to be a complication of open reduction and internal fixation.

7: Elbow Trauma, Fracture, and Reconstruction

50. Guitton TG, Zurakowski D, van Dijk NC, Ring D: Incidence and risk factors for the development of radiographic arthrosis after traumatic elbow injuries. *J Hand Surg Am* 2010;35(12):1976-1980.

   Distal humeral fractures were found to be more likely to lead to arthritis than other elbow trauma.

51. Hamid N, Ashraf N, Bosse MJ, et al: Radiation therapy for heterotopic ossification prophylaxis acutely after elbow trauma: A prospective randomized study. *J Bone Joint Surg Am* 2010;92(11):2032-2038.

   A randomized study was abandoned because preventive radiation for heterotopic ossification was causing nonunion of osteotomies and fractures.

52. Vazquez O, Rutgers M, Ring DC, Walsh M, Egol KA: Fate of the ulnar nerve after operative fixation of distal humerus fractures. *J Orthop Trauma* 2010;24(7): 395-399.

   After 69 bicolumnar distal humeral fractures were treated with plate and screw fixation, ulnar nerve dysfunction occurred in 16%, but no demographic, injury, or treatment factors were associated with a risk of postoperative ulnar nerve dysfunction.

53. Chen RC, Harris DJ, Leduc S, Borrelli JJ Jr, Tornetta P III, Ricci WM: Is ulnar nerve transposition beneficial during open reduction internal fixation of distal humerus fractures? *J Orthop Trauma* 2010;24(7): 391-394.

   A study of plate fixation of the distal humerus documented ulnar neuropathy in 33% (16 of 48) treated with transposition of the ulnar nerve and 9% (8 of 89) treated without.

54. Ruan HJ, Liu JJ, Fan CY, Jiang J, Zeng BF: Incidence, management, and prognosis of early ulnar nerve dysfunction in type C fractures of distal humerus. *J Trauma* 2009;67(6):1397-1401.

   This randomized study found a high rate of preoperative ulnar nerve symptoms (25%) in patients with a distal humeral fracture. Transposition wa considered preferable to in situ release.

55. Hwang RW, de Witte PB, Ring D: Compartment syndrome associated with distal radial fracture and ipsilateral elbow injury. *J Bone Joint Surg Am* 2009;91(3): 642-645.

   Ipsilateral unstable wrist and elbow injuries were found to have an increased risk for acute forearm compartment syndrome.

Chapter 46

Elbow Arthroscopy: Indications and Surgical Considerations

Aaron Chamberlain, MD   Ken Yamaguchi, MD

Introduction

In 1931, Burman[1] described the elbow as unsuitable for arthroscopy, based on a cadaver study. In 1985, Andrews and Carson[2] described the successful use of elbow arthroscopy in 12 patients, concluding that safe, reproducible arthroscopy of the elbow was feasible as long as the surgeon paid close attention to detail. More recent advances in surgical technique, instrumentation, and equipment have contributed to an improvement in the usefulness of elbow arthroscopy, but careful consideration of surgical indications and the surgeon's experience are imperative to safe and effective arthroscopy of the elbow.

Indications

The indications for elbow arthroscopy have broadened substantially over time. In 1985, elbow arthroscopy was described as a diagnostic and therapeutic tool that could be used to remove loose bodies and perform radial head and capitellum chondroplasties.[2] The indications for elbow arthroscopy have since broadened to include the treatment of rheumatoid arthritis, elbow osteoarthritis and associated stiffness, osteochondritis dissecans (OCD), lateral epicondylitis, some fractures, symptomatic plica, and a variety of pathologic conditions encountered by throwing athletes.

A recent literature review found only fair-quality evidence to support the use of elbow arthroscopy for the treatment of rheumatoid arthritis or lateral epicondylitis and only poor-quality evidence to support arthroscopy for plica or annular ligament excision or for the treatment of osteoarthritis, OCD lesions, posterolateral rotatory instability, loose bodies, posttraumatic arthrofibrosis, or fractures.[3] High-quality evidence is lacking

to support the use of arthroscopy in any elbow condition. Elbow arthroscopy remains a relatively new technique, and more high-quality research is needed to determine its usefulness.

Loose Body Removal

The removal of loose bodies is the most common indication for elbow arthroscopy.[4] Andrews and Carson[2] found that the removal of loose bodies was the most successful use of elbow arthroscopy compared with other indications, such as chondroplasty. In a study of 33 elbow arthroscopies for loose body removal, pain was improved in 85% of the patients, locking in 92%, and swelling in 71%.[5] Numerous published case studies have reported the clinical outcomes of loose body removal. A recent analysis of 12 case studies involving arthroscopic loose body removal found that 98 of 109 patients (90%) reported a good to excellent result or substantial improvement.[3] In nine studies of patients undergoing loose body removal during procedures such as débridement of osteophytes or chondroplasty, 110 of 150 patients (73%) had a good to excellent result or significant improvement. However, no published studies have compared arthroscopic and open loose body removal.

Synovectomy

Multiple researchers have found favorable results after arthroscopic synovectomy for rheumatoid arthritis.[6-8] In comparison with open synovectomy, arthroscopic synovectomy is less invasive, facilitates an earlier return to activity, and is associated with a lower risk of postoperative stiffness. However, two reports warned of the risk of incomplete synovectomy because of the limitations and technical challenges of the procedure.[6,9] Incomplete arthroscopic synovectomy may lead to a more rapid deterioration of results than open synovectomy. All 14 patients undergoing arthroscopic synovectomy for rheumatoid arthritis or juvenile idiopathic arthritis had mild or no pain at early postoperative follow-up, but only 8 (57%) had a good to excellent functional outcome at final follow-up (mean, 42 months).[6]

Advances in technique have improved the ability to achieve a more complete arthroscopic synovectomy. In

Dr. Yamaguchi or an immediate family member has received royalties from Tornier. Neither Dr. Chamberlain nor any immediate family member has received anything of value from or has stock or stock options held in a commercial company or institution related directly or indirectly to the subject of this chapter.

26 rheumatoid elbows undergoing arthroscopic synovectomy, the soft-spot portal and an accessory lateral portal were used to gain access to the posterior space of the radiocapitellar and proximal radioulnar joints. In addition, the standard proximal anteromedial and proximal anterolateral portals were used to gain access to the anterior joint space, and the posterolateral and posterior central portals were used for access to the posterior joint.[10] At a mean 34-month follow-up, the mean score on the visual analog pain scale had improved from 6.5 to 3.1, and the mean flexion arc had increased from 98° to 113°. For 19 elbows (73%), the patients reported good to excellent results. Clinically apparent synovitis recurred in only four elbows; two required repeat synovectomy, and one required total elbow arthroplasty. The fourth patient declined further surgery.

The overall results of arthroscopic synovectomy of the elbow are not as positive as those of arthroscopic synovectomy for other joints affected by rheumatoid arthritis. The limited case studies provide some weak evidence favoring arthroscopic synovectomy, with special attention to the need for a thorough and complete synovectomy.

Elbow Stiffness

Elbow stiffness is common and difficult to manage. Stiffness can result from a variety of traumatic and atraumatic conditions. Both intrinsic and extrinsic factors can contribute to stiffness. The intrinsic factors include pathology causing incongruity of the joint, such as arthritis, or incongruity resulting from fracture. Extrinsic causes in the context of a preserved joint include capsular tightness or contracture, heterotopic ossification, and skin or muscle contracture. Arthroscopic management of capsular contracture can be successful. Intrinsic pathology, such as arthritis with osteophyte formation, also can be treated arthroscopically with modern techniques and instrumentation.

Arthroscopic management of the stiff elbow is a challenging technical procedure. A study of the learning curve found no substantial decrease in operating time until the surgeon had completed 15 procedures.[11] Nonetheless, arthroscopic management of elbow stiffness is becoming more widely used.[11-20] A retrospective study of 14 consecutive patients with posttraumatic elbow stiffness who underwent arthroscopic capsulotomy found that only 6 of 14 patients had pain at a minimum 1-year follow-up.[12] The mean maximal pain score on the visual analog scale was 4.6. Elbow extension improved from 35.4° before surgery to 9.3° after surgery, and elbow flexion improved from 117.5° to 133°. The overall arc of motion improved from 82° to 123.6° (mean improvement, 41.6°). All patients stated they would choose to have the surgery again. A recent report described the results of arthroscopic capsular release and débridement of osteophytes in 27 elbows with posttraumatic elbow stiffness.[13] Preoperative extension and flexion were 24° and 123°, respectively.

Postoperative extension improved to 7°, flexion improved to 133°, and total range of motion improved from 99° to 125°. No neurologic complications were noted.

Only one published study has directly compared arthroscopic and open débridement. A nonrandomized controlled study of the Outerbridge-Kashiwagi procedure (open débridement of osteophytes and fenestration of the olecranon fossa) compared with arthroscopic débridement and fenestration found that both procedures were effective and led to no major complications.[21] The patients treated with arthroscopic débridement and fenestration of the olecranon fossa had a trend toward better pain relief ($P < 0.10$), and those undergoing the open Outerbridge-Kashiwagi procedure had a greater range of flexion ($P < 0.05$). A retrospective review of 20 elbows at a mean 2-year follow-up after an arthroscopic Outerbridge-Kashiwagi procedure found that the total range of motion improved from 94° to 123°, and visual analog scale pain scores improved from 5.8 to 1.8.[14] The overall results were good to excellent in 16 elbows, fair in 2, and poor in 2.

Most studies describing arthroscopic management of the stiff elbow include patients with both intrinsic and extrinsic causes of joint stiffness but exclude patients with articular incongruity or notable heterotopic ossification. No level I studies have analyzed the arthroscopic management of the stiff elbow. Despite their limitations, the existing published case studies suggest that for experienced surgeons, arthroscopic release can be a safe and effective method of managing elbow stiffness that has been refractory to nonsurgical measures.

Osteochondritis Dissecans

OCD lesions in the elbow usually are localized lesions affecting the articular surface of the capitellum. These lesions are not uncommon in young athletes. The primary factors in considering surgical management include the integrity of the articular surface, the stability of the lesion, and whether the physis is open or closed. Surgical intervention may be indicated if the patient has unstable lesions, loose bodies, and/or unsuccessful nonsurgical treatment.[22] The possible arthroscopic surgical interventions include transarticular drilling, loose body removal, drilling, microfracture, and mosaicplasty.[23] Numerous case studies have been published on the clinical results of arthroscopic management of OCD lesions.[22,24-32] A recent systematic review of nine studies evaluated arthroscopic surgery in athletes with OCD lesions in the elbow.[33] The surgical interventions in the reviewed studies included débridement, fixation of the fragment, microfracture, and osteochondral autografting. Patients returned to sport 81% to 100% of the time, and 89% to 100% were pain free. Unfortunately, studies evaluating the arthroscopic management of OCD lesions of the elbow have used varied clinical outcome measures, so direct study comparisons are difficult. No study has compared nonsurgical and arthroscopic management.

Lateral Epicondylitis

Two retrospective cohort studies have compared open and arthroscopic release of the extensor carpi radialis brevis (ECRB) for the treatment of recalcitrant lateral epicondylitis.[34,35] Neither study found a significant difference between patients treated with an open or an arthroscopic procedure. The percentage of patients with a good to excellent result ranged from 60% to 75%. One study found an earlier return to work in patients treated arthroscopically versus those treated with an open procedure (1.7 or 2.5 weeks, respectively).[34] In a recent study of 36 patients treated with arthroscopic ECRB release for persistently symptomatic lateral epicondylitis, 31% reported mild pain with strenuous activities at a mean 3.5-year follow-up.[36] Two patients (6%) received no benefit from the procedure.

Overall, the existing data on arthroscopic ECRB release reveals results similar to those of open release. Most report consistently high levels of good to excellent outcomes, but no high-quality studies have examined arthroscopic ECRB release, and there are no comparisons of arthroscopic and nonsurgical management. Nonetheless, the existing results offer support for arthroscopic management of lateral epicondylitis.[34-37]

Fractures

Arthroscopic management of fractures about the elbow is a relatively recent and evolving indication for elbow arthroscopy. Most of the published material on arthroscopic fracture management is limited to small case studies and case reports. Arthroscopic management has been described for fractures of the capitellum (excision and fixation), coronoid (excision and fixation), and radial head.[38-43] However, no studies have been published comparing open and arthroscopic management of these fractures. At this time, there is no evidence to suggest poorer outcomes with arthroscopic management or to recommend arthroscopic over open management.

The Ulnar Nerve

In patients with elbow flexion limited to 90° to 100°, the ulnar nerve must be prophylactically treated to prevent nerve compression after release and improvement in flexion.[15] The ulnar nerve is located within the cubital tunnel, the floor of which is the posterior bundle of the ulnar collateral ligament. With flexion of the elbow beyond 90°, the dimensions of the cubital tunnel decrease, thus increasing pressure on the ulnar nerve.[44] Flexion cannot be restored in an elbow that has lost a substantial amount of flexion (retains less than 90° of flexion) if contracture of the posterior bundle is not treated. In addition, injury to the ulnar nerve may occur with manipulation of the elbow into a more flexed position as the posterior bundle becomes taut.

Prior ulnar nerve transposition, especially submuscular transposition, has been considered a relative contraindication to elbow arthroscopy.[45,46] The concern is that after ulnar nerve transposition, the ulnar nerve rests anteriorly relative to its normal anatomic position at the elbow and is in close proximity to the proximal anteromedial portal commonly used to visualize the anterior compartment of the elbow. However, with experience and a standardized approach, the proximal anteromedial portal can safely be used in an elbow with a prior ulnar nerve transposition. In 59 elbows with a subluxating or previously transposed ulnar nerve, arthroscopy was done using the standard anteromedial portal.[47] If the location of the transposed nerve was unequivocal, a 1-cm incision was made away from the nerve. If the location of the nerve was equivocal, a portal incision was made approximately 1 cm away from the apparent location of the nerve. Blunt dissection was performed down to the capsule, and a blunt switching stick was used to penetrate the joint capsule. If localization of the nerve was impossible, a 2- to 4-cm incision was made, the nerve was identified, and the portal was established. There were no surgical ulnar nerve injuries related to using the proximal anteromedial portal.[47]

Contraindications

Arthroscopic management is relatively contraindicated if the elbow has severe joint incongruity, anatomy distortion, heterotopic ossification, or muscle contracture. These elbows are best managed with an open surgical approach.[15] Because of the proximity of peripheral nerves, the most important contraindication perhaps is inadequate experience in the procedure, if it is expected to be difficult. Severe elbow contractures often are associated with substantial soft-tissue adhesions and contractures of extra-articular soft tissues, which are difficult to manage arthroscopically. In an elbow with severe contracture, it can be difficult to insufflate the joint; this factor substantially increases the level of difficulty and the dangers associated with arthroscopy. Prior ulnar nerve transposition, especially submuscular transposition, is a relative contraindication and requires modification of the surgical technique to avoid nerve injury.

Surgical Considerations

Setup and Positioning

Elbow arthroscopy has the potential to cause serious injury to peripheral neurovascular structures and articular cartilage. Meticulous attention to detail is necessary in setup and positioning to minimize the risk of such complications.

Some surgeons perform elbow arthroscopy under regional anesthesia. General anesthesia is preferred, however, primarily because it allows immediate and repeated postoperative neurologic evaluation. In addition, regional anesthesia does not provide the complete relaxation of the patient that facilitates easy positioning into the lateral decubitus or prone position. Regional anesthesia may not be sufficient to prevent the patient from experiencing tourniquet pain during the procedure.

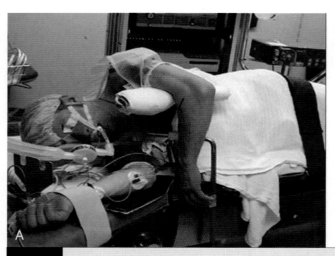
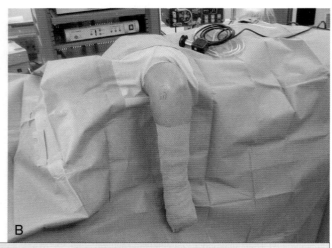

Figure 1 Intraoperative photographs showing patient positioning and setup for elbow arthroscopy before (**A**) and after (**B**) draping.

Antibiotic prophylaxis is a key consideration in elbow arthroscopy. The incidence of serious deep joint infection after elbow arthroscopy is reported to be 0.8%, and the incidence of prolonged drainage and superficial infection is reported to be 7%.[48] A first-generation cephalosporin can be used before tourniquet inflation. If an allergy must be considered, clindamycin or vancomycin can be substituted. At the conclusion of the procedure, the portal sites are closed with locked horizontal mattress stitches to prevent postoperative portal drainage and/or fistula formation. After surgery, the patient receives oral antibiotic prophylaxis for 2 weeks until the wounds are fully closed and there is very little risk of drainage.

Elbow arthroscopy can be performed with the patient in the lateral decubitus, prone, or supine position.[2,49,50] The lateral decubitus position offers the advantages of readily accessible airway management during the procedure, greater intraoperative freedom of motion of the elbow, and better access to the posterior compartment. Ready access to the posterior compartment facilitates the use of osteotomes or large burrs to excise osteophytes from the olecranon tip when aggressive débridement of osteophytes is indicated.

After the patient is positioned in the lateral decubitus position, an axillary roll or gel pad is placed. A nonsterile padded tourniquet is applied to the brachium proximally. The surgical extremity is positioned in a padded stationary arm holder with the elbow resting at approximately 90° of elbow flexion. To ensure there is enough space for instruments to fit between the elbow and the thorax, the arm should be abducted at least 90° from the body, and the elbow should be positioned slightly higher than the level of the shoulder. The patient's thorax should be positioned so that the anterior chest wall is at the edge of the bed. This positioning method allows full elbow flexion and extension during the procedure[51] (**Figure 1**).

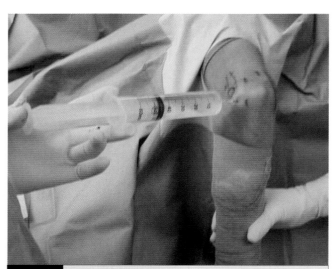

Figure 2 Intraoperative photograph showing insufflation of elbow with fluid before the arthroscopy is started.

Fluid Management

Proper fluid management is essential for the success and safety of elbow arthroscopy. Fluid distention is necessary to increase the working space in the joint. Just before a portal is created, the joint is distended with approximately 20 to 30 mL of normal saline injected with a needle through the soft spot located at the center of a triangle formed by the lateral epicondyle, the radial head, and the olecranon process (**Figure 2**). Distending the joint capsule improves safety by increasing the distance between the humerus and the joint capsule as well as nearby neurovascular structures. Capsular compliance in a very stiff elbow may be as low as 15% of that of a normal elbow; this means that joint space volume is substantially decreased, and the risk for injury is increased.[52] A lack of capsular distention (as indicated by an inability to inject more than 10 to 15 mL of normal saline) is an indication that the procedure is unusually dangerous and should be performed only by an appropriately experienced surgeon.

A pump-controlled or gravity flow fluid system can be used. A pump-controlled system is recommended, with the fluid pump pressure set to 35 mm Hg. However, it should be noted that actual pump pressures vary among products from different manufacturers. In general, the pump pressure is set approximately 30% lower for elbow arthroscopy than for shoulder arthroscopy. Low pump pressures should be used to minimize soft-tissue swelling, which can quickly occur in the elbow and can significantly impede elbow arthroscopy. Surgical time is important in elbow arthroscopy because capsular tissues quickly become edematous and inhibit the intra-articular viewing and working space. Therefore, surgical efficiency is more important in elbow arthroscopy than in arthroscopy of other major joints.

Instrumentation and Equipment Advances

The use of modern instrumentation facilitates safe, effective, and efficient elbow arthroscopy. A standard 4.5-mm joint arthroscope is commonly used for elbow arthroscopy, although the smaller 2.7-mm arthroscope can be considered. A standard 30° lens is appropriate for most procedures. However, a 70° lens can provide more complete visualization of the coronoid fossa depth, some obscure loose bodies, and occult chondral lesions.[53] Cannulas may be used for fluid outflow as well as working, although the use of cannulas is not necessary and may contribute to insufflation and edema of the surrounding soft tissues. If cannulas are used, they should be low-flow cannulas without side fenestrations, to minimize soft-tissue insufflation. A variety of working cannulas are available, generally smaller than 5.5 mm.

Arthroscopy of the elbow is much more sensitive to deviations in portal placement than arthroscopy of other major joints, and imprecise portal placement will impede the surgeon's ability to effectively perform elbow arthroscopy. Guidewires and cannulated dilators are used to accurately and safely create portal sites. The use of these instruments to create the proximal anterolateral portal avoids repeated passage of cannulas and instruments through the surrounding soft tissues and thus reduces the chance of neurovascular injury. With the arthroscope placed in the proximal anteromedial portal for viewing the radiocapitellar joint, the guidewire is placed in the joint under direct visualization. A scalpel is used to incise skin around the wire, and cannulated dilators create the precise portal. Precise portal placement with guidewires and cannulated dilators is imperative because the radial nerve is, on average, 5 to 10 mm from the proximal anterolateral portal. After proximal anteromedial and proximal anterolateral portals have been established, a blunt trochar can be used to release intra-articular adhesions and lift the anterior capsule off the anterior humerus, thus increasing the working space.

A size 4.0 oscillating shaver is useful for débriding synovium and adhesions. Care should be taken to not direct the shaver toward the capsule. Judicious use of the suction in the shaver will prevent capsular tissue from being drawn into the shaver, possibly resulting in injury to adjacent neurovascular structures. Suction is rarely used in the anterior elbow.

Small-caliber burrs are useful for resecting large osteophytes or performing more aggressive osteocapsular arthroplasty. Specially designed osteotomes are useful for aggressive osteophyte resection in the posterior compartment and resecting osteophytes at the tip of the olecranon.

A 15° up-cutting basket resector can be safely used to develop a plane between the brachialis and the anterior capsule. With the plane developed, the basket resector is used to divide the anterior capsule, proceeding from lateral to medial. If necessary, the arthroscope can be switched to the proximal anterolateral portal, and the capsulotomy can be completed from the proximal anteromedial portal. When the deep surface of the brachialis is exposed, the anterior capsulotomy is complete. This step should be done after all other work in the anterior compartment is complete because soft-tissue edema will progress rapidly after the capsulotomy is performed, decreasing the intra-articular space for working and viewing.

Specially designed elbow arthroscopy retractors can be useful for safely retracting soft tissues, such as the anterior capsule, or protecting neurovascular structures, such as the ulnar nerve, while working posteriorly in the medial gutter.

Summary

Elbow arthroscopy, once considered impossible, has evolved to become an increasingly valuable technique for treating a wide variety of elbow pathologies. Technical advances and modifications have allowed elbow arthroscopy to emerge as safe and reliable although technically demanding. A focus on surgeon education and technical advancement will be beneficial in the continuing evolution of elbow arthroscopy as a safe and beneficial technique.

Annotated References

1. Burman MS: Arthroscopy or the direct visualization of joints: An experimental cadaver study. *J Bone Joint Surg* 1931;13:669-695.

2. Andrews JR, Carson WG: Arthroscopy of the elbow. *Arthroscopy* 1985;1(2):97-107.

3. Yeoh KM, King GJ, Faber KJ, Glazebrook MA, Athwal GS: Evidence-based indications for elbow arthroscopy. *Arthroscopy* 2012;28(2):272-282.

   A recent review of the outcomes of elbow arthroscopy makes evidence-based recommendations for or against elbow arthroscopy for the treatment of various conditions. Level of evidence: IV.

4. Baker CL, Brooks AA: Arthroscopy of the elbow. *Clin Sports Med* 1996;15(2):261-281.

5. Ogilvie-Harris DJ, Schemitsch E: Arthroscopy of the elbow for removal of loose bodies. *Arthroscopy* 1993; 9(1):5-8.

6. Lee BP, Morrey BF: Arthroscopic synovectomy of the elbow for rheumatoid arthritis: A prospective study. *J Bone Joint Surg Br* 1997;79(5):770-772.

7. Nemoto K, Arino H, Yoshihara Y, Fujikawa K: Arthroscopic synovectomy for the rheumatoid elbow: A short-term outcome. *J Shoulder Elbow Surg* 2004; 13(6):652-655.

8. Tanaka N, Sakahashi H, Hirose K, Ishima T, Ishii S: Arthroscopic and open synovectomy of the elbow in rheumatoid arthritis. *J Bone Joint Surg Am* 2006; 88(3):521-525.

9. Horiuchi K, Momohara S, Tomatsu T, Inoue K, Toyama Y: Arthroscopic synovectomy of the elbow in rheumatoid arthritis. *J Bone Joint Surg Am* 2002; 84-A(3):342-347.

10. Kang HJ, Park MJ, Ahn JH, Lee SH: Arthroscopic synovectomy for the rheumatoid elbow. *Arthroscopy* 2010;26(9):1195-1202.

    Management of the rheumatoid elbow with an arthroscopic total synovectomy is described, with multiple portals and division of the elbow into the anterior, posterior, and radiocapitellar compartments. Level of evidence: IV.

11. Kim S-J, Moon H-K, Chun Y-M, Chang J-H: Arthroscopic treatment for limitation of motion of the elbow: The learning curve. *Knee Surg Sports Traumatol Arthrosc* 2011;19(6):1013-1018.

    A learning curve for elbow arthroscopy was assigned in the setting of the stiff elbow by comparing mean surgical times, mean improvement in motion, and clinical scores. Level of evidence: IV.

12. Ball CM, Meunier M, Galatz LM, Calfee R, Yamaguchi K: Arthroscopic treatment of posttraumatic elbow contracture. *J Shoulder Elbow Surg* 2002;11(6):624-629.

13. Cefo I, Eygendaal D: Arthroscopic arthrolysis for posttraumatic elbow stiffness. *J Shoulder Elbow Surg* 2011;20(3):434-439.

    The outcomes of 27 patients with posttraumatic elbow stiffness treated with arthroscopic capsular release were assessed. Level of evidence: IV.

14. DeGreef I, Samorjai N, De Smet L: The Outerbridge-Kashiwaghi procedure in elbow arthroscopy. *Acta Orthop Belg* 2010;76(4):468-471.

    The results of the arthroscopic Outerbridge-Kashiwaghi procedure were evaluated at a mean 2-year follow-up in a retrospective review of 20 elbows in 19 patients. Level of evidence: IV.

15. Keener JD, Galatz LM: Arthroscopic management of the stiff elbow. *J Am Acad Orthop Surg* 2011;19(5): 265-274.

    This review article discusses intrinsic and extrinsic causes of elbow stiffness as well as the arthroscopic management of these causes of elbow stiffness.

16. Singh H, Nam KY, Moon YL: Arthroscopic management of stiff elbow. *Orthopedics* 2011;34(6):167.

    Functional results after arthroscopic management of the stiff elbow were evaluated in a case study. Level of evidence: IV.

17. Van Zeeland NL, Yamaguchi K: Arthroscopic capsular release of the elbow. *J Shoulder Elbow Surg* 2010; 19(2, suppl):13-19.

    The reviewed technical advances and modifications have allowed arthroscopic capsular release of the elbow to emerge as a safe and reliable although technically demanding method to restore elbow motion.

18. Lapner PC, Leith JM, Regan WD: Arthroscopic debridement of the elbow for arthrofibrosis resulting from nondisplaced fracture of the radial head. *Arthroscopy* 2005;21(12):1492.

19. Nguyen D, Proper SI, MacDermid JC, King GJ, Faber KJ: Functional outcomes of arthroscopic capsular release of the elbow. *Arthroscopy* 2006;22(8):842-849.

20. Savoie FH III, Nunley PD, Field LD: Arthroscopic management of the arthritic elbow: Indications, technique, and results. *J Shoulder Elbow Surg* 1999;8(3): 214-219.

21. Cohen AP, Redden JF, Stanley D: Treatment of osteoarthritis of the elbow: A comparison of open and arthroscopic debridement. *Arthroscopy* 2000;16(7): 701-706.

22. Yadao MA, Field LD, Savoie FH III: Osteochondritis dissecans of the elbow. *Instr Course Lect* 2004;53: 599-606.

23. Ahmad CS, Vitale MA, ElAttrache NS: Elbow arthroscopy: Capitellar osteochondritis dissecans and radiocapitellar plica. *Instr Course Lect* 2011;60:181-190.

    Available arthroscopic treatment options are described for capitellar OCD and radiocapitellar plica, including mosaicplasty and transarticular drilling or removal of detached fragments or loose bodies, followed by drilling.

24. Brownlow HC, O'Connor-Read LM, Perko M: Arthroscopic treatment of osteochondritis dissecans of the capitellum. *Knee Surg Sports Traumatol Arthrosc* 2006;14(2):198-202.

25. Jones KJ, Wiesel BB, Sankar WN, Ganley TJ: Arthroscopic management of osteochondritis dissecans of the capitellum: Mid-term results in adolescent athletes. *J Pediatr Orthop* 2010;30(1):8-13.

    The mid-term results of 25 consecutive patients who underwent arthroscopic treatment of OCD of the capitellum are described. Level of evidence: IV.

26. Micheli LJ, Luke AC, Mintzer CM, Waters PM: Elbow arthroscopy in the pediatric and adolescent population. *Arthroscopy* 2001;17(7):694-699.

27. Mihara K, Suzuki K, Makiuchi D, Nishinaka N, Yamaguchi K, Tsutsui H: Surgical treatment for osteochondritis dissecans of the humeral capitellum. *J Shoulder Elbow Surg* 2010;19(1):31-37.

    Arthroscopic management of OCD of the capitellum was described in 27 male baseball players. Management consisted of drilling, fragment fixation, fragment excision, and reconstruction with osteochondral autograft. Level of evidence: IV.

28. Miyake J, Masatomi T: Arthroscopic debridement of the humeral capitellum for osteochondritis dissecans: Radiographic and clinical outcomes. *J Hand Surg Am* 2011;36(8):1333-1338.

    A retrospective review evaluated the radiographic and clinical outcomes of arthroscopic débridement of the humeral capitellum for OCD in 106 patients. Level of evidence: IV.

29. Nobuta S, Ogawa K, Sato K, Nakagawa T, Hatori M, Itoi E: Clinical outcome of fragment fixation for osteochondritis dissecans of the elbow. *Ups J Med Sci* 2008; 113(2):201-208.

    A case study assessed the efficacy of fragment fixation for OCD of the humeral capitellum. Level of evidence: IV.

30. Rahusen FT, Brinkman J-M, Eygendaal D: Results of arthroscopic debridement for osteochondritis dissecans of the elbow. *Br J Sports Med* 2006;40(12):966-969.

31. Takeda H, Watarai K, Matsushita T, Saito T, Terashima Y: A surgical treatment for unstable osteochondritis dissecans lesions of the humeral capitellum in adolescent baseball players. *Am J Sports Med* 2002; 30(5):713-717.

32. Tis JE, Edmonds EW, Bastrom T, Chambers HG: Short-term results of arthroscopic treatment of osteochondritis dissecans in skeletally immature patients. *J Pediatr Orthop* 2012;32(3):226-231.

A retrospective review evaluated a treatment regimen using arthroscopic-assisted treatments for pediatric capitellar OCD, including the removal of loose bodies, antegrade or retrograde drilling, and chondroplasty. Level of evidence: IV.

33. de Graaff F, Krijnen MR, Poolman RW, Willems WJ: Arthroscopic surgery in athletes with osteochondritis dissecans of the elbow. *Arthroscopy* 2011;27(7): 986-993.

    A systematic review evaluated studies on the results of arthroscopic surgery, including débridement, fragment fixation, microfracture, and osteochondral autografting, in athletes with OCD of the elbow. Level of evidence: III.

34. Peart RE, Strickler SS, Schweitzer KM Jr: Lateral epicondylitis: A comparative study of open and arthroscopic lateral release. *Am J Orthop (Belle Mead NJ)* 2004;33(11):565-567.

35. Rubenthaler F, Wiese M, Senge A, Keller L, Wittenberg RH: Long-term follow-up of open and endoscopic Hohmann procedures for lateral epicondylitis. *Arthroscopy* 2005;21(6):684-690.

36. Lattermann C, Romeo AA, Anbari A, et al: Arthroscopic debridement of the extensor carpi radialis brevis for recalcitrant lateral epicondylitis. *J Shoulder Elbow Surg* 2010;19(5):651-656.

    The outcome of arthroscopic release of the ECRB tendon was assessed in a consecutive series of patients. Level of evidence: IV.

37. Savoie FH III, VanSice W, O'Brien MJ: Arthroscopic tennis elbow release. *J Shoulder Elbow Surg* 2010; 19(2, suppl):31-36.

    The management of lateral epicondylitis with arthroscopic tennis elbow release was reviewed.

38. Feldman MD: Arthroscopic excision of type II capitellar fractures. *Arthroscopy* 1997;13(6):743-748.

39. Hardy P, Menguy F, Guillot S: Arthroscopic treatment of capitellum fracture of the humerus. *Arthroscopy* 2002;18(4):422-426.

40. Adams JE, Merten SM, Steinmann SP: Arthroscopic-assisted treatment of coronoid fractures. *Arthroscopy* 2007;23(10):1060-1065.

    Coronoid fractures were arthroscopically treated with screw fixation, threaded Steinmann pin fixation, and fracture débridement. Level of evidence: IV.

41. Hausman MR, Klug RA, Qureshi S, Goldstein R, Parsons BO: Arthroscopically assisted coronoid fracture fixation: A preliminary report. *Clin Orthop Relat Res* 2008;466(12):3147-3152.

    A preliminary report investigated the feasibility of arthroscopically assisted reduction and fixation of small coronoid fractures and the anterior capsule for treatment of patients with Regan-Morrey type or O'Driscoll type I or II coronoid fracture with instability of the ulnohumeral joint. Level of evidence: IV.

42. Michels F, Pouliart N, Handelberg F: Arthroscopic management of Mason type 2 radial head fractures. *Knee Surg Sports Traumatol Arthrosc* 2007;15(10): 1244-1250.

    Mid-to-long-term results were presented for an arthroscopic technique for reduction and percutaneous fixation of Mason type II radial head fractures. Level of evidence: IV.

43. Rolla PR, Surace MF, Bini A, Pilato G: Arthroscopic treatment of fractures of the radial head. *Arthroscopy* 2006;22(2):e1-e6.

44. Gelberman RH, Yamaguchi K, Hollstien SB, et al: Changes in interstitial pressure and cross-sectional area of the cubital tunnel and of the ulnar nerve with flexion of the elbow: An experimental study in human cadavera. *J Bone Joint Surg Am* 1998;80(4):492-501.

45. Dodson CC, Nho SJ, Williams RJ III, Altchek DW: Elbow arthroscopy. *J Am Acad Orthop Surg* 2008; 16(10):574-585.

    The indications for elbow arthroscopy were reviewed, with the technical advances that have expanded its indications.

46. Gramstad GD, Galatz LM: Management of elbow osteoarthritis. *J Bone Joint Surg Am* 2006;88(2): 421-430.

47. Sahajpal DT, Blonna D, O'Driscoll SW: Anteromedial elbow arthroscopy portals in patients with prior ulnar nerve transposition or subluxation. *Arthroscopy* 2010; 26(8):1045-1052.

Management strategies and complications related to the use of anteromedial portals for elbow arthroscopy were documented in a case study of patients with subluxating or previously transposed ulnar nerves. Level of evidence: IV.

48. Kelly EW, Morrey BF, O'Driscoll SW: Complications of elbow arthroscopy. *J Bone Joint Surg Am* 2001; 83-A(1):25-34.

49. O'Driscoll SW, Morrey BF: Arthroscopy of the elbow: Diagnostic and therapeutic benefits and hazards. *J Bone Joint Surg Am* 1992;74(1):84-94.

50. Poehling GG, Whipple TL, Sisco L, Goldman B: Elbow arthroscopy: A new technique. *Arthroscopy* 1989;5(3): 222-224.

51. Yamaguchi K, Tashjian RZ: *Advanced Reconstruction: Elbow*. Rosemont, IL, American Academy of Orthopaedic Surgeons, 2007, pp 3-11.

    The setup and portals used to perform elbow arthroscopy were described.

52. Gallay SH, Richards RR, O'Driscoll SW: Intraarticular capacity and compliance of stiff and normal elbows. *Arthroscopy* 1993;9(1):9-13.

53. Bedi A, Dines J, Dines DM, et al: Use of the 70° arthroscope for improved visualization with common arthroscopic procedures. *Arthroscopy* 2010;26(12): 1684-1696.

    A technique is described for using the 70° arthroscope, with the circumstances in which it offers visualization superior to that of a 30° arthroscope.

Chapter 47
Advanced Elbow Arthroscopy

James A. Hurt III, MD   Felix H. Savoie III, MD

Introduction

Elbow arthroscopy originally was used only to visualize the intra-articular anatomy and pathology of the elbow joint before open surgery or to aid in the removal of a loose body within the joint. The accepted indications for elbow arthroscopy have multiplied over the years to include treatment of arthritis, elbow stiffness and arthrofibrosis, lateral epicondylitis, posterolateral rotatory instability (PLRI), and posteromedial rotatory instability, osteochondritis dissecans (OCD), posterior impingement, intra-articular fracture, triceps repair, and septic arthritis. Although the literature supports the use of elbow arthroscopy for these conditions, the quality of the evidence generally is poor.[1] Arthroscopy of the elbow is technically demanding and requires an intimate knowledge of the surrounding anatomy and neurovascular structures.

Patient History and Examination

Every patient with elbow pain or dysfunction should have a complete history and physical examination. The patient's age, hand dominance, occupation, sports involvement, level of activity, and history of trauma should be determined. The timing of the onset of the condition, the time when symptoms are the worst, and the nature of the symptoms (pain, instability, stiffness, and mechanical symptoms) should be sought. The location of pain (anterior, posterior, medial, or lateral) and its history often lead the examiner to the diagnosis even before the physical examination or imaging.

Dr. Savoie or an immediate family member serves as a board member, owner, officer, or committee member of the Arthroscopy Association of North America, the American Shoulder and Elbow Surgeons, the American Academy of Orthopaedic Surgeons, the American Orthopaedic Society for Sports Medicine, and the International Society of Arthroscopy, Knee Surgery, and Orthopaedic Sports Medicine; serves as a paid consultant to or is an employee of Mitek, Smith & Nephew, and Exactech; serves as an unpaid consultant to Cayenne Medical; and has received research or institutional support from Mitek, Smith & Nephew, and Amp Orthopedics, Inc. Neither Dr. Hurt nor any immediate family member has received anything of value from or has stock or stock options held in a commercial company or institution related directly or indirectly to the subject of this chapter.

A thorough physical examination should include the cervical spine and the neck, the ipsilateral shoulder, the contralateral elbow, and the involved elbow. A neurovascular examination of the extremity should include pulses, reflexes, and motor and sensory testing. The range of motion (flexion, extension, pronation, and supination) should be measured and documented. Stability testing of the elbow should be performed through the arc of flexion and extension and with varus and valgus stressing. Other provocative tests should be done as dictated by the patient's history and examination.

Plain radiographs including AP, lateral, and oblique views are helpful for determining overall alignment and identifying fractures, OCD lesions, and degenerative joint disease. CT helps to define fracture patterns and identify loose bodies. MRI allows a much better assessment of the soft tissues than CT, including cartilage and ligamentous structures.

Elbow arthroscopy requires skill, experience, and detailed knowledge of the elbow and its anatomy. One of the most common and most feared complications of elbow arthroscopy is injury to a peripheral nerve. Therefore, the surgeon must be familiar with the elbow anatomy and confident of the correct placement of portals. The prone patient position is recommended for most arthroscopic surgery of the elbow. Although the lateral decubitus position is equally effective, it requires a special device to stabilize the arm.

Arthroscopically Treated Conditions

Lateral Humeral Epicondylitis
Lateral humeral epicondylitis originally was described in 1873. Its association with lawn tennis led to the commonly used name tennis elbow.[2] After 140 years, there is still a lack of consensus as to the best surgical and nonsurgical treatments of this condition. Most patients with lateral epicondylitis respond well to a variety of nonsurgical treatments, but 4% to 11% of patients require surgical intervention for continuing symptoms[3] (Figure 1).

The most commonly accepted theory of lateral epicondylitis is that repetitive use of the elbow causes microtears in the extensor carpi radialis brevis (ECRB) tendon. The absence of histologic signs of inflamma-

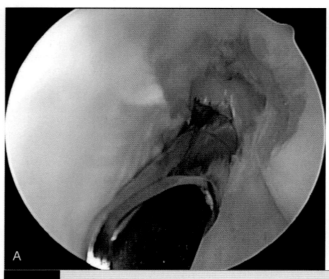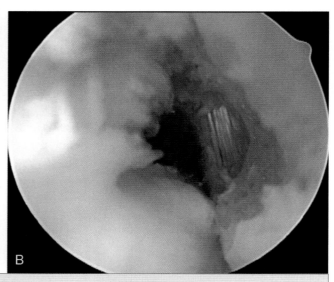

Figure 1 Arthroscopic images from the proximal anteromedial portal, showing the treatment of lateral humeral epicondylitis. **A,** The grey, amorphous angiofibrotic dysplasia of the ECRB tendon can be seen. **B,** The dysplasia has been excised, leaving the normal tendon intact.

tion led to the use of the terms angiofibroblastic hyperplasia and angiofibroblastic tendinosis to describe the condition.[4,5] Another theory is that pain is generated from impingement of the synovial fold onto the radiocapitellar joint. In a cadaver study, the synovial fold was found to be a distinct entity from the annular ligament, but it has an extremely close relationship with the common extensor enthesis.[6] It is also believed that lateral epicondylitis is caused by a combination of intra-articular and extra-articular lesions.

The exact origin of the ECRB tendon was characterized in a recent cadaver study as being just anterior to the distalmost tip of the lateral supracondylar ridge.[6,7] The tendon was found to be diamond shaped with a mean length of 13 mm (± 2 mm) and a mean width of 3 mm (± 1 mm) proximally, 7 mm (± 2 mm) in the midportion, and 4 mm (± 1 mm) distally.[6,7]

A wide assortment of percutaneous, endoscopic, and open procedures can be used to surgically treat lateral epicondylitis. Surgical intervention is indicated after unsuccessful nonsurgical treatments including activity modification, physical therapy, nonsteroidal anti-inflammatory drugs, corticosteroid and platelet-rich plasma injections, and counterforce bracing.

For arthroscopic management of lateral epicondylitis, it is helpful to create a specific tennis elbow portal 2 mm anterior to the tip of the lateral epicondyle. This portal will traverse the Nirschl lesion and allow resection from the top down rather than from the middle up, thus limiting resection to the pathologic tissue and decreasing the risk of radial nerve injury. When the portals are established, a portion of the lateral capsule is resected using a shaver to reveal the underlying common extensor origin. The ECRB origin is released completely using a shaver or an electrocautery. The lateral ligamentous structures are posterior to a line bisecting

the radial head, and the release should not be carried past this line. A 70° arthroscope can be used to obtain the best view of the ECRB insertion and lateral ligamentous structures around the corner of the capitellum.[8] An extra-articular lateral release can be done using a middle anterolateral portal that requires creating only a small hole in the joint capsule. The arthroscope is backed out of the capsule to directly visualize the diseased tissue and its débridement with a shaver entering from a proximal anterolateral portal.[9]

After the entire lesion is resected, the damaged tendon can be directly repaired to the bone or septum. This step can be done by placing a small anchor into the anterior lateral epicondyle and retrieving the sutures through the ECRB using a standard anterior lateral portal. The ECRB also can be plicated to the overlying extensor carpi radialis longus using a needle retriever technique.[10] Decortication of the underlying bone has been believed to increase healing potential. However, a recent study found that patients who underwent ECRB release and decortication had more pain postoperatively and required more time before return to work than patients who had a release alone.[3]

A case study of 36 patients who underwent arthroscopic treatment of recalcitrant lateral epicondylitis found improvement in pain, and the procedure appeared to be safe and effective.[3] A long-term follow-up study of 30 patients who underwent arthroscopic treatment of lateral epicondylitis found that no patients required further surgery, and 87% were satisfied with the outcome.[11]

Although most studies have had good results, not all patients have a favorable outcome. The results of ECRB débridement at times can be unpredictable, and some patients continue to have lateral elbow symptoms including pain.[7] Patients with a workers' compensation

Table 1

The Key Principles of Arthroscopic Release of a Posttraumatic Stiff Elbow

Use a standard and reproducible technique.

Perform a prophylactic ulnar nerve decompression.

Control the inflow of fluid to avoid excessive swelling.

Remove bone to re-create conforming joint surfaces.

Perform a capsulectomy.

Always use retractors.

Stay under the learning curve.

claim and those with a high-demand, repetitive-stress job were found to have inferior results.

Arthrofibrosis

The elbow is extremely prone to stiffness, especially after trauma, and loss of motion is the most common complication after injury to the elbow joint. The elbow with its three articulations is an extremely congruous joint. Even a small alteration in this congruity often will be magnified as a cause of stiffness. The elbow capsule can thicken and lose compliance after only a minor insult. The olecranon or coronoid fossae, if filled with loose bodies or scar tissue, limits terminal extension or flexion, respectively. Muscle contracture also can limit motion about the elbow. Pain often exacerbates posttraumatic elbow stiffness because the voluntary and involuntary guarding resulting from pain leads to worsening capsular and muscular contractures.[12] Loss of terminal extension is much more common than loss of flexion. The normal elbow range of motion is 0° to 145° of flexion and 90° of both pronation and supination. The functional range of motion is 30° to 130° of flexion and 50° of both pronation and supination.[13] A candidate for surgery should have a loss of terminal extension of 25° to 30° and/or less than 110° to 115° of flexion. Before surgical release, the patients should undergo several months of preoperative physical therapy and have a documented plateau in motion gains. Preoperative compliance is important to document, because compliance with postoperative therapy is paramount for retaining the motion gains achieved during surgery. However, overly aggressive physical therapy and manipulation can worsen the patient's symptoms and can even worsen the contracture.[12]

The arthroscopic release of a posttraumatic stiff elbow is complicated, and advanced arthroscopic skills are required to obtain motion while preserving the neurovascular structures. Heterotopic ossification is a relative contraindication to arthroscopic release. The advantages of arthroscopic treatment over open treatment include better visualization of intra-articular structures, less trauma to the surrounding tissues, and the potential for earlier postoperative motion and therapy.

Knowledge of the location of the ulnar nerve is mandatory for arthroscopy about the elbow. If there is significant loss of flexion or any doubt as to the exact location of the ulnar nerve, a separate open procedure should be performed to locate and protect the ulnar nerve.[14]

The key principles of arthroscopic release of a posttraumatic stiff elbow are listed in **Table 1**. It is the surgeon's preference as to whether to begin the procedure in the anterior or posterior compartment. Most surgeons prefer to begin in the anterior compartment, where visualization and close proximity to neurovascular structures may limit the surgeon later, as swelling increases. In the anterior compartment, a synovectomy and débridement are performed, and all loose bodies are removed. The capsule is removed from the anterior humerus. Bony osteophytes should be removed from the coronoid, the coronoid fossa, and the radial head. A complete anterior capsulectomy is performed using a biter and/or shaver without suction. Care must be taken to avoid injury to the posterior interosseous nerve at the lateral border of the brachialis.[15] Posteriorly, a synovectomy is performed, and all loose bodies are removed. Proximally, the capsule can be elevated with a retractor and any adhesions between the triceps and the humerus can be released. Osteophytes are removed as needed from the tip of the olecranon and the olecranon fossa. The capsule of the medial and lateral gutters is carefully released. Release of the medial gutter and posterior band of the medial ulnar collateral ligament is important for improving flexion.

High-grade contractures have been a relative contraindication to arthroscopic release because of the small amount of working space available for instrumentation and the decreased compliance of the capsule. In contractures of more than 50°, an extracapsular capsulectomy has been described in which a periosteal elevator is introduced through the proximal medial portal and a working space is created between the anterior humeral cortex and the anterior brachialis musculature.[12] The anterior capsule can then be dissected and excised under direct visualization.

Several recent level IV case studies reported good functional results with arthroscopic treatment of elbow arthrofibrosis.[14-16] A high percentage of patients were able to return to sports or work and were able to maintain surgical gains over a 24-month period. Patients with a traumatic etiology and those with a shorter duration of symptoms before surgical intervention had better results than other patients.

The complication rates of open and arthroscopic procedures about the elbow are similar. In comparison with open procedures, arthroscopic procedures appear to be associated with a greater risk of permanent injury. Several incidences of neurovascular injury during arthroscopy have been documented.[17] This risk necessitates the use of a careful stepwise routine during all arthroscopic elbow procedures, especially if the working space has been altered or is decreased.[17]

Degenerative Joint Disease

Elbow osteoarthritis is an uncommon condition that typically appears as weakness, pain at the extremes of motion, and loss of motion. Like arthritis in other joints, elbow arthritis typically involves bony osteophytes and loose bodies that can decrease the range of motion of the joint, with or without mechanical symptoms such as locking and catching. Unlike arthritis in other joints, elbow arthritis typically does not involve joint space narrowing or loss of cartilage.[18]

Degenerative joint disease of the elbow often is caused by rheumatoid arthritis or posttraumatic degenerative changes. Primary osteoarthritis of the elbow is almost exclusively seen in men who are athletes or do manual labor or heavy lifting. Patients with rheumatoid arthritis most often have pain throughout the range of motion, not limited to the extremes of motion. Plain radiographs are helpful in identifying arthritis in the elbow. Joint space narrowing, bony spurs, and loose bodies often are identified. When surgical intervention is being considered, CT is helpful in planning débridement, removal of loose bodies, and ulnohumeral or osteocapsular arthroplasty.

Nonsurgical treatment always should be attempted before surgical intervention. The use of NSAIDs, disease-modifying antirheumatic drugs (in patients with rheumatoid arthritis), corticosteroid injections, bracing, physical therapy, and activity modification are alternatives to surgery. Surgical intervention should be considered if nonsurgical treatments do not provide pain relief or a functional range of motion about the elbow and if the patient is limited in the ability to work or perform activities of daily living. Arthroscopic débridement of osteophytes and loose body removal, along with selective capsular release, has had good short-term to midterm results.[12]

The path of the ulnar nerve should be traced before the portals are established. There are typically several loose bodies in the anterior compartment, which can be removed if they are small. If the loose bodies are large, their removal can be deferred until a later time to preserve joint distension. A synovectomy is performed, and osteophytes are most easily removed from the coronoid with the shaver from the medial portal. The radial head is excised, at the surgeon's discretion, if the patient has radiocapitellar symptoms. A fenestration hole connecting the coronoid and olecranon fossa can then be drilled.[19]

Posteriorly, osteophytes are removed from the olecranon and the olecranon fossa. The medial and lateral gutters are débrided and cleared of loose bodies. The Outerbridge-Kashiwagi procedure is then completed by enlarging the fenestration hole to 1 to 2 cm, and the tip of the olecranon is excised broadly to achieve full extension.[19] The ulnar nerve should be decompressed or transposed in patients with a large preoperative motion loss. Motion is started immediately after surgery. The patient can be treated to prevent heterotopic ossification with 700 cGY of radiation during the first 48

hours after surgery.

The original Outerbridge-Kashiwagi procedure was open, but the arthroscopic procedure has had good results when used for elbow arthritis.[20,21] In a retrospective review, 19 patients with mild to moderate elbow arthritis underwent an arthroscopic Outerbridge-Kashiwagi procedure. The patients had improved range of motion and pain scores at a mean 2-year follow-up. A retrospective chart review of 41 patients who underwent arthroscopic osteophyte resection and capsulectomy found decreased pain and increased range of motion at a mean 176.3-week follow-up.[22] A review found that 12 of 13 patients with concurrent elbow arthritis and ulnar nerve compression at the elbow had a good or excellent result at a mean 47-month follow-up after arthroscopic ulnar nerve release, osteophyte resection, and capsulectomy.[23]

Osteochondritis Dissecans

Repetitive trauma to the lateral compartment of the immature elbow often is observed in children who participate in baseball and gymnastics, and OCD often is seen in adolescents (age 11 to 15 years) who participate in overhead sports. The disease process most likely is multifactorial; it results from repetitive microtrauma and vascular susceptibility, but the exact etiology is unknown. The blood supply to the capitellum is provided by two end arteries with minimal collateral blood flow, and the structure is predisposed to an avascular state in an elbow repeatedly subjected to microtrauma. Patients often have vague lateral elbow pain and stiffness. A 15° to 20° flexion contracture is not uncommon. Both OCD lesions and tears of the medial ulnar collateral ligament (MUCL) can be caused by valgus overload. The integrity of the MUCL should be examined. Imaging of the elbow should include AP radiographs at full extension and at 45° of flexion, as well as oblique and standard lateral views. If an OCD lesion is suspected on plain radiographs, MRI should be obtained to further delineate the lesion.

Treatment of OCD lesions depends on their size and location as well as the stability of the overlying cartilage. Lesions involving the lateral aspect of the capitellum (unconstrained or shoulder lesions) require more extensive surgery and have a worse prognosis than lesions involving only the central capitellum. A stage I OCD lesion is stable; the osteochondral lesion is intact and has not displaced. A stage I lesion often heals in 3 to 6 months and should be treated nonsurgically. Throwing and other activities that are stressful for the affected arm should be discontinued. Repeating the MRI at 2 to 3 months is helpful in monitoring healing. A stage II lesion is unstable but connected, with fractured cartilage. A stage II lesion should be treated surgically, with the size of the lesion dictating the surgical treatment. A relatively small lesion can be débrided, with good immediate pain relief.

There is debate over treatment of a stage II or larger lesion with débridement, repair, or osteochondral autograft. The location of the lesion on the capitellum can affect the treatment outcome; a lesion with lateral column involvement has a relatively poor prognosis. Fragments can be fixed using headless screws, and the use of absorbable pins has been described.[24] A stage III lesion is unstable and fully displaced, and it must be treated surgically. Débridement with drilling or microfracture or osteochondral autograft replacement is chosen, as it is for a stage II lesion.[25] Microfracture is indicated for a small stage I lesion that did not respond to nonsurgical management or a stage II lesion without lateral column involvement. Osteochondral autograft should be used for a larger lesion, a lesion that involves more than 6 to 7 mm of the lateral column, or a lesion engaged by the radial head. Short-term outcomes after surgical treatment of OCD lesions tend to be good, but long-term outcomes for stage II and III lesions are much less favorable.[26]

The angle of approach from the portal is of utmost importance for thoroughly débriding, drilling, or placing osteochondral plugs. Dual direct lateral portals do not damage the lateral ligamentous complex and allow access to 78% of the capitellum with instrumentation.[27] A distal ulnar portal also allows good exposure to the capitellum and easy access for drilling, burring, or débridement during arthroscopy.[28] A novel approach to drilling OCD lesions uses a 1.8-mm Kirschner wire drilled into the radial head from 3 cm distal. By pronating, supinating, flexing, and extending the elbow, the lesion can be drilled without the creation of a large arthrotomy.[29] Usually the lesion is best visualized through a 70° arthroscope in the proximal posterior lateral portal, using mid and distal soft-spot portals for instrumentation and retractors.

A level III review of the literature concluded that surgery is indicated when nonsurgical treatment is unsuccessful, but the published studies have a low methodologic quality.[25] The short-term results of débridement, fixation, microfracture, and autografting are promising, but the long-term results are unclear. Although evidence is lacking, autografting appears to have better results than the other surgical treatments in the long term.

A retrospective review of results in 106 patients who underwent arthroscopic débridement of OCD lesions after closure of the capitellar physis found that patients with a large lesion and an open radial physis had both poor radiographic and clinical outcomes.[25,27-30] Other patients had excellent short-term outcomes. A retrospective review of 13 patients at a minimum 1-year follow-up after débridement of an OCD lesion found subjective symptom relief and a functional elbow, although many patients reported they had ended their earlier sports activity.[30] Twenty-five consecutive patients were treated with arthroscopic débridement and drilling of an OCD lesion; 12 patients also required a miniarthrotomy for bone grafting.[26] These patients had a statistically significant postoperative increase in flexion (10°) and extension (17°), and 18 of the 21 patients

available for follow-up had returned to their sport at the preinjury level.

Triceps Injury

The triceps functions to straighten the elbow. The triceps tendon inserts on the proximal and posterior aspects of the olecranon on the proximal ulna. The incidence of injury to the triceps tendon insertion has increased as aging individuals remain active, but it is more common in individuals who lift weights. The patient often experiences an acute onset of pain at the insertion during press-type activities such as pushing up from a seated position or performing a bench-press weight lift. Partial tears tend to have a more insidious onset of pain that is more noticeable at the beginning of extension from a fully flexed position.

The physical examination often reveals swelling and ecchymosis at the triceps insertion site. Elbow extension can be completely absent in a full tear or is weakened in a partial tear. The triceps stress test reproduces pain over the site of injury when the patient attempts to extend the elbow from a fully flexed position. Surgical intervention is indicated if nonsurgical treatment is unsuccessful.

Arthroscopic fixation is a less invasive method than open repair of the triceps tendon. The patient is positioned prone or in the lateral decubitus position, and a diagnostic arthroscopy is performed. For the repair, an initial posterior central portal is placed (**Figure 2**), often through the triceps tendon tear. A posterior lateral portal is established, and the triceps tear is identified when the arthroscope is moved to this portal. The insertion at the olecranon is débrided. A dual suture anchor is inserted at the tip of the olecranon. Two mattress sutures are tied to repair the proximal aspect of the tear. A second suture anchor is placed more distally in the olecranon, and these sutures are retrieved through the tendon to complete the repair.

The ulnar nerve should be mapped out before portal placement in any arthroscopic elbow procedure (**Figure 3**). The bone in the olecranon can be extremely hard, and care must be taken to avoid breaking off the anchors during insertion. The arthroscopic repair should be converted to an open procedure if swelling becomes too great for completing the procedure arthroscopically. After surgery, the elbow should be held in full extension. Motion should be limited, with an increase in flexion slowly over a period of 6 to 8 weeks.[31]

Fractures

One of the emerging uses of elbow arthroscopy is in fracture fixation and reduction. Many innovative techniques have been developed to treat fractures with less invasive techniques that preserve the soft-tissue envelope and minimize dissection. Arthroscopically assisted fracture fixation has been described for radial head fractures, coronoid fractures, pediatric lateral condyle fractures, capitellar fractures, and epicondylar and intercondylar fractures. The ability to obtain radiographs

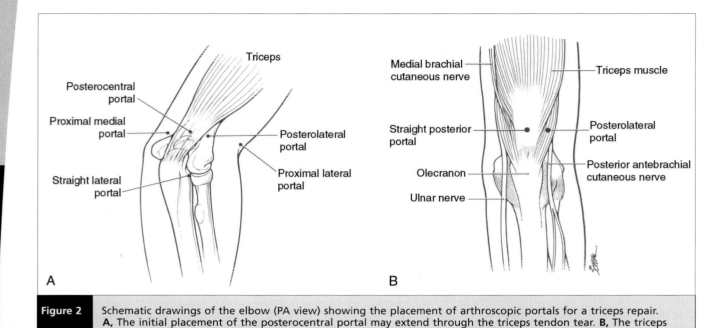

Figure 2   Schematic drawings of the elbow (PA view) showing the placement of arthroscopic portals for a triceps repair. **A,** The initial placement of the posterocentral portal may extend through the triceps tendon tear. **B,** The triceps tear is identified when the arthroscope is moved to the posterolateral portal.

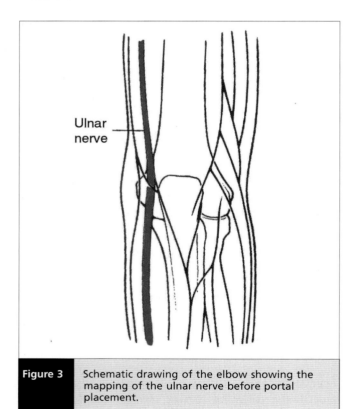

Figure 3   Schematic drawing of the elbow showing the mapping of the ulnar nerve before portal placement.

and physical examination often is limited because of the patient's pain. Aspiration of any hemarthrosis and injection of an intra-articular anesthetic can increase the ability to perform an accurate physical examination and position the extremity for radiographs, with greater patient comfort. CT and MRI should be or-

dered at the surgeon's discretion to define the fracture pattern and associated soft-tissue injuries for preoperative planning.

Unrecognized chondral injuries and other intra-articular pathology can be identified during arthroscopy. Fracture reduction can be directly visualized, thereby increasing its accuracy and decreasing the need for intraoperative fluoroscopy.

A patient with gross infection or contamination, neurovascular injury, or severely osteoporotic bone should be treated using an open procedure. The posterior interosseous nerve should be explored with an open technique in a patient with a radial head fracture that penetrates the capsule and brachialis anteriorly.[32]

Radial Head Fractures

Radial head fractures are the most common fractures about the elbow. Nondisplaced or minimally displaced Mason type I fractures often can be treated nonsurgically with early range-of-motion exercises. Mason type II and III fractures often are significantly displaced, with blocks to motion, and they are best managed surgically. During arthroscopy, a displaced two-part fracture is best visualized from the proximal anteromedial or posterolateral portal. After the fracture fragment is reduced, Kirschner wires can be placed through the anterolateral or soft-spot portal to stabilize the fracture, and the fracture then can be definitively fixed using percutaneously placed headless screws or absorbable pins. In a case study of Mason type II radial head fractures treated with arthroscopic reduction, percutaneous pinning, and placement of one or two headless screws, all 14 patients had a good to excellent result at 5.5-year follow-up.[33]

Coronoid Fractures

The coronoid plays an important role in maintaining the bony stability of the elbow joint. Fractures of the coronoid frequently are associated with axial loading and posterior dislocation of the elbow. Surgical intervention typically is recommended for a Regan-Morrey type III fracture or any fracture that interferes with joint motion or stability. Small fracture fragments or comminuted fractures not amenable to fixation with screws can be débrided or fixed using suture anchors at the fracture site. Larger coronoid fragments typically can be reduced with the aid of a tibial anterior cruciate ligament guide. The fracture can be stabilized by guidewires drilled through the guide, followed by definitive fixation with a small cannulated screw. A retrospective review of this type of arthroscopically aided coronoid fracture reduction found that all seven patients healed with a functional range of motion and were pain free.[34] A case study of four consecutive patients treated with either arthroscopically assisted screw fixation or suturing found that all patients healed with a stable elbow and achieved a functional range of motion about the elbow.[35]

Lateral Condyle Fractures

Lateral humeral condyle fractures often are seen in pediatric patients and typically are treated with a long arm cast (for a nondisplaced fracture), closed reduction and pinning, or open reduction using a Kocher approach and percutaneous pinning. These fractures often are amenable to arthroscopic evaluation and assisted reduction followed by percutaneous pinning and long arm casting. Arthroscopy avoids a large soft-tissue dissection and decreases the risk of vascular insult to the fracture fragment, which can occur with an open procedure. Two small case studies found that this technique can be used with excellent short-term results.[36,37]

Posterolateral Rotatory Instability

PLRI, first described in 1991, involves dysfunction of the lateral ligamentous structures, specifically the radial ulnohumeral ligament (RUHL).[38] The RUHL is an important elbow stabilizer during supination and extension. Injury can cause difficulty even in simple activities of daily living. The RUHL has three separate components: the radial collateral ligament, the lateral ulnar collateral ligament, and the annular ligament. There appears to be a continuum between PLRI and frank elbow dislocation.[39] Pain with lateral elbow instability can often mimic lateral epicondylitis, and PLRI may increase tension across the extensors and cause symptoms of lateral epicondylitis.[40] The close proximity of the ECRB tendon insertion and the RUHL may lead to iatrogenic PLRI during open ECRB débridement.

Arthroscopic treatment of PLRI originally was described in 2001, and several variations have more recently been described.[39,41,42] The choice of treatment depends on whether the patient has an acute dislocation, recurrent dislocation, or PLRI. In a simple dislocation,

the RUHL complex is typically avulsed from its humeral attachment and heals with nonsurgical treatment. A diagnostic arthroscopy can be performed after an anteromedial portal is established. Hematomas should be removed, and a torn annular ligament should be sutured. A posterior central portal is created, and the posterior hematoma is evacuated. The site of avulsion from the lateral humeral condyle should be identified and débrided. An anchor is then placed into the humerus in the midline of the radiocapitellar joint, and a second anchor is placed more proximally at the two primary avulsion sites of the origin of the RUHL. The suture limbs are retrieved through the ligamentous complex. To prevent overtightening, the horizontal mattress sutures should be tied with the elbow in approximately 45° to 60° of flexion.

PLRI is easily seen on arthroscopic examination as the radial head and ulna subluxate posterolaterally during a pivot shift under anesthesia. A common finding with PLRI is the drive-through sign, which is not possible in a stable elbow. In the drive-through sign the arthroscope can be moved from the posterolateral gutter across the ulnohumeral articulation from the posterior central portal.

Arthroscopic repair of PLRI involves plication of the RUHL followed by repair to the humerus. Anchors are placed at the origin sites of the RCL and the RUHL for humeral fixation, and the ligament is plicated and repaired either by using these sutures or placing additional plication sutures and repairing the plicated ligament complex to the humerus. The plication is performed by placing four to seven absorbable sutures from distal through the RUHL complex at its ulnar attachment and working proximally. The sutures are retrieved with a retrograde retriever that hooks under the radial collateral ligament from the posterolateral aspect of the lateral epicondyle. The sutures are individually retrieved percutaneously through the existing skin portals and tied sequentially. After tensioning, the drive-through sign should be eliminated.[42] The results of arthroscopic treatment of PLRI are equivalent to those of open repair.[41]

Posteromedial Impingement

Overhead athletes generate high-level valgus and extension forces through their elbow during the throwing motion. The primary constraint to valgus stress at the elbow is the anterior band of the MUCL. An incompetent MUCL gives way to valgus instability of the elbow. Over time, posteromedial impingement (called thrower's elbow), ulnar nerve symptoms, ulnar stress fractures, OCD lesions, and even capsular contractures can develop in patients with valgus elbow instability. These symptoms constitute so-called valgus extension overload. The timing of pain during the different phases of throwing can alert the physician to the possible pathologic process. Surgical intervention should be considered if symptoms become disabling (preventing the athlete from performing the sports activity) and nonsurgical measures have been unsuccessful. Radiographs and MRI should be used for preoperative planning. In a case study of nine patients with posteromedial impingement, reproducible pathology was found when preoperative MRI was compared with intraoperative arthroscopic findings.[43]

The anterior compartment should be arthroscopically examined for bony spurs, cartilage lesions, and OCD lesions of the capitellum. The anterior capsule should be evaluated if the patient has a loss of terminal elbow extension. Athletes with a loss of terminal extension are able to return to their sport at the preinjury level after arthroscopic contracture release.[44] The medial collateral ligament should be evaluated using the arthroscopic valgus stress test. In the posterior compartment, the olecranon and the olecranon fossa are visualized and débrided of osteophytes. Spurs often are found on the posteromedial aspect of the olecranon. In 16 elbows of athletes with posterior impingement who underwent arthroscopic débridement of the posterior fossa, the extension deficit decreased from 8° to 2°.[45] If the MUCL has been torn, open reconstruction should follow arthroscopy.

Summary and Future Directions

Arthroscopy of the elbow requires advanced skills and intimate knowledge of the anatomy surrounding the elbow. The indications for elbow arthroscopy appear to be expanding on an almost daily basis. Additional elbow conditions for which arthroscopy has been used include elbow chondromatosis, rheumatoid arthritis, intra-articular osteoid osteomata, septic arthritis, and medial epicondylitis.[46,47]

Annotated References

1. Yeoh KM, King GJ, Faber KJ, Glazebrook MA, Athwal GS: Evidence-based indications for elbow arthroscopy. *Arthroscopy* 2012;28(2):272-282.

   A systematic review of therapeutic studies that investigated the indications and outcomes of elbow arthroscopy found that the evidence supports elbow arthroscopy but that the quality of the evidence is poor. Level of evidence: IV.

2. Morris HP: Lawn-tennis elbow. *BMJ* 1883;2:557.

3. Kim JW, Chun CH, Shim DM, et al: Arthroscopic treatment of lateral epicondylitis: Comparison of the outcome of ECRB release with and without decortication. *Knee Surg Sports Traumatol Arthrosc* 2011; 19(7):1178-1183.

   A nonrandomized clinical study compared arthroscopic ECRB release with and without decortication. Pain and return-to-work time were greater in patients undergoing decortication, without improvement in clinical results. Level of evidence: IV.

4. Nirschl RP, Pettrone FA: Tennis elbow: The surgical treatment of lateral epicondylitis. *J Bone Joint Surg Am* 1979;61(6A):832-839.

5. Nirschl RP: Elbow tendinosis/tennis elbow. *Clin Sports Med* 1992;11(4):851-870.

6. Ando R, Arai T, Beppu M, Hirata K, Takagi M: Anatomical study of arthroscopic surgery for lateral epicondylitis. *Hand Surg* 2008;13(2):85-91.

   The anatomic and histologic relationships among the ECRB, articular capsule, and lateral collateral ligament complex, along with the number and location of synovial fringes, was studied in 100 elbows in 50 cadavers. Both extra- and intra-articular lesions were found to have a role in lateral epicondylitis.

7. Cohen MS, Romeo AA: Open and arthroscopic management of lateral epicondylitis in the athlete. *Hand Clin* 2009;25(3):331-338.

   The authors compared open and arthroscopic treatment of lateral epicondylitis and described surgical techniques. The results of surgical intervention for lateral epicondylitis can be less predictable than those of other procedures about the elbow.

8. Arrigoni P, Zottarelli L, Spennacchio P, Denti M, Cabitza P, Randelli P: Advantages of 70° arthroscope in management of ECRB tendinopathy. *Musculoskelet Surg* 2011;95(Suppl 1):S7-S11.

   A technique for arthroscopic ECRB release was described, including the use of a 70° arthroscope to visualize the tendon insertion and lateral collateral ligament during the procedure.

9. Brooks-Hill AL, Regan WD: Extra-articular arthroscopic lateral elbow release. *Arthroscopy* 2008;24(4): 483-485.

   The arthroscopic treatment of lateral epicondylitis is described, with the use of an extra-articular technique with a smaller capsulectomy.

10. Savoie FH III, VanSice W, O'Brien MJ: Arthroscopic tennis elbow release. *J Shoulder Elbow Surg* 2010; 19(2, Suppl):31-36.

    A review article outlined the history of tennis elbow and an arthroscopic release procedure that uses a modified lateral portal (the tennis elbow portal). Two additional arthroscopic repair techniques were described: plication of the ECRB to the extensor carpi radialis longus and suture anchor repair of the ECRB.

11. Baker CL Jr, Baker CL III: Long-term follow-up of arthroscopic treatment of lateral epicondylitis. *Am J Sports Med* 2008;36(2):254-260.

    A case study outlined the long-term results of 30 patients who underwent arthroscopic treatment of lateral epicondylitis. No patient required further surgery, and 87% were satisfied with their outcome. Level of evidence: IV.

12. Tucker SA, Savoie FH III, O'Brien MJ: Arthroscopic management of the post-traumatic stiff elbow. *J Shoulder Elbow Surg* 2011;20(2, suppl):S83-S89.

    A review outlined a technique for arthroscopic management of the posttraumatic stiff elbow. The authors cautioned against overly aggressive therapy and manipulation, which can worsen the symptoms and subsequently worsen the contracture.

13. Morrey BF, Askew LJ, Chao EY: A biomechanical study of normal functional elbow motion. *J Bone Joint Surg Am* 1981;63(6):872-877.

14. Van Zeeland NL, Yamaguchi K: Arthroscopic capsular release of the elbow. *J Shoulder Elbow Surg* 2010;19(2, suppl):13-19.

    A review provided an overview of arthroscopic capsular release of the stiff elbow as well as the history of the stiff elbow, physical examination and workup, surgical technique, and preferred postoperative protocols.

15. Sahajpal D, Choi T, Wright TW: Arthroscopic release of the stiff elbow. *J Hand Surg Am* 2009;34(3):540-544.

    A technique for arthroscopic release of the stiff elbow is described. The anatomy of the surgical portals and the release in a stepwise fashion are included. The focus is on safe surgical technique to avoid nerve injury.

16. Degreef I, De Smet L: Elbow arthrolysis for traumatic arthrofibrosis: A shift towards minimally invasive surgery. *Acta Orthop Belg* 2011;77(6):758-764.

    The results of 12 patients who underwent arthroscopic elbow arthrolysis were reported. On average, the patients gained 38° in range of motion. A literature review found that open and arthroscopic arthrolysis yielded gains of 44° and 31.25°, respectively. Level of evidence: IV.

17. Park JY, Cho CH, Choi JH, Lee ST, Kang CH: Radial nerve palsy after arthroscopic anterior capsular release for degenerative elbow contracture. *Arthroscopy* 2007;23(12):1360, e1-e3.

    A case report documented radial nerve palsy after an arthroscopic anterior capsular release. A 3-mm ball-tipped cautery was used instead of a 0.5-mm sharp-tipped cautery. The nerve fully recovered by one year.

18. Cheung EV, Adams R, Morrey BF: Primary osteoarthritis of the elbow: Current treatment options. *J Am Acad Orthop Surg* 2008;16(2):77-87.

    The treatment options for primary osteoarthritis of the elbow were outlined.

19. Savoie FH III, O'Brien MJ, Field LD: Arthroscopy for arthritis of the elbow. *Hand Clin* 2011;27(2):171-178, v-vi.

    The use of arthroscopy for arthritis of the elbow were outlined, including the preoperative workup and spur excision and ulnohumeral arthroplasty for elbow arthritis after unsuccessful nonsurgical treatment.

20. Kashiwagi D: Intra-articular changes and the special operative procedure, Outerbridge-Kashiwagi method, in Kashiwagi D, ed: *Elbow Joint*. Amsterdam, The Netherlands, Elsevier Science, 1985, pp 177-178.

21. Degreef I, De Smet L: The arthroscopic ulnohumeral arthroplasty: From mini-open to arthroscopic surgery. *Minim Invasive Surg* 2011;2011:798084.

    A literature review described the transition of the ulnohumeral Outerbridge-Kashiwagi procedure from open to arthroscopic, with good results.

22. Adams JE, Wolff LH III, Merten SM, Steinmann SP: Osteoarthritis of the elbow: Results of arthroscopic osteophyte resection and capsulectomy. *J Shoulder Elbow Surg* 2008;17(1):126-131.

    A retrospective chart review of 42 elbows in 41 patients at an average 176.3-week follow-up after arthroscopic osteophyte resection and capsulectomy found decreased pain and increased range of motion.

23. Kovachevich R, Steinmann SP: Arthroscopic ulnar nerve decompression in the setting of elbow osteoarthritis. *J Hand Surg Am* 2012;37(4):663-668.

    A retrospective chart review of 15 elbows in 13 patients with concurrent symptoms of arthritis and ulnar nerve compression at an average 47-month follow-up after arthroscopic ulnar nerve decompression, osteophyte resection, and capsulectomy found a good to excellent result in 12 elbows. Level of evidence: IV.

24. Takeba J, Takahashi T, Hino K, Watanabe S, Imai H, Yamamoto H: Arthroscopic technique for fragment fixation using absorbable pins for osteochondritis dissecans of the humeral capitellum: A report of 4 cases. *Knee Surg Sports Traumatol Arthrosc* 2010;18(6):831-835.

    A case study described four patients with an OCD lesion of the humeral capitellum who were treated using absorbable pins for fragment fixation. Posterolateral portals were used, and the elbow was held maximally flexed during the procedure.

25. Gonzalez-Lomas G, Ahmad C, Wanich T, ElAttrache N: Osteochondritis dissecans of the elbow, in Ryu RKN, ed: *AANA Advanced Arthroscopy: The Elbow and Wrist*. Philadelphia, PA, Saunders Elsevier, 2010, pp 40-54.

    Current treatment options for OCD lesions and Panner's disease were presented, with anatomy, patient history, and physical examination as well as treatment algorithms.

26. Jones KJ, Wiesel BB, Sankar WN, Ganley TJ: Arthroscopic management of osteochondritis dissecans of the capitellum: Mid-term results in adolescent athletes. *J Pediatr Orthop* 2010;30(1):8-13.

    A retrospective study of 25 consecutive patients treated with arthroscopic débridement and drilling for capitellar OCD lesions found a statistically significant increase in both flexion and extension. Eighteen of the 21 patients available for follow-up returned to their sport at the preinjury level.

27. Davis JT, Idjadi JA, Siskosky MJ, ElAttrache NS: Dual direct lateral portals for treatment of osteochondritis dissecans of the capitellum: An anatomic study. *Arthroscopy* 2007;23(7):723-728.

An anatomic cadaver study examined the relationship and distance of dual direct lateral portals to the lateral ligamentous complex and determined on dissection that the ligamentous complex was not damaged by dual lateral portals. Seventy-eight percent of the capitellum was accessible for instrumentation with these portals.

28. van den Ende KI, McIntosh AL, Adams JE, Steinmann SP: Osteochondritis dissecans of the capitellum: A review of the literature and a distal ulnar portal. *Arthroscopy* 2011;27(1):122-128.

The diagnosis and current treatment options for OCD of the capitellum were discussed. A new distal ulnar portal allows good in-line visualization of the OCD lesion.

29. Arai Y, Hara K, Fujiwara H, Minami G, Nakagawa S, Kubo T: A new arthroscopic-assisted drilling method through the radius in a distal-to-proximal direction for osteochondritis dissecans of the elbow. *Arthroscopy* 2008;24(2):237, e1-e4.

A novel treatment of OCD lesions is described, in which a 1.8-mm Kirschner wire is drilled from 3 cm distal to the humeroradial joint through the radial head and into the lesion. By pronating-supinating and flexing-extending, multiple holes can be drilled into the lesion without creating an arthrotomy.

30. Schoch B, Wolf BR: Osteochondritis dissecans of the capitellum: Minimum 1-year follow-up after arthroscopic debridement. *Arthroscopy* 2010;26(11):1469-1473.

A retrospective study examined the results of 13 patients who underwent arthroscopic débridement of an OCD lesion. Débridement led to a functional elbow with subjective symptom relief, but many patients ceased some sports activity. Level of evidence: IV.

31. Savoie F III, Field L, O'Brien M: *AANA Advanced Arthroscopy: The Elbow and Wrist.* Philadelphia, PA, Saunders Elsevier, 2010, pp 132-135.

An arthroscopic method of repairing partial and full-thickness triceps tendon tears using suture anchors was described.

32. Peden JP, Savoie F III, Field L: Arthroscopic treatment of elbow fractures, in Ryu RKN, ed: *AANA Advanced Arthroscopy: The Elbow and Wrist.* Philadelphia, PA, Saunders Elsevier, 2010, pp 136-143.

An arthroscopic method of assisted fracture fixation was described for a variety of intra-articular fractures about the elbow.

33. Michels F, Pouliart N, Handelberg F: Arthroscopic management of Mason type 2 radial head fractures. *Knee Surg Sports Traumatol Arthrosc* 2007;15(10):1244-1250.

A treatment technique for Mason type II radial head fractures was described, involving arthroscopic reduction and percutaneous pinning to stabilize the fracture, followed by placement of one or two headless screws. All 14 patients had a good to excellent result at an average 5.5-year follow-up. Level of evidence: IV.

34. Adams JE, Merten SM, Steinmann SP: Arthroscopic-assisted treatment of coronoid fractures. *Arthroscopy* 2007;23(10):1060-1065.

A case study examined seven coronoid fractures reduced with arthroscopic assistance and fixed using an anterior cruciate ligament guide for directional guidance and screw fixation. All patients healed with a functional range of motion and were pain free. Level of evidence: IV.

35. Hausman MR, Klug RA, Qureshi S, Goldstein R, Parsons BO: Arthroscopically assisted coronoid fracture fixation: A preliminary report. *Clin Orthop Relat Res* 2008;466(12):3147-3152.

A case study of arthroscopically assisted coronoid fracture fixation found all four consecutive patients had a stable elbow with a functional range of motion.

36. Hausman MR, Qureshi S, Goldstein R, et al: Arthroscopically-assisted treatment of pediatric lateral humeral condyle fractures. *J Pediatr Orthop* 2007;27(7):739-742.

Six skeletally immature patients with a lateral condyle fracture were treated with arthroscopic reduction and percutaneous pinning. All patients healed within 4 weeks with full range of motion. There were no malunions or nonunions. Level of evidence: IV.

37. Perez Carro L, Golano P, Vega J: Arthroscopic-assisted reduction and percutaneous external fixation of lateral condyle fractures of the humerus. *Arthroscopy* 2007;23(10):1131, e1-e4.

Arthroscopic lateral condyle fracture reduction followed by percutaneous Kirschner wire fixation was described in an 11-year-old girl.

38. O'Driscoll SW, Bell DF, Morrey BF: Posterolateral rotatory instability of the elbow. *J Bone Joint Surg Am* 1991;73(3):440-446.

39. Smith JP III, Savoie FH III, Field LD: Posterolateral rotatory instability of the elbow. *Clin Sports Med* 2001;20(1):47-58.

40. Kalainov DM, Coehn MS: Posterolateral rotatory instability of the elbow in association with lateral epicondylitis: A report of three cases. *J Bone Joint Surg Am* 2005;87(5):1120-1125.

41. Savoie FH III, Field LD, Gurley DJ: Arthroscopic and open radial ulnohumeral ligament reconstruction for posterolateral rotatory instability of the elbow. *Hand Clin* 2009;25(3):323-329.

A retrospective chart review of 61 patients treated surgically for posterolateral rotatory instability found improvement of both subjective and objective symptoms after open or arthroscopic treatment.

42. Savoie F III, Field L, Gurley DJ: Arthroscopic and open radial ulnohumeral ligament reconstruction for posterolateral rotatory instability of the elbow, in Ryu RKN, ed: *AANA Advanced Arthroscopy: The Elbow and Wrist*. Philadelphia, PA, Saunders Elsevier, 2010, pp 94-100.

Open and arthroscopic techniques for PLRI are presented, with satisfactory results.

43. Cohen SB, Valko C, Zoga A, Dodson CC, Ciccotti MG: Posteromedial elbow impingement: Magnetic resonance imaging findings in overhead throwing athletes and results of arthroscopic treatment. *Arthroscopy* 2011;27(10):1364-1370.

A case study correlated MRI findings in overhead throwing athletes with posteromedial impingement findings during arthroscopy. Reproducible pathology was seen in all nine patients, including articular surface changes at the posterior trochlea and anterior medial olecranon on MRI and posteromedial synovitis and olecranon spurring during arthroscopy. Level of evidence: IV.

44. Blonna D, Lee GC, O'Driscoll SW: Arthroscopic restoration of terminal elbow extension in high-level athletes. *Am J Sports Med* 2010;38(12):2509-2515.

In 26 elbows in 24 athletes, loss of terminal elbow extension adversely affected performance. All patients underwent arthroscopic contracture release, and 22 patients returned to the preinjury sport at the same level of intensity and performance. Level of evidence: IV.

45. Rahusen FT, Brinkman JM, Eygendaal D: Arthroscopic treatment of posterior impingement of the elbow in athletes: A medium-term follow-up in sixteen cases. *J Shoulder Elbow Surg* 2009;18(2):279-282.

A retrospective case study evaluated the results of 16 elbows in athletes who underwent arthroscopic débridement of the posterior fossa for posterior impingement. The average extension deficit decreased from 8° preoperatively to 2° postoperatively. Level of evidence: IV.

46. Flury MP, Goldhahn J, Drerup S, Simmen BR: Arthroscopic and open options for surgical treatment of chondromatosis of the elbow. *Arthroscopy* 2008;24(5):520-525, e1.

A retrospective study compared arthroscopic and open surgical treatment options for chondromatosis of the elbow. Both approaches led to satisfactory results, but the arthroscopically treated patients tended to have a shorter rehabilitation time and higher satisfaction. Level of evidence: III.

47. Kang HJ, Park MJ, Ahn JH, Lee SH: Arthroscopic synovectomy for the rheumatoid elbow. *Arthroscopy* 2010;26(9):1195-1202.

Twenty-six rheumatoid elbows in 25 patients were treated with arthroscopic synovectomy using multiple portals. Overall, patients had decreased pain and increased range of motion, and 19 had a good to excellent result. Four patients had a recurrence of synovitis. Level of evidence: IV.

Miscellaneous Shoulder and Elbow Topics

SECTION EDITOR:
EDWARD G. McFARLAND, MD

Chapter 48

Suprascapular Neuropathy

Umasuthan Srikumaran, MD   Nicholas Jarmon, MD

Introduction

Suprascapular neuropathy results from traction, entrapment, or compression of the suprascapular nerve. Most commonly, suprascapular neuropathy is considered an abnormality of the infraspinatus branch; however, the infraspinatus and supraspinatus branches can be affected independently or together. Patients typically present with posterior shoulder pain and/or weakness in forward flexion or external rotation. Suprascapular neuropathy was first described in the English literature in 1959,[1] and its true incidence and prevalence are unknown. A recent meta-analysis showed only 88 published cases between 1959 and 2001.[2] The largest case series through 2011 included 53 patients.[3]

Anatomy

The suprascapular nerve receives its primary contributions from C5 and C6, with occasional contribution from C4. Originating from the upper trunk of the brachial plexus, the nerve travels posterior to the clavicle, across the superior border of the scapula, and toward the suprascapular notch (**Figure 1**).

The suprascapular nerve runs below the transverse scapular ligament, which typically forms the roof of the suprascapular notch, a bony depression medial to the base of the coracoid; the suprascapular artery typically runs above the ligament. Various morphologies of this notch have been described, ranging from a subtle bony depression to a bony tunnel with ossification of the transverse scapular ligament.[4] After exiting the tunnel, the nerve runs posterolaterally across the bony floor of the supraspinatus fossa, where it supplies motor branches to the supraspinatus muscle and sensory branches to the acromioclavicular and glenohumeral joints. The motor branches to the supraspinatus were found to originate, on average, 3 cm from the supragle-

Dr. Srikumaran or an immediate family member is a member of a speakers' bureau or has made paid presentations on behalf of Norvartis and serves as a paid consultant to or is an employee of Abbott. Neither Dr. Jarmon nor any immediate family member has received anything of value from or has stock or stock options held in a commercial company or institution related directly or indirectly to the subject of this chapter.

noid tubercle, whereas the motor branches to the infraspinatus originate, on average, 2 cm from the posterior rim of the glenoid.[5] At the posterolateral corner of the supraspinatus fossa, the nerve enters the spinoglenoid notch, passing under the spinoglenoid (inferior transverse scapular) ligament. Anatomic analysis[6] has shown wide variations in the presence of this ligament, but a more recent study showed the ligament was present in 58 consecutive cadaver specimens[7] (**Figure 2**). A portion of this ligament inserts on the posterior capsule and becomes taut with adduction and internal rotation.[8] This position has been postulated to correspond with the follow-through phase of throwing.[8] After exiting the notch, the nerve courses medially around the base of the scapular spine, sending motor branches to the infraspinatus muscle.

Mechanism of Injury

A variety of mechanisms have been identified as the causes of suprascapular neuropathy, including repetitive traction and microtrauma, compressive lesions, local anatomic variants, glenohumeral dislocation, scapula fracture, and surgical trauma.[9]

Multiple studies have suggested that suprascapular neuropathy in overhead athletes is the result of repetitive traction and microtrauma,[10,11] possibly related to increased pressure on the nerve from tightening of the spinoglenoid ligament during the follow-through phase of the throwing motion.[8] Compression of the nerve can occur anywhere along its course. Suprascapular compression has been identified after fractures at the suprascapular notch and the distal clavicle.[12,13] Entrapment of the nerve at the spinoglenoid notch by paralabral cysts has been commonly seen.[14] Although believed to be less common, paralabral cysts can extend more medially than the spinoglenoid notch and compress the nerve at the suprascapular notch.[15] Certain anatomic variations, such as narrow suprascapular or spinoglenoid notches,[16] an anterior coracoscapular ligament,[17] ossified transverse scapular ligaments,[16] or superiorly oriented fibers of the subscapularis,[18] may predispose patients to suprascapular neuropathy. Soft-tissue and bony tumors have also been implicated in suprascapular neuropathy.[19,20] A 29% incidence of suprascapular nerve injury on electromyography (EMG) was found in patients with proximal humeral fractures or glenohumeral dislocation.[21]

The suprascapular nerve can also become entrapped at the suprascapular notch or at the base of the scapular spine with a retracted rotator cuff tear.[22] Because the motor branches of the nerve are fixed within the muscle, retracted rotator cuff tears can increase medial tension on the nerve as it courses through the suprascapular notch and around the spinoglenoid notch.[22] A cadaver study has also shown that overadvancement of a tendon (> 3 cm) can place tension on the motor branches.[5]

Suprascapular neuropathy has been described as a surgical complication secondary to direct injury. The authors of a recent study reported a patient who underwent repair of a type II superior labrum anterior to posterior (SLAP) lesion with two anchors.[23] Postoperatively, the patient had persistent pain. A repeat MRI study showed the posterior anchor protruding through cortical bone and abutting against the suprascapular nerve, and an EMG study confirmed partial denervation of the suprascapular nerve. At the second surgery, the anchor was shown to be directly compressing the nerve and was removed, after which the patient's symptoms resolved.[23] In a 2007 case report, suprascapular neuropathy caused by the penetration of screws from a Latarjet procedure into the spinoglenoid notch was described.[24] Penetration was confirmed with CT, and neuropathy was confirmed by EMG. The screws were removed, and at the time of final follow-up, the patient had complete resolution of symptoms, with a return to normal EMG findings. The suprascapular nerve is also at risk with procedures requiring a posterior approach to the scapula.[25]

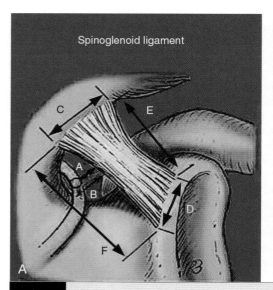

Figure 1 Anatomy of the suprascapular nerve. (Reproduced with permission from Safran MR: Nerve injury about the shoulder in athletes: Part 1. Suprascapular nerve and axillary nerve. *Am J Sports Med* 2004;32:803-819.)

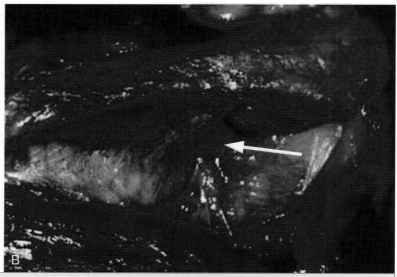

Figure 2 Anatomy of the spinoglenoid ligament from a posterior view. **A,** Artist's sketch. The lines shown are as follows: *A,* minimal distance from the ligament to the nerve; *B,* maximal distance from the ligament to bone; *C,* scapular spine insertion; *D,* glenoid insertion; *E,* superior border; and *F,* inferior border. **B,** Cadaver specimen. Arrow: spinoglenoid ligament extending from the scapular spine to the posterior capsule. (The suprascapular nerve is seen running below the ligament.) (Reproduced with permission from Plancher KD, Peterson RK, Johnston JC, Luke TA: The spinoglenoid ligament: Anatomy, morphology, and histological findings. *J Bone Joint Surg Am* 2005;87[2]: 361-365.)

History and Physical Examination

Patients with suprascapular nerve injuries may report a history of trauma or pain and/or weakness with overhead activities. The pain often is not localized, and often the patient will describe a dull or burning pain in the posterolateral, superior, or anterior aspect of the shoulder. Because this pain is often diffuse and nonlocalized, it is important to consider other potential etiologies or coexisting etiologies of pain in these patients. Cervical spine involvement of the C5 or C6 nerve roots can also simulate pain in this area and may coexist with more peripheral compressive or traction injuries to the suprascapular nerve or its branches. The suprascapular nerve does not have sensory branches to the skin, so any paresthesias in the shoulder or in the upper extremity should not be ascribed to a suprascapular nerve injury; other causes of the paresthesias should be explored.

When examining patients with shoulder pain, especially patients with suprascapular nerve or rotator cuff injury, it is important and helpful to have both of the patient's shoulders exposed for comparative anterior and posterior visualization. Bilateral comparison, especially from behind, can allow the examiner to appreciate atrophy of the supraspinatus or the infraspinatus. Simple observation of the shoulders from behind will sometimes alert the examiner to involvement of the suprascapular nerve at some level. Because the pain of suprascapular neuropathy is protean and may radiate down the arm or into the neck, neck pain may be present, and cervical spine involvement should be evaluated with the range of motion of the cervical spine. Similarly, in the presence of any suggestion of nerve injury, a neurologic evaluation of the entire upper extremity with sensory, motor, and reflex testing is required. Comparison with the opposite extremity is also helpful when performing upper extremity neurologic testing because many conditions can simulate suprascapular nerve neuropathy.

The best tests for suprascapular nerve neuropathy are resisted manual stress testing of the involved muscles. The best test for involvement of the nerve at the level of the suprascapular notch would be resisted abduction of the shoulder. If the supraspinatus and the infraspinatus are involved, one study has shown up to 75% loss of abduction and external rotation strength.[26] Some patients may have a positive external rotation lag sign, but although this test is sensitive for supraspinatus and infraspinatus weakness, it is not specific for nerve injury, and other causes for profound weakness should be considered. Resisted external rotation with the arm at the side is the best test for strength of the infraspinatus.[27]

Other provocative tests of the shoulder may shed some light on the origin of pain, but most of these tests are neither specific nor sensitive for suprascapular nerve involvement alone. In patients who have isolated infraspinatus nerve involvement, there may be signs of

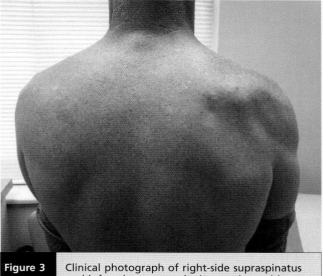

Figure 3 | Clinical photograph of right-side supraspinatus and infraspinatus atrophy in a patient with EMG-documented suprascapular neuropathy.

a coexisting SLAP lesion, but the examination for SLAP lesions remains inexact and controversial. A cadaver study has suggested that symptoms may be exacerbated with cross-arm adduction and internal rotation, but this suggestion has not been subjected to clinical verification.[8]

A detailed physical examination can help isolate the location of the lesion. Isolated atrophy of the infraspinatus is associated with injury at the spinoglenoid notch. Suprascapular neuropathy at the spinoglenoid notch will produce isolated weakness of external rotation at the side on physical examination. This weakness may be out of proportion to other physical examination, or even imaging, findings; that is, there will be no evidence of a ganglion cyst or a rotator cuff tear. Patients with atrophy of the supraspinatus and the infraspinatus are likely to have injury at the suprascapular notch (**Figure 3**). Global atrophy of the shoulder musculature suggests some other abnormality to account for a patient's symptoms. In the case of massive rotator cuff tears, the physical examination cannot determine whether the nerve is under tension based on weakness alone. In these cases, EMG and nerve conduction velocity studies are helpful.

Diagnostic Studies

Conventional radiographs are recommended in the initial evaluation of any patient with shoulder pain. Conventional radiographs are helpful for assessing the painful shoulder for fractures, previous surgically induced bone changes, tumors, dysplasia, or other bony variants that might account for nerve compression. CT defines osseous abnormalities, such as an ossified ligament or fracture callus, that may account for nerve entrapment better than does radiography.

MRI evaluation is considered the best next study for patients who have shoulder pain believed to be associated with suprascapular nerve neuropathy. The MRI study will most accurately evaluate the rotator cuff for tendon tears but will also give important information about the presence and distribution of muscle atrophy. It will potentially give information about ganglion cysts or other space-occupying lesions that might be compressing the nerve. However, MRI will not identify the suprascapular notch unless specific images of that area are requested.[28]

Multiple studies have used ultrasound to identify suprascapular nerve abnormalities.[29,30] This modality has several advantages: (1) it can be used in conjunction with diagnostic and therapeutic injections; (2) it allows for the visualization of mass lesions, including ganglions, tumors, and bony abnormalities; and (3) in thin patients, the nerve itself can be seen along its course, whereas in heavier patients, vascular structures can be seen to approximate the location of the nerve. The disadvantages of this modality are that it is heavily operator dependent, and it may be less reliable in heavier patients.

The most important test standard for the diagnosis and confirmation of suprascapular neuropathy at any level is EMG/nerve conduction velocity studies of the upper extremity. The EMG/nerve conduction velocity study should include the entire upper extremity to rule out other potential causes of the patient's symptoms, such as cervical radiculopathy, brachial plexus lesions, myopathy, or other peripheral nerve involvements. When ordering this test to evaluate the suprascapular nerve, it is often helpful to specify that the periscapular muscles, especially the infraspinatus, the supraspinatus and the deltoid muscles, should be tested.[31] EMG may help to localize the site of compression. Increased latency and fibrillation potentials, as well as decreased amplitude, suggest nerve compression and denervation. The evaluation of sensory velocities is less reliable because sensory innervation is poorly defined. Normal values for the motor nerve conduction velocity study have been established for the suprascapular nerve; what has not been clearly established is the sensitivity and the specificity of this study in detecting suprascapular neuropathy.[32]

Treatment Options

The treatment of suprascapular neuropathy depends on the severity of the symptoms and the physician's confidence that the neuropathy is the cause of the patient's symptoms. Many patients have coexisting lesions that might be contributing to the symptoms, such as symptomatic acromioclavicular arthritis or cervical spine disease. Treatment will also depend on the patient's degree of symptoms in terms of pain and disability for activities of daily living or sports participation.

In the absence of a space-occupying lesion, nonsurgical modalities, including activity modification,

NSAIDs, and physical therapy, are widely accepted as the standard initial treatment of suprascapular neuropathy. The results of nonsurgical treatment were assessed in 15 patients whose suprascapular neuropathy was diagnosed clinically and confirmed with electrodiagnostic studies.[33] The outcome was excellent in five patients and good in seven, and only three required subsequent surgery for the persistence of symptoms.[33]

However, in patients with proven compression of the nerve and a space-occupying lesion or cyst, nonsurgical treatment (although typically suggested as the initial treatment) may have less favorable results over time, and surgery will eventually be required. Of 19 patients treated nonsurgically for suprascapular neuropathy with known spinoglenoid notch cysts, only 10 were satisfied with their outcomes, whereas 26 of 27 patients treated with surgical excision of the cysts for the same abnormality were satisfied with their outcomes.[34]

In the absence of a space-occupying lesion, surgery may be considered if nonsurgical treatment fails. Ideally, an area of compression or abnormality should be localized to optimize outcomes. Data are limited with regard to determining how patients who undergo surgery fare after unsuccessful nonsurgical treatment in the absence of space-occupying lesions. Of the three patients in the aforementioned study[33] in whom nonsurgical treatment failed and who went on to have a decompression, there was one excellent, one good, and one poor result. In the case of massive rotator cuff tears, it has been shown that there is a reversal of suprascapular neuropathy, tested by EMG/nerve conduction velocity study, with repair of the tendon tear.[22] It is unclear if there is any additional benefit to decompression of the nerve at the suprascapular notch in combination with rotator cuff repair.

There are arthroscopic and open approaches to decompression of the suprascapular nerve, depending on the location and the cause of the compression. The technique used will also depend on the experience of the surgeon.

For open suprascapular notch decompression,[35] a saber or a transverse incision along the scapular spine can be used (**Figure 4**). The trapezius is then split along its fibers, and the supraspinatus is retracted posteriorly. The transverse ligament is then localized and released (**Figure 5**), taking care to preserve the vascular structures running above and the nerve running below the ligament.[35] In addition to releasing the ligament, the notch may also be widened with the use of a burr, if indicated.

An arthroscopic approach for suprascapular nerve release at the suprascapular notch has been described.[36-38] The procedure begins with the placement of standard portals for a routine diagnostic arthroscopy. After a subacromial bursectomy is performed, the anterior border of the supraspinatus is identified and traced medially when viewing from a lateral or an anterolateral portal. The coracoclavicular ligaments are then identified and serve as an anterior landmark for further

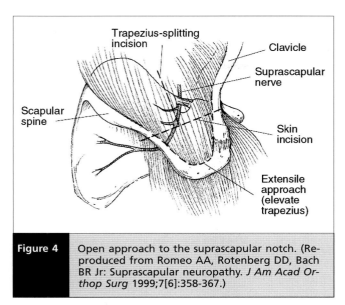

| **Figure 4** | Open approach to the suprascapular notch. (Reproduced from Romeo AA, Rotenberg DD, Bach BR Jr: Suprascapular neuropathy. *J Am Acad Orthop Surg* 1999;7[6]:358-367.) |

dissection medially and inferiorly along the coracoid base. A spinal needle is then used to localize a superior portal 1 to 2 cm medial to the acromioclavicular joint on the skin. The spinal needle should be directed toward the coracoid base and adjacent to the transverse suprascapular ligament. A blunt trocar is then placed through this portal to retract tissue medially along the transverse ligament, exposing the suprascapular nerve and vessels (**Figure 6**). A second superior portal can be made just lateral to the first, allowing for additional instrumentation to release the transverse ligament. The blunt trocar may be placed inferior to the ligament to protect the nerve while it is released. If the suprascapular transverse ligament is partially or completely ossified, small osteotomes can be introduced to release the

nerve. A Kerrison rongeur may also be used to remove bone above the nerve. This approach can be demanding for surgeons who are not familiar with the technique or the surrounding anatomy.

For open spinoglenoid notch decompression, a posterior incision is used, with a longitudinal incision 3 cm medial to the posterolateral corner of the acromion or with a vertical incision in the skin lines. The deltoid is then divided in line with its fibers, taking care not to split it too distally to avoid injury to the axillary nerve. The infraspinatus fascia is then identified and incised, and the infraspinatus muscle can then be retracted inferiorly. The dissection is then carried down the lateral aspect of the scapular spine, where the spinoglenoid ligament is identified and released.[39] An open decompression can also be accompanied by an arthroscopic examination of the joint to determine if there are any intra-articular abnormalities that might need to be addressed, such as a SLAP lesion or rotator cuff conditions.

An arthroscopic approach for suprascapular nerve release at the spinoglenoid notch was first described in a 2007 study.[40] The procedure begins with the placement of standard portals for a routine diagnostic arthroscopy. After a subacromial bursectomy is performed, the spinoglenoid notch is visualized from the subacromial space. A second posterior portal is made, and a small Langenbeck retractor is used to gently retract the infraspinatus muscle belly inferiorly, allowing better visualization of the suprascapular nerve and the paralabral cyst. The cyst can then be incised, and its contents can be aspirated with a shaver. A potential benefit of this technique is that it allows for evaluation of the intra-articular abnormality, which is often associated with cysts in this region. In some cases, it has been suggested that when a spinoglenoid cyst is found

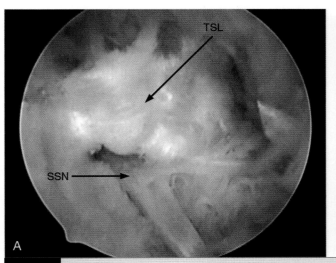

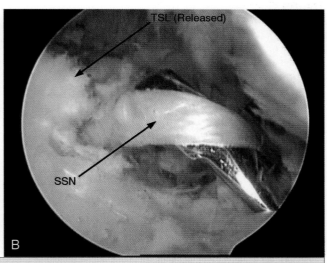

| **Figure 5** | Intraoperative arthroscopic images of the transverse scapular ligament (TSL) and suprascapular nerve (SSN) before (**A**) and after (**B**) release of the ligament. (Reproduced with permission from Boykin RE, Friedman DJ, Higgins LD, Warner JJ: Suprascapular neuropathy. *J Bone Joint Surg Am* 2010;92[13]:2348-2364.) |

8: Miscellaneous Shoulder and Elbow Topics

to be associated with a SLAP lesion or a posterior labral tear, it can be treated with labral repair alone.[41] Of 10 patients with spinoglenoid notch cysts associated with superior labral tears who underwent labral repair without cyst decompression, 4 had preoperative EMG studies confirming suprascapular neuropathy; all 4 had postoperative EMG studies showing return of normal function. Eight patients had postoperative MRI, all showing resolution of the cyst.[41]

When a single site of compression is not clearly identified on MRI, some authors have recommended empirical decompression of both notches.[42,43] Both arthroscopic[43] and open[5] techniques have been described for

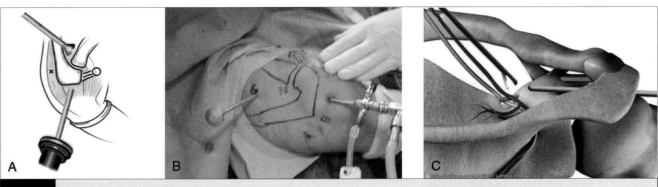

Figure 6 Portal placement for arthroscopic release of the suprascapular nerve as depicted on a right shoulder. **A**, Artist's sketch, superior view. **B**, Clinical photograph, superior view. **C**, Computer-generated image, posterior view. (Reproduced with permission from Boykin RE, Friedman DJ, Higgins LD, Warner JJ: Suprascapular neuropathy. *J Bone Joint Surg Am* 2010;92[13]:2348-2364.)

Table 1

Clinical Results

Study (Year)	No. of Patients	Mean Age (Years)	Mean Follow-up (Months; Range)	Treatment
Martin et al[33] (1997)	15	35	47 (15-54)	Physical therapy: range of motion and periscapular strengthening
Antoniou et al[3] (2001)	53	38	28 (12-91)	Surgical, 36; nonsurgical, 17
Kim et al[44] (2005)	42	41	18 (12-48)	Open decompression
Mallon et al[46] (2006)	8	68	24 (16-36)	Nonsurgical treatment, 4; partial repair of massive cuff tear with margin convergence, 4
Westerheide et al[47] (2006)	14	41	51 (24-73)	Arthroscopic decompression
Lafosse et al[38] (2007)	10	50	15 (6-27)	Arthroscopic decompression
Shah et al[45] (2011)	27	49.3	22.5 (3-44)	Arthroscopic decompression

simultaneous decompression of the nerve at both locations.

Results

Making conclusive remarks about the best treatment of suprascapular nerve neuropathy is difficult because these lesions are not common, the diagnostic criteria for making the diagnosis vary, the diagnosis is often not verified with EMG/nerve conduction velocity studies, and there are no randomized prospective studies analyzing the outcomes for the various treatment options. A meta-analysis from 2002 identified 88 cases of suprascapular nerve entrapment from 1959 to 2001.[2] Unfortunately, fewer than 50% of the studies reported clinical outcomes. Although this meta-analysis suggested that earlier surgical intervention may help limit the amount of atrophy seen, additional conclusions could not be made because of the lack of reported outcomes.

Pain relief and strength improvement were reported in 28 of 31 patients treated with an open decompression at the suprascapular notch.[44] The authors of a 2011 study[45] reported on their results of 27 patients undergoing arthroscopic decompression at the supra-

scapular and/or spinoglenoid notch: of the 24 patients available for follow-up, 71% reported pain relief, 75% had a statistically significant improvement in the American Shoulder and Elbow Surgeons score, 71% had a statistically significant improvement in subjective shoulder value scores, and 71% would have the surgery again[3,33,38,44-47] (**Table 1**).

Summary

Suprascapular neuropathy remains an uncommon diagnosis, although the true incidence is unknown. A thorough clinical evaluation is needed to properly identify this abnormality and appropriately rule out other possible conditions. After the disease process is identified and space-occupying lesions have been excluded, nonsurgical treatment remains the first line of treatment. If this treatment fails, open and arthroscopic techniques for decompression have been described. Randomized controlled trials to help guide treatment are lacking, and additional studies are needed to develop the ideal treatment algorithm.

Table 1

Clinical Results (continued)

Pre-EMG	Post-EMG	Outcome Measures	Clinical Outcomes
4 of 10 in nonsurgical group with abnormal findings	Normal after treatment	Activity, pain, strength	5 excellent, 7 good, 3 required surgery for persistent pain (1 good, 1 excellent, 1 poor).
Yes	No	Modified ASES	Compressive lesions responded to operative treatment; overuse injuries responded equally well to surgical and nonsurgical treatment.
Yes	No	Pain and strength grade	Pain improved in 7 of 8 patients presenting with persistent pain. Preoperative supraspinatus strength 0 to 2 in all patients; postoperative supraspinatus 4 or better in 90% and 2 to 3 in 10%.
All with denervation SS ± IS	2 follow-up EMGs obtained in operative group: both showed partial nerve recovery	Clinical examination	Nonsurgical group, no change; surgical group, active elevation improved in four of four patients, and spinatus atrophy remained present clinically.
11 of 11 showed denervation of IS	No	SST, Constant, strength	SST improved (4.3 to 11.5), postoperative Constant score, 94; all improved strength.
10 of 10 with findings of chronic compression	7 of 8 had complete normalization, 1 of 8 partial recovery	Constant, strength, VAS, patient satisfaction	Improved Constant score and strength in external rotation and abduction, 9 of 10 excellent with complete pain relief, 1 of 10 satisfactory with moderate pain relief.
24 of 27 had positive findings	No	VAS, subjective shoulder value, ASES	17 of 24 pain relief, 17 of 24 improved, 18 of 24 improved ASES

EMG = electromyography; ASES = American Shoulder and Elbow Surgeons score; VAS = visual analog scale; SS = supraspinatus; IS = infraspinatus; SST = simple shoulder test.

Annotated References

1. Kopell HP, Thompson WA: Pain and the frozen shoulder. *Surg Gynecol Obstet* 1959;109(1):92-96.

2. Zehetgruber H, Noske H, Lang T, Wurnig C: Suprascapular nerve entrapment: A meta-analysis. *Int Orthop* 2002;26(6):339-343.

3. Antoniou J, Tae SK, Williams GR, Bird S, Ramsey ML, Iannotti JP: Suprascapular neuropathy: Variability in the diagnosis, treatment, and outcome. *Clin Orthop Relat Res* 2001;386:131-138.

4. Edelson JG: Bony bridges and other variations of the suprascapular notch. *J Bone Joint Surg Br* 1995;77(3):505-506.

5. Warner JP, Krushell RJ, Masquelet A, Gerber C: Anatomy and relationships of the suprascapular nerve: Anatomical constraints to mobilization of the supraspinatus and infraspinatus muscles in the management of massive rotator-cuff tears. *J Bone Joint Surg Am* 1992;74(1):36-45.

6. Rengachary SS, Burr D, Lucas S, Brackett CE: Suprascapular entrapment neuropathy: A clinical, anatomical, and comparative study. Part 3: Comparative study. *Neurosurgery* 1979;5(4):452-455.

7. Plancher KD, Peterson RK, Johnston JC, Luke TA: The spinoglenoid ligament: Anatomy, morphology, and histological findings. *J Bone Joint Surg Am* 2005;87(2):361-365.

8. Plancher KD, Luke TA, Peterson RK, Yacoubian SV: Posterior shoulder pain: A dynamic study of the spinoglenoid ligament and treatment with arthroscopic release of the scapular tunnel. *Arthroscopy* 2007;23(9):991-998.

   This cadaver study sought to determine the pressure exerted on the suprascapular nerve by compression of the spinoglenoid ligament during glenohumeral range of motion. The most pressure was noted with the arm in full adduction and internal rotation.

9. Boykin RE, Friedman DJ, Higgins LD, Warner JJ: Suprascapular neuropathy. *J Bone Joint Surg Am* 2010; 92(13):2348-2364.

   This review article details the anatomy, the pathophysiology, the diagnosis, and the treatment of suprascapular neuropathy. More research is needed to determine proper etiology and treatment.

10. Ferretti A, Cerullo G, Russo G: Suprascapular neuropathy in volleyball players. *J Bone Joint Surg Am* 1987; 69(2):260-263.

11. Lajtai G, Pfirrmann CW, Aitzetmüller G, Pirkl C, Gerber C, Jost B: The shoulders of professional beach volleyball players: High prevalence of infraspinatus muscle atrophy. *Am J Sports Med* 2009;37(7):1375-1383.

    This cross-sectional study of 84 professional volleyball players found a 30% prevalence of infraspinatus muscle atrophy. Fully competitive players typically had subjectively unrecognized weakness in external rotation and frequent unspecific shoulder pain. Level of evidence: III.

12. Huang KC, Tu YK, Huang TJ, Hsu RW: Suprascapular neuropathy complicating a Neer type I distal clavicular fracture: A case report. *J Orthop Trauma* 2005; 19(5):343-345.

13. Solheim LF, Roaas A: Compression of the suprascapular nerve after fracture of the scapular notch. *Acta Orthop Scand* 1978;49(4):338-340.

14. Tirman PF, Feller JF, Janzen DL, Peterfy CG, Bergman AG: Association of glenoid labral cysts with labral tears and glenohumeral instability: Radiologic findings and clinical significance. *Radiology* 1994;190(3):653-658.

15. Moore TP, Fritts HM, Quick DC, Buss DD: Suprascapular nerve entrapment caused by supraglenoid cyst compression. *J Shoulder Elbow Surg* 1997;6(5):455-462.

16. Ticker JB, Djurasovic M, Strauch RJ, et al: The incidence of ganglion cysts and other variations in anatomy along the course of the suprascapular nerve. *J Shoulder Elbow Surg* 1998;7(5):472-478.

17. Avery BW, Pilon FM, Barclay JK: Anterior coracoscapular ligament and suprascapular nerve entrapment. *Clin Anat* 2002;15(6):383-386.

18. Bayramoglu A, Demiryürek D, Tüccar E, et al: Variations in anatomy at the suprascapular notch possibly causing suprascapular nerve entrapment: An anatomical study. *Knee Surg Sports Traumatol Arthrosc* 2003; 11(6):393-398.

19. Hazrati Y, Miller S, Moore S, Hausman M, Flatow E: Suprascapular nerve entrapment secondary to a lipoma. *Clin Orthop Relat Res* 2003;411:124-128.

20. Yi JW, Cho NS, Rhee YG: Intraosseous ganglion of the glenoid causing suprascapular nerve entrapment syndrome: A case report. *J Shoulder Elbow Surg* 2009; 18(3):e25-e27.

    A case report of an intraosseous ganglion causing a suprascapular neuropathy treated with diagnostic arthroscopy and needle aspiration of the cyst is discussed. The patient presented with pain, weakness, and tenderness to palpation at the infraspinatus fossa, all symptoms resolved at early follow-up.

21. de Laat EA, Visser CP, Coene LN, Pahlplatz PV, Tavy DL: Nerve lesions in primary shoulder dislocations and humeral neck fractures: A prospective clinical and EMG study. *J Bone Joint Surg Br* 1994;76(3):381-383.

22. Costouros JG, Porramatikul M, Lie DT, Warner JJ: Reversal of suprascapular neuropathy following arthroscopic repair of massive supraspinatus and infraspinatus rotator cuff tears. *Arthroscopy* 2007; 23(11):1152-1161.

    A case series of seven patients with massive rotator cuff tears and isolated suprascapular neuropathy who underwent arthroscopic rotator cuff tear repair is discussed. EMG/nerve conduction velocity studies 6 months postoperatively demonstrated partial or full recovery of suprascapular nerve palsy that correlated with pain relief and functional improvement. Level of evidence: IV.

23. Kim SH, Koh YG, Sung CH, Moon HK, Park YS: Iatrogenic suprascapular nerve injury after repair of type II SLAP lesion. *Arthroscopy* 2010;26(7):1005-1008.

    A case report of suprascapular nerve injury at the spinoglenoid notch after repair of a type II SLAP lesion caused by improperly inserted suture anchor is discussed.

24. Maquieira GJ, Gerber C, Schneeberger AG: Suprascapular nerve palsy after the Latarjet procedure. *J Shoulder Elbow Surg* 2007;16(2):e13-e15.

    A case report of suprascapular neuropathy after a Latarjet procedure is discussed. The diagnosis was confirmed by abnormal EMG and CT scan showing screw penetration into the spinoglenoid notch. After screw removal, the clinical and EMG findings returned to normal.

25. Wijdicks CA, Armitage BM, Anavian J, Schroder LK, Cole PA: Vulnerable neurovasculature with a posterior approach to the scapula. *Clin Orthop Relat Res* 2009; 467(8):2011-2017.

    A cadaver study of 24 specimens that defines the location of the suprascapular nerve and the circumflex scapular artery with respect to various osseous landmarks in the posterior shoulder is discussed.

26. Gerber C, Blumenthal S, Curt A, Werner CM: Effect of selective experimental suprascapular nerve block on abduction and external rotation strength of the shoulder. *J Shoulder Elbow Surg* 2007;16(6):815-820.

    The authors performed nerve blocks of the suprascapular nerve in healthy volunteers. Infraspinatus paralysis caused a loss of 70% external rotation and 45% abduction strength. Infraspinatus-supraspinatus paralysis caused a loss of 80% external rotator and 75% abduction strength.

27. Kelly BT, Kadrmas WR, Speer KP: The manual muscle examination for rotator cuff strength: An electromyographic investigation. *Am J Sports Med* 1996;24(5): 581-588.

28. Inokuchi W, Ogawa K, Horiuchi Y: Magnetic resonance imaging of suprascapular nerve palsy. *J Shoulder Elbow Surg* 1998;7(3):223-227.

29. Martinoli C, Bianchi S, Pugliese F, et al: Sonography of entrapment neuropathies in the upper limb (wrist excluded). *J Clin Ultrasound* 2004;32(9):438-450.

30. Yücesoy C, Akkaya T, Ozel O, et al: Ultrasonographic evaluation and morphometric measurements of the suprascapular notch. *Surg Radiol Anat* 2009;31(6):409-414.

    Both shoulders of each of 50 volunteers were evaluated by ultrasound to measure the width and the depth of the suprascapular notch. The skin-notch base interval and the neighboring vasculature were also imaged. Variations between the sexes are discussed.

31. Bredella MA, Tirman PF, Fritz RC, Wischer TK, Stork A, Genant HK: Denervation syndromes of the shoulder girdle: MR imaging with electrophysiologic correlation. *Skeletal Radiol* 1999;28(10):567-572.

32. Buschbacher RM, Weir SK, Bentley JG, Cottrell E: Normal motor nerve conduction studies using surface electrode recording from the supraspinatus, infraspinatus, deltoid, and biceps. *PM R* 2009;1(2):101-106.

    One hundred volunteers were recruited and completed bilateral testing using simple surface electrodes. Normal values for distal latency, amplitude, duration, and area were developed for proximal nerve conductions to the axillary, musculocutaneous, and suprascapular nerves.

33. Martin SD, Warren RF, Martin TL, Kennedy K, O'Brien SJ, Wickiewicz TL: Suprascapular neuropathy: Results of non-operative treatment. *J Bone Joint Surg Am* 1997;79(8):1159-1165.

34. Piatt BE, Hawkins RJ, Fritz RC, Ho CP, Wolf E, Schickendantz M: Clinical evaluation and treatment of spinoglenoid notch ganglion cysts. *J Shoulder Elbow Surg* 2002;11(6):600-604.

35. Post M: Diagnosis and treatment of suprascapular nerve entrapment. *Clin Orthop Relat Res* 1999;368: 92-100.

36. Bhatia DN, de Beer JF, van Rooyen KS, du Toit DF: Arthroscopic suprascapular nerve decompression at the suprascapular notch. *Arthroscopy* 2006;22(9): 1009-1013.

37. Lafosse L, Tomasi A: Technique for endoscopic release of suprascapular nerve entrapment at the suprascapular notch. *Tech Shoulder Elbow Surg* 2006;7:1-6.

38. Lafosse L, Tomasi A, Corbett S, Baier G, Willems K, Gobezie R: Arthroscopic release of suprascapular nerve entrapment at the suprascapular notch: Technique and preliminary results. *Arthroscopy* 2007; 23(1):34-42.

    A prospective series (Level IV) of 10 patients with EMG findings consistent with chronic suprascapular notch compression, posterior shoulder pain, and subjective weakness were treated with a novel arthroscopic suprascapular notch decompression. All patients had improved pain, function, and EMG findings. Level of evidence: IV.

8: Miscellaneous Shoulder and Elbow Topics

39. Piasecki DP, Romeo AA, Bach BR Jr, Nicholson GP: Suprascapular neuropathy. *J Am Acad Orthop Surg* 2009;17(11):665-676.

   This review article details the anatomy, the pathophysiology, the diagnosis, and the treatment of suprascapular neuropathy.

40. Werner CM, Nagy L, Gerber C: Combined intra- and extra-articular arthroscopic treatment of entrapment neuropathy of the infraspinatus branches of the suprascapular nerve caused by a periglenoidal ganglion cyst. *Arthroscopy* 2007;23(3):e1-e3.

   A case report of an arthroscopic technique for exposure of the spinoglenoid notch with débridement of paralabral cysts causing suprascapular neuropathy is discussed.

41. Youm T, Matthews PV, El Attrache NS: Treatment of patients with spinoglenoid cysts associated with superior labral tears without cyst aspiration, debridement, or excision. *Arthroscopy* 2006;22(5):548-552.

42. Sandow MJ, Ilic J: Suprascapular nerve rotator cuff compression syndrome in volleyball players. *J Shoulder Elbow Surg* 1998;7(5):516-521.

43. Soubeyrand M, Bauer T, Billot N, Lortat-Jacob A, Gicquelet R, Hardy P: Original portals for arthroscopic decompression of the suprascapular nerve: An anatomic study. *J Shoulder Elbow Surg* 2008;17(4):616-623.

   A cadaver study of 30 specimens is discussed. Suprascapular nerve decompressions were performed using various portals to determine the efficacy and the safety of each portal.

44. Kim DH, Murovic JA, Tiel RL, Kline DG: Management and outcomes of 42 surgical suprascapular nerve injuries and entrapments. *Neurosurgery* 2005;57(1):120-127, discussion 120-127.

45. Shah AA, Butler RB, Sung SY, Wells JH, Higgins LD, Warner JJ: Clinical outcomes of suprascapular nerve decompression. *J Shoulder Elbow Surg* 2011;20(6):975-982.

   A case series of 27 patients without rotator cuff pathology who underwent suprascapular nerve decompression is presented. At final follow-up, 71% had pain relief, 75% had an improved American Shoulder and Elbow Surgeons score, and 71% had an improved subjective shoulder value score. Level of evidence: IV.

46. Mallon WJ, Wilson RJ, Basamania CJ: The association of suprascapular neuropathy with massive rotator cuff tears: A preliminary report. *J Shoulder Elbow Surg* 2006;15(4):395-398.

47. Westerheide KJ, Dopirak RM, Karzel RP, Snyder SJ: Suprascapular nerve palsy secondary to spinoglenoid cysts: Results of arthroscopic treatment. *Arthroscopy* 2006;22(7):721-727.

Chapter 49

Scapular Kinematics, Dyskinesis, and Injuries

W. Ben Kibler, MD

Scapular Kinematics

As an integral part of the anatomy of the glenoid and the acromion, the scapula has key roles in normal shoulder and arm function. The scapula affects the movement of the glenohumeral joint and the acromioclavicular (AC) joint and is integrated with arm movement through the scapulohumeral rhythm that produces efficient kinematics. Scapular movement traditionally has been described using a single-plane, two-dimensional model in which scapular upward rotation and acromial elevation are the end points.[1,2] Upper trapezius activation to pull the acromion up and serratus anterior activation to move the inferior border laterally were described as the key muscle force couples.[1] The magnitude of the upward rotation has varied among studies but has averaged 60°, thus establishing the 1:2 scapula-humerus motion ratio for total scapulohumeral rhythm.

Research has found that scapular motion actually is multiplanar and three dimensional.[3] Motion-tracking systems and the use of indwelling bone pins have shown that total scapular movement is a composite of motions (rotations around axes) and translations (sliding motions along a surface; **Figure 1**). The three observable rotary motions are upward-downward rotation around an axis perpendicular to the scapular body, internal-external rotation around a vertical axis along the medial border, and anterior-posterior tilt around a horizontal axis along the scapular spine.[3] Two translations can occur in the presence of an intact clavicular strut and AC joint: upward-downward sliding on the thorax (resulting from clavicular upward-downward motion at the sternoclavicular [SC] joint) and anterior-posterior sliding around the curvature of the thorax (resulting from clavicular anterior-posterior motion at the SC joint).

The bony and muscular structures adjacent to the scapula determine scapular movement. The clavicle and the SC and AC joints are important for creating scapular positions, motions, and translations.[4] The anatomy of the AC and SC joints and the clavicle must be almost normal to allow normal scapular motions. The clavicle is the only bony connection of the scapula to the axial skeleton. To maximize scapular movement and scapulohumeral motion during full arm elevation, the clavicle retracts 16°, elevates 6°, and posteriorly rotates 31° on its long axis.[4] All of these motions are based on the SC joint. The AC joint motions resulting from acromial motion on the clavicle are 8° of internal rotation, 11° of upward rotation, and 19° of posterior tilting.[4] These constrained motions create a reproducible screw axis of motion between the clavicle and the scapula through the AC joint and allow the three-dimensional motions.[5]

The primary muscular factors in scapular movement involve coupling of the upper and lower fibers of the trapezius muscle with the serratus anterior and rhomboid muscles. Elevation of the scapula with arm elevation is accomplished through activation and coupling of the serratus anterior and lower trapezius with the upper trapezius and the rhomboids.[6] During this motion, the lower trapezius helps to maintain the instant center of rotation of the scapula through its attachment to the medial scapular spine.[2] The attachment of the lower trapezius to the scapular spine allows a straight line of pull as the arm elevates and the scapula upwardly rotates, and it creates a mechanical advantage for maintaining this position. The lower trapezius also has a role as a scapular stabilizer when the arm is lowered from an elevated position. The serratus anterior is multifaceted in that it contributes to all components of three-dimensional movement of the scapula; it helps to produce scapular upward rotation, posterior tilt, and external rotation while stabilizing the medial border and the inferior angle.[6]

Because these stability and mobility muscles all attach to the axial skeleton, control of posture and stability in the core is as important for maximal activation of these muscles as control of the scapula is important for maximal rotator cuff activation. Maximal activation of the muscles and force couples occurs only through patterns of activation that begin from the core and

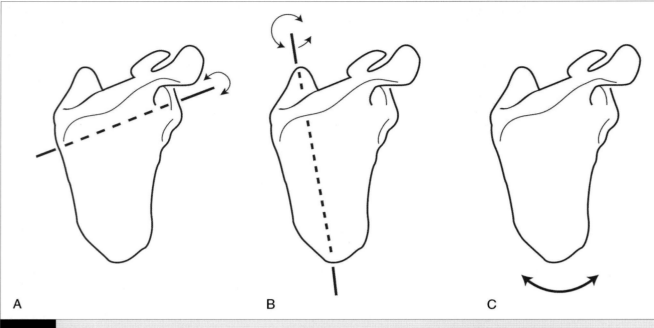

Figure 1 Schematic drawings showing three-dimensional scapular motions. **A,** The horizontal axis *(dashed line)* allows anterior and posterior tilting *(double-headed arrow).* **B,** The vertical axis *(dashed line)* allows internal and external rotation *(double-headed arrow).* **C,** The sagittal axis allows upward and downward rotation *(double-headed arrow).* (Adapted with permission from McClure PW, Bialker J, Neff N, Williams G, Karduna A: Shoulder function and 3-dimensional kinematics in people with shoulder impingement syndrome before and after a 6-week exercise program. *Phys Ther* 2004;84[9]:832-848.)

proceed to the extremities. These patterns coordinate cocontractions and force couples and synergize activation to maximize developed strength. Lower trapezius and serratus anterior activation is maximized when the recruitment is in a diagonal direction, from the contralateral hip through the lumbodorsal fascia to the lower trapezius.[7] The most stable and efficient scapular position for function is retraction.[8-10] From this position, the subacromial space is at its widest, rotator cuff activation is maximal, internal impingement is minimized, and the association with injury is lowest.[8-13]

Most scapula-related shoulder dysfunction can be traced to a loss of control of the normal resting scapular position and dynamic scapular motion, which results in alterations in position or motion that produce a position and motion of excessive protraction.[14] This protracted position causes dysfunctional symptoms or contributes to and exacerbates dysfunctional symptoms (**Figure 2**).

The altered scapular position at rest has been described as the *scapula malposition–inferior medial border prominence–coracoid pain–scapular dyskinesis* (SICK) scapula.[15] The SICK scapula is characterized by apparent inferior drooping that actually represents anterior scapular tilting. This altered position suggests alterations in pectoralis minor flexibility and serratus anterior and lower trapezius strength, and it should alert the examiner to a possible scapula-related condition.

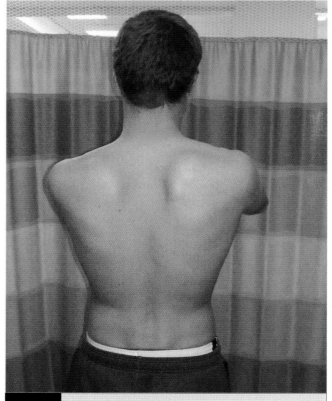

Figure 2 Photograph showing a patient with medial border prominence favoring the position of protraction.

Scapular Dyskinesis

Altered dynamic motion is called scapular dyskinesis (the term combines *dys* [alteration of] and *kinesis* [motion]). Scapular dyskinesis is characterized by medial or inferomedial scapular border prominence, early scapular elevation or shrugging when the arm is elevated, and rapid downward rotation when the arm is lowered.[14-16] The salient clinical manifestation of the dyskinetic scapula is protraction, which appears as on asymmetric prominence of the medial scapular border. Three single-plane patterns have been identified: inferomedial prominence (type I), entire medial border prominence (type II), and superomedial border prominence (type III).[17] Frequently, the pattern will appear when the arm is moved. The exact pathophysiology of each pattern and its relation to specific shoulder pathologies continue to be elucidated. It is believed that the dyskinetic patterns produce motions that alter the roles and the results of the scapula in efficient scapulohumeral rhythm.

Scapular dyskinesis is found in 67% to 100% of patients with shoulder injuries and has many causative factors.[12,13] Most often, scapular dyskinesis results from alteration in coupled muscle activation. The neurogenic causes include injury to the long thoracic or spinal accessory nerves, which appears to be relatively rare. More commonly, the muscle activation alterations are caused by inhibition of neural activation resulting from pain from a glenohumeral joint injury, a strength imbalance among the scapular stabilizers, fatigue of muscle activation, or a change in activation pattern. In almost every patient, the serratus anterior and lower trapezius are found to be weak, have lower than normal activation intensity, or are late in activation timing, and the upper trapezius has increased activation and abnormal activation timing.[18] This pattern results in less than normal posterior tilt, external rotation, and upward rotation motion, with greater than normal elevation and translation. These results have been found in patients with impingement, instability, and labral tears.[19-21]

Scapular dyskinesis also can result from muscle or glenohumeral joint stiffness. Dyskinesis is seen in almost all patients with significant degenerative arthritis of the shoulder or with adhesive capsulitis. In some patients, pectoralis minor inflexibility and tightness is believed to contribute to decreased scapular posterior tilt, upward rotation, and external rotation. Glenohumeral internal rotation deficit, which is related to posterior muscle stiffness and capsular tightness, creates dyskinesis by producing a windup of the scapula into protraction as the arm rotates into follow-through during throwing.[20]

Clavicle fracture can lead to dyskinesis if the anatomy is not almost completely restored. A malunion or a nonunion with shortening decreases the length of the strut, especially if the shortening is more than 2 cm, and it can alter the scapular position toward internal rotation and anterior tilt.[22] Similarly, a significantly angulated clavicle fracture can result in functional shortening and loss of rotation. The distal fragment in a midshaft fracture often externally rotates, thereby affecting normal kinematics by decreasing the obligatory clavicular posterior rotation and scapular posterior tilt during arm elevation.

Types III, IV and V AC joint injuries often lead to dyskinesis. These high-grade AC separations can disrupt the strut function and allow a so-called third translation, in which the scapula translates inferior to the clavicle and medial on the thorax.[23] Iatrogenic AC joint injury resulting from excessive distal clavicle resection and detachment of the AC ligaments shortens the bony strut and can allow excessive scapular internal rotation because of excessive anterior-posterior motion at the AC joint.

The final result of almost all of these causative factors is a protracted scapula at rest or an excessively protracting scapula with arm motion. This position, which usually results from increased internal rotation and anterior tilt, is unfavorable for every shoulder function except the so-called plus position in weight lifting. The malposition creates a decreased subacromial space and thereby may increase impingement symptoms.[11] In addition, the malposition decreases rotator cuff strength, and it increases strain on the anterior glenohumeral ligaments, strain on the scapula-stabilizing muscles, and the risk of internal impingement.[24] Most of the major goals of treatment of scapular dyskinesis relate to regaining functional retraction capability.

The relationship between dyskinesis and shoulder symptoms is not always clear. In a patient with nerve injury, fracture, AC separation, or muscle detachment, the injury creates the dyskinesis, which affects shoulder function. In some patients with a condition such as rotator cuff disease, labral injury, or multidirectional instability, the dyskinesis may be causative, creating pathomechanics that predispose the arm to injury. In other such patients, the dyskinesis may be a response to the injury, creating pathomechanics that increase the dysfunction. In either situation, the dyskinesis is present and must be treated with the patient's other pathologies.

The multiple causative mechanisms frequently are not isolated; several may be present in the same patient. Careful examination for the presence or the absence of scapular dyskinesis and for each of the causative mechanisms should be part of the comprehensive evaluation of a patient with shoulder injury. The clinical evaluation of the scapula should include all possible local and distant contributors to dyskinesis, with a dynamic component because scapular motion is the key component of dyskinesis.

A clinically useful and reliable examination can identify dyskinesis and serve as a basis for treatment.[14,16,25] The goals of the physical examination of the scapula are to establish the presence or the absence

8: Miscellaneous Shoulder and Elbow Topics

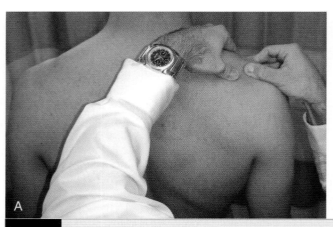
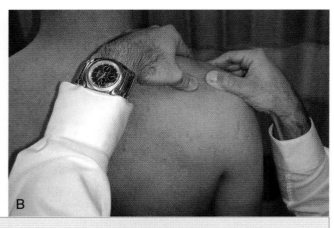

Figure 3 Photographs showing the clinical assessment of AC joint laxity. The examiner begins by stabilizing the clavicle and grasping the acromion (**A**) and then attempts to translate the acromion anteriorly and posteriorly to determine the presence and amount of joint laxity (**B**).

of a SICK scapula; identify the presence of scapular dyskinesis; evaluate joint, muscle, and bone causative factors; and use dynamic corrective maneuvers to assess the effect of correcting the dyskinesis on the patient's symptoms.[16] The results of the examination are useful in establishing the complete diagnosis of all elements of the dysfunction and in guiding treatment and rehabilitation.

Most of the scapular examination should be accomplished from the posterior aspect, with the scapula exposed for complete visualization. The patient's resting posture should be checked for side-to-side asymmetry and especially for evidence of a SICK position or inferomedial or medial border prominence. Marking the superior and inferomedial borders may be useful if it is difficult to determine the bony landmarks of the inferomedial or superomedial angles.

The SC and AC joints should be evaluated for instability, and the clavicle should be evaluated for angulation, shortening, or malrotation. Anterior and posterior AC joint laxity can be evaluated by stabilizing the clavicle with one hand and then grasping and mobilizing the acromion in an anterior-posterior direction with the other hand (**Figure 3**).

Dynamic examination of scapular motion can reliably be done by clinical observation of the motion as the arm elevates and descends when viewed from behind the patient. This motion requires activation of the muscles to maintain the closed chain mechanism of scapulohumeral rhythm. Failure to maintain this rhythm can result in increased scapular internal rotation, with consequent medial border prominence. Clinical observation of medial border prominence in patients with symptoms was correlated with biomechanically determined dyskinesis, and this method has sufficient clinical reliability to be used as the basis for determining the presence or the absence of dyskinesis.[25] The patient is asked to raise both arms in forward flex-

ion to maximal elevation and then lower the arms three to five times, while holding a 3- to 5-lb weight in each hand.[26,27] Prominence of any aspect of the medial scapular border on the symptomatic side is recorded.

The scapular assistance test (SAT), the scapular retraction test (SRT), and the scapular reposition test are corrective maneuvers that can alter the injury symptoms and provide information about the role of scapular dyskinesis in dysfunction accompanying shoulder injury.[28] The SAT is useful in evaluating scapular contributions to impingement and rotator cuff strength, and the SRT is useful in evaluating contributions to rotator cuff strength and labral symptoms. In the SAT, the examiner applies gentle pressure to assist scapular upward rotation and posterior tilt as the patient elevates one arm (**Figure 4**). The most important biomechanical effect of the SAT is to increase scapular posterior tilt by 7° to 10° throughout the entire arc of arm elevation. This test has acceptable interrater reliability.[29] A positive result occurs when the painful arc of impingement symptoms is relieved and the arc of motion is increased. In the SRT, the examiner grades supraspinatus muscle strength using standard manual muscle testing procedures (**Figure 5**) or evaluates labral injury in association with the dynamic labral shear test.[9] The examiner then places and manually stabilizes the scapula in a retracted position. The biomechanical effects are a combination of increased external rotation and posterior tilt. A positive test occurs when demonstrated supraspinatus strength is increased or the symptoms of internal impingement related to the labral injury are relieved in the retracted position. Although a positive SAT or SRT is not diagnostic for a specific form of shoulder pathology, it proves that scapular dyskinesis is directly involved in producing the symptoms and indicates the need for early scapular rehabilitation exercises to improve scapular control.

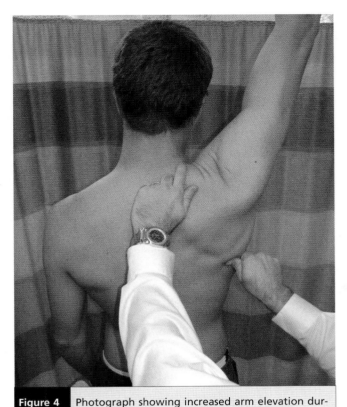

Figure 4 Photograph showing increased arm elevation during the scapular assistance test, which reveals the presence of a dysfunctional scapula.

Scapular Involvement in Shoulder Injuries

Winged Scapula

Winged scapula is a descriptive term usually used to identify the presence of an asymmetrically prominent medial scapular border at rest or with arm motion. The patient commonly has a deficit in shoulder function caused by the scapular instability. In the past, it was assumed that most incidences resulted from injury to a nerve supplying the scapula-stabilizing musculature or an underlying neuromuscular problem such as muscular dystrophy.[30-32] More recent research has shown that this biomechanical position or motion most frequently is associated with alterations in the supporting bony structure; the joints of the thoracoscapulohumeral complex; and/or in the strength, flexibility, activation sequencing, and attachment of the stabilizing musculature.[23] Therefore, the evaluation of a patient with a winged scapula must be sufficiently comprehensive to identify the factors causing the altered position and motion.

The exact frequency of neurologically based winging is poorly defined. The injury may be traumatic, iatrogenic, or idiopathic, and interpretation requires a careful patient history and examination. The long thoracic and spinal accessory nerves are most commonly involved. Long thoracic nerve injury and loss of serratus anterior muscle function lead to translation of the scapula superiorly and medially and disruption of normal scapulohumeral kinematics. Clinically, this rotation causes the inferior angle to become notably prominent in both static and dynamic examination. The diagnosis can be confirmed on electromyography at approximately 6 weeks. The initial treatment includes observation with supportive care, rehabilitation, and possibly follow-up electromyography at 3-month intervals. Rehabilitation is focused on preserving glenohumeral motion and scapular stabilization by activating the rhomboids and the lower trapezius. If there is no significant nerve recovery, maximal function is difficult to achieve because no other muscle can assume the roles of the serratus.

Surgery may be indicated for a patient with long thoracic nerve palsy after 1 year of symptoms and functional deficits, with no sign of recovery. Transfer of the sternocostal head of the pectoralis major has been the most successful procedure, with generally favorable results.[31] The selected portion of the tendon is reflected from its insertion on the humerus, tunneled ventral to the scapula, and attached to the inferior angle of the scapula by one of several techniques. The tendon length generally requires augmentation with fascia lata or other graft for length.

Scapular winging can result from injury to the spinal accessory nerve, which is susceptible to trauma from blunt force, traction, or penetrating injury. Iatrogenic injury can occur during lymph node biopsy or radical neck dissection. With loss of the trapezius activation, the scapula assumes a more inferior and lateral (drooping) posture. Winging often is less prominent than with serratus palsy, but atrophy in the upper trapezius, loss of muscle tone, and inability to shrug are easily discernible. Inability of the lower trapezius to achieve and maintain the retracted functional position of the scapula leads the patient to report pain and weakness with forward elevation and abduction. Compensatory muscle spasm in the rhomboids and levator scapula are common. The diagnosis can be corroborated by electromyography, but the findings must be carefully interpreted. Occasionally, a false-negative report results from the placement of the recording electrode in the normal underlying rhomboids instead of the thin, atrophic overlying trapezius. The treatment must be tailored to the particular cause; for neuritis or an idiopathic cause, supportive management and observation are recommended for as long as 1 year.

Surgery for spinal accessory nerve palsy can be considered if nonsurgical management is unsuccessful. In the Eden-Lange transfer, which is intended to provide a dynamic medial and superior restraint, the levator scapula and rhomboids are transferred approximately 5 cm laterally and secured through drill holes to improve mechanical advantage and a substitute for trapezius function. Substantial improvement in average American Shoulder and Elbow Surgeons Disability Index and Constant Shoulder Scores have been reported.[33]

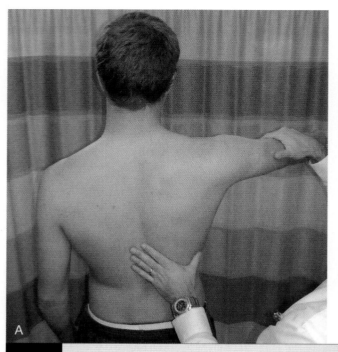
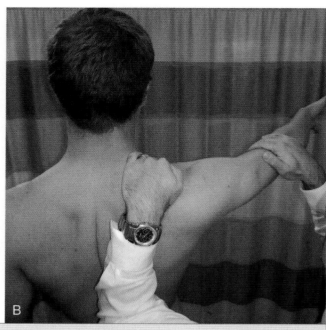

Figure 5 Photographs showing the scapular retraction test. **A,** The first component is manual muscle testing with the empty can maneuver. **B,** The second component is manual stabilization of the scapula, with the muscle test applied to the arm.

Snapping Scapula

Snapping scapula is a descriptive term for painful crepitus along the medial scapular border during arm motion. The symptoms traditionally were ascribed to osteochondromas or another bony pathology or to thickened bursitis in the thoracoscapular space, but more recent research found that alterations in normal scapulohumeral rhythm underlie most incidences of snapping scapula.[32] These alterations create increased compressive pressure along the medial border and contribute to the symptoms. The flexibility and the strength of all surrounding musculature must be comprehensively evaluated to identify the causative factors.

The diagnosis and the management of snapping scapula can be clinically challenging. Snapping scapula most frequently represents a disruption of the smooth gliding of the scapula over the thoracic cage and periscapular muscles. The normal coupled scapular motions of posterior tilt and external rotation are decreased as the arm elevates. Consequently, the normal movement of the instant center of rotation of the scapula from the superomedial border to the AC joint is disrupted, causing the scapula to rotate around the medial border, creating excessive pressure, and leading to symptoms.[23]

Patients generally report periscapular pain during overhead activities. The throwing motion, with its large scapular excursion, is particularly affected. Patients often notice an audible grinding or snapping, amplified by the thoracic cavity, which may be precipitated by active range of motion or simply by shrugging. The superomedial border is most commonly cited as the location of pain. Because of the abnormal mechanics, the cause of crepitus is believed to be the chronically inflamed bursa. In a few patients, an anatomic abnormality such as osteochondromas or a malunited rib fracture disrupts the scapulothoracic articulation and creates a predisposition to snapping scapula.

The treatment of snapping scapula should begin with comprehensive nonsurgical management directed at the individual patient's etiologic factors. The cornerstone usually is physical therapy focused on proper postural and periscapular mechanics. The lower trapezius and serratus anterior are strengthened through isometric and dynamic endurance training. The contracted anterior muscles should be mobilized by massage and stretching. Activity modification and physical therapy modalities can be included. Scapular bracing may be useful for some patients. Bursal inflammation can be treated using precise injections placed with appropriate technique and caution.

Surgery may be indicated for a patient who has undergone a thorough but unsuccessful program of nonsurgical management, is sufficiently disabled, and is willing to comply with postoperative care. Good success rates have been reported despite wide variance in the techniques.[31,32] Both open and arthroscopic techniques have been successful, although there are concerns related to morbidity and cosmesis with open procedures. Arthroscopic techniques lead to more rapid recovery but are demanding and carry a greater neurovascular risk. With either technique, the surgeon can choose a simple bursectomy or a partial scapulectomy.

Impingement and Rotator Cuff Disease

Many studies have evaluated scapular kinematics in patients with rotator cuff weakness, rotator cuff tendinopathy or impingement, or rotator cuff tear. Most of these studies have found alterations in scapular kinematics.[34] It is not clear whether the observed dyskinesis is a cause, an effect, or a compensation for the pathology. If it is a cause, decreased upward rotation and posterior tilt may be altering the size of the subacromial space and changing rotator cuff clearance under the coracoacromial arch, producing mechanical abrasion and wear. Alternatively, increased anterior tilt and internal rotation may be creating glenoid antetilting during arm motion, predisposing the rotator cuff to internal impingement; or increased strain within the rotator cuff tendon because of decreased muscle activation may be increasing the observed apoptotic changes within the tendon cells. If the dyskinesis is an effect, there may be an inhibitory effect of pain on individual muscle activation, a disruption of normal activation patterns, and an effect of pain avoidance on kinematic patterns.[34] One effect, the increased upward rotation in patients with rotator cuff tears, may represent a compensatory attempt to increase or maximize arm elevation or positioning in the face of weakened or absent rotator cuff activation. Whatever the relationship, scapular dyskinesis frequently is identified in rotator cuff disease and is associated with impaired function.

A positive SAT will show that the patient's excessive anterior scapular tilt is part of the pathophysiology producing external impingement symptoms. The treatment should include increasing the flexibility of the pectoralis minor and the short head of the biceps tendon as well as strengthening the serratus anterior as a scapular external rotator and the lower trapezius as a retractor. The scapular stability series of strengthening exercises is effective for achieving these goals (**Figure 6**). A positive SRT will show scapular involvement in the patient's muscle weakness; treatment is directed toward scapular stability in retraction, rather than the rotator cuff, as the first step in rehabilitation.

Labral Injury

Scapular dyskinesis was found to be associated with labral injury in one pathologic cascade model.[20] The altered position and motion of internal rotation and anterior tilt may change glenohumeral alignment, placing increased tensile strain on the anterior ligaments, increasing the peel-back of the biceps-labral complex on the glenoid, creating pathologic internal impingement, and weakening rotator cuff cocontraction strength. These effects are magnified in the presence of glenohumeral internal rotation deficit, which creates increased protraction because of the windup of the tight posterior structures during the follow-through phase of throwing. Evaluation of dyskinesis in a patient with suspected labral injury is key to rehabilitation. Pain during the dynamic labral shear test frequently can be eliminated or reduced by the SRT maneuver, which indicates

that dyskinesis is part of the pathophysiology. Scapular rehabilitation is required to improve scapular retraction, including mobilization of tight anterior muscles and the use of the scapular stability series of strengthening exercises. In addition, identification of scapular dyskinesis is an important part of preventing labral injury.

AC Joint Arthrosis

The bony components of the shoulder must be intact for optimal function. AC joint arthrosis with instability or high-grade AC separation alters the strut function of the clavicle on the scapula and changes the biomechanical screw axis of the scapulohumeral rhythm, allowing excessive scapular protraction and decreased dynamic acromial elevation when the arm is elevated.[5,23] This so-called third translation of the scapula allows the scapula to move in an inferomedial manner in relation to the clavicle, as is most often seen when a high-grade separation (type III, IV, or V) occurs. The protracted scapular position creates many of the dysfunctions associated with chronic AC separation, including impingement and decreased demonstrated rotator cuff strength. Scapular dyskinesis showing the third translation with arm elevation or forward flexion is a clinical examination finding that may help in determining the surgical treatment of a type III injury.

Clavicle Fracture

A fracture of the clavicle with a nonunion or shortened and rotated malunion alters the strut function and leads to a poor functional outcome. Muscle weakness and loss of range of motion are the functional deficiencies most often seen in association with a malunited or a nonunited clavicle fracture.[22] The altered strut function of the clavicle allows excessive protraction of the scapula; this position limits rotator cuff function and the ability of the humerus to fully elevate. An assessment of scapular position in a patient with an acute or a chronic fracture of the clavicle can help determine whether surgery is indicated for realigning the clavicular body and restoring the ability of the clavicle to serve as a strut.

Multidirectional Instability

One of the salient features of multidirectional instability is that symptoms and instability occur in the midranges of glenohumeral motion (where concavity-compression, bone alignment, and muscle activation play the most important roles), rather than at the end ranges of motion (where capsuloligamentous restraints are most important). Many patients with multidirectional instability simultaneously have increased protraction of the scapula and humeral head migration away from the center of the joint as the arm moves.[19,35] When the patient elevates the arm, the scapula deviates from the normal kinematic pattern of upward rotation, posterior tilting, and minimal internal rotation and instead follows a pattern of upward rotation, anterior tilting, and excessive internal rotation. This position allows the humeral head to translate inferiorly out of the

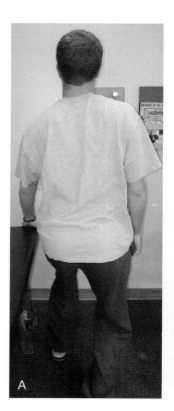
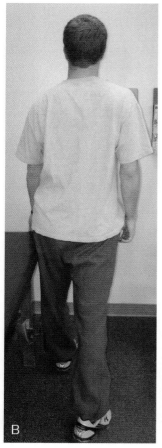
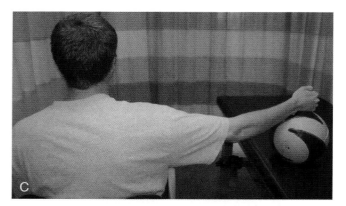
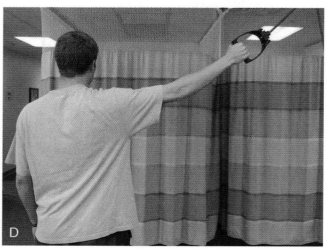
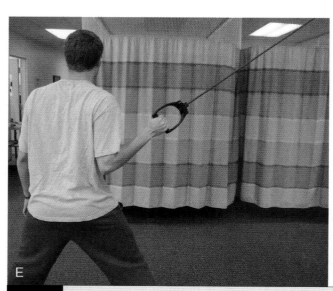
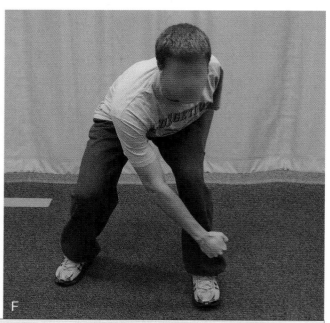

Figure 6 Photographs showing the scapular stability series of exercises. The low row in the starting position (**A**) and with extension of the hips and the trunk to facilitate scapular retraction (**B**). The active inferior glide exercise, in which co-contraction of the shoulder and scapular muscles helps depress the humerus and scapula (**C**). The fencing exercise in the starting position with the arm elevated above 90° in the frontal plane (**D**) and performed by side stepping and simultaneously retracting the scapula and adducting the arm (**E**). The lawnmower exercise (designed to integrate the lower extremity, the trunk, and the upper extremity) is shown in the starting position (**F**).

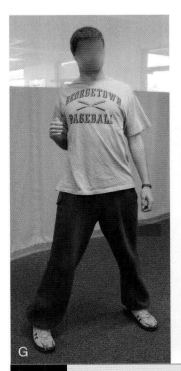
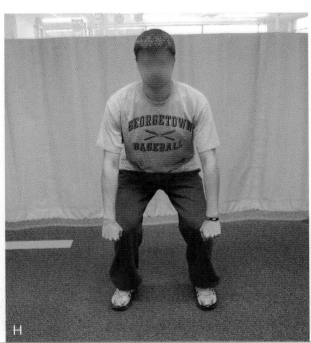
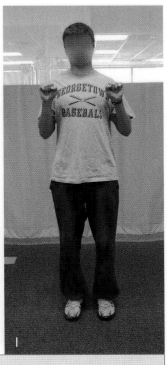

Figure 6 Photographs showing the scapular stability series of exercises (continued). The lawnmower exercise with extension of the hips and the trunk followed by rotation of the trunk to facilitate scapular retraction is shown (**G**). The robbery maneuver in the starting position, with the knees and the trunk flexed and the arms held away from the body (**H**) and with extension of the hips and trunk is shown, and the patient is instructed to attempt to "place the elbows in the back pockets (**I**)."

glenoid socket, thus creating the instability. Inhibition of the subscapularis, the lower trapezius, and serratus anterior, coupled with increased activation of the pectoralis minor and the latissimus dorsi, place the scapula in this protracted position.

In many patients with multidirectional instability, careful observation of the resting scapular position and the dynamic motion of the scapula with arm motion reveals protraction, especially in the positions associated with instability symptoms. By stabilizing the scapula in retraction, the SRT alters the glenoid position, decreases latissimus dorsi activation, and thereby decreases or eliminates the instability symptoms with arm motion. A positive SRT directs treatment toward strengthening the lower trapezius and the serratus anterior and increasing the flexibility of the pectoralis minor and the latissimus dorsi. The ability to achieve restoration of normal activation patterns accounts for the greater likelihood of successful rehabilitation in patients with multidirectional instability than in those with posttraumatic instability.

Rehabilitation of Scapular Dyskinesis

The three types of rehabilitation exercises for scapular control are proximal kinetic chain exercises to facilitate scapular muscle strength, flexibility exercises to mini-

mize traction on scapular posture, and exercises specific for periscapular activation. Kinetic chain exercises for the trunk and the hip start from and end at the ideal position of hip extension and trunk extension. Trunk and hip flexion-extension, rotation, and diagonal motions are included. The progressions include step up–step down and increasing weights. These exercises may be started before surgery when deficits have been identified and may be done while the shoulder is protected.

Flexibility exercises should focus on the anterior coracoid (pectoralis minor and biceps short head) and shoulder rotation. Tightness in these areas increases scapular protraction. The exercises include the open book and corner stretch for the coracoid muscles and the sleeper and cross-body stretches for shoulder rotation (**Figure 7**).

The goal of periscapular strengthening exercises should be to achieve a position of scapular retraction because this is the most effective position for maximizing scapular roles. Scapular retraction exercises may be done in a standing position to simulate normal activation sequences and allow kinetic chain sequencing. Scapular pinch and trunk extension–retraction exercises can be started early in rehabilitation while the shoulder is being protected because little tensile load or shear is imposed on the glenohumeral joint.

Several specific exercises are effective for activating the key scapular stabilizers (the lower trapezius and the

8: Miscellaneous Shoulder and Elbow Topics

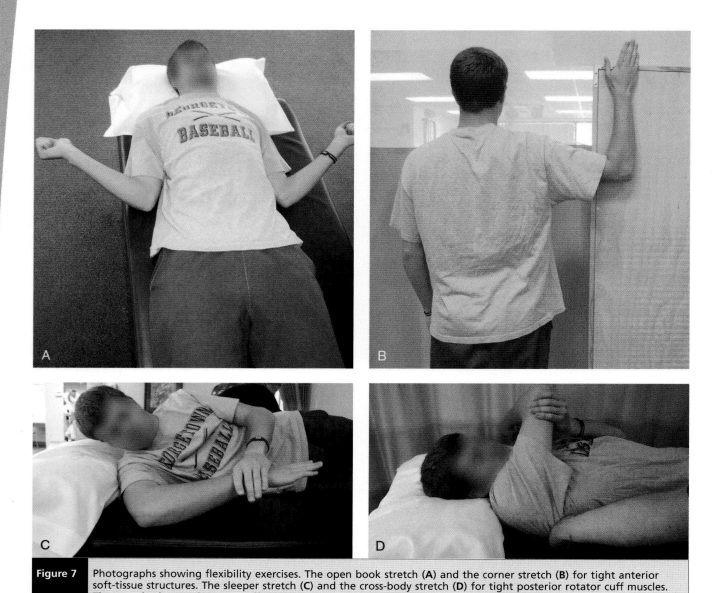

Figure 7 Photographs showing flexibility exercises. The open book stretch (**A**) and the corner stretch (**B**) for tight anterior soft-tissue structures. The sleeper stretch (**C**) and the cross-body stretch (**D**) for tight posterior rotator cuff muscles. The cross-body stretch is most effective when the scapula is stabilized.

serratus anterior) and minimizing upper trapezius activation.[36] The low row, inferior glide, fencing, lawn-mower, and robbery exercises, collectively called the scapular stability series, activate the target muscles to 18% to 30% of maximal activation[36] (**Figure 6**). This activation as well as arm angles limited to 90° abduction mean that the scapular stability exercises are particularly effective during the early stages of rehabilitation after injury or surgery.

As healing progresses and loads can be applied to the shoulder, closed chain exercises also should be emphasized to restore the normal activations of the closed chain mechanism of the shoulder that stabilize the joint.[37] In these exercises, the hand is supported on a stable or movable surface, and the arm and the scapula are loaded from distal to proximal. Rhythmic stabilization and wall washes are examples of closed chain exercises (**Figure 8**).

When scapular control is achieved, integrated scapula–rotator cuff exercises such as punches and shoulder dumps are added to stimulate rotator cuff activation from a stabilized scapula. These exercises can be done in various planes of abduction and flexion, with different amounts or types of resistance, and they can be modified to be sport specific.

Maximal integration of kinetic chain–scapula–shoulder coordination occurs when diagonal patterns of activation and loading are emphasized. Four-point, standing diagonal, and rotational exercises are used.

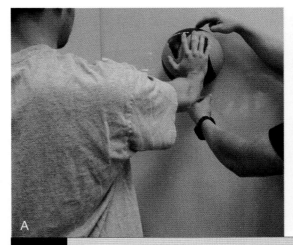
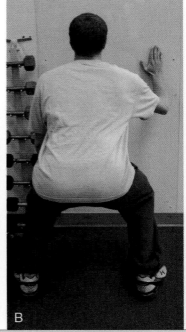
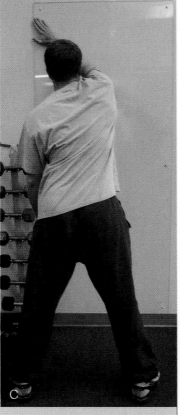

Figure 8 Photographs showing closed chain techniques, which aid in muscle reeducation and can be implemented in functional arm positions. **A,** In rhythmic stabilization, the patient attempts to stabilize a ball while the clinician applies force from various directions. In the wall wash exercise, the patient begins in a half-squat or full-squat position with the hand of the involved arm on a wall (**B**) and then stands using the legs and the trunk to drive the arm through different ranges and planes of motion (**C**).

Summary

The scapula is in a key position and plays a key role in all aspects of shoulder and arm function. Normal scapular kinematics place the glenohumeral joint in the most stable bony configuration, allow transfer of energy and force from the core to the hand, and maximize muscle activation to move the arm and stabilize the joint. Scapular dyskinesis (alteration of normal motion) is found in association with almost all shoulder pathology. It is not clear whether dyskinesis is a cause or an effect of the shoulder pathology. Dyskinesis frequently contributes to clinical dysfunction, however, and it should be evaluated and treated as part of the comprehensive evaluation and treatment of the shoulder pathology. Dyskinesis can be detected by a clinically useful and reliable examination, and the causative factors can be identified. Treatment and rehabilitation protocols then can be developed to address the deficits.

Annotated References

1. Bagg SD, Forrest WJ: Electromyographic study of the scapular rotators during arm abduction in the scapular plane. *Am J Phys Med* 1986;65(3):111-124.

2. Bagg SD, Forrest WJ: A biomechanical analysis of scapular rotation during arm abduction in the scapular plane. *Am J Phys Med Rehabil* 1988;67(6):238-245.

3. McClure PW, Michener LA, Sennett BJ, Karduna AR: Direct 3-dimensional measurement of scapular kinematics during dynamic movements in vivo. *J Shoulder Elbow Surg* 2001;10(3):269-277.

4. Ludewig PM, Phadke V, Braman JP, Hassett DR, Cieminski CJ, LaPrade RF: Motion of the shoulder complex during multiplanar humeral elevation. *J Bone Joint Surg Am* 2009;91(2):378-389.

   Bone pin placement was used to accurately categorize the exact three-dimensional motions of the clavicle, the SC and AC joints, the scapula, and the humerus. The important roles of clavicle movement and SC and AC joint motion in scapular motion were documented.

8: Miscellaneous Shoulder and Elbow Topics

Disruptions anywhere along the clavicle have deleterious effects on scapular motion and arm function.

5. Sahara W, Sugamoto K, Murai M, Yoshikawa H: Three-dimensional clavicular and acromioclavicular rotations during arm abduction using vertically open MRI. *J Orthop Res* 2007;25(9):1243-1249.

   The screw axis is the three-dimensional guide motion that defines AC motions and thereby controls coupled scapuloclaviculohumeral movement.

6. Speer KP, Garrett WE: Muscular control of motion and stability about the pectoral girdle, in Matsen FA III, Fu F, Hawkins RJ (eds): *The Shoulder: A Balance of Mobility and Stability*. Rosemont, IL, American Academy of Orthopaedic Surgeons, 1994, pp 159-173.

7. Cools AM, Dewitte V, Lanszweert F, et al: Rehabilitation of scapular muscle balance: Which exercises to prescribe? *Am J Sports Med* 2007;35(10):1744-1751.

   Some of the rehabilitation parameters that guide the restoration of muscular balance for scapular control are defined.

8. Smith J, Kotajarvi BR, Padgett DJ, Eischen JJ: Effect of scapular protraction and retraction on isometric shoulder elevation strength. *Arch Phys Med Rehabil* 2002;83(3):367-370.

9. Kibler WB, Sciascia AD, Dome DC: Evaluation of apparent and absolute supraspinatus strength in patients with shoulder injury using the scapular retraction test. *Am J Sports Med* 2006;34(10):1643-1647.

10. Tate AR, McClure PW, Kareha S, Irwin D: Effect of the scapula reposition test on shoulder impingement symptoms and elevation strength in overhead athletes. *J Orthop Sports Phys Ther* 2008;38(1):4-11.

    The use of a position of scapular retraction during clinical manual muscle testing improved rotator cuff strength. This finding confirmed earlier work by other researchers.

11. Solem-Bertoft E, Thuomas KA, Westerberg CE: The influence of scapular retraction and protraction on the width of the subacromial space: An MRI study. *Clin Orthop Relat Res* 1993;296:99-103.

12. Warner JJ, Micheli LJ, Arslanian LE, Kennedy J, Kennedy R: Patterns of flexibility, laxity, and strength in normal shoulders and shoulders with instability and impingement. *Am J Sports Med* 1990;18(4):366-375.

13. Warner JJ, Micheli LJ, Arslanian LE, Kennedy J, Kennedy R: Scapulothoracic motion in normal shoulders and shoulders with glenohumeral instability and impingement syndrome: A study using Moiré topographic analysis. *Clin Orthop Relat Res* 1992;285:191-199.

14. Kibler WB, Sciascia AD: Current concepts: Scapular dyskinesis. *Br J Sports Med* 2010;44(5):300-305.

    This is a concise review of scapular dyskinesis, including its definition, effects on shoulder function and dysfunction, relationship to all types of shoulder injuries, clinical evaluation, and treatment guidelines.

15. Burkhart SS, Morgan CD, Kibler WB: The disabled throwing shoulder: Spectrum of pathology part III. The SICK scapula, scapular dyskinesis, the kinetic chain, and rehabilitation. *Arthroscopy* 2003;19(6):641-661.

16. Kibler WB, Ludewig PM, McClure P, Uhl TL, Sciascia A: Scapular summit 2009: Introduction. July 16, 2009, Lexington, Kentucky. *J Orthop Sports Phys Ther* 2009;39(11):A1-A13.

    The results of a consensus meeting on the basic science and the clinical application of research on the scapula were presented, including current knowledge of scapular motion and dyskinesis, rehabilitation, and an evidence-based recommendation for clinical evaluation of the scapula in patients with shoulder injury.

17. Kibler WB, Uhl TL, Maddux JW, Brooks PV, Zeller B, McMullen J: Qualitative clinical evaluation of scapular dysfunction: A reliability study. *J Shoulder Elbow Surg* 2002;11(6):550-556.

18. Cools AM, Witvrouw EE, Declercq GA, Danneels LA, Cambier DC: Scapular muscle recruitment patterns: Trapezius muscle latency with and without impingement symptoms. *Am J Sports Med* 2003;31(4):542-549.

19. Ogston JB, Ludewig PM: Differences in 3-dimensional shoulder kinematics between persons with multidirectional instability and asymptomatic controls. *Am J Sports Med* 2007;35(8):1361-1370.

    Altered scapular position was found to exacerbate the symptoms typically associated with multidirectional instability. Rehabilitation for patients with this condition should focus on scapular strengthening.

20. Burkhart SS, Morgan CD, Kibler WB: The disabled throwing shoulder: Spectrum of pathology part I. Pathoanatomy and biomechanics. *Arthroscopy* 2003;19(4):404-420.

21. Michener LA, McClure PW, Karduna AR: Anatomical and biomechanical mechanisms of subacromial impingement syndrome. *Clin Biomech (Bristol, Avon)* 2003;18(5):369-379.

22. McKee MD, Pedersen EM, Jones C, et al: Deficits following nonoperative treatment of displaced midshaft clavicular fractures. *J Bone Joint Surg Am* 2006;88(1):35-40.

23. Gumina S, Carbone S, Postacchini F: Scapular dyskinesis and SICK scapula syndrome in patients with chronic type III acromioclavicular dislocation. *Arthroscopy* 2009;25(1):40-45.

    A high percentage of patients with a type III AC separation were found to have clinical evidence of scapular dyskinesis, indicating the third translation of the scapula in conjunction with AC separation.

24. Smith J, Dietrich CT, Kotajarvi BR, Kaufman KR: The effect of scapular protraction on isometric shoulder rotation strength in normal subjects. *J Shoulder Elbow Surg* 2006;15(3):339-343.

25. Uhl TL, Kibler WB, Gecewich B, Tripp BL: Evaluation of clinical assessment methods for scapular dyskinesis. *Arthroscopy* 2009;25(11):1240-1248.

    A yes-no assessment system for clinical observation of scapular dyskinesis was correlated with biomechanical evaluation of scapular motion and found to have clinically relevant utility, with sensitivities, specificities, and positive predictive values between 0.64 and 0.84.

26. McClure PW, Tate AR, Kareha S, Irwin D, Zlupko E: A clinical method for identifying scapular dyskinesis, part 1: Reliability. *J Athl Train* 2009;44(2):160-164.

    This is the first part of a two-part article on a method of visual observation found to help clinicians distinguish between the presence and the absence of scapular dyskinesis in a general population.

27. Tate AR, McClure P, Kareha S, Irwin D, Barbe MF: A clinical method for identifying scapular dyskinesis, part 2: Validity. *J Athl Train* 2009;44(2):165-173.

    This is the second part of a two-part article on a method of visual observation found to help clinicians distinguish between the presence and the absence of scapular dyskinesis in a general population.

28. Kibler WB: The role of the scapula in athletic shoulder function. *Am J Sports Med* 1998;26(2):325-337.

29. Rabin A, Irrgang JJ, Fitzgerald GK, Eubanks A: The intertester reliability of the scapular assistance test. *J Orthop Sports Phys Ther* 2006;36(9):653-660.

30. Kuhn JE, Plancher KD, Hawkins RJ: Scapular winging. *J Am Acad Orthop Surg* 1995;3(6):319-325.

31. Steinmann SP, Wood MB: Pectoralis major transfer for serratus anterior paralysis. *J Shoulder Elbow Surg* 2003;12(6):555-560.

32. Kuhne M, Boniquit N, Ghodadra N, Romeo AA, Provencher MT: The snapping scapula: Diagnosis and treatment. *Arthroscopy* 2009;25(11):1298-1311.

    This review (and a subsequent letter to the editor) discussed pathophysiology, clinical presentation, and treatment guidelines related to snapping scapula.

33. Romero J, Gerber C: Levator scapulae and rhomboid transfer for paralysis of trapezius: The Eden-Lange procedure. *J Bone Joint Surg Br* 2003;85(8):1141-1145.

34. Ludewig PM, Reynolds JF: The association of scapular kinematics and glenohumeral joint pathologies. *J Orthop Sports Phys Ther* 2009;39(2):90-104.

    The literature on scapular motion and position in relation to pathologic conditions in the shoulder shows how scapular dysfunction can influence the clinical presentation of the shoulder pathology.

35. Morris AD, Kemp GJ, Frostick SP: Shoulder electromyography in multidirectional instability. *J Shoulder Elbow Surg* 2004;13(1):24-29.

36. Kibler WB, Sciascia AD, Uhl TL, Tambay N, Cunningham T: Electromyographic analysis of specific exercises for scapular control in early phases of shoulder rehabilitation. *Am J Sports Med* 2008;36(9):1789-1798.

    A series of rehabilitation exercises was described as capable of activating scapular muscles in the early stages of rehabilitation with minimal stress on injured tissues.

37. Kibler WB, Livingston B: Closed-chain rehabilitation for upper and lower extremities. *J Am Acad Orthop Surg* 2001;9(6):412-421.

8: Miscellaneous Shoulder and Elbow Topics

Chapter 50

Complex Regional Pain Syndrome of the Shoulder and Elbow

Paul J. Christo, MD, MBA   Brian G. Wilhelmi, MD, JD

Introduction

Complex regional pain syndrome (CRPS) is a rare, debilitating neurologic condition composed of a constellation of symptoms, including exaggerated pain accompanied by sensory, autonomic, motor, and trophic dysfunction.[1] It is commonly a limb-confined chronic pain condition that may be induced by minor injury, trauma, or surgery and clinically evolves following initial presentation. The condition may complicate a surgical procedure on an extremity by creating severe pain during the postoperative period. CRPS not only adversely affects quality of life but also is associated with large personal and societal healthcare costs.[2] It is imperative for the orthopaedic practitioner to both recognize and triage patients with CRPS for appropriate care; early treatment, including medication, physical and occupational therapy, and interventional pain management, is correlated with the best outcomes.

Definition and Epidemiology

CRPS is a term standardized by the International Society for the Study of Pain to bring together a disparate, idiosyncratic set of diagnostic schemes to describe the syndrome (previously referred to as shoulder-hand syndrome, reflex sympathetic dystrophy, causalgia, or algodystrophy).[1] The diagnostic criteria for CRPS include pain disproportional to any inciting event combined with signs and symptoms of sensory, vasomotor, sudomotor (sweat gland–stimulating), and motor/trophic changes[3,4] (**Tables 1** and **2**). CRPS types 1 and 2 are subdivisions of the syndrome based on the absence or the presence of identifiable nerve injury.

Dr. Christo or an immediate family member serves as a paid consultant to or is an employee of Ameritox, Actavis, Quadrant Healthcom, Perrigo, and Cattem and has received research or institutional support from Medtronic. Neither Dr. Wilhelmi nor any immediate family member has received anything of value from or has stock or stock options held in a commercial company or institution related directly or indirectly to the subject of this chapter.

There are few epidemiologic studies in which CRPS is defined by the agreed-on criteria, but a greater understanding of the epidemiologic effect of the disease appears likely in the future as a result of clarified diagnostic criteria. CRPS is a rare disease with an estimated annual incidence between 5.46 and 26.2 per 100,000 person-years and a prevalence of 20.7-26.2 per 100,000 persons.[5] One prospective study of 596 patients documented an incidence as high as 7% following a fracture when using the revised Budapest criteria.[6] Females are disproportionately affected, with a female-to-male ratio ranging from 2.3 to 5:1.[5] There is little agreement concerning the age demographic with the greatest disease burden.[6] The disease appears to have a less severe clinical course when experienced at an older age of onset.[7] Although an individual health center's data or even multicenter epidemiologic data on CRPS are difficult to obtain, new instruments such as electronic web-based surveys or advocacy group websites may provide increased power to future studies.[7]

Table 1

International Society for the Study of Pain Orlando Criteria for Complex Regional Pain Syndrome

1. The presence of an initiating noxious event or a cause of immobilization

2. Continuing pain, allodynia, or hyperalgesia in which the pain is disproportionate to any known inciting event

3. Evidence at some time of edema, changes in skin blood flow, or abnormal sudomotor activity in the region of pain (can be a sign or a symptom)

4. Excludes the existence of other conditions that would otherwise account for the degree of pain and dysfunction

Data from Merskey H, Bogduk N: *Classification of Chronic Pain: Descriptions of Chronic Pain Syndrome and Definitions of Pain Terms*, ed 2. Seattle, WA, IASP Press, 1994.

Table 2

The Budapest Clinical Diagnostic Criteria for Complex Regional Pain Syndrome[a]

To make the clinical diagnosis, the following criteria must be met:

1. Continuing pain, which is disproportionate to any inciting event

2. Must report at least one symptom in three of the four following categories:
   Sensory: Reports of hyperesthesia and/or allodynia
   Vasomotor: Reports of temperature asymmetry and/or skin color changes and/or skin color asymmetry
   Sudomotor/edema: Reports of edema and/or sweating changes and/or sweating asymmetry
   Motor/trophic: Reports of decreased range of motion and/or motor dysfunction (weakness, tremor, dystonia) and/or trophic changes (hair, nail, skin)

3. Must display at least one sign at time of evaluation in two or more of the following categories:
   Sensory: Evidence of hyperalgesia (to pinprick) and/or allodynia (to light touch and/or temperature sensation and/or deep somatic pressure and/or joint movement)
   Vasomotor: Evidence of temperature asymmetry (> 1°C) and/or skin color changes and/or asymmetry
   Sudomotor/edema: Evidence of edema and/or sweating changes and/or sweating asymmetry
   Motor/trophic: Evidence of decreased range of motion and/or motor dysfunction (weakness, tremor, dystonia) and/or trophic changes (hair, nail, skin)

4. No other diagnosis better explains the signs and symptoms

[a]CRPS describes an array of painful conditions that are characterized by a continuing (spontaneous and/or evoked) regional pain that is seemingly disproportionate in time or degree to the usual course of any known trauma or other lesion. The pain is regional (not in a specific nerve territory or dermatome) and usually has a distal predominance of abnormal sensory, motor, sudomotor, vasomotor, and/or trophic findings. The syndrome shows variable progression over time. Data from Harden RN, Bruehl S, Perez RS, et al: Validation of proposed diagnostic criteria (the "Budapest Criteria") for complex regional pain syndrome. *Pain* 2010;150(2):268-274.

Pathophysiology

Although the exact mechanisms of CRPS have yet to be discovered, the scientific understanding of the pathophysiologic basis of the syndrome has increased greatly over the past decade.[8] Research has led to the theory that multiple pathologic mechanisms likely play a role in the initiation and the propagation of CRPS, and the variable expression of these mechanisms in various patients (and within the same patient over time) account for differences in clinical presentation.[1]

A neuronal injury trigger, however imperceptible, has been implicated with the development of CRPS (including CRPS type 1) and is part of the revised diagnostic criteria.[8] This trigger appears to alter the peripheral nervous system, given that patients with CRPS demonstrate fewer C-type and Aδ-type cutaneous afferent nerve fibers within the affected region as opposed to nonaffected regions of the body. Trauma to a limb also causes the peripheral nerves to increase the release of neuropeptides substance P, bradykinin, and glutamate, which sensitize and increase the activity of local peripheral and secondary central nociceptive neurons and increase pain.

Repetitive stimulation and sensitization of nociceptors in the peripheral nervous system lead to changes in central nervous system (CNS) nociceptive processing. Patients with CRPS demonstrate wind-up, or increased excitability of wide-dynamic range central neurons. The windup of central sensitization is thought to be responsible for pain in response to nonnoxious stimuli (allodynia) and increased pain from noxious stimuli (hyperalgesia). Several cortical activity mapping techniques, including functional magnetic resonance imaging (fMRI), have demonstrated cortical reorganization in patients with CRPS.[9] These studies have shown a reduction in the cortical distance between discrete activation areas of the thumb and the fifth finger in response to tactile stimulation and widespread cortical activation in response to pin-prick hyperalgesia and mechanical allodynia.[9] Follow-up of patients with cortical changes demonstrated a reversal of changes in patients who experienced a reduction of pain through therapy. These findings suggest that induced CNS changes may be responsible for reduced tactile discrimination and enhanced pain signaling in CRPS.

The clinical presentation of the acute phase of CRPS stimulates hypotheses about the role that inflammatory pathways play in the development of the syndrome.[10] The initial warm, erythematous, and edematous extremity is likely caused by plasma and protein extravasation accompanied by vasodilation. These tissue processes may be induced by proinflammatory cytokines such as interleukins-1β, -2, -6, and tumor necrosis factor (TNF)-α as well as the neuropeptides calcitonin gene-related peptide (CGRP), bradykinin, and substance P. Studies of patients with CRPS have demonstrated increased proinflammatory cytokines in blister fluid, plasma, and cerebrospinal fluid. Proinflammatory neuropeptides may play a specific role in inflammatory pain because they not only directly increase nociceptive firing but also stimulate vasodilation, protein extravasation, and further release of other proinflammatory cytokines.

Sympathetic nervous system (SNS) dysfunction has long been theorized to be a core component of CRPS pathophysiology.[8] During the acute or warm phase of clinical presentation, the affected limb is vasodilated and fails to vasoconstrict with cold stimuli, and sweating is often decreased. The limb concomitantly demonstrates decreased circulating plasma levels of norepinephrine. In time, transition to the chronic or cold phase of clinical presentation is that of vasoconstriction and sweating, even in the presence of decreased circulating plasma norepinephrine levels. This presentation suggests that adrenergic receptors are upregulated during the transition from acute to chronic disease, and the

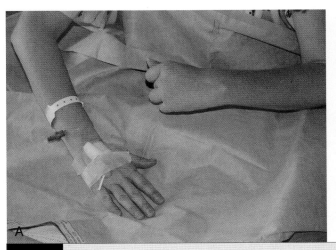
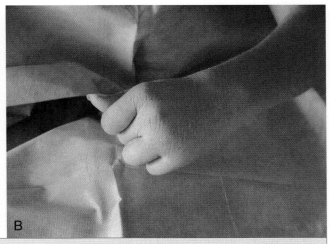

Figure 1 **A** and **B**, Photographs showing a hand with cold type CRPS. Contractures, changes in skin color, muscle wasting, and trophic changes to skin and nails are seen.

limb becomes hyperreactive to adrenergic stimulation in the chronic phase. Pain experienced by patients with CRPS also appears to be SNS mediated because stimuli such as cold or extreme emotion aggravate the pain experienced, and sympathetic blockade has been demonstrated to provide pain relief. Animal studies demonstrating adrenergic receptor expression on nociceptive fibers following nerve trauma have fueled speculation that such receptor expression in humans may be the mechanism of sympathetically mediated pain.

Research on predisposing factors that could predict which patients are susceptible to CRPS continues.[8] Recent genetic research on familial cases of CRPS has focused on the HLA molecules on the major histocompatibility complex gene and promoter regions of the TNF-α inflammatory cytokines. Additional research has focused on the genetic inhibition of the successful transcription of angiotensin-converting enzyme, which aids in the degradation of bradykinin. No genetic factors have yet been proven to be a definitive link to CRPS.

Studies of the serum of patients with CRPS have demonstrated the presence of autoantibodies directed against surface antigens found on autonomic neurons.[10] In a small pilot trial, intravenous immunoglobulin treatment led to a significant reduction in pain symptoms of patients with CRPS when compared with placebo.[11] These findings, along with the potential of predisposing HLA genotypes, support the belief that CRPS has an autoimmune pathology.

Psychopathologic factors also have been examined for their role in the predisposition or propagation of CRPS because of the prevalence of anxiety and depression within this population.[8] No definitive causation has yet been demonstrated.

Clinical Features

CRPS is a clinical entity that has historically been described as an evolution of stages.[12] A recent study, however, demonstrates a variable initial clinical presentation and variety in the subsequent clinical course among patients.[7] Despite this, the use of the classically described stages may someday provide phenotypic subgrouping for treatment tailored to the patient's current pathology and symptoms.[7]

Following neurologic injury, the most common initial presentation of CRPS is considered the acute or warm stage, in which the limb experiences exaggerated pain (both allodynia and hyperalgesia) warmth, erythema, decreased sweating, and extra-articular edema.[12] The second stage is the intermediate dystrophic stage, in which increased pain, sensory dysfunction, and continued evidence of vasomotor dysfunction are accompanied by significant motor and trophic changes (skin becomes glossy or thickened, nails become thickened or striated, and hair growth increases or decreases).[12] The third stage is the chronic, cold, or atrophic stage typified by decreased blood flow to the affected limb, thinning skin, muscle atrophy, decreased joint range of motion and contractures, and demineralization of bone[12] (**Figure 1**).

The onset of CRPS symptoms follows a neurologic insult that may result from mechanical, thermal, chemical, or ischemic events.[13] It is difficult for a surgeon to predict which upper extremity procedures are more likely to initiate CRPS, but any surgery or injury to the upper extremity could be considered a potential inciting event. Initial symptoms include temperature differences, edema, skin color or texture variations, sweat alterations, hair or nail texture changes, and motor weakness. Almost all individuals with CRPS experience

8: Miscellaneous Shoulder and Elbow Topics

constant pain with a burning, tearing, stinging, aching, or throbbing quality.[7] Exacerbations of constant pain occur with physical and emotional stress, cold weather, movement of the affected limb, and work. The pain is associated with the signs and the symptoms that define the disease, namely hypersensitivity (both allodynia and hyperalgesia), temperature differences, and swelling. Evolution of the clinical symptoms experienced by patients is common. The location and the extent of pain in an affected area tends to spread following the onset of symptoms. Clinical symptoms experienced also evolve as hypersensitivity, temperature differences, color variation, and swelling may decrease while motor weakness and disability of the affected limb may increase. There are patients in whom symptoms have been reported to resolve, but many of those experiencing resolution may experience subsequent relapse.

Approximately one third of patients will suffer from sympathetically mediated pain, which is pain that is exacerbated by the increased release of catecholamines from the sympathetic nervous system.[14] The proposed mechanism is a pathologic coupling of the somatic afferent system and SNS systems, as discussed previously. These patients will experience pain triggered by cold, light mechanical stimulation, and emotional arousal. Sympathetically mediated pain has been singled out as a symptom of special interest in CRPS because of the possibility of either medical or surgical sympatholysis to provide relief.

The individual psychological, social, and financial toll of CRPS is substantial.[7] Pain negatively affects sleep, mobility, self-care, and activities of daily living. The disease is costly to diagnose and treat; an average patient will see more than four physicians before diagnosis and may undergo expensive diagnostic testing before establishing the diagnosis and the therapy plan. The costs of care are more difficult to bear because patients typically suffer loss of income due to impaired job performance and frequent unemployment. Psychiatric illness including anxiety and depression is common, and suicidal ideation may be reported in up to one half of affected individuals at one point during the course of their disease.

Evaluation of the Patient Suspected of Having Upper Extremity CRPS

Orthopaedic practitioners are asked to evaluate upper extremity pain of various etiologies, and the ability to recognize the CRPS diagnostic pattern and initiate basic treatment is an important skill. CRPS is a rare diagnosis that may have subtle initial signs. A high index of suspicion is necessary in the setting of exaggerated pain following a recognized noxious event (such as trauma or surgery) or peripheral nerve injury. CRPS is a clinical diagnosis; therefore, a complete history and physical examination documenting the signs and the symptoms of CRPS provide the basis of diagnosis. Diagnostic testing

provide additional evidence of the sequelae of CRPS, but it is often useful in ruling out other pathology.

The physical examination of an upper extremity for signs of CRPS is an evaluation aimed at distinguishing expected inflammatory, neurologic, and orthopaedic changes from injury or surgery from those indicating a likely case of CRPS. The clinician should always have a high index of suspicion for CRPS when examining patients after an upper extremity injury or surgical procedure when the patient is describing disproportionate pain severity or a failure of pain to improve as predicted. Orthopaedic surgeons should conduct a full neurologic examination of the extremity, documenting sensory deficits, motor weakness, edema, spontaneous pain, or allodynia. Orthopaedic evaluation should document range of motion of joints proximal and distal to the injury and joint deformity. Limbs should be compared for asymmetric skin color or texture and hair or nail patterns, and changes in sweat patterns (an abnormally dry limb) should be questioned.

One of the simplest diagnostic tests for CRPS is the application of ice to the affected limb. The arm affected by CRPS is frequently sensitive to cold, and cooling the affected limb produces an increase in burning pain.[1] The use of the ice test is a simple, quick, in-office diagnostic test that should be performed during a first evaluation.

Electromyography (EMG) and nerve conduction velocity studies (NCS) quantify the amplitude and the transmission speed of neuronal signaling. Neurologic conditions such as diabetic peripheral neuropathy, ulnar nerve entrapment, myasthenia gravis, and Lambert-Eaton syndrome may be differentiated from CRPS on the basis of EMG/NCS. Nerve injury after shoulder or elbow surgery, even if just neurapraxia, can initiate CRPS, and these individuals should be considered at risk after the nerve injury is appreciated by the clinician.

Radiographs are typically used to evaluate limb pain and may reveal osteopenia in chronic CRPS. CT or MRI of the cervical spine may reveal other causes of upper extremity neuropathic pain, including cervical stenosis or radiculopathy.[7] MRI of the painful limb may reveal brachial plexopathy, adhesive capsulitis, or other neurologic injury. MRI of the affected limb may demonstrate soft-tissue or marrow edema from acute CRPS, or the atrophy associated with chronic CRPS.

A variety of methods have been used to measure autonomic and sudomotor dysfunction in the patient with CRPS. Infrared thermography involves the use of infrared cameras to produce color mapping of the temperature of the skin of the affected limb for comparison with the unaffected limbs and normative control limbs.[15] A difference in temperature of 1°C between the affected and unaffected limbs is considered significant. A second quantitative test used in assessing sudomotor sweat production is the quantitative sudomotor axon reflex test. This test compares sweat produced following the topical application of a sweat-inducing agent, such as acetylcholine.

Table 3

Sensitivity, Specificity, Positive Predictive Value, and Negative Predictive Value of Selected Diagnostic Procedures Following Distal Radial Fracture

	Sensitivity (%)	Specificity (%)	Positive Predictive Value (%)	Negative Predictive Value (%)
2 weeks after trauma				
Thermography	45	50	17	79
8 weeks after trauma				
Thermography	50	67	26	85
Radiography – bilateral	36	94	58	86
MRI	43	78	31	85
Triple phase bone scan (TPBS)	19	96	58	86
16 weeks after trauma				
Thermography	29	89	38	84
MRI	13	98	60	83
TPBS	14	100	100	83

Reproduced with permission from Schurmann M, Zaspel J, Löhr P, et al: Imaging in early posttraumatic complex regional pain syndrome: A comparison of diagnostic methods *Clin J Pain* 2007;23(5):449-457.

Sympathetically mediated pain is suggestive of but not necessary for a diagnosis of CRPS. Intravenous regional blockade with α-adrenergic receptor antagonists or local anesthetic blockade of the stellate ganglion, lumbar sympathetic chain, or thoracic sympathetic chain that relieves pain is considered a positive test for sympathetically mediated pain.

Triple phase bone scan is a series of radiographic images taken in a timed sequence following the injection of a radionuclide tracer.[15] The series demonstrates arterial blood, regional blood pooling, and bone uptake of the tracer in sequential fashion. Increased periarticular uptake of the tracer is associated with the acute phase of CRPS. This finding occurs as a result of increased blood flow and bone turnover during the acute phase of the disease. This scan can supplement rather than establish the diagnosis of CRPS.

Despite the potential benefits of diagnostic testing, diagnostic tests should be considered supplemental information to establishing a definitive diagnosis.[15] Recent prospective analyses of 158 patients for the first 16 weeks following a radial fracture found that thermography, plain radiographs, MRI, and TPBS lacked sufficient sensitivity and specificity to provide appropriate positive predictive value or negative predictive value for diagnosis[15] (Table 3).

Treatment

CRPS is a complex disease likely consisting of several pathologic mechanisms; therefore, multidisciplinary treatment involves physical, pharmaceutical, psycho-logical, and possibly surgical/procedural intervention[2,3,13,16-40] (Table 4). All practitioners should strive to establish rapport with patients early because building a long-term strategy for intervention will be based on trust in the patient-physician relationship. Treatment is focused on the restoration of extremity function. Early initiation of CRPS therapy is a key component of therapy. Early range of motion of joints not affected directly by the surgery (for example, the elbow, the wrist, and fingers in the case of shoulder procedures) should be encouraged. Patients who delay treatment for longer than 6 months have a poorer long-term prognosis, and it is generally believed that early-stage CRPS symptoms may be reversible.[41]

Physical and Occupational Therapy

Physical medicine, including physical and occupational therapy, is a core component of rehabilitation designed to ensure positive functional outcomes. Pain can create a barrier of fear in the patient with CRPS who is attempting to use the affected limb (a condition known as kinesophobia). The goals of physical and occupational therapy are to overcome this fear of pain and return the patient to the best functional use of the limb. To accomplish this, physical therapists develop an incremental program designed to desensitize the affected limb and increase range of motion, flexibility, posture, and muscle strength.[3] Common modalities include contrast baths, alternating hot and cold water soaks, isometric exercises, and stress loading.[13] Occupational therapists encourage everyday use of the limb in activities of daily living. Specialized garments or wrappings may be enlisted to reduce edema and sensory overload

Table 4

Treatment Strategies for CRPS and Available Evidence

Treatment Class	Methods	Evidence
Pharmacologic (oral, intravenous, and transdermal)[16-27]	Varied	See Table 5.
Physical and occupational therapy[3,13]	Contrast baths Stress loading Isometric exercises Hot and cold water soaks Edema stockings	Physical therapy and occupational therapy provide improved quality of life and function to the affected limb.
Psychologic therapy[28]	Relaxation Biofeedback	Insufficient evidence of efficacy for recommendation, but expert opinion encourages treatment of non-organic contributions to chronic pain.
Sympathetic blockade and regional anesthesia[29-33]	Stellate ganglion block Interscalene block	Small retrospective studies demonstrate benefit when paired with physical therapy.
Intraveous regional blocks[34]	Guanethidine Lidocaine Clonidine Droperidol Reserpine	No evidence of benefit demonstrated when compared with placebo.
Neuromodulation[35,36]	Spinal cord stimulator Transcurtaneous electrical nerve stimulation (TENS)	Provides pain reduction and improved quality of life in carefully selected patients with refractory disease who have undergone successful trial stimulation. Insufficient evidence of efficacy for the use of TENS in CRPS.
Intrathecal medications[37-39]	Baclofen	Some evidence of efficacy for CRPS-related dystonia and improvement of function.
Surgical ablation[26,40]	Surgical sympathectomy Radiofrequency sympathectomy Chemical sympathectomy	Insufficient evidence of efficacy for pain relief in CRPS. Anecdotal reports of pain relief but with documented incidents of new neuropathic pain following sympathectomy.

of the affected limb. Mirror box therapy is a technique that has demonstrated promise in reducing neuropathic pain. All physical medicine should allow for incremental increases in stress and patient breaks as needed to prevent catastrophic pain.

Psychological Therapy

The emotional burden of unrelieved chronic pain despite best therapeutic interventions creates a need for psychological therapy in the CRPS population.[28] At minimum, a patient with a new CRPS diagnosis should have a discussion with a psychological care provider to outline what is known about the pathophysiology and the course of the disease process and explain the need for active self-management and participation in a care plan. Psychological therapy is designed to reconstruct dysfunctional cognitive patterns and behaviors about CRPS pain into thought patterns that facilitate rehabilitation (cognitive-behavioral therapy). Further goals include skills in relaxation and biofeedback to be implemented when pain exacerbations occur. Assessment and treatment of concomitant axis I disorders, such as major depression, generalized anxiety disorder, or post-traumatic stress disorder, are important because these disorders complicate the goal of return to function.

Pharmacologic Therapy

Pharmacotherapy for CRPS is used in situations where the severity of pain is limiting participation in functional rehabilitation. The evidence for the use of pharmacologic agents is limited by a lack of prospective randomized controlled trials (RCTs).[16] Clinicians are currently guided by available clinical trial data on CRPS and data from RCTs in neuropathic pain conditions to guide a sequential trial of medications.

Corticosteroids and NSAIDs have been used to treat the inflammation associated with CRPS. Randomized clinical trials have demonstrated that an oral regimen of corticosteroids has a clinically positive effect when taken during the acute phase following insult.[17] The only controlled trial of corticosteroids used in CRPS treatment trialed 30 mg oral prednisone daily (10 mg, three times daily) for up to 12 weeks.[17] In open trials, clinicians trialed initial doses of 40-60 mg oral prednisone with rapid taper over 4 weeks.[18] No studies have provided significant decrement of neuropathic pain from NSAIDs.[16]

Antioxidants have been used based on the perception that oxygen free radicals created by inflammation may be a key component of CRPS propagation. A trial of vitamin C following a wrist fracture was found to lessen the incidence of postfracture CRPS development.[19] Dimethyl sulfoxide (DMSO) and N-acetylcysteine have been demonstrated to provide significant pain relief in prospective trials when applied topically for 17 and 52 weeks.[20]

Anticonvulsant medications, such as gabapentin and pregabalin, have good evidence for effectiveness in neuropathic pain disorders, and this has prompted their use in CRPS. One prospective study of gabapentin in CRPS type 1 failed to provide significant benefit in pain reduction with this population, but sensory deficits improved.[21] A second study demonstrated a significant reduction of spontaneous and provoked pain in patients with CRPS with a mean disease duration of 2.7 months.[22]

Upregulation of inflammatory pathways sensitizes excitatory nociceptive pathways that use N-methyl-D-aspartic acid (NMDA) as a neurotransmitter.[23] Ketamine, a NMDA receptor blocker, is an attractive medication for the possible reversal of central sensitization and alteration of neural plasticity. Subanesthetic intravenous infusions, ketamine-induced comas, and topical ketamine ointments have proven effective at reducing numeric pain scores, although the duration of the effect remains uncertain.[23] Topical and subanesthetic ketamine currently have as good if not stronger support and are less intrusive.[23]

Adrenergic antagonists, such as phenoxybenzamine and phentolamine, have been used in the treatment of CRPS to block sympathetically mediated pain. Studies of oral use of adrenergic antagonists have shown promise in relieving pain based on retrospective review, but further prospective study is needed.[24] Intravenous regional phentolamine may be useful in the diagnosis of sympathetically mediated pain. Topically applied clonidine, an α-2 adrenergic agonist, has been demonstrated to relieve localized hyperalgesia in patients with sympathetically mediated pain.[25]

During CRPS progression, localized bone resorption occurs in the affected limb and is observable through TPBS (described previously). Bisphosphonates and calcitonin have their clinical effect through the inhibition of the osteoclast bone resorption.[26] The use of bisphosphonate therapy has proven to be superior to placebo in pilot studies for the relief of subjective pain. Calcitonin has generated conflicting data with regard to its ability to reduce average pain scores.[26]

Opioid therapy for the treatment of CRPS may be needed and is a topic of debate among physicians. Although potentially useful in the acute phases of tissue injury, the long-term use of opioids for either peripheral or central neuropathic pain is less efficacious or at minimum is required in a large dosage.[27] At higher doses, adverse effects such as tolerance, addiction, immunosuppression, or endocrine dysfunction, may become more prevalent[17,18-21,26,27,37-39,42-48] (**Table 5**).

Sympathetic Blockade and Regional Anesthesia

The presence of sympathetically mediated pain has led to blockade of the primary sympathetic ganglion (the stellate ganglion), which provides sympathetic innervation for the upper extremity for both diagnosis and treatment of sympathetically mediated pain. Current prospective studies support the use of stellate ganglion blocks with local anesthetic or botulinum toxin to reduce pain on a visual analog scale and increase participation in rehabilitation, especially when blocks are performed early (< 16 weeks) following the onset of symptoms. Several questions remain concerning stellate ganglion blocks, including duration of pain relief and whether intermittent single-dose or continuous infusion administration are more effective.[29] Sympathetic blocks for diagnostic purposes have created large numbers of false-positive and false-negative results.[30] Although no positive predictors of sympathetic blockade are demonstrable, allodynia and hypoesthesia may be negative predictors for blockade success.[31]

Regional blockade of the brachial plexus has been demonstrated to provide pain relief and allow the medication-refractory patients with CRPS to participate in shoulder rehabilitation by blockade of somatic Aδ and C afferent nerve fibers.[32] The technique has been effective when used in continuous infusion settings lasting approximately 1 week. Although this technique has been used when sympathetic blockade fails, a recent pilot study comparing continuous stellate ganglion block to a continuous infraclavicular brachial plexus block demonstrated significant reduction in background neuropathic pain and pain exacerbations in both groups.[33]

Intravenous regional sympathetic blockade using the Bier block technique with various medications has been studied. Guanethidine, ketanserin, bretylium, atropine, droperidol, and reserpine have all been used as agents, but none have proven to have significant clinical benefit in decreasing pain over a significant length of time following meta-analysis.[34]

Surgical and Procedural Intervention

Neuromodulation through implantation of spinal cord stimulators in the epidural space has been effective in decreasing the burning pain associated with chronic or cold CRPS (up to 70% success) and has been considered a positive treatment by patients undergoing this therapy at long-term follow-up appointments.[35] Undesirable outcomes may occur in up to 34% of patients with permanent stimulator implantations.[36] Most commonly, the revision is due to electrode repositioning rather than other complications, including equipment failure or infection.[36] Long-term follow-up has demonstrated diminishing relief at approximately 5 years.[35]

8. Miscellaneous Shoulder and Elbow Topics

Table 5

Pharmacologic Treatments of CRPS

Pharmaceutical	Mechanism of Action	Dosage Range Studied	Evidence for Effectiveness
Anti-inflammatory Medications			
Corticosteroids[17,18]	Reduction in transcription of inflammatory cytokines	Oral prednisone 10 mg PO TID Methylprednisolone 32 mg PO QID x 14 days with 14-day taper	Improvement on CRPS rating scale Improvement on CRPS rating scale at 6 months following
Parecoxib[43]	Inhibition of cyclooxygenase 2 Reduction of prostaglandin formation	5 mg IV in combination with 1 mg/kg lidocaine/30 mg clonidine IV regional block once per week x 3 weeks	Reduction in daily rescue medication and VAS pain score compared with control
Free-Radical Scavengers			
Vitamin C[19]	Free-radical scavenging	500 mg PO daily x 50 days	Reduction in incidence of CRPS.
DMSO[20]	Free-radical scavenging	50% DMSO cream topically to the affected area 5 times daily x 52 weeks	Greater improvement than treatment with N-acetylcysteine in patients with warm CRPS Lower total treatment costs when compared to N-acetylcysteine Improvement in range of motion and vasomotor instability
N-acetylcysteine[20]	Free-radical scavenging	600 mg PO TID x 52 weeks	Greater improvement than treatment with DMSO in patients with cold CRPS
Pain Medications			
Gabapentin[21]	Blocks calcium channels in neurons	600 mg PO daily x 2 days, then 600 mg BID x 2 days, then 600 mg TID x 17 days	No difference in treatment group versus placebo group after 3-week course in pain scores but improvement versus placebo in global perceived pain
Opioids[27,44]	Activation of opioid receptors	90 mg PO daily sustained-release oral morphine Approximately 8.9 mg PO levorphanol	No significant data demonstrating a reduction of pain High-dose opioid therapy demonstrating a significant global reduction in neuropathic pain
Ketamine[45-47]	Antagonism of NMDA receptor	10% ketamine cream transdermally Intravenous ketamine–sub-anesthetic 30 mg/h x 4.2 days Intravenous ketamine coma 7mg/kg/h + 0.15-0.4 mg/kg/h IV midazolam x 5 days	Reduction in mechanoallodynia and hyperalgesia Significant pain relief at up to 11 weeks follow-upComplete remission of symptoms in 50% of patients at 10 years post-treatment
Antispasmotic Agents			
Baclofen[37-39]	Inhibition of GABA-β receptors	Intrathecal baclofen up to 450 µg/d	Reduced dystonia and pain and increased quality of life

IV = intravenous; PO = by mouth; ROM = range of motion; VAS = visual analog scale; BID = twice daily; TID = three times daily; QID = four times daily.; DMSO = dimethyl sulfoxide; NMDA = N-methyl-D-aspartic acid.

Table 5

Pharmacologic Treatments of CRPS (continued)

Pharmaceutical	Mechanism of Action	Dosage Range Studied	Evidence for Effectiveness
Osteoclast Inhibitors			
Bisphosphonates[26,48]	Inhibition of osteoclasts/bone remodeling	Ibandronate 6 mg IV daily × 3 days Alendronate 40 mg PO daily × 8 weeks 7.5 mg IV daily × 3 days Pamidronate 60 mg IV once Clodronate 300 mg IV daily × 10 days	Improvement in average and worst pain ratings Improvement in spontaneous pain, pressure tolerance, and joint mobility Significant reduction in spontaneous pain, tenderness, and swelling along with improvement in motion of involved extremity at 2 and 4 weeks Improvement in pain score, global assessment of disease severity score, and physical function Improvement in pain score and clinical global assessment at 40 days
Calcitonin[26]	Release of β-endorphin Inhibition of osteoclasts/bone remodeling	200 IU intranasal daily 100 IU intramuscular 100 IU TID × 3 weeks 100 IU BID × 4 weeks 100 IU TID × 3 weeks	No statistically significant benefits Significant reduction in pain scores and ROM Significant improvement in pain and ROM, significant improvement in upper extremity CRPS patients, no difference in level of edema No difference in improvement in pain scores, stiffness, swelling, and vascular instability Improvement in pain scores at 1 week

IV = intravenous, PO = by mouth, ROM = range of motion, VAS = Visual Analog Scale, BID = twice daily, TID = three times daily, QID = four times daily

Intrathecal medications have been suggested as a viable treatment to the central nervous system component of CRPS pain. Baclofen, a gamma-aminobutyric acid-β (GABA) agonist, has been shown to reduce the dystonia and pain associated with chronic CRPS in prospective trials.[37-39]

Surgical sympathectomy involves the surgical severance of the sympathetic trunks or the stellate ganglion using chemical, radiofrequency, or open surgical techniques to reduce sympathetically mediated pain. These techniques are extensions of the temporary sympathetic block techniques described previously and may be used to prolong pain relief. A retrospective review of radiofrequency stellate ganglion sympathectomies identified 40% of patients with a greater than 50% reduction in pain at follow-up of approximately 1 year.[40] Despite positive findings, controversy over the long-term efficacy of surgical sympathectomy remains.[26]

Prevention

Primary prevention and prevention of secondary reactivation of CRPS in the postoperative/posttrauma patient are areas of ongoing study. One study documented administration of vitamin C for 50 days following wrist fracture and demonstrated a substantial decrement in the incidence of CRPS observed (7% vitamin C versus 22% control).[19] Surgery on a limb previously affected by CRPS has been shown to cause exacerbation or relapse of symptoms. Perioperative calcitonin, stellate ganglion blockade, intravenous blockade, and multimodal anesthesia have all shown initial promise in reducing relapse.[16] Current recommendations support postponement of surgery until CRPS signs are minimal.[16]

Summary

CRPS is a disease with a complex pathophysiologic basis. The orthopaedic surgeon should be aware of its implications preceding or following surgery of the shoulder and elbow to recognize and properly treat this debilitating illness. Through early recognition and intervention, orthopaedic surgeons can provide their patients with the best multimodal team-based approach and thereby the best chance for positive long-term outcomes.

Annotated References

1. Marinus J, Moseley GL, Birklein F, et al: Clinical features and pathophysiology of complex regional pain syndrome. *Lancet Neurol* 2011;10(7):637-648.

   This review article summarizes the basic and clinical research into the epidemiology and pathophysiological mechanisms of CRPS. The authors emphasize multiple mechanisms to explain the complex clinical presentation of CRPS.

2. Goebel A: Complex regional pain syndrome in adults. *Rheumatology (Oxford)* 2011;50(10):1739-1750.

   This review article summarizes the epidemiology, pathophysiology, clinical presentation, and treatment of CRPS. It provides additional information on the economics of CRPS, initiatives for treatment, and opportunities for future research.

3. Merskey H, Bogduk N: *Classification of Chronic Pain. Descriptions of Chronic Pain Syndromes and Definitions of Pain Terms*, ed 2. Seattle, WA, IASP Press, 1994.

4. Harden RN, Bruehl S, Perez RS, et al: Validation of proposed diagnostic criteria (the "Budapest Criteria") for complex regional pain syndrome. *Pain* 2010; 150(2):268-274.

   This study applied the older Orlando criteria and the more recent Budapest criteria to a cohort of 113 CRPS and 47 non-CRPS neuropathic pain patients to compare specificity and sensitivity. The Orlando criteria had a sensitivity of 1.0 and a specificity of 0.41 while the Budapest criteria had a sensitivity of 0.99 and a specificity of 0.68.

5. Sethna NF, Meier PM, Zurakowski D, Berde CB: Cutaneous sensory abnormalities in children and adolescents with complex regional pain syndromes. *Pain* 2007;131(1-2):153-161.

   This study examined 42 patients with CRPS for standardized neurologic examination and quantitative sensory testing. Twenty-one patients exhibited allodynia in response to cold, and 26 patients exhibited allodynia in response to dynamic and static mechanical stimulation.

6. Beerthuizen A, Stronks DL, Van't Spijker A, et al: Demographic and medical parameters in the development of complex regional pain syndrome type 1 (CRPS1): Prospective study on 596 patients with a fracture. *Pain* 2012;153(6):1187-1192.

   This study reviewed 596 patients with a single fracture. There were 7% in whom CRPS was later diagnosed. An analysis of these patients demonstrated they more often had intra-articular fracture, fracture-dislocations, rheumatoid arthritis, or musculoskeletal comorbidities.

7. Sharma A, Agarwal S, Broatch J, Raja SN: A web-based cross-sectional epidemiological survey of complex regional pain syndrome. *Reg Anesth Pain Med* 2009;34(2):110-115.

   This study was a survey of 75 questions posted on the Reflex Sympathetic Dystrophy Syndrome Association of America website. There were 888 responses that were accepted for analysis of demographic and symptomatic review.

8. Bruehl S: An update on the pathophysiology of complex regional pain syndrome. *Anesthesiology* 2010; 113(3):713-725.

   This review article summarizes the basic and clinical research into the epidemiology and pathophysiologic mechanisms of CRPS. The authors emphasize multiple mechanisms to explain the complex clinical presentation of CRPS.

9. Cappello ZJ, Kasdan ML, Louis DS: Meta-analysis of imaging techniques for the diagnosis of complex regional pain syndrome type I. *J Hand Surg Am* 2012; 37(2):288-296.

   The results of MRI, plain films, and TPBS were examined by meta-analysis. TPBS was found to have greatest sensitivity and higher negative predictive value.

10. Kohr D, Tschernatsch M, Schmitz K, et al: Autoantibodies in complex regional pain syndrome bind to a differentiation-dependent neuronal surface autoantigen. *Pain* 2009;143(3):246-251.

    Serum of the patients with CRPS and control patients were screened for the presence of autoantibodies. Thirteen of 30 patients with CRPS demonstrated specific surface binding to autonomic neurons.

11. Goebel A, Baranowski A, Maurer K, Ghiai A, McCabe C, Ambler G: Intravenous immunoglobulin treatment of the complex regional pain syndrome: A randomized trial. *Ann Intern Med* 2010;152(3):152-158.

    A randomized, double-blind, placebo-controlled crossover trial of 12 patients is presented. The average pain intensity score was 1.55 units lower on the visual analog scale following intravenous immunoglobulin treatment.

12. Bonica JJ: *The Management of Pain, With Special Emphasis on the Use of Analgesic Block in Diagnosis, Prognosis and Therapy.* Philadelphia, PA, Lee and Feibeger; 1953.

13. Patterson RW, Li Z, Smith BP, Smith TL, Koman LA: Complex regional pain syndrome of the upper extremity. *J Hand Surg Am* 2011;36(9):1553-1562.

    This review article summarizes the epidemiology, pathophysiology, clinical presentation, and treatment of CRPS. It emphasizes the viewpoint of the hand surgeon in describing potential functional limitations to the hand and therapeutic surgical interventions.

14. Drummond PD: Sensory disturbances in complex regional pain syndrome: Clinical observations, autonomic interactions, and possible mechanisms. *Pain Med* 2010;11(8):1257-1266.

    This review article describes the sensory disturbances found in CRPS and potential pathophysiologic mechanisms. A special focus of the article involves the clinical presentation of sensory disturbances.

15. Schürmann M, Zaspel J, Löhr P, et al: Imaging in early posttraumatic complex regional pain syndrome: A comparison of diagnostic methods. *Clin J Pain* 2007; 23(5):449-457.

    One hundred fifty-eight consecutive patients were followed for 16 weeks following trauma with bilateral thermography, plain films, MRI, and TPBS. All studies were demonstrated to have a low positive predictive value (17% to 60%) and moderate negative predictive value (79 to 86%).

16. Perez RS, Zollinger PE, Dijkstra PU, et al; CRPS I task force: Evidence based guidelines for complex regional pain syndrome type 1. *BMC Neurol* 2010;10:20.

    This article presents a multidisciplinary task force's review of the literature to provide evidence-based recommendations for care. It classifies the evidence found in the literature according to objective standards.

17. Christensen K, Jensen EM, Noer I: The reflex dystrophy syndrome response to treatment with systemic corticosteroids. *Acta Chir Scand* 1982;148(8):653-655.

18. Kozin F, Ryan LM, Carerra GF, Soin JS, Wortmann RL: The reflex sympathetic dystrophy syndrome (RSDS): III. Scintigraphic studies, further evidence for the therapeutic efficacy of systemic corticosteroids, and proposed diagnostic criteria. *Am J Med* 1981; 70(1):23-30.

19. Zollinger PE, Tuinebreijer WE, Kreis RW, Breederveld RS: Effect of vitamin C on frequency of reflex sympathetic dystrophy in wrist fractures: A randomised trial. *Lancet* 1999;354(9195):2025-2028.

20. Perez RS, Zuurmond WW, Bezemer PD, et al: The treatment of complex regional pain syndrome type I with free radical scavengers: A randomized controlled study. *Pain* 2003;102(3):297-307.

21. van de Vusse AC, Stomp-van den Berg SG, Kessels AH, Weber WE: Randomised controlled trial of gabapentin in complex regional pain syndrome type 1 [IS-RCTN84121379]. *BMC Neurol* 2004;4:13-22.

22. Tan AK, Duman I, Taşkaynatan MA, Hazneci B, Kalyon TA: The effect of gabapentin in earlier stage of reflex sympathetic dystrophy. *Clin Rheumatol* 2007; 26(4):561-565.

    Twenty-two patients with CRPS were enrolled to take an average of 1,145 mg of gabapentin daily. At 6 weeks, there was statistically significant improvement in spontaneous and provoked pain.

23. Schwartzman RJ, Alexander GM, Grothusen JR: The use of ketamine in complex regional pain syndrome: Possible mechanisms. *Expert Rev Neurother* 2011; 11(5):719-734.

    This review article describes the clinical experience using differing protocols of ketamine dosing for the treatment of chronic pain in CRPS. It provides possible explanations of the physiological mechanism of the relief provided by ketamine to patients with CRPS.

24. Muizelaar JP, Kleyer M, Hertogs IA, DeLange DC: Complex regional pain syndrome (reflex sympathetic dystrophy and causalgia): Management with the calcium channel blocker nifedipine and/or the alpha-sympathetic blocker phenoxybenzamine in 59 patients. *Clin Neurol Neurosurg* 1997;99(1):26-30.

25. Davis KD, Treede RD, Raja SN, Meyer RA, Campbell JN: Topical application of clonidine relieves hyperalgesia in patients with sympathetically maintained pain. *Pain* 1991;47(3):309-317.

26. Sharma A, Williams K, Raja SN: Advances in treatment of complex regional pain syndrome: Recent insights on a perplexing disease. *Curr Opin Anaesthesiol* 2006;19(5):566-572.

27. Rowbotham MC, Twilling L, Davies PS, Reisner L, Taylor K, Mohr D: Oral opioid therapy for chronic peripheral and central neuropathic pain. *N Engl J Med* 2003;348(13):1223-1232.

28. Bruehl S, Chung OY: Psychological and behavioral aspects of complex regional pain syndrome management. *Clin J Pain* 2006;22(5):430-437.

29. Yucel I, Demiraran Y, Ozturan K, Degirmenci E: Complex regional pain syndrome type I: Efficacy of stellate ganglion blockade. *J Orthop Traumatol* 2009;10(4): 179-183.

    The authors discuss a prospective study of 22 patients following administration of three stellate ganglion blocks separated by 1-week intervals. A significant decrease in VAS pain scores and increased range of motion were documented.

30. Krumova EK, Gussone C, Regeniter S, Westermann A, Zenz M, Maier C: Are sympathetic blocks useful for diagnostic purposes? *Reg Anesth Pain Med* 2011; 36(6):560-567.

    The authors discuss a pilot study of 19 patients with chronic neuropathic pain where sympathetic block was used in diagnosis. Of the 12 with sufficient temperature change following sympathetic block, 3 were diagnosed with CRPS.

31. van Eijs F, Geurts J, van Kleef M, et al: Predictors of pain relieving response to sympathetic blockade in complex regional pain syndrome type 1. *Anesthesiology* 2012;116(1):113-121.

    The authors discuss a prospective study of 49 patients with CRPS for less than 1 year duration before stellate ganglion block. Allodynia and hypoesthesia were negative predictors for treatment success.

32. Detaille V, Busnel F, Ravary H, Jacquot A, Katz D, Allano G: Use of continuous interscalene brachial plexus block and rehabilitation to treat complex regional pain

8. Miscellaneous Shoulder and Elbow Topics

syndrome of the shoulder. *Ann Phys Rehabil Med* 2010;53(6-7):406-416.

The authors present a prospective trial of a 1-week continuous interscalene brachial plexus on 59 patients with treatment-refractory CRPS type 1.

33. Toshniwal G, Sunder R, Thomas R, Dureja GP: Management of complex regional pain syndrome type I in upper extremity-evaluation of continuous stellate ganglion block and continuous infraclavicular brachial plexus block: A pilot study. *Pain Med* 2012;13(1): 96-106.

The authors present a randomized prospective trial of 1 week of either continuous stellate ganglion block or continuous infraclavicular block. At 4-week follow-up, both groups demonstrated improvement in edema and range of motion.

34. Kingery WS: A critical review of controlled clinical trials for peripheral neuropathic pain and complex regional pain syndromes. *Pain* 1997;73(2):123-139.

35. Kemler MA, de Vet HC, Barendse GA, van den Wildenberg FA, van Kleef M: Effect of spinal cord stimulation for chronic complex regional pain syndrome Type I: Five-year final follow-up of patients in a randomized controlled trial. *J Neurosurg* 2008;108(2): 292-298.

A randomized controlled trial involving 36 patients with implanted spinal cord stimulators with 5-year follow-up is discussed. Despite diminishing efficacy at 5 years, 19 patients indicated a willingness to repeat treatment of the same result.

36. Turner JA, Loeser JD, Deyo RA, Sanders SB: Spinal cord stimulation for patients with failed back surgery syndrome or complex regional pain syndrome: A systematic review of effectiveness and complications. *Pain* 2004;108(1-2):137-147.

37. van Rijn MA, Munts AG, Marinus J, et al: Intrathecal baclofen for dystonia of complex regional pain syndrome. *Pain* 2009;143(1-2):41-47.

A single-blind, placebo-run-in, dose-escalation study enrolling 36 patients is presented. Intention-to-treat analysis revealed a substantial improvement in dystonia, pain, disability, and quality of life.

38. van der Plas AA, van Rijn MA, Marinus J, Putter H, van Hilten JJ: Efficacy of intrathecal baclofen on different pain qualities in complex regional pain syndrome. *Anesth Analg* 2013;116(1):211-215.

A prospective study examining the effects of intrathecal baclofen infusion pumps in 6 women. Three of six women had complete resolution of hand dystonia, 4 women had reduced painful muscle spasms, and 2 had marked reduction in myoclonic jerks.

39. van Hilten BJ, van de Beek WJ, Hoff JI, Voormolen JH, Delhaas EM: Intrathecal baclofen for the treatment of dystonia in patients with reflex sympathetic dystrophy. *N Engl J Med* 2000;343(9):625-630.

The authors present a prospective study of 42 patients with intrathecal baclofen pumps and one or more limbs affected by CRPS for 1 year. Of these patients, more than 60% had a reduction in pain score and global dystonia severity.

40. Forouzanfar T, van Kleef M, Weber WE: Radiofrequency lesions of the stellate ganglion in chronic pain syndromes: Retrospective analysis of clinical efficacy in 86 patients. *Clin J Pain* 2000;16(2):164-168.

A retrospective review of 86 patients treated with radiofrequency ablation of the stellate ganglion is discussed. There were 40.7% of patients who experienced > 50% reduction of pain, 54.7% who noted no effect, and 4.7% who experienced worsening of pain.

41. Varitimidis SE, Papatheodorou LK, Dailiana ZH, Poultsides L, Malizos KN: Complex regional pain syndrome type I as a consequence of trauma or surgery to upper extremity: Management with intravenous regional anaesthesia, using lidocaine and methylprednisolone. *J Hand Surg Eur Vol* 2011;36(9):771-777.

One hundred sixty-eight patients with CRPS-1 of the upper extremity were treated with intravenous lidocaine and methylprednisolone. The reported results were 88% of patients with minimal or no pain, and a complete absence of pain in 92% of patients at 5-year follow-up.

42. Braus DF, Krauss JK, Strobel J: The shoulder-hand syndrome after stroke: A prospective clinical trial. *Ann Neurol* 1994;36(5):728-733.

43. Frade LC, Lauretti GR, Lima IC, Pereira NL: The antinociceptive effect of local or systemic parecoxib combined with lidocaine/clonidine intravenous regional analgesia for complex regional pain syndrome type I in the arm. *Anesth Analg* 2005;101(3):807-811.

Thirty patients with CRPS were randomized into either intravenous regional analgesia with lidocaine/clonidine or intravenous regional analgesia with oral parecoxib. Patients on intravenous regional analgesia/parecoxib consumed less rescue medication.

44. Harke H, Gretenkort P, Ladleif HU, Rahman S, Harke O: The response of neuropathic pain and pain in complex regional pain syndrome I to carbamazepine and sustained-release morphine in patients pretreated with spinal cord stimulation: A double-blinded randomized study. *Anesth Analg* 2001;92(2):488-495.

45. Finch PM, Knudsen L, Drummond PD: Reduction of allodynia in patients with complex regional pain syndrome: A double-blind placebo-controlled trial of topical ketamine. *Pain* 2009;146(1-2):18-25.

Twenty patients received 10% topical ketamine on two occasions separated by 1 week. Ketamine was found to inhibit allodynia to light brushing and hyperalgesia punctate stimuli.

46. Sigtermans M, Dahan A, Mooren R, et al: S(+)-ketamine effect on experimental pain and cardiac output: A population pharmacokinetic-pharmacodynamic

modeling study in healthy volunteers. *Anesthesiology* 2009;111(4):892-903.

Sixty CRPS type 1 patients were administered sub-anesthetic ketamine for 4.2 days. Significant pain relief was demonstrated against placebo at up to 11 weeks follow-up.

47. Kiefer RT, Rohr P, Ploppa A, et al: Efficacy of ketamine in anesthetic dosage for the treatment of refractory complex regional pain syndrome: An open-label phase II study. *Pain Med* 2008;9(8):1173-1201.

A prospective study of 20 American Society of Anesthesiologists I-III patients using anesthetic dosage ketamine is presented. Significant pain relief was observed at 1, 3, and 6 months following treatment.

48. Breuer B, Pappagallo M, Ongseng F, Chen CI, Goldfarb R: An open-label pilot trial of ibandronate for complex regional pain syndrome. *Clin J Pain* 2008; 24(8):685-689.

An open-label three day trial of ibandronate is presented. A significant improvement in average and worst pain ratings was observed.

Chapter 51

Frozen Shoulder

Douglas Scott, MD   Andrew Green, MD

Introduction

The term frozen shoulder is commonly used by medical professionals and the lay public to refer to conditions of shoulder pain and stiffness. The term periarthritis was first used in 1872 to refer to shoulders that had both limited active and passive shoulder motion.[1] Codman introduced the term frozen shoulder in 1934 to refer to a constellation of symptoms, and not necessarily a specific disease entity.[2] Many conditions result in shoulder pain and limited motion. The term adhesive capsulitis was popularized by Neviaser and was based on surgical and autopsy findings of cases of frozen shoulder.[3] The differences between the various etiologies of frozen shoulder have been highlighted, and idiopathic adhesive capsulitis is defined as "a condition of uncertain etiology characterized by substantial reduction of both active and passive shoulder motion that occurs in the absence of a known intrinsic shoulder disorder."[4] Despite the prevalence of the condition and the extensive research on the subject, general practitioners and even orthopaedic surgeons are often confused about the diagnosis and treatment, and the underlying pathophysiology has not been identified. Identifiable causes and underlying conditions of shoulder pain and stiffness must be considered before treating a patient for frozen shoulder. Nonsurgical management provides the mainstay of treatment, with surgical intervention showing improved outcomes in refractory cases.

Dr. Green or an immediate family member has received royalties from Tornier; is a member of a speakers' bureau or has made paid presentations on behalf of DJ Orthopaedics; serves as a paid consultant to or is an employee of Tornier; has stock or stock options held in IlluminOss Medical and Pfizer; has received research or institutional support from DJ Orthopaedics and Synthes; has received nonincome support (such as equipment or services), commercially derived honoraria, or other non–research-related funding (such as paid travel) from Arthrex and Smith & Nephew; and serves as a board member, owner, officer, or committee member of the American Academy of Orthopaedic Surgeons and the American Shoulder and Elbow Surgeons. Neither Dr. Scott nor any immediate family member has received anything of value from or has stock or stock options held in a commercial company or institution related directly or indirectly to the subject of this chapter.

Epidemiology

The incidence of frozen shoulder is difficult to estimate because of the lack of strict diagnostic criteria, insidious onset, and confusion with other shoulder disorders. Most studies on the subject report an incidence of 2% to 5% in the general population, although these figures may be inflated.[5] A study of female patients noted a prevalence of approximately 10% to 12%.[6] Although recurrence in the same shoulder is rare, the condition develops in the contralateral shoulder in up to 20% of patients. Approximately 60% to 80% of patients are female and most patients are between 40 and 60 years of age.[7] The nondominant arm is involved in about 60% of cases, with left shoulder involvement in approximately 60% of cases.

Etiology and Pathophysiology

Many primary disease processes in the shoulder can ultimately result in painful loss of motion. Rotator cuff disease, primary glenohumeral arthritis, posttraumatic (soft-tissue injuries and fractures) contractures, postoperative contractures, inflammatory joint and systemic diseases, and sequelae of neurologic conditions are among the many acquired causes of shoulder stiffness. In contrast, idiopathic adhesive capsulitis occurs in the absence of major trauma, previous surgery, or other identifiable intrinsic or extrinsic pathology. The process that triggers idiopathic adhesive capsulitis has been difficult for researchers to define, leaving the true underlying etiology unknown.

Analyses of tissue obtained during arthroscopy show the presence of fibroblasts, proliferating fibroblasts, and myofibroblasts.[8] Some consider the process to be histologically similar to that seen in Dupuytren disease, and the two diseases are thought to share a common biochemical pathway that leads to contracture and fibrosis. The cell types identified have been shown to deposit a dense type III collagen matrix in the shoulder capsule. In a 2007 study, an infiltration of chronic inflammatory cells, including mast cells, T cells, B cells, and macrophages, was observed, as well as increased vascularity from angiogenesis suggested by staining with CD34 antibodies.[8] The authors of this study found positive results for S100 staining consistent with the presence of nerve cells. In contrast to other studies, they found little evidence of a myofibroblast population.

The findings of studies investigating the pathophysiology of frozen shoulder are likely affected by the clinical stage of the patients from whom tissue is obtained. Because these studies generally involve tissue samples that are obtained from patients in the later stages of disease who have not responded to early nonsurgical treatment, the findings may not directly relate to or identify the actual underlying etiology of the pathophysiologic process of adhesive capsulitis. Associating the findings of basic science studies with the natural history of idiopathic adhesive capsulitis suggests the following summary: a triggering event or process leads to the initial freezing phase, which involves a painful, inflammatory process that gradually progresses to a chronic, contracted frozen phase.

Cadaver studies have investigated the pathoanatomy implicated in frozen shoulder. A simulation of localized capsular contractures was done by performing selective capsular plication and the resultant restrictions defined in passive range of glenohumeral motion.[9] The authors found that closure of the rotator interval, including the coracohumeral and superior glenohumeral ligaments, can restrict external rotation, particularly with the shoulder in an adducted position. The authors also found that tightening of the anteroinferior aspect of the capsule, including the anteroinferior glenohumeral ligament complex, restricts motion with increasing abduction of the arm. These findings are consistent with the intraoperative findings of patients with adhesive capsulitis and shoulder contracture and provide a rationale for the selective release of specific anatomic structures during surgical treatment.

A genetic heritability has been defined in a classic twin model comparing the prevalence of frozen shoulder among female monozygotic and dizygotic twins to assess the relative genetic and environmental contributions to frozen shoulder.[6] A greater concordance was found among monozygotic than dizygotic twins, suggesting a genetic factor in the etiology of frozen shoulder.

Clinical Evaluation

Frozen shoulder is a clinical diagnosis based on patient history and the physical examination findings. Typically, the patient recalls either a trivial traumatic event or none at all. Initially, pain is the primary complaint, with subsequent gradual loss of shoulder motion. Pain at night is a common complaint. The shoulder is often comfortable during rest or when sedentary, with pain associated with reaching to the extreme of any motion. Most patients eventually exhibit a marked loss of active and passive shoulder motion relative to the contralateral shoulder, particularity with the shoulder in 90° of abduction. Often, a loss of external rotation of 50% or greater is present. Manual stretching of the shoulder capsule at the extremes of motion reveals a firm end point and causes pain. Similarly, the capsular contracture results in global limitation of translation of the shoulder.

A thorough evaluation includes standard plain radiographs (true anterior, axillary lateral, and outlet views) of the shoulder to exclude signs of other causes of shoulder pain and stiffness such as glenohumeral arthritis, acromioclavicular arthritis, and calcific tendinitis. Advanced imaging studies are not typically warranted in the early evaluation of frozen shoulder. Nevertheless, the imaging literature includes descriptions of typical findings seen on MRI and magnetic resonance arthrography.[10,11] Thickening of the coracohumeral ligament, thickening and gadolinium enhancement of the capsule in the axillary recess, decreased overall capsular volume, and subcoracoid fat obliteration in the rotator cuff interval are seen in patients with frozen shoulder. Specifically, the thickness of the coracohumeral ligament has also been shown to correlate with the clinical loss of internal and external rotation.[10] Overuse of advanced imaging should be avoided because the diagnosis usually can be readily determined based on the history, physical examination, and plain radiography. Unnecessary advanced imaging has potentially deleterious clinical ramifications. A recent study reported a high false-positive rate of rotator cuff tears, especially partial-thickness tears, being interpreted from MRIs obtained in patients undergoing capsular release for frozen shoulder.[12]

Recent literature suggests that coracoid and acromioclavicular pain are associated with frozen shoulder. Coracoid tenderness was found to be a highly sensitive and specific finding after evaluating 830 consecutive patients, and the authors hypothesized that it resulted from the nearby coracohumeral ligament and the rotator cuff interval tissues that are involved.[13] The authors of a 2011 study hypothesized that compensatory pathologic scapulothoracic and acromioclavicular motion resulting from limitation of glenohumeral motion is the cause of acromioclavicular joint pain.[14] After treatment of the frozen shoulder and restoration of glenohumeral motion, the associated acromioclavicular pain resolved in most patients.

Clinically, the natural history of frozen shoulder is divided into three phases (**Table 1**). The frequent delay in presentation, its insidious nature, and its variable course and severity make such definitions somewhat inexact. However, although it can sometimes be difficult to pinpoint a patient's exact position on a clinical spectrum, the phases can be a helpful, general guide to expectations of the anticipated clinical course.

Associated Conditions

The importance of obtaining a thorough patient history is highlighted by the medical conditions found to be associated with primary frozen shoulder. Diabetes mellitus is the most notable and extensively studied medical comorbidity related to frozen shoulder. Various reports have shown the incidence of frozen shoulder to be as high as 10% to 36% in individuals with diabetes, and the disease is thought to have profound implications for the natural progression and outcomes of nonsurgical as well as surgical outcomes.[15,16] It is commonly believed that these patients are at greater risk for failure of nonsurgical treatment and recurrence after surgical treatment or manipulation, often resulting in a protracted course. Nevertheless, the authors of a 2012 study reported no significant difference in improvement after manipulation under anesthesia of patients with diabetes compared with nondiabetic patients, even though the patients with diabetes had a greater recurrence rate and more frequently required repeat manipulation.[17]

Although a recent study illustrated the coincidence between diabetes and frozen shoulder, the researchers failed to show a direct correlation between glycemic control, evaluated by patients' hemoglobin A1c level, and the actual prevalence of frozen shoulder.[18] However, the prevalence of frozen shoulder in individuals with type I diabetes was found to be nearly twice that of patients with type II diabetes, and the duration of diabetes correlated with the development of frozen shoulder.

Other medical conditions associated with frozen shoulder include thyroid disease, stroke, peripheral neuropathy, brachial plexus lesions, and cardiopulmonary disease. Approximately 10% of patients are reported to have hypothyroidism.[7] In addition, frozen shoulder can develop in patients with neurologic conditions and ipsilateral upper extremity trauma not involving the shoulder. There is a tendency for the development of stiffness in patients with proximal humeral fractures and associated axillary nerve or brachial plexus injuries.

Nonsurgical Treatment

Nonsurgical management is the mainstay of treatment of frozen shoulder, and much evidence has been reported to support its role. Many studies, including randomized clinical trials, have investigated a variety of nonsurgical treatments of frozen shoulder—both compared with placebo and other treatments. Most have focused on the treatment of idiopathic adhesive capsulitis, which is by far the most common problem.

Corticosteroids

Multiple studies support the role of corticosteroids in the treatment of frozen shoulder. A randomized clinical trial reported that intra-articular corticosteroid injection, combined with physiotherapy consisting of modalities and exercises, resulted in significantly greater improvement of Shoulder Pain and Disability Index

Table 1	
Phases of Frozen Shoulder	
Phase	**Characteristics**
Freezing	Severe, acute pain and stiffness
Frozen	Decreased pain but residual stiffness
Thawing	Protracted course of resolution of symptoms

scores and range of motion at 6-week follow-up compared with injection alone, saline injection with physiotherapy, and saline injection alone.[19] After 3 months, patients in the corticosteroid groups had greater improvement in the Shoulder Pain and Disability Index score. Nevertheless, at 12-month follow-up, no difference was reported between the groups. A more recent prospective study compared a course of oral glucocorticoids with a series of three fluoroscopically guided intra-articular corticosteroid injections.[20] Patients in both groups were also supplemented with a physical therapy program. Patients in the cohort with intra-articular injections showed superior Constant-Murley scores at all times up to the 1-year follow-up. Patients in the injection group also had consistently better range of motion at up to 8 weeks and variable differences beyond that. Visual analog scale scores for pain and function were no different, and the scores for patient satisfaction were better for those in the injection group. In a 2012 study, the use of corticosteroid injections was specifically investigated in a randomized clinical trial of 45 patients with diabetes mellitus who were recognized to have a poor prognosis.[21] Although improvements in the patients in the injection group were reported for pain at 4 weeks and function at 12 weeks after injection, no significant differences were reported at 24-week follow-up.

A 2010 systematic review of randomized trials that compared corticosteroid injections with physiotherapeutic interventions concluded that there was evidence of a medium effect in the short term that decreased to a small effect over time in favor of corticosteroid injections.[22] Another study analyzed the benefit of multiple corticosteroid injections.[23] Of four studies rated high in quality, three showed that multiple injections were beneficial with reduced pain, improved function, and increased shoulder motion. There was no evidence that more than three injections were beneficial.

Several studies have highlighted the point that in clinical practice, the accuracy of intra-articular injections in the glenohumeral joint can be unpredictable. One study determined that the accuracy of intra-articular glenohumeral injection from an anterior approach without radiographic guidance was only 26%.[24] Another study reported accuracies of glenohumeral injection of 65% for an anterior approach, 46% for a posterior approach, and 46% for a superior approach.[25] A third

8. Miscellaneous Shoulder and Elbow Topics

study compared the short-term efficacy of ultrasonographically guided glenohumeral and subacromial corticosteroid injections and found that although greater improvement in pain after glenohumeral injection was reported at 3-week follow-up, there was no difference at 6- and 12-week follow-ups.[26] In addition, there was no significant difference between the effect of subacromial and glenohumeral injections with respect to the Constant-Murley score or range of motion at any time point. A fourth study compared the efficacy of corticosteroid injection for treatment of intra-articular pathology, including adhesive capsulitis, and found that the short-term response was independent of the location of the injection (intra-articular versus extra-articular).[27] They did not evaluate longer-term outcomes.

Evidence appears to support the use of intra-articular glenohumeral corticosteroid injections for the short-term management of symptoms. However, if the effect is indeed dependent on injection accuracy, then imaging-assisted guidance should be used to ensure the location of the injection. Nonetheless, corticosteroid injections do not appear to cure the condition or have any additional long-term benefit over the natural history of idiopathic adhesive capsulitis.

Physiotherapy

In addition to traditional physical therapy exercises, interest has increased in alternative treatments and the use of modalities in the management of frozen shoulder. A report in 2011 summarized the findings of Cochrane reviews as recent as 2008, as well as other more recent randomized clinical trials of nonsurgical and surgical treatments.[28] The authors found moderate evidence for mobilization techniques in short-term and long-term follow-up. The authors also found that when compared with placebo, laser treatment and both electroacupuncture and interferential acupuncture had a significantly positive short-term effect on pain, function, and range of motion.

The authors of a 2009 study reported on the effect of dynasplint treatment of adhesive capsulitis.[29] The relatively small study demonstrated that the outcomes were comparable to those of corticosteroid injection and standardized physical therapy. Data were insufficient to conclude that there was no difference.

Physical therapy programs focusing on a home-based program of shoulder stretching exercises are well accepted as treatment of frozen shoulder. Pendulum circumduction and passive shoulder stretching exercises, including forward elevation, external rotation, horizontal adduction, and internal rotation, were performed by patients in a prospective study in which 90% the of patients were satisfied with their therapy at long-term follow-up.[7] Diabetes and male sex were factors associated with a poor outcome. Although no studies exist that compare stretching exercises with benign neglect, it seems logical that there are only minimal risks and disadvantages to attempting exercises in all cases.

A retrospective study reported on 89 shoulders that underwent treatment with a supervised stretching program as well as corticosteroid injection in 47 of the shoulders.[30] Twenty-five shoulders underwent manipulation under anesthesia combined with arthroscopic capsular release in 23. Stepwise logistic regression analysis demonstrated that younger age and greater initial internal rotation deficits most significantly predicted the need for surgical treatment. In addition, the presence of diabetes mellitus did not predict the need for surgery in their cohort.

Viscosupplementation

Hyaluron is a major component of hyaline articular cartilage and synovial fluid and is FDA approved for the treatment of knee arthritis. Utilization for the treatment of shoulder disorders has been less extensive. Basic science investigations suggest a possible basis for using viscosupplementation to treat adhesive capsulitis. The effect of hyaluron on fibroblasts harvested from the glenohumeral capsule of patients with idiopathic and secondary adhesive capsulitis was studied; a significant and dose-dependent inhibitory effect was found on cell proliferation, messenger RNA expression of adhesion-related procollagen, and cytokines.[31]

The authors of a 2012 study assessed intra-articular hyaluronic acid injection in a prospective randomized clinical trial of 70 patients with adhesive capsulitis.[32] After 3 months, patients in both groups had improvement in pain, disability, and quality of life, and both active and passive range of motion improved linearly. However, the investigators did not identify a significant effect of hyaluronic acid injection.

A systematic review of four Level I and three Level IV published studies investigating the use of hyaluronic acid found that at short-term follow-up (mean, 9 weeks), shoulder range of motion, Constant scores, and pain were significantly improved.[33] The authors also reported that isolated intra-articular hyaluronate injection had equivalent clinical outcomes and range of motion compared with intra-articular corticosteroid injection.

Arthrodilatation

The goal of arthrodilatation, or arthrographic distention, is to inject fluid under pressure into the contracted shoulder to disrupt the capsule. Several studies support the use of this treatment. A recent Cochrane review concluded that some evidence, although not strong, supports that arthrographic distension with saline and steroids provides short-term benefits in pain, range of motion, and function in adhesive capsulitis. However, it is uncertain whether this method is better than alternative interventions.[34]

Suprascapular Nerve Block

In addition to motor innervation of the supraspinatus and infraspinatus muscles, the suprascapular nerve provides sensory innervation to the glenohumeral joint capsule.

Recent areas of investigation include suprascapular nerve blockade to provide pain relief and allow for a more aggressive and tolerable stretching program.[35] Although limited current data show short-term pain relief, future research is needed to qualify long-term benefits in pain, disability, and patient satisfaction.

Surgical Treatment

Manipulation Under Anesthesia

At least 95% of patients with idiopathic adhesive capsulitis can be successfully treated nonsurgically. Most authors recommend at least 6 months of nonsurgical treatment before considering surgical intervention. Multiple studies have illustrated the benefits of manual manipulation under anesthesia for the treatment of frozen shoulder that is refractory to nonsurgical treatment. Most literature for manipulation report short-term and midterm benefits. A study from the Mayo Clinic also reported that improvements in pain relief, range of motion, and satisfaction were maintained after manipulation under anesthesia for patients followed for an average of 15 years.[36] Patients with frozen shoulder and diabetes do not respond as readily or successfully to nonsurgical treatment as those without diabetes. A retrospective case-control study compared the outcome of manipulation under anesthesia during the frozen stage in patients with diabetes with that of a control group of patients with frozen shoulder.[17] The authors included patients with primary and secondary frozen shoulder and found that 50% of the patients with diabetes and primary frozen shoulder required additional manipulation, compared with 14% of the patients without diabetes who had primary frozen shoulder. Despite the high rate of secondary manipulation in the diabetic cohort, 85% of those patients were satisfied with the final outcome, and, overall, the end-point range of motion and outcome scores were not statistically different from their counterparts without diabetes.

When electing to proceed with manipulation under anesthesia after a trial of nonsurgical treatment has failed, the clinician should understand the importance of delaying such intervention until the frozen phase. Manipulation during the inflammatory, or freezing phase, can exacerbate patients' symptoms and ultimately can be counterproductive. Most manipulations currently are performed under a supplemental regional nerve block to ensure muscle paralysis and provide postprocedural analgesia. The scapula should be stabilized to isolate true glenohumeral motion, and gradual stretching maneuvers are performed. Care must be taken to prevent iatrogenic injury, including glenohumeral dislocation, rotator cuff tear, and fracture, especially in older patients and patients with osteopenia. A sequence of traction and flexion, cross-body adduction, external rotation, and abduction with external and internal rotation is safe and reliable to see measurable differences between premanipulation and postmanipulation passive range-of-motion measurements. The importance of maintaining a diligent stretching program after manipulation cannot be overemphasized. Plain radiographs should be obtained after manipulation under anesthesia to rule out bony injury. In a prospective study, 30 patients who underwent manipulation under anesthesia for primary frozen shoulder were examined with arthroscopy.[37] Manipulation successfully restored passive range of shoulder motion in all cases. The capsule was seen to be ruptured superiorly in 11 patients, anteriorly down to the infraglenoid pole in 24 patients, and 16 patients had posterior capsular tearing. In 18 patients, no additional joint damage was found after manipulation. Iatrogenic lesions included four patients with superior labrum anterior to posterior lesions, three fresh partial tears of the subscapularis tendon, four anterior labral detachments (one with a small osteochondral defect), and two tears of the middle glenohumeral ligament. The authors confirmed the general understanding that although manipulation under anesthesia can effectively restore joint motion, there is a risk of iatrogenic injury, and a careful technique should be used.

Capsular Release

Arthroscopic capsular release is now an established means of providing consistent clinical improvement in the treatment of recalcitrant frozen shoulder. The procedure is increasingly replacing closed manipulation alone because it provides a diagnostic inspection of the joint, a more precise capsulotomy, and minimizes the risk of iatrogenic injury. Arthroscopy in the presence of a severe contracture can be technically difficult. Entering into the glenohumeral joint is more difficult because of the thickened and contracted capsule as well as the limited joint volume. The reduced joint volume and synovitis can make standard diagnostic arthroscopy difficult. The procedure usually begins with a synovectomy of the rotator cuff interval to facilitate visualization of the biceps, the subscapularis tendon, and the anterior capsule. Capsular release can be performed with arthroscopic punches or cautery devices. Confirmation of complete release is achieved via manipulation, during which the tearing of any remaining contracted capsule can be palpated. The authors of a 2012 study described a modification of the usual technique of capsular release that began in the subacromial space rather than the glenohumeral joint.[38] The literature is conflicted as to whether release of the posterior capsule and the posteroinferior humeral ligament should be routinely performed, effecting a "360-degree release."[39,40]

Arthroscopy has eliminated the need for open capsular releases in the treatment of idiopathic adhesive capsulitis. Nevertheless, open release still has a role in some cases of secondary shoulder stiffness related to an extrinsic cause, such as an overly tight repair for instability or a proximal humeral fracture. An open approach is required if lengthening of the subscapularis tendon is needed to achieve external rotation. In addition, extensive subdeltoid scarring is frequently not amenable to arthroscopic capsular release. The disadvantages of an open approach include the need to protect the repaired or lengthened subscapularis tendon, which is counterproductive to the aggressive postoperative therapy needed to maintain range of motion.

The results of a prospective study of arthroscopic capsular release in 73 patients who were followed for 1 year postoperatively were reported.[41] Pain diminished at at an average of 2.24 weeks, range of motion was within 10% of the contralateral shoulder at an average of 5.5 weeks, and patients were well enough to be discharged at an average of 8.9 weeks. Nevertheless, 37% of the patients received a steroid injection for postoperative management, and 11% of the patients eventually developed recurrence of symptoms, the latter finding being consistent with multiple other studies. The results of a retrospective study of the long-term outcomes of arthroscopic capsular release indicated significant improvement in pain, function, and range of motion. The range of motion was equivalent to that of the contralateral unaffected shoulder.[42]

Although shoulder stiffness and loss of motion are relatively common sequelae of traumatic shoulder injuries and shoulder surgery, surgical releases are not frequently required or performed. One study reported that 3 of 345 patients who underwent rotator cuff repair were treated with arthroscopic capsular release.[43] Another study reported on 21 patients, 14 with proximal humeral fractures, who underwent arthroscopic capsular and subacromial release for posttraumatic frozen shoulder.[44] Substantial improvements were seen in shoulder motion and outcome. Patients with isolated soft-tissue injury without fracture had better results. In a 2010 study, the effect of etiology of frozen shoulder on the outcome of arthroscopic capsular release was evaluated, and no differences were found between idiopathic and posttraumatic stiffness.[5] In contrast, patients with postoperative contracture had significantly worse outcomes.

Evidence Review

Many studies have used systematic literature review and meta-analysis to analyze the evidence for treatment of adhesive capsulitis. More of these studies have been reported in the past few years than original investigations of the various treatment modalities. These reviews present the various previously reported studies in an organized fashion, assess the quality of the studies, and summarize the findings.

The authors of a 2011 study reviewed the effectiveness of nonsurgical and surgical management of frozen shoulder and included the findings from 5 Cochrane reviews and 18 randomized controlled trials.[28] Short-term pain, range of motion, and overall outcome scores in patients with frozen shoulder were found to be improved by corticosteroid injections, laser therapy, mobilization techniques, arthrographic distension, and suprascapular nerve block. Physiotherapy was found to have longer-term effects. The authors concluded that

the assessment of the effectiveness of the many available treatment options is limited by a paucity of high-level evidence studies as well as inconsistencies in the methodology of reported studies.

The evidence for the nonsurgical treatment of adhesive capsulitis appears to demonstrate that pharmacologic intervention with oral and injected corticosteroids has a greater early effect on pain and function. Nevertheless, no study has demonstrated a difference in the effect of any treatment at long-term follow-up. The evidence for the use of surgical treatment is limited to case series and demonstrates significant improvements in shoulder motion, reduction in pain, and improvement of function without substantial risk of complications.

Summary

Idiopathic adhesive capsulitis is characterized by shoulder pain and limitation of glenohumeral motion. Although the natural history of the condition is well known, the etiology and pathophysiology are not understood. Most patients recover with nonsurgical treatment but should be advised that a protracted course is typical. The efficacies of the various nonsurgical treatments are not clear. Surgical intervention, including arthroscopic capsular release, provides reliable clinical improvement for refractory cases. The true natural history of the disease and corresponding basic science findings are still debated, making it difficult to predict which patients will be unresponsive to nonsurgical treatment. Researchers hope that studying the characteristics and sequelae of frozen shoulder will lead to a better understanding of its etiology.

Annotated References

1. Duplay S: De la péri-arthrite scapula-humérale et des raideurs de l'épaule qui en sont al consequence. *Arch gen méd* 1872;20:513-542.

2. Codman EA: *The Shoulder: Rupture of the Supraspinatus Tendon and Other Lesions in or About the Subacromial Bursa.* Boston, MA, Thomas Todd and Co, 1934, pp 216-224.

3. Neviaser JS: Adhesive capsulitis of the shoulder: A study of pathological findings in periarthritis of the shoulder. *J Bone Joint Surg Am* 1945;27-A(2): 211-222.

4. Zuckerman JD, Cuomo F: Frozen shoulder, in Matsen FA III, Fu FH, Hawkins RJ, eds: *The Shoulder: A Balance of Mobility and Stability.* Rosemont, IL, American Academy of Orthopaedic Surgeons. 1993, pp 253-267.

5. Elhassan B, Ozbaydar M, Massimini D, Higgins L, Warner JJ: Arthroscopic capsular release for refractory

shoulder stiffness: A critical analysis of effectiveness in specific etiologies. *J Shoulder Elbow Surg* 2010;19(4): 580-587.

This retrospective case series found that arthroscopic capsular release is an effective treatment of refractory shoulder stiffness and showed that patients with idiopathic and posttraumatic shoulder stiffness have better outcomes than patients with postsurgical stiffness. Level of evidence: IV.

6. Hakim AJ, Cherkas LF, Spector TD, MacGregor AJ: Genetic associations between frozen shoulder and tennis elbow: A female twin study. *Rheumatology (Oxford)* 2003;42(6):739-742.

7. Griggs SM, Ahn A, Green A: Idiopathic adhesive capsulitis: A prospective functional outcome study of nonoperative treatment. *J Bone Joint Surg Am* 2000; 82-A(10):1398-1407.

8. Hand GC, Athanasou NA, Matthews T, Carr AJ: The pathology of frozen shoulder. *J Bone Joint Surg Br* 2007;89(7):928-932.

Biopsies obtained from tissues of the rotator cuff interval during arthroscopic release were analyzed and found to include fibroblasts, proliferating fibroblasts, and chronic inflammatory cells, including mast cells, T cells, B cells, and macrophages. In addition, the authors found increased vascularity from angiogenesis and positive results from S100 staining consistent with the presence of nerve cells.

9. Gerber C, Werner CM, Macy JC, Jacob HA, Nyffeler RW: Effect of selective capsulorrhaphy on the passive range of motion of the glenohumeral joint. *J Bone Joint Surg Am* 2003;85-A(1):48-55.

10. Lee SY, Park J, Song SW: Correlation of MR arthrographic findings and range of shoulder motions in patients with frozen shoulder. *AJR Am J Roentgenol* 2012;198(1):173-179.

The thickness of the coracohumeral ligament and the capsule in axillary recess seen with MR arthrography were significantly greater in patients with frozen shoulder than in patients in a control group. Additionally, coracohumeral ligament thickness correlated with clinical range-of-motion limitations. Level of evidence: IV.

11. Song KD, Kwon JW, Yoon YC, Choi SH: Indirect MR arthrographic findings of adhesive capsulitis. *AJR Am J Roentgenol* 2011;197(6):W1105-9.

An abundance of enhancing tissue in the rotator cuff interval and thickening and enhancement of the axillary recess were found to be signs suggesting adhesive capsulitis on indirect magnetic resonance arthrography. Level of evidence: IV.

12. Loeffler BJ, Brown SL, D'Alessandro DF, Fleischli JE, Connor PM: Incidence of false positive rotator cuff pathology in MRIs of patients with adhesive capsulitis. *Orthopedics* 2011;34(5):362.

MRI interpretation of the rotator cuff was compared with the rotator cuff status intraoperatively for patients who underwent capsular release for frozen shoulder. MRI interpretations predicted a 57.9% incidence of rotator cuff pathology compared with a true incidence of 13.2%. Level of evidence: IV.

13. Carbone S, Gumina S, Vestri AR, Postacchini R: Coracoid pain test: A new clinical sign of shoulder adhesive capsulitis. *Int Orthop* 2010;34(3):385-388.

Patients with adhesive capsulitis were clinically evaluated to establish whether pain elicited by pressure on the coracoid may be considered a sign of this condition. With respect to patients in a control group, the sensitivity and the specificity were 0.99 and 0.98, respectively. Level of evidence: IV.

14. Anakwenze OA, Hsu JE, Kim JS, Abboud JA: Acromioclavicular joint pain in patients with adhesive capsulitis: A prospective outcome study. *Orthopedics* 2011;34(9):e556-e560.

In adhesive capsulitis, there is not only compensatory scapulothoracic motion but also acromioclavicular motion. The authors hypothesized this would result in transient symptoms at the acromioclavicular joint, which abated as the adhesive capsulitis resolved and glenohumeral motion improved. Level of evidence: III.

15. Bridgman JF: Periarthritis of the shoulder and diabetes mellitus. *Ann Rheum Dis* 1972;31(1):69-71.

16. Walker-Bone K, Palmer KT, Reading I, Coggon D, Cooper C: Prevalence and impact of musculoskeletal disorders of the upper limb in the general population. *Arthritis Rheum* 2004;51(4):642-651.

17. Jenkins EF, Thomas WJ, Corcoran JP, et al: The outcome of manipulation under general anesthesia for the management of frozen shoulder in patients with diabetes mellitus. *J Shoulder Elbow Surg* 2012;21(11): 1492-1498.

This retrospective case-control study showed improvement, including no difference between patients with and without diabetes treated with manipulation for frozen shoulder. However, a repeat procedure was required in 36% of the patients with diabetes compared with 15% of the control patients. Level of evidence: III.

18. Yian EH, Contreras R, Sodl JF: Effects of glycemic control on prevalence of diabetic frozen shoulder. *J Bone Joint Surg Am* 2012;94(10):919-923.

This retrospective analysis with statistical review showed no association between the hemoglobin A1c level and the prevalence of frozen shoulder in the studied diabetic population. Level of evidence: II.

19. Carette S, Moffet H, Tardif J, et al: Intraarticular corticosteroids, supervised physiotherapy, or a combination of the two in the treatment of adhesive capsulitis of the shoulder: A placebo-controlled trial. *Arthritis Rheum* 2003;48(3):829-838.

20. Lorbach O, Anagnostakos K, Scherf C, Seil R, Kohn D, Pape D: Nonoperative management of adhesive capsulitis of the shoulder: Oral cortisone application versus intra-articular cortisone injections. *J Shoulder Elbow Surg* 2010;19(2):172-179.

Intra-articular injections of glucocorticoids showed superior results in shoulder outcome scores, range of motion, and patient satisfaction compared with a short course of oral corticosteroids for the treatment of adhesive capsulitis in this randomized controlled trial. Level of evidence: I.

21. Roh YH, Yi SR, Noh JH, et al: Intra-articular corticosteroid injection in diabetic patients with adhesive capsulitis: A randomized controlled trial. *Knee Surg Sports Traumatol Arthrosc* 2012;20(10):1947-1952.

This randomized clinical trial concluded that a corticosteroid injection decreased pain and functional outcome scores in the early treatment of adhesive capsulitis in patients with diabetes compared with a control group of patients. Level of evidence: II.

22. Blanchard V, Barr S, Cerisola FL: The effectiveness of corticosteroid injections compared with physiotherapeutic interventions for adhesive capsulitis: A systematic review. *Physiotherapy* 2010;96(2):95-107.

Six studies were included in this systematic review, which suggests that corticosteroid injections have greater effect compared with physical therapy interventions in short-term treatments of adhesive capsulitis. This finding decreased over time, however, with only a small effect in favor of injections at longer time points studied.

23. Shah N, Lewis M: Shoulder adhesive capsulitis: Systematic review of randomised trials using multiple corticosteroid injections. *Br J Gen Pract* 2007;57(541):662-667.

This systematic review of randomized clinical trials concluded that multiple additional corticosteroid injections provided pain reduction, improved function, and increased range of shoulder motion in the treatment of adhesive capsulitis for up to 16 weeks after the initial injection. Level of evidence: I.

24. Sethi PM, Kingston S, ElAttrache N: Accuracy of anterior intra-articular injection of the glenohumeral joint. *Arthroscopy* 2005;21(1):77-80.

25. Tobola A, Cook C, Cassas KJ, et al : Accuracy of glenohumeral joint injections: Comparing approach and experience of provider. *J Shoulder Elbow Surg* 2011;20(7):1147-1154.

The accuracies of posterior, supraclavicular, and anterior approaches used for glenohumeral injections were compared in a case-controlled study. The anterior approach was the most accurate, but neither provider experience nor confidence was associated with success. Level of evidence: III.

26. Oh JH, Oh CH, Choi JA, Kim SH, Kim JH, Yoon JP: Comparison of glenohumeral and subacromial steroid injection in primary frozen shoulder: A prospective, randomized short-term comparison study. *J Shoulder Elbow Surg* 2011;20(7):1034-1040.

This randomized controlled trial showed that although patients with frozen shoulder treated with intra-articular glenohumeral injection showed lower pain visual analog scale scores at 3 weeks, no difference was seen at 6 and 12 weeks between these patients and those being administered subacromial injections. Level of evidence: I.

27. Hegedus EJ, Zavala J, Kissenberth M, et al: Positive outcomes with intra-articular glenohumeral injections are independent of accuracy. *J Shoulder Elbow Surg* 2010;19(6):795-801.

This prospective cohort demonstrated that despite documented inaccuracy of glenohumeral injections, short-term follow-up showed improvement in pain and Disabilities of the Arm, Shoulder and Hand scores in patients with various shoulder pathologies. Level of evidence: II.

28. Favejee MM, Huisstede BM, Koes BW: Frozen shoulder: The effectiveness of conservative and surgical interventions—systematic review. *Br J Sports Med* 2011;45(1):49-56.

This review found strong evidence for the short-term effectiveness of steroid injections and laser therapy in frozen shoulder. Moderate evidence was found for steroid injections in midterm follow-up, mobilization techniques in the long term, and the effectiveness of arthrographic distension. Level of evidence: III.

29. Gaspar PD, Willis FB: Adhesive capsulitis and dynamic splinting: A controlled, cohort study. *BMC Musculoskel Disord* 2009;10:111.

This controlled cohort study showed the efficacy of dynamic splinting as an effective home therapy adjunct to physical therapy. This additional end-range stretching combined with standardized physical therapy was considered to be responsible for the greatest change in external rotation. Level of evidence: II.

30. Rill BK, Fleckenstein CM, Levy MS, Nagesh V, Hasan SS: Predictors of outcome after nonoperative and operative treatment of adhesive capsulitis. *Am J Sports Med* 2011;39(3):567-574.

This cohort study concurrently evaluated patients with adhesive capsulitis who were treated surgically and nonsurgically. The two cohorts showed similar improvement in final outcomes scores, illustrating that although most patients improved with nonsurgical treatment, refractory cases responded well to surgical intervention. Level of evidence: III.

31. Nago M, Mitsui Y, Gotoh M, et al: Hyaluronan modulates cell proliferation and mRNA expression of adhesion-related procollagens and cytokines in glenohumeral synovial/capsular fibroblasts in adhesive capsulitis. *J Orthop Res* 2010;28(6):726-731.

This in vitro study examined the effects of hyaluronan on glenohumeral synovial and capsular fibroblasts from patients with frozen shoulder. Hyaluronan modulated cell proliferation and the expression of adhesion-related procollagens and cytokines, suggesting it may prevent the progression of adhesion formation.

32. Hsieh LF, Hsu WC, Lin YJ, Chang H-L, Chen C-C, Huang V: Addition of intra-articular hyaluronate injection to physical therapy program produces no extra benefits in patients with adhesive capsulitis of the shoulder: A randomized controlled trial. *Arch Phys Med Rehabil* 2012;93(6):957-964.

    This randomized clinical trial found that hyaluronate injections did not significantly change active or passive range of motion, pain, disability, or quality of life outcomes for adhesive capsulitis patients treated with physical therapy. Level of evidence: I.

33. Harris JD, Griesser MJ, Copelan A, Jones GL: Treatment of adhesive capsulitis with intra-articular hyaluronate: A systematic review. *Int J Shoulder Surg* 2011;5(2):31-37.

    This systematic review concluded that short-term clinical outcomes for patients with adhesive capsulitis treated with hyaluronate injections are better than control groups but equivalent to intra-articular corticosteroid injection. Level of evidence: IV.

34. Buchbinder R, Green S, Youd JM, Johnston RV, Cumpston M: Arthrographic distension for adhesive capsulitis (frozen shoulder). *Cochrane Database Syst Rev* 2008;1:CD007005.

35. Dahan TH, Fortin L, Pelletier M, Petit M, Vadeboncoeur R, Suissa S: Double blind randomized clinical trial examining the efficacy of bupivacaine suprascapular nerve blocks in frozen shoulder. *J Rheumatol* 2000;27(6):1464-1469.

36. Farrell CM, Sperling JW, Cofield RH: Manipulation for frozen shoulder: Long-term results. *J Shoulder Elbow Surg* 2005;14(5):480-484.

37. Loew M, Heichel TO, Lehner B: Intraarticular lesions in primary frozen shoulder after manipulation under general anesthesia. *J Shoulder Elbow Surg* 2005;14(1):16-21.

38. Lafosse L, Boyle S, Kordasiewicz B, Guttierez-Arramberi M, Fritsch B, Meller R: Arthroscopic arthrolysis for recalcitrant frozen shoulder: A lateral approach. *Arthroscopy* 2012;28(7):916-923.

    The authors describe a technique for arthroscopic capsular release that begins in the subacromial space followed by intra-articular entry to perform a 360° capsular release. Level of evidence: IV.

39. Chen J, Chen S, Li Y, Hua Y, Li H: Is the extended release of the inferior glenohumeral ligament necessary for frozen shoulder? *Arthroscopy* 2010;26(4):529-535.

    This randomized controlled study compared arthroscopic capsular with and without posterior capsular release. The addition of posterior release did not improve patient function or range of motion at 6 months. However, extended release did improve range of motion more rapidly in the short term. Level of evidence: I.

40. Jerosch J: 360 degrees arthroscopic capsular release in patients with adhesive capsulitis of the glenohumeral joint—indication, surgical technique, results. *Knee Surg Sports Traumatol Arthrosc* 2001;9(3):178-186.

41. Watson L, Dalziel R, Story I: Frozen shoulder: A 12-month clinical outcome trial. *J Shoulder Elbow Surg* 2000;9(1):16-22.

42. Le Lievre HM, Murrell GA: Long-term outcomes after arthroscopic capsular release for idiopathic adhesive capsulitis. *J Bone Joint Surg Am* 2012;94(13):1208-1216.

    Patients with idiopathic adhesive capsulitis treated with an arthroscopic capsular release had significant improvements in shoulder range of motion, pain frequency and severity, and function. These improvements were maintained and/or enhanced at 7-year follow-up. Level of evidence: IV.

43. Namdari S, Green A: Range of motion limitation after rotator cuff repair. *J Shoulder Elbow Surg* 2010;19(2):290-296.

    This case-control study followed patients after rotator cuff repair and found that preoperative limited range of motion, diabetes, and worker's compensation claims were all associated with postoperative loss of motion. Level of evidence: III.

44. Levy O, Webb M, Even T, Venkateswaran B, Funk L, Copeland SA: Arthroscopic capsular release for posttraumatic shoulder stiffness. *J Shoulder Elbow Surg* 2008;17(3):410-414.

    This study reports the results of arthroscopic capsular release in 21 patients who presented with posttraumatic stiff shoulders resistant to nonsurgical therapy. Improvements were observed in range of motion and patient satisfaction. Level of evidence: IV.

8: Miscellaneous Shoulder and Elbow Topics

Chapter 52

Anesthesia and Analgesia for Shoulder and Elbow Surgery

E. David Bravos, MD

Introduction

Patients who require shoulder and elbow surgery can present several challenges for the perioperative team. Given the wide variety of patient ages, comorbidities and the concern for neurologic evaluation, careful planning between the surgeon and the anesthesiologist is essential. One of the most significant concerns is managing postoperative pain. In addition to the traditional use of opioid and nonopioid analgesic agents, peripheral nerve blockade (PNB) of the brachial plexus is an excellent choice for postoperative analgesia because most surgeries can be covered with a single approach to the brachial plexus. The use of PNB has increased over the past several years, secondary to the advancement of ultrasound guidance to perform it. When used as an analgesic agent, PNB can provide superior analgesia, decrease opioid-related adverse effects, and lead to greater patient satisfaction compared to intravenous opioids alone.[1,2] For certain surgeries of the elbow, PNB may serve as the intraoperative anesthetic, but for surgeries of the shoulder, it is commonly used as a postoperative analgesic and combined with a general anesthetic or heavy sedation. In cases where postoperative pain is expected to be moderate or severe, continuous peripheral nerve blockade (CPNB) can be used. More recently, CPNB is being used in the outpatient setting and for inpatients where it can be used to facilitate early physical therapy and manipulate frozen joints.

General Considerations for Preoperative Management

Given the wide range of patients who present for shoulder and elbow surgery, from the young healthy athlete to the elderly patient with significant comorbidities, careful preoperative evaluation must occur. In addition to the well-known contraindications to PNB, certain coexisting diseases may preclude their use. Patients known to have significant pulmonary disease may not

be the best candidates for a brachial plexus block that can cause phrenic nerve paralysis. An interscalene block has been shown to cause blockade of the phrenic nerve 100% of the time and a supraclavicular block up to 80% of the time.[3-5] This can result in up to a 27% reduction in pulmonary mechanics, such as forced vital capacity and forced expiratory volume in the first second.[6] Additionally, patients with a contralateral diaphragmatic paresis would not be candidates for a brachial plexus block affecting the phrenic nerve. Other contraindications would include a recurrent laryngeal nerve palsy because of the potential blockade of the recurrent laryngeal nerve that can occur with interscalene or supraclavicular nerve blocks.

Patients with a preexisting nerve injury must be evaluated to determine if they are appropriate candidates for PNB. Careful communication between the anesthesiologist and the surgeon must take place if there is concern for potential nerve injury during the procedure or the need for immediate or ongoing postoperative neurologic examination.

Other preoperative considerations include whether patients will receive medications for preventive analgesia. Celecoxib, gabapentin, and acetaminophen have all been used.

General Considerations for Intraoperative Management

Intraoperative anesthetic management for shoulder and elbow surgery may be achieved with general anesthesia, regional anesthesia, or a combination of both. There are several factors that dictate whether a patient can have a regional technique alone as the intraoperative anesthetic or whether this must be combined with a general anesthetic requiring airway management with an endotracheal tube, a laryngeal mask airway, or heavy sedation. Understanding not only the anatomy and innervation of the upper extremity, but also the clinical distribution of the different blocks of the brachial plexus is essential.

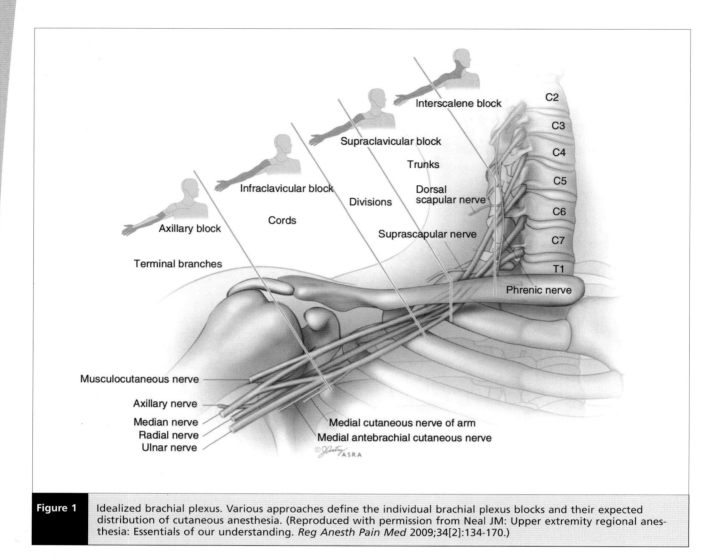

Figure 1 Idealized brachial plexus. Various approaches define the individual brachial plexus blocks and their expected distribution of cutaneous anesthesia. (Reproduced with permission from Neal JM: Upper extremity regional anesthesia: Essentials of our understanding. *Reg Anesth Pain Med* 2009;34[2]:134-170.)

Appropriate Selection of PNB

There are four major blocks of the brachial plexus, which are named according to the anatomic location of where these blocks are performed (**Figure 1**). Given that these blocks are located at different levels of the brachial plexus, they subsequently have different clinical distributions of anesthesia and analgesia of the upper extremity. Surgeries of the shoulder and the proximal humerus are best served by an interscalene block. This is because of blockade of the C3 and C4 nerve roots, which are not part of the brachial plexus, but rather help form the superficial cervical plexus. This, in turn, gives rise to the supraclavicular nerves, which provide sensation to the cape of the shoulder. These nerves are typically blocked by spread of a larger volume of local anesthetic when this block is performed at the level of C6. This will cover incisions that extend into the cape of the shoulder. A single-shot supraclavicular block has been used for surgery of the shoulder if enough volume of local anesthetic is given; however, it may not be the best block choice if CPNB is used because this type of block typically is run at a lower vol-

ume of local anesthetic postoperatively. Infraclavicular and axillary blocks are not appropriate for surgery of the shoulder or the proximal humerus. For surgeries of the distal humerus and the elbow, an infraclavicular block or a supraclavicular block would appropriately cover this area. An interscalene block may not be the best choice because of ulnar sparing caused by missing the C8 and T1 nerve roots. However, a low interscalene approach with a large enough local anesthetic volume may provide coverage. Axillary blocks are best suited for procedures below the elbow.

Other Local Anesthetic Techniques

In addition to PNB of the brachial plexus, other local anesthetic techniques may include subacromial (bursal) or intra-articular infiltration of local anesthetic, as well as suprascapular with or without axillary (circumflex) nerve blocks. In a recent systematic review, different local anesthetic techniques were studied to determine their efficacy and potential for opioid sparing.[7]

It is unclear if there is significant analgesic efficacy of subacromial/intra-articular infiltration. More importantly, concern for iatrogenic chondrolysis of continuous infusion of local anesthetic has caused this modality to fall out of favor. Suprascapular nerve blockade may provide clinically significant analgesia compared with placebo. The addition of an axillary nerve block may improve the analgesic efficacy of this technique. Although less efficacious compared to an interscalene nerve block, it may be used in patients with significant pulmonary disease in whom avoidance of phrenic nerve paralysis is preferred. A continuous interscalene block with a basal rate infusion, along with patient-controlled boluses, is the most efficacious of all local anesthetic techniques for surgery of the shoulder.

Intraoperative Anesthetic Technique

For surgery of the shoulder, innervaton of cutaneous and bony structures may not be covered by a brachial plexus block alone. Therefore, PNB is commonly performed for postoperative analgesia and combined with general anesthesia or heavy sedation. This is usually determined by the position in which the patient is placed (beach chair versus lateral) and the ability of the anesthesiologist to have access to the patients' airway.

For surgery of the elbow, a brachial plexus block may provide complete anesthesia of all the areas of surgical stimulation and may be used as the sole anesthetic technique, depending on the patient's position. This approach may allow the patient to be awake or minimally sedated if desired. For patients placed in a lateral or a prone position, more definitive airway management may be necessary.

Positioning

Position for surgery of the shoulder typically takes place in the beach chair or the lateral decubitus position. Regardless of technique, care in positioning and an understanding of the potential complications is paramount. Some advantages of the beach chair position include ease of setup, decreased risk of nerve injury from traction, and ease of conversion to an open procedure.[8] Patients in the beach chair position are supine, with the head of the bed raised from 20° to 30° and up to 80° depending on the specific procedure. The table can also be positioned such that the hips are in a flexed position from 45°-60° and the knees flexed to 30°. Alternatively, the legs may be kept in a more straight position at the knees to decrease venous pooling and increase venous return and cardiac output. Patients in the beach chair position may experience sudden and profound hypotension and bradycardia with reports of cardiovascular collapse.[9,10] This is thought to be a result of the Bezold-Jarisch reflex (**Figure 2**), whereby venous pooling in the lower extremities decreases venous return. Compensatory increases in heart rate and contractility can lead to the activation of receptors within the heart that paradoxically increase parasympathetic and decrease sympathetic output, leading to bradycardia, vasodilation, and resultant hypotension or cardiovascular collapse. This may be exacerbated by epineph-

rine containing local anesthetic solutions used for PNB.[11] Treatment may include adequate hydration, beta-blockers if the patient becomes reflexively tachycardic, and atropine or epinephrine for severe bradycardia.[12] Additionally, there is concern for central nervous system end-organ ischemia, including cerebral ischemia, opthalmoplegia, and visual loss in the beach chair position.[13,14] The exact mechanism is unknown, but has been purported to be from postural hypotension that can occur with the blood pressure being monitored from the patients' calf.[15] Cerebral perfusion pressure can be significantly different from what is measured intraoperatively because of the hydrostatic pressure difference from the head and the lower extremity. Exacerbation of this pressure can occur during arthroscopy, when the blood pressure may be further lowered to improve visualization in the surgical field. Another mechanism may include manipulation or positioning of the head, causing mechanical obstruction of the neck vessels.

The advantages of the lateral position include better visualization with arm traction, increased cerebral perfusion, and better access to the superior and posterior portals. The disadvantages of this position include the need for airway management and general anesthesia, risk of traction neuropathy, and difficulty with conversion to an open procedure.[8] Positioning for elbow surgery can be performed in the supine, lateral, or prone positions depending on the approach needed.

Neurologic Complications

Nerve injury can vary from a minor paresthesia to complete loss of motor function. Injury can be related to surgical, patient, or anesthesia-related factors. The overall incidence is low, but when it occurs, nerve injury can cause significant distress to the patient and the perioperative team. The nerves most commonly injured from shoulder surgery include the axillary, musculocutaneous, suprascapular, and subscapular nerves. Injuries to these nerves most commonly occur during joint arthroplasty and surgery for anterior joint instability. The reported incidence is 1% to 2% in patients undergoing rotator cuff surgery, 1% to 8% in patients undergoing surgery for anterior instability, and 1% to 4% in patients undergoing arthroplasty.[16-19] Confounding any type of neurologic complication is the use of PNB. More specifically, an interscalene block is typically performed at the level of C6. The nerves most vulnerable during shoulder surgery come from the C5, C6, and C7 nerve roots. The incidence of nerve injury for PNB has been estimated to be less than 3%.[20] Therefore, open communication between the surgeon and the anesthesiologist is imperative if the patient is at increased risk of nerve injury. A thorough preoperative neurologic examination should be performed. If there is concern for neurologic injury or the need for postoperative neurologic monitoring, a single-shot nerve block can be performed postoperatively or a peripheral nerve catheter can be placed preoperatively, but not dosed until a nor-

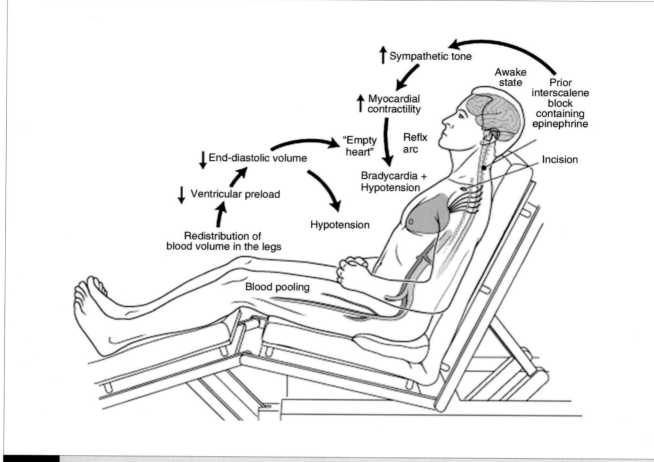

Figure 2 Mechanisms of hypotension/bradycardia. Patients who receive interscalene brachial plexus block, are sedated, and are placed in the beach chair position may develop hypotension and bradycardia during their anesthetic course. The proposed mechanism for this phenomenon is a relative preload deficit from the sitting position, combined with a hypercontractile ventricle, which occurs as a consequence of exogenous and endogenous epinephrine. The vigorously contracting "empty" heart causes reflex bradycardia and hypotension. (Reproduced with permission from Neal JM: Upper Extremity regional anesthesia: Essentials of our understanding. *Reg Anesth Pain Med* 2009;34[2]:134-170.)

mal postoperative neurologic examination has been documented.

Postoperative Analgesia

In addition to the unwanted psychological and physiologic effects of suboptimally treated pain, a lack of adequate postoperative analgesia can interfere with early physical therapy and rehabilitation, and possibly increase the risk of chronic postsurgical pain.[21-23] Perioperative opioids have been a mainstay for the treatment of pain despite many of the well-known adverse effects of nausea, vomiting, pruritis, sedation, constipation, and respiratory depression. In addition to these well-known adverse effects, surgeries with moderate to severe postoperative pain requiring larger amounts of opioids can delay discharge and create unanticipated hospital admissions in the outpatient setting. Using sev-

eral types of analgesic agents with different mechanisms and employing multimodal and preventative analgesic strategies may minimize some of the unwanted effects.

Preventive and Multimodal Analgesia

Preventive analgesia refers to preventing or attenuating central sensitization that can occur after a traumatic insult and the inflammatory response that ensues.[24] Although it was initially thought that initiating analgesia before the insult was more efficacious than afterward, clinical trials have not consistently supported this finding.[25,26] More recently, it is thought that the most efficacious approach is to use a multimodal analgesic regimen during the entire perioperative period that can attenuate the firing of nociceptive input to the central nervous system before, during, and after a surgical procedure.[27] In turn, multimodal analgesia employs two or more analgesic agents with different mechanisms of action whose overall analgesic effects become additive or synergistic while decreasing the adverse effects of any one agent.[28] Greater emphasis has been placed on using regional analgesic techniques with opioid and nonopioid analgesic agents for breakthrough pain.[29]

Opioids

Opioids are one of the most common analgesic agents used that have the benefit of being delivered by multiple routes (oral, intravenous, intramuscular, subcutaneous, intranasal, transmucosal, and neuraxial). They have no analgesic ceiling effect; however, their analgesic efficacy can be limited by the adverse effects of nausea, vomiting, sedation, pruritis, ileus, and respiratory depression. Patients undergoing shoulder and elbow surgery are typically treated with intravenous, oral, or intramuscular regimens.

Parenteral Administration

Administration through the intravenous route produces a relatively rapid onset and reliable analgesia that can be quickly titrated compared with other routes. Patients with moderate to severe pain may require intravenous opioids, most commonly delivered in the form of intravenous patient-controlled analgesia (IV PCA). This method of delivery likely provides better pain relief and improved patient satisfaction compared with dosing as required by nursing staff.[30]

The variables that can be programmed into an IV PCA include the bolus or demand dose, lockout interval, and background infusion (**Table 1**). The optimal settings are not known, but following a few basic principles may increase analgesic efficacy and decrease the risk of potential overdosing. The optimal bolus or demand dose is based on the potency of the opioid and should be sufficient to decrease pain after a few patient-controlled doses. Too small of a dose can lead to inadequate analgesia, whereas too large of a dose can lead to increased adverse effects, including respiratory depression. The lockout interval should be based on the analgesic onset and the peak effect of the opioid and should allow the patient to determine the efficacy of the prior dose before another dose is self-administered. Too long of a lockout interval can lead to inadequate analgesia, and too short an interval can lead to "stacking" of doses. Continuous or background infusions are not typically recommended for opiate-naïve patients. It was thought that running a continuous infusion during periods of sleep while patients could not self-administer a dose may improve analgesia. However, this may lead to increased adverse events, such as respiratory depression, without a proven benefit of improved analgesia.[31,32] Continuous infusions may be of benefit in opioid-tolerant patients.

An important concept to realize when using an IV PCA is that one size does not fit all.[33] The process of treating a patient's pain is dynamic. Individuals may have different analgesic requirements, and these analgesic requirements may change during the perioperative period. This is especially true during the first 24 to 48 hours after surgery. A constant reassessment of a patient's pain control needs to be performed with adjustment of the analgesic regimen.

Enteral Administration

Oral opioids can be used to treat moderate to severe pain once a patient can tolerate oral administration, but they

Table 1

Intravenous Opioid Patient-Controlled Analgesic Regimens

Opioid Lockout	Demand Dose	Interval	Infusion Rate[a]
Morphine	0.5-2.5 mg	5-10 min	1-10 mg/h
Fentanyl	10-20 µg	5-10 min	20-100 µg/h
Hydromorphone	0.1-0.2 mg	5-10 min	0.1-0.2 mg/h

[a] Continuous infusions are not recommended for opiate-naïve patients

Table 2

Oral Opioid Analgesic Agents

Opioid	Dose	Interval	Comments
Oxycodone (IR)	5-10 mg	4-6 h	More than 4 doses should not be exceeded in a 24-h period to avoid the stacking of doses with risk of adverse opioid side effects
Oxycodone (ER)	10-20 mg	12 h	May be combined with acetaminophen or aspirin
Morphine (ER)	15-30 mg	8-12 h	More than 4 doses should not be exceeded in a 24-h period to avoid the stacking of doses with risk of adverse opioid side effects
Hydrocodone	5-10 mg	4-6 h	Combined with acetaminophen
Hydromorphone	2-4 mg	4-6 h	
Codeine	30-60 mg	4 h	May be combined with acetaminophen or aspirin
Tramadol	50-100 mg	6 h	

8: Miscellaneous Shoulder and Elbow Topics

Table 3

Nonopioid Analgesic Agents

Analgesic	Dose	Interval	24-h Maximum Dose	Comments
Aspirin	325-1,000 mg	4-6 h	4000 mg	
Acetaminophen	500-100 mg	4-6 h	4000 mg	
Ibuprofen	200-800 mg	4-6 h	3200 mg	
Naproxen	500 mg	12 h	1000 mg	
Celecoxib	200-400 mg	12 h	800 mg	
Ketorolac	15-30 mg	6 h	60-120 mg	15 mg if < 50 kg or > 65 years; 30 mg if > 50 kg or < 65 years; should not be given for more than 5 days
Gabapentin	300-1200 mg			Ideal analgesic dosing not known
Pregabalin	150- 300 mg			Ideal analgesic dosing not known

can be less reliable and titratable compared to intravenous opioids. They are available in both immediate-release and controlled-release formulations (**Table 2**). Although the immediate-release form has the ability to control moderate to severe pain, it needs to be given every 4 to 6 hours to maintain adequate plasma levels. Delays in administration when these medications are given as needed can result in an unnecessary increase in pain. Guidelines have been developed that recommend a fixed dosing schedule when using this formulation.[34] Controlled-release formulations may provide a more stable plasma level of opioid and extended period of pain relief with less fluctuations. Using scheduled dosing of controlled-release formulations with as-needed immediate-release doses for breakthrough pain has been used.

Tramadol

Tramadol is a synthetic analgesic agent that is structurally related to codeine and morphine. It is thought to act directly on μ receptors as well as prevent the uptake of norepinephrine and serotonin, which are involved in spinal inhibition of pain.[35,36] Tramadol is less potent than morphine, but it has the benefit of a lower incidence of adverse effects such as respiratory depression, constipation, and dependence.[37,38] Its use has been shown to have a beneficial effect that is comparable to other opioids in managing patients with moderate postoperative pain. It may be used as part of a multimodal analgesic regimen or in patients who may not tolerate opioids.

Nonopioid Analgesic Agents

In congruency with a multimodal analgesic regimen, nonopioid analgesic agents play an important role in providing postoperative analgesia. A balanced regimen of nonopioid analgesic agents may lead to opioid sparing, decreased opioid-related adverse effects, and increased analgesic efficacy (**Table 3**).

Nonsteroidal Anti-inflammatory Drugs

NSAIDs have effectively been used for treating nonsurgical pain because of their analgesic, anti-inflammatory, and antipyretic effects. Their role has increased in postoperative patients with the introduction of intravenous formulations such as ketorolac and diclofenac, which have been shown to have similar analgesic efficacy compared to that of opioids.[39,40] These drugs act through inhibition of cyclooxygenase (COX) enzymes and ultimately the production of prostaglandins, which are chemical mediators of the acute inflammatory and pain response. The main site of action is in the peripheral nervous system, but there may also be a central effect in nociception.[41] The COX-1 enzyme is constitutively expressed and is involved in gastric mucosal protection through prostaglandin E_2 and has a thromboxane-mediated effect on platelet aggregation. The COX-2 isoform is an inducible enzyme produced during inflammation and fever. Nonspecific COX inhibitors, such as ketorolac, block COX-1 and COX-2 isoenzymes, whereas selective COX inhibitors, such as celecoxib, inhibit only the COX-2 isoenzyme. COX-2 inhibitors have minimal effect on the coagulation system, allowing them to be safely used in the perioperative period with less concern for bleeding.

Although the use of NSAIDs as an analgesic agent has been shown to be beneficial, their use may be limited by some of their adverse effects. Of these, the most concerning for perioperative patients are platelet dysfunction, renal dysfunction, and gastrointestinal bleeding. Additionally, some concern for bone healing may exist when NSAIDs are used in orthopaedic procedures where an inflammatory response and prostaglandin production play a role in this process.[42] The adverse effects are due to the inhibition of COX enzymes. Inhibition of thromboxane synthesis can inhibit platelet aggregation and potentially increase surgical bleeding. Inhibition of prostaglandin production can lead to gastrointestinal bleeding through loss of mucosal protection and renal dysfunction from renal arteriolar vasoconstriction. The use of all COX inhibitors can lead to renal dysfunction; however, the use of selective COX-2 inhibitors can limit the risk of platelet dysfunction and gastrointestinal bleeding. The use of NSAIDs should be dictated by individual patients and the particular surgery they are having.

Acetaminophen

Acetaminophen is a nonopioid analgesic agent that is thought to act by inhibiting COX enzymes and decreasing central prostaglandin production.[43] Until recently, acetaminophen was available only in oral and rectal form in the United States, but it is now available in an intravenous formulation. Although it has weak anti-inflammatory properties, acetaminophen has significant analgesic and antipyretic properties with minimal gastrointestinal, renal, and platelet adverse effects. The use of acetaminophen has been studied in several surgery types, including orthopaedic surgery. When compared with placebo, acetaminophen decreased overall 24-hour morphine consumption, with improved pain scores and patient satisfaction.[44,45] Additionally, the combination of acetaminophen and NSAIDs has been shown to be more effective than either NSAIDs or acetaminophen alone[46] and more effective when given in scheduled doses rather than on an as-needed basis.[47] Despite its opioid-sparing and analgesic effect, acetaminophen has not been consistently shown to decrease opioid-related adverse effects.[48,49]

Gabapentin and Pregabalin

Gabapentin and pregabalin are gamma-aminobutyric analogues whose mechanism is thought to act on voltage-gated calcium channels, but whose true analgesic effect is unknown. Several studies suggest gabapentin, when given in a single preoperative dose, may have an opioid-sparing effect and may improve pain scores at rest and movement.[50-53] Additionally, one study has shown a decrease in opioid-related adverse effects, such as vomiting, but was not significantly reduced in others. Similarly, pregabalin has been shown to have a significant reduction in pain relief, pain intensity difference, and pain relief intensity difference compared to placebo and 400 mg ibuprofen with dental pain from tooth extraction.[54,55]

Ketamine

Ketamine is an N-methyl-D-aspartic acid receptor antagonist and has mostly been used as an anesthetic in the operating room. With the discovery of the N-methyl-D-aspartic acid receptor and its possible role in central sensitization and chronic postsurgical pain, there has been renewed interest in its role as a postop-

erative analgesic.[56] However, its use has been limited out of concern for the psychomimetic and cardiovascular effects that may occur with anesthetic doses. More recently, several studies have shown a possible analgesic and opioid-sparing effect when ketamine has been used in subanesthetic doses.[57] Patients undergoing total knee replacement under general anesthesia who received low-dose ketamine intraoperatively and postoperatively for the first 48 hours had lower pain scores at rest and with movement, along with decreased time for flexion to 90° compared to placebo.[58]

Summary

Anesthesia and analgesia for shoulder and elbow surgery can be approached in several ways. Continuous communication between the anesthesiologist and the surgeon is essential to provide the best intraoperative and postoperative care. Using a multimodal analgesic approach with local anesthetic in the form of PNB and nonopioid analgesic agents while reserving opioids for rescue analgesia may be optimal. Patients may likely have superior analgesia, fewer opioid-related adverse effects, and overall greater satisfaction. This, in turn, can help the patient reach the ultimate goal of striving for the best functional and clinical outcome.

Annotated References

1. Richman JM, Liu SS, Courpas G, et al: Does continuous peripheral nerve block provide superior pain control to opioids? A meta-analysis. *Anesth Analg* 2006; 102(1):248-257.

2. Pogatzki-Zahn EM, Zahn PK: From preemptive to preventive analgesia. *Curr Opin Anaesthesiol* 2006; 19(5):551-555.

3. Urmey WF, Talts KH, Sharrock NE: One hundred percent incidence of hemidiaphragmatic paresis associated with interscalene brachial plexus anesthesia as diagnosed by ultrasonography. *Anesth Analg* 1991;72(4): 498-503.

4. Knoblanche GE: The incidence and aetiology of phrenic nerve blockade associated with supraclavicular brachial plexus block. *Anaesth Intensive Care* 1979; 7(4):346-349.

5. Dhuner KG, Moberg E, Onne L: Paresis of the phrenic nerve during brachial plexus block analgesia and its importance. *Acta Chir Scand* 1955;109(1):53-57.

6. Urmey WF, McDonald M: Hemidiaphragmatic paresis during interscalene brachial plexus block: Effects on pulmonary function and chest wall mechanics. *Anesth Analg* 1992;74(3):352-357.

8: Miscellaneous Shoulder and Elbow Topics

7. Fredrickson MJ, Krishnan S, Chen CY: Postoperative analgesia for shoulder surgery: A critical appraisal and review of current techniques. *Anaesthesia* 2010;65(6): 608-624.

This review critically assesses the evidence relating to the efficacy of different local anesthetic-based techniques for postoperative analgesia following shoulder surgery.

8. Peruto CM, Ciccotti MG, Cohen SB: Shoulder arthroscopy positioning: Lateral decubitus versus beach chair. *Arthroscopy* 2009;25(8):891-896.

The authors review the advantages and the disadvantages of the lateral decubitus and beach chair positions, including setup, surgical visualization, access, and patient risk.

9. Aviado DM, Guevara Aviado D: The Bezold-Jarisch reflex: A historical perspective of cardiopulmonary reflexes. *Ann N Y Acad Sci* 2001;940:48-58.

10. Campagna JA, Carter C: Clinical relevance of the Bezold-Jarisch reflex. *Anesthesiology* 2003;98(5): 1250-1260.

11. D'Alessio JG, Weller RS, Rosenblum M: Activation of the Bezold-Jarisch reflex in the sitting position for shoulder arthroscopy using interscalene block. *Anesth Analg* 1995;80(6):1158-1162.

12. Liguori GA, Kahn RL, Gordon J, Gordon MA, Urban MK: The use of metoprolol and glycopyrrolate to prevent hypotensive/bradycardic events during shoulder arthroscopy in the sitting position under interscalene block. *Anesth Analg* 1998;87(6):1320-1325.

13. Bhatti MT, Enneking FK: Visual loss and ophthalmoplegia after shoulder surgery. *Anesth Analg* 2003; 96(3):899-902.

14. Pohl A, Cullen DJ: Cerebral ischemia during shoulder surgery in the upright position: A case series. *J Clin Anesth* 2005;17(6):463-469.

15. Rains DD, Rooke GA, Wahl CJ: Pathomechanisms and complications related to patient positioning and anesthesia during shoulder arthroscopy. *Arthroscopy* 2011; 27(4):532-541.

The authors comprehensively review case reports and studies looking at complications related to patient positioning (lateral decubitus versus beach chair) for shoulder surgery and the possible pathophysiologic mechanisms associated with them.

16. Boardman ND III, Cofield RH: Neurologic complications of shoulder surgery. *Clin Orthop Relat Res* 1999; 368:44-53.

17. Wirth MA, Rockwood CA Jr: Complications of shoulder arthroplasty. *Clin Orthop Relat Res* 1994;307: 47-69.

18. Wirth MA, Rockwood CA Jr: Complications of total shoulder-replacement arthroplasty. *J Bone Joint Surg Am* 1996;78(4):603-616.

19. Zanotti RM, Carpenter JE, Blasier RB, Greenfield ML, Adler RS, Bromberg MB: The low incidence of suprascapular nerve injury after primary repair of massive rotator cuff tears. *J Shoulder Elbow Surg* 1997;6(3): 258-264.

20. Brull R, McCartney CJ, Chan VW, El-Beheiry H: Neurological complications after regional anesthesia: Contemporary estimates of risk. *Anesth Analg* 2007; 104(4):965-974.

The authors report an estimate for risk of neurologic complications associated with regional anesthetic techniques by retrospectively reviewing 32 studies over a 10-year period.

21. Perkins FM, Kehlet H: Chronic pain as an outcome of surgery: A review of predictive factors. *Anesthesiology* 2000;93(4):1123-1133.

22. Wu CL, Fleisher LA: Outcomes research in regional anesthesia and analgesia. *Anesth Analg* 2000;91(5): 1232-1242.

23. Wu CL, Rowlingson AJ, Partin AW, et al: Correlation of postoperative pain to quality of recovery in the immediate postoperative period. *Reg Anesth Pain Med* 2005;30(6):516-522.

24. Kissin I: Preemptive analgesia. *Anesthesiology* 2000; 93(4):1138-1143.

25. Woolf CJ, Chong MS: Preemptive analgesia—treating postoperative pain by preventing the establishment of central sensitization. *Anesth Analg* 1993;77(2): 362-379.

26. Kissin I: Preemptive analgesia: Why its effect is not always obvious. *Anesthesiology* 1996;84(5):1015-1019.

27. Pogatzki-Zahn EM, Zahn PK: From preemptive to preventive analgesia. *Curr Opin Anaesthesiol* 2006; 19(5):551-555.

28. Buvanendran A, Kroin JS: Multimodal analgesia for controlling acute postoperative pain. *Curr Opin Anaesthesiol* 2009;22(5):588-593.

The authors review and evaluate recent studies that explore new and improved methods of multimodal anesthesia for relieving moderate to severe postoperative pain.

29. Elvir-Lazo OL, White PF: The role of multimodal analgesia in pain management after ambulatory surgery. *Curr Opin Anaesthesiol* 2010;23(6):697-703.

This review article discusses the role of multimodal analgesia in the ambulatory setting and, more specifically, the role and use of nonopioid analgesic agents.

30. Rathmell JP, Wu CL, Sinatra RS, et al: Acute post-surgical pain management: A critical appraisal of current practice, December 2-4, 2005. *Reg Anesth Pain Med* 2006;31(4, suppl 1):1-42.

31. Macintyre PE: Safety and efficacy of patient-controlled analgesia. *Br J Anaesth* 2001;87(1):36-46.

32. Smythe MA, MB Zak, O'Donnell MP, Schad RF, Dmuchowski CF: Patient-controlled analgesia versus patient-controlled analgesia plus continuous infusion after hip replacement surgery. *Ann Pharmacother* 1996;30(3):224-227.

33. Etches RC: Patient-controlled analgesia. *Surg Clin North Am* 1999;79(2):297-312.

34. *Acute Pain Management: Operative or Medical Procedures and Trauma.* (Clinical Practice Guideline). Publication No. AHCPR 92-0032. Rockville, MD: Agency for Health Care Policy and Research, Public Health Service, U.S. Department of Health and Human Services, February 1992.

35. Halfpenny DM, Callado LF, Hopwood SE, Bamigbade TA, Langford RM, Stamford JA: Effects of tramadol stereoisomers on norepinephrine efflux and uptake in the rat locus coeruleus measured by real time voltammetry. *Br J Anaesth* 1999;83(6):909-915.

36. Bamigbade TA, Davidson C, Langford RM, Stamford JA: Actions of tramadol, its enantiomers and principal metabolite, O-desmethyltramadol, on serotonin (5-HT) efflux and uptake in the rat dorsal raphe nucleus. *Br J Anaesth* 1997;79(3):352-356.

37. Scott LJ, Perry CM: Tramadol: A review of its use in perioperative pain. *Drugs* 2000;60(1):139-176.

38. Edwards JE, McQuay HJ, Moore RA: Combination analgesic efficacy: Individual patient data meta-analysis of single-dose oral tramadol plus acetaminophen in acute postoperative pain. *J Pain Symptom Manage* 2002;23(2):121-130.

39. Ding Y, White PF: Comparative effects of ketorolac, dezocine, and fentanyl as adjuvants during outpatient anesthesia. *Anesth Analg* 1992;75(4):566-571.

40. McLoughlin C, McKinney MS, Fee JP, Boules Z: Diclofenac for day-care arthroscopy surgery: Comparison with a standard opioid therapy. *Br J Anaesth* 1990;65(5):620-623.

41. Møiniche S, Kehlet H, Dahl JB: A qualitative and quantitative systematic review of preemptive analgesia for postoperative pain relief: The role of timing of analgesia. *Anesthesiology* 2002;96(3):725-741.

42. Harder AT, An YH: The mechanisms of the inhibitory effects of nonsteroidal anti-inflammatory drugs on bone healing: A concise review. *J Clin Pharmacol* 2003;43(8):807-815.

43. Duggan ST, Scott LJ: Intravenous paracetamol (acetaminophen). *Drugs* 2009;69(1):101-113.

    This article discusses the analgesic efficacy of acetaminophen when given in single or multiple doses compared with that of placebo.

44. Sinatra RS, Jahr JS, Reynolds LW, Viscusi ER, Groudine SB, Payen-Champenois C: Efficacy and safety of single and repeated administration of 1 gram intravenous acetaminophen injection (paracetamol) for pain management after major orthopedic surgery. *Anesthesiology* 2005;102(4):822-831.

45. Sinatra RS, Jahr JS, Reynolds L, et al: Intravenous acetaminophen for pain after major orthopedic surgery: An expanded analysis. *Pain Pract* 2012;12(5):357-365.

    This article reexamines the analgesic efficacy of intravenous acetaminophen since its approval by the FDA showing a statistically significant difference compared with that of placebo.

46. Ong CK, Seymour RA, Lirk P, Merry AF: Combining paracetamol (acetaminophen) with nonsteroidal anti-inflammatory drugs: A qualitative systematic review of analgesic efficacy for acute postoperative pain. *Anesth Analg* 2010;110(4):1170-1179.

    This systematic review looks at the efficacy of combining paracetamol with NSAIDs and comparing the analgesic efficacy of the combination of each alone. The review suggests that a combination of paracetamol and an NSAID may offer superior analgesia compared with either drug alone.

47. Sutters KA, Miaskowski C, Holdridge-Zeuner D, et al: A randomized clinical trial of the efficacy of scheduled dosing of acetaminophen and hydrocodone for the management of postoperative pain in children after tonsillectomy. *Clin J Pain* 2010;26(2):95-103.

    This study shows the increased analgesic efficacy of around-the-clock dosing of acetaminophen compared with as-needed dosing in children after tonsillectomy.

48. Remy C, Marret E, Bonnet F: Effects of acetaminophen on morphine side-effects and consumption after major surgery: Meta-analysis of randomized controlled trials. *Br J Anaesth* 2005;94(4):505-513.

49. Maund E, McDaid C, Rice S, Wright K, Jenkins B, Woolacott N: Paracetamol and selective and nonselective non-steroidal anti-inflammatory drugs for the reduction in morphine-related side-effects after major surgery: A systematic review. *Br J Anaesth* 2011;106(3):292-297.

    This systematic review shows that the addition of paracetamol or other NSAIDs decreases opioid consumption after major surgery. There was not a significant difference between the different classes of these analgesic adjuncts in doing so.

50. Dirks J, Fredensborg BB, Christensen D, Fomsgaard JS, Flyger H, Dahl JB: A randomized study of the effects of single-dose gabapentin versus placebo on

postoperative pain and morphine consumption after mastectomy. *Anesthesiology* 2002;97(3):560-564.

51. Dierking G, Duedahl TH, Rasmussen ML, et al: Effects of gabapentin on postoperative morphine consumption and pain after abdominal hysterectomy: A randomized, double-blind trial. *Acta Anaesthesiol Scand* 2004;48(3):322-327.

52. Rorarius MG, Mennander S, Suominen P, et al: Gabapentin for the prevention of postoperative pain after vaginal hysterectomy. *Pain* 2004;110(1-2):175-181.

53. Dahl JB, Mathiesen O, Møiniche S: "Protective premedication": An option with gabapentin and related drugs? A review of gabapentin and pregabalin in in the treatment of post-operative pain. *Acta Anaesthesiol Scand* 2004;48(9):1130-1136.

54. Hill CM, Balkenohl M, Thomas DW, Walker R, Mathé H, Murray G: Pregabalin in patients with postoperative dental pain. *Eur J Pain* 2001;5(2):119-124.

55. Agarwal A, Gautam S, Gupta D, Agarwal S, Singh PK, Singh U: Evaluation of a single preoperative dose of pregabalin for attenuation of postoperative pain after laparoscopic cholecystectomy. *Br J Anaesth* 2008; 101(5):700-704.

This study shows that a single preoperative dose of pregabalin decreases both static and dynamic pain as well as opioid consumption after laparascopic surgery.

56. Schmid RL, Sandler AN, Katz J: Use and efficacy of low-dose ketamine in the management of acute postoperative pain: A review of current techniques and outcomes. *Pain* 1999;82(2):111-125.

57. Subramaniam K, Subramaniam B, Steinbrook RA: Ketamine as adjuvant analgesic to opioids: A quantitative and qualitative systematic review. *Anesth Analg* 2004;99(2):482-495.

58. Aveline C, Gautier JF, Vautier P, et al: Postoperative analgesia and early rehabilitation after total knee replacement: A comparison of continuous low-dose intravenous ketamine versus nefopam. *Eur J Pain* 2009; 13(6):613-619.

This study shows that ketamine produces opioid sparing, decreases pain intensity, and improves mobilization after total knee replacement to a greater degree than that of nefopam.

Chapter 53

Advanced Imaging of the Shoulder and Elbow

John A. Carrino, MD, MPH   Rashmi S. Thakkar, MD

Introduction

Various abnormalities of the shoulder and elbow joints can cause pain and/or dysfunction. Consequently, the demand for imaging these complex joints has increased in the past few years. Standard radiographs are considered to represent the basis of all imaging. Radiography is the initial imaging technique because of its lower cost, wide availability, and ability to detect certain key conditions, such as fractures, calcific tendinitis, moderate to severe degenerative disease, and some neoplastic tumor-like conditions. However, for more detailed diagnoses, especially with regard to soft tissues, advanced imaging techniques are required.

In this chapter, advanced imaging techniques such as MRI, magnetic resonance arthrography (MRA), CT, computed tomographic arthrography (CTA), and ultrasound will be discussed, along with various pathologies of the shoulder and elbow.

MRI and MRA

Musculoskeletal MRI at 3.0 T has moved steadily from research into routine clinical practice in the past few years. The most important advantage of high-field MRI is the higher signal-to-noise ratio (SNR), which allows acquisitions in the musculoskeletal system with higher spatial resolution within the same scan time.[1] The increased SNR may enable imaging with a higher resolution and a faster acquisition of the musculoskeletal and nervous structures. The maximum contrast-to-noise ra-

---

Dr. Carrino or an immediate family member serves as a paid consultant to or is an employee of Quality Medical Metrics, Medtronic, General Electric Healthcare, Vital Images, and Siemens Medical Systems; serves as an unpaid consultant to General Electronic Healthcare, Carestream Health, and Siemens Medical Systems; has stock or stock options held in Merge; and has received research or institutional support from Siemens Medical Systems, Carestream Health, and Toshiba Medical. Neither Dr. Thakkar nor any immediate family member has received anything of value from or has stock or stock options held in a commercial company or institution related directly or indirectly to the subject of this chapter.

tios (CNRs) also depend on the strength of the magnetic field. It has been shown that the CNRs between muscle and bone, between bone and cartilage, and between cartilage and fluid may all be higher at 3.0 T than at 1.5 T. The potential advantages have aroused anticipation of better image quality and higher diagnostic accuracy. Small joints, such as the elbow, and the visualization of fibrocartilaginous anatomy and pathology in the shoulder and elbow joints benefit from higher resolution protocols.

Musculoskeletal magnetic resonance protocols used at most institutions consist of two-dimensional fast/turbo spin-echo sequences in multiple planes. These sequences have good SNR, high tissue contrast, and high in-plane resolution. However, they have relatively thick slices and small gaps between the slices, which can obscure pathology secondary to partial volume averaging. Three-dimensional sequences may reduce partial volume averaging by acquiring thin, continuous slices through the joints.[2] Three-dimensional sequences can also be used to create multiplanar reformat images that allow joints to be evaluated in any orientation following a single acquisition.

Shoulder Joint

MRI is the imaging modality of choice for many indications, primarily because of its free choice of imaging planes and excellent soft-tissue contrast resolution. MRI provides the most detailed diagnosis with regard to abnormalities of the rotator cuff, capsulolabral structures, tendons, muscles, occult fractures, articular surfaces, and abnormalities of instability in the shoulder joint. It can help to detect bone and soft-tissue abnormalities associated with shoulder impingement. Lesions of the supraspinatus tendons, the subacromial bursa, and the biceps tendon can be disclosed, along with morphologic abnormalities of the acromion, the acromioclavicular joint, and the coracoacromial ligament.

On unenhanced MRI, the rotator cuff, the labrum, the joint capsule, and cortical bone normally appear dark on all pulse sequences. Because of their close proximity and abutment, they may be difficult to distinguish from one another. The presence of either a

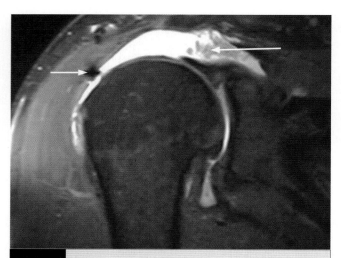

Figure 1 A coronal fat-suppressed intermediate weighted MRI (repetition time/echo time-3200/44) of the shoulder of a 36-year-old man is shown. The patient underwent rotator cuff repair 1 year prior to this image and reported right shoulder pain following an injury. A recurrent full-thickness, full-width tear of the supraspinatus with retraction of the fibers to the glenohumeral joint is seen (long arrow), along with a susceptibility artifact from the previous surgery (short arrow).

joint effusion or intra-articular gadolinium contrast helps to separate these structures and improve tissue contrast, outlining the structures with a material that is of substantially different signal characteristic.[3]

A recent study reported on the diagnostic sensitivity of 3-T conventional MRI versus MRA of the shoulder in the same patient population.[4] On conventional MRI, sensitivities and specificities, respectively, compared with arthroscopy were as follows: anterior labral tear, 83% and 100%; posterior labral tear, 84% and 100%; superior labrum anterior to posterior (SLAP) tear, 83% and 99%; supraspinatus tendon tear, 92% and 100%; partial-thickness articular surface tear, 68% and 100%; and partial-thickness bursal surface tear, 84% and 100%. On MRA, sensitivities and specificities, respectively, compared with arthroscopy were as follows: anterior labral tear, 98% and 100%; posterior labral tear, 95% and 100%; SLAP tear, 98% and 99%; supraspinatus tendon tear, 100% and 100%; partial-thickness articular surface tear, 97% and 100%; and partial-thickness bursal surface tear, 84% and 100%. MRA showed a statistical improvement in sensitivity ($P < 0.05$) for detecting partial-thickness articular surface supraspinatus tears, anterior labral tears, and SLAP tears at 3.0 T.

In the shoulder joint, two-dimensional fast spin-echo sequences are currently the sequence of choice for noncontrast MRI. However, three-dimensional sequences, such as gradient echo steady-state free precession, have been attempted at many institutions. Recently, three-dimensional isotropic resolution fast spin-echo se-

quences have been used to decrease the time required to evaluate the shoulder joint during noncontrast MRI. Also, three-dimensional T1-weighted isotropic resolution sequences have been used to provide rapid and comprehensive shoulder joint assessment during MRA.

Rotator Cuff

Axial, sagittal oblique, and coronal oblique planes are typically used for imaging the rotator cuff. The sagittal oblique and coronal oblique planes are in reference to the supraspinatus tendon, not the anatomic axis. A combination of sequences is used for routine MRI of the shoulder. In general, short-echo time sequences (T1 and proton density weighted) provide delineation of anatomic detail and help quantify fatty atrophy, whereas fluid-sensitive sequences (proton density fat-suppressed, T2 fat-suppressed images) are most sensitive to an abnormal increase in water signal that accompanies most pathologic conditions of the tendons. Full-thickness tears of the rotator cuff tendons can be accurately identified using conventional MRI with high sensitivity and specificity. Increased signal intensity extending from the inferior to the superior surface of the tendon on all imaging sequences is an accurate sign of a full-thickness rotator cuff tear. The morphologic changes that might be associated with the tear are tendon retraction, muscle atrophy, and fatty infiltrations, which are also important prognostic factors (**Figure 1**). This type of information can be useful for treatment decisions regarding nonsurgical versus surgical repair, the type of surgical repair (open or arthroscopic; substitute or muscle transfer), and postoperative prognosis.

MRA is recommended if there is any question concerning the distinction between a full-thickness and a partial-thickness tear.[5] It is particularly important if the abnormal signal intensity extends along the undersurface of the tendon. The detection of these partial-thickness tears can be optimized with the help of certain technical aspects of imaging. First, abduction and external rotation positioning has been shown to increase the conspicuity of partial-thickness articular surface tears by lifting the tendon off the humeral head and reducing the compression of the articular surface fibers; also, the anterior stabilizing structures are placed under tension with the arm in this position. Second, partial volume averaging related to the course of the tendon can be reduced by external rotation of the humerus for coronal oblique imaging, bringing the tendon course in plane.

A 2009 study compared the diagnostic accuracy of MRI, MRA, and ultrasound for the diagnosis of rotator cuff tears through a meta-analysis of literature studies.[6] Sixty-five articles met the inclusion criteria for this meta-analysis. In diagnosing a full-thickness tear or a partial-thickness rotator cuff tear, MRA is more sensitive and specific than either MRI or ultrasound ($P < 0.05$). There are no significant differences in either sensitivity or specificity between MRI and ultrasound in the diagnosis of partial- or full-thickness rotator cuff tears ($P > 0.05$). Summary receiver operating characteristic (ROC) curves for MRA, MRI, and ultrasound for all tears show the area under the ROC curve is greatest for MRA (0.935), followed by ultrasound (0.889) and MRI (0.878); however, pairwise comparisons of these curves show no significant differences between MRI and ultrasound ($P > 0.05$).

Capsulolabral Pathology

Direct MRA with intra-articular injection of a dilute gadolinium solution because of its ability to distend the joint helps to outline labral and capsular structures, aiding in the diagnosis as well as therapeutic planning and follow-up (**Figure 2**).

Patients undergo 3-T MRA if anterior labral tears, SLAP tears, and partial-thickness supraspinatus tears are suspected clinically. MRA could help with accurate identification and demonstration of the integrity of the glenohumeral ligaments, the capsule, and the labrum and could help in staging abnormalities.[7] It is sensitive and specific for detecting a detached labral fragment, labral degeneration, and lesions of the inferior part of labrum and the inferior glenohumeral ligament.

SLAP injuries of the superior labrum are best demonstrated in the oblique coronal plane. Fluid or contrast extending between the labrum and the superior glenoid is diagnostic. Ancillary findings to support a true SLAP tear include lateral extension of abnormal signal intensity into the substance of the labrum, irregularity of the labral margin, and extension of the signal into the proximal biceps tendon. In distinguishing true labral pathology from variants such as a sublabral hole, the sublabral recess tends to be more medial than SLAP tears and is located between the biceps tendon and the glenoid articular cartilage. Conversely, SLAP tears will often extend posterior to the biceps tendon and more laterally than a sublabral recess. They are most likely to demonstrate laterally curved, high signal intensity on oblique coronal images, and anteroposterior extension on axial images.

The anterior and posterior portions of the labrum are best evaluated on axial images. Magnetic resonance findings of a labral tear include abnormal signal within the labrum or interposed between the labrum and the glenoid. Assessment of anterior capsule stripping is much more difficult because of extreme variability of the normal capsular attachments along the anterior glenoid.

Cartilage of the Shoulder Joint

The optimal evaluation of cartilage is challenging, especially in the shoulder joint. Improving spatial resolution on two-dimensional sequences and obtaining different planes or arm positioning to better cover different areas of the curved humeral head all are possible improvements. Tissue contrast can be improved by obtaining sequences, such as intermediate-weighted proton density sequences, that are tailored for cartilage imaging.

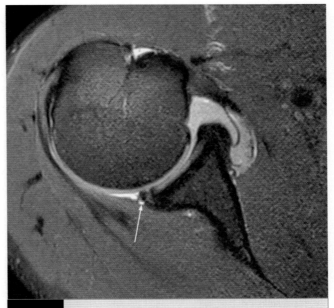

| **Figure 2** | MRI of the shoulder of a 40-year-old man with shoulder pain is shown. The direct magnetic resonance arthrography fat-suppressed axial T1-weighted image (repletion time/echo time-850/18) shows a posterior labral tear with a small paralabral cyst (arrow). |

Elbow Joint

The patient undergoing MRI of the elbow can be positioned either supine with the arm extended at the side or prone with the arm extended overhead. The prone position is often preferable so that the elbow is near the isocenter for homogeneous signal and uniform fat suppression, although sometimes this position is not well tolerated by the patient.

The protocol for elbow MRI includes a fast spin-echo T1-weighted or proton density sequence and fluid sensitive sequence using either a fast spin-echo T2-weighted sequence or a short T1 inversion recovery sequence. For diagnosis of pathology in the lateral and medial compartments of the elbow, imaging studies performed in the axial and coronal planes are evaluated, where as pathologies of the anterior and posterior compartments are best evaluated in the axial and sagittal planes.[8]

In the elbow joint, three-dimensional sequences can acquire much thinner slices than two-dimensional sequences, allowing better visualization of the collateral ligaments in the coronal plane. Three-dimensional sequences also can be used to obtain multiplanar reformat images, which allow the collateral ligaments to be evaluated in any orientation. This is especially important when assessing the ulnar band of the lateral collateral ligament, which can be best visualized in its entirety by using a 20° posterior oblique coronal plane. Recently developed three-dimensional isotropic resolution fast spin-echo sequences combine the most optimal tissue contrast with the ability to acquire thin continu-

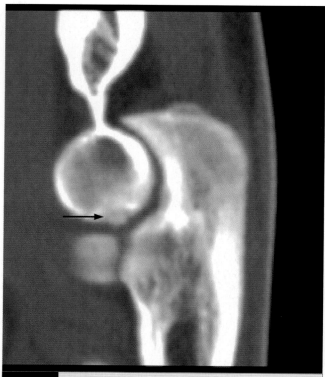

Figure 3 A sagittal CT scan of the elbow of a man with elbow pain shows a small osteochondral defect (arrow) involving the capitellum.

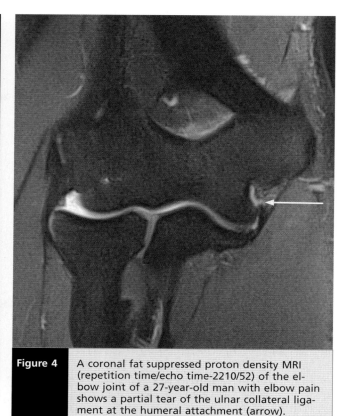

Figure 4 A coronal fat suppressed proton density MRI (repetition time/echo time-2210/52) of the elbow joint of a 27-year-old man with elbow pain shows a partial tear of the ulnar collateral ligament at the humeral attachment (arrow).

ous slices through the elbow joint, which may improve the detection of collateral ligament tears. The intermediate-weighted tissue contrast and multiplanar capabilities of these sequences may also be useful for evaluating tendons, muscles, and osseous structures of the elbow joint, especially when combined with fat suppression to improve fluid sensitivity.

Intra-articular contrast can be helpful in the evaluation of a ligament injury or when evaluating for the presence and suspicion of loose bodies that are not identified on conventional radiographs.

Osteochondral Injury

The osteochondroses of the elbow represent a group of disorders that are well evaluated by MRI. Panner disease is of uncertain etiology but is thought to originate from repetitive valgus stress resulting in compressive and shear forces, which lead to vascular compromise in throwing athletes (usually adolescent boys). On a radiograph, the epiphysis appears mottled and fragmented. On MRI, it appears as patchy hypointensities on T1-weighted sequences. Loose bodies are not a prominent feature of Panner disease.

Osteochondritis dissecans of the capitellum generally affects older athletes (age 12 to 16 years) and is more common in baseball players and gymnasts. They experience chronic lateral impaction forces due to repetitive microtrauma, leading to lesions affecting both sub-

chondral bone and overlying cartilage. Initial radiographs are normal, but MRI picks up the abnormality earlier. MRA with intra-articular contrast is especially useful for localizing the defect and demonstrating fragment stability. Fragments are considered unstable when any of the following findings exist: T2 hyperintensity surrounding the fragment, cysts are seen deep to the fragment, or T2 hyperintense edema is seen within the fragment. The bony defect can also be identified on CT (**Figure 3**).

MRI in Collateral Ligament Injury

Avulsion of the ulnar collateral ligament at the insertion site on the ulna is a source of chronic medial elbow pain in the throwing athlete and is best evaluated with a combination of radiographs and MRI.[9] MRI shows increased signal intensity of the ligament and can appear discontinuous if completely torn (**Figure 4**). Associated findings, such as a bone contusion in the lateral compartment and/or injury to the common extensor tendons, may be seen. Thickening or attenuation of the ligament, with or without abnormal intrinsic signal intensity, and calcification or ossification is seen in chronic injury. MRA is excellent in distinguishing partial and complete tears of the ulnar collateral ligament. Diagnosis of a partial tear is made when the "T" sign of contrast, saline, or joint fluid is seen extending in a linear fashion along the medial margin of the coronoid process, through the disrupted deep ulnar collateral lig-

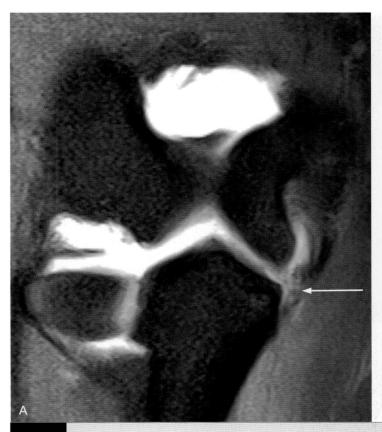 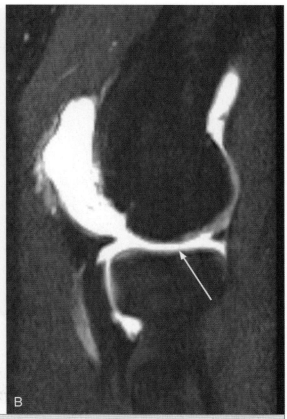

Figure 5 Imaging studies of the elbow of a 21-year-old male baseball pitcher. **A**, A direct magnetic resonance arthrography fat-suppressed coronal T1-weighted image (repetition time/echo time (TR/TE)-800/21) shows a full-thickness tear of the anterior band of the ulnar collateral ligament from the ulnar attachment (arrow). **B**, A fat-suppressed sagittal SPACE image (TR/TE-1020/60) shows a high-grade cartilage defect at the radiocapitellar joint (arrow).

ament fibers, but confined by the intact joint capsule. MRA also can help identify any cartilage abnormality present in the elbow joint (**Figure 5**).

Laterally, the radial collateral ligament complex includes the radial collateral ligament proper, the annular ligament, the lateral ulnar collateral ligament, and the accessory collateral ligament. The radial collateral ligament complex is less commonly injured than the ulnar collateral ligament. If the complex is sprained or partially torn, MRI demonstrates high signal intensity, representing periligamentous edema and hemorrhage, surrounding an intact ligament. Torn ligaments may be seen as discontinuous fibers.

MRI in Muscle and Tendon Injury

Normal tendons appear as uniform low signal intensity on all pulse sequences. The tendon affected by tendinopathy usually demonstrates areas of thickening with intermediate T1 and T2 signals. Partial or complete tears can occur as a result of acute traumatic events or as sequelae of chronic advanced tendinopathy. Partial tears can be seen with tendon thinning surrounded by T2 hyperintense fluid signal. In complete tears, the torn tendons are separated by T2 hyperintense fluid signal.

Lateral epicondylitis is an overuse syndrome in which the tendons involved are tendinopathic. The primary tendons involved are the extensor tendons, with the extensor carpi radialis brevis involved first. The anterior edge of the extensor digitorum communis is involved 50% of the time, followed by extensor carpi radialis longus and extensor carpi ulnaris. As the degree of injury increases, the underlying collateral ligaments are assessed for injury, especially the lateral ulnar collateral ligament.

The most common condition to affect the medial elbow is medial epicondylitis, also known as medial tennis elbow, golfer's elbow, and pitcher's elbow. The tendons involved originate from the pronator teres, the flexor carpi radialis, and/or the palmaris longus. There may be secondary involvement of the flexor carpi ulnaris and the flexor digitorum superficialis tendons. As the degree of injury increases, the underlying anterior band of the medial collateral ligmanent should also be assessed.

In the skeletally immature athlete with medial elbow pain, MRI plays an important role in identifying the pathology. The medial epicondyle physis is weaker than the anterior band of the medial collateral ligament. This condition, combined with the tensile forces generated by the

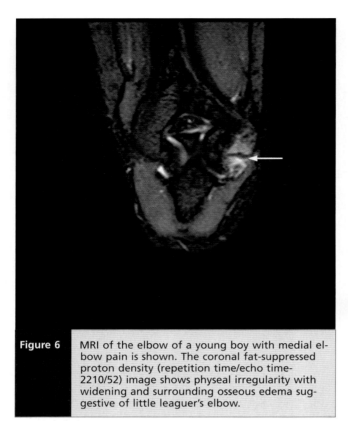

Figure 6 MRI of the elbow of a young boy with medial elbow pain is shown. The coronal fat-suppressed proton density (repetition time/echo time-2210/52) image shows physeal irregularity with widening and surrounding osseous edema suggestive of little leaguer's elbow.

common flexor tendon origin during valgus stress, can lead to the physeal injury known as little leaguer's elbow. MRI demonstrates physeal irregularity with widening and surrounding osseous edema (**Figure 6**).

In the anterior compartment of the elbow, rupture of the distal biceps tendon is rare, accounting for fewer than 5% of biceps tendon injuries. Partial tears can be seen with increased T2 signal within an abnormally thickened or thinned tendon associated with an osseous finding of edema within the radial tuberosity and fluid within the radiobicipital bursa. In a complete tear with retraction, the torn tendons are lax and separated by T2 hyperintense fluid signal. When it is difficult to assess the insertion of the tendon on the radial tuberosity, a flexed elbow, abducted shoulder, forearms supinated position may be helpful. Sagittal images are then acquired of the humerus extending into the forearm, resulting in longitudinal images of the distal biceps tendon, including its insertion. Isolated brachialis muscle tears are extremely rare. Brachialis musculotendinous strain/tears have been described in rock climbers and are referred to as climber's elbow.

The most common condition to affect the posterior elbow is posterior epicondylitis, an overuse syndrome in which the triceps tendon is tendinopathic and leads to a partial tear.

MRI in Nerve Entrapment

The three primary nerves at the elbow joint are the ulnar, radial, and median nerves. Among these, the nerve most commonly entrapped is the ulnar nerve at the cubital tunnel. Ulnar nerve compression is the most frequently seen peripheral neuropathy around the elbow and commonly occurs in throwing athletes. MRI can be helpful in assessing the integrity of nerves and evaluating the muscle groups supplied by nerves for normal morphology and signal intensity. Axial T1-weighted imaging depicts the size and the shape of the ulnar nerve, whereas T2-weighted imaging may show increased signal intensity of the nerve in case of entrapment. When an entrapment syndrome is present, the muscle group supplied in the acute phase demonstrates abnormally increased T2-weighted signal intensity on fat-suppressed images. When the process is chronic, the muscles will undergo atrophy and decrease in muscle bulk with fatty infiltration, which is best seen on T1-weighted sequences.

CT and CTA

CT depicts osseous detail, and combined with arthrography, intra-articular pathologies, capsulolabral pathologies, and pathologies related to tendons, a diagnosis of joint ligaments can be made. Modern multislice CT scanners provide excellent spatial and contrast resolution. Images can be reconstructed in any arbitrary oblique plane that best shows complex joint anatomy. Three-dimensional models also can be constructed from the raw data, which are helpful for surgical planning.

CT is advantageous because of its ability to evaluate soft-tissue calcification, myositis ossificans, and intra-articular bodies more readily than MRI. Osteoarthritis is readily apparent when the subchondral bone is involved. The disadvantages of CT include the resultant radiation dose, which may be a consideration if multiple examinations are necessary or if a patient is pregnant. CT has poor soft-tissue characterization, which can make the detection of subtle soft-tissue injuries challenging. Metallic hardware within the bone or periarticular soft tissues can cause significant beam hardening artifacts, which limits the evaluation of the surrounding bone and soft tissues.

CTA of the joint requires two steps: intra-articular injection of the contrast media and acquisition of the CT images. The introduction of submillimeter isotropic multidetector computed tomography (MDCT) technology provided the crucial solution for excellent spatial resolution and multiplanar capability, which markedly improved the diagnostic power of CTA of the joint. The general indications for MDCT arthrography are usually related to inability to perform MRI or the failure of MRI in evaluating the shoulder.[10] Such indications include the presence of metal hardware close to the joint (postoperative shoulder), the presence of MRI-incompatible implanted medical devices, and some general indications, such as claustrophobia and obesity of the patient.

CTA has several advantages, including isotropic sub-millimeter spatial resolution with improved longitudinal resolution. The scan time is substantially reduced with decreased motion artifact, which renders it useful for trauma and pediatric patients. The disadvantages of CTA include its invasive nature of arthrography and exposure to ionizing radiation. Contrast resolution is less for bone marrow edema and soft-tissue lesions.

A study was performed to evaluate the diagnostic accuracy and indications of arthrography with MDCT arthrography of the shoulder in patients with absolute or relative contraindications to MRI and in patients with periarticular metal implants using diagnostic arthroscopy as the gold standard.[11] In the 42 nonsurgically treated patients, the comparison between MDCT arthrography and arthroscopy showed sensitivity and specificity ranging between 87% and 100%. In the 28 surgically treated shoulders, MDCT arthrography had an accuracy of 94% compared with 25% with MRI. Interobserver agreement was almost perfect (kappa = 0.95) in the evaluation of all types of lesions, both on MDCT and MRI. When MDCT arthrography was compared with MRI in the postoperative patients by a McNemar test, a significant difference ($P < 0.05$) was found between these two techniques.

Shoulder Joint

Specific indications for arthrography of the shoulder involve increasing the contrast resolution of images of the intra-articular soft tissues, which are not adequately present on unenhanced images. The indications include evaluation of the rotator cuff, the capsulolabral-ligamentous complex, and the articular cartilage, especially in postoperative cases where the metal artifact interferes with MRI[12] (**Figure 7**).

Elbow Joint

CT is widely used to evaluate elbow fractures around the joint and show intra-articular extension or small fracture fragments within the joint. Intravenous iodinated contrast can be administered to determine any vascular injury adjacent to the joint. CTA with intra-articular injections of iodinated contrast is an excellent method of detecting disease in the overlying articular cartilage, although internal structural changes are not detected if the cartilage surface is intact. CTA is generally performed when there are contraindications in performing MRI.

Ultrasound

With the availability of high-frequency linear transducers in the range of 10 to 18 MHz, musculoskeletal ultrasound is a rapidly growing field. Musculoskeletal ultrasound has several advantages over MRI, including availability, quick scan time, and opportunity to perform dynamic scanning.[13] Ultrasound is also noninvasive with no ionizing radiation and allows easy, safe,

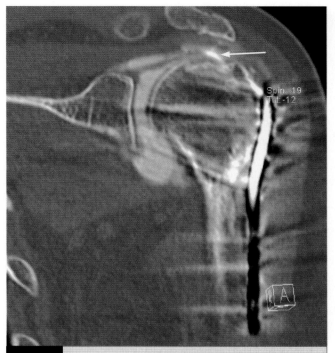

Figure 7 Computed tomography arthrography of the left proximal shoulder of a 60-year-old woman with a history of fracture fixation in 2005 is shown. The patient reports pain during lifting. The coronal section shows an intermediate grade undersurface tear of the supraspinatus with a small pinhole full-thickness perforation (arrow). Healed fracture deformity of the left greater tuberosity with surgical fixation of the humeral head and neck with lateral plate and screws is seen. Cyst formation and bony productive changes at the greater tuberosity compatible with chronic enthesopathy also are seen.

and contralateral comparison. However, it is an operator-dependent modality, and training in musculoskeletal ultrasound is necessary because of a steep learning curve. It also is limited in providing a comprehensive image of the shoulder and elbow joint. It has limited field of view and poor osseous penetration. It is best used to answer a focused, specific question. Ultrasound is less useful for the evaluation of deeper structures, such as bony abnormalities or osteochondral pathologies.

Technologic developments, including panoramic imaging, video storage, and three-dimensional probes, help to bridge the gap between stored static ultrasound and MRI.

Shoulder Joint

Ultrasound can be used to evaluate tendons of the rotator cuff and biceps, diagnose bursitis, and serve as a real-time tool for guiding procedures.

A 2011 study sought to determine the diagnostic accuracy of ultrasound to detect partial and complete-thickness rotator cuff tears based on all available clini-

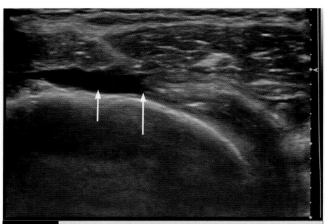

Figure 8 An ultrasound (high resolution, 12 MHz transducer) of the shoulder of a 67-year-old man with chronic pain and inability to abduct his shoulder is shown. A full-thickness tear of the supraspinatus muscle and retracted tendons (long arrow) with presence of anechoic fluid in the subacromial subdeltoid bursa (short arrow) are seen.

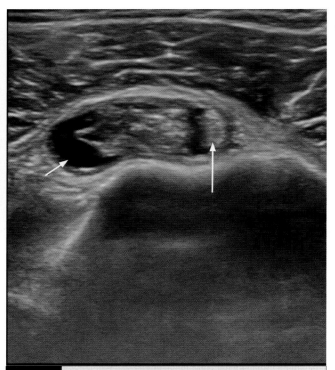

Figure 9 A high-resolution ultrasound of the painful left shoulder joint of a 65-year-old man shows thickening of the biceps tendon (long arrow) with fluid (short arrow) surrounding the biceps tendon, suggestive of biceps tendinitis.

cal trials.[14] Sixty-two studies assessing 6,007 patients and 6,066 shoulders were included. Ultrasonography had good sensitivity and specificity for the assessment of partial-thickness (sensitivity, 0.84; specificity, 0.89) and full-thickness rotator cuff tears (sensitivity, 0.96; specificity, 0.93).

Ultrasonographic evaluation of the tendons should be performed in the longitudinal and transverse planes. For each rotator cuff tendon, there is a particular arm position required to optimally interpret the tendon. The normal rotator cuff tendons appear as hyperechoic structures with a pattern of parallel fibrillary lines in the longitudinal plane and a hyperechoic ovoid structure in the transverse plane. It can distinguish between partial-thickness and full-thickness rotator cuff tears where it appears hypoechoic to anechoic. Signs of a partial-thickness tear include focal anechoic or hypoechoic defects in the bursal or joint surface of the tendon (**Figures 8** and **9**). Tissue harmonic imaging, by showing intratendinous tears as a hypoechoic line, and three-dimensional ultrasound may improve the conspicuity of partial-thickness tears.[15]

Rotator cuff impingement on ultrasound is diagnosed when in addition to evidence of rotator cuff damage or bursal thickening, dynamic scanning during abduction may show bursal distension, pooling of fluid in the bursa, or buckling of bursa. Many radiologists perform an ultrasound impingement test by injecting a long-acting local anesthetic, such as bupivacaine, usually combined with a therapeutic injection of long-acting steroids, such as methylprednisolone, into the subdeltoid bursa under ultrasound guidance.

Elbow Joint

Ultrasound is commonly used to evaluate soft-tissue disease around the elbow, enabling high-resolution imaging of superficial structures, such as ligaments, tendons, and nerves.[16] Ultrasound can be used to detect joint effusion, ligamentous or tendon tears, and ulnar nerve abnormalities as well as to guide various interventions around the elbow.

Dynamic ultrasound also can be used to assess pathologic conditions that may be apparent only when the limb is moved, such as ulnar nerve subluxation or muscle hernias. Ultrasound also has the ability to detect subtle calcification or foreign bodies that may not be easily apparent on a radiograph or MRI. Ultrasound serves as a guiding modality to perform procedures such as steroid injections in the tendon. With the help of Doppler imaging, injury to the vessel can be avoided when the procedure is performed under ultrasound guidance.

Summary

For shoulder impingement syndrome and rotator cuff tears, either MRI or ultrasound could be used to detect of rotator cuff tears. Both MRA and CTA are effective methods for detecting labral tears. **Table 1** depicts appropriate assessment of various pathologies of the shoulder joint on various imaging modalities.

Table 1

Appropriate Assessment of Anatomic Regions of the Shoulder Joint on Various Imaging Modalities

	MRI	MRA	CT	CTA	US
Labral tears	++	+++	—	+ ++	—
Rotator cuff—partial tear (bursal surface)	+++	++	—	++	+
Rotator cuff— partial tear (articular surface)	+++	+++	—	+++	+
Rotator cuff— full tear	+++	+++	—	+++	+
Cartilage defects	++	+++	—	+++	—
Bone marrow edema	+++	+++	+	+	—

CTA = computed tomography arthrography; MRA = magnetic resonance arthrography; US = ultrasound.

For elbow pathologies, plain MRI using appropriate sequences is better for the assessment of occult bone injuries and cartilage abnormalities and the diagnosis of soft-tissue pathologies in tendons, ligaments, and nerves.

Annotated References

1. Bolog N, Nanz D, Weishaupt D: Muskuloskeletal MR imaging at 3.0 T: Current status and future perspectives. *Eur Radiol* 2006;16(6):1298-1307.

2. Kijowski R, Gold GE: Routine 3D magnetic resonance imaging of joints. *J Magn Reson Imaging* 2011;33(4):758-771.

   This article describes various three dimensional sequences used in musculoskeltal MRI, along with their clinical application in various joints.

3. Osinski T, Malfair D, Steinbach L: Magnetic resonance arthrography. *Orthop Clin North Am* 2006;37(3):299-319, vi.

   This article describes the technique of performing MRA as well as its advantages and disadvantages over conventional MRI.

4. Magee T: 3-T MRI of the shoulder: Is MR arthrography necessary? *AJR Am J Roentgenol* 2009;192(1):86-92.

   The purpose of this study is to report the diagnostic sensitivity of 3-T conventional MRI versus MRA of the shoulder in the same patient population.

5. Shahabpour M, Kichouh M, Laridon E, Gielen JL, De Mey J: The effectiveness of diagnostic imaging methods for the assessment of soft tissue and articular disorders of the shoulder and elbow. *Eur J Radiol* 2008;65(2):194-200.

   In this article, a meta-analyisis was performed of the relevant literature, and the role of MRI of the shoulder and elbow discussed, along with a comparison of other diagnostic modalities. Level of evidence: III.

6. de Jesus JO, Parker L, Frangos AJ, Nazarian LN: Accuracy of MRI, MR arthrography, and ultrasound in the diagnosis of rotator cuff tears: A meta-analysis. *AJR Am J Roentgenol* 2009;192(6):1701-1707.

   The authors of this study compared the diagnostic accuracy of MRI, MRA, and ultrasound for the diagnosis of rotator cuff tears through a meta-analysis of literature studies. Sixty-five articles met the inclusion criteria for this meta-analysis.

7. Shah N, Tung GA: Imaging signs of posterior glenohumeral instability. *AJR Am J Roentgenol* 2009;192(3):730-735.

   The purpose of this article is to review mechanisms of injury leading to posterior glenohumeral instability and the correlated imaging findings on CT and MRI. In patients with suspected posterior glenohumeral instability, imaging of the affected shoulder can show abnormalities of the bone, the labrum, and the joint capsule. Accurate detection and characterization of these lesions aid in both diagnosis and management.

8. Brunton LM, Anderson MW, Pannunzio ME, Khanna AJ, Chhabra AB: Magnetic resonance imaging of the elbow: Update on current techniques and indications. *J Hand Surg Am* 2006;31(6):1001-1011.

9. Stevens KJ, McNally EG: Magnetic resonance imaging of the elbow in athletes. *Clin Sports Med* 2010;29(4):521-553.

   This article reviews imaging of common disease conditions occurring around the elbow in athletes, with an emphasis on MRI.

10. Fritz J, Fishman EK, Small KM, et al: MDCT arthrography of the shoulder with datasets of isotropic resolution: Indications, technique, and applications. *AJR Am J Roentgenol* 2012;198(3):635-646.

    The purposes of this review were to summarize the indications MDCT arthrography of the shoulder, highlight the features of MDCT acquisition, and describe the normal and abnormal MDCT arthrographic appearances of the shoulder. MDCT arthrography is a valid alternative for shoulder imaging of patients with

8. Miscellaneous Shoulder and Elbow Topics

contraindications to MRI or after failed MRI. MDCT arthrography is accurate for assessming a variety of shoulder abnormalities and, with further validation, may become the imaging test of choice for evaluating the postoperative shoulder.

11. De Filippo M, Bertellini A, Sverzellati N, et al: Multidetector computed tomography arthrography of the shoulder: Diagnostic accuracy and indications. *Acta Radiol* 2008;49(5):540-549.

   In this study, diagnostic accuracy and indications of arthrography and MDCT arthrography of the shoulder with absolute and relative contraindications to MRI of the shoulder in patients with periarticular metal implants were evaluated using diagnostic arthroscopy as the gold standard. The results showed that MDCT arthrography of the shoulder is a safe technique that provides accurate diagnosis in identifying chondral, fibrocartilaginous, and intra-articular ligamentous lesions in patients who cannot be evaluated by MRI and in patients after surgery.

12. Oh JH, Kim JY, Choi JA, Kim WS: Effectiveness of multidetector CTA for assessing shoulder pathology: Comparison with magnetic resonance imaging with arthroscopic correlation. *J Shoulder Elbow Surg* 2010; 19(1):14-20.

   This study evaluated the diagnostic efficacy of CTA in the assessment of various shoulder pathologies with arthroscopic correlation. It was hypothesized that CTA would be cost-effective and comparable with MRA for assessing labral detachments and full-thickness rotator cuff tears. The sensitivity, specificity, and agreement were comparable in each imaging study for Bankart lesions, SLAP lesions, Hill-Sachs lesions, and full-thickness rotator cuff tears, but those of CTA were significantly lower than MRA for partial-thickness cuff tears. The ROC curves for CTA and MRA were not significantly different for any of the pathologies, except partial-thickness cuff tears. Level of evidence: I.

13. Jacobson JA: Musculoskeletal ultrasound: Focused impact on MRI. *AJR Am J Roentgenol* 2009;193(3): 619-627.

   This article compares image interpretation, accuracy, observer variability, economic effect, and education with regard to musculoskeletal ultrasound and MRI because these factors will influence the growth of musculoskeletal ultrasound and the effect on MRI. The development of less expensive portable ultrasound machines has opened the market to nonradiologists, and applications for musculoskeletal ultrasound have broadened. Selective substitution of musculoskeletal ultrasound for MRI can result in significant cost saving to the healthcare system.

14. Smith TO, Back T, Toms AP, Hing CB: Diagnostic accuracy of ultrasound for rotator cuff tears in adults: A systematic review and meta-analysis. *Clin Radiol* 2011;66(11):1036-1048.

   This study was performed to determine the diagnostic accuracy of ultrasound to detect partial- and full thickness rotator cuff tears based on all available clinical trials. Sixty-two studies assessing 6,007 patients and 6,066 shoulders were included. Ultrasonography had good sensitivity and specificity for the assessment of partial-thickness (sensitivity, 0.84; specificity, 0.89), and full-thickness rotator cuff tears (sensitivity, 0.96; specificity, 0.93). However, the literature poorly described population characteristics and assessor blinding and was based on limited sample sizes.

15. Parker L, Nazarian LN, Carrino JA, et al: Musculoskeletal imaging: Medicare use, costs, and potential for cost substitution. *J Am Coll Radiol* 2008;5(3): 182-188.

   This study explores the substitution of ultrasound for MRI of musculoskeletal disorders by describing the recent use and costs of musculoskeletal imaging in the Medicare population, projecting these trends from 2006 to 2020, and estimating cost savings involved in substituting musculoskeletal ultrasound for musculoskeletal MRI, when appropriate.

16. Lee KS, Rosas HG, Craig JG: Musculoskeletal ultrasound: Elbow imaging and procedures. *Semin Musculoskelet Radiol* 2010;14(4):449-460.

   This article discusses the unique application of ultrasound in evaluating common elbow pathology and in advanced ultrasound-guided treatments.

Index